Thieme

Imaging of Bones and Joints

A Concise, Multimodality Approach

Klaus Bohndorf, MD
Professor of Radiology
MR Highfield Center
Department of Biomedical Imaging and Image-guided Therapy
Medical University of Vienna
Vienna, Austria

Mark W. Anderson, MD
Professor of Radiology
MSK Imaging
Department of Radiology
University of Virginia
Charlottesville, Virginia, USA

Mark Davies, MRCP, FRCR
Professor of Radiology
Department of Radiology
Royal Orthopaedic Hospital
Birmingham, UK

Herwig Imhof, MD
Professor of Radiology
Formerly Department of Biomedical Imaging and Image-guided Therapy
Medical University of Vienna
Vienna, Austria

Klaus Woertler, MD
Professor of Radiology
Department of Radiology
Technical University of Munich
Munich, Germany

2181 illustrations, including 338 on the Thieme MediaCenter

Thieme
Stuttgart · New York · Delhi · Rio de Janeiro

Library of Congress Cataloging-in-Publication Data
is available from the publisher.

This book is an authorized, adapted, and revised version of the 3rd German edition published and copyrighted 2014 by Georg Thieme Verlag, Stuttgart. Title of the German edition: Radiologische Diagnostik der Knochen und Gelenke

Translator: Grahame Larkin, Stuttgart, Germany
Illustrator: Christiane and Dr. Michael von Solodkoff, Neckargemünd, Germany

3rd German edition 2014
1st Italian edition 2003
1st Portuguese edition 2006

Thieme Publishers Stuttgart
Rüdigerstrasse 14, 70469 Stuttgart, Germany
+49 [0]711 8931 421, customerservice@thieme.de

Thieme Publishers New York
333 Seventh Avenue, New York, NY 10001, USA
+1-800-782-3488, customerservice@thieme.com

Thieme Publishers Delhi
A-12, Second Floor, Sector-2, Noida-201301,
Uttar Pradesh, India
+91 120 45 566 00, customerservice@thieme.in

Thieme Publishers Rio, Thieme Publicações Ltda.
Edifício Rodolpho de Paoli, 25° andar, Av. Nilo Peçanha,
50 – Sala 2508
Rio de Janeiro 20020-906 Brasil
+55 21 3172 2297/+55 21 3172 1896

Cover design: Thieme Publishing Group
Typesetting by Ziegler + Müller, Kirchentellinsfurt, Germany
Printed in Germany by Aprinta GmbH, Wemding

ISBN 978-3-13-240647-6

Also available as an e-book:
eISBN 978-3-13-240876-0

Important note: Medicine is an ever-changing science undergoing continual development. Research and clinical experience are continually expanding our knowledge, in particular our knowledge of proper treatment and drug therapy. Insofar as this book mentions any dosage or application, readers may rest assured that the authors, editors, and publishers have made every effort to ensure that such references are in accordance with **the state of knowledge at the time of production of the book.**

Nevertheless, this does not involve, imply, or express any guarantee or responsibility on the part of the publishers in respect to any dosage instructions and forms of applications stated in the book. **Every user is requested to examine carefully** the manufacturers' leaflets accompanying each drug and to check, if necessary in consultation with a physician or specialist, whether the dosage schedules mentioned therein or the contraindications stated by the manufacturers differ from the statements made in the present book. Such examination is particularly important with drugs that are either rarely used or have been newly released on the market. Every dosage schedule or every form of application used is entirely at the user's own risk and responsibility. The authors and publishers request every user to report to the publishers any discrepancies or inaccuracies noticed. If errors in this work are found after publication, errata will be posted at www.thieme.com on the product description page.

Some of the product names, patents, and registered designs referred to in this book are in fact registered trademarks or proprietary names even though specific reference to this fact is not always made in the text. Therefore, the appearance of a name without designation as proprietary is not to be construed as a representation by the publisher that it is in the public domain.

MIX
Paper from responsible sources
FSC® C004592
www.fsc.org

Contents

Preface

Brevity is the soul of wit
William Shakespeare, *Hamlet*

This book is a concise, practically oriented textbook that concentrates on the essentials of musculoskeletal imaging. It is intended to provide an overview of the subject and also to serve as an aid for getting started, as a reference book, and as a faithful companion right up to board examinations and beyond. That is why the book is organized around clinical disorders, describing the imaging findings of all modalities relevant to each disorder. It is not intended to replace more detailed subspecialty textbooks.

Thirty-five authors have contributed to the text and images. It should not, however, read as a multi-authored book because it follows the principle of "many authors but only one style." The editors have carefully revised, harmonized, supplemented, or sometimes trimmed the text and images to produce a book that is "cast from a single mold"—that is its claim. In this it honors the ethos and form of its "progenitor," the third edition of Thieme's *Radiologische Diagnostik der Knochen und Gelenke*, through the careful review and adaption by the editors Mark Anderson (USA) and Mark Davies (Great Britain), of the English rendition by Grahame Larkin.

Comprehensive books, whether printed or electronically rendered, in our view continue to be the ideal tool for gaining an overview, learning the basic principles, and acquiring knowledge of the field of musculoskeletal radiology. Research has shown that text and images must relate to and support each other to maximize comprehension and memorization. As a result, the format we have chosen is to present the material in units of two facing pages wherever possible, with the left-hand page for text and the right-hand page for images. Many images have been annotated to avoid the need for long, exhaustive captions.

The book has been designed and composed with this principle in mind. Nevertheless, considerable additional information has been placed on the Thieme MediaCenter, accessible via the internet (see "How to Use This Book"). This is intended not simply as a tribute to the technological spirit of the times, but also as a practical way to expand the book's contents. In this way the problem of squaring the circle—of producing an affordable, compact book while at the same time making available even more images and information—has been elegantly solved. The web-based supplementary material is clearly indicated in the book by the use of the MediaCenter icon ► so that the reader can decide whether or not it will be useful to take advantage of it.

The support of the Thieme publishing house for this book has been exemplary in every way. This publisher has a history of producing esthetically beautiful yet challenging books, without excluding themselves from modern-day media. That is a stroke of luck for editors and authors like us who hope to see many of our ideas and intentions put into practice. We would like to express our thanks to Stephan Konnry for supporting this endeavor. We are also grateful to the editorial team, in particular Gabriele Kuhn-Giovannini and Jo Stead, and to Len Cegielka, the copy editor, for their skills, patience, empathy, and tenacity during the realization of our joint project.

Klaus Bohndorf, MD
Mark W. Anderson, MD
Mark Davies, MRCP, FRCR
Herwig Imhof, MD
Klaus Woertler, MD

Acknowledgments

Armin Seifarth, MD, Augsburg, for editing and reviewing all chapters on ultrasound. Where deemed necessary, he has added material to the chapters and supplied more images.

Walter Braun, MD, Professor of Surgery, Augsburg, for his competent and prompt advice on Chapters 1 and 2 from the traumatologist's standpoint.

Thomas Naumann, MD, former head of the Department of Orthopedic Surgery I, Hessing Klinik, Augsburg, for improvements to Chapter 9.3.

Martin Seidler, MD, Augsburg, and Mr. Ulf Wolkenstein, Augsburg, for providing and giving advice on the necessary IT requirements.

Many colleagues have kindly and generously supplied image material. In particular the sterling work by Thomas Grieser, MD (Augsburg), Herbert Rosenthal, MD (Hanover), and Dr. Bjoern Jobke (Heidelberg) deserves particular acknowledgment. The names of the contributors are noted below the images; this information has been omitted for images that originate from the archives of the editors.

The Editors

Contributors

Editors and Authors

Klaus Bohndorf, MD
Professor of Radiology
MR Highfield Center
Department of Biomedical Imaging
and Image-guided Therapy
Medical University of Vienna
Vienna, Austria

Mark W. Anderson, MD
Professor of Radiology
MSK Imaging
Department of Radiology
University of Virginia
Charlottesville, VA, USA

Mark Davies, MRCP, FRCR
Professor of Radiology
Department of Radiology
Royal Orthopedic Hospital
Birmingham, UK

Herwig Imhof, MD
Professor of Radiology
Formerly Department of Biomedical Imaging
and Image-guided Therapy
Medical University of Vienna
Vienna, Austria

Klaus Woertler, MD
Professor of Radiology
Department of Radiology
Technical University of Munich
Munich, Germany

Contributors

Amadeus Altenburger, MD
Staff Radiologist
Department of Radiology and Neuroradiology
Klinikum Augsburg
Augsburg, Germany

Rainer Braunschweig, MD
Chairman and Radiologist
Department of Diagnostic Imaging
and Interventional Radiology
BG Klinik Bergmannstrost
Halle, Germany

Hassan Douis, MRCP, FRCR
Consultant Musculoskeletal Radiologist
Department of Radiology
University of Birmingham
Birmingham, UK

Andreas Peter Erler, MD
Staff Radiologist
Department of Diagnostic Imaging
and Interventional Radiology
BG Hospital Bergmannstrost
Halle, Germany

Oliver Ertl, MD
Radiologist
Diagnostic Center Vinzentinum
Augsburg, Germany

Robert Fessl, MD
Staff Neuroradiologist
Department of Radiology and Neuroradiology
Klinikum Augsburg
Augsburg, Germany

Wolfgang Fischer, MD
Radiologist
MRI Center
Hessingpark Klinik
Augsburg, Germany

Klaus M. Friedrich, MD
Associate Professor of Radiology
Neuroradiology and MSK Radiology
Department of Biomedical Imaging
and Image-guided Therapy
Medical University of Vienna
Vienna, Austria

Michael Gebhard, MD
Staff Radiologist
Department of Radiology and Neuroradiology
Klinikum Augsburg
Augsburg, Germany

Thomas Grieser, MD
Staff Radiologist
Department of Radiology and Neuroradiology
Klinikum Augsburg
Augsburg, Germany

Bjoern Jobke, MD
Staff Radiologist
Department of Radiology
German Cancer Center
Heidelberg, Germany

Nicolas Jorden, MD
Department of Radiology and Neuroradiology
Klinikum Augsburg
Augsburg, Germany

Franz M. Kainberger, MD
Professor of Radiology
Neuroradiology and MSK Radiology
Department of Biomedical Imaging
and Image-guided Therapy
Medical University of Vienna
Vienna, Austria

Egbert Knoepfle, MD
Staff Radiologist
Department of Radiology and Neuroradiology
Klinikum Augsburg
Augsburg, Germany

Gerwin M. Lingg, MD
Radiologist
Formerly Acura-SanHa Rheumatology Centre
Bad Kreuznach, Germany

Edgar Johann Mayr, MD
Professor of Orthopaedic Surgery
Department of Trauma, Hand
and Reconstructive Surgery
Klinikum Augsburg
Augsburg, Germany

Eugene McNally, FRCR
Consultant Musculoskeletal Radiologist
The Oxford Clinic
Oxford, UK

Wolfgang Michl, MD
Pedriatric Radiologist
Formerly Department of Radiology
and Neuroradiology
Klinikum Augsburg
Augsburg, Germany

Iris Melanie Noebauer-Huhmann, MD
Associate Professor of Radiology
Neuroradiology and MSK Radiology
Department of Biomedical Imaging
and Image-guided Therapy
Medical University of Vienna
Vienna, Austria

Christian W.A. Pfirrmann, MD
Professor of Radiology
Chairman
Balgrist Hospital
University of Zurich
Zurich, Switzerland

Frank Roemer, MD
Associate Professor of Radiology
Institute of Radiology
University of Erlangen
Erlangen, Germany

Herbert Rosenthal, MD
Professor of Radiology
Chairman
Department of Diagnostic and Interventional Radiology
KRH Klinikum
Hannover, Germany

Fabian Sauerwald, MD
Staff Orthopaedic Surgeon
Department of Trauma, Hand
and Reconstructive Surgery
Klinikum Augsburg
Augsburg, Germany

Armin Seifarth, MD
Radiologist
Radiologie im Zentrum
Munich, Germany

Reto Sutter, MD
Staff Radiologist
Balgrist Hospital
University of Zurich
Radiology
Zurich, Switzerland

Siegfried Trattnig, MD
Professor of Radiology
Chairman
MR Highfield Center
Department of Biomedical Imaging
and Image-guided Therapy
Medical University of Vienna
Vienna, Austria

Eva-Maria Wagner, MD
Staff Radiologist
Department of Radiology and Neuroradiology
Klinikum Augsburg
Augsburg, Germany

Richard Whitehouse, FRCR
Consultant Musculoskeletal Radiologist
Department of Clinical Radiology
Manchester Royal Infirmary
Manchester, United Kingdom

Walter A. Wohlgemuth, MD
Professor of Radiology
Department of Diagnostic Radiology
University of Regensburg
Regensburg, Germany

Joachim Zentner, MD
Radiologist
Radiology Center Friedberg
Friedberg, Germany

Abbreviations

ABC aneurysmal bone cyst
ABER abduction and external rotation
ACL anterior cruciate ligament
ALIF anterior lumbar interbody fusion
ALPSA anterior labroligamentous periosteal sleeve avulsion (lesion)
ANA antinuclear antibody
ANCA antineutrophil cytoplasmic antibody
anti-CCP anti-cyclic citrullinated peptides
AP anteroposterior
ARCO Association Internationale de Recherche sur la Circulation Osseuse
ASPED angel-shaped phalangoepiphyseal dysplasia
AT antetorsion angle (angle between the prosthetic neck and the stem
ATAF anterior talofibular (ligament)
ATR Achilles tendon reflex
AV anteversion angle (angle between the acetabular axis and the vertical line)
AVM arteriovenous malformation
AVN avascular necrosis
BMD bone mineral density
BPOP bizarre parosteal osteochondromatous proliferation (Nora lesion)
BTR biceps tendon reflex
cANCA classic antineutrophil cytoplasmic antibody
cCT cranial CT
CF calcaneofibular (ligament)
CHL coracohumeral ligament
CID Concealed Intratendinous Delamination (lesion)
CPPD calcium pyrophosphate deposition disease
CREST calcinosis, Raynaud's phenomenon, esophageal dysmotility, sclerodactyly, and telangiectasia (syndrome)
CRITOL capitulum—radial head—internal epicondyle—trochlea—olecranon—external epicondyle
CRMO chronic recurrent multifocal osteomyelitis
CRP C-reactive protein
CRPS complex regional pain syndrome
CSF cerebrospinal fluid
CT computed tomography
DCP dynamic compression plate
DESS double echo steady state (sequence)
DEXA dual energy X-ray absorptiometry
DIP distal interphalangeal (joint)
DISH diffuse idiopathic skeletal hyperostosis
DISI dorsal intercalated segment instability deformity
DOMS delayed onset muscle soreness
DRUJ distal radioulnar joint
DSA digital subtraction angiography
dSSc diffuse systemic sclerosis
DWI diffusion weighted imaging
ECU extensor carpi ulnaris (tendon)
eILW extended interlaminar window
ELPS extensive lateral compression syndrome
ESR erythrocyte sedimentation rate
FABS flexed elbow, abducted shoulder, forearm supinated
FAI femoroacetabular impingement
FDG fluorodeoxyglucose
FDP flexor digitorum profundus
FFE fast field echo (sequence)
FLAIR fluid attenuated inversion recovery
FLASH fast low-angle shot (sequence)
FSE fast spin echo
GE, GRE gradient echo
GLAD glenolabral articular disruption (lesion)
HAGL humeral avulsion of glenohumeral ligament (lesion)
IASP International Association for the Study of Pain
IGHL inferior glenohumeral ligament
ILW interlaminar windowing
INR International Normalized Tatio
ISP infraspinatus muscle
ISSVA International Society for the Study of Vascular Anomalies
IV intravenous
IVS intervertebral space
LBT long biceps tendon
LC-DCP low-contact DCP
LCP locking compression plate
LISS less invasive stabilization system
LLC labroligamentous complex
lSSc limited systemic sclerosis
LT lunotriquetral
LUCL lateral ulnar collateral ligament
MACT matrix-associated autologous chondrocyte implantation
MCL medial collateral ligament
MDT multidisciplinary team
MEN multiple endocrine neoplasia
MGHL middle glenohumeral ligament
MGUS monoclonal gammopathy of undetermined clinical significance
MIP maximum intensity projection
MOCART Magnetic Resonance Observation of Cartilage Repair Tissue (classification)
MPFL medial patellofemoral ligament
MPR multiplanar reconstruction
MR magnetic resonance
MRA magnetic resonance arthrography
MRI magnetic resonance imaging
MTP metatarsophalangeal
OATS osteochondral autograft transfer system
PAINT Partial Articular-sided tear with INTratendinous extension (lesion)
PASTA Partial Articular-sided Supraspinatus Tendon Avulsion (lesion)
PCL posterior cruciate ligament
PD proton density
PDW proton density–weighted

PEST papilledema, extravascular volume overload, sclerotic bone lesions, and thrombocytosis/erythrocytosis
PET positron emission tomography
PIP proximal interphalangeal (joint)
PLIF posterior lumbar interbody fusion
POEMS polyneuropathy, organomegaly, endocrinopathy, M-proteins, skin changes
POLPSA posterior labrocapsular periosteal sleeve avulsion
PT posterior tibial (tendon)
PTAF posterior talofibular (ligament)
PTR patellar tendon reflex
PTT partial thromboplastin time
PVNS pigmented villonodular synovitis
PWI perfusion-weighted imaging
RANK receptor activator of nuclear factor κB
RL radiolunate angle
RSL radioscapholunate
SAPHO synovitis, acne, pustulosis, hyperostosis, and osteitis (syndrome)
SCIWORA spinal cord injury without radiographic abnormality (syndrome)
SE spin echo
SGHL superior glenohumeral ligament
SIJ sacroiliac joint
SL scapholunate
SLAC scapholunate advanced collapse
SLAP superior labral anterior-to-posterior (lesion)
SNAC scaphoid nonunion advanced collapse
SONK spontaneous osteonecrosis of the knee
SPGR spoiled gradient recalled acquisition (sequence)
SSC subscapularis muscle
SSC subscapularis muscle
SSP supraspinatus muscle
SST supraspinatus tendon
STAS supraspinatus tendon articular-sided (lesion)
STIR short-tau inversion recovery
STJ subtalar joint
STT scaphoid, trapezium, and trapezoideum
T1W T1-weighted
T2W T2-weighted
TE echo time
TE echo time
TFCC triangular fibrocartilage complex
TILT triquetral impingement ligament tear
TIRM turbo inversion recovery magnitude (sequence)
TJR total joint replacement
TLICS Thoracolumbar Injury Classification and Severity Score
TLIF transforaminal interbody lumbar fusion
TTR triceps tendon reflex
TT–TG tibial tuberosity–trochlear groove (distance)
UPS undifferentiated high-grade pleomorphic sarcoma
USP ulnar styloid process
UTE ultrashort echo time
VISI volar intercalated segmental instability
WE water-excitation (sequence)
XLIF extreme lateral interbody fusion

How to Use This Book

Structure of the Chapters

The chapters have been constructed in a common, consistent format to help organize the information and facilitate navigation within the text. Chapters are divided into sections under the following headings:

▶ **Anatomy.** Here you will find the most important anatomical features of a particular region. To help streamline the text, some of the anatomy chapters have been placed on the ▶ Thieme MediaCenter.

▶ **Pathology.** The pathology and pathophysiology of each disease entity are briefly presented here.

▶ **Clinical presentation.** Important features of the clinical presentation of a patient with the condition are described here.

▶ **Radiology/US/CT/MRI.** Findings on each modality are listed in this section. Modalities that do not provide additional information are not included.

▶ **NUC MED.** When appropriate, the findings of radionuclide studies will be described here.

▶ **Important findings.** This deals with information of importance to the clinician that should be included in the imaging report.

▶ **Special features in children.** Important features of childhood disorders are listed.

> **Note**
> Here you will find important take-home messages in each chapter.

> **Caution**
> Warnings regarding possible imaging pitfalls.

▶ **DD.** The most common and most important differential diagnoses are listed here along with brief differentiating criteria.

References

Indexes of the recommended literature referenced in the book are provided on the ▶ Thieme MediaCenter.

Layout of the Text and Images

A special feature of this book is that the **images** referred to in the text are found on the same double page spread (sometimes on the same page as the text, usually on the facing page) or occasionally on the next page, avoiding the need to thumb through the book to find a referenced image. In addition, **labels** have been largely integrated within the images, avoiding extensive captions.

In the top left corner of CT and MR images are noted details relating to the imaging plane ("ax", "cor", "sag", etc.), and in the case of MR images the imaging sequence. The sequence details have intentionally been kept simple. For example, all images with fat suppression have been labeled with "fs" (regardless of whether a spectral fat saturation or inversion recovery technique was used), and all images with intravenous contrast material administration are labeled "CM".

We hope you will enjoy reading and using this book!

Nicolas Jorden, MD
on behalf of the editors

In addition to the book there is an ▶ online supplement on the Thieme MediaCenter containing additional images, text, and references. You will be able to access this material using the individual access code printed in the front of the book.

Chapter 1

Acute Trauma and Overuse Injuries: Essentials

1

1 Acute Trauma and Overuse Injuries: Essentials

1.1 Normal Skeletal Development, Variations, and Transitions to Pathologic Conditions

1.1.1 Normal Skeletal Development

▶ **Anatomy.** Normal skeletal development involves growth and maturation of the epiphyseal and metaphyseal growth zones as well as changes involving the medullary cavity. Of all imaging modalities available, magnetic resonance imaging (MRI) is best suited for demonstrating these processes. It allows imaging of the epiphysis (which is formed entirely as a cartilaginous precursor or anlage), the conversion of epiphyseal cartilage into bone, the growth plate (= physis, epiphyseal plate), and the age-related conversion of the bone marrow (▶ Fig. 1.1).

Postnatal skeletal development unfolds in **three steps** leading to ossification of the bone, between which the bone undergoes periods of longitudinal growth:

- Development and growth of the ossification centers in the preformed cartilaginous epiphyses of the short and long tubular bones as well as in the carpal and tarsal bones.
- Development and growth of the apophyseal ossification centers.
- Bony epiphyseal closure.

Only two **epiphyseal ossification centers** are present in the mature newborn: the distal femoral epiphyseal ossification center and usually also the proximal tibial epiphyseal ossification center. The order in which other ossification centers become visible is age dependent. Once an ossification center has appeared, ossification then progresses toward the margins of the cartilaginous precursor.

The **physis** or **growth plate** has a decisive role in the maturation process. Not only is it responsible for eventual height and body mass, it also contributes to resilience and elasticity of the skeleton during growth. It consists of five zones separating the secondary ossification center (the so called chondroepiphysis) from the metaphysis. The growth plate is especially prone to injury (see Chapter 1.3). The cartilaginous plate between the bony epiphysis and the shaft is obliterated and replaced by bone by the time the epiphysis closes; only the joint cartilage remains as a narrow cartilaginous layer.

Apophyseal ossification centers appear shortly before or during puberty. Fusion of the apophyses with the bones starts after puberty and is usually complete by the age of 25 years. The time of appearance of the ossification centers, their growth, and fusion of the epiphysis and apophysis with the bone are constant within a certain range of variation, allowing assessment of skeletal maturity and skeletal age.

During postnatal skeletal development, remodeling of the bone marrow proceeds in parallel with the ossification steps. The medullary cavity of the fetus is still filled with hemato-

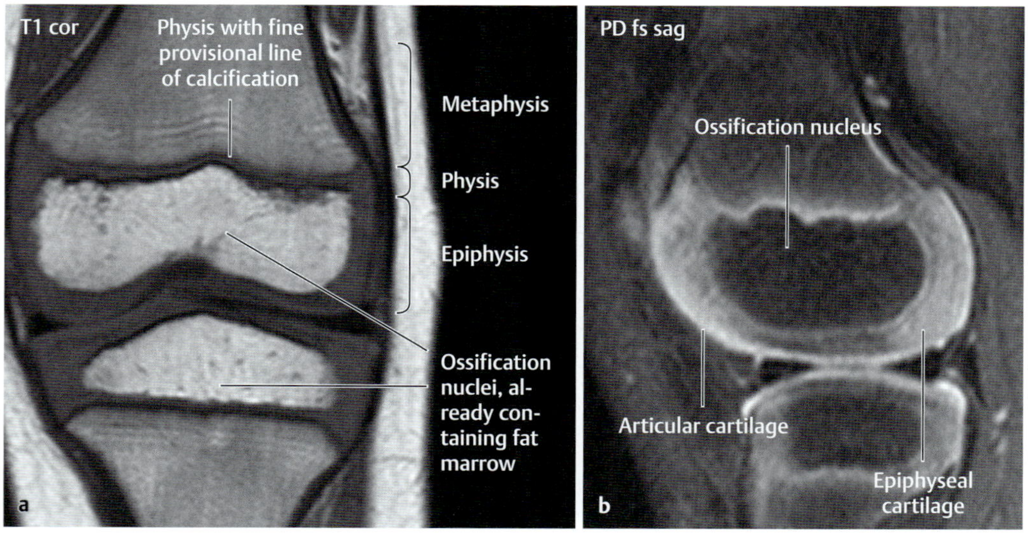

Fig. 1.1 MRI of the knee joint of a 5-year-old child. **(a)** Fat marrow signal in the ossification nucleus of the epiphysis. On the T1W image, the signal intensity in the metaphysis is intermediate between fat and muscle, the classic appearance of red bone marrow. **(b)** On the PDW fat-saturated image, it is possible to differentiate between epiphyseal cartilage and articular cartilage. It is physiologic for epiphyseal cartilage to demonstrate somewhat heterogeneous signal intensity.

poietic red marrow. Shortly before birth, conversion to fat marrow begins in the limbs in a centripetal direction, starting in the distal phalanges. In early adulthood, hematopoietic marrow is still mainly present in the skull, the sternum, the ribs, the pelvis, and the proximal humerus and femur; fat marrow is found in the rest of the skeleton (Chapter 5).

1.1.2 Variations and Disturbances of Skeletal Development

The ossification centers within the preformed cartilaginous epiphyses and apophyses can exhibit numerous anatomical variations during skeletal growth; for example, two or several ossification nuclei may later fuse to form a single ossification center. During this phase, the ossification centers often demonstrate irregular margins, fragmentation and irregular mineralization on radiographs (▶ Figs. 1.2 – 1.4).

Among frequently encountered epiphyseal and apophyseal "variants" are the following:

- **Cone-shaped epiphyses** of the bones of the hand are often associated with disturbances of endochondral growth of the affected phalanges (▶ Fig. 1.5). In contrast, cone-shaped epiphyses and disturbances of epiphyseal and metaphyseal growth of the long bones are always regarded as pathologic, likely the result of early epiphyseal and metaphyseal disturbances of circulation of various etiologies. A common feature is fusion between epiphysis and metaphysis (▶ Fig. 1.6).
- **Pseudoepiphyses** or atypical epiphyses occur in healthy children or more often in children with systemic abnormalities of skeletal development in the proximal metacarpals II–IV and the distal metacarpal I and are of no clinical significance.

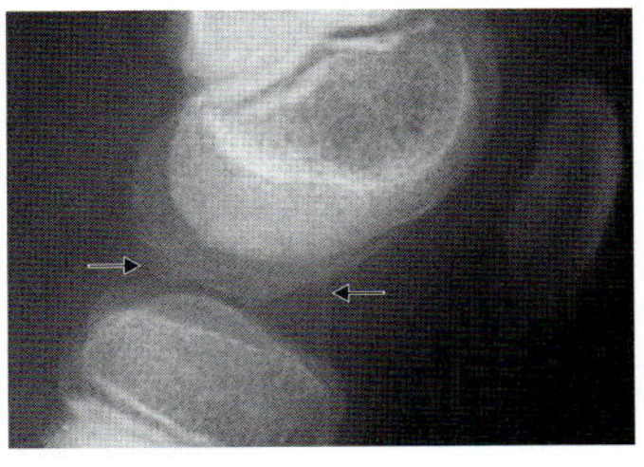

Fig. 1.2 Physiological irregular marginal contour (arrows) of the ossification center of the condylar epiphysis. Variant within the normal range. This most typically involves the posterior aspect of the femoral condyle.

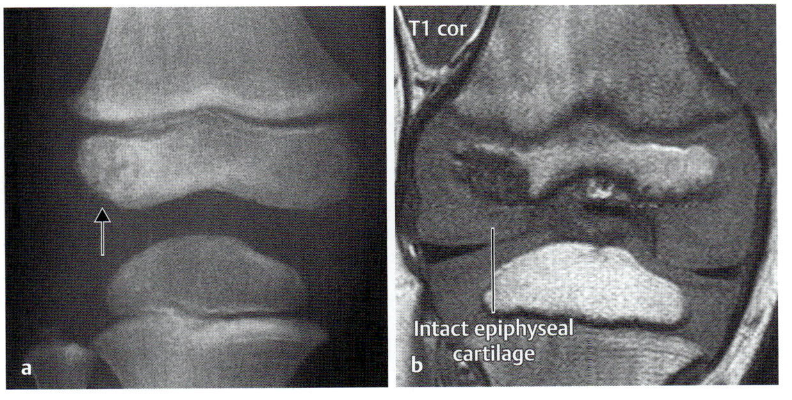

Fig. 1.3 Variant of the ossification nucleus of the distal femoral epiphysis. **(a)** Heterogeneous calcification of the epiphysis (arrow). **(b)** This MRI scan shows an area of low signal intensity in that region as a sign of increased sclerosis.

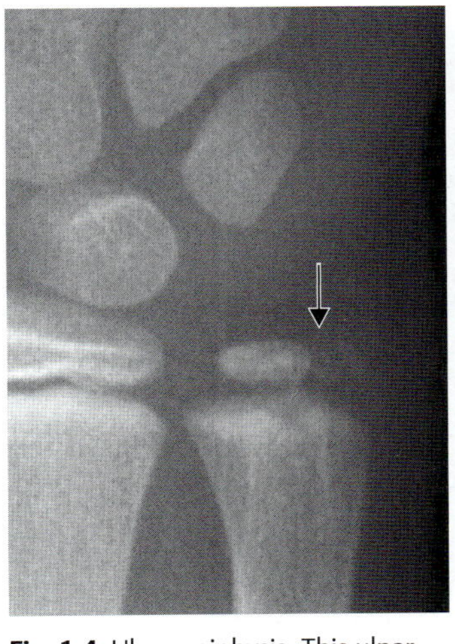

Fig. 1.4 Ulnar epiphysis. This ulnar epiphysis consists of three ossification nuclei (arrow) which will later fuse together.

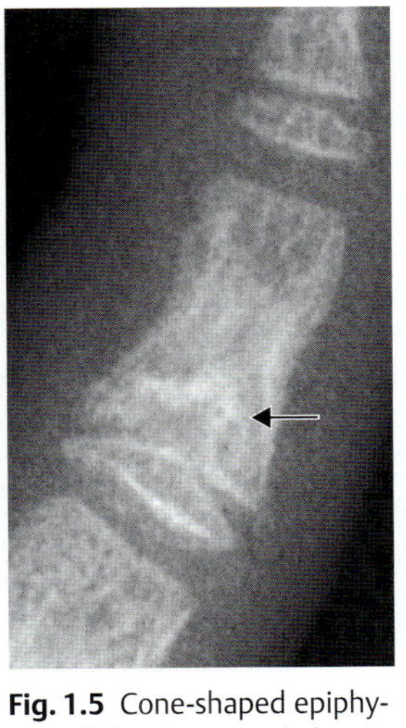

Fig. 1.5 Cone-shaped epiphysis with brachymesophalangia (arrow), a normal variant with mild disturbance of endochondral bone growth.

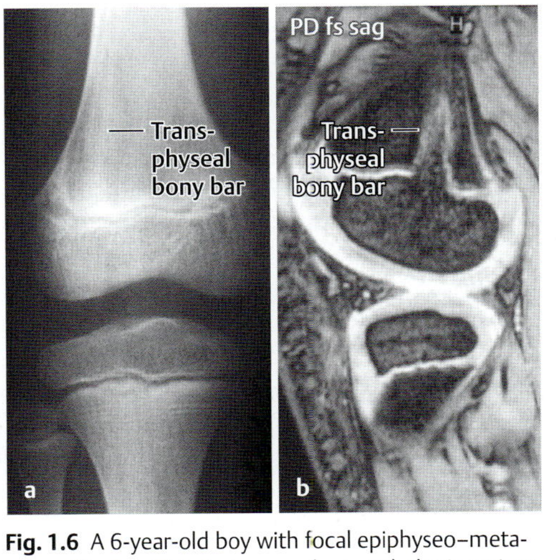

Fig. 1.6 A 6-year-old boy with focal epiphyseo–metaphyseal fusion. This fusion may be a pathologic variant of the cone-shaped epiphysis, which leads to in interference with growth. **(a)** The irregularity of the epiphyseal plate and the metaphysis on the radiograph suggest that fusion has taken place. **(b)** The MRI scan confirms a bony bar extending across the distal femoral physis.

1

- **Increased mineralization** of the epiphyseal ossification nucleus may present in healthy children, most often in the distal phalanges. These ivory or marble-bone epiphyses (▶ Fig. 1.7), as they are called, must be distinguished from other skeletal disorders with increased sclerosis, such as osteopoikilosis.

The radiological appearance of ossification centers can vary, especially in the carpal and tarsal bones and may include:
- The appearance of the ossification nuclei at different ages.
- Irregular mineralization.
- Fusion with an adjacent ossification nucleus.
- The occasional appearance of accessory ossification nuclei.

1.1.3 Transitions to Pathologic States

It is sometimes difficult to draw a line between a normal developmental variant and an alteration with clinical significance, especially when it is accompanied by transient local pain and/or a joint effusion. In these cases the presence of a developmental variant must be confirmed and a pathologic condition excluded.

▶ **Radiography.** Epiphyseal or apophyseal variants can create difficulties in accurate diagnosis, and include:
- **Epiphyseal** or **apophyseal fracture** in the presence of several atypical ossification centers (▶ Figs. 1.8 and ▶ 1.9).
- Avascular **necrosis** with irregular sclerosis and narrowing of the ossification nuclei (▶ Fig. 1.10).
- **Osteochondritis dissecans** or **osteochondral fracture** associated with an irregular peripheral contour of the epiphysis (▶ Fig. 1.11).
- **Congenital disorder of skeletal development** associated with an atypical appearance of the epiphysis (▶ Fig. 1.12).

▶ **US.** Differentiation between a traumatic epiphyseal dislocation in infancy and a normal bone is possible by identifying the ossification center within the epiphyseal cartilage and its position relative to the ossified metaphysis. If a subchondral fracture, osteochondritis dissecans, or avascular necrosis is suspected in early to mid-childhood, an associated effusion—which is always present with these conditions—combined with a history of pain will prompt further diagnostic investigation. If no joint effusion is present, then true pathology is unlikely.

▶ **MRI.** MRI findings in most cases allow a distinction to be made between traumatic injury and a variant or disturbance of ossification. Today, MRI is routinely used as a supplemental modality in cases with equivocal findings on ultrasound, and is the diagnostic method of choice for evaluating the bone marrow. Knowledge of age-related bone marrow conversion is a prerequisite for evaluating pathologic bone marrow findings (Chapter 5.1).

Note

Anatomical variants or disturbances in the radiological appearance of the epiphyses and apophyses can be found in all areas of the pediatric skeleton. These are dealt with in detail in the relevant literature, which should be accessed by the radiologist when an unfamiliar finding is encountered.

1.2 Fractures: Definition, Types, and Classifications

1.2.1 Definition and Classification

A fracture (from the Latin: "frangere" = to break) is an interruption in the continuity of bone whether it involves cortical or trabecular bone. In everyday (surgical) language, the term is synonymous with radiographically visible fractures.

However, there are fractures that are not revealed on conventional radiographs, although CT (computed tomography), MRI, and, at certain anatomical sites, even ultrasound can identify the fracture. These fractures are considered "radiographically occult." The lowest level of traumatic bone damage is the purely trabecular fracture. It is only detectable on an MRI scan where fracture-related bone marrow edema (also known as "bone contusion" or "bone bruise") will be evident. These lesions are indeed painful, but they generally heal spontaneously with rest and a short period of immobilization.

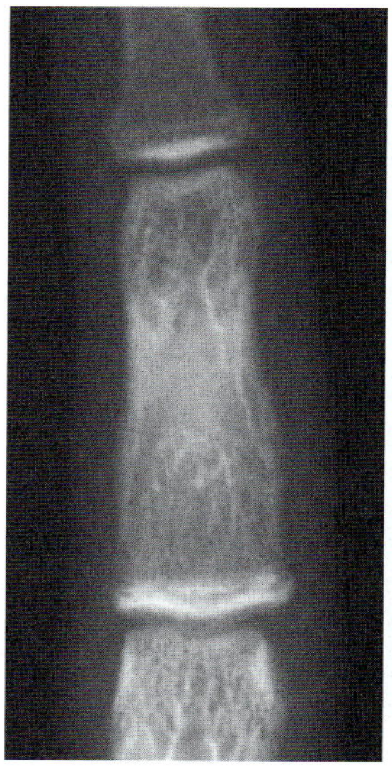

Fig. 1.7 Increased sclerosis of the phalangeal epiphyses (known as ivory or marble-bone epiphysis), a normal variant.

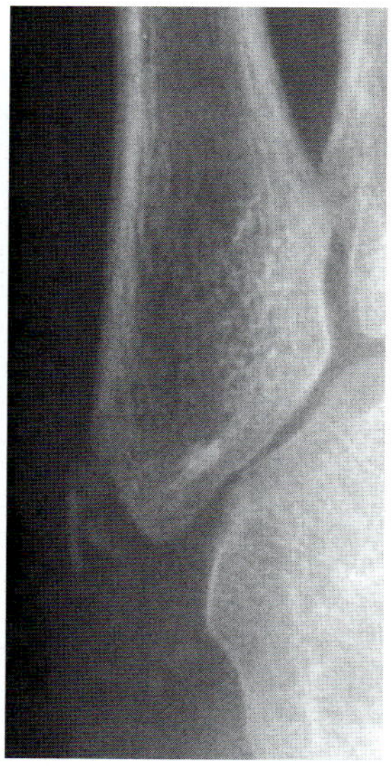

Fig. 1.8 Two shell-like ossification centers at the base of the fifth metatarsal, a normal variant.

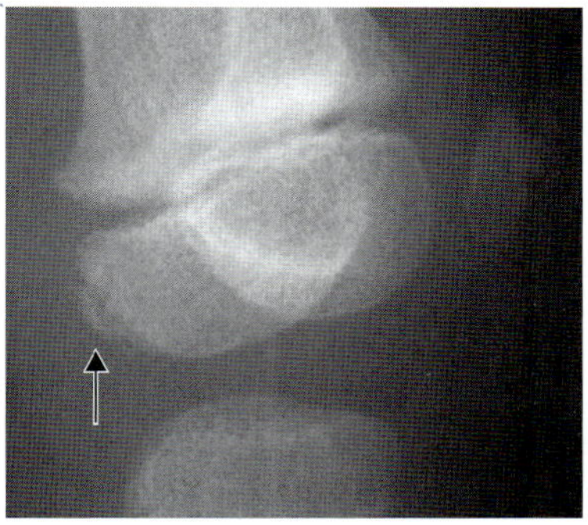

Fig. 1.9

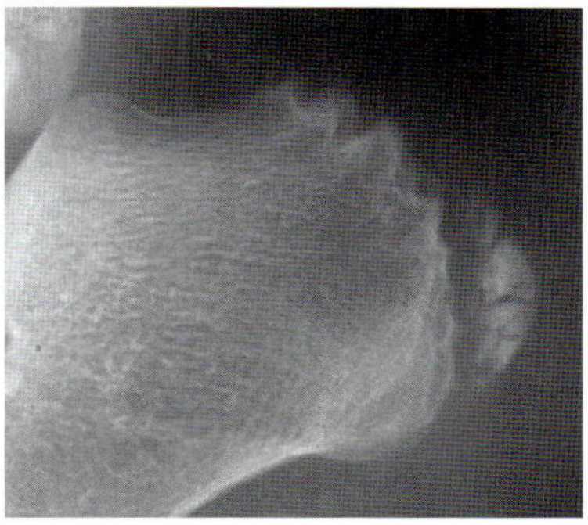

Fig. 1.10

Fig. 1.9 Shell-like ossification nucleus posteriorly at the medial femoral condyle, a normal variant.

Fig. 1.10 Fragmented and sclerotic appearance of the calcaneal apophysis, a normal variant.

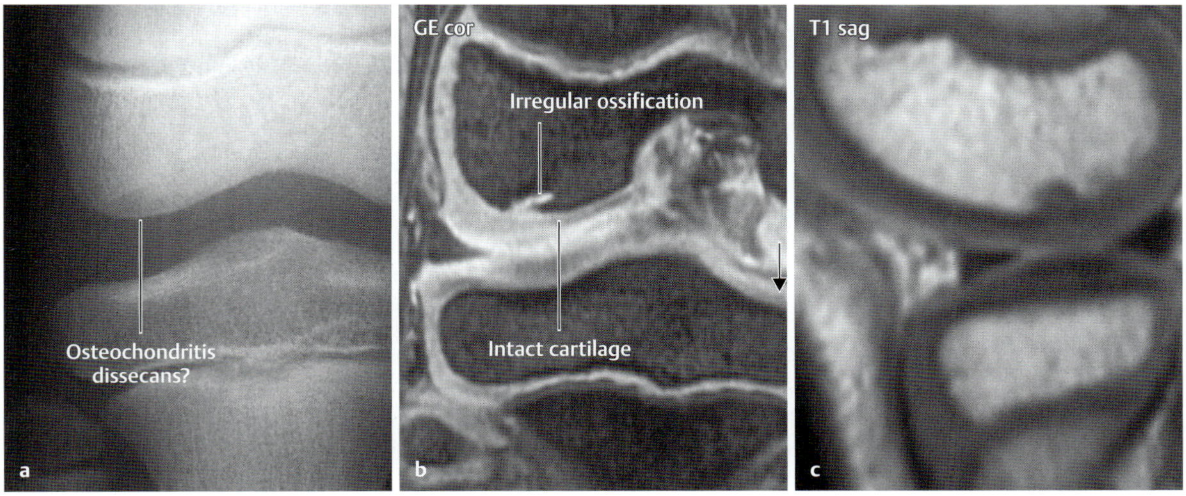

Fig. 1.11 Irregular epiphyseal marginal contour. **(a)** Small subchondral lucency along the lateral condylar epiphysis. **(b)** Corresponding MRI shows a focus of irregular ossification. **(c)** Without evidence of a cartilage defect or a surrounding bone marrow reaction.

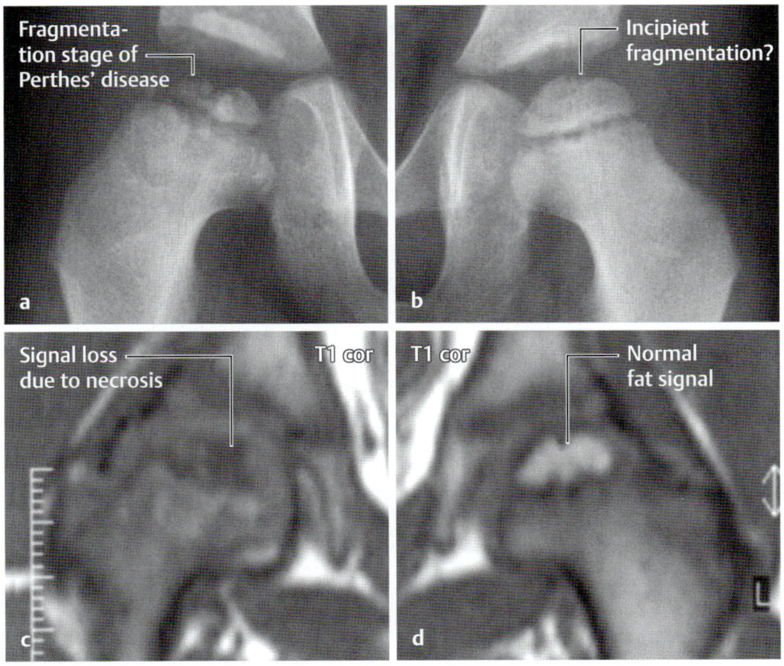

Fig. 1.12 Comparison between Perthes' disease and a normal developmental variant (Meyer's dysplasia). **(a)** Perthes' disease in the fragmentation stage. **(b)** Irregularly contoured epiphysis comprising several "fragments." **(c)** Loss of signal of the epiphysis on the native T1W scan in a case of Perthes' disease. **(d)** Normal fat signal intensity within the multiple ossification centers (= Meyer's dysplasia).

With regard to the underlying cause, a distinction is made between traumatic, stress, and pathologic fractures:

Traumatic fracture. Loading and overloading of a bone can occur directly through a blunt or penetrating injury, or indirectly. Indirect injury may result from traction, compression, shearing or torsional forces.

Stress fractures. There are two types of stress fractures: *fatigue fractures* and *insufficiency fractures. Fatigue fractures* result from repeated overloading of normal bone and are distinguished from *insufficiency fractures*, which occur in abnormal bone that is more prone to injury, even from normal loading. The bone in the latter case is already weakened (usually by osteoporosis) and will fracture after a mild injury or with repetitive loading.

Pathologic fracture. Pathologic fractures are fractures that arise as a result of preexisting *cortical* destruction when even an otherwise low-magnitude force is applied to the bone. These therefore represent a variant of insufficiency fracture. The most common causes are metastases, myeloma, and bone cysts.

1.2.2 Fracture Types

The morphology of the fracture reflects the direction, type, and extent of the forces acting upon the bone at the time of injury. In addition to the type of fracture, other important features include involvement of a joint and any associated subluxation or dislocation. ▸Fig. 1.13 provides a simple overview of the most important fracture types.

Definitions

Nondisplaced fracture (hairline fracture). This is a fine fracture line without any fragment displacement. It can be either incomplete or complete (passing through the whole bone).

Impacted fracture. One fragment is wedged (firmly driven) into the other, e.g., in the hip.

Depression fracture. This arises from the impact of a circumscribed force on the bone (e.g., on the skull). Avulsions of articular margins by opposing bones are a variation of depression fractures.

Compression fracture. There is very little distinction between the terms "impacted fracture" and "compression fracture," especially when the spine is involved.

Avulsion fracture. These are fractures in which a small fragment of bone is torn away at the site of attachment of a ligament or tendon. Typical sites are the base of the fifth metatarsal bone, the tibial tubercle (patellar tendon), the superior pole of the patella (quadriceps tendon), the lesser trochanter (iliopsoas tendon), and the proximal phalanx of the first ray of the hand. These are more common in the skeletally immature patient.

Dislocation. Dislocation involves complete loss of congruency between the articulating joint surfaces. An additional intra- or periarticular fracture may also be present. Subluxation is a joint malalignment where the articular surfaces still have some degree of contact with one another.

Open fracture. In an open fracture, the soft tissue covering the bone has been violated.

1.2.3 Classifications

Fracture classification systems have practical purposes:
- To determine the severity of the injury.
- To select appropriate treatment.
- To assess prognosis.
- To have easy application and be easily reproducible.

The **classification systems for fractures** in individual anatomical regions are dealt with in detail in Chapter 2. The AO Classification (AO Foundation, Switzerland; see http://aofoundation.org), is one of the best known and will be highlighted in the subsequent chapters.

The **AO classification** distinguishes the following criteria:
- Anatomical region (which bone is involved?).
- Part (which segment of the bone is involved?).
- Fracture type (letters are used to indicate either joint involvement or the complexity of shaft fractures; the digit after the letter defines the fracture more precisely).

The AO-OTA classification combines the AO classification and the 1996 OTA classification. The OTA classification adopts the principles of the AO classification and completes it by coding some of the bones hitherto not classified by the AO system.

▸ References for Chapter 1.2.

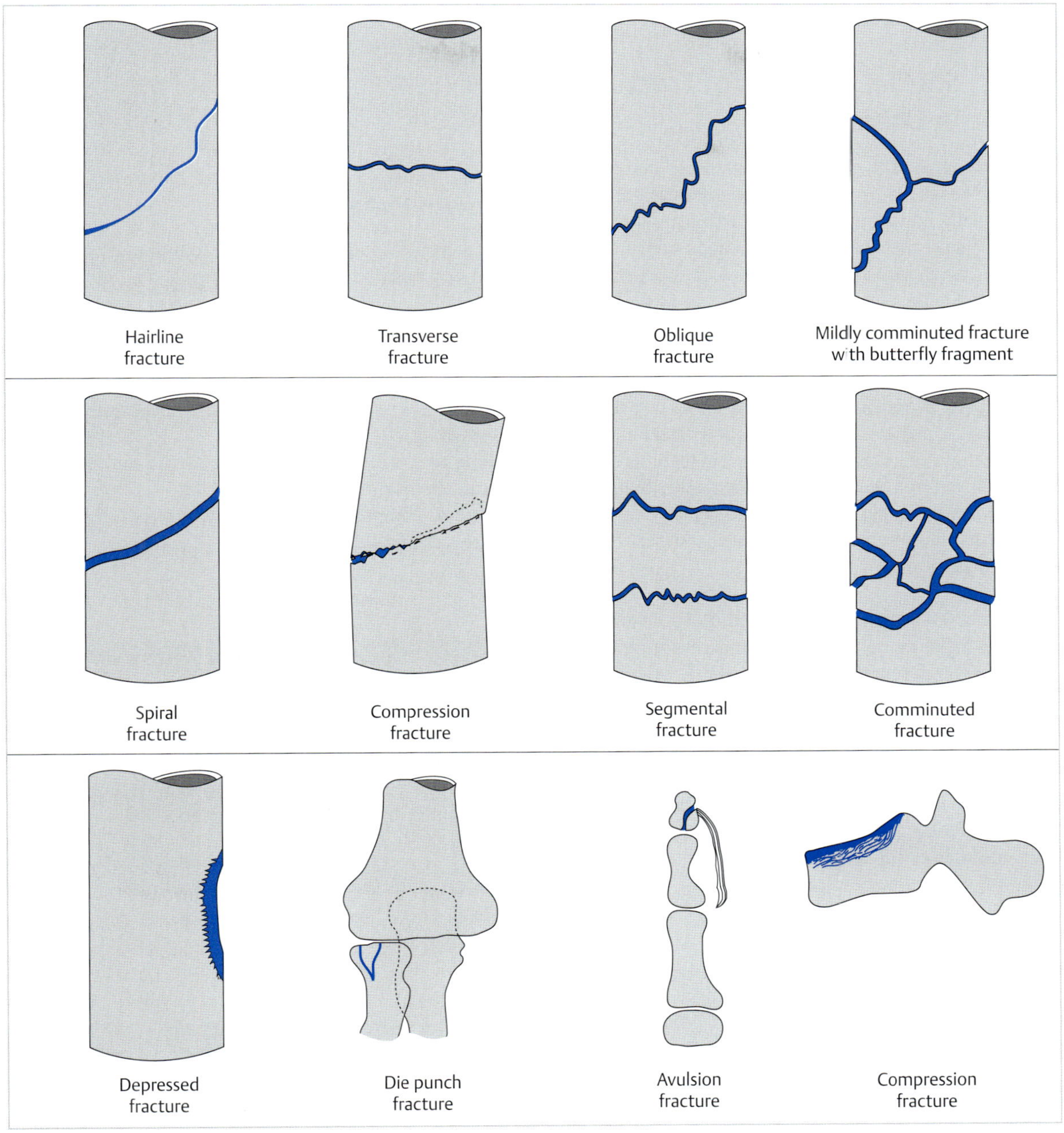

Fig. 1.13 The most important fractures types.

1.3 Fractures in Children

1.3.1 Special Features of Fractures in Children

The most important anatomical difference between the adult and the pediatric skeleton is the open growth plate in the skeletally immature patient. Growth plate injuries can result in disturbances of bone development, from premature physeal closure (arrest). The thicker and stronger periosteum found in the developing skeleton also allows the child to readily form callus, which can in some cases be very exuberant.

The elasticity of pediatric bone allows for greater deformation before a complete fracture occurs and the strong periosteum often prevents any major displacement of the fracture fragments. Because the growth plate is weaker than the adjacent bone and supporting ligaments, epiphyseal separation occurs more frequently than do nonphyseal fractures or joint dislocations.

From a physiological view, the skeleton of a child has the tendency for more rapid healing and excellent remodeling such that the development of nonunion is extremely uncommon.

The normal classifications for adult fractures cannot usually be applied to the pediatric skeleton. Specific classifications, such as the PCCF–**AO classification** (see http://aofoundation.org), were accordingly developed for fractures in children. A simple classification according to location is usually sufficient for everyday clinical purposes:

- Diaphyseal.
- Metaphyseal.
- Epiphyseal.
- Combined injuries.

Special Fracture Types in Children

Buckle or torus fracture. This is caused by compression in the region of the metaphysis. The cortex bulges out on one side. Changes on the opposite side of the bone are either absent or very subtle (▶ Fig. 1.14).

Greenstick fracture. This is an incomplete fracture that often involves only one side of the bone (▶ Fig. 1.15). The special feature of this fracture is that the periosteal sleeve remains intact.

Bowing fracture. This refers to a plastic bending of the bone due to its increased elasticity in childhood, without the presence of a true fracture line (▶ Fig. 1.16).

Transition fracture. This involves injury to the growth plate that is in the process of closing (▶ Fig. 1.17; Chapter 2.14.1).

> **Note**
> The term *transition fracture* is not used in some countries (e.g., USA). This fracture is just described and should be considered a subtype of the Salter–Harris classification.

Growth Plate Injuries

The Salter–Harris classification system is most commonly used for describing injuries involving the growth plate (▶ Fig. 1.18):

- **Type I:** Epiphyseal separation.
- **Type II:** Metaphyseal fracture with involvement of the growth plate.
- **Type III:** Epiphyseal fracture with involvement of the growth plate.
- **Type IV:** Fracture through the epiphysis and metaphysis, crossing the growth plate (▶ Fig. 1.19).
- **Type V:** Compression of the growth plate (crush injury) (see ▶ Fig. 1.18).

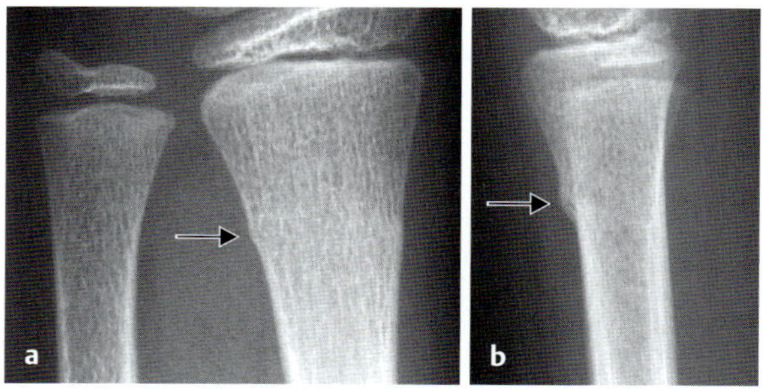

Fig. 1.14 Buckle fracture (arrows) in a 9-year-old girl. **(a)** PA radiograph. **(b)** Lateral radiograph.

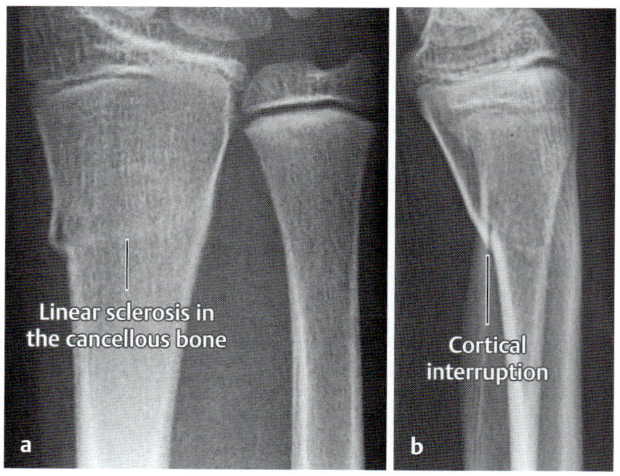

Fig. 1.15 Greenstick fracture in a 13-year-old boy (asymmetric cortical disruption). **(a)** Transverse sclerotic line in the trabecular bone with disruption of the lateral cortex. **(b)** The cortex is disrupted only on the palmar aspect.

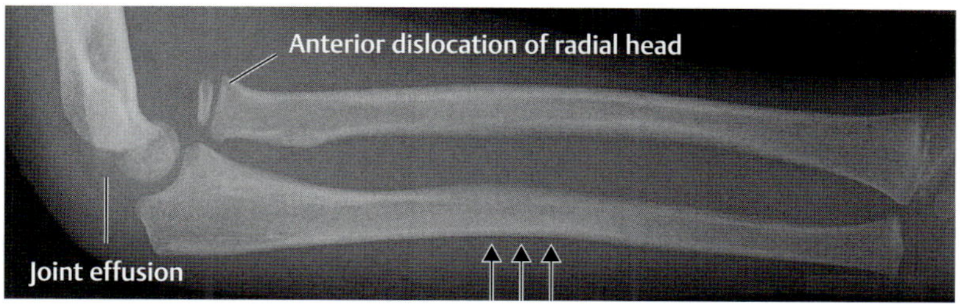

Fig. 1.16 Bowing fracture (arrows) of the ulna with subluxation of the radial head. There is no evidence of a fracture line. This is a case of a Monteggia-type injury (Chapter 2.8.3).

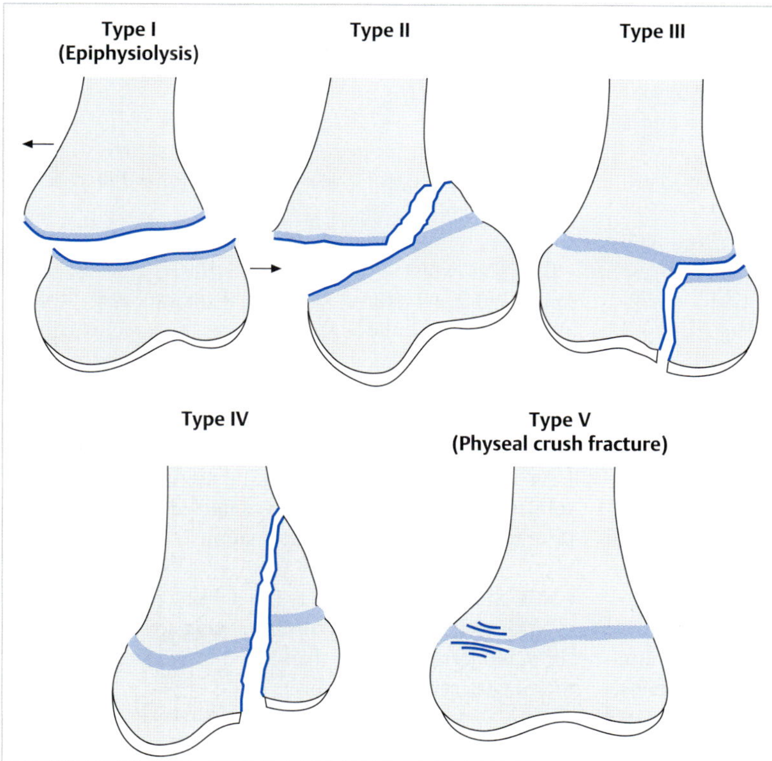

Fig. 1.18 Salter–Harris classification of fractures involving the growth plate.

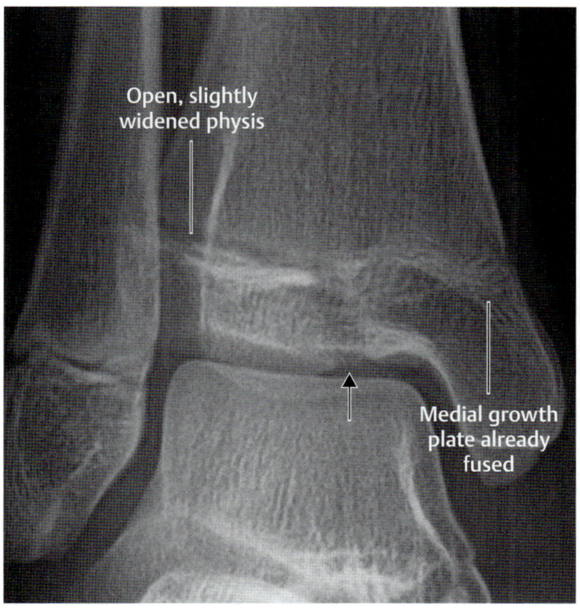

Fig. 1.17 Salter–Harris III fracture in a partially closed physis. Fracture at the transition (arrow) between the closed and open epiphyseal plate.

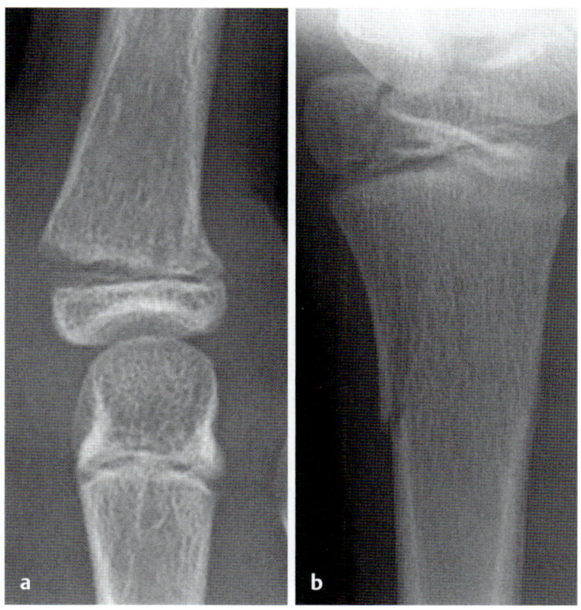

Fig. 1.19 Growth plate injuries. **(a)** Salter–Harris II injury. **(b)** Salter–Harris IV injury.

1

1.3.2 Battered-Child Syndrome

Battered-child syndrome (synonym: child abuse) encompasses all types of harm to a child, such as physical and mental traumatization, neglect, and sexual abuse. Usually neonates, babies, and infants have been subjected to physical abuse. Despite figures for suspected cases that are alarmingly high, only a small percentage of cases are brought to court, but the radiologist plays a decisive role in those cases in diagnosing physical abuse, which may be life-saving for the child.

▸ **Clinical presentation.** Significant grounds for suspicion:

- Hematomas, abrasions, and burns of varying age and at unusual sites.
- Inadequate history for the type of injury and delayed presentation of the child to the doctor.
- Multiple skeletal injuries of varying age and fracture types that are "pathognomonic" for child abuse.
- Subdural hematomas; cerebral contusions with or without skull fracture.
- Patient age usually under 2 years.

Skeletal injuries may present as single or multiple fractures in varying stages of healing and associated with marked periosteal reaction and callus formation. Older fractures are typically asymptomatic by the time the child presents. Fractures of the limbs present as metaphyseal and diaphyseal lesions in equal numbers. Brain injuries occur in the form of subdural hematomas and brain contusions as a result of direct force or hyperextension–hyperflexion injury with or without skull fracture. Shaking injuries result in subdural hematomas secondary to tears in bridging veins. Retinal hemorrhages are concomitant features in shaking injuries. If a head injury is suspected, ultrasound up to the first year of life and cCT (cranial CT) or MRI are the diagnostic methods of choice (▸ Fig. W1.1).

▸ **Radiography.** Conventional radiograph is usually the first imaging examination.

Rib fractures, especially posteriorly, are rare in early childhood. They are therefore very suspicious for physical abuse, as are fractures of the scapula, sternum, and spinous processes of the spine.

Metaphyseal corner (chip) fractures are *pathognomonic* for the use of physical force. The radiological appearance comprises small rim fragments ("corner sign"), often with a fine, shell-like fragment along the metaphyseal ossification zone. This type of injury is caused by an abrupt jerk or twist of the limb. The periosteum and the insertion of the joint capsule in the region of the ossification zone are very firmly attached to the metaphysis, so that a sudden traction force will result in a metaphyseal fragment breaking away, along with the epiphysis (▸ Figs. 1.20 – 1.23).

Periosteal new bone formation—even without a visible fracture—is a common finding. In early childhood, the periosteum of the diaphysis is only loosely attached to the cortex, unlike the periosteum of the metaphysis. An injury can therefore easily produce a subperiosteal hematoma. In babies and infants, periosteal new bone formation becomes visible on radiographs between days 6 and 8, after injury (▸ Figs. 1.24 and ▸ 1.25).

Multiple bone lesions of varying age are indicative of abuse (▸ Fig. 1.26). They are also of forensic significance since the radiological appearances can be used for estimating when the abuse occurred.

If child abuse is suspected, then a full skeletal survey is obligatory up to the age of 2 years, and each limb should be imaged in two planes.

▸ **US.** The extent of damage, especially in cases of metaphyseal corner fractures, is difficult if not impossible to visualize radiographically as the epiphyses are largely cartilaginous in early childhood. The position of the already ossified metaphysis relative to the cartilaginous epiphysis is recognizable on ultrasound, which allows the extent of damage and any possible epiphyseal dislocation to be assessed (see ▸ Fig. 1.22). Joint effusions are easily detected. Additionally, subperiosteal hematomas can be detected at an early stage, prior to periosteal new bone formation.

▸ **NUC MED.** A bone scan is a reliable screening method, even for clinically silent or uncertain bony lesions. Skull fractures and fractures older than 3 to 5 months cannot be detected with certainty, however.

▸ **MRI.** In individual cases an MRI scan allows a better differentiation between Salter–Harris II and Salter–Harris IV fractures involving complex joints, such as the elbow. Its broader overview provides an advantage over ultrasound for preoperative planning. In addition, a whole-body MRI allows the detection of soft tissue lesions which may also be of forensic importance. Whole-body MRI is not associated with radiation exposure and therefore, as a screening method, has an advantage over skeletal survey radiography and radionuclide scanning; however, it has low sensitivity with a high degree of specificity, particularly for metaphyseal lesions.

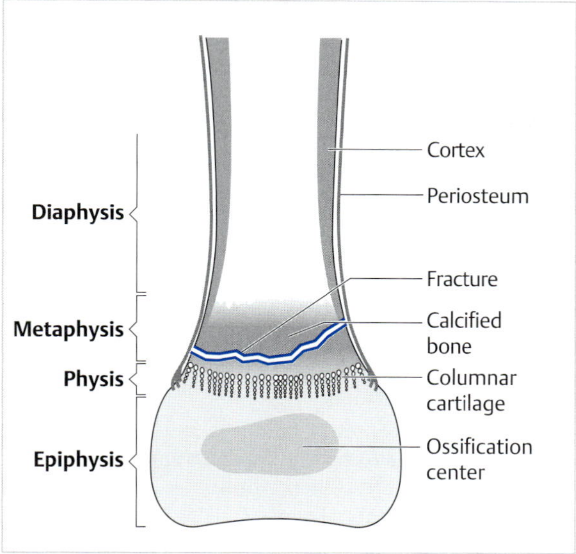

Fig. 1.20 Actual course of the fracture line in the case of a radiologically visible, metaphyseal corner or chip fracture.

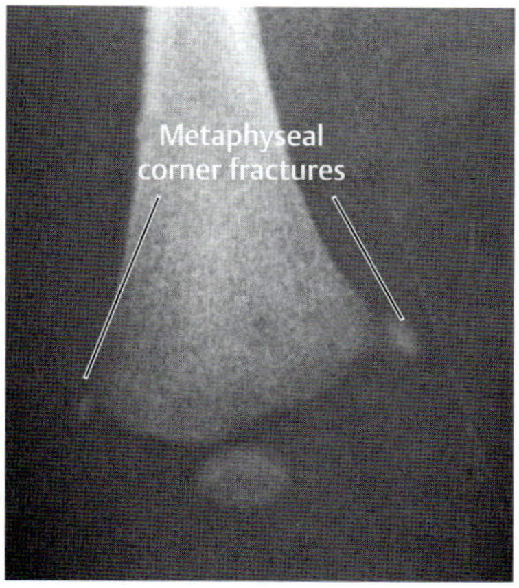

Fig. 1.21 Battered child. Nine-day-old neonate.

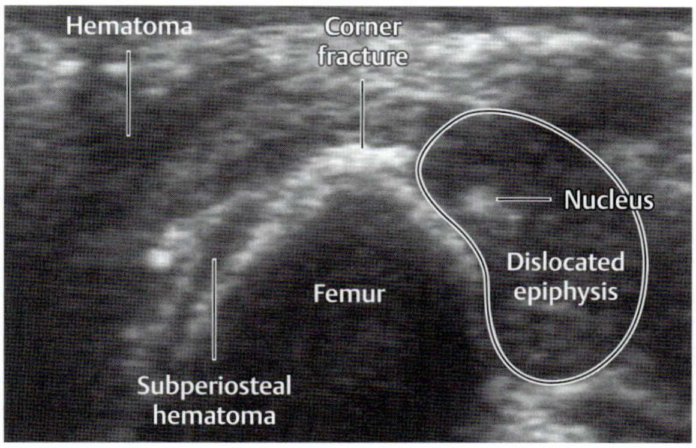

Fig. 1.22 Epiphyseal dislocation of the distal femur in a battered child (transverse sonogram).

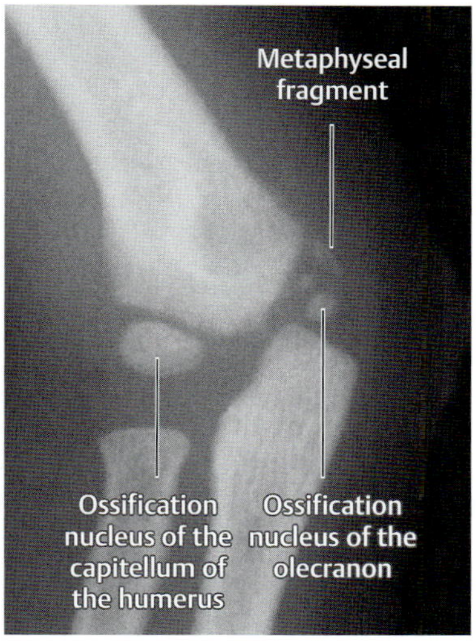

Fig. 1.23 Battered child. Six-month-old infant with protective posture of the elbow.

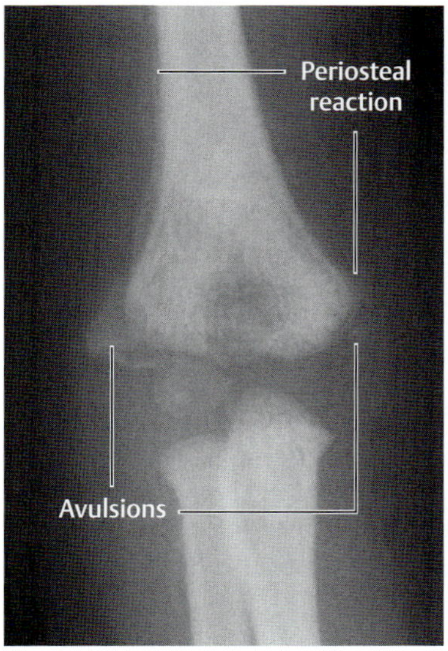

Fig. 1.24 Battered child. Same child as in ▶ Fig. 1.23. Three weeks later. Obvious periosteal new bone formation as a reaction to bilateral metaphyseal corner fractures.

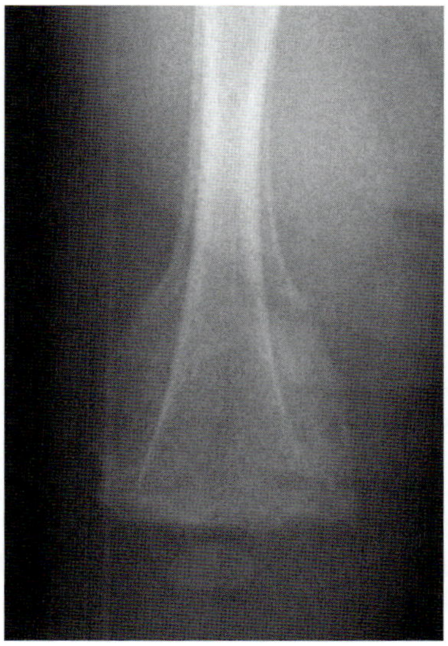

Fig. 1.25 Battered child. Periosteal new bone formation encasing the diametaphyseal region after a distal metaphyseal fracture with a subperiosteal hematoma, 3 weeks after injury.

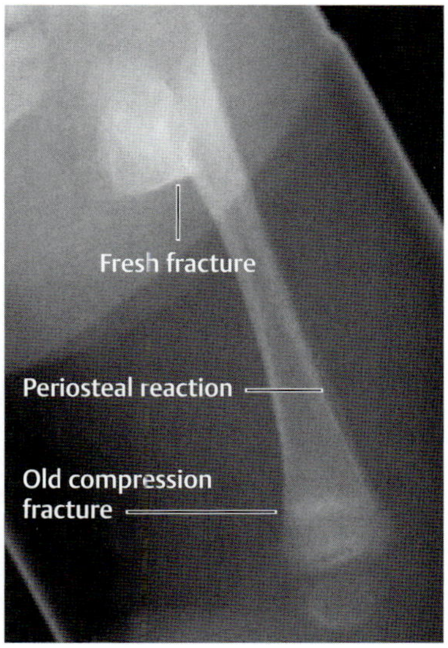

Fig. 1.26 Battered child. Two-month-old infant.

> **Note**
> If the suspicion of child abuse is substantiated, a complete diagnostic imaging examination is necessary for the protection of the child (for detailed review see the consensus recommendations by the American College of Radiology, 2011, referenced in the web material); this has both therapeutic and forensic implications. Injury to the central nervous system in particular requires prompt treatment, while findings of skeletal injury patterns indicative of abuse provide critical forensic evidence.

► **DD.** The diagnosis is not difficult to establish in cases demonstrating typical skeletal changes. Disorders with a similar appearance must be excluded, however, given the consequences of this grave diagnosis. Similar bony lesions are seen in the following disorders:

- Obstetric and accidental fractures, e.g., sustained during very boisterous play with parents and relatives.
- Neurological disorders, e.g., meningomyelocele, associated with fractures sustained during physiotherapy or otherwise.
- Osteogenesis imperfecta, achondroplasia.
- Metabolic disorders (rickets, Menkes' syndrome).
- Prostaglandin therapy.
- Infantile cortical hyperostosis.

1.4 Fractures of the Articular Surfaces: Subchondral, Chondral, and Osteochondral Fractures

Fractures of the articular surfaces are confined to the cartilage; those of the subchondral plate are confined to the cancellous subchondral bone. They run more or less parallel to the joint surface, and should be distinguished from fractures of the underlying bone which *also* extend into the joint (fractures with joint involvement). They are B or C fractures according to the AO classification (Chapter 1.2.3).

► **Anatomy.** The important biomechanical properties of hyaline cartilage include its load-bearing capacity, its elasticity, smoothness of its gliding surface, and its durability. Hyaline cartilage is arranged in various layers. The deep calcified zone and subchondral bone are closely interlinked. Avulsion of the cartilage (traumatic separation) occurs between the deep calcified part of the cartilage and the noncalcified part adjacent to the joint. Traumatic injury to the joint surface is caused by sudden abnormal contact of the articular surfaces with one another and may take the form of shearing forces, rotational forces, or vertical impaction, depending on the mechanism of injury.

> **Note**
> Cartilage is more elastic than the subchondral trabecular structure of the bone. Subchondral bone therefore tends to fracture under abnormal force where cartilage rapidly recovers and "bounces back" to a normal state. As a rule, a distinction can be made between four stages of injury to articular surfaces (► Figs. W1.2–W1.5).

Classification of fractures involving joint surfaces (► Fig. 1.27):

- Subchondral fractures.
- Chondral fractures.
- Osteochondral fractures.

► **Clinical presentation.** Clinical symptoms are typically nonspecific in nature. A hemarthrosis is often associated with an osteochondral fracture.

Location: The tibiotalar joint and the knee joint, including the patellofemoral compartment, are most commonly involved, but other locations, such as the femoral head and humeral head, may be affected.

► **Radiography.** A search should be made for contour irregularities and abnormal subchondral densities. Small circumscribed areas of radiolucency are suspicious for an "empty" fragment bed after dislodgement of the fragment; in those cases, radiopaque loose bodies should be looked for (► Figs. 1.28–1.30). Views in two planes are not always sufficient, so oblique views (of the knee, elbow, fingers, and foot) or axial views (of the patella) will often increase the diagnostic yield.

> **Note**
> A radiographic examination has a relatively high rate of false-negative findings in fractures involving joint surfaces, despite imaging in more than two planes. In the case of the tibiotalar joint, for example, missed fractures are to be expected in up to 30% of cases.

► **CT.** CT is a very sensitive method for establishing the diagnosis of an osteochondral fracture of the joint surface. In some centers, CT arthrography, a very sensitive method, has become an established technique for diagnosing fine chondral injuries (► Fig. 1.31). CT is also the technique of choice for detecting intra-articular loose bodies.

► **MRI.** MRI is the imaging modality of choice for making a definitive diagnosis of osteochondral injuries. Common forms of injury to cartilage and subchondral bone include:

- Simple longitudinal or transverse fissures.
- Stellate type.
- Chondral flap.
- Full-thickness cartilage defect secondary to a punched-out fragment with relatively sharply defined margins.

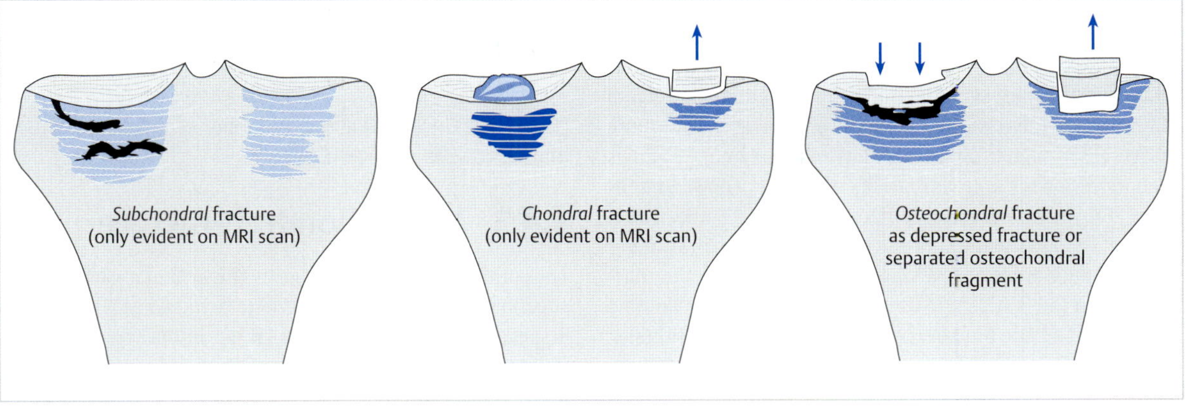

Fig. 1.27 Classification of fractures involving joint surfaces.

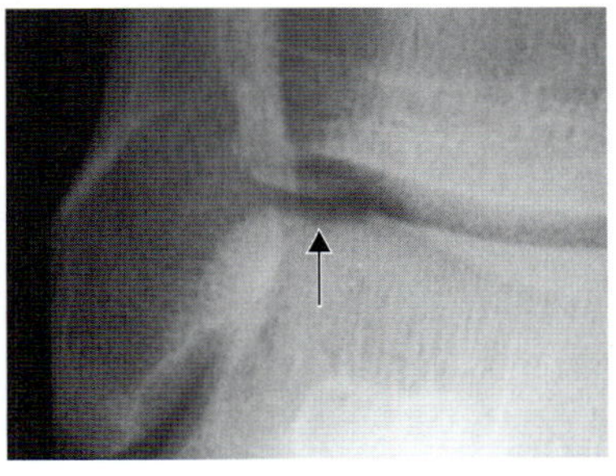

Fig. 1.28

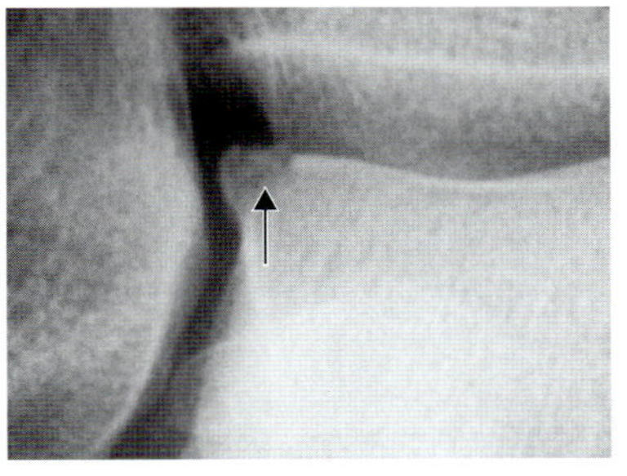

Fig. 1.29

Fig. 1.28 Osteochondral fracture (arrow) of the lateral talar dome.

Fig. 1.29 Osteochondral fracture (arrow) of the lateral talar dome.

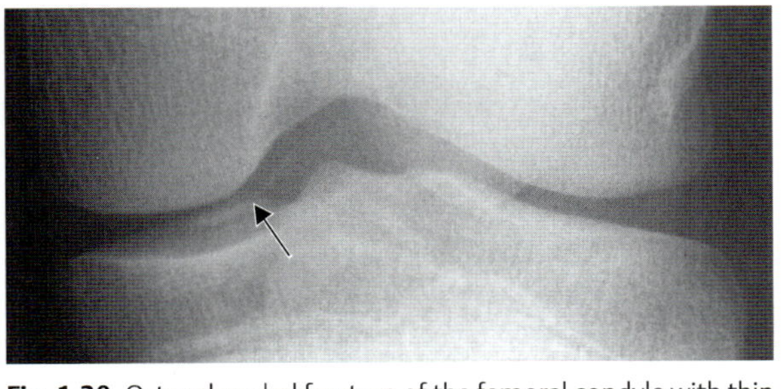

Fig. 1.30 Osteochondral fracture of the femoral condyle with thin and long loose fragment (arrow).

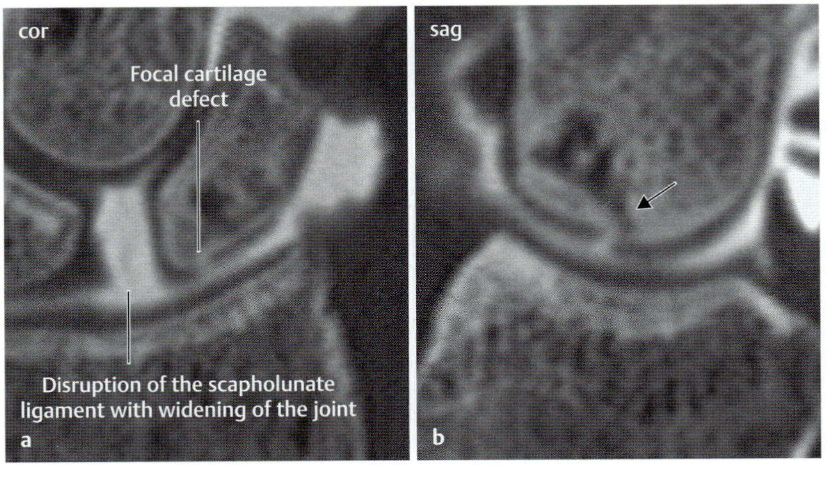

Fig. 1.31 Osteochondral fracture of the proximal pole of the scaphoid as seen on CT arthrography. **(a)** Scapholunate (SL) dissociation. Focal defect of the articular cartilage at the proximal scaphoid pole. **(b)** There is a subchondral fracture (arrow) extending through the subchondral plate into the joint space.

1.4.1 Subchondral Fracture

In the case of a subchondral injury, the articular cartilage is intact and the joint surface not depressed. Edemalike signal intensity is evident in the subchondral bone as a vague area of decreased signal on T1W (T1-weighted) images and is even more conspicuous as high signal intensity on fluid-sensitive (T2W) MR sequences, especially when fat saturation is applied. Associated fracture lines may be detected as linear or curvilinear areas of low signal intensity within the marrow edema (▶ Fig. 1.32); in the absence of a fracture line the diagnosis of a bone marrow contusion is made. Occasionally, a subchondral contusion may present as a very circumscribed hypointense area on T1W scans, reminiscent of a focus of osteonecrosis, but ultimately heal.

1.4.2 Chondral Fracture

A chondral fracture may be associated with a **cartilage defect** with relatively sharply defined margins secondary to a displaced fragment (▶ Fig. 1.33). Chondral fissures may be **longitudinal, oblique**, or **transverse** and may extend to the subchondral bone plate (▶ Fig. 1.34). Associated **subchondral edema** is very often, but *not always*, seen below a defect.

A very important type of chondral pathology known as **delamination** occurs when the hyaline cartilage separates from the subchondral bone plate. If there is an associated vertical fissure, a cartilage "flap" will occur, but if not, the delamination may not be detectable at arthroscopy unless the area is probed (▶ Fig. 1.35).

Abnormal **signal intensity**, with or without thickening of the cartilage, is sometimes the only indication of chondral pathology. In this case, chondromalacia is the most appropriate term.

Osteoarthritis, rather than trauma, should be considered as an etiology for chondral abnormalities in older people, but the distinction is sometimes difficult.

▶ Figs. W1.6 – W1.10 show a number of different cartilage injuries as seen on 3-tesla (3 T) MRI.

1.4.3 Osteochondral Fracture

These injuries involve damage to the articular cartilage and subchondral bone and are often detected on MRI because of associated edema within the underlying marrow (▶ Figs. 1.36 – 1.39). It is important to look for a fracture or depression of the subchondral plate. In some cases an osteochondral fragment may be displaced into the joint.

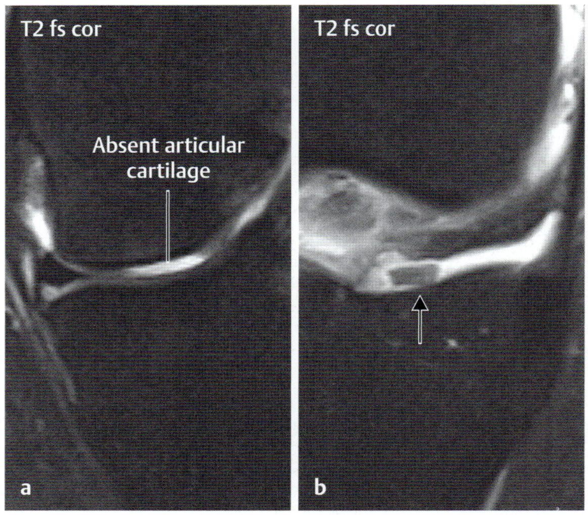

Fig. 1.33 Chondral fracture. **(a)** Focal cartilage defect. The absence of other signs of osteoarthritis suggests that this is related to an acute chondral fracture. **(b)** The cartilage fragment (arrow) is located in the lateral joint compartment.

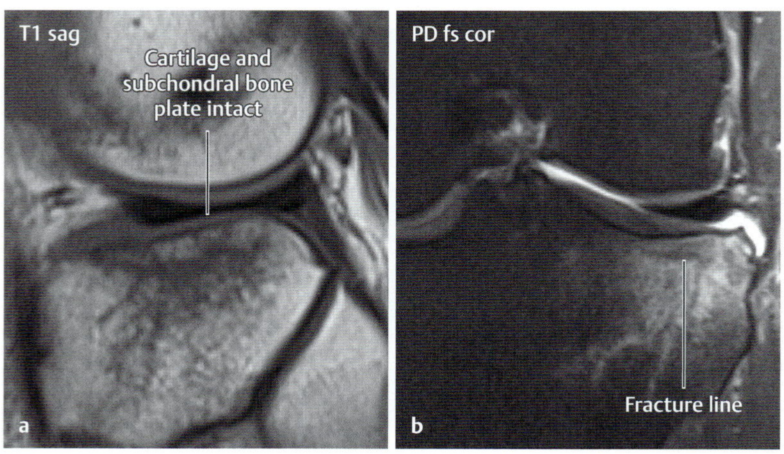

Fig. 1.32 Subchondral fracture of the lateral tibial plateau. **(a)** Hypointense trabecular fracture lines. **(b)** A fracture line is definable within the marrow edema.

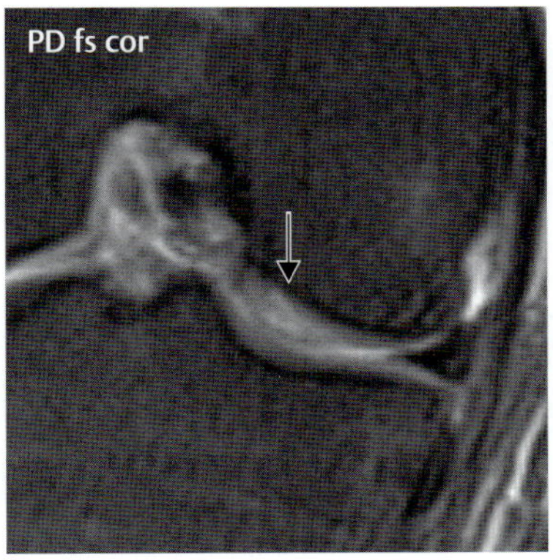

Fig. 1.34

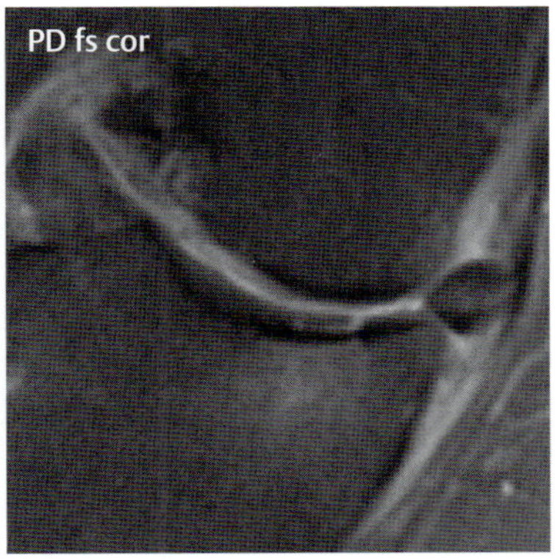

Fig. 1.35

Fig. 1.34 Traumatic cartilage injury (arrow) of the femoral condyle.

Fig. 1.35 Chondral delamination injury of tibial plateau. Note the high signal intensity extending between the cartilage and subchondral plate.

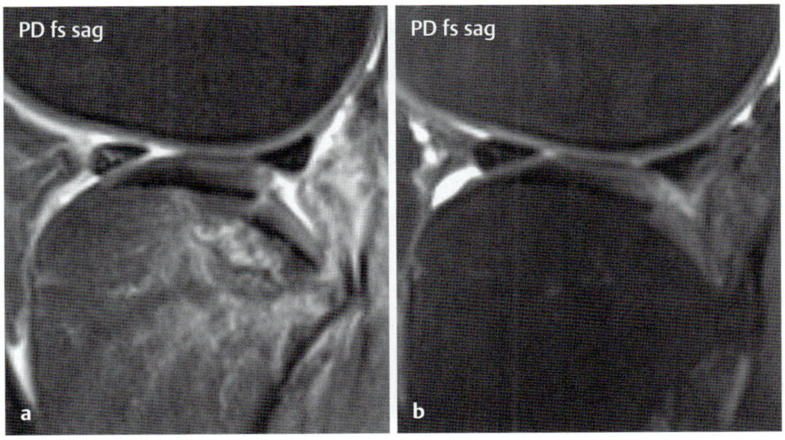

Fig. 1.36 Serial scans of an osteochondral fracture of the tibial plateau. **(a)** Immediately after injury. **(b)** Five months later. The marrow edema is no longer evident but the depression of the articular surface persists.

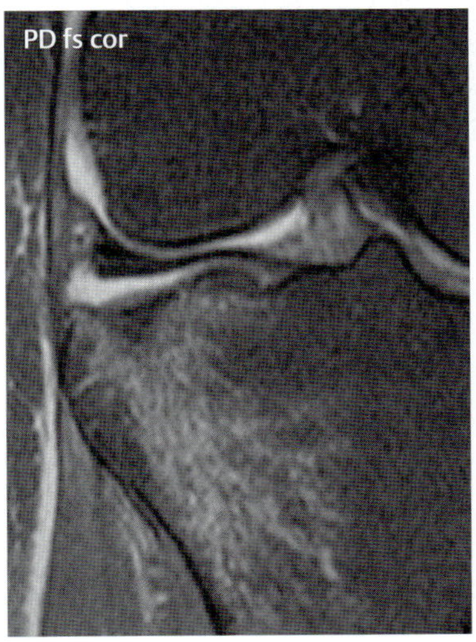

Fig. 1.37 Osteochondral fracture of the tibial plateau. Joint effusion.

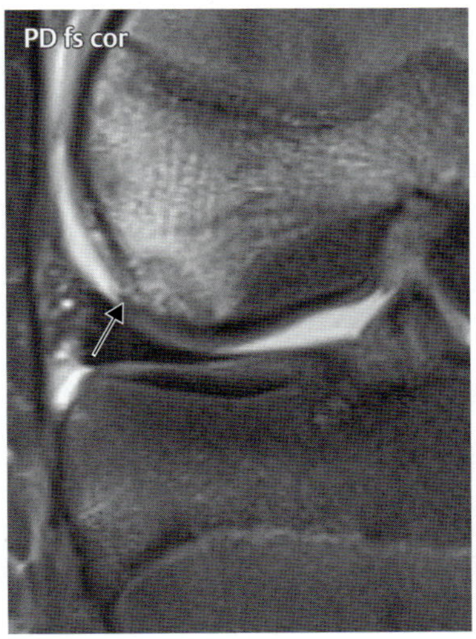

Fig. 1.38 Osteochondral fracture of the lateral femoral condyle. Only discrete step-off in the lateral cortex at the periphery of the articular surface (arrow).

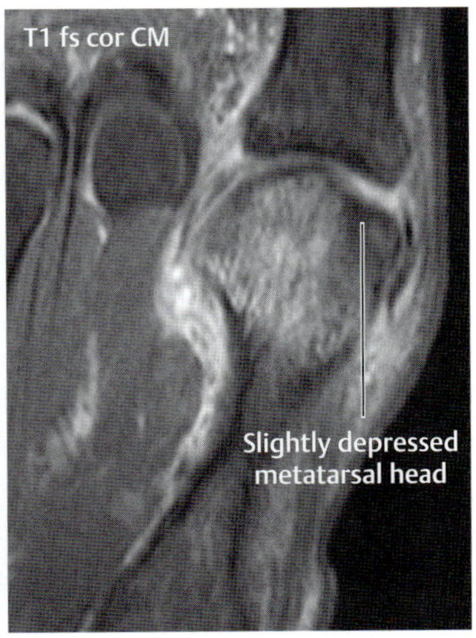

Fig. 1.39 Mildly depressed osteochondral impression fracture of the first metatarsal head.

1.5 Stress and Insufficiency Fractures

▸ **Pathology.** "Stress" refers to a force or a load exerted on a bone that is the result of muscular activity and/or body weight. Bone is a dynamic tissue that needs stress for normal development. If normal stress is removed from the bone, a rapid osteoclastic absorption of cancellous and cortical bone will automatically ensue; in addition, osteoblastic activity ceases, resulting in disuse osteoporosis.

It is not fully understood how stress causes the bone to adapt to its mechanical function, but there are indications that this adaptation occurs primarily by way of **microfractures**. The initial response to increased stress is osteoclastic resorption. Osteoclastic resorption cavities are subsequently filled with lamellar bone over the course of weeks to months. In the meantime, if the excessive stresses continue, an imbalance between bone resorption and formation occurs and results in a temporary weakening of the bone. Periosteal and endosteal new bone formation provides some support for the temporarily weakened bone, but if the bone is not given sufficient rest, fatigue fractures of the trabecular and/or cortical bone may occur.

1.5.1 Classification

Stress fractures are divided into two categories, depending on the initial state of the bone:

Fatigue fractures. Bone density and structure are normal in these patients. A (reversible) weakening of the bone develops in response to increased activity. These are most common in athletes.

Insufficiency fractures. In bone of abnormal density or structure, a fracture may develop even with only the stresses of normal daily activities. Osteoporosis is the most common etiology. A pathologic fracture (Chapter 1.5.3) is a type of insufficiency fracture that occurs in bone that has been weakened by underlying tumor. The most common type of insufficiency fracture is the osteoporotic vertebral compression fracture (Chapter 8.1.3).

> **Note**
> Insufficiency fractures of the pelvis are commonly the result of pelvic radiotherapy.

▸ **Clinical presentation.** The clinical hallmark of a stress fracture is activity-related localized pain and soft tissue swelling that is relieved with rest. Insufficiency fractures of the femoral neck or spine may remain asymptomatic for a very long time.

▸ **Radiography.**

- Classic fracture line (rare).
- Lamellar to solid periosteal reaction as a sign of the repair process (see ▸ Fig. 1.40).
- Ill-defined line of density between cancellous bone and cortex (late stage; ▸ Figs. 1.40 and ▸ 1.41).
- Callus formation (late stage; ▸ Figs. 1.42 and ▸ 1.43).

> **Note**
> Radiographic findings are often absent in the early stages of a stress or insufficiency fracture and may never develop if the causative activity is curtailed.

▸ **NUC MED.** A bone scan is well suited for detecting stress and insufficiency fractures in the presence of negative radiological findings. A false-negative finding is a rarity in adults.

▸ **CT.** CT is suitable for detecting the early findings of periosteal and/or endosteal new bone formation as well as any fracture lines (▸ Figs. 1.44 and ▸ 1.45). Identification of a fracture line, together with reactive sclerotic bony changes, usually allows a specific diagnosis (see ▸ Fig. 1.47b).

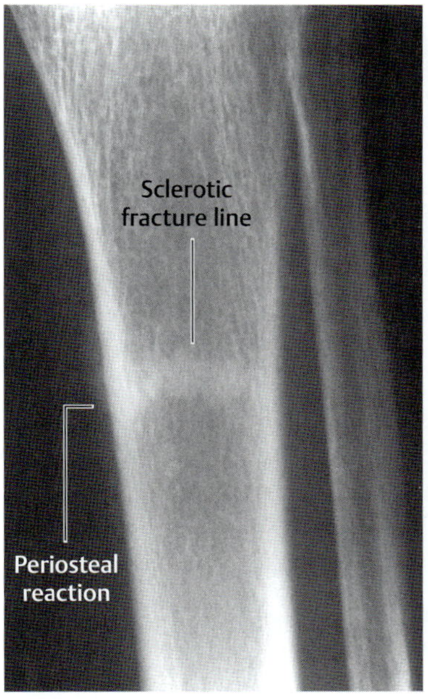

Fig. 1.40 Stress fracture of the tibia in a marathon runner.

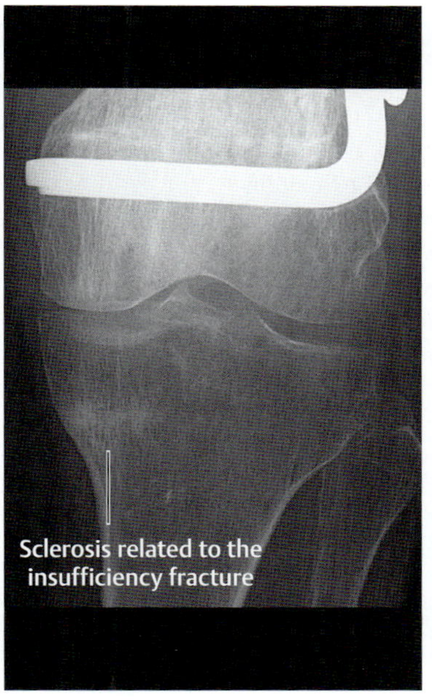

Fig. 1.41 Insufficiency fracture of the tibial plateau in a case of disuse osteoporosis secondary to a distal femoral fracture.

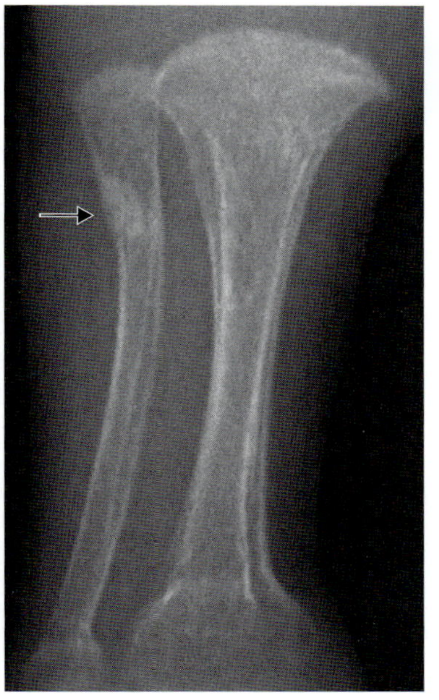

Fig. 1.42 Insufficiency fracture (arrow) of the fibula in a 4-month-old boy with rickets.

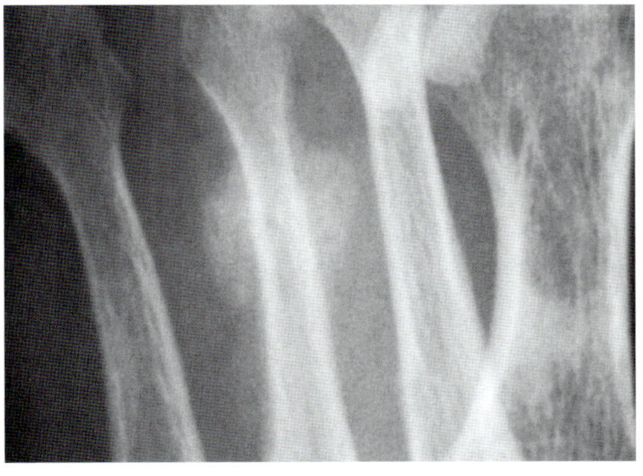

Fig. 1.43 Metatarsal insufficiency fracture with marked callus formation in an elderly patient with osteoporosis.

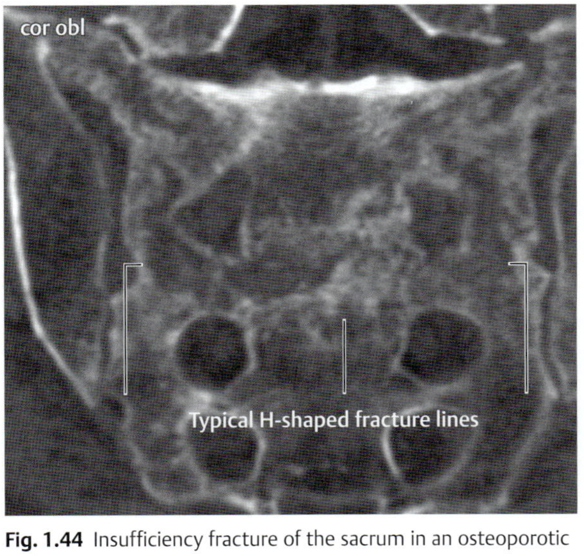

Fig. 1.44 Insufficiency fracture of the sacrum in an osteoporotic patient.

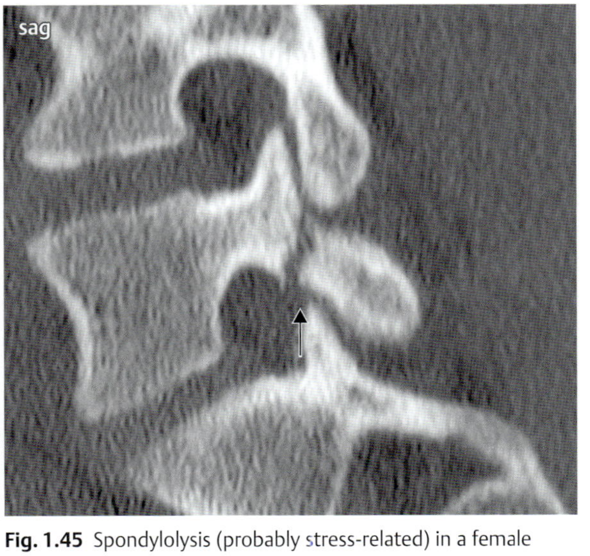

Fig. 1.45 Spondylolysis (probably stress-related) in a female competitive swimmer.

▸ **MRI.** MRI is an extremely sensitive method for detecting stress and insufficiency fractures, primarily because of the associated bone marrow edema that is very conspicuous on fat-saturated fluid-sensitive sequences (▸ Figs. 1.46 – 1.49). A fracture line may also be evident (see ▸ Figs. 1.46, ▸ 1.48, and ▸ 1.49). It may be hypointense on T1W, T2W, or gadolinium-enhanced images or, occasionally as a hyperintense line on T2W images (see ▸ Fig. 1.46). The low-signal intensity marrow edema may be relatively inconspicuous on T1W scans, such that more confluent low signal intensity should raise the possibility of tumor or osteomyelitis. Stress fractures may be associated with markedly increased edema within the surrounding soft tissues.

> **Note**
> If no fracture line is detectable on the MRI scan in cases of stress or insufficiency fractures, then this is referred to as a stress reaction (▸ Figs. 1.50 and ▶ W1.11).

▸ **DD.**

Osteoid osteoma. This lesion typically demonstrates intense cortical/periosteal thickening on radiographs with a central, rounded radiolucency (that may only be detectable on CT or MR images). Evidence of a linear structure is absent in an osteoid osteoma. Other tumors rarely mimic a stress injury.

Osteomyelitis. Osteomyelitis (acute, subacute, and chronic) can also produce significant periosteal new bone formation and cortical thickening and even a central lucency (Brodie's abscess). An associated sinus tract and clinical findings of infection may help distinguish infection from stress injury or osteoid osteoma.

Diabetic foot. A warm, swollen foot in a diabetic patient may be secondary to osteomyelitis or an insufficiency fracture. In both cases, radiography may reveal only osteopenia, while MRI demonstrates diffuse marrow edema within the bone. In the absence of an adjacent skin ulceration, cortical destruction, sinus tract or abscess, marrow edema alone (with or without a demonstrable fracture line) is more suggestive of a stress injury than of infection (Chapter 3.1).

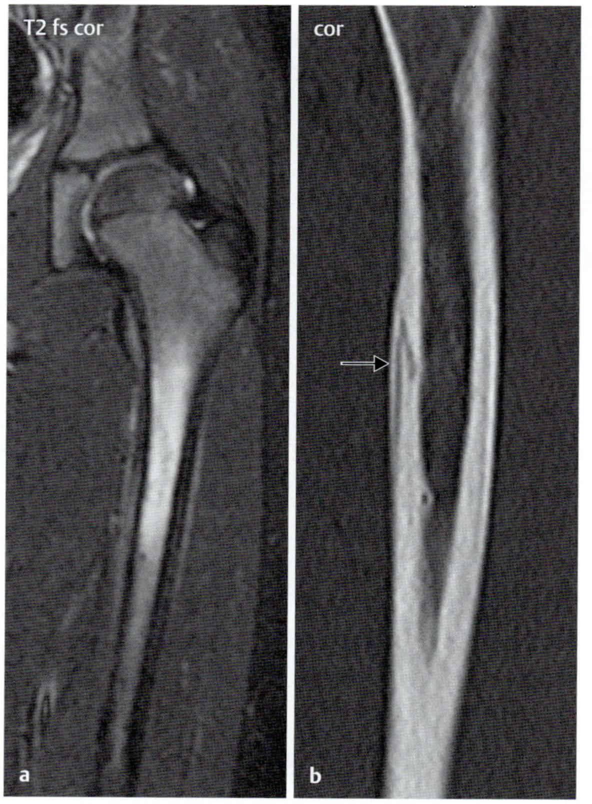

Fig. 1.47 Stress fracture of the left femur secondary to excessive sports activity. **(a)** Bone marrow edema and discrete periosteal edema. **(b)** The CT scan confirms the fracture (arrow) and excludes inflammatory or tumorous differential diagnoses.

Fig. 1.49 Subchondral insufficiency fracture of the femoral head. ▶ **(a)** Hypointense subchondral fracture line (arrow). **(b)** The fracture line is more conspicuous after contrast administration. Note also the small area of reduced subchondral perfusion, which is of no prognostic significance.

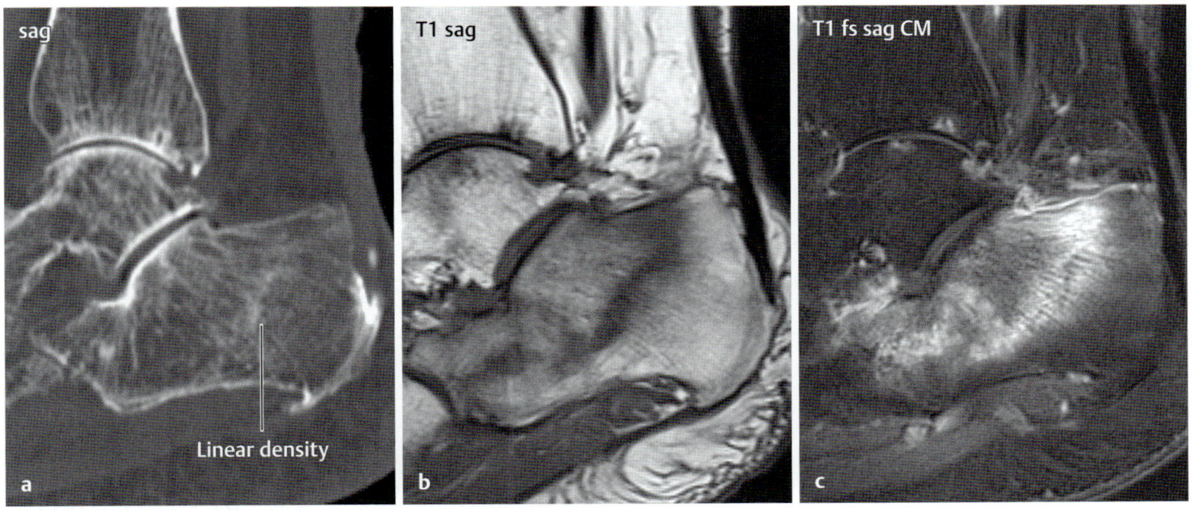

Fig. 1.46 Insufficiency fracture of the calcaneus in a patient with a history of steroid therapy for long-standing rheumatoid arthritis. **(a)** Sclerotic fracture line in the trabecular bone on a CT scan; the cortical bone is intact. **(b)** Hypointense fracture line and adjacent edema on a T1W scan. **(c)** Prominent enhancement is present around the fracture, which does not take up contrast.

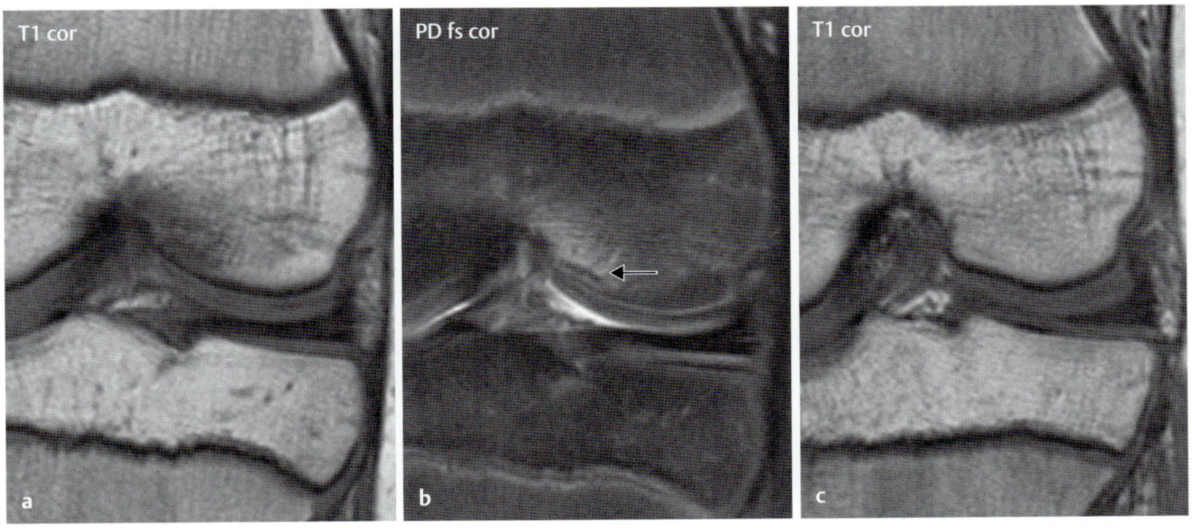

Fig. 1.48 Subchondral stress fracture after excessive jogging. **(a)** Subchondral edema of the medial femoral condyle. **(b)** The hypointense fracture line (arrow) is demonstrated within the area of edema. **(c)** Near complete resolution after 2 months' rest.

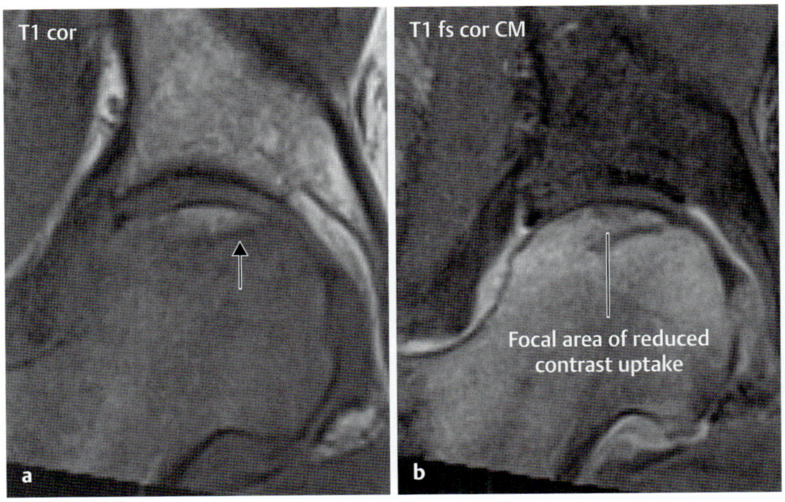

Fig. 1.49

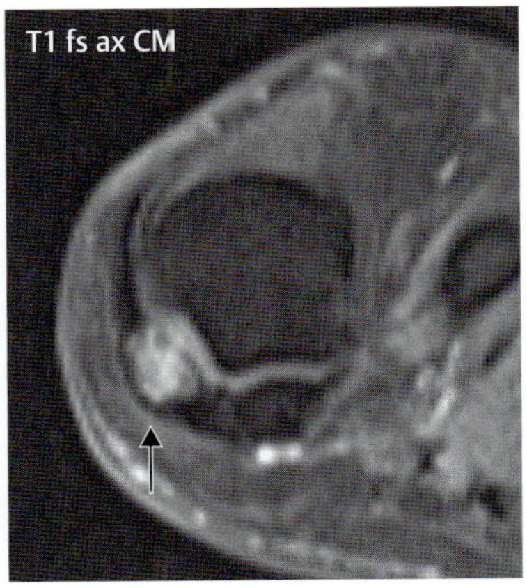

Fig. 1.50 Stress reaction of the medial sesamoid (arrow) of the first metatarsophalangeal joint.

1.5.2 Insufficiency Fractures and Destructive Arthropathy

Fundamental histological research has demonstrated the association between insufficiency fractures of articular bones (femoral head, femoral condyles, metatarsal bone) and destructive arthropathy (see references in the web material). Older, obese women with osteoporosis or patients under long-term steroid medication are primarily affected. The sudden onset of pain with an essentially normal radiograph should raise concern for a subchondral insufficiency fracture. Use of MRI is decisive. T1W scans demonstrate an area of low signal intensity, which is confined to the subchondral bone, and bone marrow edema on fluid-sensitive sequences (▶ Fig. 1.51), often with bandlike foci running parallel to the articular surface (▶ Fig. 1.52a). Findings after administration of intravenous contrast vary: If the subchondral bone takes up contrast well, then the diagnosis of an insufficiency fracture is established. If subchondral contrast enhancement is absent, this indicates a sclerotic area of fractured trabeculae that are no longer perfused (▶ Fig. 1.51b; see also ▶ Fig. 1.52b). In these cases, a transition to osteonecrosis may occur (cf. Chapter 6).

If the articular surfaces of long bones are involved, the bone may "melt away" in the late stage of an unhealed insufficiency fracture (▶ Fig. 1.52c and d).

1.5.3 Pathologic Fractures

Pathologic fracture is an insufficiency fracture variant that occurs in a bone that is already weakened by a tumor or tumorlike condition (▶ Fig. 1.53). Pathologic fractures are most often related to juvenile bone cyst or osteolytic metastasis (▶ Fig. 1.54).

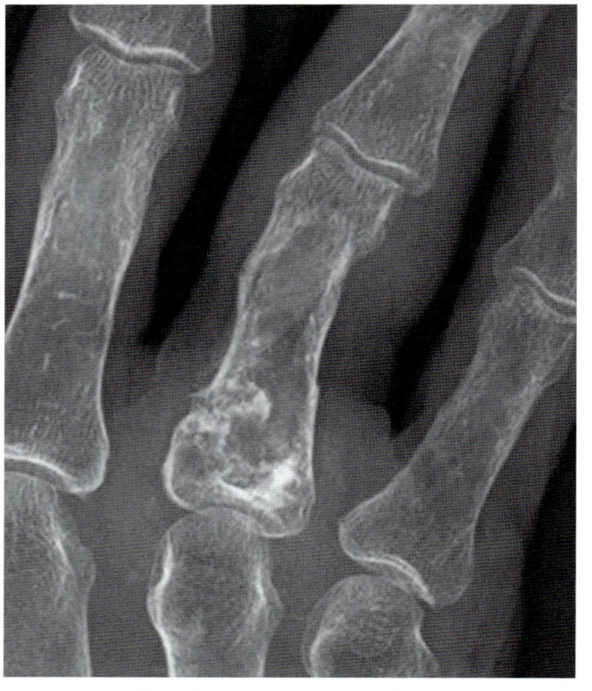

Fig. 1.53 Pathologic fracture of the proximal phalanx secondary to an underlying enchondroma.

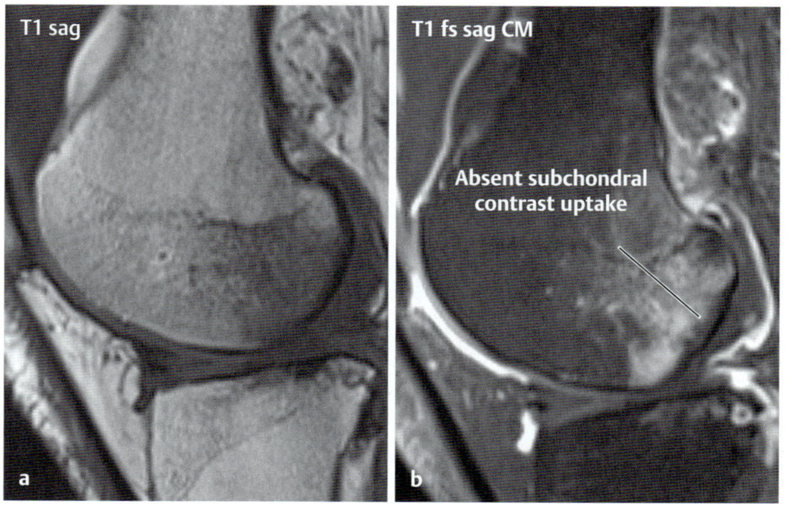

Fig. 1.51 Insufficiency fracture of the dorsal femoral condyle with incipient infraction of the joint surface. Progression of the process will result in classic Ahlback's disease (Chapter 6.5). **(a)** Mild dorsal impression. **(b)** Absent subchondral contrast uptake with adjacent edema. No distinct fracture line is evident.

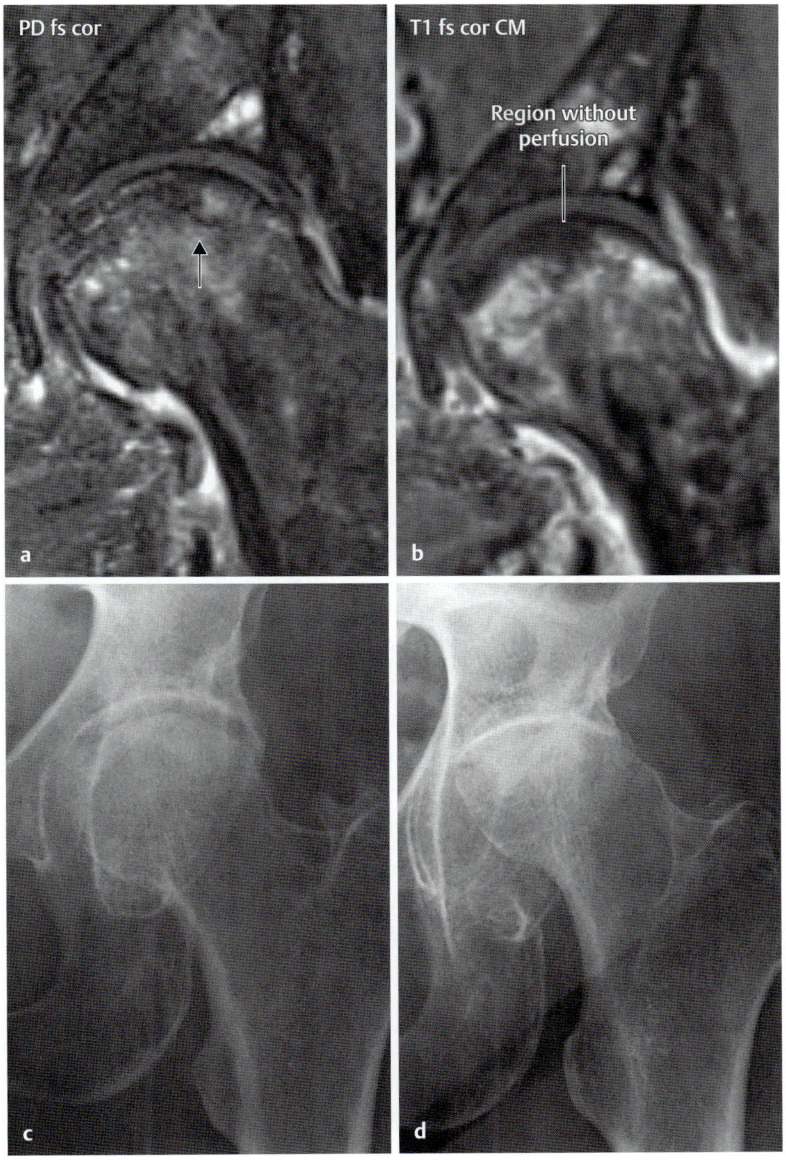

Fig. 1.52 Destructive arthropathy secondary to an insufficiency fracture. **(a)** Bone marrow edema, with thin fracture lines (arrows). **(b)** Above the fracture line there is compressed, nonperfused bone on this postcontrast image. **(c)** Radiographic finding at the time of the MRI scan. **(d)** Radiographic finding 1 month later. Rapidly progressive "melting away" of the femoral head.

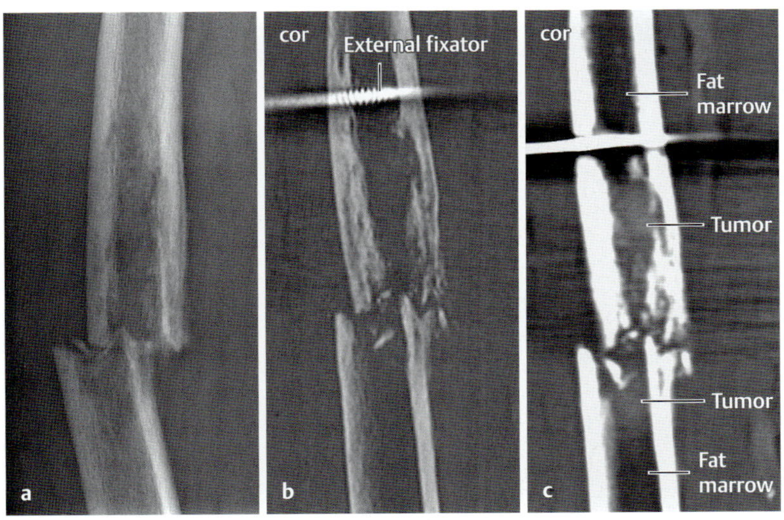

Fig. 1.54 Pathologic fracture of the femur due to radiation sarcoma. **(a)** Radiograph showing permeative osteolysis above and below the fracture. **(b)** CT scan depicting well the permeative type of cortical bone destruction. **(c)** Using soft tissue windowing, tumor-related soft tissue density rather than normal fatty marrow is well demonstrated on the CT scan.

1.5.4 Transient Osteoporosis and Transient Bone Marrow Edema

Transient osteoporosis is a rare bone disorder, the etiology of which is still unclear, located within a juxta-articular location, especially the ends of the long bones of the lower extremities. This condition is characterized on radiographs by regional osteopenia. As its name implies, it is a transient, self-limiting condition.

On MR images transient osteoporosis exhibits diffuse edemalike signal intensity within the marrow at the end of a long bone ("**transient bone marrow edema syndrome**"). The clinical and imaging findings will typically resolve over the course of 6 to 12 months.

> **Note**
> Transient osteoporosis and transient bone marrow edema differ only inasmuch as they are detected by different imaging techniques. All patients with findings of transient osteoporosis on radiography will exhibit bone marrow edema on MRI. The converse does not apply, since MRI is more sensitive than radiography in this condition.

▸ **Pathology.** The etiology and pathophysiology are still not fully understood. The possibility of venous stasis as an etiology has been suggested. Ischemia or some form of complex regional pain syndrome (CRPS—formerly known as Sudeck's disease) have also been suggested (without convincing proof). Some of the patients suffering from this regional abnormality do have generalized osteoporosis, and increased body weight also appears to play a role. The condition may be related to juxta-articular cancellous fractures that develop cortical disruption only in individual cases. Histologically there are corresponding focal areas of thin, partly interrupted bony trabeculae, covered with osteoid and osteoblasts.

> **Note**
> Cases of transient osteoporosis or transient bone marrow edema do not show imaging signs of osteonecrosis.

▸ **Clinical presentation.** Transient osteoporosis mainly affects men of middle age and women in the third trimester of pregnancy. The classic symptom is pain. The disorder most commonly affects the hips (75% of cases) and can, in rare cases, develop bilaterally. Other locations are the femoral condyles and tarsal bones. Treatment is conservative and includes analgesics and partial weight-bearing.

▸ **Radiography/CT.** Some weeks after onset of symptoms, a regional reduction in bone density of the juxta-articular bone becomes evident (▸ Fig. 1.55). The subchondral bone plate loses density and image clarity. Joint space width remains normal. Radiographic findings lag behind those of MRI. Areas of mild, patchy osteosclerosis may develop months after onset.

▸ **NUC MED.** A bone scan is a sensitive method for detecting this condition but it is no longer routinely used for diagnosis because the findings are nonspecific.

▸ **MRI.** On T1W images, a diffuse, ill-defined area of decreased signal intensity is evident, which is particularly marked in the subchondral and epiphyseal regions and can extend toward the metaphysis (▸ Figs. 1.56, ▸ 1.57, and ▶ W1.12). These areas demonstrate diffusely increased, edemalike signal intensity on fluid-sensitive sequences and homogeneous enhancement after intravenous contrast administration. Associated joint effusion is typically present and concomitant edema may be seen in the adjacent soft tissues. A fracture line is not present. The marrow signal intensity then returns to normal after some months, although streaky areas of hypointense signal can persist for a very long time.

Migratory transient osteoporosis and migratory transient bone marrow edema. This type of transitory marrow edema can "migrate": from one femoral head to the other, from the femoral head to the acetabulum, from one femoral condyle to the other, or within the tarsal bones. There is currently no explanation for this, although an association with complex regional pain syndrome has been suggested.

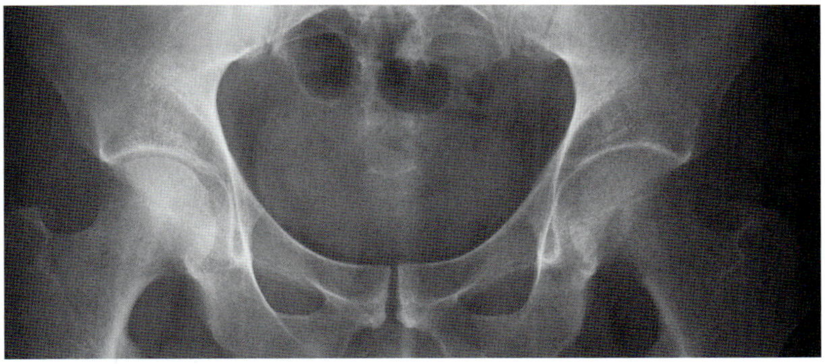

Fig. 1.55 Transient osteoporosis of the left femoral head. (Image courtesy of R. Whitehouse, Manchester.)

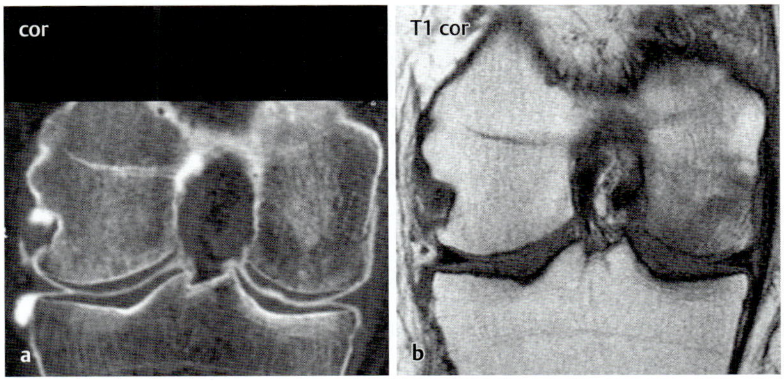

Fig. 1.56 Transient bone marrow edema/ transient osteoporosis of the knee joint. **(a)** Juxta-articular demineralization of the medial femoral condyle. **(b)** Corresponding ill-defined edema on a T1W MR image.

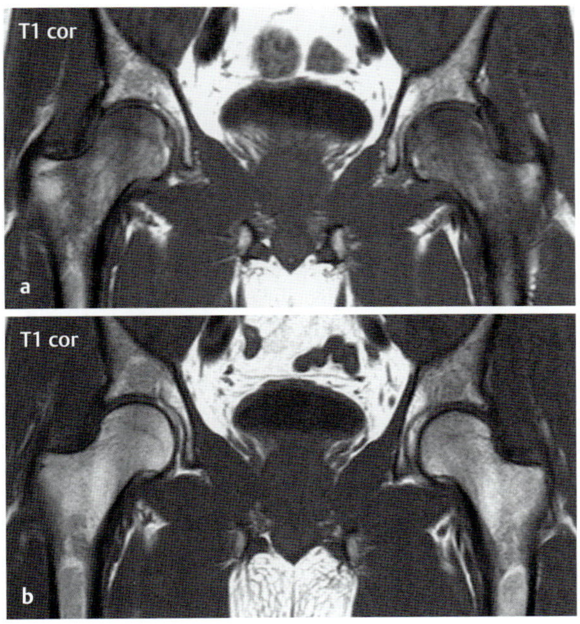

Fig. 1.57 Transient bilateral bone marrow edema of the proximal femur. ▶ For additional images see ▸ Fig. W1.12. **(a)** Hypointense bone marrow edema is present within both proximal femurs at the time of presentation. **(b)** The marrow has returned to normal after 10 months.

▸ DD.

Stress or insufficiency fracture. Stress injuries may produce a similar imaging appearance; however, a visible fracture line is usually absent in cases of transitory osteoporosis.

Atrophic form of arthritis deformans. Osteoarthritis may result in marrow edema but it also demonstrates associated joint-space narrowing.

Osteonecrosis. In the case of osteonecrosis, an area of subchondral signal abnormality is present, typically with a characteristic low-signal intensity serpentine margin. The abnormality should demonstrate a thickness of at least 4 mm on T2W images (differentiating it from a subchondral insufficiency fracture. Collapse of the articular surface is a late finding in osteonecrosis.

> **Note**
>
> Transient osteoporosis is a diagnosis of exclusion. The diagnosis should only be made if there is no history to suggest a stress injury. If the patient is significantly osteoporotic then insufficiency fracture should be the favored diagnosis.

1.6 Fracture Healing

Primary (direct) and secondary (indirect) fracture healing mean that stability of the bone is restored by regeneration of the original tissue. Immobilization is the most important factor in fracture healing.

1.6.1 Primary Fracture Healing (Direct Cortical Reconstruction)

Primary fracture healing is characterized by the absence of callus and presupposes the following factors:

- Contact between the fragments with a maximal gap of 0.5 mm (fixation of the fragments together under pressure improves the chances of primary fracture healing).
- Immobilization of the fracture (e.g., by fracture fixation).
- Adequate blood supply and viability of the fragments.

Union of the fracture ends begins with the activation of osteoclasts and proceeds via the direct ingrowth of haversian systems from one fragment into the other (contact healing), after which trabecular bone fills the fracture gap and is later replaced by osteons (gap healing). Activation of periosteal or endosteal mesenchymal cells does not occur.

► **Radiography.** Characteristic features include blurring of cortical margins and a nonvisible or "fading" fracture gap (► Fig. 1.58a). Widening of the fracture gap or the "reappearance" of one, secondary to resorption of the fragment ends, is a sign of disruption of primary bone healing.

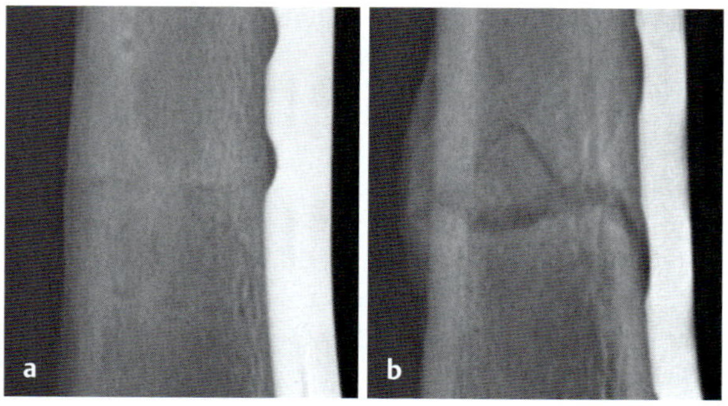

Fig. 1.58 Types of fracture healing (in each case after plate fixation). **(a)** Primary fracture healing after osteotomy: direct bone-fragment contact, no callus formation. **(b)** Secondary fracture healing after a fracture: clearly visible callus formation.

1.6.2 Secondary Fracture Healing (Fracture Healing by Callus Formation)

Secondary bone healing occurs in the presence of dehiscence or inadequate mechanical fixation of the fracture ends (► Fig. 1.58b). A callus cuff forms around the fracture gap, initially as "instability callus" and then as "fixation callus." Mesenchymal cells convert the fracture hematoma into fibrous tissue as well as fibrous and hyaline cartilage. This immature reparative tissue is then converted secondarily into bone. This conversion starts peripherally, slightly away from the actual fracture line, and proceeds in a central direction into the fracture gap. Secondary fracture healing is similar in its course to normal endochondral ossification.

► **Radiography.** Secondary fracture healing progresses along a characteristic staged course, which is presented in ► Table 1.1 where it is correlated with radiographic findings.

Fracture Healing

Bony fracture healing should be primarily assessed *clinically*. Because mineralization only takes place during later stages, radiological signs always lag behind. **Clinical signs** of fracture healing (which should not be equated with complete fracture healing) include:

- Stability during clinical examination.
- Absence of pain.
- A capacity for loading of the bone.

► **Radiography.** Radiological signs of fracture healing include the following features:

- The fracture is completely bridged over.
- The fracture callus demonstrates homogenous density and is sharply demarcated.
- These signs must be visible in at least two projections.

> **Caution**
> Underexposed (too "bright") radiographs will exaggerate the degree of fracture healing.

Table 1.1 Stages of secondary bone healing. Correlation of pathological anatomical findings with the radiograph

Time after fracture			
First days	**Up to 3rd–4th week**	**From 3rd–4th week to 3rd–4th month**	**From 4th month to 24 months**
Stage			
Inflammatory phase:	**Granulation phase:**	**Callus hardening:**	**Remodeling and modeling:**
• Hematoma secondary to the disruption of the periosteum, the bone, the bone marrow, and the surrounding soft tissue	• Fibrous transformation of the hematoma by proliferating tissue with collagen fibers and capillary ingrowth	• Mineralization of ground substance	• Conversion of woven bone into lamellar bone (remodeling)
• Activation and inflow of multiple cell types	• Differentiation (migration) of osteoclasts and osteoblasts (→ bone formation) and chondroblasts (→ cartilage formation) • Formation of a “soft” callus	• Formation of woven bone	• Restoration of normal bone contour and medullary cavity (modeling; this process can even correct abnormal angulation)
Radiography			
3rd–14th day: Reduced density of bone; the fracture line becomes more clearly visible (due to bone resorption) **From the 10th day:** new periosteal bone formation	**From the 14th day:** Slowly increasing density within the fracture gap; ill-defined fragment margins	**From the 6th–8th week:** Osseous bridging and consolidation (the callus is sharply contoured, the fracture gap becomes increasingly less visible; isolated gaps may remain longer)	Osseous bridging is usually completed before consolidation; complete remodeling takes varying lengths of time (depending upon age among other things)
Example			
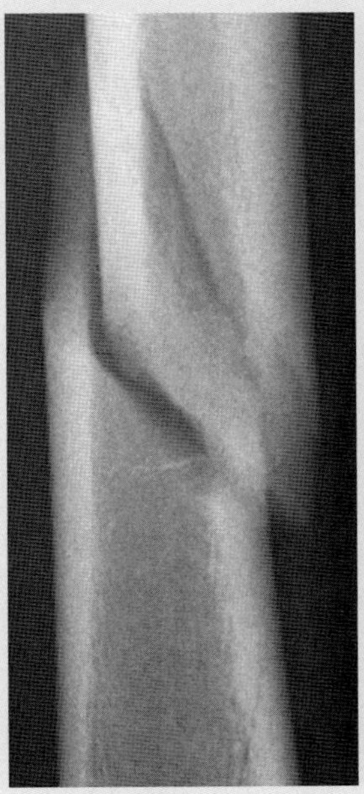	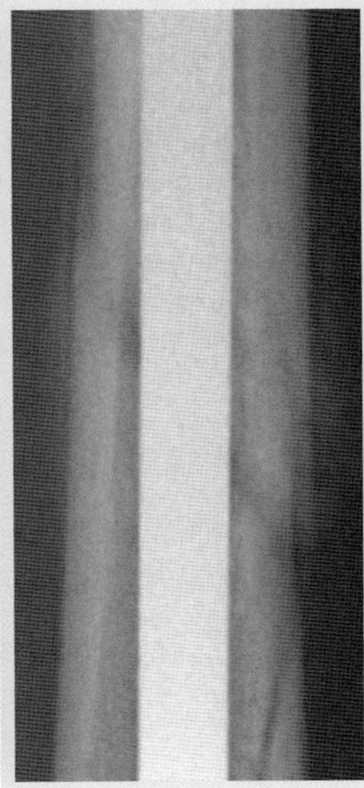	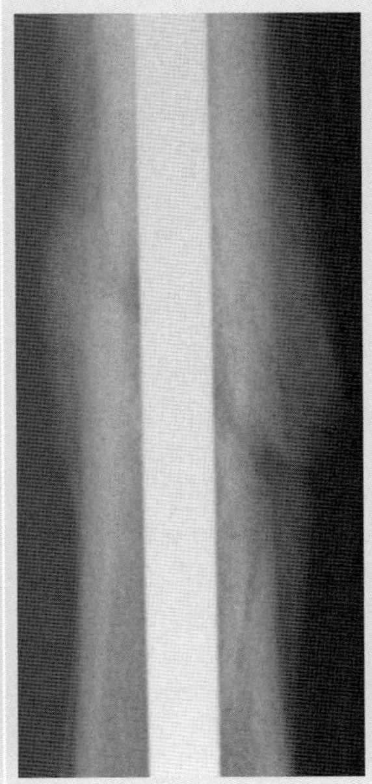	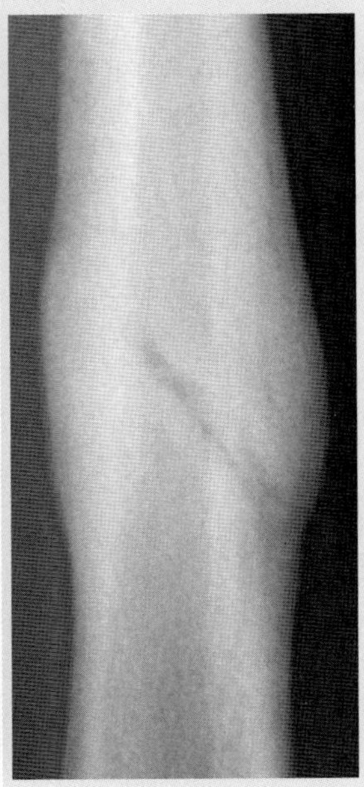

1.6.3 Radiological Assessment after Fracture Fixation of the Peripheral Skeleton

The aim of any form of fracture fixation is to secure the result of reduction, immobilization of the fragments, and, in many methods of fracture fixation, interfragmentary compression to promote fracture healing. The numerous fracture fixation techniques can be assigned to one of the following categories: external fixation, screw fixation, plate fixation, intramedullary nailing and cerclage wiring.

External Fixation

Schanz screws are inserted through small incisions and screwed to an external connecting rod (or several rods) via clamps (▶ Fig. 1.59). Usually two Schanz screws each are inserted into major fragments or across joints. Adequate stability is only achieved if purchase is gained in the far cortex and there is sufficient distance between the screws on either side of the fracture.

A variation of the external fixator is the spatial frame fixator. This involves drilling metal pins (Steinmann pins) instead of Schanz screws through the bone and stabilizing them with rods.

The external fixator is used for higher-grade open fractures, in fractures with significant soft tissue damage, in long-segment fractures, or in fractures with joint damage, particularly in patients with multiple injuries, and is usually an interim solution until definitive management can be carried out.

Screw Fixation

With pure screw fixation, the fragments are usually stabilized with two or three lag screws. A distinction is made between cancellous and cortical bone screws. The **cancellous screw** requires a deep thread for adequate purchase in cancellous bone. The **cortical screw** needs only a shallow thread due to the higher stability of cortical bone (▶ Fig. 1.60). It is either self-tapping (i.e., it can be screwed into the cortex without prior thread cutting) or self-drilling (i.e., the screw has a drill head to breach the cortex). A large number of screws are also available as cannulated screws, which enables them to be inserted directly over a Kirschner wire.

In order to achieve compression between the fragments, partial-thread screws are commonly used. These screws have no threads in the fracture fragment situated on the side of the screw head. Alternatively, the fragment at the head end may be overdrilled to produce a gliding hole for the fully threaded screw. These screws are often used with fractures of the radial styloid process, fractures of the neck of femur in young patients, or fractures of the femoral condyles or the proximal tibia. The double-thread screw (Herbert screw; ▶ Fig. 1.61) has distal and proximal threads (with different pitches). This allows interfragmentary compression to be exerted at sites where a prominent screw head would not normally be tolerated, such as the scaphoid bone or the ulnar styloid process.

Plate Fixation

Numerous types of plate are available; these are often named according to their form (e.g., clover plate, T-plate) or their profile (e.g., one-third tubular plate), but this conveys nothing about their function. To understand these devices, it is important to be acquainted with the basic principles of fixation plates.

Compression plate. This plate is secured onto the bone in such a way that axial compression is exerted across the fracture. This can be achieved with the aid of a tension device or a dynamic compression plate (DCP). The DCP has oval-shaped holes with sloped edges and an inclined glide plane in the hole, while the corresponding screw has a conical head. The screws may be inserted eccentrically. The head of the screw is pressed against the edge of the hole on tightening; this results in an axial force across the screw. Cortical screws are used in the shaft region (predrilled or self-tapping) and are also anchored in the far cortex. Cancellous screws are used where there is inadequate thickness of the far cortex (epiphysis or metaphysis). Pressing the plate onto the bone reduces periosteal perfusion, which in turn impairs fracture healing. The LC-DCP (low-contact DCP) reduces the contact surface with the periosteum by its undercut surface (▶ Fig. 1.62).

Functional tension band plating. The plate is placed across the fracture and experiences a traction force on physiological loading, while the bone on the side opposite the plate experiences a compression force. A typical example is the femoral shaft fracture: body weight places medial compression on the femur that counteracts the tensile load on the lateral-sided plate.

Neutralization plate. If interfragmentary compression is achieved by insertion of a screw, the addition of a plate can neutralize detrimental forces that could otherwise result in dislocation of the fragments. The interfragmentary compression screw can also pass through a plate hole. Typical uses of this technique include a fracture of the lateral malleolus or corrective osteotomy of the ulna (▶ Fig. 1.63).

As well as compromising periosteal perfusion, the plate fixation techniques described above have another potential disadvantage: manipulation around the fracture site for exact reduction and screw fixation of the relevant fragments is required to achieve interfragmentary compression. This involves more intraoperative manipulation, which can result in additional interference with vascularization and subsequent fracture healing.

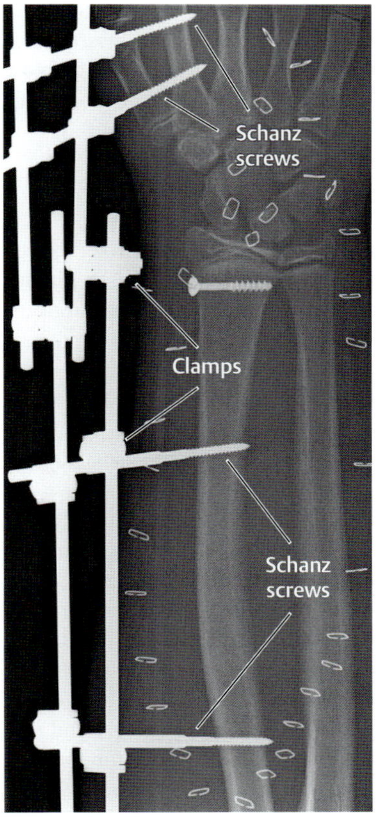

Fig. 1.59 External fixator. Multiple skin staples in the presence of extensive soft tissue damage.

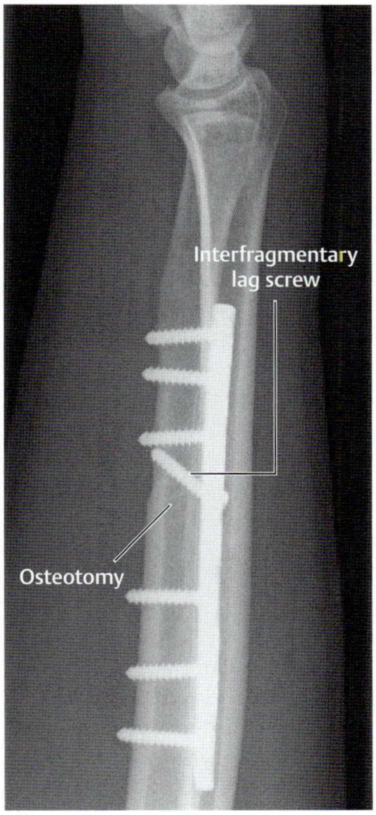

Fig. 1.63 Neutralization plate. This ulnar shortening osteotomy was stabilized under compression using a cortical screw (overdrilled in the proximal fragment). The plate "neutralizes" the forces that would otherwise have led to failure of screw fixation alone.

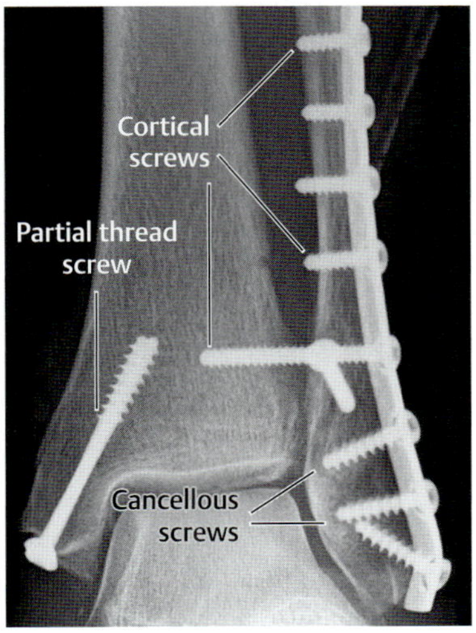

Fig. 1.60 Various types of screws. Cortical screws obtain purchase by penetrating the far cortex; cancellous screws in contrast have a greater thread depth.

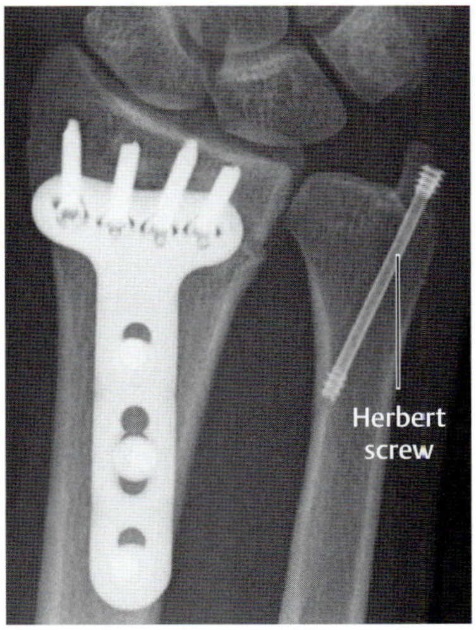

Fig. 1.61 Double-thread screws. Note the different pitches of the two threads and the central lucency of the cannulated screw. The radius was stabilized with an angle-stable plate.

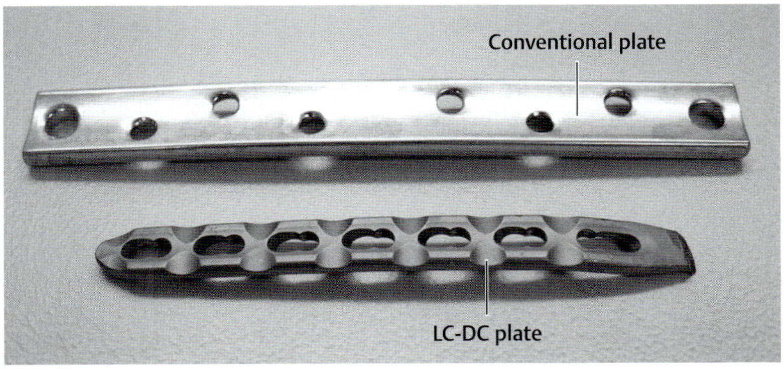

Fig. 1.62 LC-DCP (below). The notches on the undersurface reduce the contact surface with the bone and periosteum.

Angle-stable plate fixation. With this technique, the screw (known as a locking-head screw) with a threaded head is secured to the plate in such a way as to prevent both a tilting movement ("angle-stable") and axial migration ("axis-stable"). The plate does not need to be compressed onto the underlying bone, but acts instead as an internal fixator that does not rest against the cortex. This does not achieve interfragmentary compression, so fracture healing is not primary but due to interfragmentary callus formation. An exact reduction of the fracture fragments is not necessary provided there is no joint involvement. This type of plate is used, for example, in the distal femur or proximal tibia (▶ Fig. 1.64). The LCP (locking compression plate; ▶ Fig. 1.65) is a further development and is characterized by the presence of combination holes. These combine threaded with threadless holes. Conventional screws can also be inserted into the threadless holes at an oblique angle. They must then press the fragment against the plate.

Intramedullary Fixation (Intramedullary Nailing)

Certain fractures can be stabilized with one or several nails inserted into the medullary cavity. A distinction is made between reamed and unreamed nails: **reamed intramedullary nails** are inserted after reaming the medullary cavity and achieve surface contact with the inner cortex. Traumatization of the medullary cavity with compromise of endosteal vascularization is a potential disadvantage. **Unreamed medullary nails** are less prone to this complication with their thinner caliber, and can be inserted more quickly (▶ Fig. 1.66). Both types of nails have round and sometimes also slotted holes at their tips through which interlocking screws can be inserted into the far cortex with the aid of a targeting device. This ensures rotational stability and allows for static interlocking (screws inserted into the round holes) or dynamic interlocking (screws inserted only into the slotted gliding holes, resulting in compression with loading). With unreamed intramedullary nails the interlocking screws may be anchored with partial angle stability. Specially designed nails may be used to treat not only shaft fractures of large long bones but also juxta-articular or articular fractures (e.g., of the proximal humerus or femur).

In addition to these, **thin elastic nails** of various forms and sizes are used, especially in children. They are inserted singly (radius, ulna) or as a pair (humerus, femur), using almost the entire length of the shaft so that they wedge themselves in the medullary cavity (▶ Fig. 1.67).

Wire Fixation

A simple and less invasive form of fracture fixation is osteosynthetic wiring (e.g., the **Kirschner wire** with or without thread). One or several wires cross the fracture gap and create stability for secondary fracture healing. This procedure is frequently used in the hand or distal forearm. The wires should be drilled as far as the opposite cortex, but should not penetrate it. To ensure rotational stability, the wires should not cross each other at the level of the fracture (▶ Fig. 1.68).

Cerclage wires are drawn around or through the fragments, before being twisted or sealed at their ends. Typical uses include additional fixation of an oblique shaft fracture or loose fragment, as a supplement to plate fixation, or for fixation of an iatrogenic shaft avulsion (see ▶ Figs. 1.64 and ▶ 1.68).

Tension band wiring is a combination of straight and cerclage wires. Two fragments are held together by a wire loop; displacement is prevented by (usually two) Kirschner wires placed perpendicular to the fracture plane. The fragments are pressed together on one side by muscular traction; this results in primary fracture healing. Classic uses include olecranon fractures and osteotomies, as well as transverse patellar fractures (▶ Fig. 1.69).

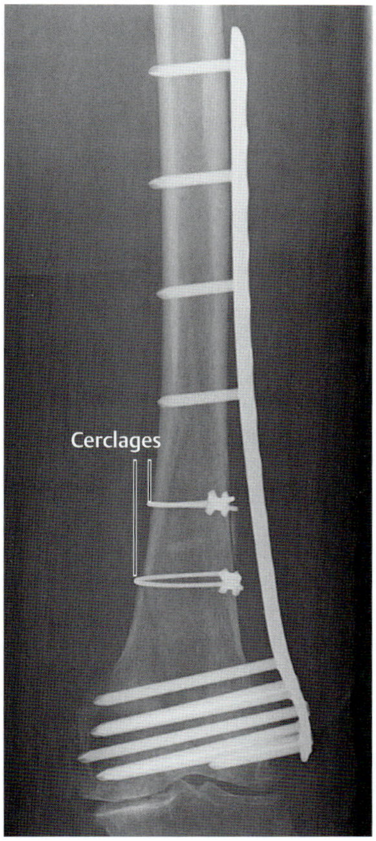

Fig. 1.64 LISS ("less invasive stabilization system") plate for a distal femoral fracture. Two additional cerclage wires have been applied.

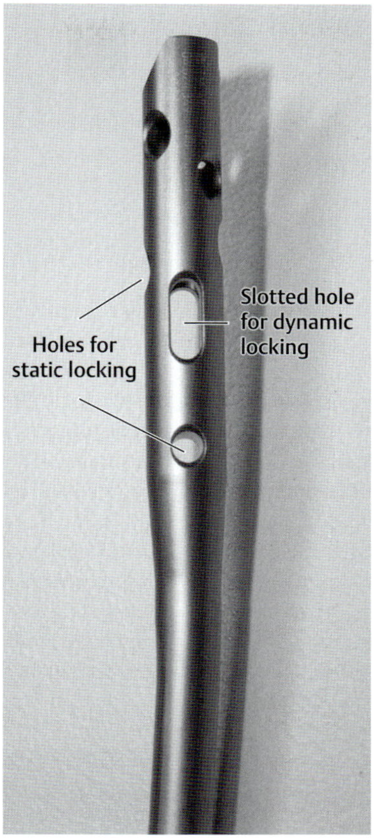

Fig. 1.66 Upper end of an unreamed tibial nail. The interlocking screws are introduced with the aid of a targeting device.

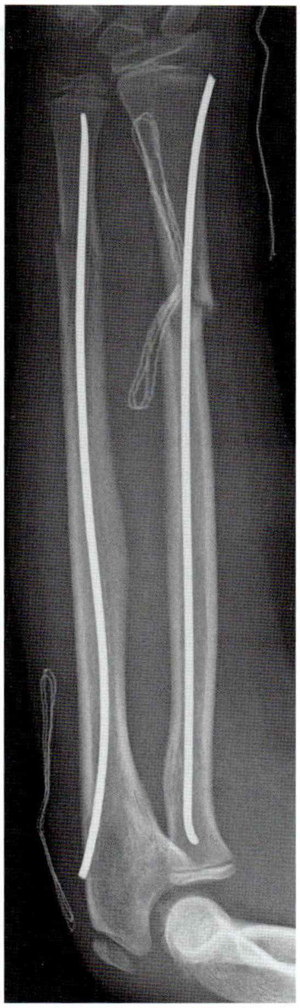

Fig. 1.67 Elastic intramedullary nailing of radial and ulnar shaft fractures in a child.

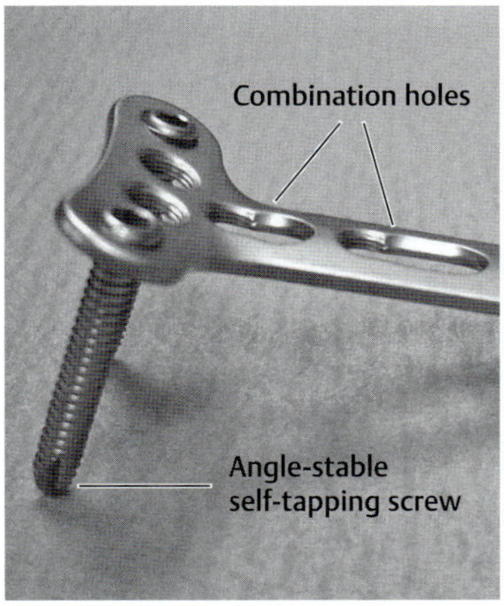

Fig. 1.65 LCP for the distal radius (palmar). Locking-head screws are inserted into the threaded proximal holes, while there also is the option of placing conventional screws in the combination holes.

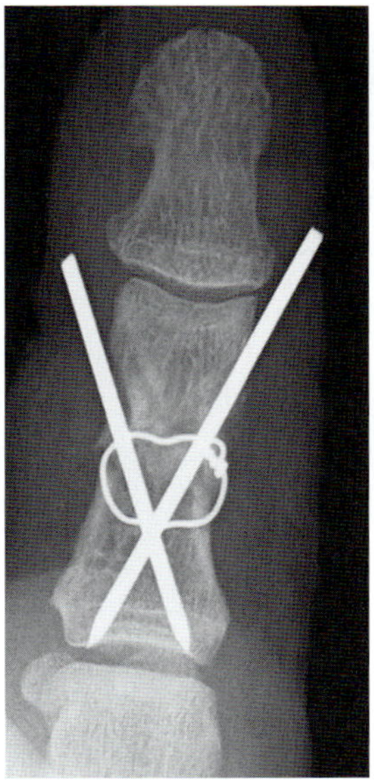

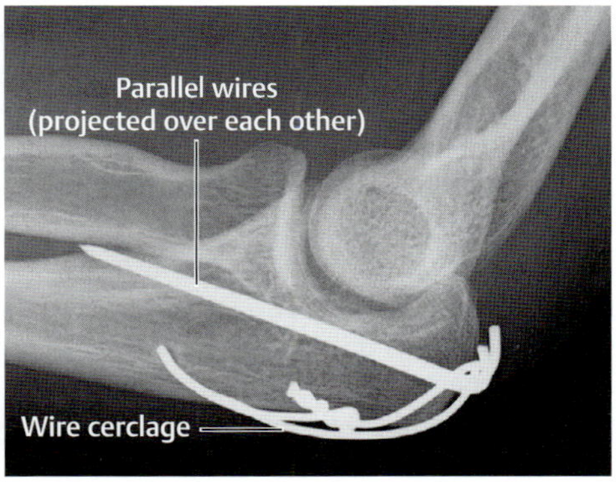

Fig. 1.69 Tension band wiring of the olecranon. Traction of the triceps tendon "rotates" the olecranon in a counterclockwise direction; this results in compression of the fracture surfaces on the joint side.

Fig. 1.68 Wire fixation. The shaft fracture of the proximal phalanx is stabilized with two Kirschner wires and a wire cerclage. Perfect position of the K-wires: The subchondral bone plate is not quite breached; there is no crossing of the wires at the level of the fracture site.

Further Methods of Fracture Fixation

Dynamic plate and screw fixation. A typical example of this type of fracture fixation is the dynamic hip screw (▶ Fig. 1.70). The technique can also be used for fractures of the femoral condyles (dynamic condylar screw).

Buttress plate. After reduction, the juxta-articular fragments of an epiphyseal or metaphyseal fracture can be screwed to a plate that flares out toward the joint. This prevents dislocation by providing buttress support to these fragments.

Angled or blade plate. The blade plate is angled (synonym: angled plate). The blade is hammered into the medullary cavity and the plate screwed onto the metaphyseal cortex. It is used in the distal femur or proximal tibia. Over recent years this type of plate has been used less frequently and is currently used almost exclusively for corrective osteotomies.

Reconstruction plate. This plate has deep lateral notches between the holes that allow the plate to be contoured along bones that are not straight (e.g., the pelvis). The plate can be easily pre-bent in all three planes and/or twisted (▶ Fig. 1.71).

Postoperative Radiographic Evaluation

The degree of fracture reduction, the stability of the fracture fixation, iatrogenic or otherwise unrecognized fractures, and malpositioning of implants should be assessed on the **initial postoperative radiograph**.

Result of fracture reduction. It is necessary to describe alignment of the fracture fragments. Abnormalities such as angulation malrotation, displacement, impaction, or distraction/dehiscence should be described. In the case of an intra-articular fracture, the degree of incongruity of the articular surface must be assessed. Even if there is good reduction of the fracture fragments, ultimate healing requires that the fixation method is able to maintain the position of the fragments during the healing process. A variety of problems may result in suboptimal fixation, such as fixation plate screws not finding purchase in the far cortex, a plate being too short, or the pins of an external fixator being placed too close together (▶ Fig. 1.72). Accurate assessment of postoperative radiographs requires a working knowledge of the various techniques of fracture fixation and potential complications.

> **Note**
> Evaluation of the adequacy of fracture fixation requires experience and at least a basic understanding of fixation techniques. Other factors such as clinical factors before and during surgery may not be evident on imaging studies and therefore caution should be exercised when contemplating the use of words such as "good," "poor," or "adequate" when describing postoperative images.

Malpositioning. If any fixation hardware protrudes across an articular surface, then osteoarthritis will inevitably develop (▶ Fig. 1.73). If it extends too far into the joint on the extension or flexion side, then it may restrict joint motion. Screws that extend too far beyond the opposite cortex may produce symptoms related to injury of adjacent soft tissues (e.g., tendons; ▶ Fig. 1.74).

Serial follow-up radiographs should be assessed for ongoing fracture reduction, progressive fracture healing, and evidence of failure of hardware or fracture fixation. Radiographic signs indicating a postoperative complication are summarized in ▶ Table 1.2.

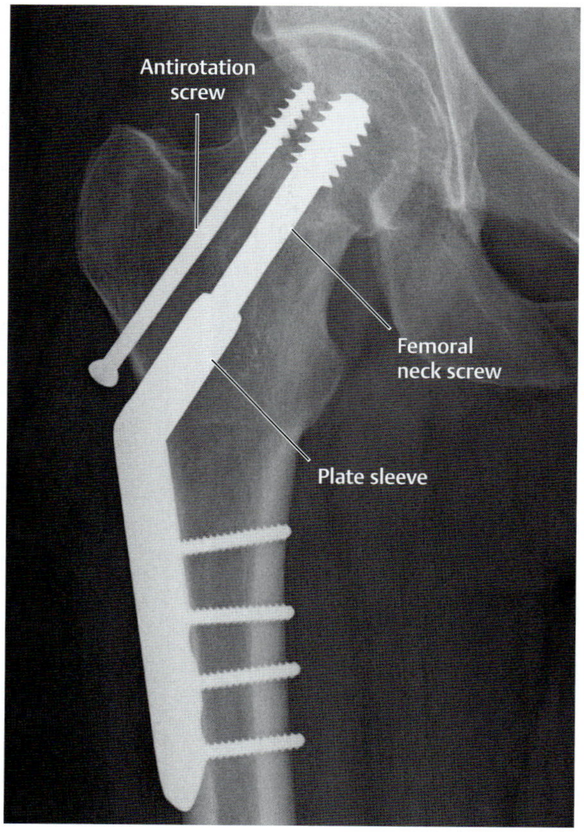

Fig. 1.70 Dynamic hip screw. The screw glides in the plate sleeve; loading of the leg subsequently results in compression of the fragments. The antirotation screw is inserted in a parallel direction and prevents secondary malrotation.

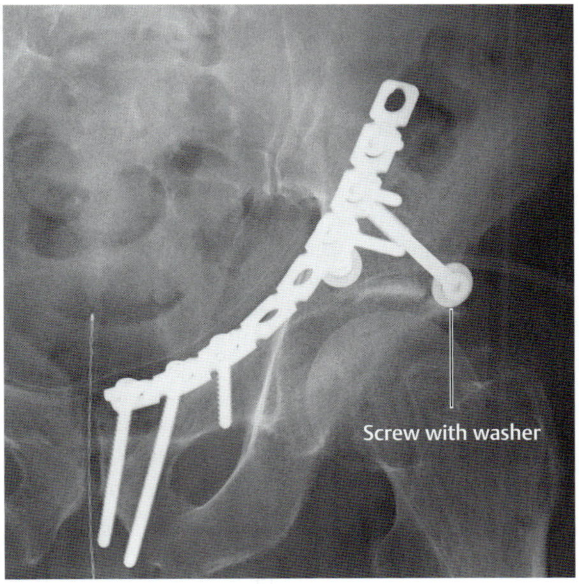

Fig. 1.71 Reconstruction plate. This anterior column fracture has been stabilized with a reconstruction plate that was contoured along the iliac and pubic bones. A posterior transverse fracture has also been secured with two lag screws (plus washers).

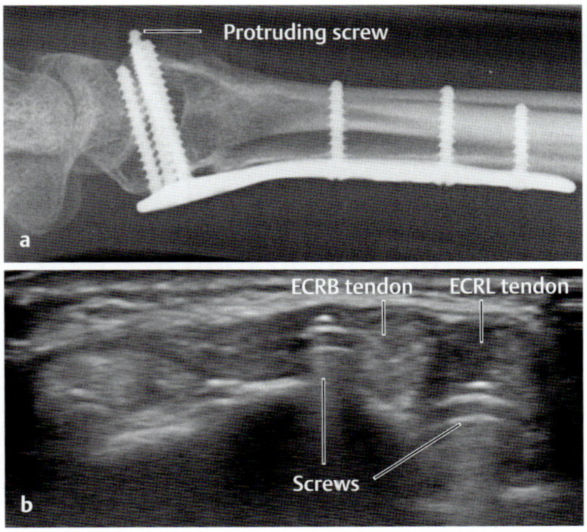

Fig. 1.74 Abnormal contact of protruding screws with extensor tendons over the dorsal wrist. **(a)** Screw protrusion distal to Lister's tubercle. **(b)** Ultrasound (dorsum of the wrist in cross section): The contact between the screws and extensor tendons is clearly documented.
ECRB = extensor carpi radialis brevis.
ECRL = extensor carpi radialis longus.

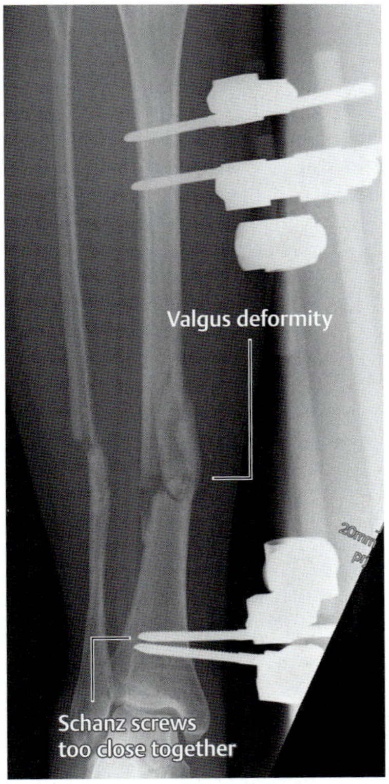

Fig. 1.72 External fixator. The proximal Schanz screws reach the far cortex; the distal screws cannot be assessed on this film because they do not lie parallel on this projection plane. Inadequate distance between the screw pairs (insufficient stability). There is valgus alignment of the tibial fracture.

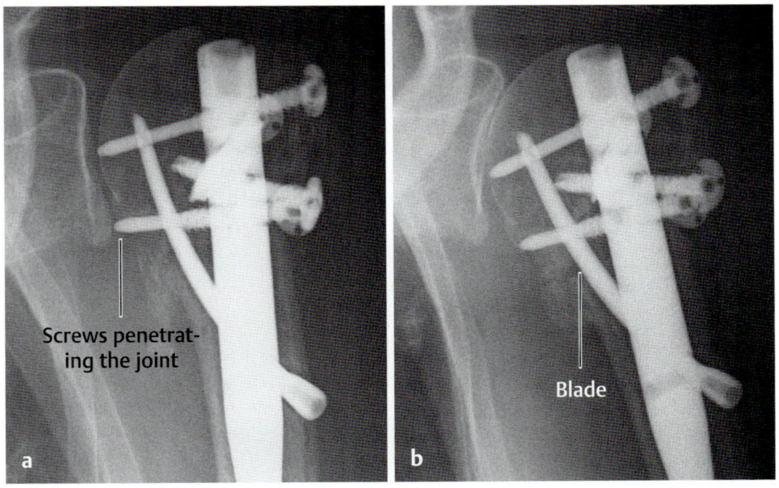

Fig. 1.73 Management of a subcapital humerus fracture with a locking blade nail. A blade inserted through the nail provides additional stabilization. **(a)** Two of the screws just breach the subchondral bone plate and violate the articular surface. **(b)** Over time, significant joint-space narrowing has developed as a sign of cartilage damage.

Radiographs obtained after hardware removal should reveal the absence of retained hardware, evidence of fracture healing, and the absence of a recurrent or new fracture. If fixation hardware obscures the fracture site, its removal will allow for optimal assessment of fracture healing (e.g., in the finger).

1.6.4 Radiological Assessment after Implantation of a Joint Prosthesis in the Peripheral Skeleton

Total joint replacement (TJR) of the hip is the most frequently performed and most extensively studied type of arthroplasty. The principles of imaging assessment of joint prostheses will therefore be described with special reference to the hip.

Radiological Findings after Total Hip Replacement

The acetabular cup and femoral prostheses are each usually composed of two components: the cup with a polyethylene liner (▶ Fig. 1.76) and the femoral prosthesis with stem and attachable head (metal or ceramic). The acetabular cup may be cementless (screwed in via a self-tapping thread: "threaded cup") or pressed into the acetabular bed ("press-fit cup," with or without additional spikes or screws).

> **Caution**
> Only radiographic views with identical alignment should be used to compare pre- and postoperative hips after total joint replacement since even slight differences in projection may lead to spurious findings.

The position of the acetabular component is described using the acetabular angle (synonym: inclination; normal ~40°; ▶ Fig. 1.77) and the anteversion angle (normal ~15°; ▶ Fig. 1.78). The acetabular angle is the angle between the transischial line (reference line) and the lateral opening of the acetabulum (normal: ~40°). A change in the acetabular angle by 4° or more is an indication of acetabular cup loosening. The distance between the tip of the greater tuberosity and the reference line increases with cranial migration of the cup. If the stem migrates distally, a fixed point on the prosthetic stem will move toward the lesser trochanter ("subsidence").

Depending on the choice of implant and insertion technique, the prosthesis can produce leg-length discrepancy. The difference in leg length can be quantified on radiographs by documenting asymmetry of height of the lesser trochanter in comparison with the contralateral side.

The angle between the prosthetic neck and stem (stem antetorsion) should amount to about 10° in the axial plane. The stem anteversion angle may appear to be increased if the femur is externally rotated against the stem prosthesis. The greater trochanter, which normally faces in a dorsal direction, is then no longer prominent in the axial plane. If both trochanters disappear in the AP (anteroposterior) view, then there is an internal rotational error.

> **Caution**
> The stem anteversion angle may also appear to be increased if the leg is excessively internally rotated for the axial projection. Conversely, both trochanters can disappear behind (or in front of) the stem in the AP view as a result of malpositioning of the patient (externally rotated leg).

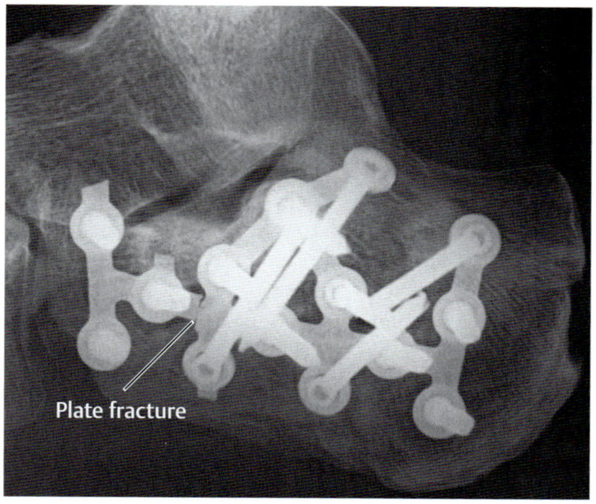

Fig. 1.75 Hardware failure of a reconstruction plate 3 months after fracture fixation. This is a radiographic sign of motion at an unconsolidated fracture.

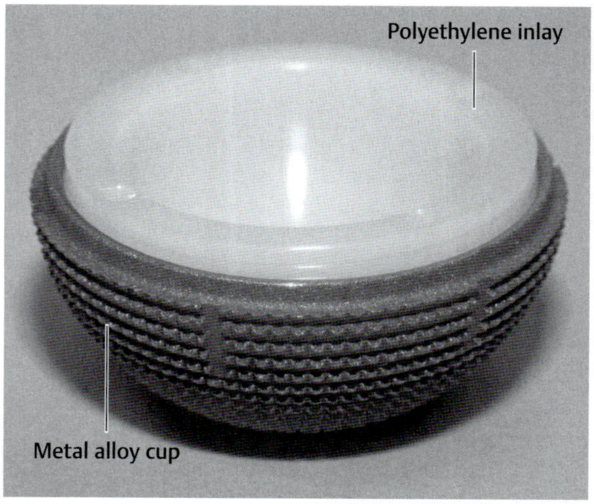

Fig. 1.76 Acetabular cup prosthesis. This model has a rough surface (press-fit technique).

Table 1.2 Findings to be attentive for on follow-up radiographs after fracture studies

Radiographic sign	(Potential) Complication
Hardware failure or distortion	Failure of fracture fixation, instability (► Fig. 1.75)
New fracture or fissure	Failure of fracture fixation, previously unrecognized fracture, iatrogenic fracture
Lucent zone around the implant	Osteomyelitis, aseptic loosening
Dislocation of implant components	Failure of fracture fixation, osteomyelitis
Secondary fragment dislocation	Failure of fracture fixation, osteomyelitis, refracture, osteonecrosis
Loose body in a joint	Failure of fracture fixation, refracture, previously unrecognized fragment
New defects in the trabecular bone, cortex, or subchondral bone plate	Osteomyelitis, empyema, hypotrophic nonunion, osteonecrosis
Focal density	Bone infarction, osteonecrosis, subsidence, osteomyelitis, osteoarthritis
Collapse of an epiphyseal fragment	Osteonecrosis, subchondral fracture
Subchondral lucent line	Osteonecrosis, subchondral fracture
Demineralization	CRPS, osteomyelitis, disuse osteoporosis
Exuberant callus formation	Hypertrophic nonunion, limitation of motion, nerve or vascular compression
Periosteal reaction	Osteomyelitis, bone infarction
Joint-space narrowing	Osteoarthritis, inflammatory arthritis, septic arthritis, chondrolysis
Juxta-articular osteophytes	Osteoarthritis
Air inclusions	Soft tissue infection/cellulitis, iatrogenic introduction of air (joint aspiration/ injection, surgery)
Extensive heterotopic ossification	Limitation of motion, nerve or vascular compression
Soft tissue swelling, joint effusion	Osteomyelitis, septic arthritis, soft tissue infection/cellulitis, postoperative bleeding

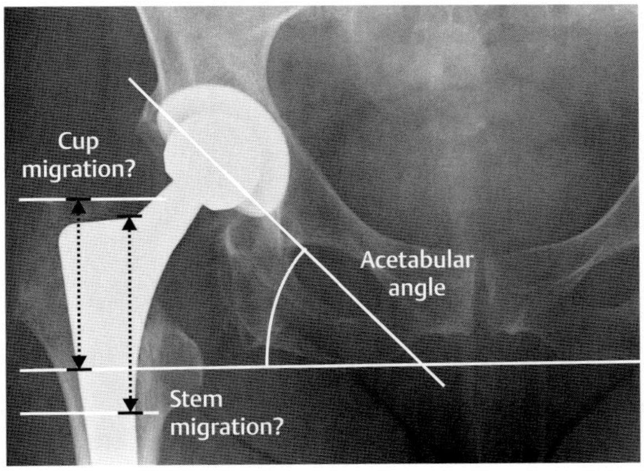

Fig. 1.77 Normal radiographic findings after total hip replacement. The transischial line is used as a reference (see Chapter 1.6.4).

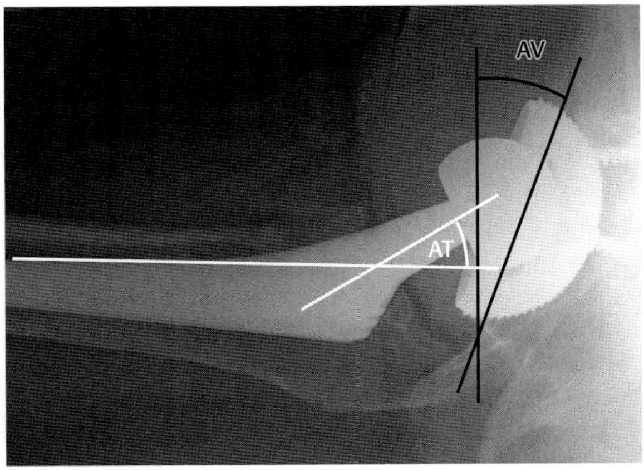

Fig. 1.78 Normal finding after total hip replacement; cross-table lateral view. AV = anteversion angle = angle between the acetabular axis and the vertical line (ideally ~ 15°). AT = antetorsion angle = angle between the prosthetic neck and the stem (ideally ~ 10°).

Loosening of the Prosthesis

▸ **Clinical presentation.** Patients with prosthesis loosening complain about pain on weight bearing and on rotation, which is referred to the thigh (stem loosening) or the groin/ buttock (acetabular cup loosening). When assessing joint prostheses it is important to analyze the bone–prosthesis interface as this will provide important information about the stability of the prosthesis. A margin of lucency between prosthesis and bone and/or between the cement and bone (with or without a fine sclerotic line) of up to 2 mm is of no significance; wider margins are an indication of prosthesis loosening. A prosthesis that has no firm fit in its prosthetic bed causes pain and impairment of or even complete loss of function. Unequivocal signs of loosening are component fractures (prosthesis or cement) and periprosthetic fractures occurring over time; on the other hand, iatrogenic fractures sustained during prosthesis implantation that are immediately recognized and treated usually heal without any problems.

A distinction must be made between a cemented and an uncemented prosthetic component The **cemented implant** should demonstrate immediate evidence of stability as evidenced by the smooth cement fixation between prosthesis and bone. Essential criteria for loosening include prosthesis migration and a pathological margin of lucency.

- *Component migration* of at least 4 mm is suspicious (▸ Fig. 1.79), as are cup rotation of at least 4° of central cup migration and varus or valgus migration of the stem (▸ Fig. 1.80). If the stem subsides by 2 mm, that is also suspicious.
- A *zone of periprosthetic lucency* is suspicious if it is wider that 2 mm or appears wedge-shaped (▸ Fig. 1.81). Lucency between prosthesis and cement is also noteworthy, as is cement degradation. The wider, longer, or more circumferential the lucent zone is, the greater is the risk of loosening. The same applies even if this sign appears after many years. An initially narrower marginal lucency (less than 2 mm) or an incomplete cement mantle may indicate an increased risk of loosening, especially if the stem tip is not closely approximated by adjacent bone.

With an **uncemented prosthesis**, primary stability of the stem is achieved with the press-fit technique, in which, ideally, the stem obtains good cortical fixation and becomes wedged. This provides an even transfer of force from implant to bone. The specially structured surface is supposed to ensure the ingrowth of bone, known as secondary stability. Alternatively, this may also be accomplished by fibrous fixation alone. Various forces can exert their effect on the metal–bone interface if primary stability is suboptimal. This produces different reactions in the bone:

- Periprosthetic osteolysis of the cortex, a periprosthetic margin of lucency, calcar resorption or conversion of compact bone to cancellous bone can appear in stress-shielded areas (▸ Fig. 1.82).
- Periosteal reaction (especially at the level of the implant tip), sclerotic lines along the margin of lucency, sclerosis of the lucent margin, including pedestal formation, and new trabecular formation within the lucent margin can develop in areas of increased loading or secondary to repair processes (▸ Fig. 1.83).

In a favorable case, these adaptive changes lead to secondary stability; however, if these mechanisms fail then the prosthesis becomes loose or does not set. Suspicion of loosening is particularly probable if a margin of sclerotic lucency measures more than 2 mm, if it is located proximally or at a sclerotic pedestal, if it widens over time, or if the sclerosis disappears. Acceleration of prosthesis migration or migration after initial stability is at any rate suspicious of loosening.

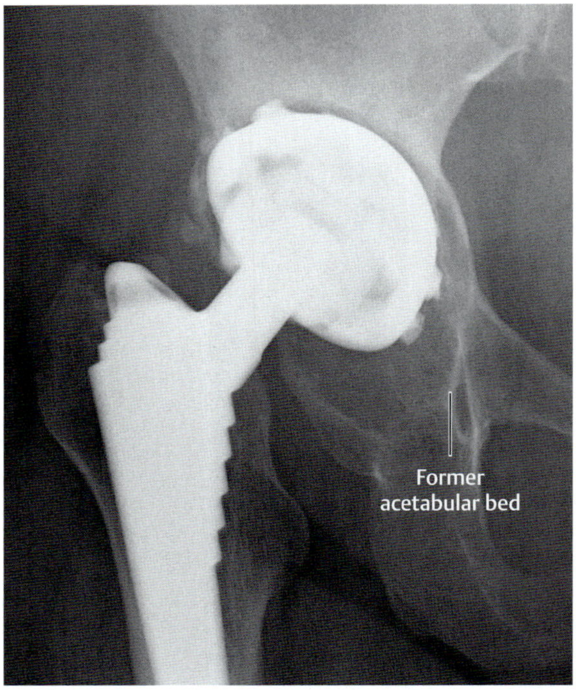

Fig. 1.79 Acetabular cup loosening. Cranial to the acetabular cup there is a narrow margin of lucency with a wide sclerotic zone tapering off in a cranial direction. There is a very wide lucent margin medially; the cup has migrated considerably in a cranial direction. Note also the proximal position of the lesser trochanter relative to the ischium.

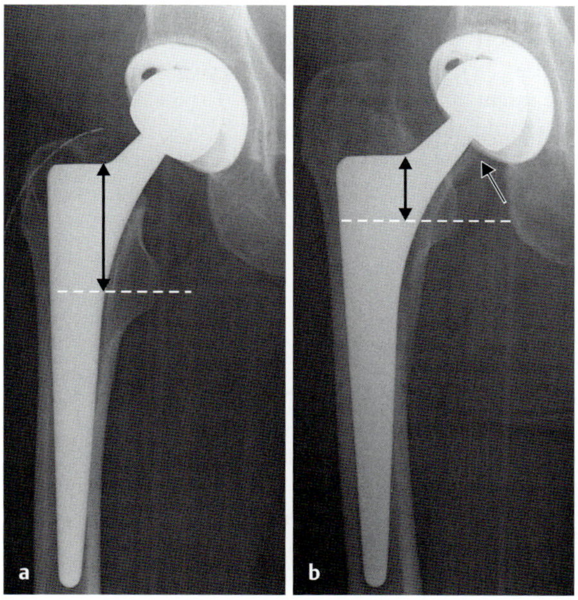

Fig. 1.80 Prosthesis subsidence. **(a)** Initial postoperative study. **(b)** Prosthesis loosening after 4 months: The stem prosthesis has clearly subsided; furthermore, the stem tip has migrated laterally (varus migration). The calcar femorale already reaches as far as the cup (arrow).

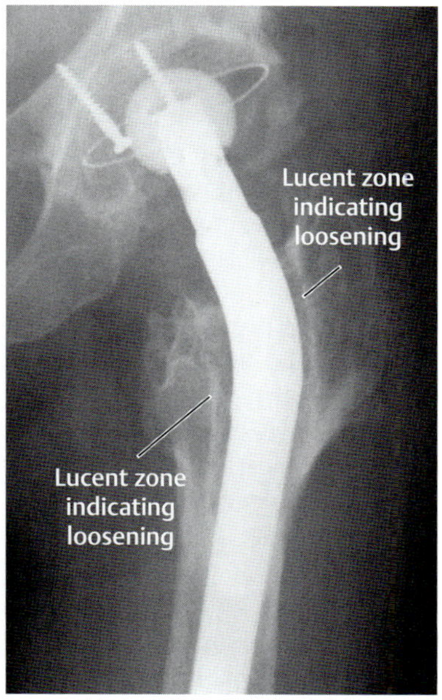

Fig. 1.81 Loose prosthesis stem. There is a considerable (3–6 mm) circumferential lucent zone proximally.

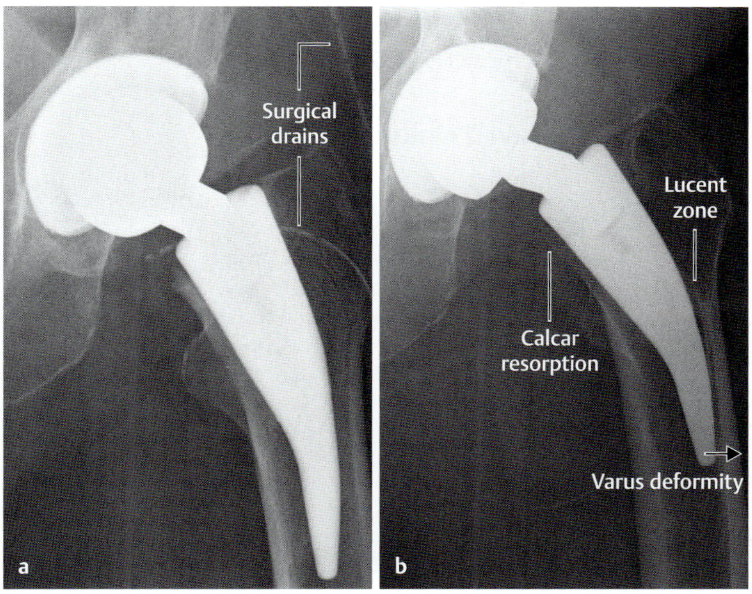

Fig. 1.82 Signs of inadequate secondary stability at the prosthesis stem. **(a)** Initial postoperative radiograph after uncemented joint replacement. **(b)** Six months after surgery: cancellous bone formation with resorption of the calcar femorale, curved sclerotic margin lateral to the implant, and varus position of the stem.

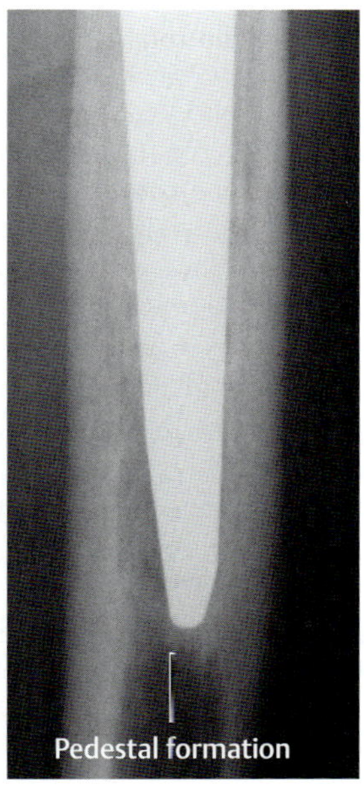

Fig. 1.83 Pedestal formation is visible as sclerosis at the femoral stem tip.

Further Complications

Centrifugal forces are exerted on the cortex during insertion of a femoral stem component and may result in **splitting of the shaft** (▶ Fig. 1.84). Nutrient canals can pose challenges for differential diagnosis. They are usually easily differentiated by their morphology (marginal sclerosis) and position (proximal to middle third of the dorsal femoral cortex).

Prosthetic hip dislocation is not rare and is usually clearly identified in the AP view (▶ Fig. 1.85). In the case of a bipolar hip arthroplasty, the entire implant typically dislocates out of the native acetabular cup, whereas the prosthetic head usually dislocates out of the acetabular cup component of a total hip arthroplasty. Only rarely does the cup prosthesis dislocate out of the pelvis.

Postoperative infection can develop after joint replacement. Furthermore, **late infection** is a special complication of joint replacement and can present clinically with an insidious onset (osteomyelitis) or in an acute manner (septic joint). Periprosthetic osteomyelitis may not be evident on radiographs or may demonstrate destruction of periprosthetic bone and cement. An infection must always be considered in the case of prosthetic loosening.

Infectious destruction of the bone must be distinguished from osteolysis secondary to **foreign-body reactions ("wear disease")** in which fine particles of metal, cement, or polyethylene can cause osteolysis at all prosthetic interfaces. The particles can also destroy cement and are distinguishable from areas of infectious osteolysis by their round or oval form with a honeycomb-like or expansile appearance and well-defined margins (▶ Fig. 1.86). Wear disease may result in prosthetic loosening if the osteolysis is particularly severe or progresses rapidly.

Fracture of the metal components of joint prostheses is very rare. The polyethylene acetabular liner, on the other hand, is subject to **wear** and resulting asymmetric thinning (appearing as asymmetry of the femoral head within the cup on radiographs, ▶ Fig. 1.87).

Periprosthetic heterotopic **soft tissue ossification** is a relatively common occurrence after a hip replacement (▶ Fig. 1.88), typically developing over a period of months. Clinical findings will depend on the extent of ossification and range from no symptoms to restriction of movement or even to complete immobility of the joint. Extruded cement may rarely produce similar symptoms.

Conclusion

Conventional radiography plays an essential role in the assessment of prosthetic joint replacements. CT scanning can be helpful, especially for the evaluation of prosthetic loosening or possible iatrogenic fractures. Both bone scanning and PET (positron emission tomography) can be of help in differentiating between septic and aseptic loosening. MRI is playing a more important role in assessing joint prostheses, especially for detecting perioprosthetic collections or defining the extent of a superficial infection. Fistulography can provide further information in certain cases (▶ Fig. 1.89). Ultrasound may reveal perioprosthetic abscesses or seromas and is able to assess the position of hardware relative to adjacent soft tissue structures, with the added option of dynamic assessment.

1.7 Complications after Fractures

Infection and **osteonecrosis** are possible fracture-related complications, but may also result from numerous other causes, and will therefore be dealt with in the relevant chapters (Chapters 3 and 6).

Heterotopic ossification is also occasionally seen after a fracture, but is basically a separate disorder that can develop without a fracture or even without apparent injury. The reader is therefore referred to the relevant chapter (see Chapter 11.5.2).

1.7.1 Delayed Union, Nonunion, and Posttraumatic Bone Cyst Formation

Delayed Union

> **Note**
> The definition of a fracture healing as "slow," "delayed," or even (without any further intervention) as "nonunion" is highly subjective. All concepts regarding the "normal" timing of fracture healing and its complications are only rough estimates. Radiologists should use such terms with great caution.

Slowed bone healing may be normal in any of the following conditions:

- Extension of the fracture into the articular surface.
- Slow bone metabolism in elderly patients.
- Poor approximation of the bone fragments.
- Inconsistent immobilization of the fragment ends.
- Major soft tissue damage (resulting in poor perfusion).

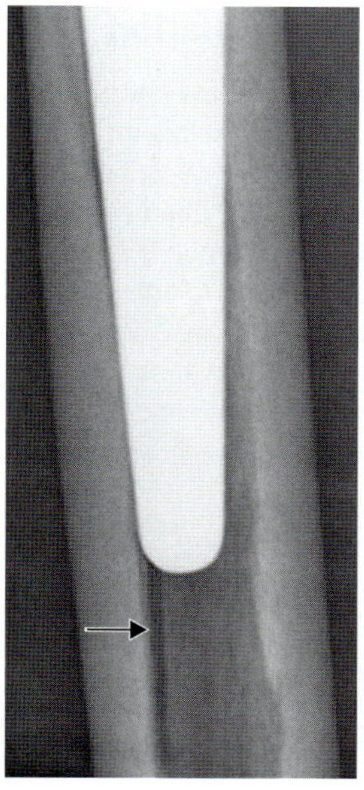

Fig. 1.84 Intra-operative splitting of the femoral shaft. A longitudinal fracture in the shaft (arrow) was not noticed during implantation of the stem component.

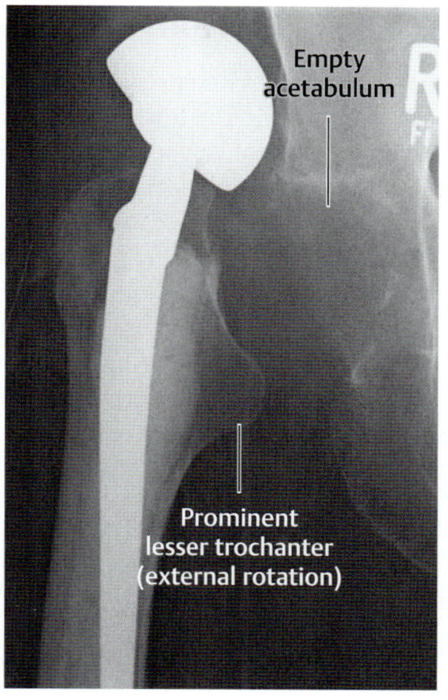

Fig. 1.85 Dislocation of a cemented bipolar implant out of the acetabulum.

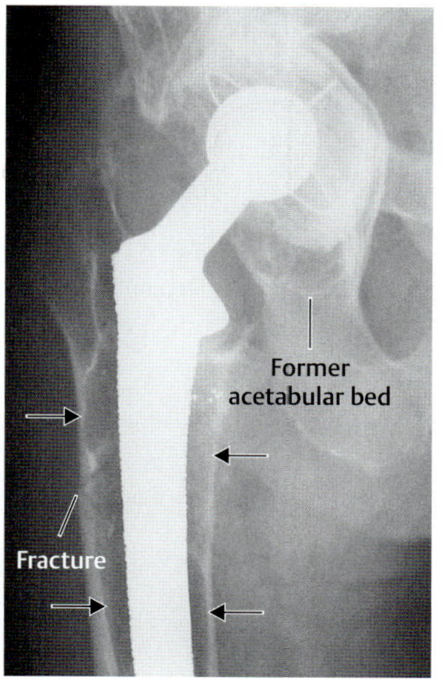

Fig. 1.86 Granulomatous foreign-body reaction. Prominent areas of osteolysis (arrows) have developed along the stem component and have already resulted in a fracture of the proximal femoral shaft. Note also the central migration of the acetabular component.

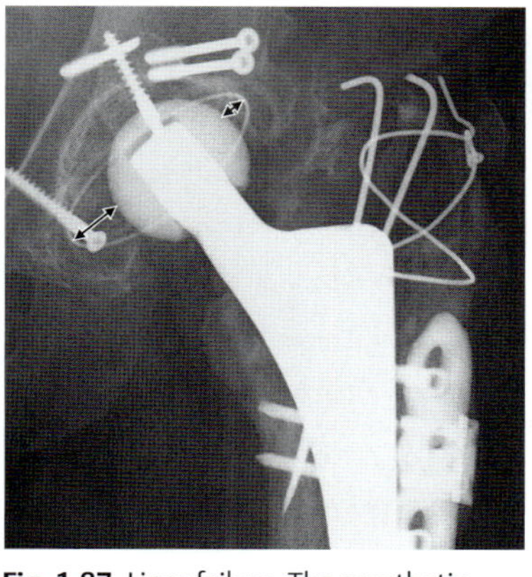

Fig. 1.87 Liner failure. The prosthetic head is positioned asymmetrically in the cup (arrows) indicating either wear or fracture of the polyethylene liner.

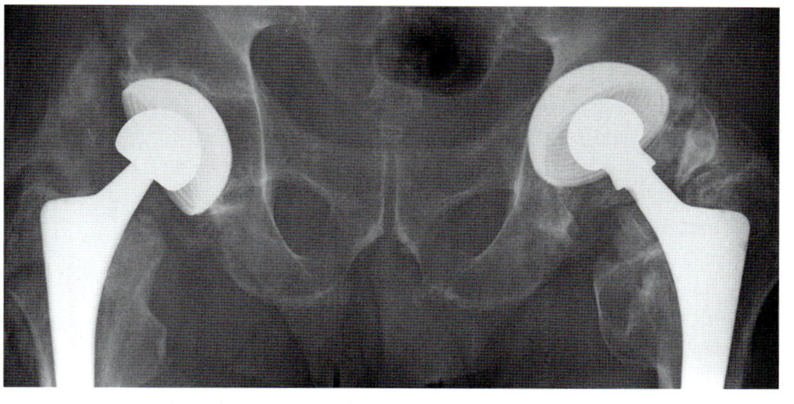

Fig. 1.88 Periprosthetic heterotopic soft tissue ossification. This patient with DISH (diffuse idiopathic skeletal hyperostosis) developed extensive, functionally impairing heterotopic ossification adjacent to both hip arthroplasties.

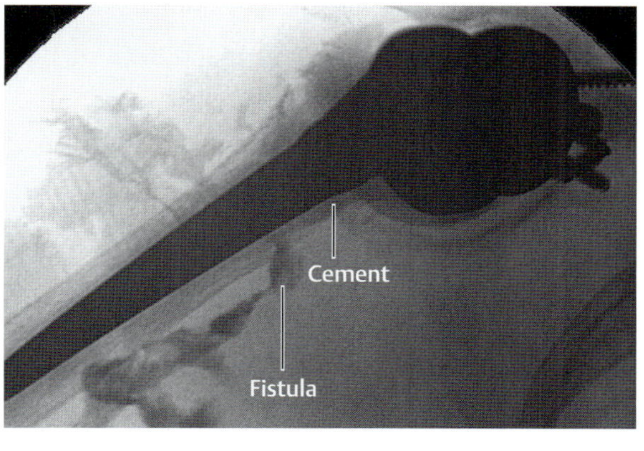

Fig. 1.89 Fluoroscopy-assisted contrast radiography of a skin fistula years after implantation of a reverse shoulder prosthesis. The fistula extends up to the cement.

Delayed (disturbed) bone healing may be assumed—with caution—when the fracture healing time has been exceeded by as much as double the typical time span (▶Table 1.3). Causes include:

- Inadequate immobilization.
- Poor blood supply.
- Infection.

Delayed bone healing can, but need not, lead to nonunion.

Nonunion

Absence of fracture healing may be assumed after 8 to 9 months. Problems with either primary or secondary fracture healing can lead to nonunion. Causes include:

- Inadequate immobilization.
- Interposition of fibrous tissue in the fracture gap.
- Significant loss of bone substance.
- Inadequate blood supply.
- Infection with sequestration.

There are a number of different classifications of nonunions and the imaging appearance may provide clues as to the etiology:

- **Hypertrophic form:** "elephant foot," "horse hoof"; inadequate immobilization of the fracture.
- **Atrophic form:** poor perfusion.
- **Defect nonunions:** segmental loss of bone, which no longer allows osseous bridging and consolidation.

▶ **Radiography.**

Hypertrophic type (▶Fig. 1.90a)

- The fragment ends are widened (elephant foot, horse hoof), have irregular margins and are sclerotic.
- The surrounding bone is eburnated.
- There is absent or incomplete osseous bridging.
- The fragment ends may be rounded off.

Atrophic type (▶Fig. 1.90b)

- There is little or no sclerosis at the fracture margins.
- The fragment ends usually demonstrate smooth margins.
- Osteopenia is prominent.
- There is increasing bone loss over time.

▶ **CT.** CT scanning has today become an indispensable modality for evaluating the degree of healing. It helps in distinguishing between posttraumatic or postoperative defects from nonunions (▶Fig. 1.91).

Assessment of the fracture margins, unobscured by overlying structures, is needed in cases of equivocal healing, particularly in the hypertrophic type, before any surgical intervention is performed. The same imaging criteria apply as for conventional radiography. Consolidation of 5 to 10% of the fragment surface or even smaller areas of peripheral bridging does not preclude the diagnosis of nonunion (▶Fig. 1.92).

Posttraumatic Bone-Cyst Formation

Large circumscribed hematomas can become encapsulated within the fracture zones and are then excluded from the normal course of fracture healing. In rare cases, large lytic bone defects may develop, even though the fracture is stable and capable of load bearing. This phenomenon is often seen in greenstick fractures, but may also occur in other types of fractures. The radiologically apparent lucency is found both centrally and near the cortex. An MRI scan will clarify its origin if there are any differential-diagnostic concerns. Posttraumatic cysts resolve slowly and spontaneously over the course of years (▶Fig. 1.93).

Table 1.3 Approximate reference values for normal fracture healing times in adults with normal bone density

Mean duration of healing	Fracture site
3–6 weeks	• Skull • Clavicle, scapula • Sternum, ribs • Head of humerus • Distal humerus • Elbow • Radial head • Distal forearm • Metacarpals/fingers • Metatarsals/toes
6–8 weeks	• Humeral shaft • Forearm shaft • Distal lower leg
8–10 weeks	• Tibial shaft • Femoral shaft
10–14 weeks	• Carpus • Neck of femur • Pelvis • Distal femur • Tibial plateau • Tarsus/calcaneus

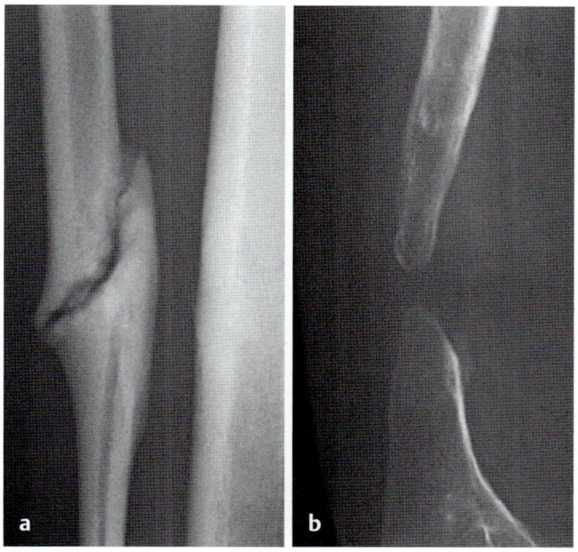

Fig. 1.90 Nonunions. **(a)** Hypertrophic nonunion of the fibula. **(b)** Atrophic nonunion of the humerus.

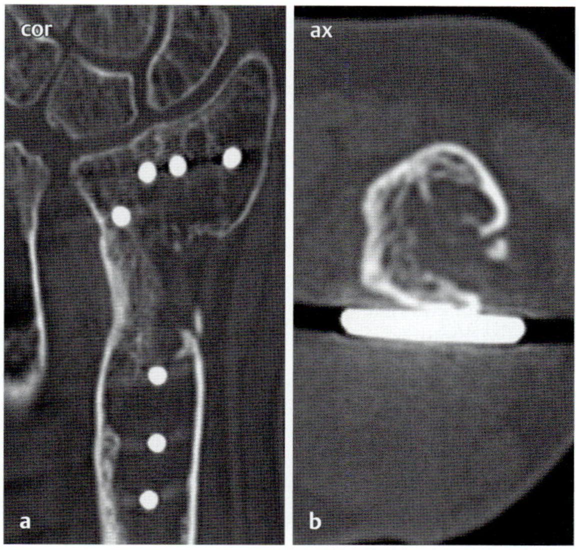

Fig. 1.91 Posttraumatic cortical defect. **(a)** This coronal image shows a large area of absent bone. **(b)** The corresponding axial image, however, demonstrates that the actual amount of absent cortex is much smaller.

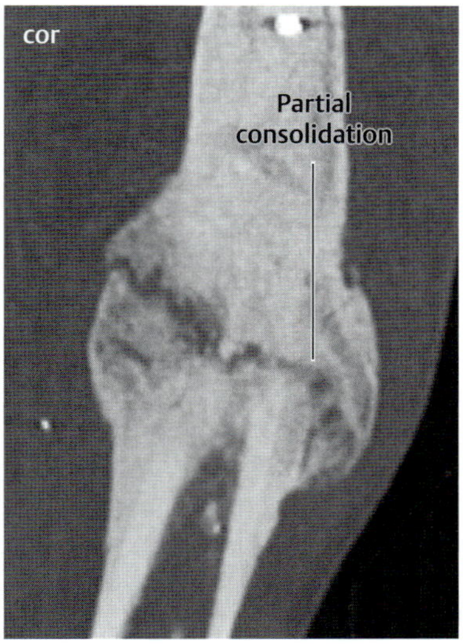

Fig. 1.92 Long-standing hypertrophic nonunion.

Fig. 1.93 Posttraumatic cyst in the distal ulna. (Images courtesy of H. Rosenthal, Medical University Hannover.) **(a)** Initial finding: distal forearm fractures. **(b)** Normal callus formation initially. **(c)** Four years later: evidence of a posttraumatic cyst within the ulna. **(d)** Seven years later: extensive sclerosis of the healed lesion.

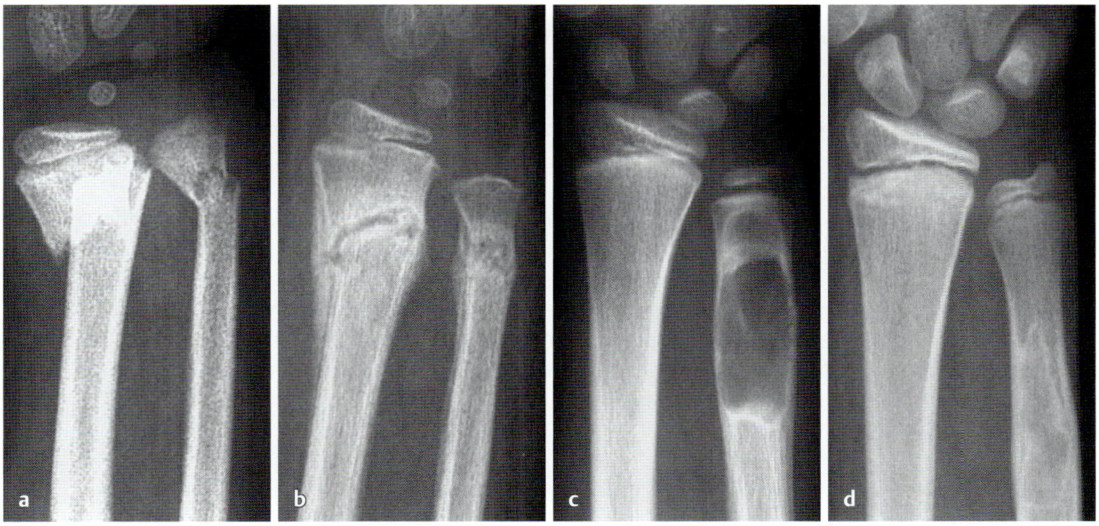

1.7.2 Posttraumatic Disturbances of Growth in Children and Adolescents

Longitudinal growth of tubular bones is controlled by the physis, whereas growth in diameter is produced by the periosteum and endosteum. Traumatic disturbances of growth in bone diameter (e.g., nonunions) are very rare in childhood due to the high capability for regeneration, but disturbances of longitudinal growth related to physeal injury secondary to fractures involving the growth plate are common (Chapter 1.3.1).

Both growth acceleration and growth retardation can occur as a response to traumatic injury to the physis:

- **Growth acceleration** is due to marked hyperemia in the region of the growth plate in reaction to an injury. If the injury is sustained during the physiological growth period, then abnormally increased longitudinal growth of the affected tubular bone will occur. If the injury occurs in the period before or during physiological closure of the growth plate, then hyperemia will lead to early maturation of the growth plate and result in (usually) mild shortening of the tubular bone.
- **Growth retardation** occurs as a result of premature closure of the growth plate after severe damage to the epiphysis. Premature closure may be complete or partial (▶ Fig. 1.94). The greater the residual potential for growth (i.e., the younger the child), the more pronounced is the degree of shortening. If the damage is only partial, then an osseous bridge ("physeal bar") develops between the epiphysis and the metaphysis. Growth ceases in this area, and if this bridge forms asymmetrically within the growth plate, it will result in axial malalignment. A central position of this osseous bridge will result in cupping of the metaphysis and a cone-shaped form of the epiphysis, i.e., there is an appearance of invagination of the epiphysis into the metaphysis (cf. ▶ Figs. 1.5 and ▶ 1.6).

Interference with growth can also occur after **greenstick fractures**, in which the cortex on the convex side is completely disrupted while the cortex on the concave side is only partially disrupted and the periosteal sleeve is intact. The fracture consolidates quickly on the concave side while consolidation is delayed or lacking on the convex side, resulting in a risk of refracture and/or axial malalignment.

However, in the skeletally immature, these posttraumatic growth disturbances may be offset—unlike with adults—by **corrective mechanisms** that help to restore normal bone morphology. The younger the child is, the more marked are these self-correction mechanisms. For example, in a maligned shaft fracture, periosteal new bone will be produced on the side of greatest static load while endosteal erosion will occur on the unloaded side, thereby resulting in correction of the abnormal angulation and restoration of the original morphology.

1.7.3 Disuse Osteoporosis

This is a form of osteopenia that results from reduced bone mass and altered bone architecture secondary to immobilization of a limb. It is typically not radiographically apparent until at least 14 days after immobilization, but in children it may be recognized after only a few days.

▶ **Radiography/CT.** The changes associated with disuse osteoporosis initially affect cancellous bone. **Patchy demineralization** develops with oval, rounded, or irregularly configured lucencies (▶ Figs. 1.95 and ▶ 1.96). Over time, thinning of the cortex and enlargement of the haversian canals is also visible.

As well as this predominantly patchy form of demineralization, **bandlike demineralization** may also develop. This latter form is found preferentially in the region of former growth plates and subchondral bone. Such radiolucent lines are usually found in younger adults. In children, demineralization can produce such homogeneous osteopenia that it is sometimes only recognizable in comparison with the contralateral side.

▶ **MRI.** The bone marrow may be unremarkable in the setting of osteopenia or may demonstrate foci of linear or punctuate signal intensity on fluid-sensitive or postcontrast images, particularly in subchondral bone. These foci are often detectable on fluid-sensitive sequences and also after contrast administration, most likely as a reflection of hyperperfusion (▶ Fig. 1.97).

▶ **DD.**

Generalized osteoporosis. This not only develops in a limb (regional, local) but also diffusely, particularly in the axial skeleton.

CRPS. This is primarily a clinical diagnosis (see Chapter 1.7.4). The associated radiological findings are more or less identical with those of disuse osteoporosis.

1.7.4 Complex Regional Pain Syndrome

Complex regional pain syndrome (CRPS) is a disorder of unknown etiology classically characterized initially by painful soft tissue swelling and later by soft tissue atrophy and patchy osteoporosis. It often occurs after an injury to an extremity.

Nomenclature. Originally known as "Sudeck's disease," this disorder has also been known by numerous names—algodystrophy, chronic traumatic edema, sympathetic dystrophy, and reflex sympathetic dystrophy. In 1994, the IASP (International Association for the Study of Pain) defined the disorder as "CRPS" and this is now the preferred term.

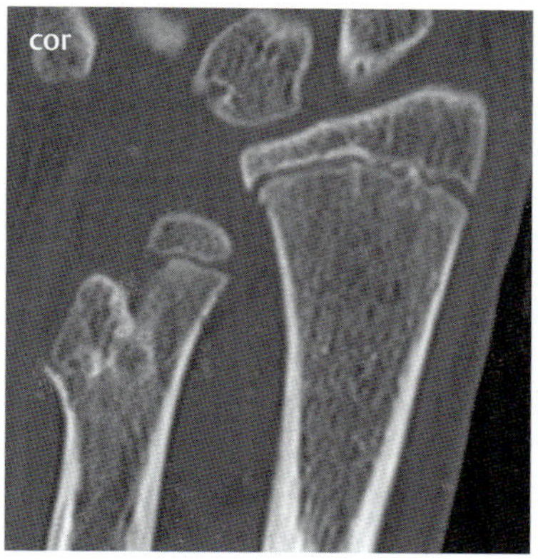

Fig. 1.94 Deformation of the distal ulna with partial, premature closure of the growth plate in this boy (14 years old) who sustained a distal forearm fracture 6 years previously, at which time there was no deformity.

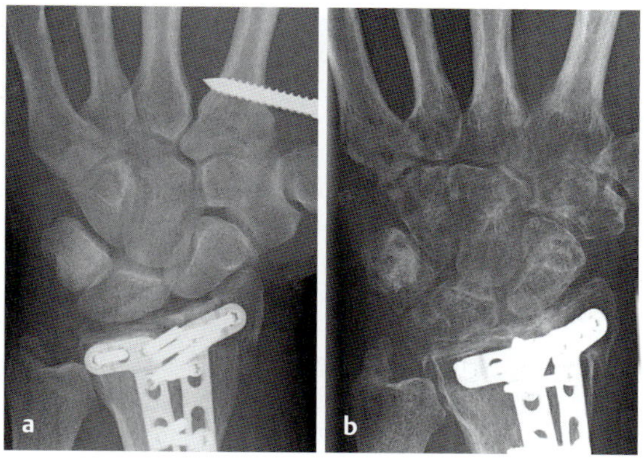

Fig. 1.95 Disuse osteoporosis. **(a)** Initial appearance of the wrist after operative fixation of a comminuted distal radius fracture. **(b)** Massive demineralization 2 months later.

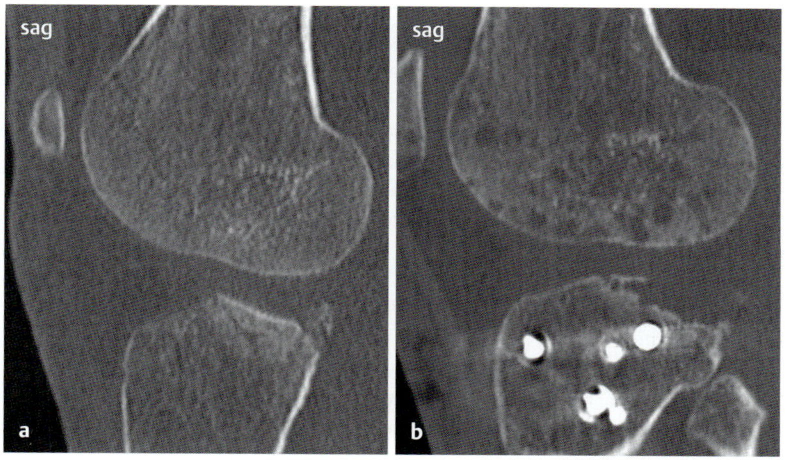

Fig. 1.96 Disuse osteoporosis. **(a)** Initial finding: fracture of the tibial plateau. **(b)** Patchy demineralization 7 months later after internal fixation.

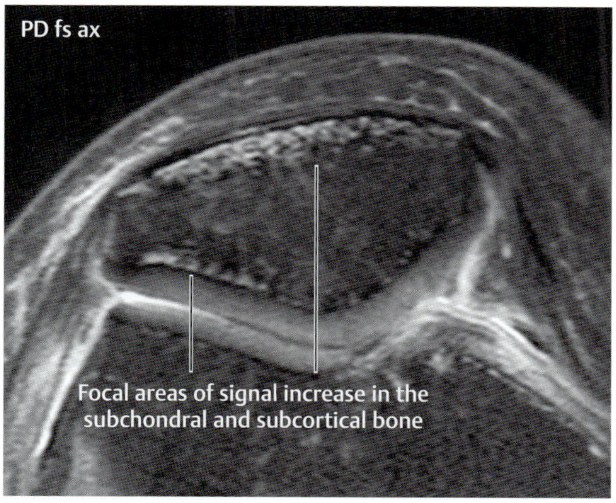

Fig. 1.97 Disuse osteoporosis of the patella after cruciate ligament reconstruction.

▶ **Pathology.** In about 10% of cases, no initiating event is apparent; 90% are the result of trauma, most frequently after a fracture of the distal radius or tibia. However, there is no correlation between the severity of the initiating event and the degree of impaired function and pain. It is thought that disturbances of the sympathetic nervous system and microcirculation may be involved in the development of CRPS but the exact pathomechanics of the disorder is unclear.

▶ **Clinical presentation.** CRPS is characterized by a triad of symptoms comprising sensory, sympathetic, and motor disturbances. The classic case progresses through three phases:

1. **Inflammatory phase:** spontaneous burning pain, soft tissue swelling, skin reddish-blue, moist and warm, painful stiffness; hyperesthesia and hyperalgesia; acute onset within hours to days after the initiating event.
2. **Dystrophic phase:** pain on motion and increasing stiffness, but less pain at rest; skin pale-bluish, cool and dry, trophic skin changes (fibrosis, changes in hair and nail growth), contractures: typically develops over the course of weeks to months.
3. **(Irreversible) atrophic phase:** atrophic, dry "wax skin," contractures, complete loss of function.

The course of the disease, however, does not always progress through these stages. The onset can be especially insidious and redness and increased warmth may initially be absent.

▶ **Radiography.** At first, only soft tissue swelling is evident. Radiographic changes in the bones are not to be expected until at least 4 weeks after symptom onset. A patchy or sometimes bandlike demineralization then develops, which becomes more homogeneous over time (▶ Fig. 1.98). Fading of the subchondral bone plate and thinning of the cortex due to subperiosteal, intracortical and endosteal absorption can also appear (▶ Fig. 1.99b). Absence of radiologically recognizable changes, however, does not exclude the disorder. In children, the bones may appear normal throughout the course of the disorder.

A few weeks after the disorder has subsided, the bony changes usually disappear again. However, in severe cases remineralization may be incomplete. In this case, streaky coarse trabecular bone and a narrow cortex remain.

▶ **NUC MED.** In Stage I, the bone scan demonstrates typical changes in the soft tissue phase (5–15 minutes after injection of radiotracer) *and* in the early bone phase: There is significantly increased tracer uptake near the joints, although this pattern may also appear over the entire affected limb, with a primarily distal emphasis. In Stage II, tracer uptake of the soft tissue is reduced, while uptake within the bone remains high. In the stage of atrophy, the scintigraphic image of the bone may return to normal.

▶ **MRI.** In the inflammatory phase, MRI shows soft tissue edema, corresponding to the clinical picture, with increased contrast uptake within the affected regions. In the majority of cases, the bones appear unremarkable over the entire course of the disease. When abnormal marrow signal findings are present, these usually present as solitary or multifocal edemalike regions predominantly within the subchondral bone (▶ Fig. 1.99a). Low-signal intensity lines may be apparent within the edema, suggesting that these are in fact insufficiency fractures as a secondary manifestation of CRPS. MRI is therefore used only to exclude other disorders and cannot provide a specific diagnosis of CRPS.

▶ **DD.**

Arthritis. In most arthritides, periarticular osteoporosis is confined to the affected joints, and other findings such as periarticular soft tissue swelling, joint-space narrowing, and bone erosions are helpful discriminators.

Disuse osteoporosis. The demineralization pattern on radiographs does not allow for differentiation. However, associated pain and soft tissue swelling are absent in the case of disuse osteoporosis.

Transient bone marrow edema syndrome. MR imaging reveals marked bone marrow edema, but the clinical picture lacks any dystrophic components.

Acute or chronic osteomyelitis. With osteomyelitis, extensive bone marrow abnormality is always present on MR images, unlike in CRPS. Associated abscesses may also be present (Chapter 3.1).

1.7.5 Posttraumatic Osteoarthritis

Posttraumatic, early-onset osteoarthritis is not uncommon, especially in cases where there is involvement of an articular surface. Traumatic disruption of the cartilage results in its early degeneration and development of classic osteoarthritis deformans. Posttraumatic articular incongruity may also result in osteoarthritis due to the unequal loading of the joint surface. Posttraumatic malalignment or leg-length discrepancy may result in abnormal weight-bearing in adjacent joints and/or the spine and may cause early osteoarthritis at these sites.

Posttraumatic osteoarthritis is a **secondary osteoarthritis**, although it does have the same clinical course as primary osteoarthritis (Chapter 10.2).

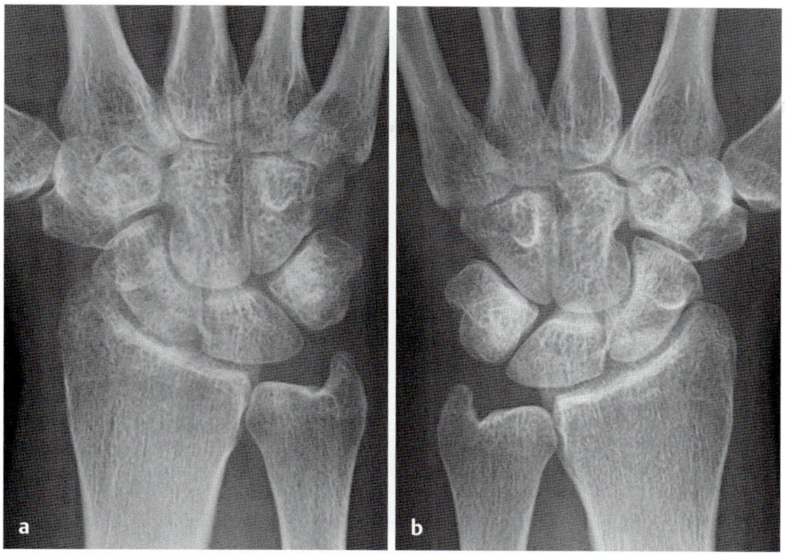

Fig. 1.98 Stage II complex regional pain syndrome (CPRS) following a crush injury 4 months previously. The patient was a 47-year-old woman. **(a)** Diffuse reduction in bone density. **(b)** Healthy contralateral side for comparison.

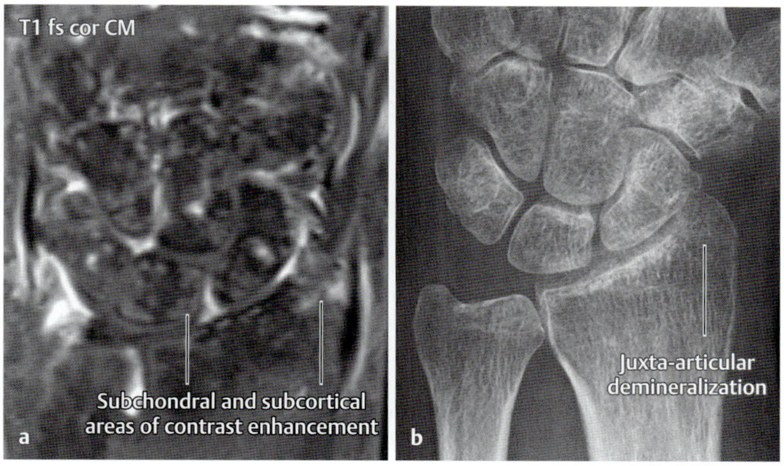

Fig. 1.99 Stage I–II CRPS. No trauma recalled. **(a)** Bone marrow edema of the subchondral bone and the periarticular soft tissues. **(b)** Predominantly periarticular decalcification.

1.8 Traumatic and Overuse Injuries to Muscles, Tendons, and Tendon Insertions

Muscle, tendon, and the tendon insertion form an anatomical unit. Tears always develop at the weakest point of this chain, which will differ depending on the patient's age, the extent of previous damage, and the type of strain. In childhood and adolescence, the insertion of tendons on bone is prone to strain injuries or a bony avulsion. Tears of muscle and at the musculotendinous junction are more likely to be seen in young adulthood. Tears within a tendon do not usually occur unless it has been previously damaged or weakened by age-related degeneration, chronic overloading, or previous injury, all of which are more common in older patients. Tendon rupture in these patients is therefore usually the final step of a long process.

For didactic reasons, the unit "muscle/tendon/tendon insertion on bone" will be dealt with in this chapter in separate sections, beginning with the muscle.

1.8.1 Muscles

▸ Pathology. Injuries to muscles arise as a result of fatigue, neurogenic factors (faulty innervation due to disturbances at the level of the lumbar spine and/or sacroiliac joints), and overstretching to various degrees. Muscle contusions (from a direct blow or crush injury) or lacerations are the result of direct blunt and sharp trauma, respectively. What is known as muscle stiffness (DOMS = delayed onset muscle soreness) is due to disruption of muscle fibrils.

Muscle injuries are typically **graded** in a simple three-level scheme:

- Grade 1: strain.
- Grade 2: partial tear (▸ Fig. W1.13).
- Grade 3: full-thickness tear.

▸ US. A muscle strain may demonstrate subtle decreased echogenicity on US, but these are often undetectable. With partial and full-thickness tears, US will often reveal an anechoic to hypoechoic hematoma (▸ Fig. 1.100). Subacute and chronic hematomas often have a stratified or "onion-skin" appearance. It should be noted that a hemorrhage is typically echogenic in the initial days after injury and often difficult to distinguish from the surrounding muscle. Rolled muscle fiber ends extending into the hematoma (known as the bell-clapper sign) are pathognomonic.

▸ MRI. Signs of edema or hemorrhage are found in *all* grades of injury on fat-saturated T2W scans and T1W sequences after contrast application (▸ Figs. 1.101 – 1.104). A simple grading system of muscle injuries on MRI is listed in ▸ Table 1.4.

▸ Sequelae of muscle injuries:

- Posttraumatic heterotopic ossification.
- Posttraumatic inflammatory pseudotumors.
- Fascial hernias, which are usually far better detected by dynamic clinical examination than by imaging techniques.
- Acute compartment syndrome (Chapter 11.6).
- Nerve compression syndromes (entrapment neuropathies; Chapter 11.8).

1.8.2 Tendons

▸ Pathology. Degenerative tendon disorders are caused either by repetitive overloading related to muscular traction forces or by the effects of compression, usually at the site where the tendon changes direction. This may involve the peritenon, the tendon sheath, or the tendon itself. Histologically, "angiofibroblastic" hyperplasia involving fibroblasts and granulation-like tissue predominates in (noninflammatory/nonrheumatic) tendon degeneration. These changes within the tendon can result in calcification. An overview of the most commonly affected sites is found in ▸ Table 1.5.

The **nomenclature for describing tendon pathologies** is inconsistent. This book follows the terms proposed by Donald Resnick:

- **Paratendinitis.** This refers to inflammation of the soft tissues (irrespective of whether degenerative or rheumatic) surrounding the tendon. A classic example is paratendinitis in the adipose connective tissue around the Achilles tendon.
- **Peritendinitis.** This is usually associated with paratendinitis. The term defines inflammation of the peritenon (of tendons that have no sheath, also known as peritenonitis).
- **Tenosynovitis.** This results from inflammation of the tendon sheath. If in addition there are fibrous exudation and adhesions within the tendon sheath, then this may also be referred to as "stenosing tenosynovitis."
- **Tendinosis** (synonym: tendinopathy). This refers to intrinsic degeneration disturbance of the tendon based on aging and/or strain.

Both tendinosis and tenosynovitis can result in a partial or complete **rupture** of the tendon.

Table 1.4 MRI grading system for muscle injuries

Grade	MRI finding
I	On fluid-sensitive sequences, edema and hemorrhage result in focal or diffuse increase in signal intensity within the muscle and along the muscle fascia; macroscopically, continuity of the fibers is not interrupted (see ▶ Fig. 1.101 and ▶ Fig. 1.102)
II	In addition to the findings of Grade I, *partial* disruption of muscle fibers is evident, which may be further subdivided according to severity (II a < ⅓; II b ⅓–⅔; II c > ⅔, but not complete); partial ruptures most often involve the musculotendinous junction (▶ Fig. W1.13; see also ▶ Fig. 1.103, ▶ Fig. 1.104)
III	Discontinuity involves the *entire* diameter of the muscle; a hematoma fills the gap; a variant is complete disruption of the intramuscular tendon

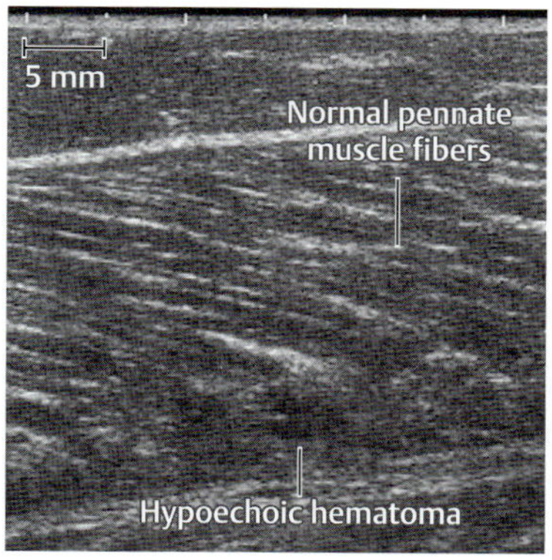

Fig. 1.100 Small (< 5 mm) tear within the gastrocnemius muscle.

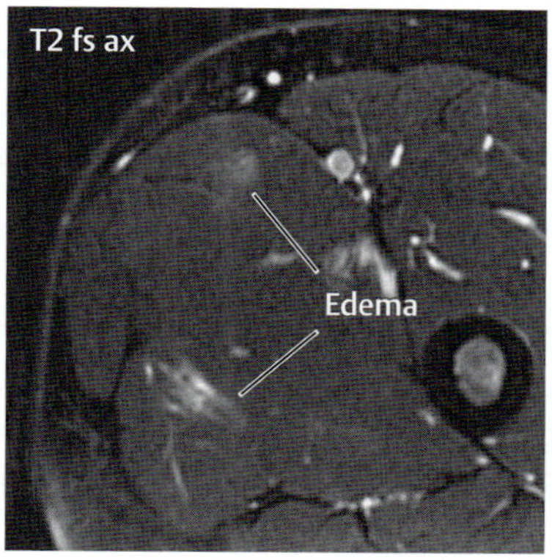

Fig. 1.101 Injuries of the adductor muscles (Grade I, MRI grading) in the proximal thigh.

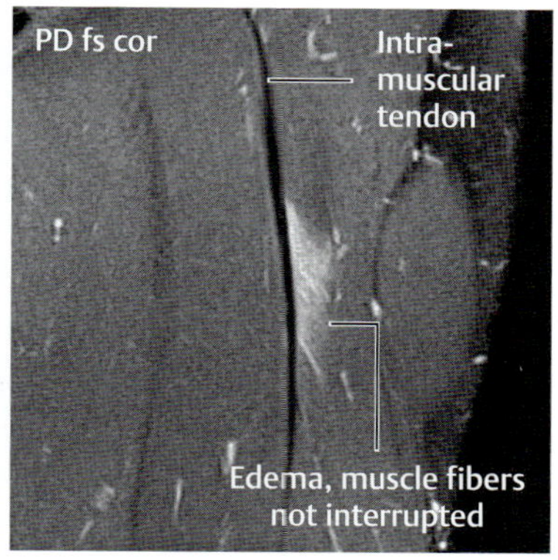

Fig. 1.102 Muscle injury (Grade I, MRI grading) of biceps femoris.

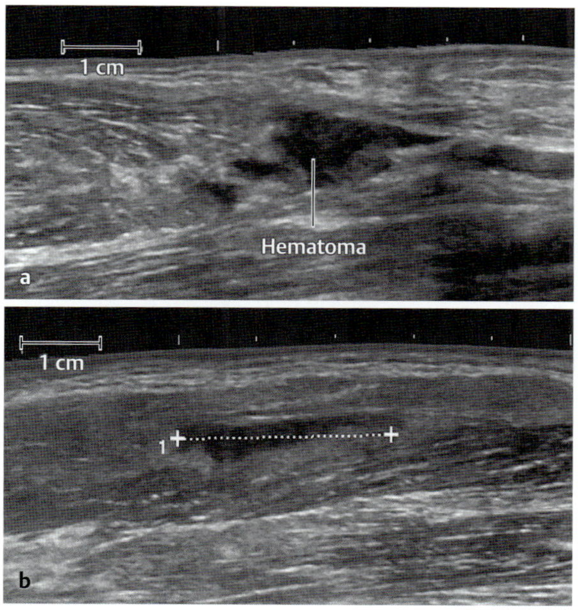

Fig. 1.103 Large (> 5 mm) muscle tear of the biceps brachii secondary to a crush injury. **(a)** Longitudinal ultrasound showing extensive muscle fiber disruption. **(b)** The fibers are only partially disrupted.

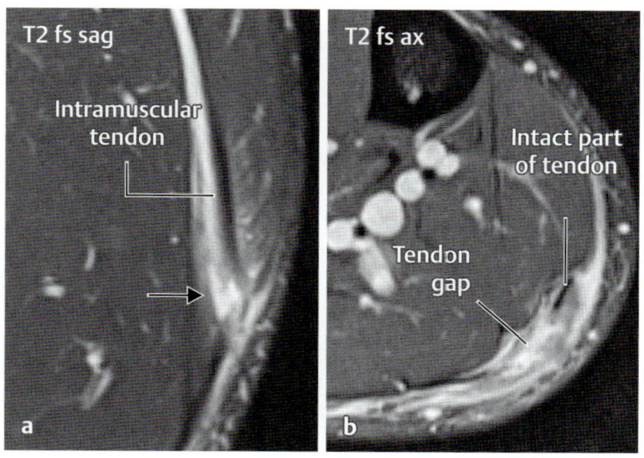

Fig. 1.104 Partial tendon rupture (Grade II, MRI grading) at the myotendinous junction. **(a)** Hyperintense hematoma and edema along the tendon with partial tearing of the tendon (arrow). **(b)** The disrupted portion of the tendon is evident on this axial section.

Table 1.5 Sites commonly affected by strain-related tendon injury

Site	Tendon injury	Description
Shoulder and upper arm	Rotator cuff secondary to subacromial impingement	Pathology of the rotator cuff tendons (see ▶ Fig. 1.108) and the subacromial bursa due to narrowing of the subacromial space or functional compression of the supraspinatus tendon during overhead movements
Hand and fingers	de Quervain's stenosing tenosynovitis	Tendinosis and tenosynovitis of abductor pollicis longus and extensor pollicis brevis tendons at the level of the radial styloid process
Hip and thigh	Iliotibial band syndrome	Friction of the iliotibial band and the greater trochanter (see ▶ Fig. 1.110)
Knee	Iliotibial band friction syndrome at the knee (known as runner's knee)	Friction of the iliotibial band and the lateral femoral epicondyle
Ankle and foot	Achillodynia	Tendinosis of the Achilles tendon as a result of chronic strain, excessive stretching or torsion
	Tibialis posterior dysfunction	Tendinosis of the tibialis posterior tendon

▶ **Radiography/CT.** Radiographs can reveal anatomical features that may predispose to tendon pathology, such as valgus hindfoot, which predisposes to Achilles tendon pathology, or pes equinovarus (clubfoot), which overloads the tibialis posterior tendon. Amorphous calcifications in the tendons usually indicate chronic tendon pathology and may be detected with radiographs, but in general ultrasound and MRI are the modalities of choice for tendon evaluation.

▶ **US.** In the case of tendinosis, the tendon will appear thickened and hypoechoic on ultrasound. The more chronic the finding, the more heterogeneous the echotexture of the tendon (▶ Fig. 1.105). Tendon calcifications can be identified earlier than with routine radiography. With tenosynovitis, hypoechoic fluid and/or hypertrophic, hypoechoic tissue is present around the tendon (▶ Fig. 1.106). Differentiation between effusion and thickened, hypoechoic tenosynovial tissue is not always easy. The additional use of Doppler ultrasound has proven useful by demonstrating increased perfusion of the hypertrophied tendon sheath.

Tendons without a tendon sheath (the Achilles tendon in particular) demonstrate focal hypoechogenicity (focal tendinosis), hypoechoic reaction of the peritendinous tissue (acute peritenonitis), fusiform swelling and an inhomogeneous echo pattern. Ruptures are characterized by dehiscence of fibers (the tendon may be completely absent) and, in the acute stage, by an associated hypoechoic or heterogeneous hematoma (▶ Fig. 1.107). In a full-thickness tear, a dynamic examination can be used to better reveal the torn margins of the tendon during attempted plantar flexion of the foot.

▶ **MRI.** Normal tendons give little or no signal using SE sequences; they appear very dark or even black. This is because normal tendons mainly consist of well-structured collagen. The result is a very short T2 relaxation time (on average below 2 milliseconds). SE sequences, either T2 or PD weighted (PDW), use echo times that are longer than 10 milliseconds. Consequently, a signal of normal tendon tissue cannot be revealed. The use of Ultrashort echo time (UTE) imaging solves the problem but its clinical use is still in its infancy.

The tendon sheath, in contrast, is a two-layered structure (fibrotic and synovial), resembling the MR characteristics of the joint capsule.

Tendinosis results primarily in hypertrophy of the tendon. The signal increase in the tendon is strongly related to the degree of collagen disorganization, the change of the intrasubstance water content, and the number of vessels. Circumscribed or more diffuse increase of signal intensity on water-sensitive (best with fat suppression) PDW and T2W sequences is the general finding (▶ Figs. 1.108 – 1.110).

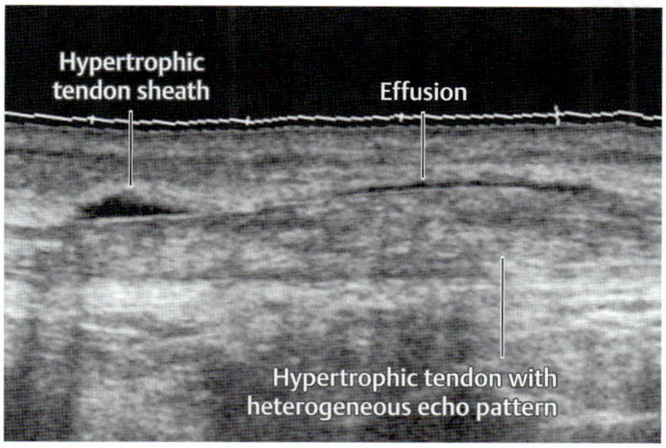

Fig. 1.105 Chronic tendinosis of the tibialis anterior tendon with tenosynovitis. The cause was gout; imaging does not allow differentiation from other causes of tendinosis.

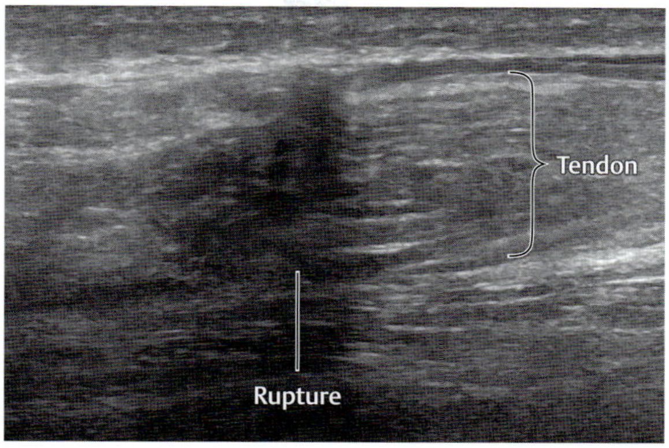

Fig. 1.107 Complete rupture of the Achilles tendon.

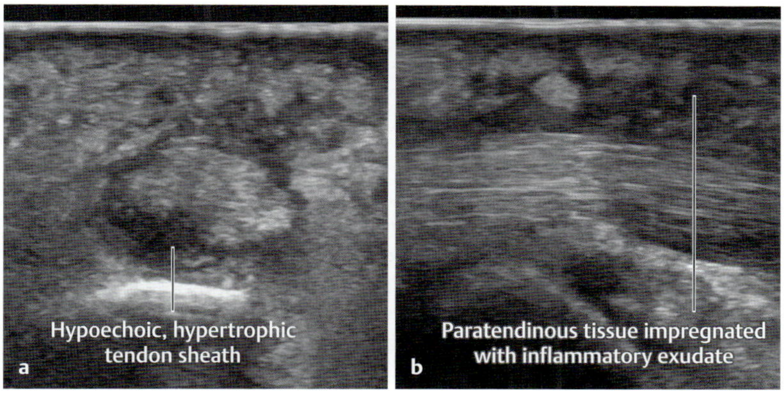

Fig. 1.106 Inflammatory tenosynovitis of the finger flexor tendons at the metacarpophalangeal joint on ultrasound. **(a)** Cross section. **(b)** Longitudinal section.

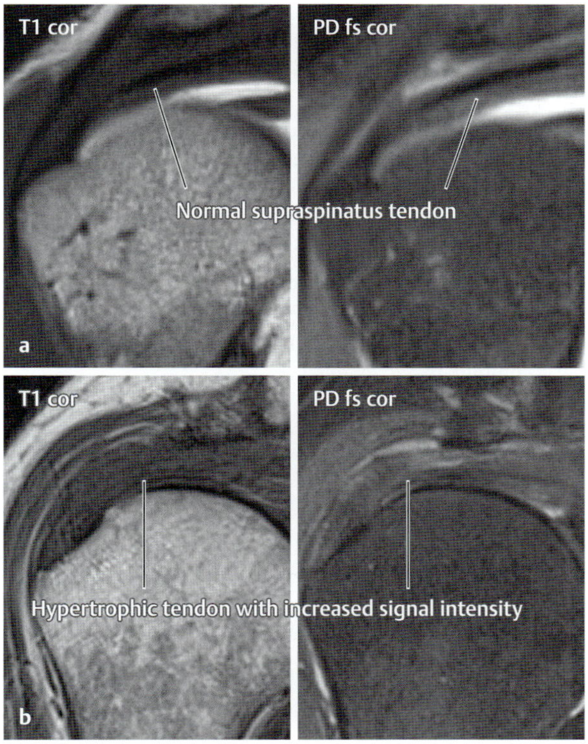

Fig. 1.108 Comparison between a normal supraspinatus tendon and one affected by tendinosis. **(a)** Normal finding (MR arthrography). **(b)** Tendinosis.

Partial tendon tears may demonstrate many forms including attenuation, focal defect or a longitudinal split type of tear. A full-thickness tear is diagnosed when high-signal intensity fluid is seen separating the torn tendon margins on T2W sequences. The torn tendon may also retract (▶ Fig. 1.111). Partial tendon tears can develop within the tendon (intrasubstance) or extend to the surface of the tendon (▶ Fig. 1.112).

Paratendinitis and peritendinitis appear on fluid-sensitive sequences as hyperintense, edematous tissue around the affected tendon. Tenosynovitis will reveal thickening of the sheath and often fluid within the sheath.

Pathologic changes of the tendon itself, but especially of the paratenon and the tendon sheath, can be particularly well demonstrated after intravenous administration of contrast medium.

▶ DD.
Rheumatic disorders. The most important differential diagnosis of degenerative and/or overuse tendinosis and tenosynovitis is the inflammatory tendon pathology related to rheumatic diseases. On purely morphological grounds, these tendon changes are often indistinguishable from age-related degeneration and damage from overuse. For this reason, the clinical history and the evidence of other inflammatory manifestations (laboratory results, erosive arthropathy) are extremely important. The simultaneous identification of synovitis and joint erosions is highly suggestive of an underlying rheumatic cause (▶ Fig. W1.14).
Metabolic toxic effects. Tendon damage can also develop secondary to toxic metabolic effects (steroid treatment, familial hyperlipoproteinemia, diabetes mellitus).
Xanthoma. Xanthoma of the Achilles tendon in patients with familial hyperlipidemia results in tendon hypertrophy and intratendinous signal alterations. Contrast administration helps in distinguishing tendinopathy from xanthomas as the latter do not take up contrast.
CPPD (calcium pyrophosphate dihydrate arthropathy) and hydroxyapatite deposits. These disorders can also cause calcification of the tendons. Differentiation is very difficult using imaging alone, and these types of calcifications may be simply related to advanced age (cf. Chapter 10.9).

1.8.3 Tendon Insertions (Enthesopathy)

The general term for damage at the insertions of tendons, ligaments and capsule to bone is "enthesopathy" (Greek: "énthesis" = to see into, to insert; synonym: insertional tendinopathy). Chronic strain and aging are important causes of enthesopathies, which may result in the development of bone spurs and/or erosions. Bone spurs are particularly marked in cases of a congenital tendency toward excessive ossification such as diffuse idiopathic skeletal hyperostosis (DISH). An acute injury at the enthesis can also result in tendon avulsion often with an associated bone fragment.

> **Caution**
> Systemic inflammatory rheumatic diseases, such as ankylosing spondylitis and psoriasis, also lead to prominent enthesopathies (Chapter 10).

▶ **Anatomy.** There is no periosteum at the epiphyseal and apophyseal insertions of tendons, ligaments, and joint capsules. The fibers of these structures do not merge directly into the bone substance at these insertion sites. Instead, there is a zone of fibrous cartilage interposed between the firm fibrous tissue and bone. This **fibrous cartilage** is mineralized toward the bone. By contrast, at the diaphysis, tendon fibers radiate in a fanlike fashion into the periosteum and intertwine with the periosteal fibers and only then do they connect with the bone. There are, therefore, distinct morphological differences although the function of these attachments of tendon, ligament, and capsule is identical.

▶ **Pathology.** Repetitive injury at an enthesis results in an "inflammatory" reaction with lymphocytic infiltration, edema, and resorptive changes at the bone. The calcaneus, ischium, olecranon, and iliac crest are most often affected. Typical locations and manifestations are summarized in ▶ Table 1.6. There is a difference between damage resulting from chronic avulsive injuries and an acute traumatic avulsion of the tendon insertion resulting in a bony avulsion, which is particularly common in adolescence.

> **Note**
> Since the enthesis always maintains the ability to form new bone, traumatic-reparative, degenerative, inflammatory, or metabolic processes can lead to new bone formation at this site.

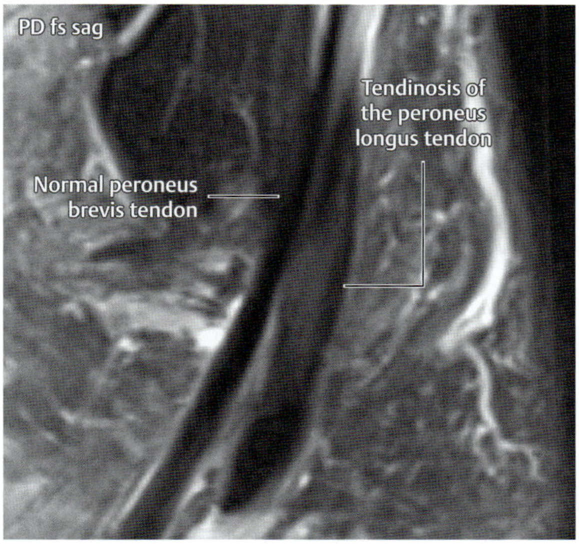

Fig. 1.109 Tendinosis of the peroneus longus tendon.

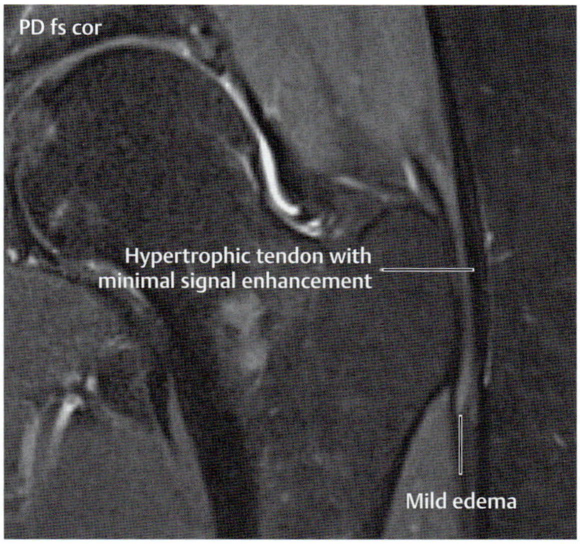

Fig. 1.110 Iliotibial band syndrome with a "snapping" hip due to incorrect weight-bearing secondary to hip cysplasia.

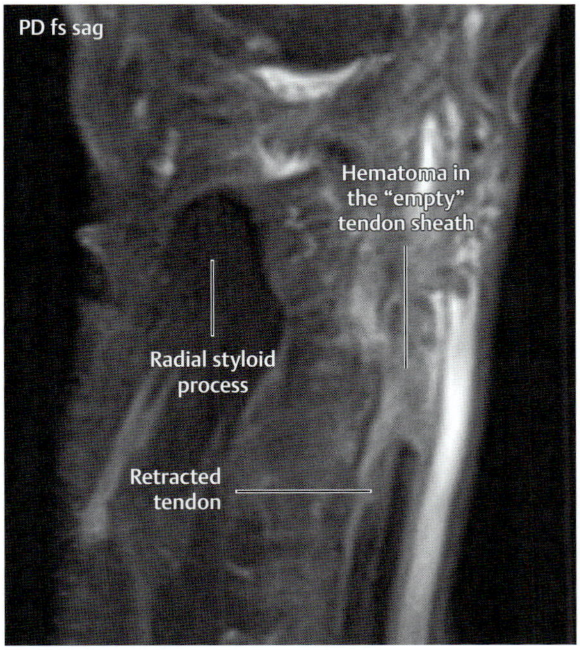

Fig. 1.111 Rupture of the flexor carpi radialis tendon with retraction.

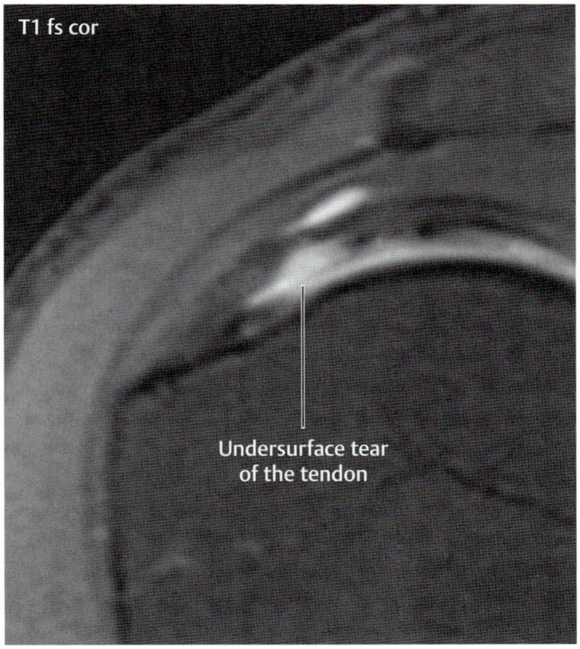

Fig. 1.112 Partial tear of the supraspinatus tendon. MR arthrography.

Table 1.6 Sites commonly affected by strain-related enthesopathies

Region	Manifestation
Shoulder	Rotator cuff insertions (Chapter 2.4)
Elbow	E.g., tennis elbow (Chapter 2.7)
Hip and thigh	E.g., greater trochanteric pain syndrome (Chapter 2.11)
Knee	E.g., patellar pole, tibial tuberosity, pes anserinus (Chapter 2.13)
Upper ankle joint and foot	E.g., heel spur, Haglund's deformity (Chapter 2.15)

▶ **Radiography/CT.** New bone formation (spur, spike, ridge; ▶ Fig. 1.113) as well as bone defects (rarefactions, resorption zones; ▶ Fig. 1.114) may appear at tendon insertion sites. The defects are usually surrounded by a sclerotic margin of varying width.

At the diaphysis, chronic or acute avulsive forces may result in periosteal elevation and/or calcification at the affected enthesis (▶ Fig. 1.115). Flakes of bone may be identified in the presence of a true tendon avulsion.

Caution

Radiological differentiation between bone spurs and dystrophic calcifications within a tendon (especially those lying near the tendon insertions) is not always easy. Radiography and ultrasound will show a lack of continuity with the bone in cases of dystrophic calcification (see ▶ Fig. 1.113b).

▶ **US.** The prerequisite for an effective ultrasound examination of tendon insertions is a comparison with the contralateral side. This will allow a better identification of even subtle changes. Strain injuries demonstrate hypertrophy and fraying of the tendons at the junction with the bone. Tendons tend to be hypoechoic. Hyperechoic embedded particles are detectable in the presence of calcifications. Generally speaking, the older the alteration, the more heterogeneous is the echo pattern. In the case of a rupture at the tendon insertion (avulsions), the tendon margins can be detected usually with interposed hypoechoic tissue compatible with an associated hematoma. Separation of the tendon margins under dynamic conditions is confirmatory. It is often difficult to distinguish traumatic partial ruptures from chronic degeneration or strain injuries. Color-coded duplex sonography typically demonstrates hypervascularization in cases of enthesopathy (e.g., "epicondylitis").

▶ **MRI.** The classic finding on fat-saturated, fluid-sensitive sequences and on T1W sequences after IV administration of gadolinium is an increase in signal intensity within the hypertrophic insertion of a tendon (▶ Figs. 1.116–1.118). If there is an anatomical bursa near the tendon insertion it is almost always involved. Also, the paratendinous tissue and bone adjacent to the tendon insertion often exhibit increased signal intensity (especially in the painful, acute inflammatory stage). Ruptures at the tendon insertions are easily recognized on PDW or T2W scans as absence of the tendon and demonstration of tortuous or folded tendon ends. Small bony avulsions are easily missed on MR images, and are often more easily seen on radiographs.

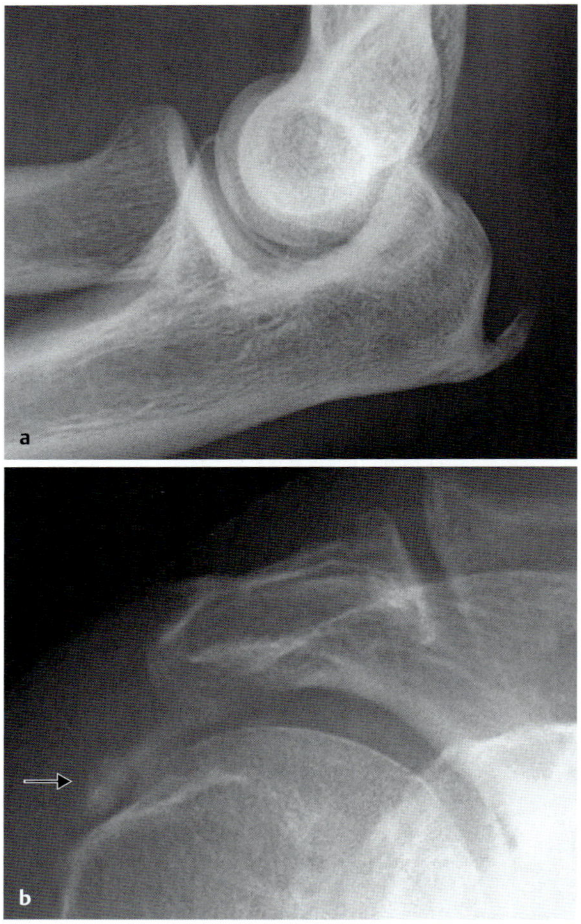

Fig. 1.113 Two types of calcification. **(a)** Spur ("enthesophyte") at the insertion of the triceps tendon on the olecranon. **(b)** Hydroxyapatite deposit (arrow) in the supraspinatus tendon.

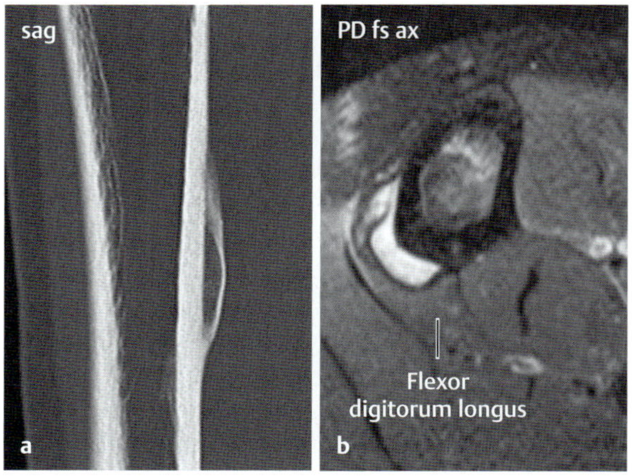

Fig. 1.115 Posttraumatic periosteal elevation. **(a)** Lamellar calcification at the tibial insertion of the flexor digitorum longus. **(b)** The MRI scan demonstrates fluid between cortex and elevated periosteum.

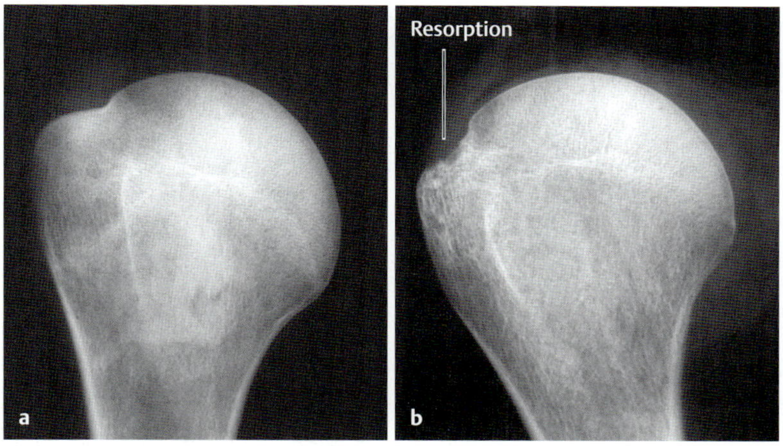

Fig. 1.114 Small enthesopathic defects at the insertion of the supraspinatus tendon. Specimen radiographs. **(a)** Normal finding for comparison. **(b)** Small area of resorption.

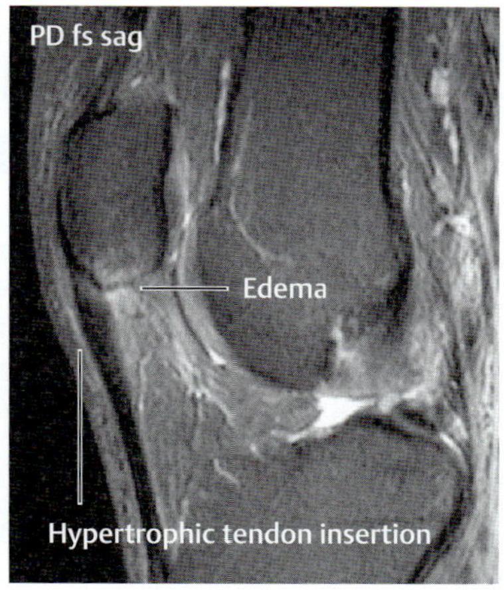

Fig. 1.116 Enthesopathy of the inferior patella and tendinosis of the proximal patellar tendon (known as jumper's knee).

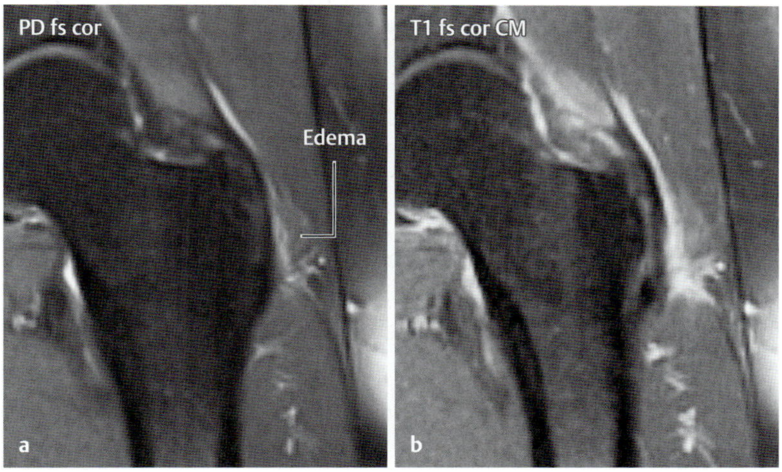

Fig. 1.117 Nonspecific enthesopathy at the left greater trochanter. This was presumably related to strain, but the patient also had a known history of rheumatoid arthritis. **(a)** Edema at the insertion of gluteus medius tendon. **(b)** Prominent contrast uptake at the tendon insertion.

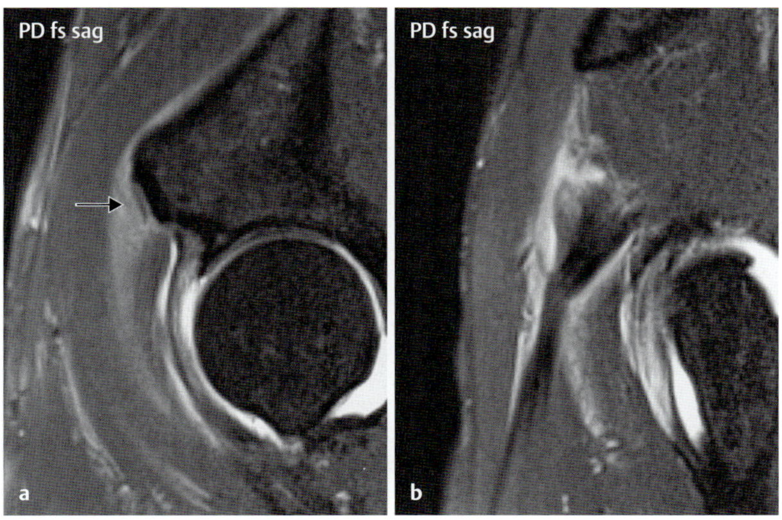

Fig. 1.118 Avulsion of the rectus femoris tendon from its origin at the anterior inferior iliac spine. **(a)** Avulsion of a small bone fragment (arrow). **(b)** Prominent intra- and peritendinous edema is evident on this image obtained just lateral to **(a)**.

1.9 Practical Advice on Diagnostic Radiography in Traumatology

- As a rule, imaging of a bone after trauma must be performed in **at least two planes**. It is often difficult to meet this requirement at a number of anatomical sites (e.g., shoulder, hip). Special views have been described for each anatomical region (see specialist literature on radiological views).
- Involvement of an articular surface must be specifically looked for if a fracture is located near a **joint**. In addition to the standard two views, other projections are often helpful. CT scanning is especially useful for evaluating possible involvement of an articular surface and is often used in lieu of obtaining additional radiographic views.
- If one of the two **bones** of the forearm or lower leg is fractured, then it is imperative to specifically look for a fracture or dislocation of the other bone. Identification of a proximal fibular injury is particularly important if there is a facture involving the distal tibia.
- To be adequately assessed, the entirety of a bone must be imaged. Additionally, the joints proximal and distal to a long bone need to be visualized.
- It is important to understand that radiographs cannot exclude a fracture with certainty ("radiologically occult fracture") and if there is a strong clinical suspicion of a fracture in the setting of negative radiographs, then **further imaging with CT, or preferably MRI** should be considered. This recommendation should be documented in the written report.
- When should **particular caution** be exercised?
  - Femoral neck fractures are often radiographically occult, especially in osteoporotic bones. Because of the clinical consequences of an occult fracture becoming displaced, further evaluation with MRI should be strongly considered in an osteoporotic patient with a suspected hip fracture and negative radiographs.
  - In sprains of the ankle joint, radiographs do not always depict associated osteochondral fractures of the talus.
  - One should be aware that **rotational malalignment of a fracture is** often difficult to assess on radiographs and, when it is suspected, further evaluation with CT or MRI should be considered.
- In most countries the use of ionizing radiation must be "justified," and it is the radiologist's responsibility to ensure that this is the case. The radiologist should also confirm that the requested examination is suited to answer the clinical question. If information regarding the clinical reason for the examination is inadequate or vague, the radiologist is **obliged** to obtain more **clinical information** prior to the radiographic examination.
- The radiology report must be documented contemporaneously **in writing**. If any portion of the report is later amended or corrected, then this must be noted clearly in the report, including the date the modification was made.

1.9.1 Report of Findings

The radiology report should include the following features:

- *Where is the fracture?* In long bones, the bone is divided into thirds. The level of the fracture should be noted accordingly (e.g., at the junction of the middle and distal thirds).
- *What is the type of fracture?* The principal fracture types (transverse, oblique, spiral, etc.) should be noted as well as whether there are multiple fragments ("comminuted").
- *Alignment of the fracture?* It should be noted that, with malalignment, the position of the distal fragment is described in relation to the proximal fragment. The angulation of the fragments should be expressed in degrees to provide a rough indication. Varus angulation refers to deviation of the distal fragment toward the midline of the body. With valgus angulation the distal fragment is directed away from the midline. The orthogonal radiograph demonstrates whether there is any anterior or posterior malalignment. Congenital or chronic axial malalignment of the axial skeleton or the distal limb demonstrated on radiographs taken in a recumbent position should only be described as "suspected." Weight-bearing radiographs will provide more reliable information and allow for better quantification.
- *Displacement of fragments?* Displacement of fragments should be described if the fracture fragments are maligned in a medial, lateral, anterior, or posterior direction (again using the distal fragment when describing the direction of displacement). The amount of displacement may be described with an actual measurement or relative to the bone itself (e.g., "one half bone width medial displacement").
- *Involvement of a joint surface?* This feature is of critical importance to the orthopaedist.
- *Is there an associated subluxation or dislocation of an adjacent joint?*

1.9.2 Follow-Up Reviews

Important features to be assessed on follow-up studies include:

- Position of the fracture and the fragments compared with the initial and the most recent radiographs.
- Signs of osseous bridging and consolidation.
- Hardware complications (such as a fractured screw or plate).
- In a case of superimposed osteomyelitis, have any new areas of lysis appeared? Are there any areas of increasing lucency around fixation hardware?
- Are there any signs of osteonecrosis?

1.9.3 What to Avoid

- Terms such as "good," "adequate," "acceptable" should be avoided when assessing the results of surgery or the healing process.
- Description of a fracture as demonstrating "delayed union" or "nonunion" should also be avoided. The use of these terms requires a full knowledge of the clinical picture. Instead, imaging signs of healing should be described such as the amount of callous present and whether there is evidence of osseous bridging or not. It should also be stated whether any or all of the fracture line is still visible.

2 Acute Trauma and Chronic Overuse (According to Region)

2.1 Cranial Vault, Facial Bones, and Skull Base

Intracranial sequelae of trauma are of paramount concern, clinically and prognostically, when it comes to diagnostic imaging of acute traumatic brain injury. The diagnostic algorithm depends primarily upon the mechanism of the trauma (impact force, impact site) and upon the clinical findings. Conventional diagnostic radiography is only useful for examining the region of the facial bones. Otherwise, potential bony injuries of the skull should be evaluated with high-resolution multidetector CT. MRI can be complementary in certain clinical settings such as a subacute traumatic brain injury or brainstem lesion.

2.1.1 Fractures of the Cranial Vault

▸ **Pathology.** Depending on the type of force, cranial vault fractures may be linear, comminuted, segmental (often associated with fragment dislocation), or depressed. Variants include separation of the cranial sutures (diastatic fractures) in patients up to the age of 30 years and "ping-pong" fractures in infants, which resemble the elastic and reversible dents of a ping-pong (table tennis) ball.

Complications include cerebrospinal fluid fistula (in some cases associated with pneumocephalus), brain contusions, and brain herniation. Temporal fractures often result in intracranial hemorrhage (middle meningeal artery, venous sinuses). In rare cases involving children, a leptomeningeal cyst may develop that presents as a "growing" skull fracture.

▸ **Radiography.** Conventional radiographs are obsolete for evaluating skull trauma as they may demonstrate fractures but not associated intracranial pathology. Furthermore, studies have shown that only approximately 50% of patients with intracranial hemorrhage also have a fracture. When radiographs are obtained, confusion can arise from normal variants that may simulate fractures including vascular grooves, sutures, synchondroses, and irregularities of the internal table. Fracture lines may cross these normal structures and their lack of sclerotic margins is often helpful in diagnosis (▸ Fig. 2.1).

▸ **CT.** Indications for obtaining a CT examination after head injury include impaired consciousness, persisting vomiting, retrograde amnesia, seizure, severe (penetrating) trauma, multiple injuries, or signs of a basilar skull fracture.

Indirect signs of a fracture should be noted: opacification or air–fluid levels in the paranasal sinuses, the mastoid cells, and the middle ear cavity, or air in the subarachnoid space.

▸ **US.** Ultrasound is only used in children. Palpable cephalohematomas associated with skull contusions can be well assessed using ultrasound, as can possible skull fractures. In these cases it is important to distinguish between fractures and cranial sutures. An adjacent epidural or subdural hematoma must be excluded in the presence of a displaced or impacted skull fracture, if necessary with the use of a CT scan.

▸ **MRI.** MRI has little if any role in the diagnostic work-up of acute head injury.

▸ **Special features in children.** Strict criteria must be applied when considering the use of radiography in children, especially after mild head injury Guidelines on the use of imaging of children after mild head trauma are issued by national societies in many countries and should be consulted. Moderate and severe head injuries, however, require immediate diagnostic imaging with CT.

2.1.2 Basilar Skull Fractures

▸ **Pathology.** Basilar skull fractures commonly occur with head trauma. They preferentially involve the orbital roof, cribriform plate, petrous pyramid of the temporal bone, or the occipital bone. The central parts of the skull base are less frequently involved. These fractures may be associated with injuries to the neurovascular structures passing through this region (cranial nerve injuries, cerebrospinal fluid fistulas, carotid aneurysms, sinus cavernosus fistulas, etc.; ▸ Figs. 2.2 and ▸ 2.3). Lesions of the optic nerves or chiasm are common complications of injuries of the middle or anterior skull base. Posttraumatic cerebrospinal fluid fistulas are most commonly found in the region of the cribriform plate where the fractures typically course along the thin parts of the bone. Fractures of the posterior skull base often extend from elsewhere in the skull, but primary fractures in this region often result in a fatal brainstem injury.

▸ **Radiography.** Conventional radiographs have no role in evaluating this type of injury.

▸ **CT.** High-resolution multidetector CT with a slice thickness of 0.5 to 1.0 mm (with or without 3D reconstructions) is the standard imaging technique in this clinical scenario.

▶ **MRI.** MRI is employed as a supplementary modality when injury to neurovascular structures is suspected. Absolute indications for its use are brainstem injuries and contradictory or equivocal findings on CT.

2.1.3 Fractures of the Petrous Bone

The classification of fractures of the petrous bone into transverse and longitudinal fractures is somewhat arbitrary as many cases involve more than one fracture orientation.

Longitudinal fractures of the petrous bone are more common, representing 70 to 80% of all petrous bone fractures. They course along the longitudinal axis of the temporal bone and through the roof of the middle ear cavity, to end in the region of the tensor tympani muscle (▶ Fig. 2.4). The region around the geniculate ganglion is often involved (10–20% of these cases are associated with facial nerve injuries). They often result in dislocation of the ossicular chain and conductive hearing loss. These carry a risk of an associated ascending infection from the external auditory canal, found in 20% of all fractures of the petrous bone.

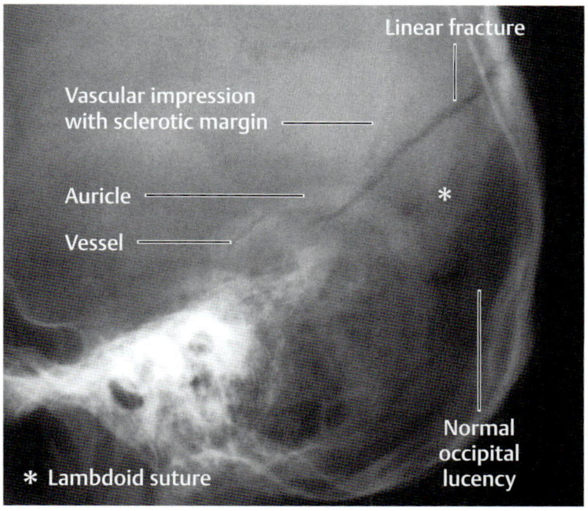

Fig. 2.1 Typical linear skull fracture. Note the sharp contour of the fracture line and the absent marginal sclerosis in contrast with the cranial suture and the vascular channel.

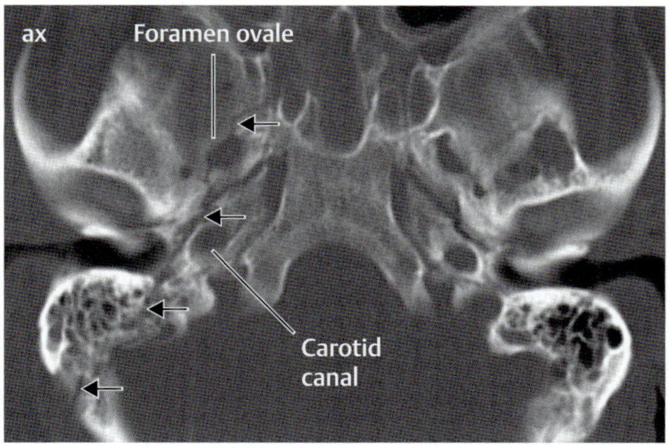

Fig. 2.2 Long-segment basilar skull fracture (arrows).

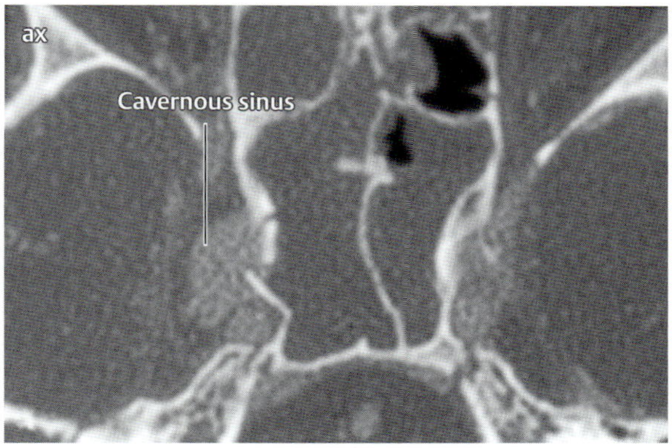

Fig. 2.3 Basilar skull fracture involving the cavernous sinus secondary to fracture of the lateral wall of the sphenoid sinus. The patient had exophthalmos on the right side. CT after contrast administration.

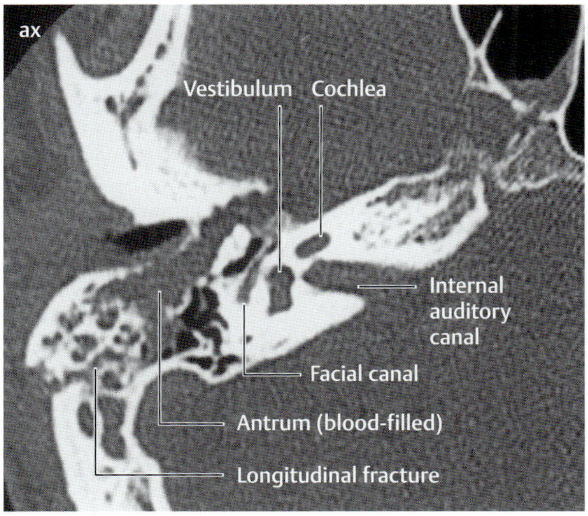

Fig. 2.4 Longitudinal fracture of the petrous bone.

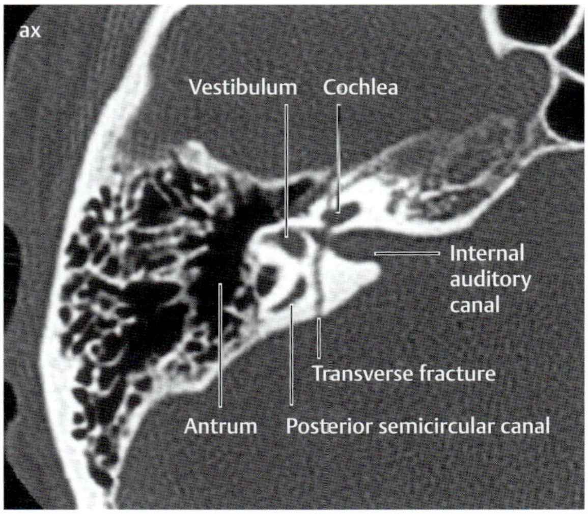

Fig. 2.5 Transverse fracture of the petrous bone.

Transverse fractures of the petrous bone begin at the posterior surface of the pyramid, traverse the roof of the internal auditory canal and also proceed toward the geniculate ganglion. They usually terminate in the musculotubal canal (▶ Figs. 2.5 and ▶ 2.6). Symptoms depend on the course of the fracture and may include sensorineural deafness and/or vertigo and spontaneous nystagmus. The facial nerve is injured in up to 50% of cases.

▶ **CT.** Using the data from axial thin-slice CT scanning, coronal reconstructions are usually helpful for assessing the course of the fracture. Indirect signs of a fracture are opacification of the mastoid cells and/or the tympanon.

▶ **MRI.** If hearing loss and/or facial nerve paralysis is present, MRI is indicated to directly evaluate the facial nerve and exclude a hematoma.

▶ **Important findings.** It is important to search particularly for fractures involving the labyrinth, the internal auditory canal, and the facial nerve as well as dislocation of the ossicular chain.

2.1.4 Facial Bone Fractures

A distinction is made between midfacial, orbital, and mandibular fractures. Facial bone fractures are primarily the result of motor vehicle accidents and, less commonly, physical altercations.

High-resolution CT using a low-dose technique (if necessary with 3D reconstructions) is the standard imaging modality, especially for fractures of the midface and orbit. Mandibular fractures (usually multiple), dental fractures, etc. may be evaluated with conventional radiographs, orthopantomography, or low-dose CT.

Typical **direct fracture signs:**
- Interruption in contour (with or without step-off).
- Double contour or increased density (fragment superimposition).
- Radiolucent line.

Typical **indirect fracture signs:**
- Soft tissue swelling.
- Opacification or air–fluid levels in the paranasal sinuses.
- "Hanging drop" sign of an orbital floor fracture.
- Intraorbital and/or intracranial air.

Isolated Facial Bone Fractures

Nasal fractures. This is the most common isolated fracture. Radiographs are not usually necessary. Lateral views of the nasal bone and possibly paranasal sinus views may be helpful in equivocal cases.

> **Caution**
> There is the risk of confusing fractures of the nose with normal sutures; fractures are usually situated more peripherally (▶ Fig. 2.7).

Fracture of zygomatic arch. This is best visualized with the axial view (so called bucket-handle view) (▶ Fig. 2.8). More displaced fractures are of therapeutic relevance. In small children, the zygomatic arch should be assessed primarily by ultrasound.

Fracture of the zygoma. A common injury is the *tripod fracture,* in which the bony connections of the zygoma with the adjacent bones are disrupted or fractured (▶ Figs. 2.9 and ▶ 2.10). Its depiction is achieved with paranasal sinus views and/or lateral views. CT is used in equivocal cases.

Orbital fracture. Fractures of the thin orbital floor and the thin medial lamina papyracea are common. Herniation of orbital contents (fat, inferior rectus muscle) into the maxillary sinus may complicate this type of fracture (▶ Figs. 2.11–2.13). Typical indirect signs of a fracture include the "hanging drop" sign (see ▶ Figs. 2.11 and ▶ 2.12) and orbital emphysema. The term *blow-in fracture* is used when an orbital wall fracture results in bone being displaced into the orbit. Diagnostic imaging typically begins with orbital radiographs; a CT scan is indicated when a fracture has been detected (to search for other fractures, define the extent of the fracture, or assess for an associated hematoma) and in equivocal cases.

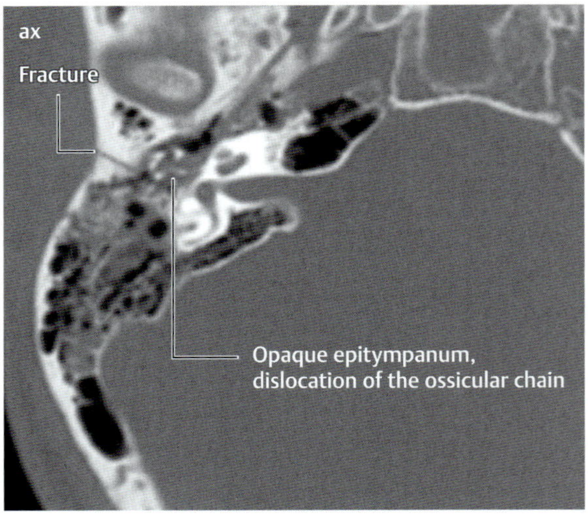

Fig. 2.6 Transverse fracture of the petrous bone extending through the epitympanum. Shadowing prevents demarcation of the facial nerve. Dislocation of the ossicular chain is also evident.

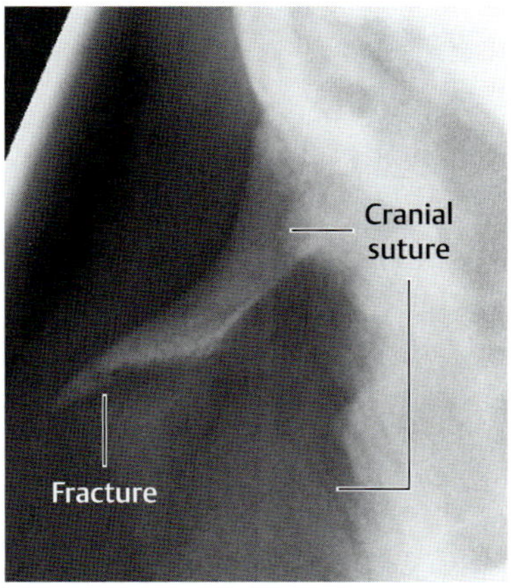

Fig. 2.7 Nasal fracture.

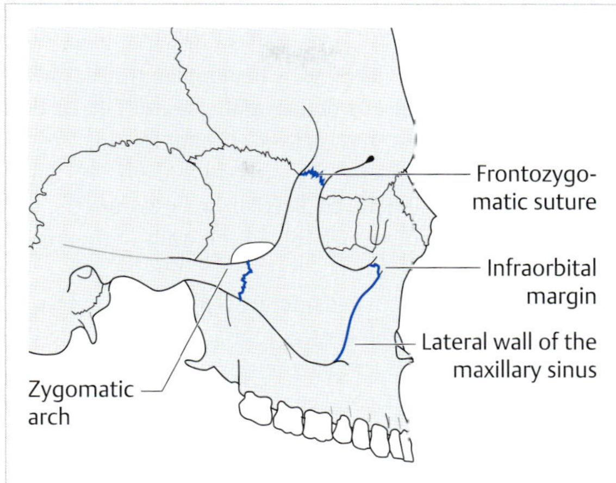

Fig. 2.9 Schematic presentation of the zygoma showing the typical fracture sites (blue).

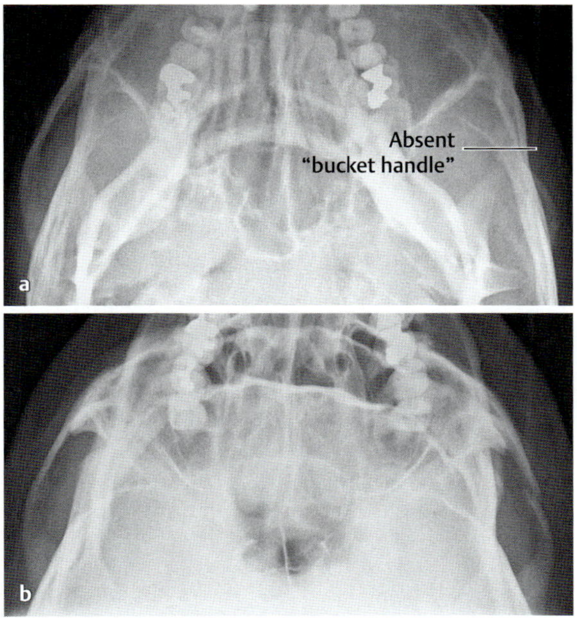

Fig. 2.8 Zygomatic arch fracture. **(a)** Loss of the physiological contour indicating the significant impression. **(b)** After surgical reduction.

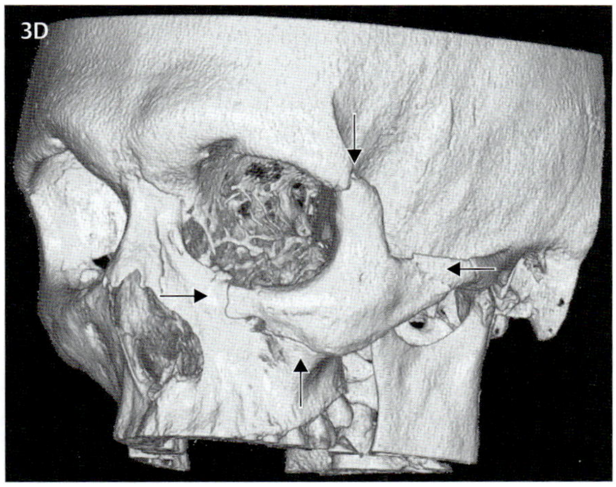

Fig. 2.10 Classic tripod fracture. Fractures are marked by arrows. Surface reconstruction using CT data set

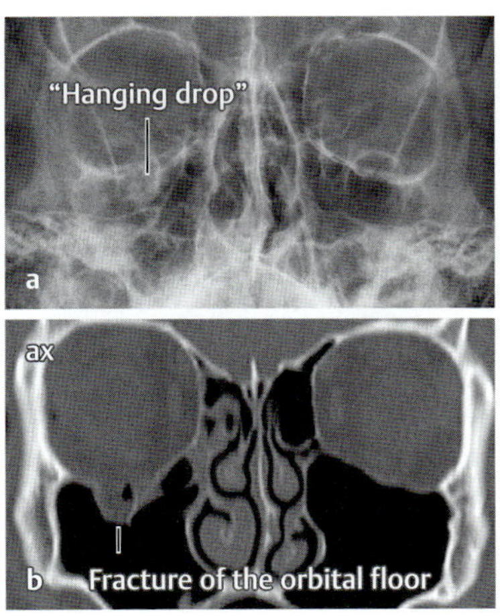

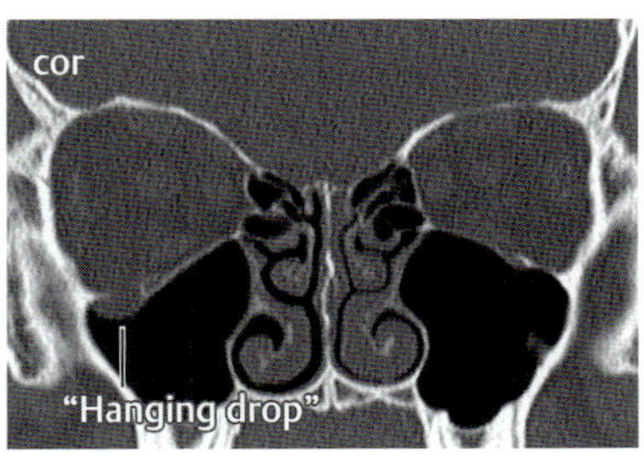

Fig. 2.12 Minimally displaced orbital floor fracture.

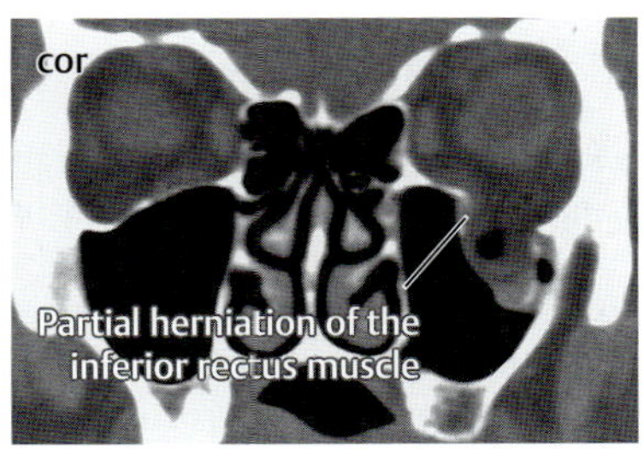

Fig. 2.13 Orbital floor fracture.

Fig. 2.11 Orbital floor fracture. **(a)** Typical shadowing of the cranial part of the maxillary sinus. **(b)** The fracture is better seen on CT scan, unobscured by overlying structures.

Midfacial Fractures

Severe facial trauma often results in complex transfacial injuries that are difficult to define and classify. The **Le Fort classification system** has proven useful in this regard (▶ Fig. 2.14):

- **Le Fort I:** Separation of the alveolar process from the rest of the maxilla (floating palate). All the walls of the maxillary sinuses are fractured.
- **Le Fort II:** Pyramid-shaped fracture ("pyramidal fracture") with separation of the central midface. The fracture line courses through the root of the nose, the medial orbital wall, and the orbital floor. The medial wall of the maxillary sinus is preserved.
- **Le Fort III:** This fracture results in separation of the face from the skull. The fracture line courses bilaterally through the root of the nose, medial orbital wall, orbital floor, and lateral orbital wall. There are additional fractures of the zygomatic arches.

The common feature of all Le Fort fractures is **involvement of the pterygoid processes** (▶ Fig. 2.15).

It is very common to find combinations of different (Le Fort) fracture types in one or even both halves of the midface (▶ Fig. 2.16). Particular attention should be paid to possible associated injuries (anterior skull base, mandible, etc.).

▶ **CT.** High-resolution CT is the modality of choice for suspected complex midfacial injuries. 3D reconstructions are often helpful for providing better visualization.

▶ **MRI.** When associated cranial nerve injury and/or brain injury are suspected, MRI is indicated.

Mandibular Fractures

Mandibular fractures are commonly multiple (50–60% of cases). Fractures that course through the dental alveolus are regarded as open fractures. A differentiation is made between fractures of the mandibular body, the mandibular angle, and the mandibular ramus as well as those that involve the mandibular joint.

▶ **Radiography.** Standard radiographs are typically obtained. An orthopantomogram may be helpful.

▶ **CT.** CT offers the most exact fracture depiction, which is often essential for an optimal treatment outcome (▶ Fig. W2.1). In addition to 3D reconstructions (▶ Fig. W2.2), orthopantomograms can also be generated from the CT data set. A more recent technique, known as cone beam CT, is also proving to be useful (▶ Fig. W2.3).

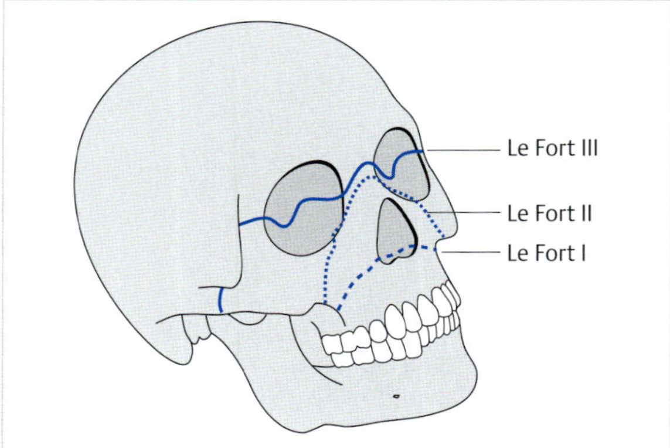

Fig. 2.14 Classification of midfacial fractures according to Le Fort.

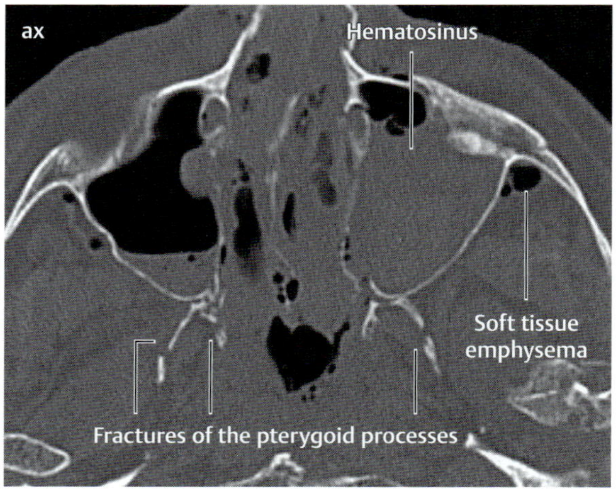

Fig. 2.15 Fracture involving the pterygoid process of the sphenoid. All Le Fort fractures involve the pterygoid process.

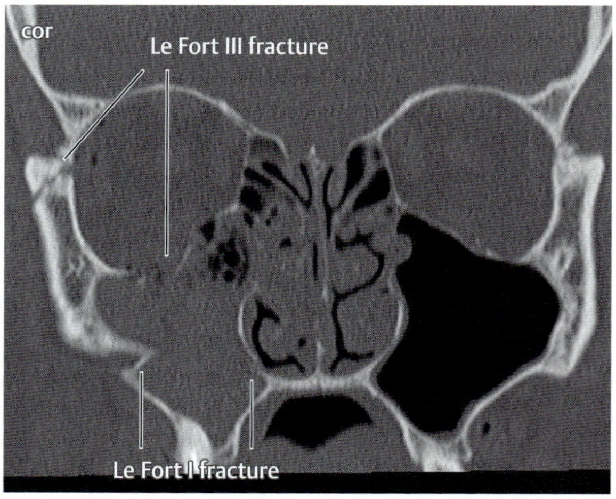

Fig. 2.16 Complex midfacial injury with a combined Le Fort I and Le Fort III injury on the right.

2.2 Spine

2.2.1 Anatomy, Variants, Technique, and Indications

▸ **Anatomy.** See Chapter 2.2.1 and ▸ Fig. W2.4.

Technique and Indications

▸ **Radiography.** Radiographs are still commonly used for screening in cases of mild spinal trauma. The lateral view is the most important. It should be performed without repositioning the patient. Severe spinal injuries should be immediately investigated with CT because the extent of injury is often underestimated on conventional radiographs. The need for lateral and swimmer oblique views, and above all functional studies, should be assessed critically with regard to their diagnostic value. If a multislice CT unit is available, then conventional radiographs of the spine should be dispensed with in the patient who has sustained significant trauma.

Apart from evidence of fracture lines and/or fragments, **indirect signs** of spinal injury include:

- Loss of vertebral height.
- Widening or deformity of the vertebral body.
- Linear sclerosis within a vertebral body.
- Irregularity or interruption of reference lines (▸ Figs. 2.17 and ▸ 2.18).
- Segmental malalignment (this is best recognized by observing the posterior vertebral line; segmental fanning of the facet joints and spinal processes is a very helpful sign of significant injury (▸ Fig. 2.19).
- Widening or narrowing of an intervertebral disk space relative to adjacent levels.
- Widened prevertebral soft tissues (in the cervical spine this should not exceed 7 mm in adults at the level of the inferior margin of C2) (▸ Fig. 2.20; see also ▸ Fig. 2.17). However, a normal appearance of the prevertebral soft tissues does not exclude significant underlying bone or ligament injury. Attention should also be paid to any displacement of the prevertebral fat stripe or contour of the trachea.

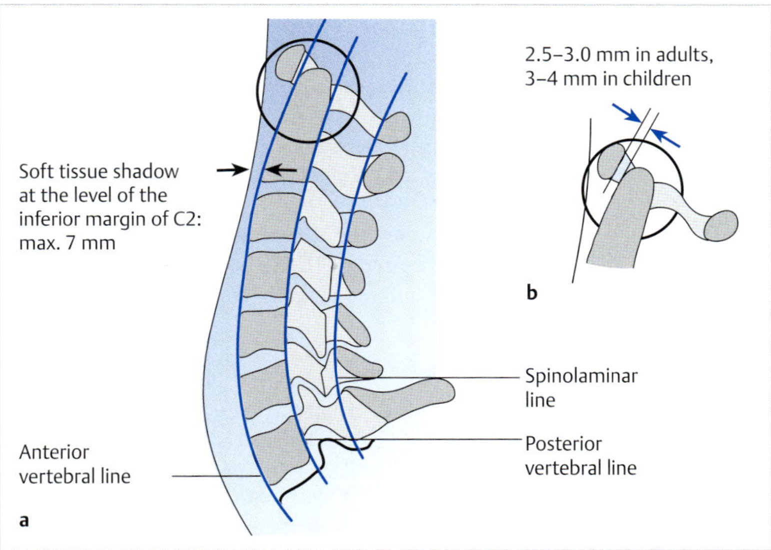

Fig. 2.17 Criteria for assessing the lateral view of the cervical spine. **(a)** Reference lines for assessing alignment and physiological width of the prevertebral soft tissue shadow. **(b)** Physiological width of the atlantodental interval.

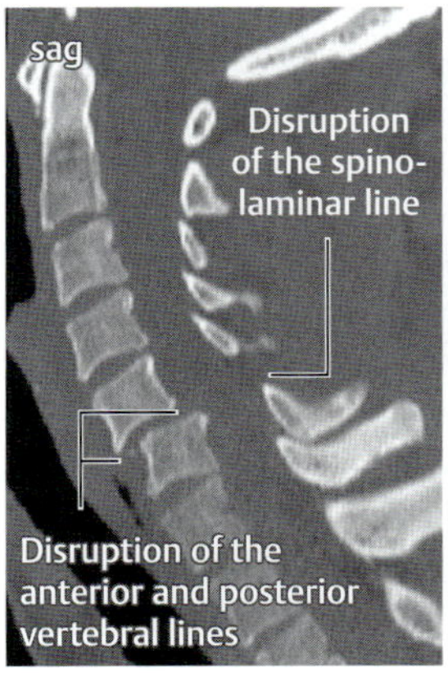

Fig. 2.18

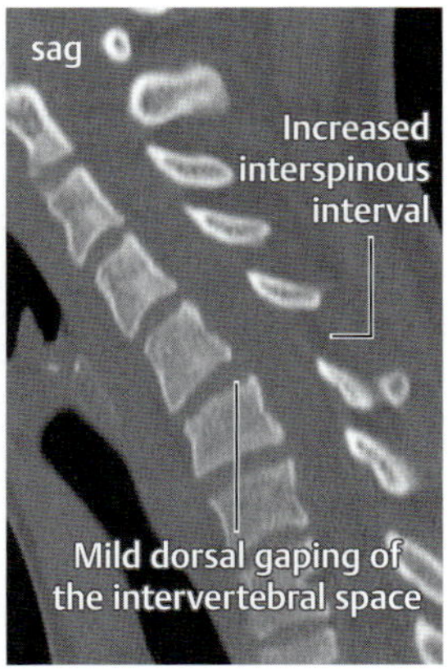

Fig. 2.19

Fig. 2.18 Disruption of all three reference lines in the presence of anterior subluxation of C5. The disruption is secondary to discoligamentous rupture and bilateral facet joint dislocation (flexion–distraction injury).

Fig. 2.19 Segmental interspinous gaping and widening of the dorsal intervertebral space at C5/C6 after a flexion–distraction injury.

Caution

It should always be kept in mind that any attempt to classify an injury on the basis of radiographs alone should be done with the utmost caution since high-grade, unstable injuries can be easily underestimated with radiographs and may even be present despite an unremarkable radiographic series.

► CT. CT of the spine has become the imaging modality of choice for evaluating patients after significant trauma (e.g., high-speed motor vehicle accident, fall from a height, and the like). The use of CT is obligatory for possible unstable fractures detected with radiography and in cases with suspected canal compromise due to displaced fragments or hematoma.

► MRI. The advantages of MRI are its ability to display discoligamentous injuries (especially in an obtunded patient), spinal cord injuries (edema, hematomyelia, transection, vascular occlusion), and bone bruises. Its use is indicated in all patients who present with neurologic findings.

2.2.2 Mechanisms of Injury and Classifications

► Pathology. Fractures, dislocations, and soft tissue injuries are most commonly located at the level of the lower cervical spine and the thoracolumbar junction. In many cases clinical signs and symptoms together with radiographic findings will allow a prompt and correct diagnosis. However, factors such as poor-quality radiographs (portable technique, overlying structures, especially in the lower cervical and upper thoracic regions) or inexperience of the imager result in a relatively high rate of radiologically unrecognized spinal injuries (~ 15–30 %).

As well as the use of anatomical aspects (such as the location within the spine), spinal injuries are classified according to the type of forces involved:

- Compression.
- Flexion.
- Extension.
- Rotation.
- Translation (shearing).

One of the most commonly used classification systems for spinal injuries is that of **Magerl**, which is based on the current **AO classification system** (► Fig. 2.21). It also attempts to take into consideration discoligamentous injury patterns as evident on MRI scans. With the Magerl classification, the severity of the injury increases from Types A through C as well as within the types from groups 1 through 3. Type A and Type B injuries are often combined.

In the United States, the **Thoracolumbar Injury Classification and Severity Score (TLICS)**, published in 2005 by A. R. Vaccaro et al. is currently used (► see references in Chapter 2.2.2).

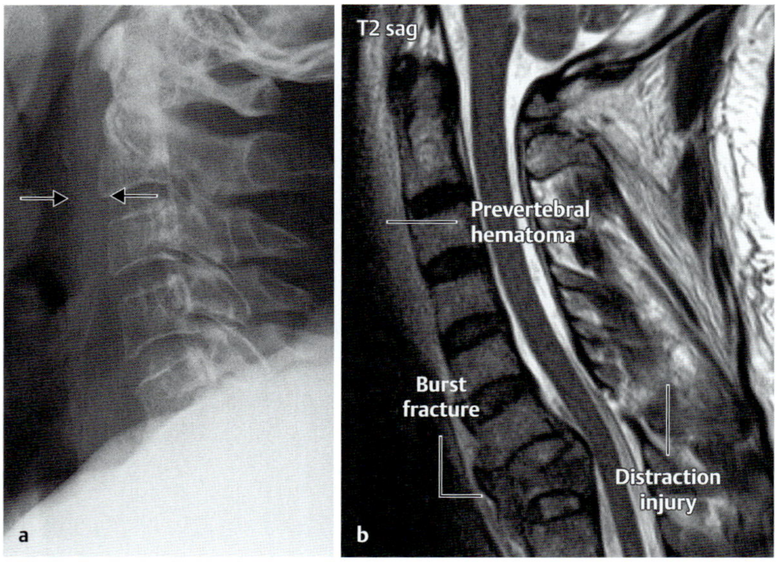

Fig. 2.20 Widening of the prevertebral shadow should raise concern for injury. **(a)** Because it was not possible to evaluate the lower cervical spine adequately on radiographs due to superimposition of the shoulder girdle, clarification must be achieved using sectional imaging. **(b)** MRI reveals an (unstable) C6/C7 flexion injury as the cause of the prevertebral hematoma.

Type A **Mechanism:** Compression **Radiological signs:** • Reduced vertebral height • Split vertebral body • Widening of interpedicular distance	**A1: Impaction fractures[1]** 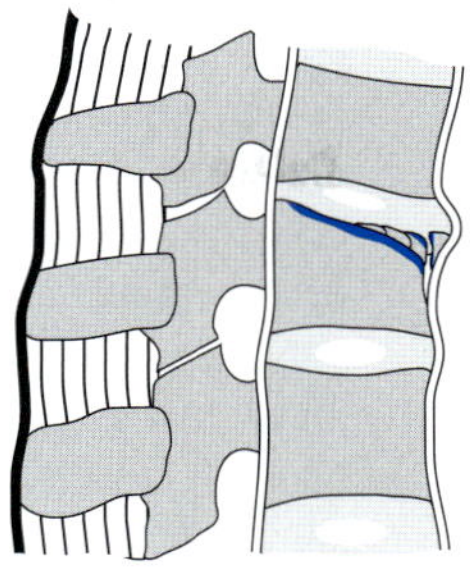	**A2: Split fractures[2]** 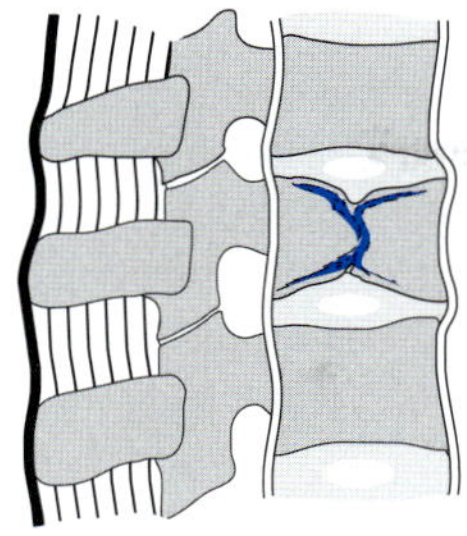	**A3: Burst fractures[3]** 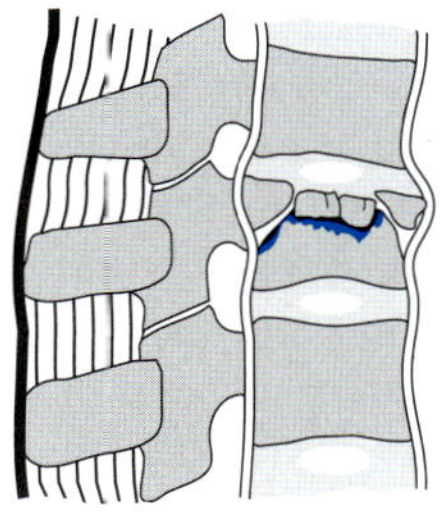
Stability:	Stable	Usually stable	See subgroups
Subgroups Type A3 **Characteristics:** • Typical superior, dorsally displaced, posterior marginal fragment • Fracture of the arch or spinous process • Injury to one or both adjacent discs • Intact posterior ligamentous complex	**A3.1: Incomplete burst fracture** 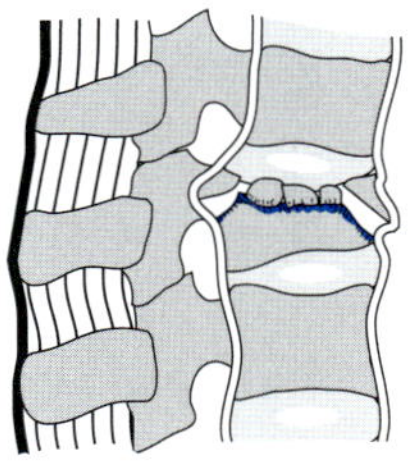	**A3.2: Burst-split fracture** 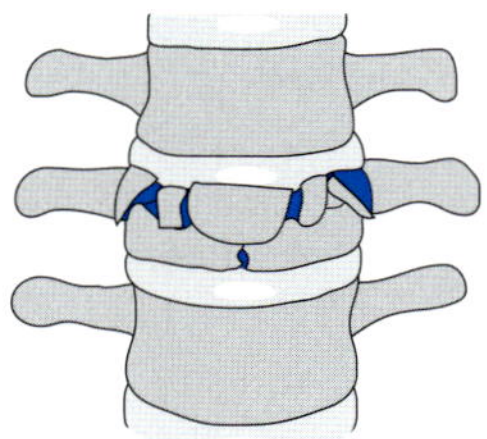	**A3.3: Complete burst fracture** 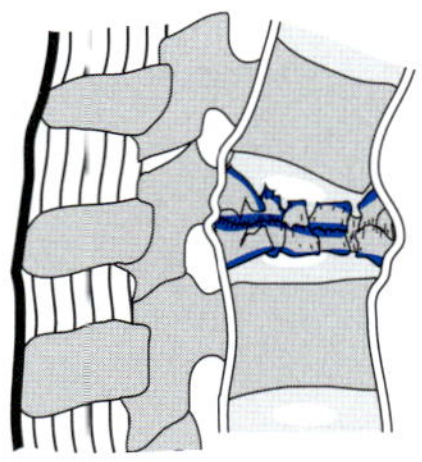
Stability:	Unclear, probably stable	Unclear, probably stable	Unclear, probably unstable
Type B **Mechanism:** Distraction **Radiological signs:** • Increased interspinous distance • Subluxation/dislocation of the facet joints • Elevation of posterior vertebral margin • Transverse fractures • Avulsion fragments of vertebral body rim	**B1: Posterior ligamentous disruption with ...[3]** 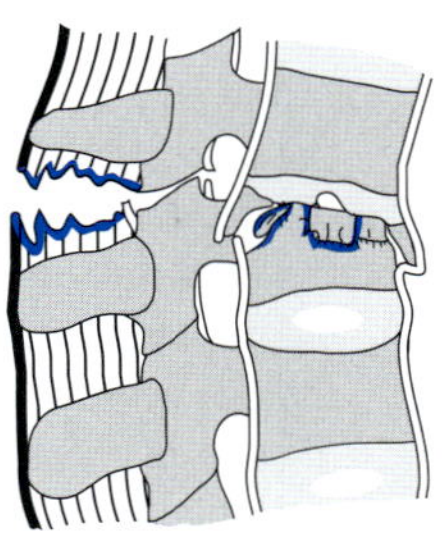	**B2: Posterior osseous disruption with ...[4]** 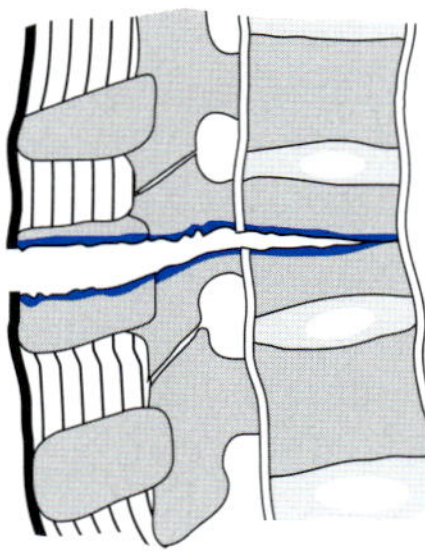	**B3: Disruption through the disk with ...[5]** 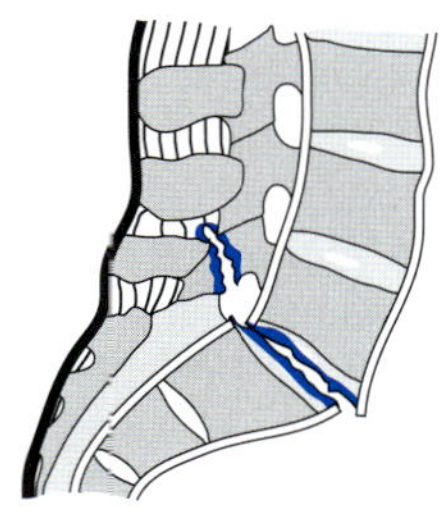
Stability:	Unstable		
Type C **Mechanism:** Rotation **Radiological signs:** • Lateralization of the vertebral body • Pedicle asymmetry • Dislocation of the spinous processes • Fractures of the transverse processes • Unilateral subluxation/dislocation fracture of the posterior vertebral segments • Unilateral rib fracture/exarticulation	**C1: Type A injury with rotation** 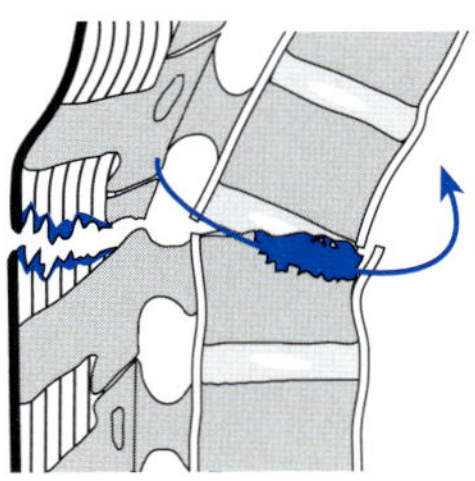	**C2: Type B injury with rotation** 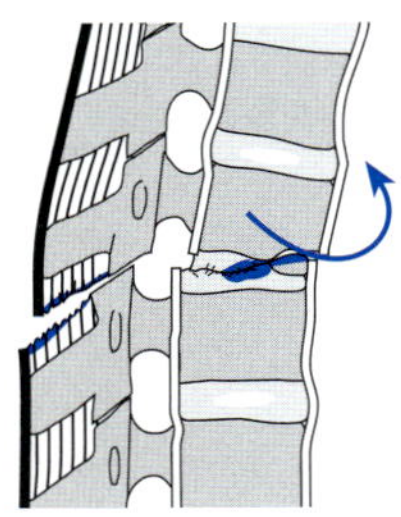	**C3: Rotation shear fractures** 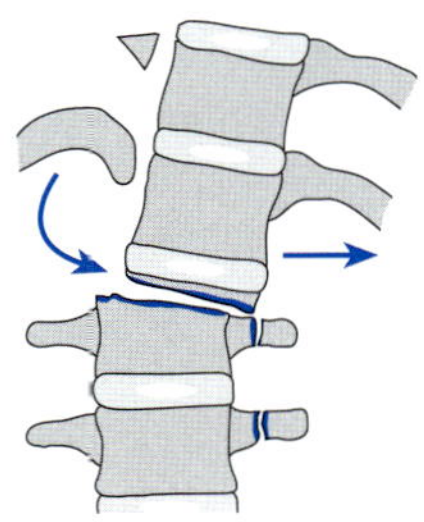
Stability:	Highly unstable		

[1]Variants: End plate impression (A1.1), wedge fracture (A1.2), vertebral impaction ("fish vertebra", A1.3)
[2]Sagittal (A2.1) and frontal (A2.2) are regarded as stable; frontal split fractures with simultaneous vertebral comminution and disruption of disk material ("pincer fracture", A2.3) are regarded as unstable
[3]With disruption of the disk (B1.1) or associated Type A fracture (B1.2)
[4]With disruption of the vertebral body (B2.1) or disk (B2.2) or associated Type A fracture (B2.3)
[5]With subluxation or fracture of the articular process (B3.1), with spondylosis (B3.2) or posterior dislocation (B3.3)

Fig. 2.21 Classification of spinal injuries according to Magerl (AO).

2

Compression Injuries

Compression injuries result from vertical forces impacting on the vertebra from a cranial or caudal direction. The fracture is usually located in the thoracolumbar region and characterized by widening of the vertebral body and loss of vertebral height as well as by disruption of the vertebral cortex. The Type A1 lesion (▶ Fig. 2.21) is a failure of the anterior column resulting in an isolated vertebral body injury. *Subgroups* of A1 fractures include

- A1.1: a pure impact fracture of the superior end plate.
- A1.2: a wedge type fracture.
- A1.3: a vertebral body collapse.

A1.3 fractures are typical osteoporotic compression fractures that result in compression of both end plates with an intact posterior wall (the so-called “fish” or “fish mouth” vertebra).

Whereas A1 and A2 fractures are usually stable injuries (▶ Figs. 2.21 and ▶ 2.22),

A3 burst fractures (▶ Figs. 2.23 and ▶ 2.24) are often considered to be unstable due to involvement of the posterior wall and contiguous intervertebral disks and in some cases may require surgical stabilization, especially when the burst fracture is complete (A3.3) (see ▶ Fig. 2.24). Comminuted fractures with displacement fracture fragments in the spinal canal often result in associated neurologic complications. If the neurologic deficit does not correlate with the extent of the spinal canal stenosis, then a search should be made for an associated epidural hematoma, intervertebral disk protrusion or spinal cord injury, in which case an MRI scan is the diagnostic modality of choice. CT myelography is an alternative for a patient with a contraindication for MRI or if MR scanning is unavailable.

> **Caution**
> Widening of the interspinous distance and/or fractures of the posterior spinal segments are indications of a higher-grade injury (▶ Fig. 2.25); it is imperative that these structures are assessed on the radiographic examination, and CT may be needed for complete evaluation.

Extension Injuries

Extension injuries are less common than those related to flexion but are frequently overlooked or underestimated due to the often subtle associated radiographic findings. They result in neurologic damage less commonly than do flexion injuries. They often occur in older patients who sustain a ground-level fall, striking their head, producing hyperextension of the cervical spine. The cervical spine is particularly susceptible to hyperextension injuries due to its exposed position and its high degree of sagittal mobility with the center of rotation at the level of the articular processes. Vertebral alignment, including the spinolaminar line, may be normal after injury.

> **Caution**
> Any (segmental) widening of an intervertebral space is highly suspect of a hyperextension injury; a segmentally *widened* intervertebral space is *never* a normal finding!

Extension teardrop fracture. A hyperextension injury (typical case: a dive head-first into shallow water) results in a genuine avulsion of bone at the attachment of the anterior longitudinal ligament (▶ Figs. 2.26–2.28). Typical levels of injury include the lower cervical spine (often in young patients) as well as in the C2 region (especially in older patients). An important point is the fact that the teardrop fragment represents the fixed point because it has remained firmly attached to the anterior longitudinal ligament, while the associated vertebral body has torn away, resulting in a triangular fragment along the anterior inferior margin of the involved vertebra on radiographs. However, neither radiography nor CT reflects the full degree of soft tissue pathology associated with such injuries, and MR imaging is indicated in these cases to identify ligamentous and spinal cord injuries.

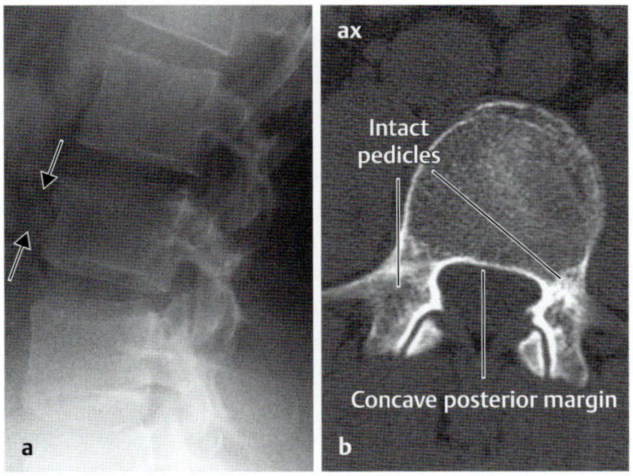

Fig. 2.22 Magerl Type A1 compression fracture. **(a)** Anterior reduction of height (arrows) as compared with the adjacent vertebrae. **(b)** The CT scan shows that only the anterior parts of the vertebra are involved.

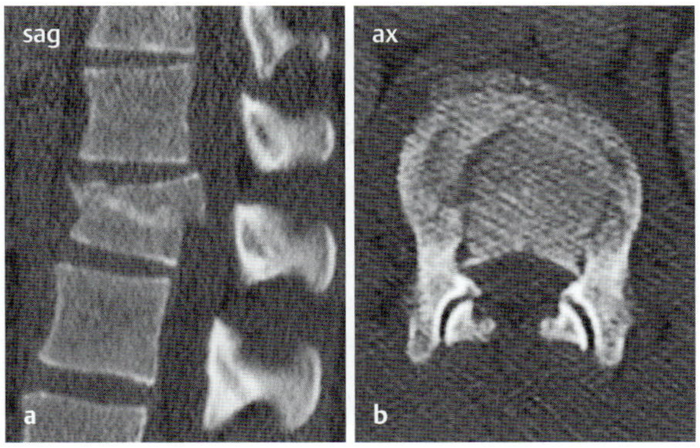

Fig. 2.23 Partial burst fracture (Type A3.1 compression fracture). **(a)** The cranial part of the vertebral body has burst; the inferior end plate is intact. **(b)** Spinal canal stenosis secondary to dorsal displacement of a posterior fragment.

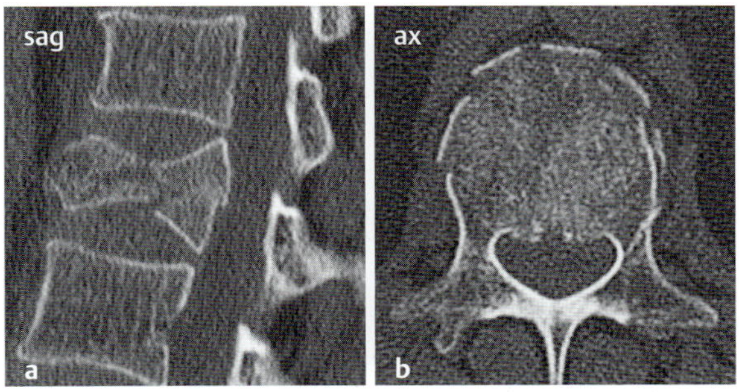

Fig. 2.24 Complete burst fracture (Type A3.3 compression fracture). **(a)** Inferior and superior end plates are fractured. **(b)** The vertebral body has multiple fracture lines running through it.

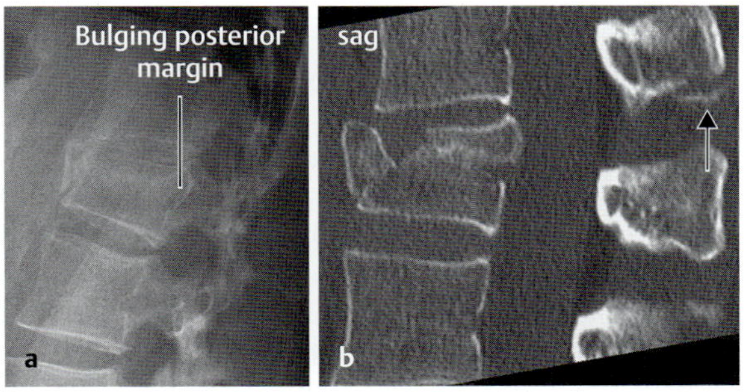

Fig. 2.25 Higher-grade injury? Always look at the posterior parts of the vertebra! **(a)** The radiograph shows a compression fracture of L1 with involvement of the posterior margin (most likely Type A3.1), but the spinous processes have been cropped from the film. **(b)** A bony avulsion of the interspinous ligament at T12 (arrow) is apparent on this CT image; this confirms an (unstable!) Type B1 flexion injury.

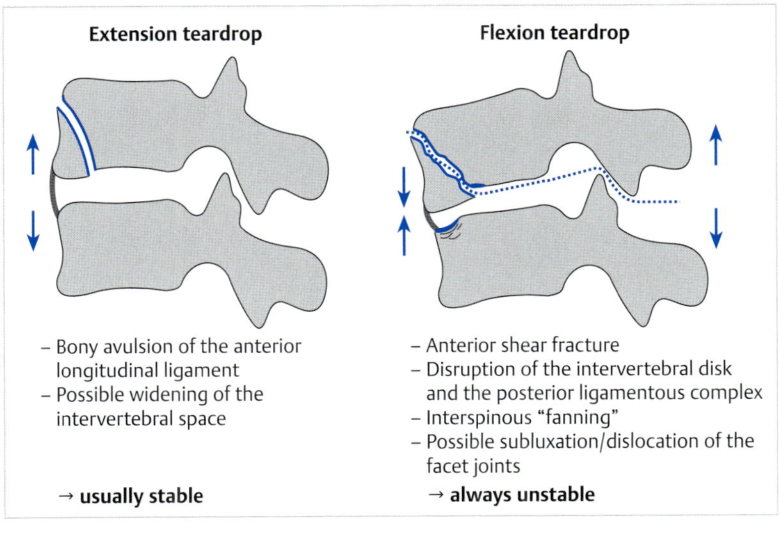

Fig. 2.26 Mechanism of injury of teardrop fractures.

Posterior subluxation/dislocation. Rupture of the anterior and (rarely) the posterior longitudinal ligaments as well as the intervertebral disk, combined with dislocation/subluxation of the facet joints and, in some cases, additional fractures through the neural arches results in transient posterior translation of the vertebra (▶ Fig. 2.29). This injury is highly unstable and is associated with severe neurologic deficits. It most often occurs in the mid-cervical region (C4–C6) and at the thoracolumbar junction. Because the vertebra frequently reduces spontaneously, spinal alignment may appear normal on radiographs. Indirect, often subtle, findings such as anterior soft tissue swelling or anterior widening of a disk space should prompt further evaluation with MRI to assess the degree of ligamentous and spinal cord injury. Such hyperextension injuries are particularly common in older patients with degenerative spines in whom the canal is already narrowed by osteophytes and redundant ligaments (Chapter 2.2.4). These patients often present with a **central cord syndrome** in which the neurologic symptoms are more pronounced in the upper than in the lower extremities.

Flexion Injuries

Flexion injuries are the most commonly encountered in the spine. They are the result of excessive flexion of the spine in which the axis of rotation is usually at the level of the dorsal third of the intervertebral disk space. The anterior vertebral segments are maximally compressed, while the posterior are distracted. Typical compression/distraction injuries can develop as a result of this mechanism such as transverse disruption of the posterior ligamentous complex (Type B1 injury) or transverse bony disruption (spinous processes, pedicles, pars interarticularis; Type B2) (▶ Figs. 2.30–2.33).

With high-velocity flexion loading, subluxation/dislocation of the facet joints occurs, resulting in some cases in complete bilateral dislocation and locked facets. This may result from pure discoligamentous disruptions without an associated fracture (see ▶ Fig. 2.33).

Unilateral facet joint dislocations or fractures occur when there is an additional rotational force, which is often underestimated on radiographs. Spontaneous fracture reduction can occur with the patient in a supine position. Pure anterior compression fractures are stable, whereas all flexion–distraction injuries are potentially unstable.

Anterior wedge fracture. The mildest form of flexion injury involves anterior compression of the vertebral end plate, which remains intact posteriorly. A stronger force produces more extensive compression with more marked formation of a wedge-shaped vertebra and possible involvement of the posterior body (middle column). A wedge-shaped vertebra can develop not only anteriorly but also laterally. The osteoporotic wedge-shaped vertebra will be discussed in Chapter 8.

> **Note**
> In general, care should be taken not to exclude middle column involvement in a compression injury on the basis of conventional radiographs. With wedging of more than 15 to 20° relative to the opposite end plate, involvement of the middle column should certainly be excluded by CT.

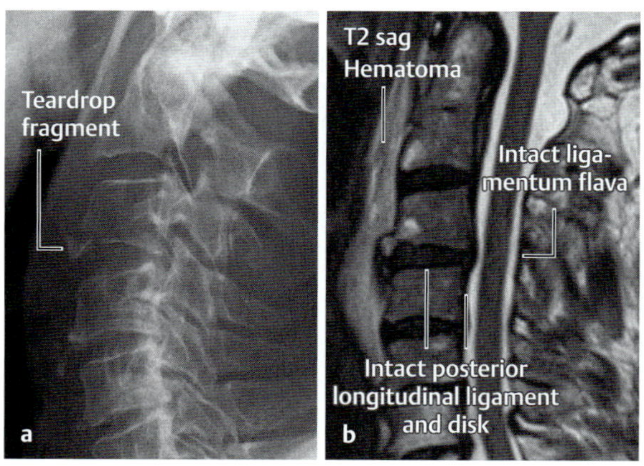

Fig. 2.27 Teardrop injury, at a typical site in the upper cervical spine. **(a)** Triangular fragment arising from the anterior inferior margin of C3. Alignment maintained; no interspinous gaping. **(b)** No spinal cord injury. On the whole, the findings are most compatible with a (stable) extension injury.

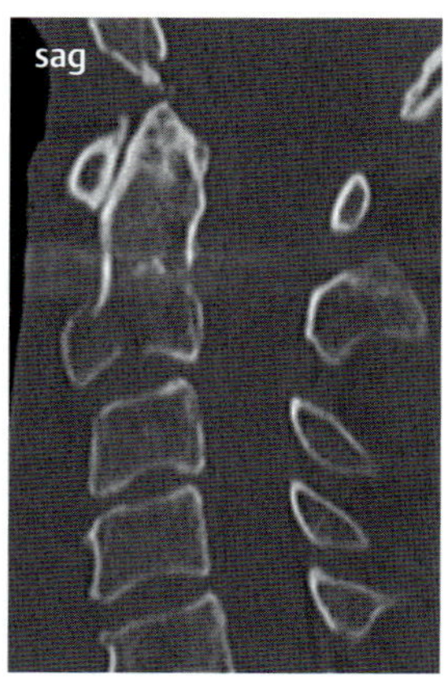

Fig. 2.28 Extension teardrop fracture at a typical site: C2 in this case.

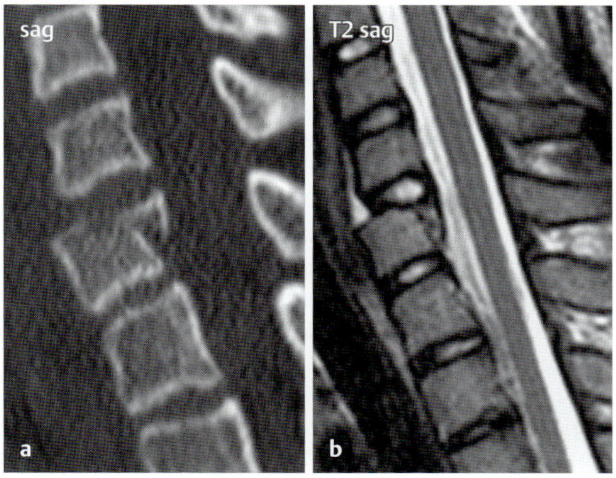

Fig. 2.29 Posterior subluxation. **(a)** Posterior teardrop fragment of C7. **(b)** Anterior discoligamentous detachment of the anulus fibrosus.

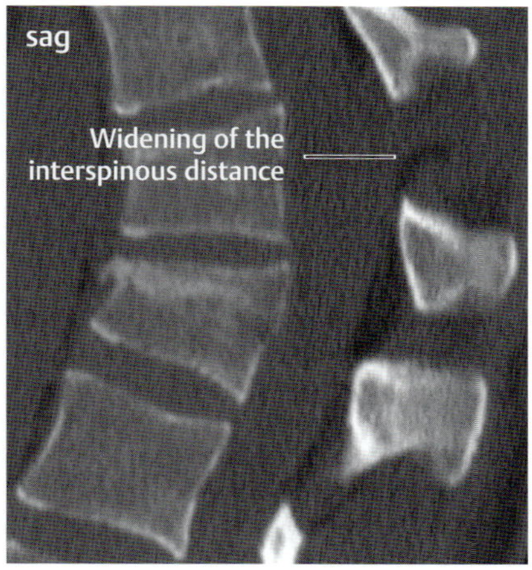

Fig. 2.30 Flexion injury. The posterior margin of the wedge-shaped fractured thoracic vertebra is disrupted, and widening of the interspinous distance one segment higher is evidence of an unstable Type B1 injury.

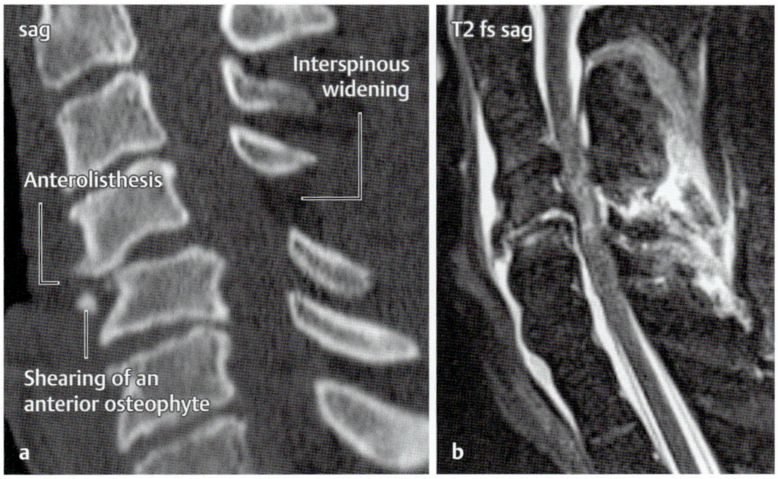

Fig. 2.31 Flexion injury in the presence of cervical spine degeneration. **(a)** Typical dorsal interspinous widening with avulsion of the anterior osteophyte. **(b)** MRI demonstrates complete discoligamentous disruption, indicating a high-grade unstable flexion–distraction injury.

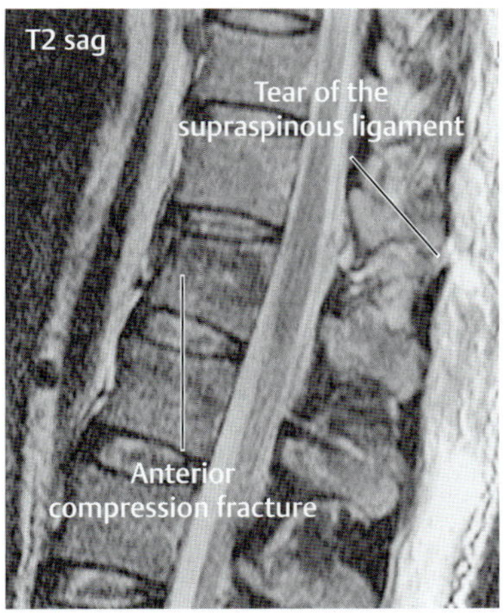

Fig. 2.32

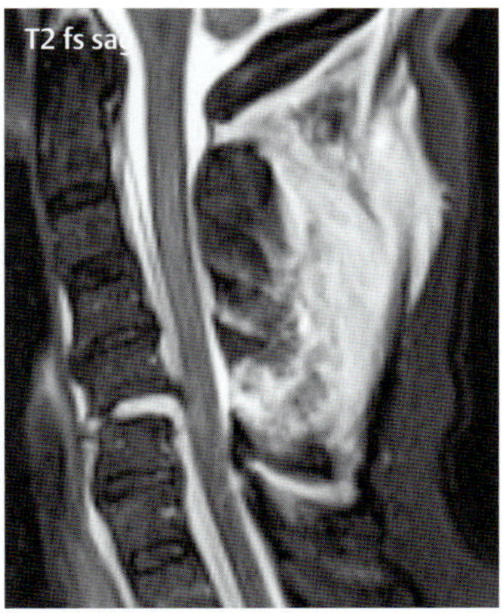

Fig. 2.33

Fig. 2.32 Lumbar Type B1 injury. Disruption of the dorsal ligamentous structures (ligamenta flava and ligamentum supraspinale) with concomitant anterior compression fracture.

Fig. 2.33 Purely discoligamentous flexion injury.

Flexion teardrop fracture. In this type of fracture flexion has resulted in separation of a triangular, or "teardrop," fragment from the anteroinferior corner of the vertebral body (▶ Fig. 2.34; see also ▶ Figs. 2.26 and ▶ 2.35). The vertebral body is split in the coronal plane, with the posterior fragment protruding into the spinal canal. The fracture is most frequently located at the lower cervical spine (70% at C5). The most important feature of this injury, however, is that it results in disruption of the posterior longitudinal ligament and is therefore extremely unstable. It also commonly results in spinal cord injury.

Chance fracture. A flexion injury with the center of rotation moved to the anterior abdominal wall (as is seen with a lap seatbelt) results in significantly magnified tensile forces in the spine and a horizontally orientated disruption of the vertebral column. These fractures most commonly involve the mid-thoracic to mid-lumbar vertebra with fractures involving not only the vertebral body but also the pedicle and other posterior elements, rendering these highly unstable (▶ Figs. 2.35 and ▶ 2.36). Of note, the disruption may predominantly involve the soft tissues (disk, ligaments) which will be best evaluated with MR imaging. These fractures may also be associated with anterior vertebral compressions (Type A fracture) and angular hyperkyphosis.

Anterior subluxation/dislocation. This is a severe form of flexion–distraction injury that is characterized by disruption of the posterior ligamentous complex together with a tear of the posterior longitudinal ligament. The intervertebral disk is also commonly involved (discoligamentous disruption). This injury is highly unstable. Rupture of the posterior anulus fibrosus can in rare cases result in traumatic disk extrusion. This results in anterior tilting of the vertebra over the underlying vertebra with fanning of the spinous processes, incomplete articulation of the facet joints, and anterior displacement of the subluxed vertebra by more than 50%. In marked cases, **unilateral or bilateral facet dislocation** can also develop (known as **locked facets**; ▶ Fig. 2.37). This is found predominantly at the lower cervical spine. It involves the tip of the dislocated inferior articular facet (superior vertebral body) being locked in front of the superior facet of the inferior vertebral body. A pure unilateral facet dislocation is a relatively stable injury as a result of **interlocking** of the dislocated facet joints and neurologic symptoms are uncommon. Nevertheless, the rotatory malalignment requires correction. The reverse hamburger-bun sign and the headphone sign on axial images are helpful imaging findings in these cases (▶ Fig. 2.38). Bilateral facet dislocation commonly results in traumatic spinal canal stenosis with neurologic deficits, which can occasionally develop after some delay.

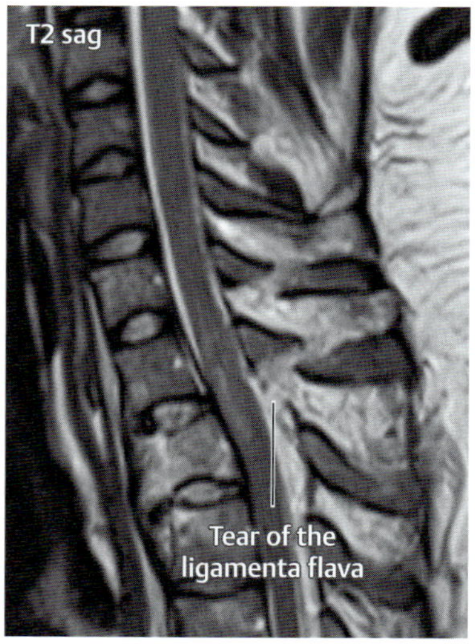

Fig. 2.34 Flexion injury of the upper thoracic spine. Fractures of the spinous processes with disruption of the posterior ligamentous complex. Additional vertical fracture of the anterior third of T2 (large flexion teardrop fragment).

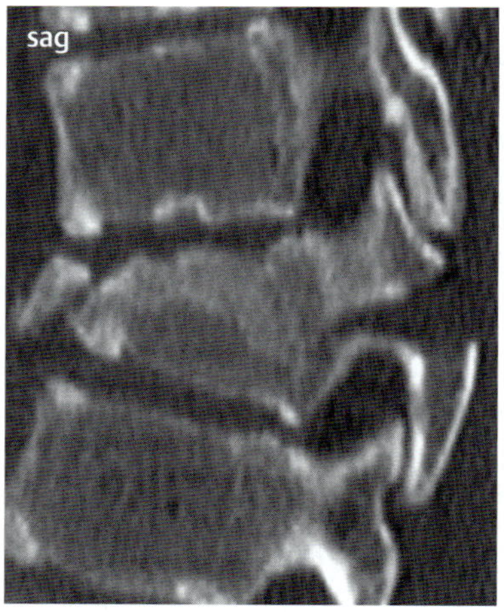

Fig. 2.35 Chance fracture. Fracture with disruption of the posterior bony vertebral elements as well as compression of the anterior vertebra with a flexion teardrop.

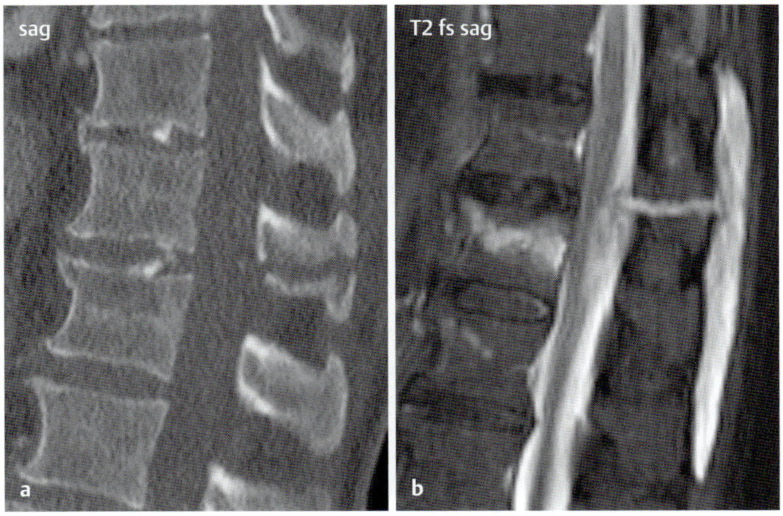

Fig. 2.36 Chance fracture. **(a)** Dorsal bony disruption is evident on this CT scan. **(b)** The MRI scan also demonstrates the anterior bony disruption.

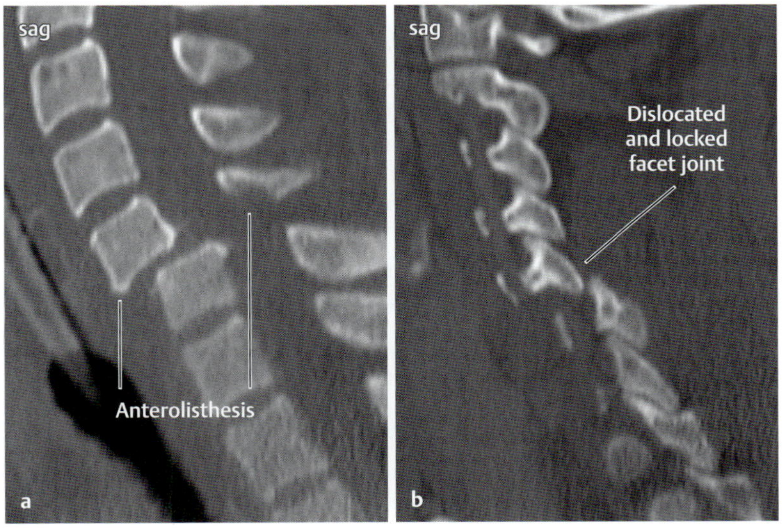

Fig. 2.37 Appearance after a flexion injury. **(a)** Anterior subluxation. **(b)** Locked facet.

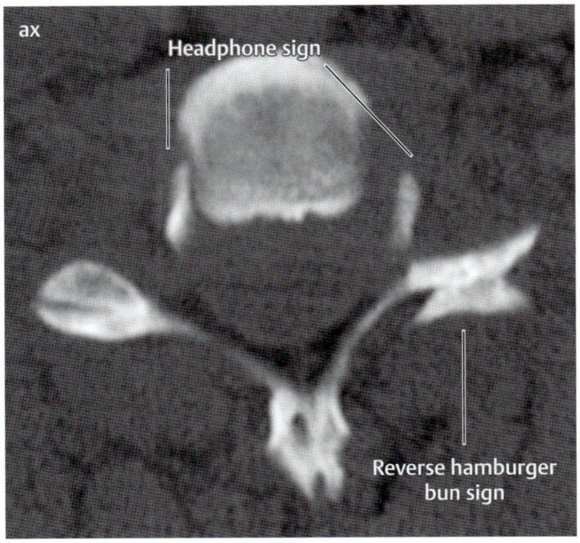

Fig. 2.38 Typical findings of a dislocation injury of the cervical spine as demonstrated on axial imaging. Depiction of unilateral facet dislocation secondary to a rotational injury. Headphone sign: uncovertebral dislocation and step-off: reverse hamburger bun sign: loss of the regular facet contact; in each case empty joint surfaces are positioned "back to back."

Rotational Injuries

Sites of predilection for typical rotational injuries are found at the atlantoaxial level and the thoracolumbar junction.

Rotational injuries usually originate from severe flexion trauma combined with a torsional vector that leads to rupture of the posterior ligamentous and/or discoligamentous complex and/or fracture of the facet joints, resulting in rotational malalignment of the spinal axis. The discoligamentous involvement produces **unstable spinal injuries** that are associated with a high incidence of concomitant spinal cord injuries. The findings of asymmetrical dislocation or fracture of the facet joints and/or juxta-articular neural arch fractures point to a rotational component (▶ Fig. 2.39). Furthermore, fractures of the proximal parts of the ribs, transverse processes, and spinous processes are indirect signs of a rotational injury. Because of the risk of long-term rotatory and translational malalignment it is imperative to carefully assess images of spinal injuries (burst fractures in particular) for rotational malalignments. Rotational injuries —albeit uncommon—tend to be underestimated and underdiagnosed in multiply injured patients.

Unilateral facet dislocation occurs as a result of a combination of hyperflexion with rotation and is found predominantly in the lower cervical spine (see ▶ Fig. 2.39). In only one-third of cases is it associated with a fracture of an articular process. There is often neurologic compromise due to associated foraminal narrowing.

Caution

MRI should be performed before treatment of unilateral facet dislocation to exclude disk injury. Any manipulation to reduce the dislocated facet joint can result in posterior displacement of an existing disk protrusion leading to neurologic complications.

Translational Injuries (Shearing Injuries)

These injuries are the result of enormous horizontal or oblique forces. Usually the lower half of the body is fixed while the upper segment moves relative to it. The ligaments are always disrupted, even without associated fracture, if the superior spinal components are displaced dorsally. The vertebroligamentous injury pattern is complex. These are usually Grade C3 injuries according to the AO Classification (see ▶ Fig. 2.21), even though the rotational component is not always apparent (effect of positioning, spontaneous reduction in immobilization devices; ▶ Figs. 2.40 and ▶ 2.41). These injuries are often associated with severe neurologic symptoms, and multilevel injuries are commonly found in the rigid spine (Chapter 2.2.4).

Special Fracture Types That Do Not Threaten Spinal Stability

Transverse process fracture. Fractures of the lumbar transverse processes are predominantly the result of direct blows and usually of no clinical relevance. However, they are important as warning signs because these fractures are often associated with concomitant injuries such as other spinal injuries (possibly at a significant distance), and especially injuries to abdominal and retroperitoneal organs (e.g., renal lacerations) (▶ Fig. 2.42).

Clay-shoveler's fracture. This fracture of the tip of a spinous process occurs as a result of an abrupt flexion of the head and neck relative to the tight nuchal ligaments. It is a bony avulsion fracture at the attachment of the supraspinatus ligament at the cervicothoracic junction level, such that both this ligament and the posterior longitudinal ligament remain intact. The line of fracture is usually vertical through the dorsal portion of the spinous process and it is often a chronic, incidental finding (evidenced by sclerotic margins with or without associated calcification of the nuchal ligament; ▶ Fig. 2.43). However, clay-shoveler's fractures must not be confused with an oblique Chance fracture of the spinous process or with fractures of the spinous process, which are indication of a severe dorsal distraction injury.

Sequelae of Trauma to the Sacral and Coccygeal Bones

Fractures of the sacrum. These are usually the result of a direct trauma (fall). The majority occur in combination with pelvic fractures. Denis distinguishes three types:

- **Type I**: Lateral to the neural foramina, no neurologic symptoms.
- **Type II**: Transforaminal sacral fractures, commonly associated with neurologic symptoms (▶ Fig. 2.44).
- **Type III**: Central fractures involving the sacral canal; neurologic symptoms are common.

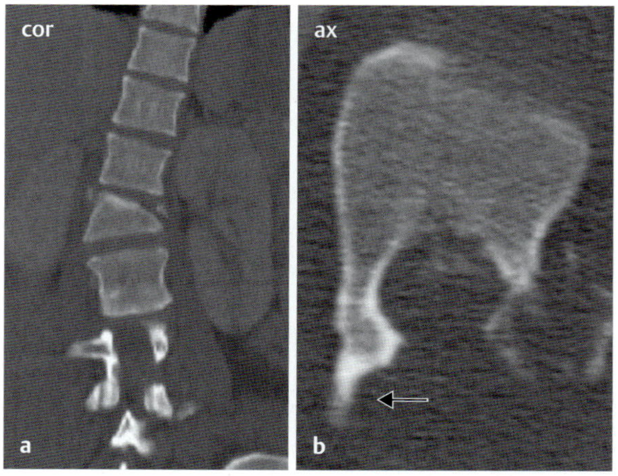

Fig. 2.39 Rotational injury of the thoracolumbar junction. **(a)** Obvious segmental angulation. **(b)** Concave fracture of the facet joint: "empty" facet joint on the convex side (arrow), indicating facet dislocation.

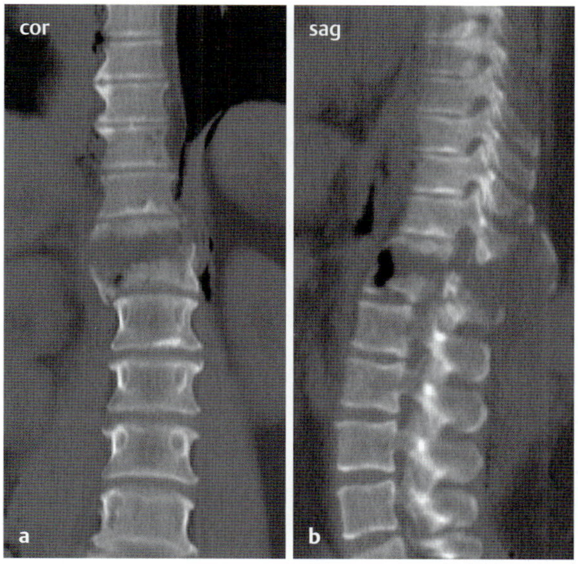

Fig. 2.40 Translational shear-type injury of the thoracolumbar junction. **(a)** Complete osteoligamentous disruption with lateral subluxation. **(b)** Prominent distraction with dorsal dislocation.

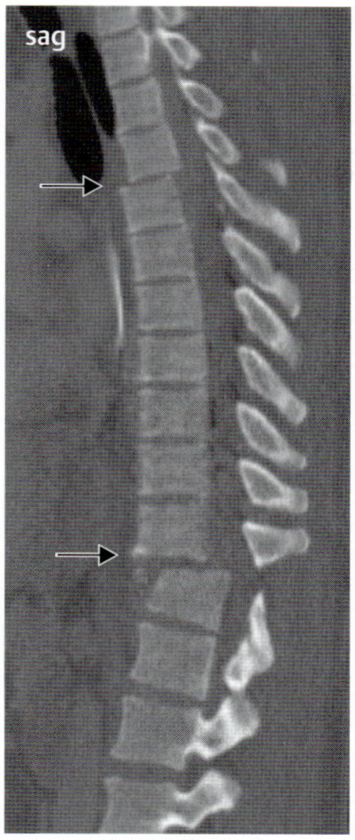

Fig. 2.41 A rare case of discontinuous and considerably separated thoracic and thoracolumbar fractures/dislocations with bony avulsion of the anterosuperior margin of T12. The corresponding axial slices (not shown here) illustrated slight rotatory malalignment of the involved segments.

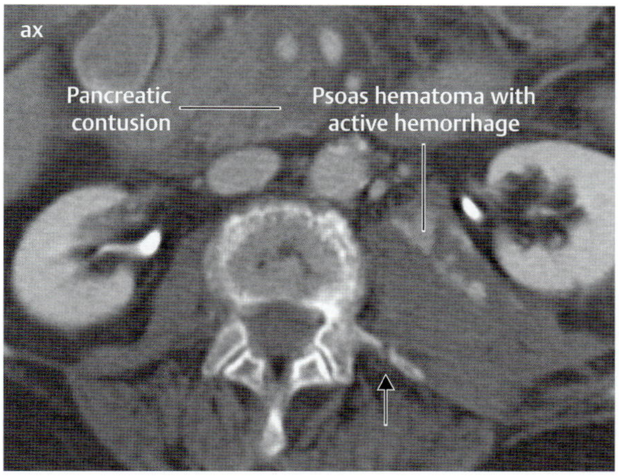

Fig. 2.42 Fracture of the transverse process (arrow). In itself it is of no clinical significance, but is often an important indicator of associated injuries.

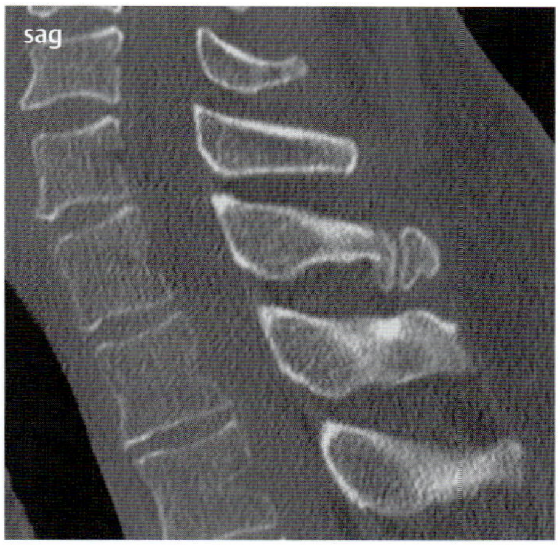

Fig. 2.43 Old fracture of the spinous process (clay-shoveler's fracture) of T2.

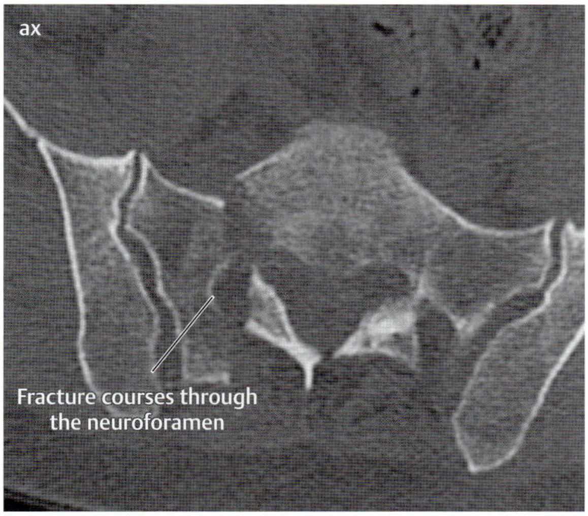

Fig. 2.44 Transforaminal fracture of the sacrum (Type II).

Sacral fractures are overlooked on survey radiographs in up to 50% of cases. A CT scan is therefore always indicated if there is a high degree of clinical suspicion or there are indirect radiographic signs (transverse process fractures of L5, anterior pelvic ring fracture, symphysis disruption).

Fractures of the coccyx. Radiographic assessment of the sacrococcygeal region is difficult due to the wide range of individual anatomical variability. Ventral angulation at the sacrococcygeal junction is an extremely common variant. A fracture may be identified using sectional imaging modalities (CT, MRI), but this rarely results in a change in subsequent management. Even so, chronic posttraumatic coccydynia may develop in some cases.

2.2.3 Special Traumatology of the Cervical Spine and the Craniocervical Junction

The Magerl classification system (based on the AO system) is used for classifying fractures of the subaxial cervical, thoracic, and lumbar spine (the latter two may also be classified according to the TLICS system, see Chapter 2.2.2). Other classification systems have been developed for the upper cervical region (from the craniocervical junction to C2).

Fractures of the Occipital Condyles

Fractures of the occipital condyles are rare and are usually the result of axial blows to the head; they are best classified using the **Anderson and Montesano system:**

- **Type I:** Compression fracture of the occipital condyles.
- **Type II:** Basilar skull fracture that extends to involve the occipital condyle region. These fractures are usually stable and only identified on appropriate CT scan sections (▶ Fig. 2.45).
- **Type III:** Avulsion fractures with bony ligamentous avulsions (alar and cruciform ligaments of the atlas) on the inner surface of the condyles; these injuries are potentially unstable. They often occur in combination with brainstem injuries and are the result of severe trauma. The often subtle avulsion fragments must be carefully looked for on multiplanar CT images since they are often the only signs of severe craniocervical ligament disruption (▶ Fig. 2.46). MRI may be used to assess associated ligamentous and/or cord injury.

Craniocervical Dissociation

The infrequently encountered disruption of all ligaments at the craniocervical junction represents the ultimate form of craniocervical dissociation. This injury is seen after high-velocity trauma from considerable whiplash movement of the head with the body restrained; it is especially common in children owing to their large head-to-body ratio and lax craniocervical ligaments. (see the subsection "Special features of pediatric cervical spine injuries"). This injury is almost always fatal due to severe spinal cord damage, and if the patient does survive it is typically with a severe neurologic deficit.

Fractures of the Atlas

The angled position of the occipital condyles and atlantoaxial articular surfaces as well as the ring configuration of the atlas predispose the atlas to a burst fracture of its arch during axial compression (the so-called burst effect). Isolated fractures of the anterior and posterior arch of the atlas, on the other hand, are caused by hyperextension injuries. Neurologic deficits are rather rare with fractures of the atlas since they tend to result in enlargement of the diameter of the spinal canal.

The following **modified fracture classification system according to Jefferson** is currently in use:

- **Type I**: Fracture of the anterior ring of the atlas; there is often an additional fracture of the dens. Extension mechanism, usually stable.
- **Type II:** Fracture of the posterior ring of the atlas; the most common form. The posterior ring of the atlas is wedged between occiput and C2, resulting in the fracture. Extension mechanism, usually stable.
- **Type III:** Fracture of the ring involving both the anterior and posterior arches (Jefferson's fracture; ▶ Fig. 2.47a). It occurs as a result of abnormal axial loading of the occipital condyles on the atlas with the head extended (compression fracture). This fracture is unstable if it is associated with a rupture of the transverse atlantal ligament. An indirect sign of ligament disruption on the odontoid view or on reformatted coronal CT images is bilateral displacement of the lateral articular masses of the atlas beyond the articular margins of the axis by more than 7 mm combined (▶ Fig. 2.47b). However, this sign may be masked in the presence of concomitant rotation, rendering a CT examination necessary for an exact assessment of the fracture.
- **Type IV:** Unilateral or bilateral compression fracture of the lateral masses of the atlas; stable but unfavorable prognosis with regard to the development of posttraumatic osteoarthritis of the occipital-atlantal joints.
- **Type V:** Fracture of a transverse process of the atlas (stable).

> **Caution**
> Traumatic dissection of the vertebral artery is a possible complication of a Type V Jefferson fracture.

In addition there are a number of other nonclassified fracture types, such as a horizontal fracture of the anterior arch of the atlas due to traction of the anterior longitudinal ligament and the longus colli muscle, and the bilateral, vertical fracture of the posterior arch due to forced hyperextension of the head (which should be differentiated from a congenital unfused posterior arch of the atlas).

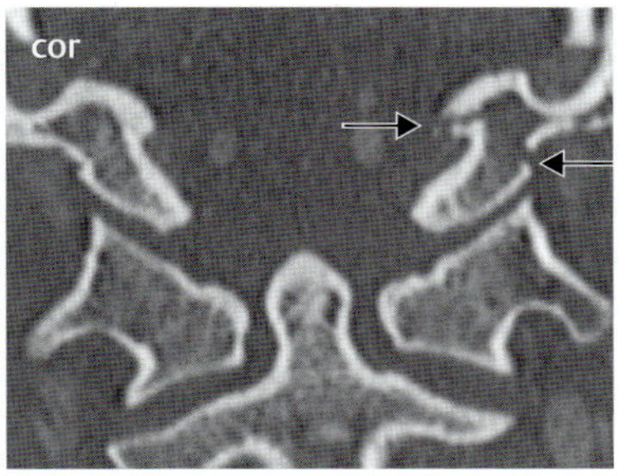

Fig. 2.45 Fracture of the occipital condyle (Anderson and Montesano Type II; arrows).

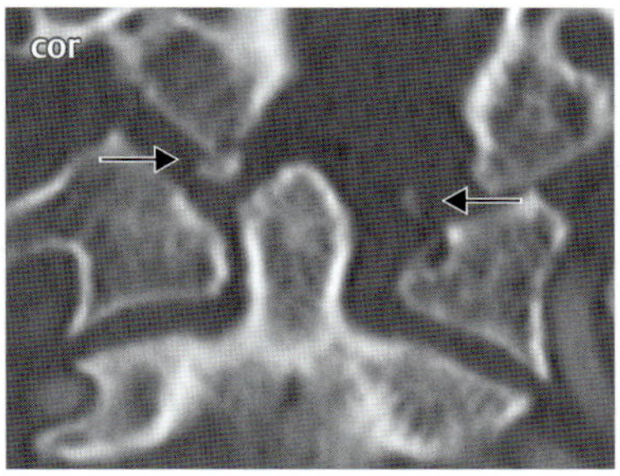

Fig. 2.46 Anderson and Montesano Type III injury. Bony avulsion of the alar ligaments (arrows).

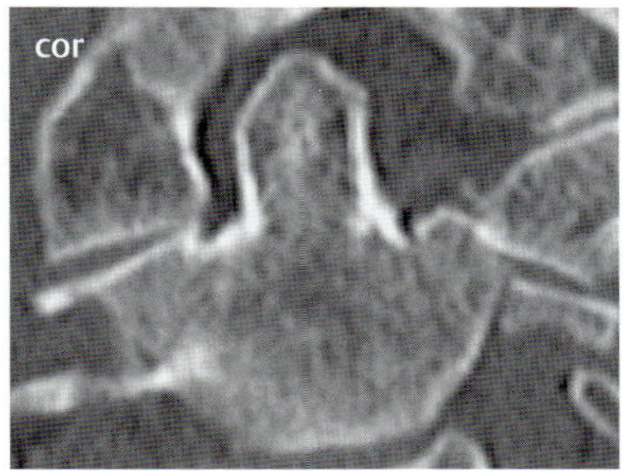

Fig. 2.48 Asymmetry of the atlantodental intervals and the atlantoaxial joint spaces (known as the wink sign on the radiograph) as an indication of a rotational atlantoaxial injury.

Atlantoaxial Dislocation and Atlantoaxial Rotational Dissociation

This traumatic dislocation occurs as a result of disruption of the transverse ligament of the atlas and/or the alar ligaments and is very rare. A distinction is made between anterior, posterior, and lateral dislocations of the atlas over the stable C2. The diagnosis is best made by CT or conventional radiography, which includes an open-mouth odontoid view. The atlantodental interval must not exceed 3 mm in adults and 5 mm in children (known as Spence's rule). However, it should also be kept in mind that patients with congenital craniocervical junction abnormalities can develop atlantoaxial instability (e.g., unstable os odontoideum), while chronic inflammatory arthritides, such as rheumatoid arthritis, can also result in craniocervical and atlantoaxial ligamentous laxity.

The assessment of traumatic rotational, atlantoaxial malalignment (subluxation or dislocation) and its differentiation from voluntary, postural rotation in the superior cranial joints are difficult. Clues for rotational injuries can include asymmetry on the AP odontoid view; in particular unilateral (rarely bilateral) loss of the atlantoaxial joint space on a correctly adjusted view (known as the wink sign; ▶ Fig. 2.48). The degree of rotation can be determined on axial CT sections (up to 45° is normal at maximum rotation), at which time pathologic anterior displacement of the atlas over the axis may also be detected.

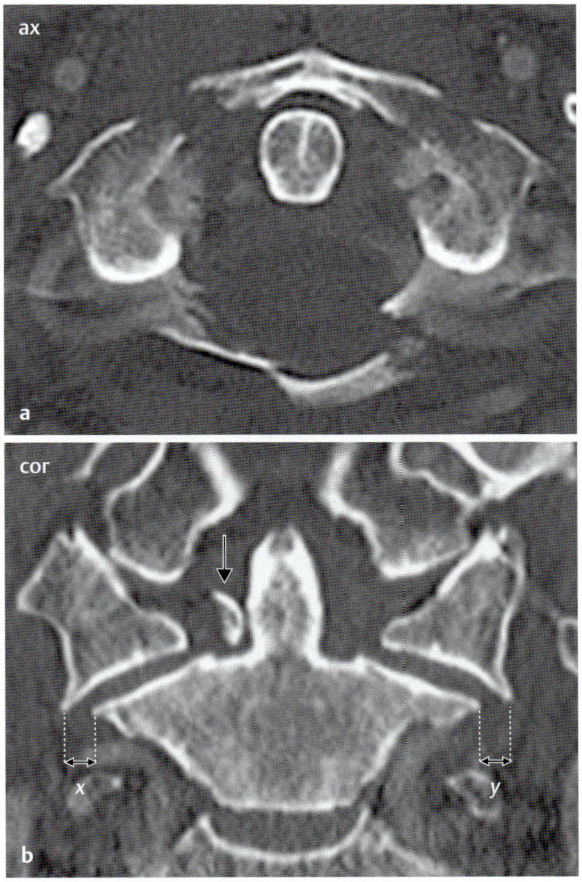

Fig. 2.47 Classic four-part burst fracture according to Jefferson (Type III). **(a)** Burst fracture of the atlas ring. Note the spatial proximity of the fracture of the atlas to the course of the vertebral arteries. **(b)** Indirect sign of a Type III fracture of the atlas: lateral displacement of the lateral masses of the atlas ($x + y > 7$ mm) relative to those of the axis. In addition, there is a bony avulsion of the transverse ligament of the atlas (arrow): unstable fracture.

Classification System According to Fielding and Hawkins

- **Type I:** Pure rotatory, unilateral atlantoaxial dislocation (▶ Fig. 2.49); without fracture, it is impossible to differentiate from a voluntary rotation of the head on a static CT image. Only after a dynamic examination is it possible to demonstrate a fixed rotational malalignment (when it is impossible to return the malalignment to the neutral position by turning the head to the opposite side).
- **Type II:** Atlantoaxial rotatory abnormality with anterior dislocation and an atlantodental interval of less than 5 mm. The transverse ligament of the atlas may be ruptured.
- **Type III:** Atlantoaxial rotatory abnormality with anterior dislocation and an atlantodental interval of less than 5 mm. Disruption of the transverse ligament of the atlas with instability.
- **Type IV:** Atlantoaxial rotatory abnormality, with the atlas displaced unilaterally or bilaterally in a posterior direction in relation to the axis (posterior dislocation); usually in the presence of a Type II fracture of the dens or an unstable dens nonunion.

Fractures of the Axis and Dens

Dens fractures are common and constitute approximately 20% of all cervical fractures. Hyperextension mechanisms are most commonly responsible for these fractures. Whereas more forceful accidents are mainly responsible in young adults, these fractures occur in the aged as a result of simple falls. Associated neurologic deficits are present in up to 30% of cases. A CT scan is best suited for assessing the fracture. Dens fractures are classified by **Anderson and D'Alonzo** into three types (▶ Fig. 2.50):

- **Type I:** Obliquely through the *tip of the dens;* actually an avulsion fracture of the alar ligaments; an extremely rare fracture.
- **Type II:** Transversely through the *base (waist) of the dens,* unstable, the most common fracture type (▶ Fig. 2.51). Nonunion develops in ~ 30% of cases.
- **Type III:** Fracture of the *body of C2,* commonly with involvement of an atlantoaxial joint surface; anterior dislocation in 90% of cases. This fracture is also mechanically unstable, but does not tend to proceed to nonunion.

Caution

- A dens fracture is often simulated on conventional radiographs (AP targeted dens view) by what is known as the *Mach effect* (▶ Fig. 2.52). This is a linear lucency passing across the base of the dens that is an artifact (edge effect) occurring when two radiodense structures overlap (e.g., overlapping of the dens by the arch of the atlas).
- The dens and body of the axis normally fuse between the ages of 3 and 7 years (▶ Fig. 2.53); however, fusion may be delayed or completely absent, thus creating the impression of a Type II fracture. Differential diagnostic aid: An os odontoideum develops when fusion is absent and, unlike a fracture, typically has a smooth margin, shows marginal sclerosis, and is usually rounded (▶ Fig. W2.5; see also ▶ Fig. 2.53). Often, the anterior arch of C1 is also hypertrophied in the presence of an os odontoideum, while the dens is hypoplastic.
- Fusion of the ossiculum terminale of the dens, which is normally complete by the age of 12 years, may fail to occur. This simulates a Type I fracture (see ▶ Fig. 2.53).

Traumatic Spondylolisthesis of the Axis

Also termed a "hangman's fracture", this injury occurs as a result of extension with simultaneous vertical compression, such as that which occurs in rear-end collisions. However, other mechanisms can also result in this injury, such as a pure flexion. The most commonly used **classification system** is that of **Effendi:**

- **Type I:** Nondislocated fracture with intact intervertebral disk, stable.
- **Type II:** Involvement of the C2–C3 intervertebral disk, sagittal displacement of the body of the axis by more than 3 mm, or angulation of the dens by more than 11°, unstable (▶ Figs. 2.54–2.56).
- **Type III:** In addition to the findings with a Type II fracture, the facet joints at C2–C3 are dislocated and locked.

Neurologic complications are less common than with other injuries due to the relatively large width of the spinal canal at this level.

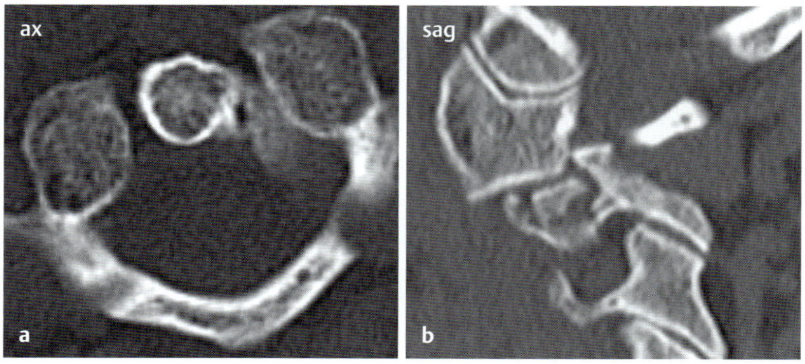

Fig. 2.49 Fielding and Hawkins Type I injury. **(a)** Unilateral atlantoaxial rotatory subluxation. **(b)** Locking of the atlantoaxial joint with a burst fracture of the lateral mass of C2.

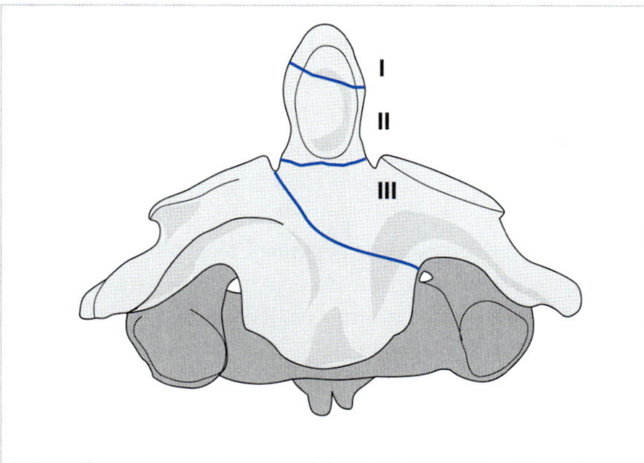

Fig. 2.50 Schematic presentation of types of dens fractures.

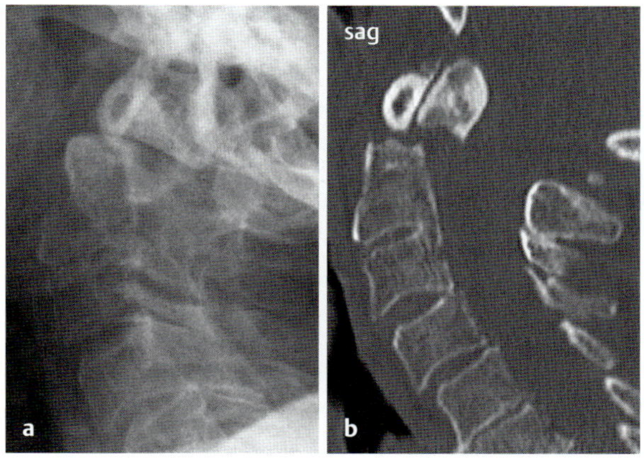

Fig. 2.51 Dislocated Anderson and D'Alonzo Type II dens fracture. **(a)** The anterior arch of the atlas rests upon the base of the dens. **(b)** The tip of the dens is clearly dislocated dorsally and may compress the adjacent cervical cord.

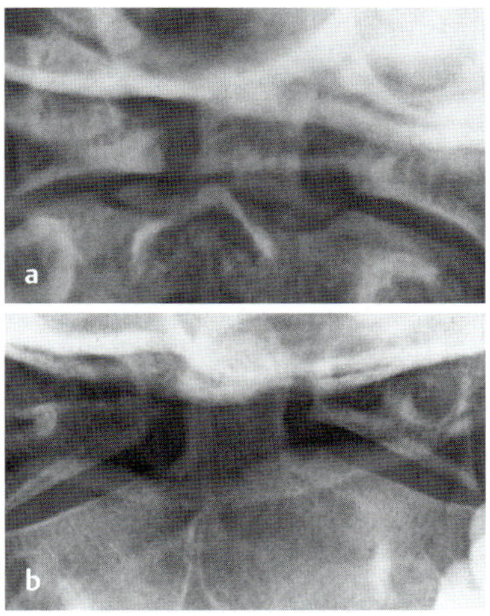

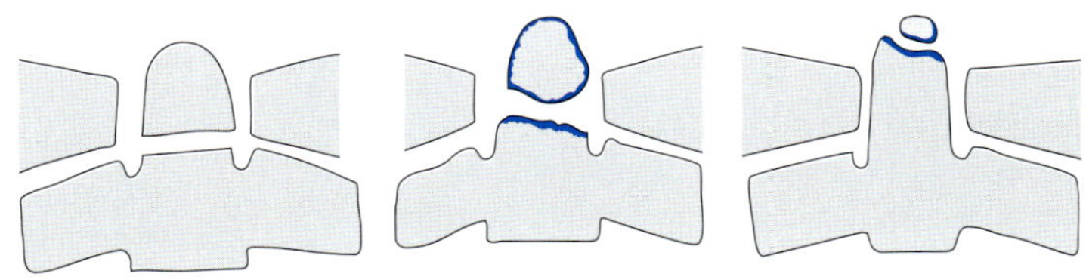

Fig. 2.53 Special features associated with the dens axis.

◀ **Fig. 2.52** The Mach effect as an imaging pitfall. **(a)** Anderson and D'Alonzo Type III dens fracture. **(b)** No fracture! The radiolucent line is a Mach effect due to overlapping of the arch of the atlas.

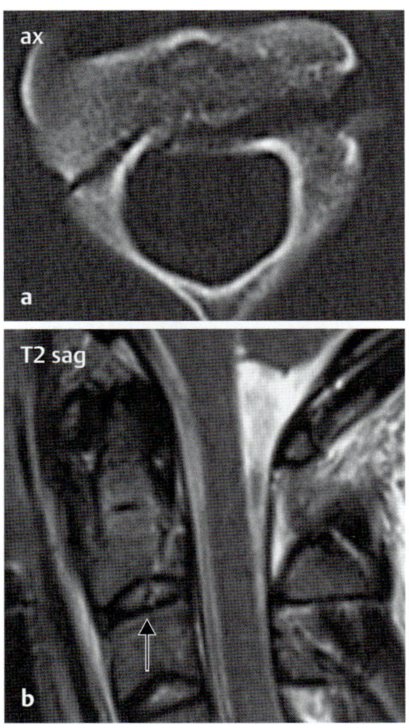

Fig. 2.54 Traumatic spondylolisthesis of C2 (hangman's fracture). **(a)** Course of the fracture line through the body of the axis. **(b)** Involvement of the intervertebral disk (arrow): therefore an Effendi Type II injury.

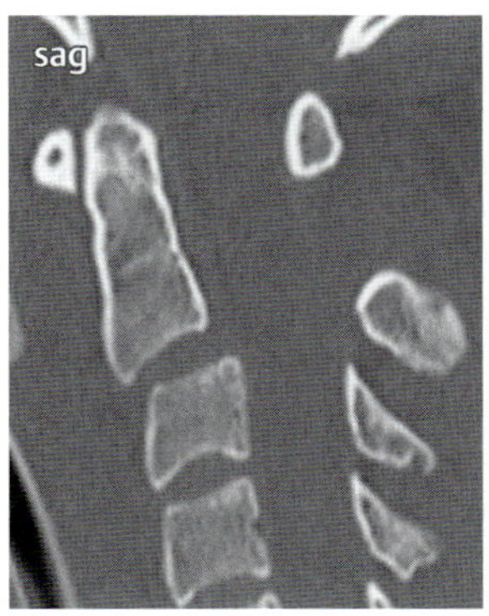

Fig. 2.55 Traumatic spondylolisthesis at C2. Anterior angulation of the C2 vertebra.

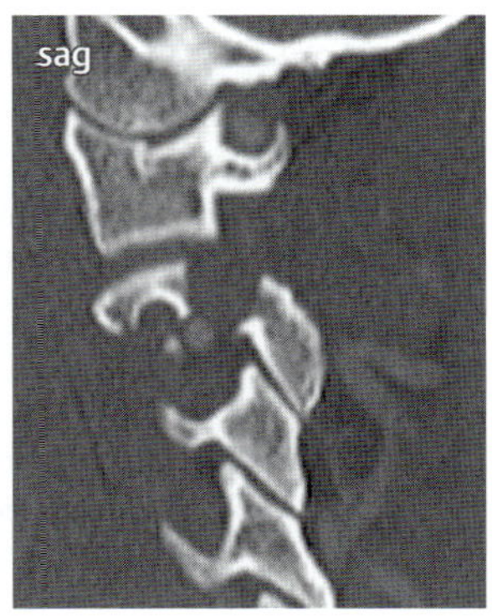

Fig. 2.56 Traumatic spondylolisthesis at C2. Spondylolysis of more than 3 mm: therefore an Effendi Type II injury.

2

Whiplash Injury of the Cervical Spine

There are numerous definitions for the term "whiplash injury" including, in many cases, any form of acceleration/ deceleration injury of the cervical spine. The Quebec Task Force defined symptoms following a whiplash injury as **"whiplash-associated disorder."** It may occur with mechanisms other than rear-impact collisions, such as a side-impact collision. If injuries to the bony structures or the soft tissues are detected on diagnostic imaging, then this is referred to as a **"whiplash injury."**

▸ **Radiography.** Radiographic examination is performed to exclude bony injury or segmental malalignment.

▸ **MRI.** Use of MRI is only indicated for cases with radicular symptoms or of unusually severe pain, in which case this should be done early to establish osseous and soft tissue edema or discoligamentous injuries. The value of MRI for evaluating the alar ligaments is a matter of great controversy and its routine use in this scenario is not recommended.

> **Caution**
> Loss of normal cervical lordosis does not necessarily indicate underlying pathology; it may merely be a positional abnormality of the cervical spine. When found in isolation it should not be regarded as pathologic.

Special Features of Pediatric Cervical Spine Injuries

In children, skeletal structures still possess a high degree of elasticity. For this reason, bony injuries to the spine are relatively rare, even in the presence of accident-related neurologic deficits. This special feature is subsumed under the acronym **"SCIWORA syndrome"** (spinal cord injury without radiographic abnormality). Ligamentous laxity in childhood with associated discoligamentous flexibility results in significant degrees of movement, which can bruise, overstretch, and even disrupt the spinal cord. Intramedullary hemorrhage can also occur (▸ Fig. 2.57).

The decisive point is that radiological signs (fractures, dislocations) are absent despite a severe neurologic deficit. This explains the central role of MRI in such cases. Children less than 10 years of age are mostly affected, especially those under the age of 3 years. The most common site of the spinal cord injury is at the level of C2.

Another special feature of pediatric cervical injury is the vulnerability of the occipitoatlantal junction: The occipitoatlantal ligaments and membranes are unable to stabilize the still relatively large head of the child during severe deceleration events, resulting in disruption of the atlantoaxial complex and, in some cases, fatal occipitoatlantal dissociation.

Incomplete ossification or fusion of the ossification centers must not be confused with a fracture. The following are important time points of ossification (▸ cf. also "Variants" in Chapter 2.2.1):

- **Atlas:** ossification of the posterior arch at age 4 years, complete fusion during the 7th to 10th years.
- **Axis:** fusion of the posterior arches between the ages of 2 and 3 years with fusion with the body of C2 by the age of 7 years. The ossiculum terminale of the dens fuses with the body of the dens around the age of 11 to 12 years. Subdental synchondrosis can persist until adolescence and may be confused with a Type II fracture of the dens. An MRI scan helps in equivocal cases since true injuries are typically associated with edema in the marrow and adjacent tissues.

Anterior displacement of C2 on C3 or of C3 on C4 is a physiologic variant in ~ 20% of children up to the age of 5 years. However, alignment of the spinolaminar line is maintained in this "pseudo subluxation."

Inadequate distension of the pharynx can often produce a prevertebral soft tissue shadow on conventional radiographs that can be mistaken for a hematoma. MRI can help in equivocal cases.

2.2.4 Injury Patterns of the "Stiff" Spine

Both acquired and degenerative block vertebrae (synostoses) extending over several segments of the spine, e.g., in **diffuse idiopathic skeletal hyperostosis** (**DISH**) or **ankylosing spondylitis**) lead to long-segment loss of the normal excursion of the spine. This results in reduced flexibility during trauma, as well as a reduction in actual bone stability secondary to severe demineralization, particularly with ankylosing spondylitis.

Because of absent segmental mobility, long rigid leverages, and vertebral osteoporosis, even apparently harmless falls can result in severe fractures with discoligamentous disruptions, subluxations, or dislocations (▸ Fig. 2.58). The fractures often course horizontally or obliquely through an entire vertebral body, adjacent disk space and into the posterior elements; consequently all three columns of the axial skeleton are typically involved (▸ Fig. 2.59). Fractures are often encountered at multiple levels.

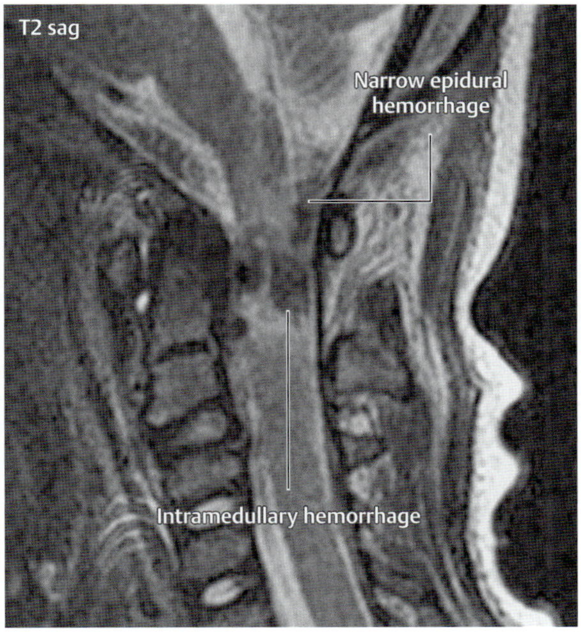

Fig. 2.57 SCIWORA syndrome in a 6-year-old boy following a car accident. The radiograph was unremarkable.

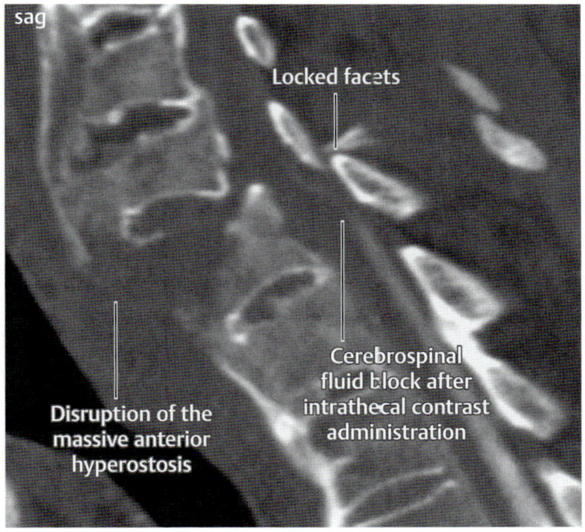

Fig. 2.58 Cervical extension fracture-dislocation of a stiff spine. Combined discovertebral injury with anterior malalignment and "pincerlike" compression of the spinal cord.

These fractures are highly unstable because they result in disruption of all bony and often discoligamentous structures.

Three factors make diagnosis of these fractures difficult:

- Overlapping spondylophytes (e.g., DISH) and marked osteoporosis (e.g., ankylosing spondylitis) make it difficult to recognize the fractures on survey radiographs (▶ Fig. W2.6).
- Fractures may occur at a distance from the site of impact or even at multiple sites (e.g., cervicothoracic *and* thoracolumbar in patients with ankylosing spondylitis).
- Even traumatic events judged to be only mild (e.g., striking the head during a ground-level fall) can result in a significant vertebral injury.

Conclusions. If the clinical history and clinical examination in a patient with a "stiff spine" suggest a spinal injury that is not evident on survey radiographs, a CT scan is indicated and should include long segments at potential risk of fracture. Given the above propensity for instability with these fractures and often coincidental spinal stenoses in elderly patients, an MRI should also be subsequently performed to better evaluate any spinal cord injury.

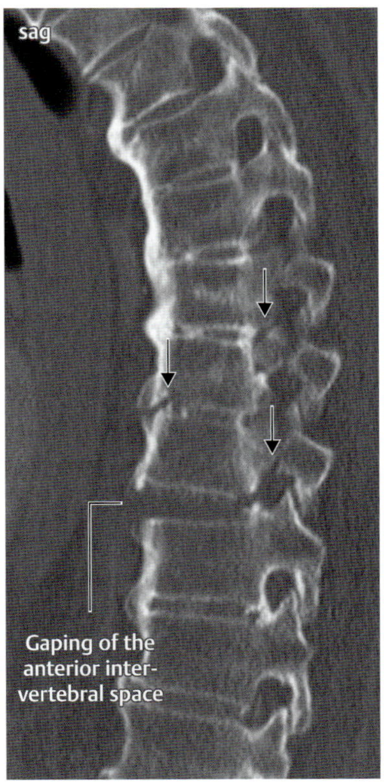

Fig. 2.59 Extension injury following a fall from a ladder. Preexisting stiff vertebral column in ankylosing spondylitis. The fractures (arrows) traverse the anterior and posterior spinal segments.

2.2.5 Stable or Unstable Fracture?

What is Meant by "Stable"?

"Stability" with respect to spinal injuries means the spine's capability for resistance to physiological loads without damage or progressive compromise to the spinal cord or nerve roots and without the development or progression of deformities or structural changes.

Assessment of stability of the spinal column remains challenging in daily practice. The problem of assessing spinal stability using objective criteria has not been satisfactorily solved.

Upper Cervical Spine

Assessment of stability of fractures of atlas and odontoid has been discussed in the sections describing those injuries (Chapter 2.2.3).

Middle and Lower Cervical Spine

There are no universally recognized classification systems for assessing the stability of injuries involving the subaxial cervical spine, but the classification system according to Magerl is increasingly being applied to this portion of the spine. While there are no absolute criteria for diagnosing instability, the following criteria may serve as guidelines:

- Horizontal translation of more than 3.5 mm between adjacent spinal segments (if the anterolisthesis or retrolisthesis is interpreted as being degenerative, then additional signs of degeneration should be clearly evident, e.g. disk space narrowing, osteophytes, etc.).
- Angulation between two adjacent vertebrae of more than 11°.
- Widening of a disk space.
- Facet joint subluxation resulting in less than 50% overlap.
- Increased interspinous distance.

> **Caution**
> If an unclear anterior wedge avulsion is evident in a cervical spine injury, it is extremely important to ascertain whether this is in fact a teardrop fracture. This injury is always unstable. A complete burst fracture (Type A3.3) is almost always associated with disruption of the posterior ligamentous structures and is considered to be an unstable Type B injury.

Thoracic and Lumbar Spine

There is currently broad agreement with regard to criteria for assessing the stability of thoracolumbar fractures, in particular with respect to *osseous* injury patterns, which can be assessed using the **classification system according to Magerl** (Chapter 2.2.2).

Type A fractures are generally regarded as stable with the exception of Type A3, although this does not mean that they should necessarily be treated conservatively. There has been a tendency over recent years to regard Type A3 fractures as unstable (progressive collapse with malalignment of the axial skeleton and also, in the case of a large, avulsed posterior wall fragment, a possible neurologic deficit). The paradigm of the intact posterior wall as an exclusive discriminator of stability has been abandoned (▶ see "Anatomy" in Chapter 2.2.1).

Type B fractures are unstable due to their potential for discoligamentous disruptions secondary to flexion or extension forces. However, these can be very difficult to identify using radiography or CT when bony injuries are either absent or extremely subtle in nature. This applies, for example, to small teardrop fragments, which are an indication of a severe flexion/extension injury. It may well be helpful to postulate instability using certain metric criteria (e.g., segment angulation by more than 11°, sagittal translation by more than 3.5 mm, subluxation of the facet joints by more than 50%), but it may not always apply in particular cases. Apart from confirming the integrity of sagittal alignment, it is also very important to confirm *uniformity of disk heights and interspinous distances.* Additionally, congruence of the facets on either side of the spine must be confirmed when using CT.

> **Caution**
> Any focal segmental change in the morphological criteria in a Type B injury described above demands a plausible explanation and—following significant trauma—must be regarded as a discoligamentous injury until proven otherwise, typically with MRI.

Type C injuries pose a diagnostic challenge due to the subtle imaging findings in some of these cases. Type C injuries are rotational injuries and always result in significant instability; initially or over time, possibly resulting in a neurologic deficit. Any *unilateral facet joint fracture or dislocation* indicates a rotational injury. Fractures of proximal ribs and transverse processes may also reflect prior rotational trauma. The difficulty in identifying such rotational and shear injuries lies in the fact that they often reduce spontaneously during positioning and transport, thus masking the true nature of the injury.

2.2.6 Fresh or Old Fracture?

Determination of the age of a fracture appears simple but it can be problematic, or even impossible in some cases. First, there should be a clinical correlation between a vertebral deformity and pain at that site. If this is not the case, then the acuity of the fracture becomes doubtful. However, it must be remembered that osteoporotic fractures in particular can be clinically silent.

▶ **Radiography.** Differentiation using radiography is unreliable. The finding of vertebral deformity with sharp-edged fragments but without evidence of reactive osteophyte formation suggests an acute fracture. However, this is only valid for traumatic vertebral fractures; the age of an osteoporotic compression fracture, in particular, usually cannot be estimated with certainty unless there are recent radiographs available for comparison.

▶ **CT.** CT allows a better assessment of the integrity of the vertebral cortex in acute fractures (▶ Fig. 2.60). Evaluation of trabecular bone is problematic, however, because trabecular injuries are often not apparent until the development of microcallus that produces bandlike sclerotic patterns in later stages (see ▶ Fig. 2.60). The presence of thin linear cancellous densities parallel to the end plates is suggestive of an acute trabecular injury, whereas during subacute stages resorption bands may also become evident.

▶ **MRI.** MRI provides the most reliable way to differentiate between acute and older fractures, irrespective of their etiology. Fluid-sensitive sequences with fat suppression are well suited for detecting fracture-related edema in an acute injury. The hyperintense edema on these sequences is often bandlike, extending parallel to the superior or inferior end plates (▶ Fig. 2.61a). Similarly, T1W sequences will reveal corresponding hypointense fracture lines, but some normal, hyperintense fatty marrow should always be observed (▶ Fig. 2.61b). When the entire vertebral body is involved, the possibility of a pathologic fracture related to underlying neoplasm must be considered! IV contrast administration sometimes improves fracture line delineation.

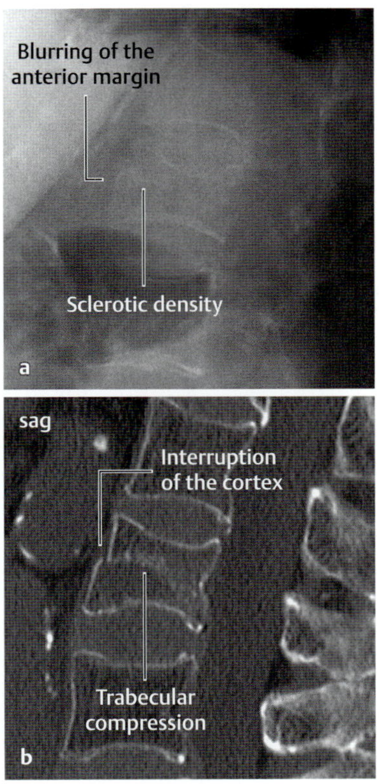

Fig. 2.60 Acute traumatic L2 fracture. **(a)** Equivocal features on the radiograph in the presence of severe osteoporosis. **(b)** The CT image confirms the acute fracture.

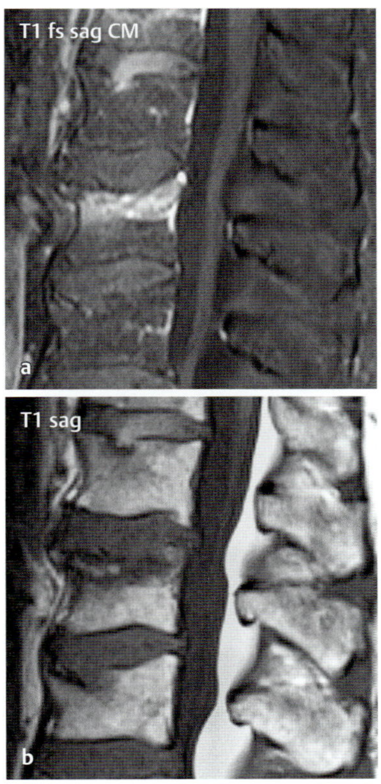

Fig. 2.61 Acute osteoporotic fracture of the end plate. **(a)** Edema and contrast uptake are typically evident in a bandlike fashion along the involved end plate. **(b)** Multilevel end plate irregularities.

2.2.7 Differential Diagnosis "Osteoporotic Versus Pathologic Fracture"

▸Table 2.1 provides an overview of radiological decision aids and important radiological signs. Image examples with explanations of the radiological signs may be found in ▸Figs. 2.62–2.65.

> **Note**
> Osteoporotic fractures are not classified as pathologic fractures. Pathologic fractures are usually related to malignant bone lesions; in rare cases, benign primary bone tumors within the spine will result in vertebral fractures (e.g., Langerhans' cell histiocytosis, vertebral hemangioma, aneurysmal bone cyst).

2.2.8 Stress Phenomena in the Spine: Stress Reaction and Stress Fracture (Spondylolysis) of the Neural Arches

Stress reaction of the neural arches caused by repetitive trauma represents a chronic form of spinal injury. Physically active children and adolescents who participate in sports involving repetitive hyperlordosis (e.g., gymnastics, tennis, swimming) are at particular risk and are most commonly affected. Continued overloading may result in a true stress fracture of the interarticular portion of the neural arches (the pars intra-articularis), also known as spondylolysis.

> **Note**
> Persistent, low lumbar back pain is not physiologic in childhood and adolescence and should be investigated by MRI, which can detect a stress reaction or true spondylolysis of the affected pars intra-articularis (▸Fig. 2.66).

> **Caution**
> A stress fracture of the vertebral arch is sometimes difficult to identify on MRI as the defect can be misinterpreted as a facet joint. Apart from the associated edemalike signal intensity, indirect signs may be helpful, such as widening of the spinal canal in the sagittal diameter and a horizontal or hourglass configuration of the neuroforamen.

Insufficiency fractures, e.g., due to osteoporosis or associated with pregnancy, are common in the sacrum (see also Chapter 2.3.3).

2.2.9 Value of MRI in Acute Trauma

The diagnostic evaluation of the trauma patient is undergoing a paradigm shift due to the increasing availability, better accessibility, and hardware improvements of MRI scanners. Although MRI is still not the diagnostic modality of choice for the multiply injured patient, it is becoming increasingly important in the post-primary phase for assessing discoligamentous and spinal injuries.

Table 2.1 How to differentiate different etiologies of vertebral fractures

Imaging finding	Traumatic	(Benign) osteoporotic	Malignant
Involvement of the pedicles and other posterior elements	Possible	Virtually never	Often present
Convex bulging/destruction of the posterior wall	Possible fragment displacement into the spinal canal	No	Typical
Surrounding paravertebral soft tissue	No	No	Often present
Vertebral body edema	Linear, bandlike, also irregular in the fracture region	Often bandlike, rarely affecting the entire vertebral body	Focal, irregular, diffuse
Contrast enhancement	Possible in the fracture region	Usually linear, bandlike	Focal, irregular, diffuse
Intravertebral fatty marrow (on T1W images)	Always detectable	Usually detectable	Fat marrow signal completely or irregularly replaced or rounded low-intensity foci
Cleft sign/fluid sign	Possible	Typical, if present	Very rare
Intravertebral vacuum phenomenon (on radiographs)	Rare	Very typical	Atypical

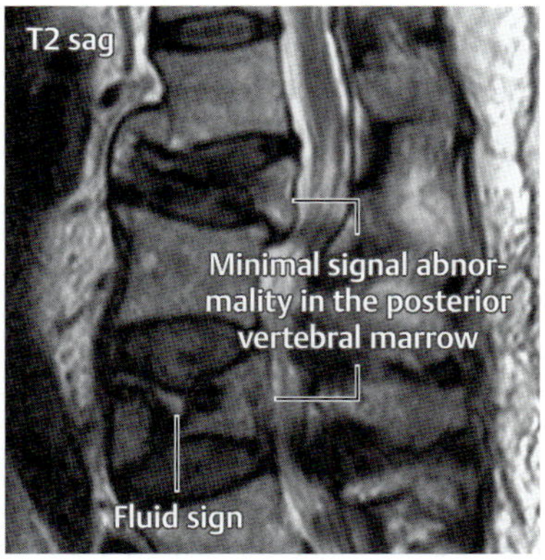

Fig. 2.62 Typical signs of osteoporotic vertebral fractures.

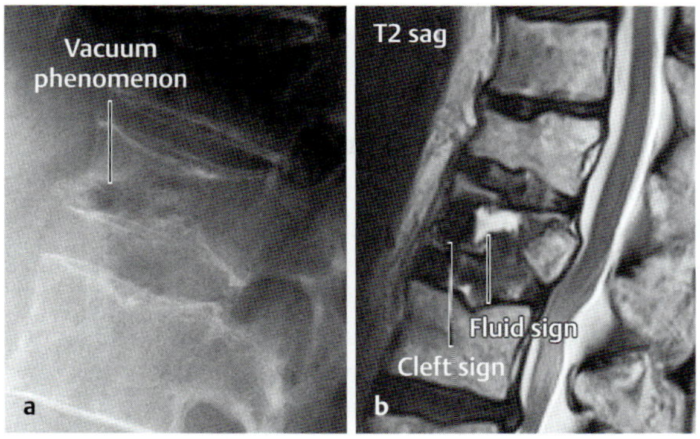

Fig. 2.63 Osteoporotic vertebral fracture with intravertebral cleft formation (cleft sign). **(a)** Vacuum phenomenon visible on the radiograph. **(b)** MRI demonstrates fluid in the intravertebral cleft (fluid sign), with an air–fluid level within the cleft related to the supine position of the patient.

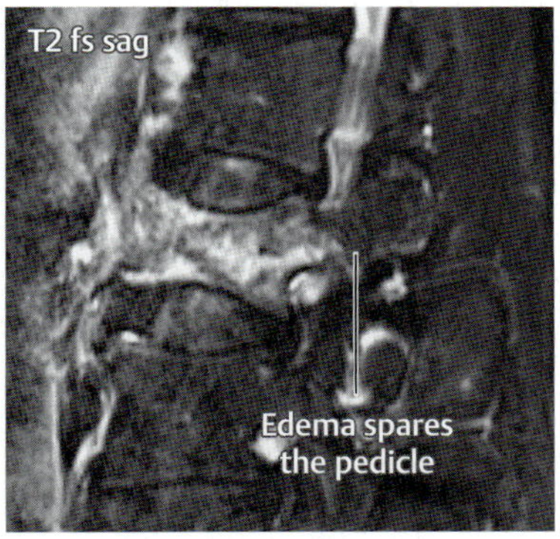

Fig. 2.64 Osteoporotic vertebral fracture. The edema typically involves only the vertebral body.

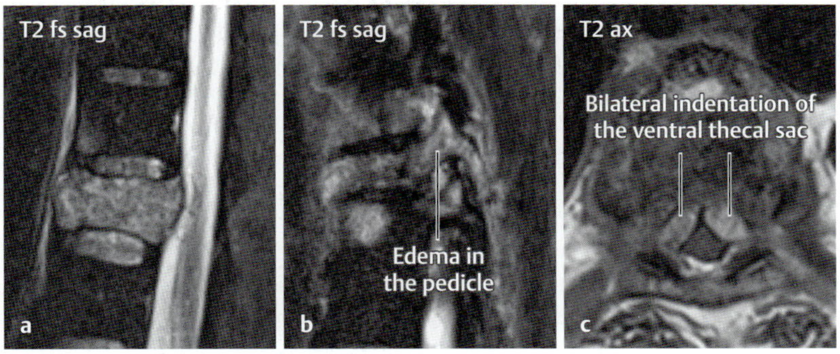

Fig. 2.65 Typical signs of a pathologic tumor-related fracture. **(a)** Convex eccentric dorsal displacement of the posterior margin. **(b)** The edema also involves the pedicles. **(c)** Bilateral indentation of the ventral thecal sac by tumor extending into the epidural space.

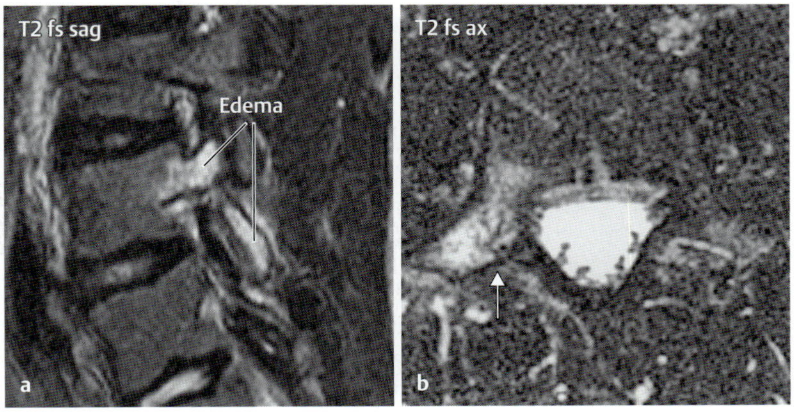

Fig. 2.66 Incipient, stress-related spondylolysis in a competitive gymnast. **(a)** Bone marrow edema of the vertebral arch and articular processes. **(b)** The hypointense line (arrow) represents an incipient stress fracture.

Indication for MRI

After interdisciplinary consultation (trauma surgeon, anesthetist, neurologist/neurosurgeon, and radiologist) it must be decided whether and when an MRI scan should be performed for a case of spinal injury. Essentially, we regard the following situations as indications for MRI scanning:

- The patient presents an unclear, posttraumatic **spinal neurologic deficit** that is not sufficiently explained by CT.
- CT shows a **specific injury pattern** that indicates a potentially unstable discoligamentous lesion (e.g., teardrop fractures, subluxations, or dislocations in hyperflexion injuries; widened disk spaces secondary to hyperextension mechanisms).
- It is not possible to conduct a neurologic examination on a patient (obtunded, altered mental status) in whom there is a **high suspicion of ligamentous or cord damage** based on the mechanism of injury.
- Spinal MRI should be more readily considered in **children** because, radiographs may appear normal despite severe trauma (SCIWORA), and CT of the entire axial skeleton should be avoided for reasons of radiation safety.
- MRI may play an important role in the preoperative assessment and subsequent surgical planning by defining extent and site of spinal cord compression, presence of intraspinal hematomas, occult vertebral fractures, etc.

However, MRI should not be undertaken if it will lead to a delay of essential therapeutic measures (e.g., emergent spinal decompression). Also, in cases where MRI is contraindicated, CT myelography may be considered as an alternative modality.

Ligamentous Injuries

In addition to assessment of the spinal cord, MRI is excellent for demonstrating discoligamentous injuries, which is critical given the potential for associated instability and poor healing if they are left untreated.

Critical ligamentous structures include:

- Anterior and posterior longitudinal ligaments.
- Ligamenta flava.
- Interspinous ligaments.

The critical ligamentous structures of the upper cervical spine and the craniocervical junction worthy of particular mention are the transverse atlantal ligament, the tectorial membrane, and the posterior atlanto-occipital membrane. Evaluation of the alar ligaments requires great care due to their variability of morphology and signal intensity.

Ligament disruptions are best recognized on fat-suppressed T2W or STIR sequences (STIR = short-tau inversion recovery). Hyperflexion injuries are often associated with disruptions of the posterior ligamentous complex and can be well identified by extensive edema within the interspinous tissues (▸ Figs. 2.31 and ▸ 2.33). It is often possible to identify directly discontinuity and tears of the longitudinal ligaments and the ligamenta flava (see ▸ Figs. 2.33 and ▸ 2.34). Hemorrhage and dislocations of vertebral fragments can elevate, or even obscure, the longitudinal ligaments.

Disk Injury

The effects of disk injury remain uncertain, despite various staging proposals.

Traumatic disk prolapse. The occurrence of traumatic disk herniation is the focus of intense discussion—especially in the insurance law literature. Given adequate trauma, it can occur, albeit rarely (▸ Figs. 2.67 and ▸ 2.68). Associated findings suggesting an acute injury (soft tissue edema, ligament tears, hematomas, bone bruises) should be observed in these cases. Traumatic disk prolapse, along with the hyperflexion injury itself, may result in spinal cord injury (cord contusion or even intramedullary hemorrhage), especially in the cervical region.

Hematomas

Trauma-related spinal hemorrhage predominantly involves the **epidural** space; subdural subarachnoid hemorrhages are extremely rare.

Epidural hematomas are found between the periosteum of the vertebrae or vertebral arches and the dura mater of the thecal sac and extend a significant craniocaudal distance—usually over several segments. They are most commonly encountered in the ventral epidural space. In addition to uncomplicated epidural hemorrhages associated with traumatic vertebral fractures, hemorrhages associated with the epidural venous plexus will often form space-occupying hematomas that may result in compression of the cord or, less frequently the cauda equina. Rapidly progressive paraplegia makes an epidural hemorrhage an emergency situation demanding immediate intervention.

In addition to traumatic epidural hematomas, spinal hemorrhages may develop during anticoagulant therapy either spontaneously (▸ Fig. 2.69) or after minimal trauma. Other possible causes of epidural hematomas include spinal interventional procedures or surgery.

▸ **MRI.** The MRI appearance of hemorrhage varies depending on its age. Fresh hematomas are often isointense to, and difficult to differentiate from, cerebrospinal fluid on T1W sequences, while on T2W sequences they can still appear hypointense in the acute phase but change rapidly to an intermediate or even hyperintense appearance. Typical methemoglobin formation occurs after a few days (the subacute phase) and is characterized by hyperintensity on T1W images. GRE (gradient echo) sequences can be helpful in identifying hemorrhage giving rise to typical susceptibility artifacts related to the iron content of the blood. Contrast administration can be dispensed with in the acute stage.

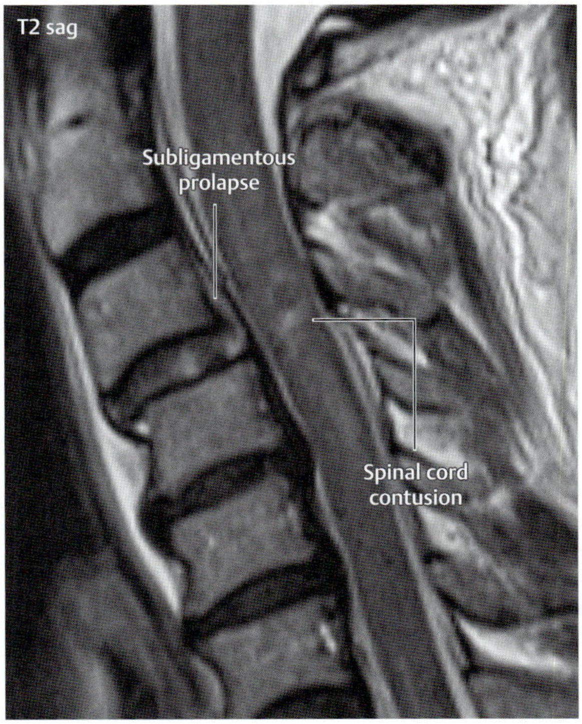

Fig. 2.67 Disk prolapse.

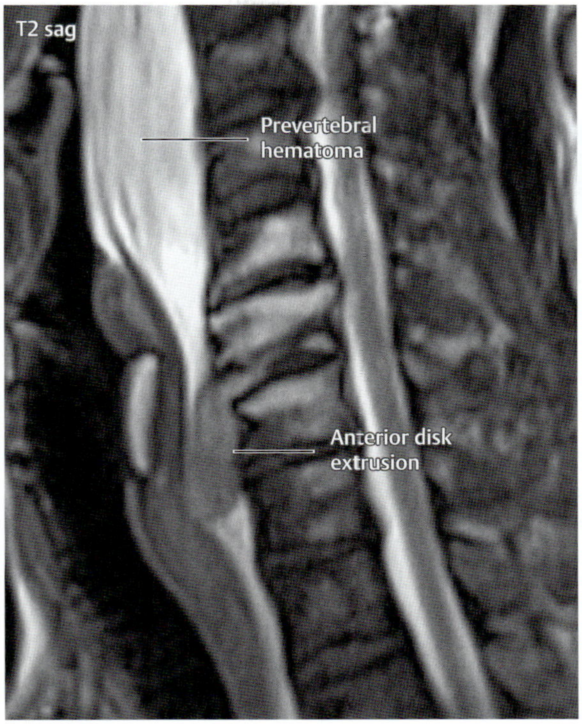

Fig. 2.68 Traumatic disk rupture with massive anterior disk extrusion.

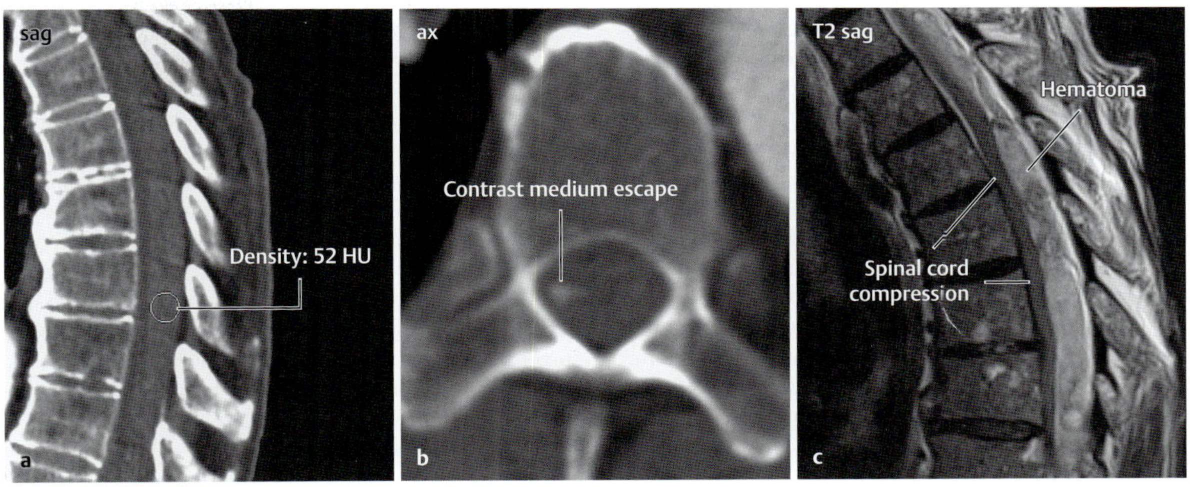

Fig. 2.69 Spontaneous epidural hematoma in a patient on anticoagulants. **(a)** Only increased intraspinal density, which can be easily overlooked, is evident on the plain CT image. **(b)** Active hemorrhage in the region of the thoracic spine is evident after contrast administration. **(c)** MRI demonstrates the space-occupying, epidural hematoma.

Chronic epidural hematomas display marginal contrast enhancement. Epidural hemorrhages related to intermittent bleeding are characterized by marked signal heterogeneity.

> **Caution**
> Despite a suspicious clinical picture, epidural hematomas can be difficult to identify. Clues such as subtle disturbances of the epidural fat or mass effect upon the thecal sac must be searched for since even long-segment epidural hematomas can readily escape the cursory glance!

Traumatic Spinal Cord Injuries

In addition to the discoligamentous injuries already discussed, spinal cord lesions play an important prognostic role in patients with spine injuries. A distinction must be made between hemorrhagic and nonhemorrhagic spinal cord contusions. This differentiation is important because hemorrhagic contusions are typically associated with a poor neurologic outcome.

▸ **MRI.** Spinal cord contusions are evident on T2W sequences as hyperintense intramedullary lesions (▸ Fig. 2.67). The spinal cord signal abnormality can be either subtle and situated very distinctly at the level of the vertebral injury or occupy extensive cross-sectional areas of the cord and extend over several segmental levels. Attention should be paid to features of preexisting degenerative spinal canal stenosis (osteophytes, etc.) as these can result in cord contusion even after minor injuries. The degree of spinal cord signal abnormality (swelling, edema) correlates significantly with the ultimate prognosis. Intramedullary hemorrhage is evident as focal, sometimes only punctate alterations. Susceptibility-weighted sequences (DWI [diffusion weighted imaging], gradient echo [T2*W], or even FLAIR [fluid attenuated inversion recovery]) are therefore best suited to demonstrate intramedullary hemorrhage. Extensive intramedullary hemorrhage tends to be rare after trauma and raises the possibility of other conditions such as a cord tumor or vascular malformation but is associated with a severe neurologic deficit (symptoms of complete spinal cord injury), which aids in the diagnosis. The most severe form of traumatic cord damage is spinal cord disruption, which—provided the patient survives—is associated with spastic paraplegia or tetraplegia and the entire spectrum of autonomic dysfunction in addition to pain.

Sequelae resulting from traumatic spinal cord injuries include myelomalacia, syringohydromyelia, medullary cyst formation, tethered cord syndrome of varying degrees (posttraumatic synechiae of the thecal sac), and spinal cord atrophy.

2.2.10 Radiological Assessment after Surgery of the Spine

Indication and Value of Imaging Modalities

▸ **Radiography.** Survey radiography in standard projections is the primary modality for evaluating the postoperative spine. Improper placement of implants may thus be assessed before more sophisticated imaging procedures are undertaken. Additional functional studies of the spine can detect postoperative or adjacent degenerative instability, e.g., in adjacent segments after long-segment fusions. Provided the examination has been correctly performed, displacement in the sagittal plane by more than 3.5 mm or angulation of the adjacent level by more than 11° are considered signs of segmental instability.

▸ **Myelography.** With the ever improving availability of MRI, myelography in the postoperative patient increasingly serves as a back-up modality, especially in patients who are unable to undergo an MRI examination. In the late postoperative phase it may be a supportive diagnostic tool for identifying scar formation, e.g., in what is known as postnucleotomy syndrome. With the option of performing dynamic, "functional," examinations, myelography is also well suited for demonstrating postoperative instability and secondary segmental hypermobility and their effect on cerebrospinal spaces and neural structures.

▸ **CT.** CT provides high-resolution depiction of bony structures and assessment of the location of implants. Secondary reconstructions with bone and soft tissue technique should be generated in all cases. Evaluation of the soft tissues, especially in the spinal canal, is limited in the postoperative setting. This can be improved by combining it with myelography (CT myelography). CT angiography is indicated for vascular issues (e.g., injury to the vertebral artery during surgery of the cervical spine). All paravertebral structures included on the images (e.g., pneumothorax secondary to lung injuries) must also be assessed.

▸ **MRI.** MRI is the best method for evaluating soft tissue structures of the spine. This applies to the spinal canal when looking for hemorrhage, recurrent disk extrusion, spinal canal injuries, myelopathy, or inflammatory conditions, as well as in assessing paravertebral soft tissues for hematoma, inflammatory changes, musculoligamentous injuries, or vascular issues (often with the aid of MR angiography). The ability to assess bone marrow is especially useful for demonstrating postoperative vertebral body edema or in cases of secondary fractures. The MRI protocol includes at least sagittal T1W and T2W sequences, axial T2W, and fat-suppressed coronal and/or sagittal T2W sequences. Obtaining additional heavily T2-weighted 3D sequences with MIP (maximum intensity projection) reconstructions can be helpful ("MR myelography"). Within the first 2 to 4 weeks postoperatively, intravenous contrast administration often leads to difficulties in interpretation due to postoperative changes and should therefore only be administered in specific situations, e.g., for suspected infection or abscess formation. Fat-suppressed sequences are often limited due to field heterogeneity caused by metallic implants, so other techniques such as inversion recovery (STIR) or subtraction imaging may be helpful. Susceptibility-weighted sequences are useful for suspected hemorrhage, and DWI sequences for suspected ischemia.

Complications of Spinal Surgery

Direct sequelae. This refers to postoperative complications involving the structures surrounding the spine, such as adjacent neurovascular structures (▶ Fig. 2.70). In the cervicothoracic region, the trachea, the esophagus (▶ Fig. 2.71), or the pleural cavity may be affected by direct trauma or indirectly as a result of swelling or space-occupying hematomas.

Indirect sequelae. These include malpositioning or loosening of surgical implants and their effect on bony structures, iatrogenic instability caused by extensive resection of the posterior elements, and cement leakage during cement augmentations.

In the **late postoperative stage**, infection of the vertebrae, disks, paravertebral space, and especially within the spinal canal poses a challenge for diagnostic examinations.

After fusion of vertebral segments, accelerated degeneration develops in adjacent motion segments due to mechanical overuse and altered biomechanics ("junctional disease").

Adjacent segment instability in its proper sense refers to the detection of pathologic hypermobility of motion segments above and below a fusion. It does not develop immediately after surgery but usually appears years later and is more commonly situated above the fused segments.

The diagnostic value of lateral flexion/extension studies is controversial because hypermobility is underestimated if movement is limited by pain and, conversely, translational movements of 4 mm are found in up to one-third of asymptomatic persons.

See the specialized literature for the complex topic of postoperative symptoms secondary to scarring (**postnucleotomy syndrome**).

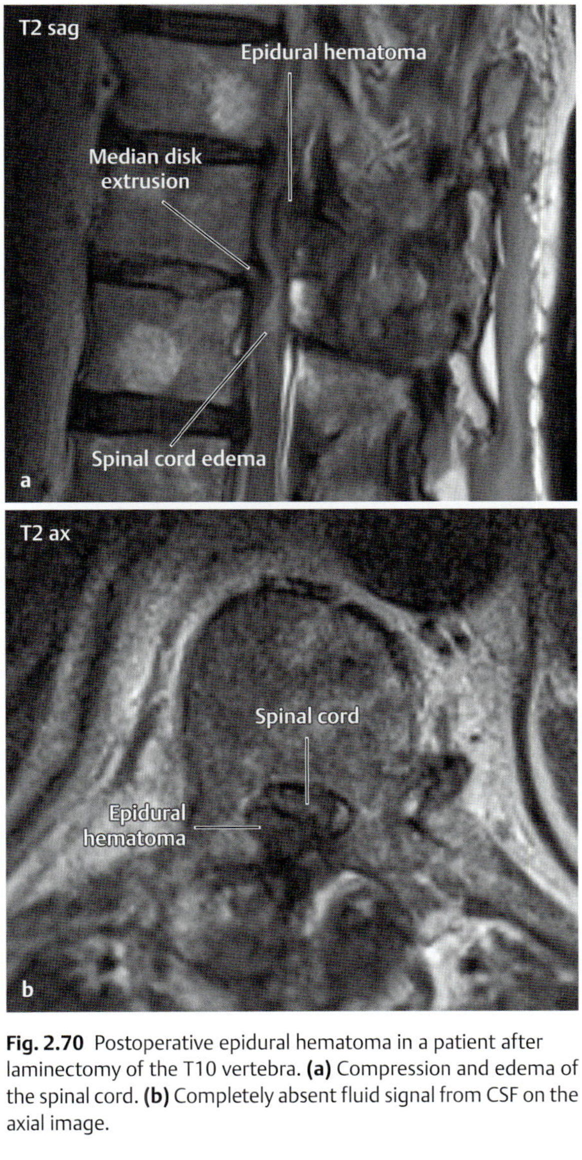

Fig. 2.70 Postoperative epidural hematoma in a patient after laminectomy of the T10 vertebra. **(a)** Compression and edema of the spinal cord. **(b)** Completely absent fluid signal from CSF on the axial image.

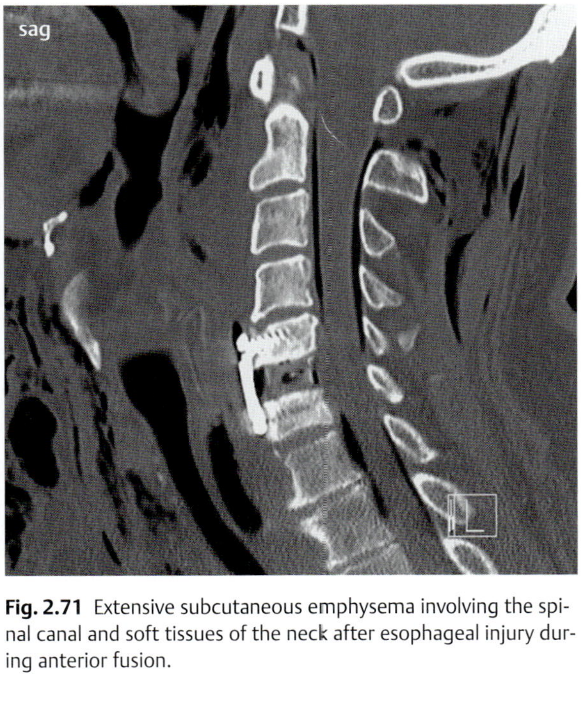

Fig. 2.71 Extensive subcutaneous emphysema involving the spinal canal and soft tissues of the neck after esophageal injury during anterior fusion.

Expressions Used by Surgeons

Posterior approach to the spinal canal. The classic approaches for disk surgery are *access via interlaminar windowing (ILW)* without the need to resect bony structures and, alternatively, *extended interlaminar window (eILW)*. The term refers to extension of bony access to the spinal canal in addition to resection of the ligamentum flavum, sometimes extended even further for a *medial facetotomy*. *Hemilaminectomy*—the unilateral resection of the lamina of the vertebral arch—may be necessary in cases of more extensive disk sequestration or bony stenosis of the spinal canal; the spinous process remains untouched. A *laminectomy* involves the complete resection of the posterior vertebral elements together with removal of the spinous process.

Fusion procedures. Procedures which are intended to create a permanent bony union of two vertebrae are included in the term "fusion." Established procedures here are *anterior lumbar interbody fusion (ALIF), posterior lumbar interbody fusion (PLIF), transforaminal interbody lumbar fusion (TLIF)*, and *extreme lateral interbody fusion (XLIF)*, which differ in their respective approaches (see specialist literature).

Posterior instrumentation. This term describes posterior stabilization with the aid of an internal fixator.

Postoperative Assessment of the Position of Spinal Implants

Disk implants. The majority of implants have radiopaque markers that allow assessment of their position relative to the adjacent vertebrae, especially relative to the anterior and posterior margins, on survey radiographs. For evaluation of individual implants, consider consulting a surgeon or obtaining information from the manufacturer.

Cages and vertebral body replacement. Tilting or even penetration of cages or vertebral replacements into the adjacent vertebral end plates must be noted (▶ Fig. 2.72). This is particularly relevant in spines weakened by osteoporosis and not stabilized by other means, where progressive penetration by implants can ensue. Implants that are not flush with the adjacent end plates can result in progressive malalignment and should be documented.

Screws. "Suboptimal" screw positioning—such as penetration of the anterior vertebral cortex by a few millimeters; a lateral rather than concentrically medial course of the screw in the vertebral body; or injury to the medial or lateral pedicle wall—is generally of no clinical relevance. On the other hand, extrapedicular malposition of the screws through the spinal canal should be reported as it will usually require revision. Screws that impinge on the course of vessels must be mentioned and may need to be examined further by supplementary CT angiography (▶ Fig. 2.73). A lucent rim of more than 2 mm with sclerotic margins and/or a change of direction or penetration into the end plate over time suggest screw loosening (▶ Fig. 2.74).

Cement. Cement leakage into intervertebral spaces becomes possible as soon as the cement abuts the end plates of the vertebra (see ▶ Fig. 2.74c). Mild cement leakage into the paravertebral space, paravertebral veins, or the epidural venous plexus is usually asymptomatic, whereas leakage into the spinal canal with a space-occupying effect or leakage into the venous system as far as the vena cava or the azygos/hemiazygos venous system, with the associated risk of pulmonary embolism, is to be regarded as a complication (▶ Figs. 2.75 and ▶ W2.7).

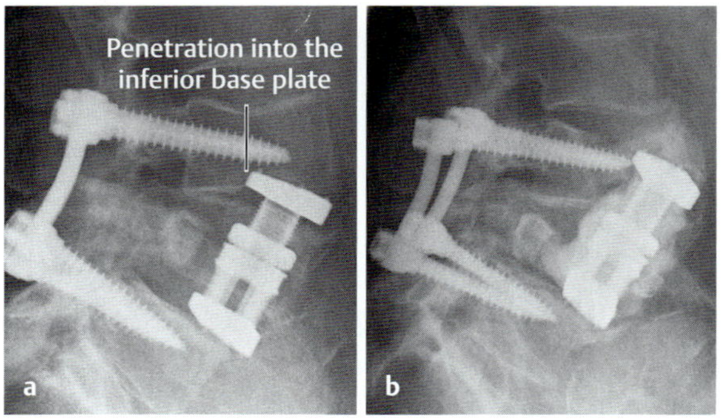

Fig. 2.72 Implant migration following vertebral replacement and posterior instrumentation. **(a)** The superior margin of the vertebral replacement device does not run parallel to the inferior base plate and is impacted into the plate. **(b)** Follow-up after 5 months: despite the use of cement, migration of the vertebral replacement has occurred with subsequent destruction of the overlying vertebra.

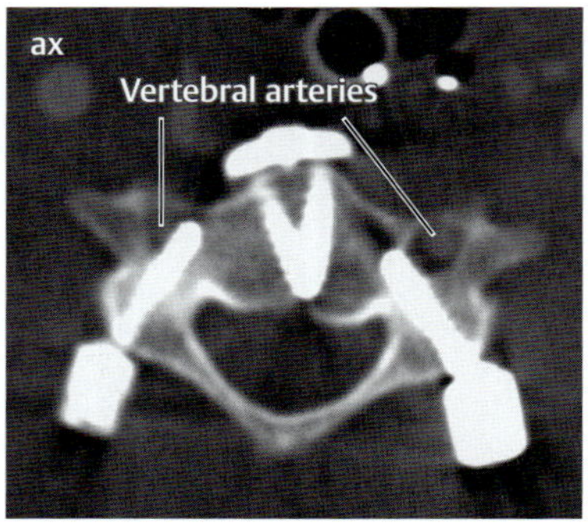

Fig. 2.73 Pedicle screw. The course of the right pedicle screw puts the vertebral artery at risk. CT angiography.

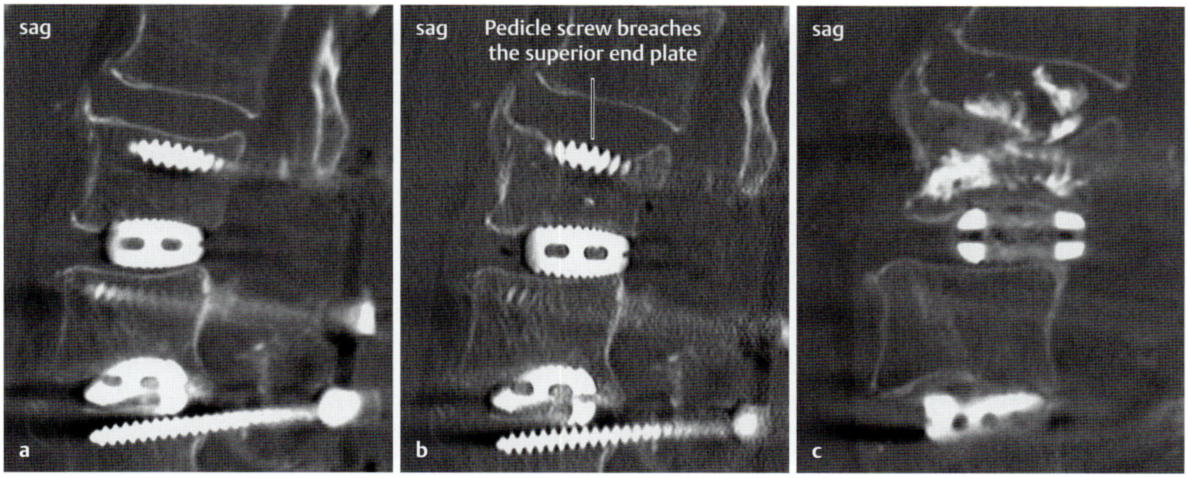

Fig. 2.74 Complications after posterior lumbar interbody fusion and dorsal instrumentation at L2–3 and L3–4. **(a)** Unremarkable postoperative CT. **(b)** Follow-up 2 weeks later: superior end plate insufficiency fracture at L2 with breakthrough of a pedicle screw. **(c)** After vertebroplasty: cement leakage into the disk space as far as the inferior end plate of L1.

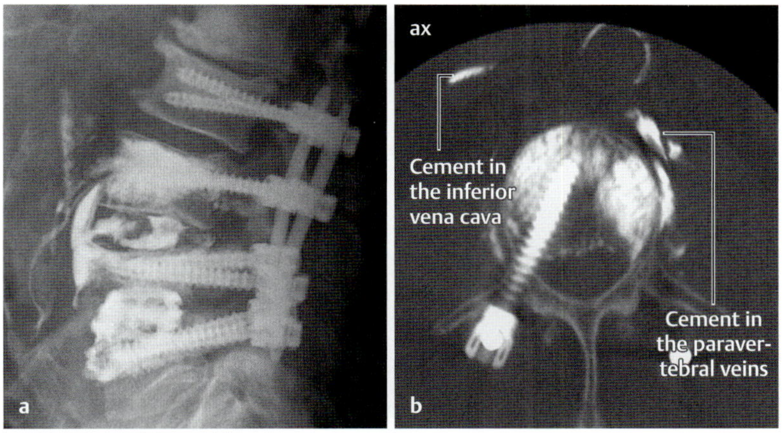

Fig. 2.75 Cement leakage as a complication after posterior instrumentation with cement-augmented pedicular screws. Fig. W2.7 shows the chest radiograph of a patient with multiple pulmonary artery cement emboli. **(a)** Considerable leakage of cement into paravertebral and prevertebral vessels. **(b)** CT scan confirms cement in the inferior vena cava.

2.3 Pelvis

2.3.1 Fractures of the Pelvic Ring

▸ **Anatomy.** See Chapter 2.3.1 including ▸ Fig. W2.8.

▸ **Pathology.** Injuries to the pelvic ring usually result from falls or direct impact injury. Whereas minor injuries predominate at an older age, pelvic ring fractures in younger patients are usually the result of high-energy trauma. Consequently, a host of associated injuries should be expected and are often the reason for the high mortality associated with complex pelvic fractures. Typical associated injuries include injuries to the genitourinary tract with bladder rupture and urethral avulsion, and vascular damage.

The most established classification system for pelvic ring fractures, the **AO classification**, is based on the classification by **Tile**, who subdivides the fractures into three groups:

- Stable fractures.
- Rotationally unstable fractures.
- Rotationally and vertically unstable fractures.

The history of the injury with regard to energy and force vector are important features in addition to the imaging findings (see Radiography and CT).

Classification

Type A: stable fractures of the pelvic ring (▸ Fig. 2.76).

- *A1:* Fractures of this type result from spontaneous violent muscle contractions and are most commonly found in adolescent athletes (▸ Fig. 2.77).
- *A2:* These are fractures of the iliac wing or fractures of the anterior pelvic ring and are usually due to a lateral compression injury. The CT scan often reveals associated compression fractures of the anterior sacrum. These A2 fractures typically do not become unstable (▸ Fig. 2.78).
- *A3:* These are transverse fractures of the inferior end of the sacrum, including the coccyx.

Type B: Fractures with rotational instability but preserved vertical stability (▸ Fig. 2.79).

- *B1:* Unilateral external rotation injury with disruption of the symphysis pubis. The trauma impact mostly comes from anterior impact, so that the hemipelvises are forced apart (referred to as an open-book injury). A classic example of this injury is that of a motorcyclist involved in a head-on collision that results in the two halves of the pelvis being separated by the bike's tank at the time of impact (▸ Figs. 2.80 and ▸ 2.81).
- *B2: Unilateral* internal rotation injury with disruption of the symphysis pubis and overriding of the anterior pelvic ring. The impact comes from the side, causing the struck side of the pelvic to rotate inward. This results in a fracture of the anterior pelvic ring with internal rotation of the involved half of the pelvis. Here too, the opposing hemipelvises are forced apart, potentially resulting in disruption of the sacroiliac joints anteriorly due to rupture of the anterior sacroiliac ligaments. A typical example is a side-impact collision into the driver-side door of a car.
- *B3:* Bilateral rotational instability due to bilateral B1 or B2 injuries.

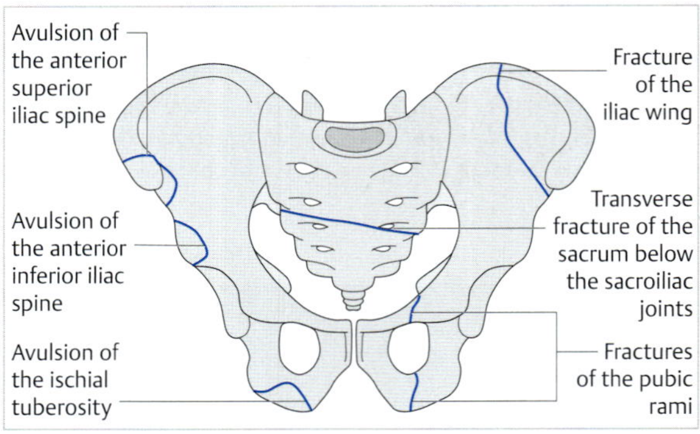

Fig. 2.76 Fractures of Types A1–3. For further details see the text.

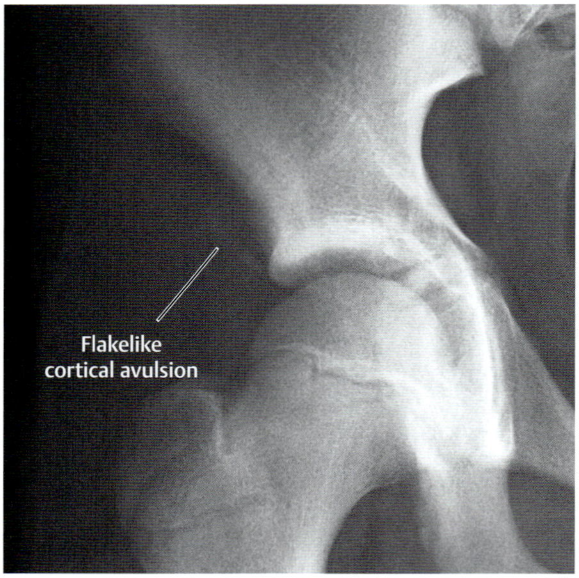

Fig. 2.77 Avulsion fracture at the anterior inferior iliac spine (Type A1) due to traction of the rectus femoris.

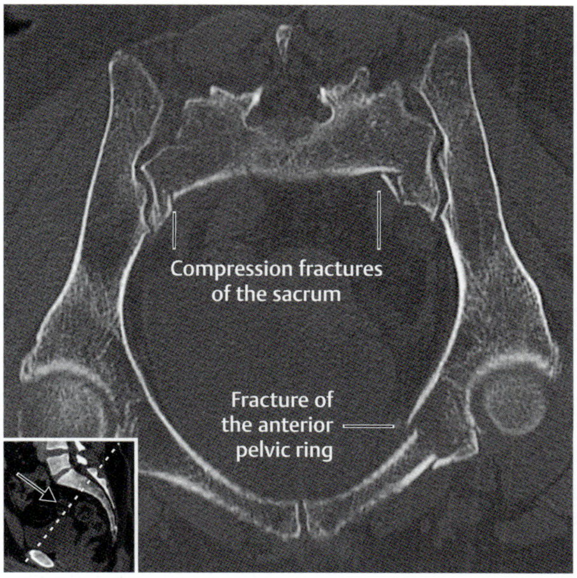

Fig. 2.78 Type A2 fracture. Fracture of the anterior pelvic ring with associated anterior compression fracture of the sacrum; no instability. Oblique-axial reconstruction CT; for slice level see the small inset image.

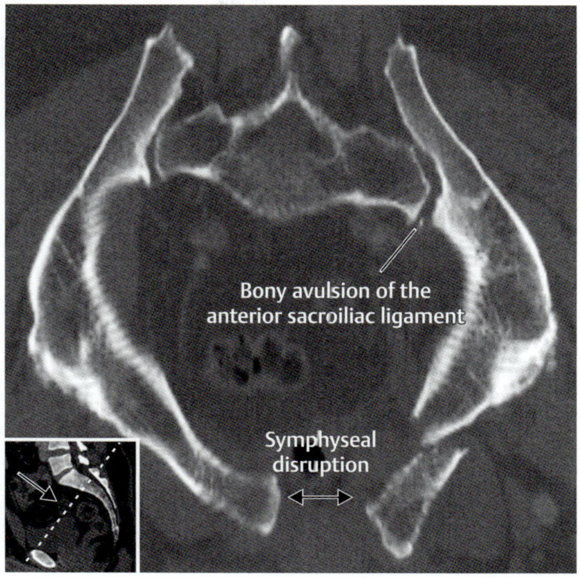

Fig. 2.81 Open-book injury (Type B1). Anterior gaping of the right sacroiliac joint.

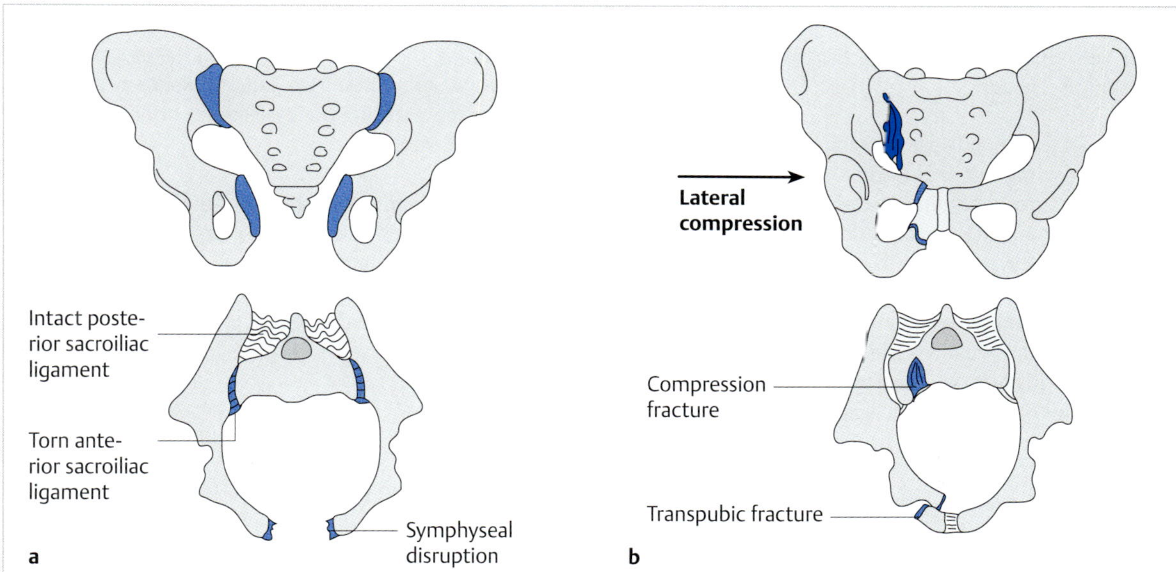

Fig. 2.79 Type B injuries. **(a)** Type B1 injury (open book) due to impact force in a sagittal plane; rotational instability. **(b)** Type B2 injury due to lateral compression; rotational instability.

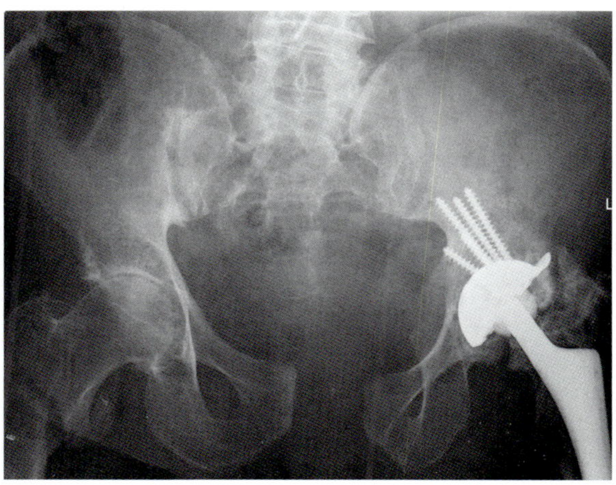

Fig. 2.80 Open-book injury (Type B1).

2

Type C: Fractures with combined rotational and vertical instability. These injuries are commonly caused by being run over or buried. Falls from very great heights can also result in complete disruption of the anterior and posterior pelvic ring:

- *C1:* This injury is associated with a complete disruption of one hemipelvis, with a stable contralateral side (▶ Figs. 2.82 and ▶ 2.83).
- *C2:* This is a Type C1 injury of one hemipelvis combined with a Type B injury of the contralateral side.
- *C3:* This is a bilateral Type C1 injury (▶ Fig 2.84).

One fracture type not included in the AO classification system is the suicidal jumper's fracture, in which an axial compression injury results in separation of the spinal column from the pelvis (▶ Fig. 2.85).

Imaging

▶ **Radiography.** Despite the current widespread availability of CT imaging, AP views of the pelvis are still the first study obtained not only for acute assessment but also because they can be used for comparison with postoperative radiographs. Inlet views of the pelvis allow for assessment of AP and rotational malalignment of the pelvic ring, while the outlet view demonstrates any vertical malalignment of the pelvic ring (▶ Fig. 2.86).

▶ **CT.** Apart from nondisplaced fractures of the anterior pelvic ring following minimal trauma and typical apophyseal avulsion fractures, CT is typically indicated for all pelvic fractures and multiplanar reconstructions should always be generated. When evaluating the CT, attention should be paid to the course of the fractures as well as to indirect signs of instability such as widening of one or both sacroiliac joints. Small bony avulsions from the caudal sacrum correspond in the majority of cases to avulsion fractures of the sacrotuberous or sacrospinous ligaments and indicate vertical instability.

▶ **MRI.** MRI has no role in the diagnostic work-up of acute trauma to the bony pelvis but plays an important role in the detection of fatigue fractures (Chapter 2.3.3).

Stress-Related Apophyseal Avulsion Fractures

Apophyseal avulsions may result from a single injury or from chronic repetitive microtrauma in athletes. This affects primarily the ischial tuberosity (origin of the hamstrings), the anterior inferior iliac spine (rectus femoris; see ▶ Fig. 2.77), anterior superior iliac spine (sartorius and tensor fasciae latae), and less frequently also the pubic bone (adductors). An avulsion fracture of the lesser trochanter (iliopsoas) is also possible, especially in the younger patient. Untreated apophyseal injuries can result in exuberant ossification that may resemble that of a cartilaginous exostosis (osteochondroma) or other bone-forming tumor.

▶ **Radiography.** If the apophysis is already mineralized and sufficiently retracted then it can be readily seen on the radiograph.

▶ **US.** Separation of the apophyses can be easily evaluated by US in the majority of cases.

▶ **MRI.** An MRI scan will demonstrate edema of the apophyseal growth plate and the adjacent soft tissues.

2.3.2 Acetabular Fractures

Acetabular fractures are almost invariably the result of high energy trauma. The position of the femur in the hip joint at the time of the accident and the vector of the transmitted force determine the type of fracture.

▶ **Anatomy.** The acetabulum arises from the innominate bone (os coxa), which forms from three ossification centers: the ilium, ischium, and pubis. These three segments join at the tri-radiate cartilage, a Y-shaped synchondrosis centered on the acetabulum. Complete fusion of the innominate bone occurs in the late teens.

Seen from outside, the acetabulum is divided by a longer limb, forming the anterior column and a shorter one, the posterior column. These two columns serve as struts, mechanically representing the coalescence of bony trabeculae along lines of stress.

The anterior column is composed of both pubic rami and a large portion of the ilium, extending from the iliac crest down the iliac wing and through the superior pubic ramus towards the pubic symphysis. The posterior column is composed mainly of the ischium and a small part of the ilium.

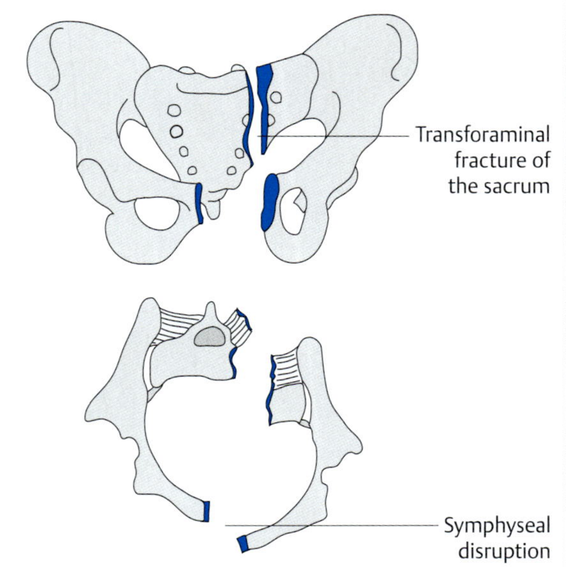

Fig. 2.82 Type C1 injury. Combined rotational and vertical instability; complete dissociation of the left hemipelvis.

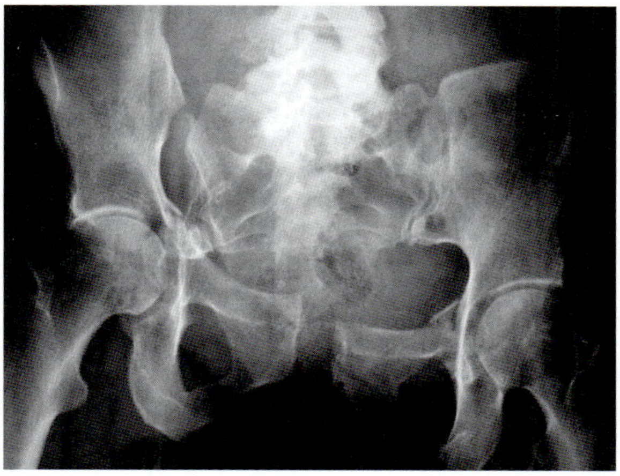

Fig. 2.83 Type C1 injury with vertically displaced separation of the sacroiliac joint plus symphysis disruption. In addition, there is an anterior pelvic ring fracture on the left side.

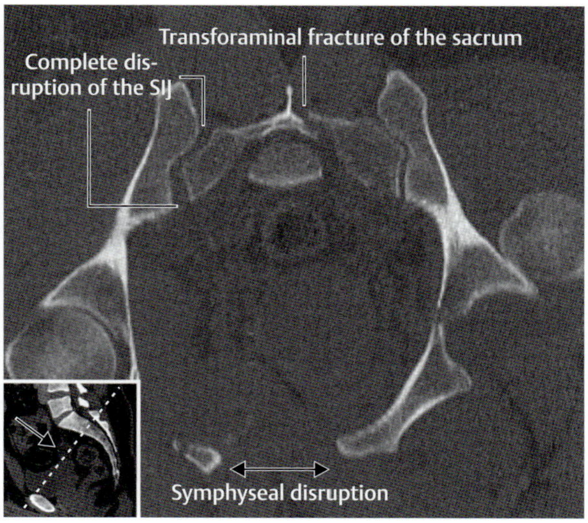

Fig. 2.84 Type C3 fracture with bilateral complete disruption of the posterior pelvic ring and symphysis diastasis. There is additional posterior dislocation of the left femoral head. For slice level see the small inset image. SIJ, sacroiliac joint.

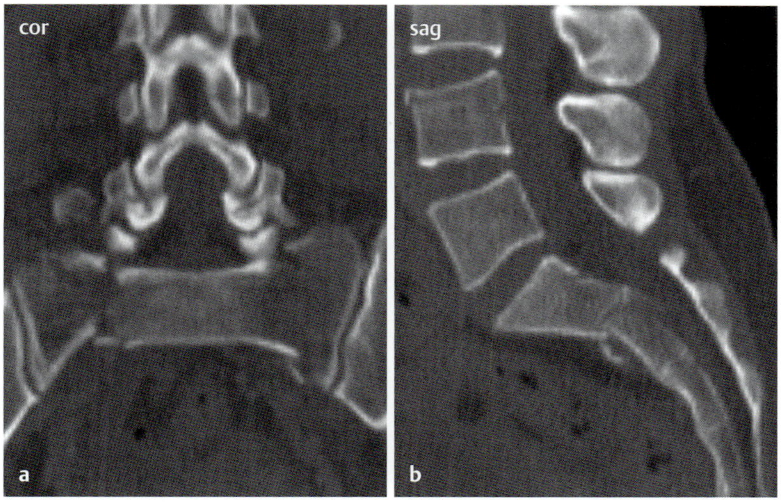

Fig. 2.85 Suicidal jumper's fracture. Axial compression forces the spine out of the sacrum. **(a)** Bilateral longitudinal fracture of the sacrum. **(b)** Combined with a transverse fracture of the sacrum.

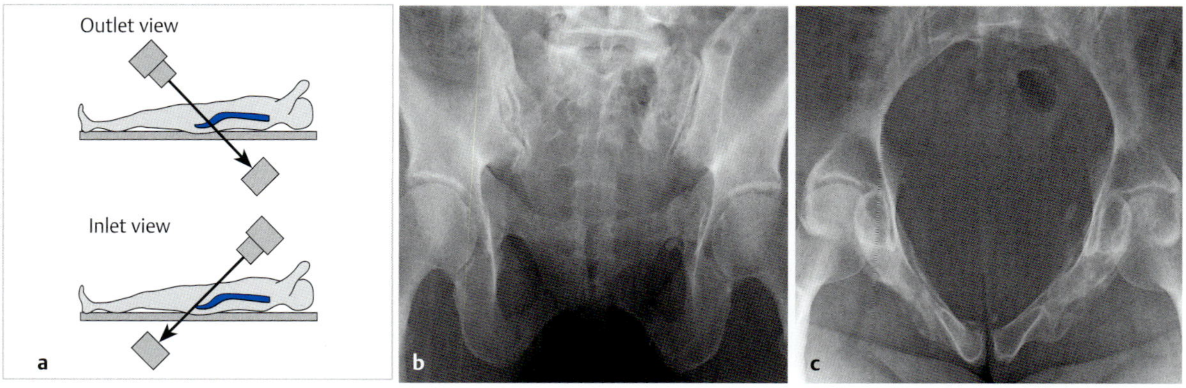

Fig. 2.86 Inlet and outlet views of the pelvis. **(a)** Schematic diagram. **(b)** Outlet view. **(c)** Inlet view.

The anterior and posterior acetabular walls are outward projections of their respective columns.

The **AO classification** of acetabulum fractures (▸ Fig. 2.87) is closely based on the classification proposed by **Judet and Letournel** (▸ Fig. W2.9), which takes into account the embryonic development of the acetabulum and distinguishes between anterior and posterior columns (see Anatomy above).

- **Type A fracture:** Only one column is involved; the main part of the joint is intact.
- **Type B fracture:** Involvement of both columns; one part of the acetabular roof remains attached to the ilium.
- **Type C fracture:** Complete detachment of the acetabulum from the ilium; both columns are involved.

▸ **Radiography.** Conventional radiographs are still used to evaluate acetabular fractures despite the availability of CT. In addition to the AP radiograph, iliac and obturator oblique (Judet) views are obtained. Classification is best done using these projections (▸ Figs. 2.88 and ▸ W2.10).

Caution

The term "both-column fracture" often leads to a misunderstanding. This is a clearly defined entity and does not mean that the fracture involves both columns. Instead, the classic both-column fracture involves a **separation** of both columns and discontinuity of all weight-bearing parts of the acetabulum from the posterior pelvic ring (▸ Fig. 2.89). The classic cause of a both-column fracture is a lateral collision trauma. The femoral head takes virtually all parts of the acetabulum medially with it, resulting in a central dislocation of the head of the femur; all articular fragments remain more or less congruent with the femoral head (see ▸ Fig. 2.89). The phenomenon is known as "secondary congruence." The medial dislocation of the acetabulum brings the ilium into profile on the obturator view, giving rise to the spur sign, which is pathognomonic for a both-column fracture (▸ Figs. 2.90 and ▸ W2.11).

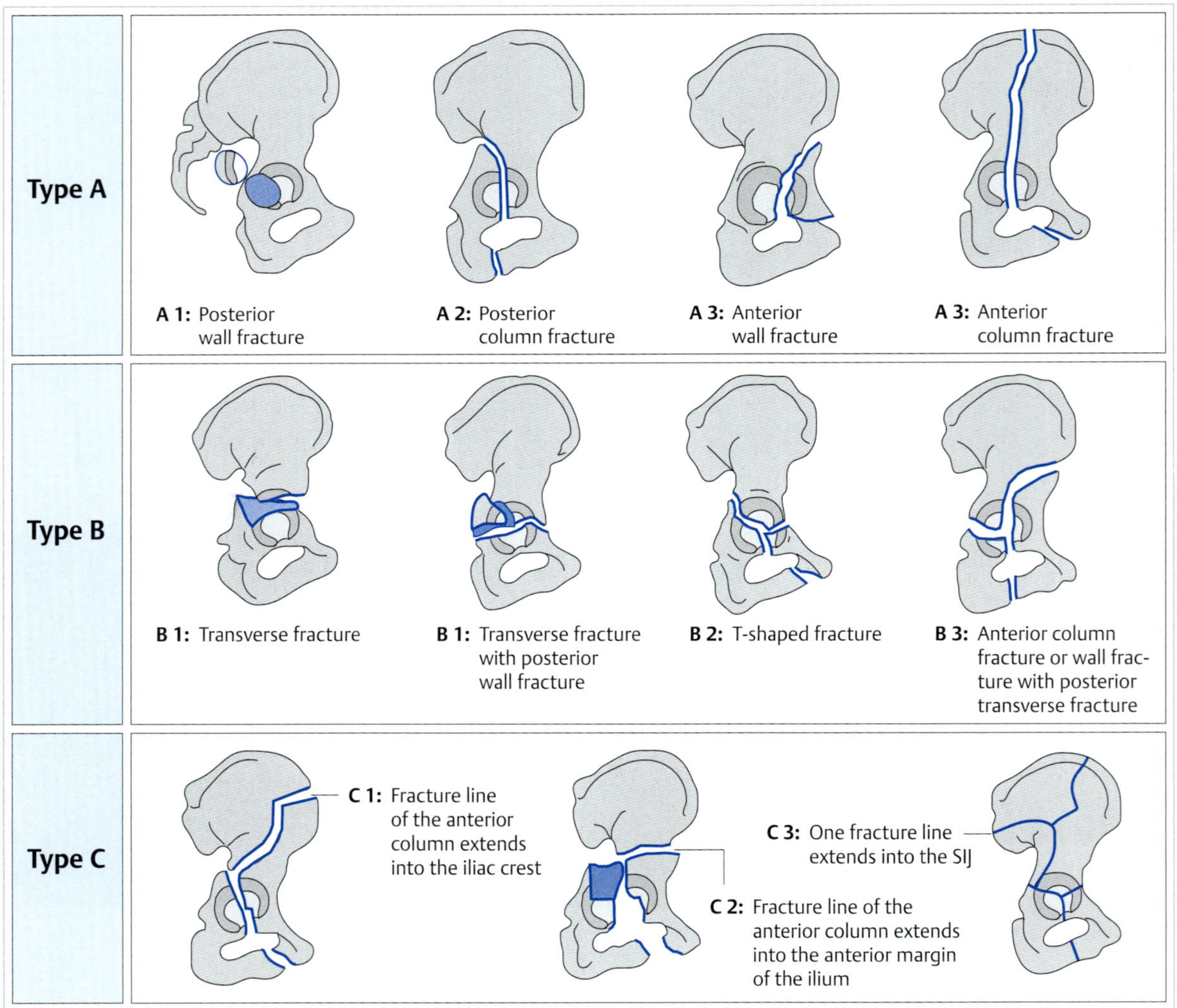

Fig. 2.87 AO classification of acetabular fractures. SIJ, sacroiliac joint.

▸ **CT.** Currently, CT is an integral part of the diagnostic investigation of acetabular fractures. Although fracture classification is more difficult using CT, it provides for detailed assessment of fracture morphology. Small fragments that become entrapped in the joint space are readily evident (▸ Fig. 2.91). CT is also of crucial importance for optimal preoperative planning.

2.3.3 Fatigue Fractures of the Pelvis

Fatigue fractures of the pelvis occur predominantly at the pubic rami and the parasymphyseal region. Stress fractures of the sacrum are also found in children, athletes, and pregnant women (▸ Fig. 2.92); osteoporosis-related insufficiency fractures also occur frequently at this location. Other common sites for an insufficiency fracture include the supra-acetabular region, the ilium, the pubic rami, and the parasymphyseal bone.

Changes due to insufficiency fractures are often very subtle on conventional radiographs and are easily overlooked. CT and especially MRI are very well suited for detecting these fractures. Sacral insufficiency fractures (unilateral or bilateral) typically display vertical fracture lines near to the sacroiliac joint. Horizontal fracture lines are also found in the midsacrum (known as the H-pattern or Honda sign; ▸ Fig. 2.93).

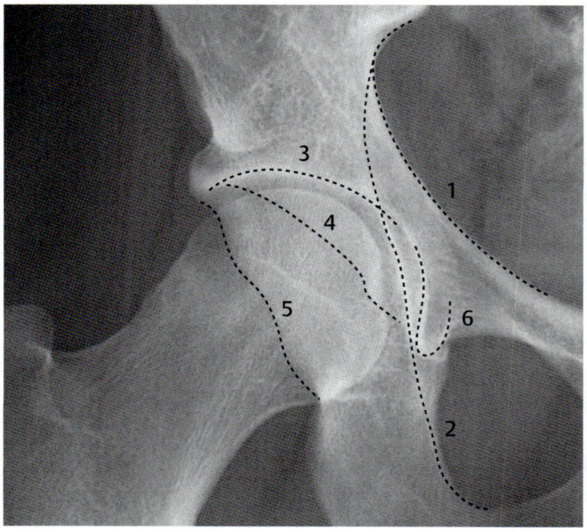

Fig. 2.88 Reference lines of the acetabulum on the AP projection. 1, iliopectineal line (anterior column); 2, ilioischial line (posterior column); 3, acetabular roof; 4, anterior acetabular rim; 5, posterior acetabular rim; 6, Koehler's teardrop.

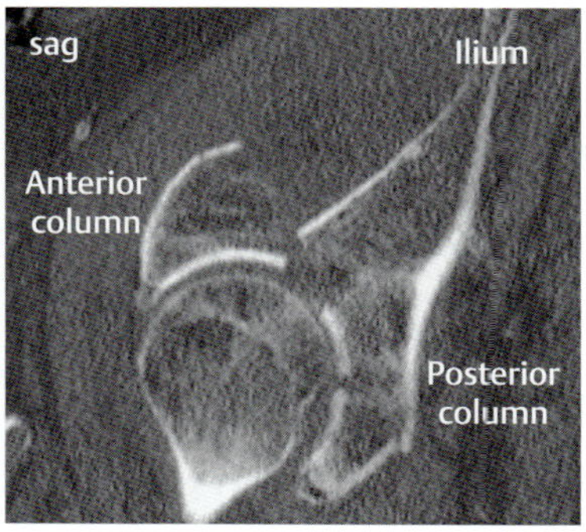

Fig. 2.89 Both-column fracture. All weight-bearing parts are dissociated from the posterior pelvic ring.

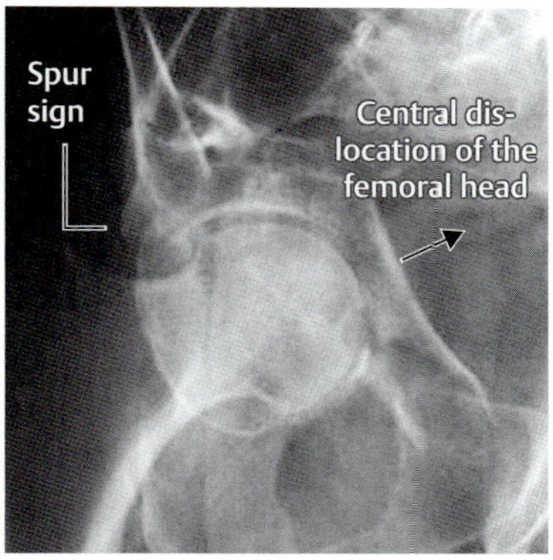

Fig. 2.90 Spur sign of the both-column fracture.

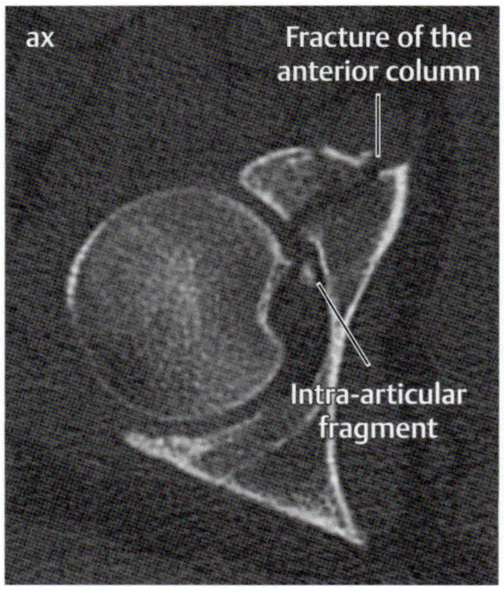

Fig. 2.91 Anterior column fracture. The CT scan demonstrates a loose joint body.

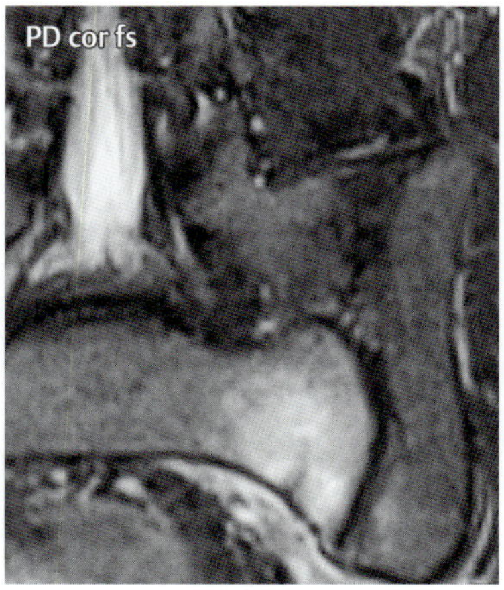

Fig. 2.92 Sacral fracture in a pregnant patient. MRI. This is most likely a combination of insufficiency and fatigue fractures.

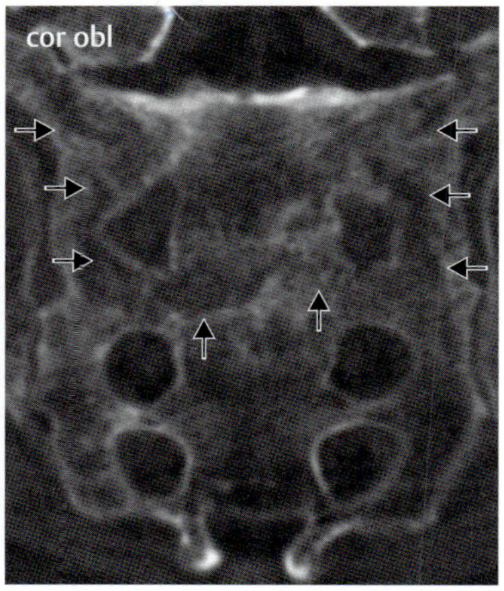

Fig. 2.93 Osteoporotic insufficiency fractures of the sacrum. Also termed "H fracture" because of the course of the fractures (arrows). Oblique coronal MPR (multiplanar reformatting) from one CT dataset.

2.3.4 Hip Dislocation/Fracture Dislocations of the Hip

Dislocation of the hip joint is usually due to high-energy axial compression. Hip dislocations also occur from extreme muscle convulsions, such as during an epileptic seizure or an electrical accident. We differentiate between various types of dislocation (posterior: iliac and ischiadic; anterior: pubic and obturator).

In rare cases fracture of the femoral head may occur during dislocation of the hip joint, either in the form of an avulsion fracture of the ligamentum teres or in the form of a shearing fracture related to the posterior acetabular rim. Such fractures of the femoral head are classified according to **Pipkin** (▶ Fig. 2.94).

CT is essential for assessing Pipkin fractures and provides the only method for correctly assessing the size of the sheared fragment and of the defect within the femoral head (▶ Fig. W2.12).

2.3.5 Pubalgia (Osteitis Pubis)

▶ **Anatomy.** ▶ See Chapter 2.3.5 including ▶ Fig. W2.13.

▶ **Pathology.** Osteitis (symphysitis) pubis is a chronic overuse injury of the symphysis and the adjacent pubic rami. This stress reaction may also be associated with adductor pathology. It is often the cause of groin pain in athletes and affects football players in particular.

> **Caution**
> The majority of patients (athletes) with osteitis pubis present with the clinical diagnosis "inguinal hernia."

▶ **Radiography/CT.** The appearance depends on the chronicity of the stress reaction. Initially, resorptive changes may predominate, in which case the joint space is widened (▶ Figs. 2.95a and ▶ 2.96). In more chronic cases, subchondral sclerosis and osteophytes predominate, often with joint space narrowing (▶ Fig. 2.95b).

▶ **MRI.** MRI allows differentiation of osteitis pubis from adductor injuries and other causes of groin pain.

Findings in osteitis pubis:

- Increased signal intensity on water-sensitive sequences or enhancement (after IV administration of gadolinium) in the bones adjacent to the symphysis and in the symphyseal joint space (▶ Fig. 2.97).
- Concomitant involvement of the adjacent adductor entheses (in ~ 60% of cases; see ▶ Fig. 2.97).
- Osteophytes.
- Cysts or geodes (in ~ 80% of cases; ▶ Fig. 2.98)
- Erosions at the insertions of the pubic ligament.
- So-called secondary cleft sign (a bright line between bone and the joint space; ▶ Fig. 2.99).

▶ **US.** Ultrasound is helpful for injuries of the nearby tendon insertions of the rectus abdominis and the adductors but is unable to demonstrate stress changes within the bones.

▶ **DD.**

Infections. In cases of infection, MRI should be used to detect intra-articular or para-articular abscesses (▶ Fig. 2.100). Laboratory results should also be examined.

Rheumatic disorders. Seronegative spondylarthropathies can also affect the symphysis. The underlying condition is almost always known, so there are rarely any differential diagnostic difficulties.

Inguinal hernia. A sound physical examination and, in some cases, the use of ultrasound should allow for accurate diagnosis.

Tendinopathy of the adductors or rectus abdominis. The use of ultrasound or MRI will provide an accurate diagnosis (▶ Fig. 2.101).

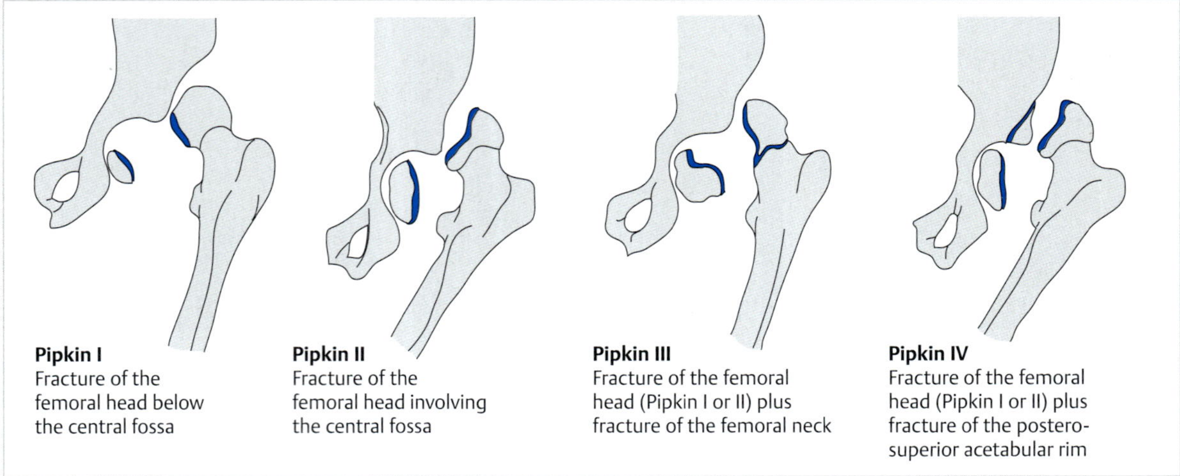

Fig. 2.94 Pipkin classification of dislocation fractures of the femoral head.

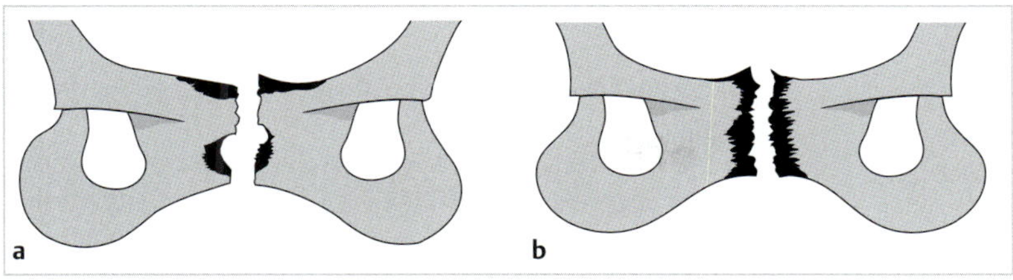

Fig. 2.95 Clinical forms of osteitis pubis. **(a)** Predominantly erosive changes with bone resorption, often in the early phase. **(b)** Increased sclerosis and osteophyte formations, commonly in the late phase.

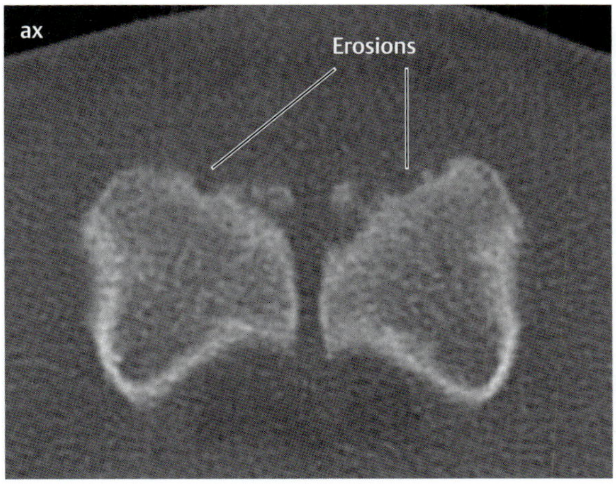

Fig. 2.96 Osteitis pubis with erosive changes and bone resorption anteriorly at the symphysis.

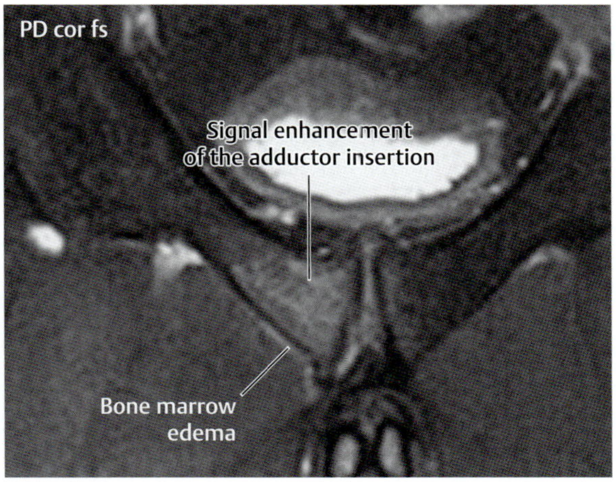

Fig. 2.97 Osteitis pubis.

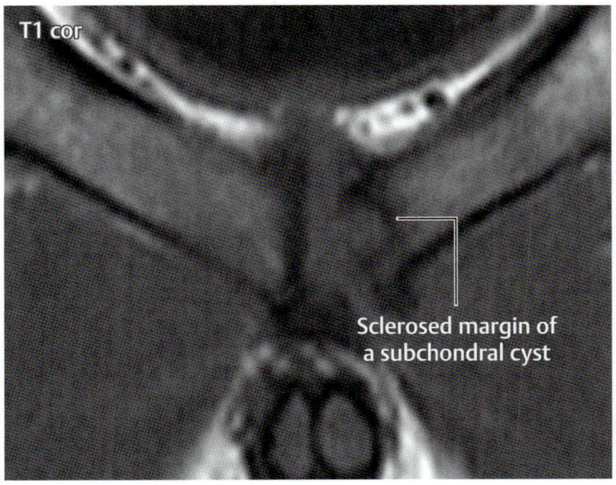

Fig. 2.98 Subchondral cyst (geode) in osteitis pubis.

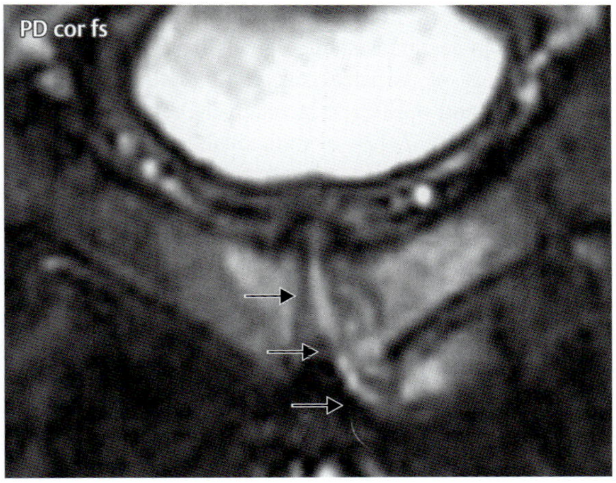

Fig. 2.99 Osteitis pubis. Hyperintense line (arrows) between bone and cartilage (secondary cleft sign). Osteophyte at the upper and lower margins of the left pubis.

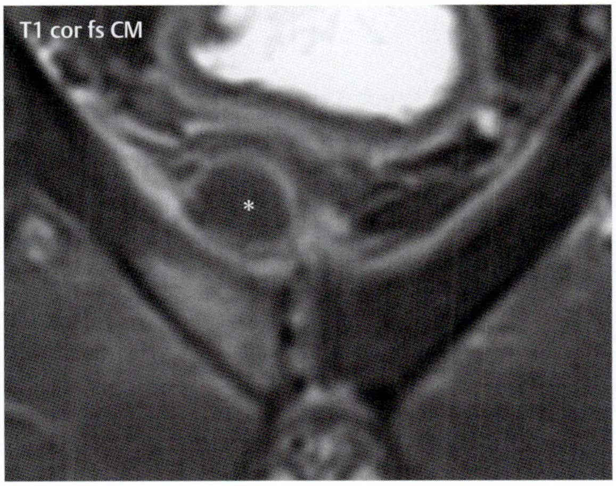

Fig. 2.100 Infectious symphysitis associated with parapubic abscess (asterisk).

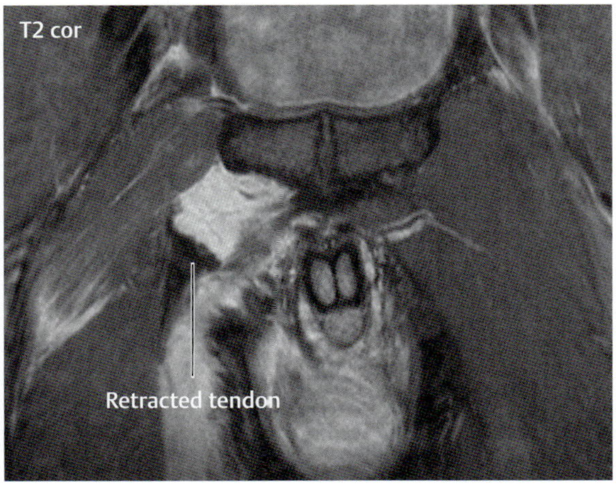

Fig. 2.101 Avulsion of the adductor tendon from the pubic bone.

2

2.4 Shoulder Joint

2.4.1 Anatomy, Variants, and Technique

▸**Anatomy.** See Chapter 2.4.1 including ▸Figs. W2.13–▸W2.19.

Variants

The **shape of the acromion** demonstrates considerable variation. The variants reported by Bigliani and Gagey (▸Fig. 2.102) refer to the differences in morphology of the acromion in the sagittal plane, but this provides an incomplete definition of the geometry of the subacromial space because of additional variation in acromial morphology in the coronal plane.

Os acromiale (▸Fig. 2.103) refers to a persistent ossification center of the anterior acromion. The finding occurs bilaterally in about 60% of cases and must not be mistaken for a fracture of the acromion. It should be kept in mind that fusion of the acromial ossification center is not complete until relatively late (between 21 and 25 years of age).

Anatomically, the **glenoid labrum** is a highly variable structure. Its cross-sectional shape ranges from triangular to round and is of variable size. A **sublabral foramen** (▸Figs. 2.104 and ▸2.105) is a relatively common normal variant (incidence: 7–12% of individuals). This refers to a lack of attachment of the labrum to the anterosuperior part at the glenoid (at the 1 to 3 o'clock position). A **"Buford complex"** refers to absence of the labrum in this region associated with a thickened, cordlike middle glenohumeral ligament, which may rarely insert on the long biceps tendon. This anomaly is less common, with an incidence of 1.5 to 2% (see ▸Fig. 2.104). The anteroinferior labrum is normal in both of these variants.

The anatomy of the **biceps tendon anchor** varies considerably. A firm attachment of the superior labrum to the glenoid margin is evident in only 30% of individuals (▸Fig. 2.106a). A sublabral cleft of variable depth (2–10 mm), lined with a synovial membrane, is commonly found and known as a sublabral recess (▸Fig. 2.106b). In the presence of a deep recess, the superior labrum may be meniscoid and hypermobile. A sublabral recess may extend anteriorly into a sublabral foramen.

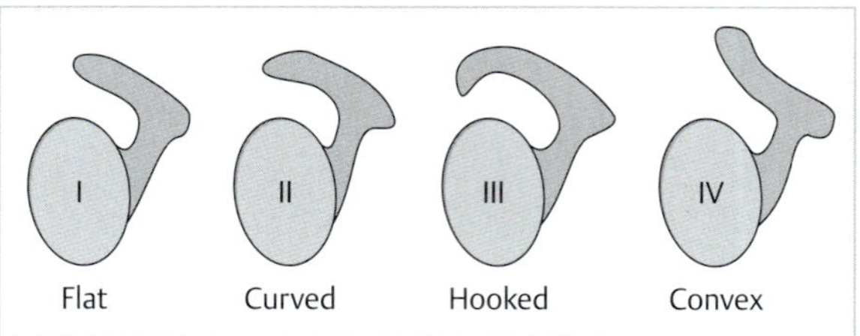

Fig. 2.102 Morphologic variants of the acromion according to Bigliani and Gagey.

Technique

The following rules should be observed for MRI of the shoulder:

- The examination should include **three planes**: *transverse*, *oblique coronal* (parallel to the supraspinatus tendon), and *oblique sagittal* (parallel to the surface of the glenoid surface).
- **Routine sequences** include a PDW sequence with fat saturation (oblique coronal, transverse), as well as a T1W (oblique coronal) and a T2W (oblique sagittal) FSE sequence (fast spin echo sequence). GRE sequences are reserved for special cases. The slice thickness should not exceed 3 mm.
- The arm should be placed in the **neutral position**.
- An advantage of an **additional sequence in abduction and external rotation (ABER position)** with MR arthrography is the better assessment of the anteroinferior labrum and anterior labroligamentous complex. For this position, the hand is placed behind the head or neck of the patient. Oblique sagittal slices parallel to the proximal humerus are then obtained.

Primary indications for MR arthrography (following the intra-articular injection of a gadolinium-containing solution)

- All forms of shoulder instability.
- Suspected SLAP lesion (superior labral anterior-to-posterior lesion; see relevant part of Chapter 2.4.6).
- Diagnostic work-up for shoulder pain in competitive athletes.

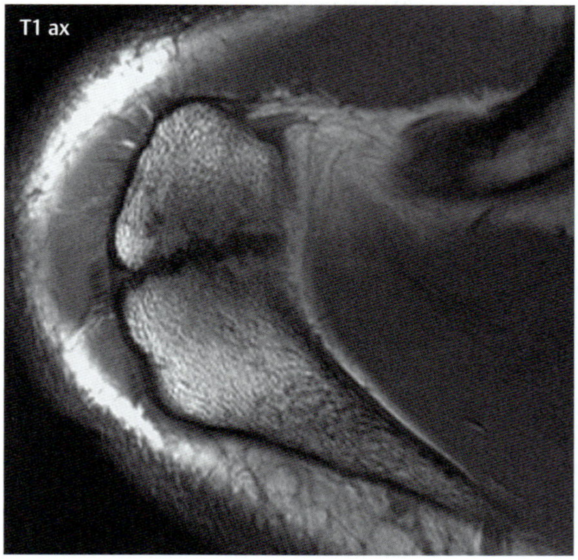

Fig. 2.103 Os acromiale.

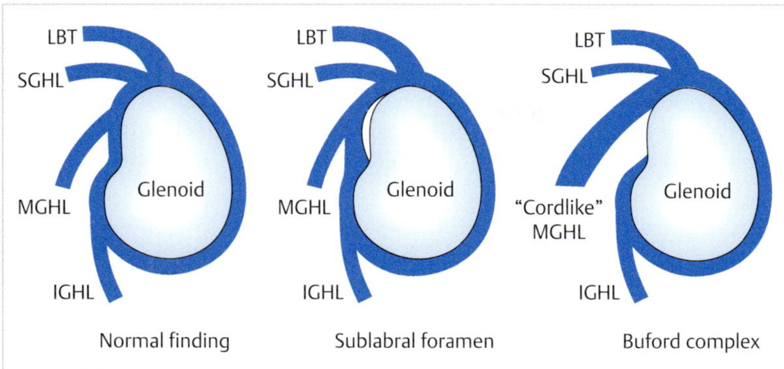

Fig. 2.104 Variants of the anterior glenoid labrum. Sagittal schematic diagrams. IGHL, inferior glenohumeral ligament; LBT, long biceps tendon; MGHL, middle glenohumeral ligament; SGHL, superior glenohumeral ligament.

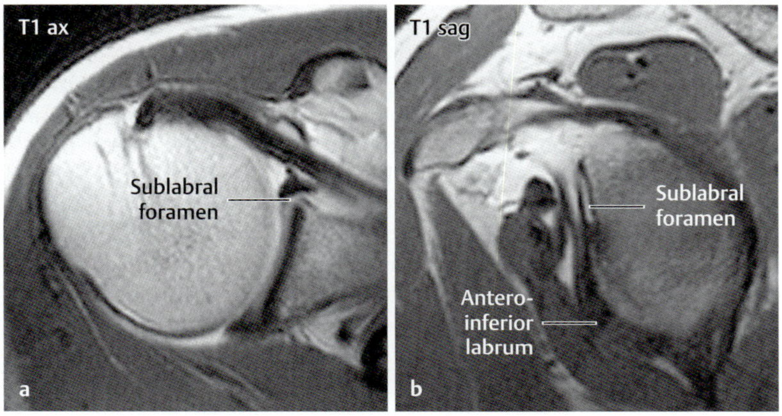

Fig. 2.105 Sublabral foramen. MR arthrography. **(a)** Transverse plane. **(b)** Coronal plane.

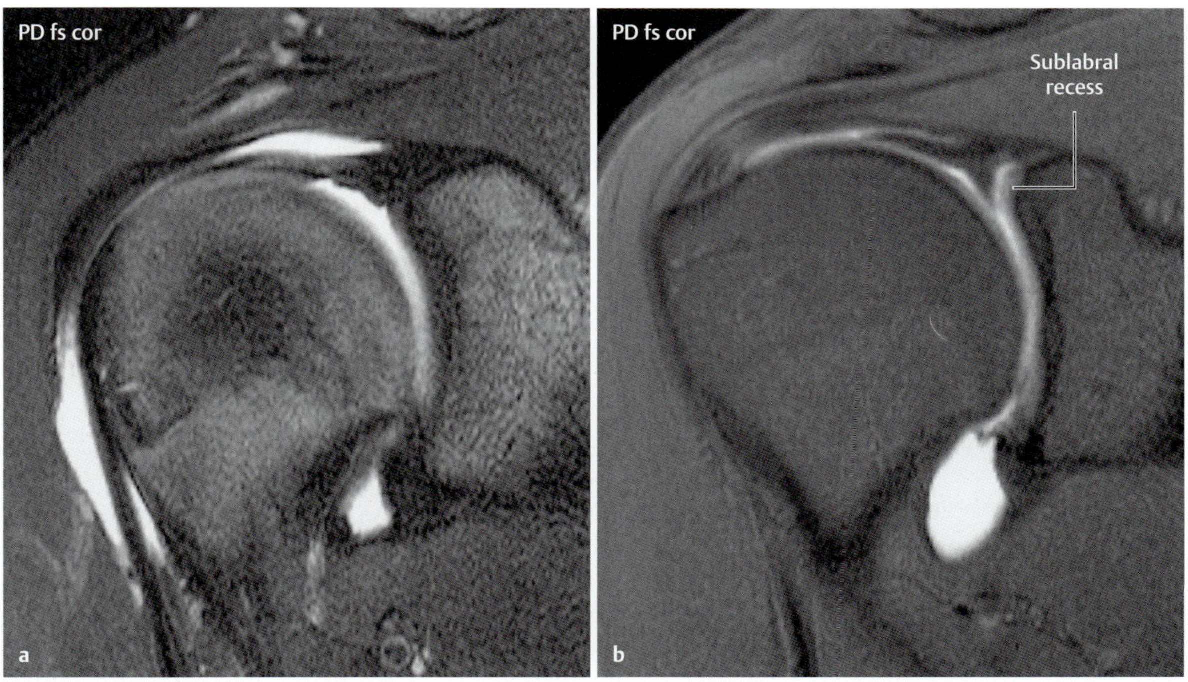

Fig. 2.106 Superior labrum and biceps anchor. MR arthrography. **(a)** Firm attachment. **(b)** Sublabral recess and meniscoid labrum.

2.4.2 Impingement

Impingement syndromes are among the most common types of pathology of the shoulder joint. A distinction is made between primary and secondary extrinsic, and secondary intrinsic impingement syndromes (▶ Table 2.2).

Primary Extrinsic Impingement

Subacromial Impingement

▶ Pathology. Primary extrinsic impingement (i.e., outlet impingement) is due to narrowing of the **subacromial** space. Impingement of the supraspinatus tendon and the subacromial bursa between the anterior acromion and the head of the humerus causes chronic bursitis and tendinopathy of the supraspinatus. A tendon tear may develop over time. Affected patients are typically older than 40 years of age and do not present with shoulder instability.

Predisposing factors for subacromial impingement include a Bigliani Type 3 acromion (see ▶ Fig. 2.102), subacromial osteophytes, a laterally downsloping acromion, a thickened coracoacromial ligament, and an (unstable) os acromiale. Osteoarthritis of the acromioclavicular joint with marked osteophytes and hypertrophy of the rotator cuff are rare causes.

▶ Clinical presentation. Classic symptoms are nocturnal pain, pain on elevation of the arm between 60 and 120° ("painful arc"), shoulder stiffness, and weakness.

▶ Radiography. Assessment of acromial morphology is best accomplished on an outlet view (SST [supraspinatus tendon] view, Neer view). Subacromial osteophytes are found at the anterior margin of the acromion in the region of the insertion of the coracoacromial ligament; strictly speaking, therefore, they are enthesophytes. Narrowing of the acromiohumeral interval to less than 7 mm is considered pathologic and is suggestive of a rotator cuff tear (▶ Fig. 2.107). Tendon calcification is not part of the subacromial impingement syndrome, but instead indicates calcific tendinitis secondary to calcium hydroxyapatite deposition disease (Chapter 10.9.3).

▶ MRI. Subacromial impingement is a clinical diagnosis. MRI (▶ Figs. 2.108 and ▶ 2.109) may demonstrate a typical constellation of findings but is unable to establish the diagnosis. The task of MRI is to define the stage of disease, especially with regard to rotator cuff integrity. Fluid-sensitive images may demonstrate increased fluid content and/or thickening of the wall of the subacromial bursa, which is often the only finding in early stages of the disorder. Over time, tendinopathy of the supraspinatus develops (Chapter 2.4.3). Thickening of the tendon will further narrow the subacromial space. Rotator cuff tears typically involve the anterior fibers of the supraspinatus tendon from where they can progress further. The morphology of the acromion can be well appreciated on oblique sagittal and oblique coronal views, while an os acromiale is best seen on transverse slices. Commonly reported, but less meaningful, findings include thickening or a convex course of the coracoacromial ligament and the absence of the subacromial fat pad.

▶ US. Ultrasound demonstrates thickening of the wall of the subacromial/subdeltoid bursa, which may be partially fluid-filled. A recognizable sign of subacromial impingement during abduction of the arm is a "ballooning" of the lateral part of the subdeltoid bursa, which results from fluid being pressed out of the medial part of the bursa as the bursa glides beneath the acromion. Signs of tendinopathy are thickening of the tendon, decreased and somewhat heterogeneous echogenicity, and loss of the normal fibrillar structure of the tendon; comparison with the contralateral side is sometimes helpful. Identification of tendinopathy, however, does not prove the presence of a subacromial impingement syndrome.

Table 2.2 Classification of impingement at the shoulder

Type	Etiology	Affected soft tissue structures
Primary extrinsic impingement		
• Subacromial impingement	• Subacromial narrowing	• Subacromial bursa, supraspinatus tendon (anterior)
• Subcoracoid impingement	• Subcoracoid narrowing	• Subscapularis tendon
Secondary extrinsic impingement	Instability	Supraspinatus tendon
Secondary intrinsic impingement		
• Posterosuperior impingement	• Microinstability	• Supraspinatus tendon (posterior), infraspinatus tendon, posterosuperior labrum
• Anterosuperior impingement	• Microinstability	• Subscapularis tendon, pulley system

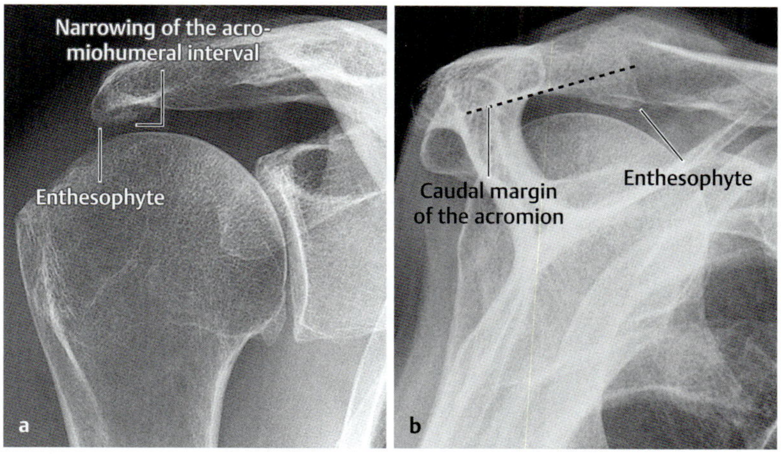

Fig. 2.107 Radiographic findings in subacromial impingement. **(a)** AP radiograph. **(b)** Outlet view.

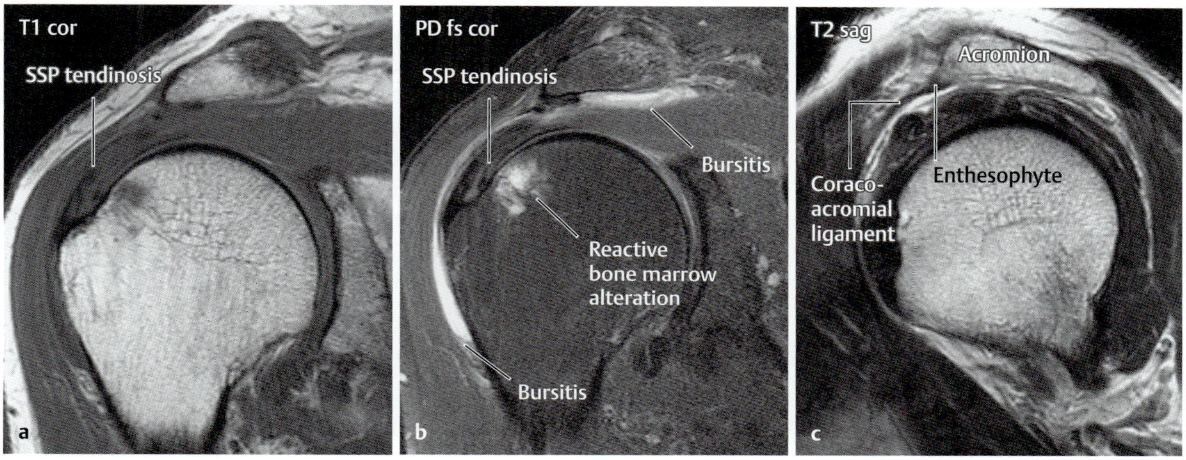

Fig. 2.108 MRI findings in subacromial impingement. SSP, supraspinatus. **(a)** Heterogeneous increased signal intensity within the supraspinatus tendon. **(b)** Bone marrow edema and evidence of subacromial/subdeltoid bursitis (thickening of bursal wall and bursal fluid). **(c)** Enthesophyte at the insertion of the coracoacromial ligament.

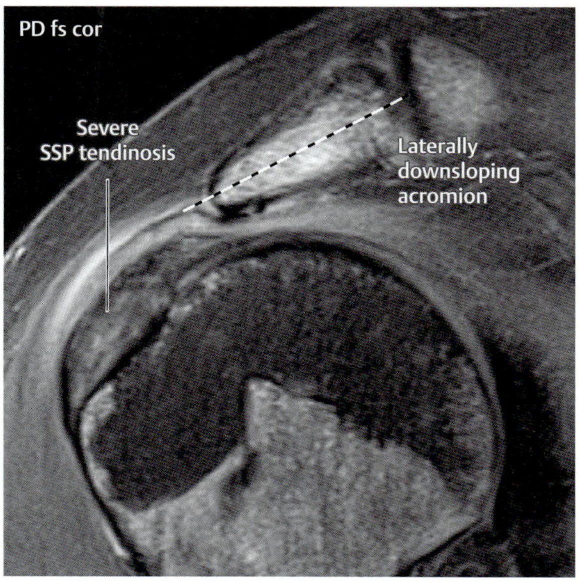

Fig. 2.109 Subacromial impingement with laterally downsloping acromion.

2

Subcoracoid Impingement

▶ **Pathology.** Subcoracoid impingement arises when the subscapularis tendon becomes impinged between the coracoid process and humeral head, resulting in tendon pathology. The syndrome is rare and occurs predominantly with acquired alterations of the coracoid (fracture, surgery) and sometimes as a result of a congenital deformity of the coracoid. Other cases may be related to unrecognized shoulder instability and are more appropriately placed into the group of secondary impingement syndromes.

▶ **Radiography/CT.** Radiographs may demonstrate abnormal coracoid morphology, but equivocal cases will require CT.

▶ **MRI.** MRI is useful for revealing lesions of the subscapularis tendon or to exclude other pathology. From measurement of the width of the coracohumeral interval various authors have reported that measurements of less than 6 to 11 mm are pathologic, but these measurements are not considered to be reliable.

▶ **US.** Abnormalities of the subscapularis tendon are readily assessed by ultrasound and may be an indication of subcoracoid impingement.

Secondary Extrinsic Impingement

▶ **Pathology.** Secondary extrinsic impingement is the result of shoulder instability. Impingement of the soft tissue structures between the acromion and head of the humerus is due to the abnormal mobility of the humeral head. Distinction of this from primary impingement cannot be made on the basis of imaging findings and requires correlation with the clinical examination.

▶ **MRI.** MRI findings of instability impingement do not differ from those of primary subacromial impingement with respect to the changes of the subacromial space (see Subacromial Impingement at the beginning of Chapter 2.4.2).

Secondary Intrinsic Impingement

See also Chapter 2.4.5.

2.4.3 Rotator Cuff Pathology and Biceps Tendinopathy

Rotator Cuff Lesions

▶ **Pathology.** The vast majority of lesions of the rotator cuff are caused by tendon failure secondary to chronic overuse. The actual tendon tear is the final event of this chronic process due to various intrinsic and extrinsic factors. Older individuals with a history of subacromial impingement syndrome are usually affected. Whereas younger patients are more likely to suffer a bony avulsion secondary to an acute injury rather than a tendon rupture, repetitive eccentric overuse associated with chronic microtrauma and intrinsic impingement can lead to tendon lesions in young athletes, especially those participating in overhead sports (pitchers, tennis players, etc.).

Classification of Rotator Cuff Lesions

A basic distinction is made between **tendinopathy, partial-thickness and full-thickness tears**. With tendinopathy only degenerative changes of the tendon are present, without macroscopically evident interruption of continuity. Partial-thickness tears involve only a portion of the tendon, whereas full-thickness tears extend across the entire thickness of the tendon, at least at one site (▶ Fig. 2.110). Full-thickness tears are therefore “transtendinous” and result in a communication between the joint cavity and the subacromial bursa.

Table 2.3 Variants of partial lesions of the rotator cuff

Term	Meaning of the acronym	Morphology
PASTA lesion, also known as rim-rent tear	Partial articular-sided supraspinatus tendon avulsion	Articular-sided partial-thickness tear of the supraspinatus tendon with extension to the tendon insertion (footprint lesion), delamination of the tendon with variable retraction of the articular-sided layer (see ▶ Fig. 2.115a)
CID lesion	Concealed intratendinous delamination	Concealed intratendinous partial-thickness tear (delamination)
PAINT lesion, also known as a delamination tear	Partial articular-sided tear with intratendinous extension	Articular-sided partial tear with intratendinous component (see ▶ Fig. 2.115b)
STAS lesion	Supraspinatus tendon articular-sided but not at footprint	Articular-sided lesion of the supraspinatus tendon outside the footprint region

Caution

With regard to tendon tears, the terms “partial-thickness” (partial) and “full-thickness” (complete) do not state (as is often erroneously assumed) whether the rupture involves the entire tendon or only a part of the tendon.

Partial-thickness Tears

These are classified according to their location as articular-sided (most common type), bursal-sided, or intratendinous. In recent years, several variants of partial tears have been reported (▶ Table 2.3; see also ▶ Fig. 2.110). The depth of articular- or bursal-sided partial tears may be classified according to Ellman (▶ Table W2.1 in Chapter 2.4.3).

Full-thickness Tears

Full-thickness tears typically result from progression of a partial-thickness tear over time. A distinction is made between small (≤ 1 cm), intermediate (1–3 cm), large (3–5 cm), and massive tears (larger than 5 cm in the sagittal plane). Larger defects may be associated with retraction of the proximal tendon stump in a medial direction. The extent of the retraction may be classified according to Patte (▶ Fig. 2.111).

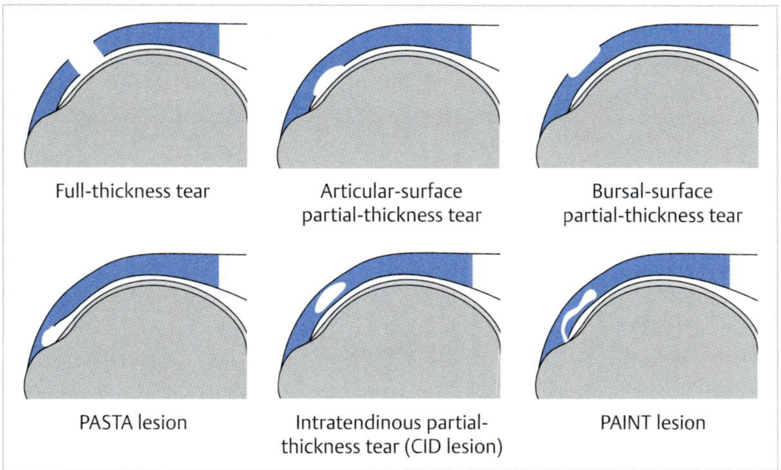

Fig. 2.110 Classification of rotator cuff tears. Compare ▶ Table 2.3.

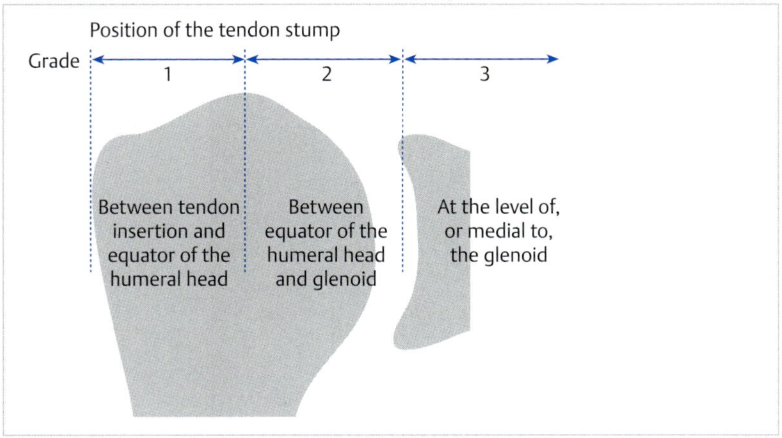

Fig. 2.111 Extent of retraction of full-thickness rotator cuff tears according to Patte.

2

Tears of the Subscapularis Tendon

The subscapularis tendon is often involved in cases of extensive degenerative rotator cuff lesions. Isolated tears are less common and occur, for example, after traumatic anterior shoulder dislocation. Because defects of the subscapularis tendon typically progress in a cranial to caudal direction, Fox and Romeo have proposed a specific classification system (▸ Table 2.4).

▸ **Radiography.** It is not possible to diagnose focal lesions of the rotator cuff on radiographs. Cranial migration of the humeral head with an acromiohumeral distance of less than 7 mm indicates a large defect of the supraspinatus and infraspinatus tendons. The term "defect arthropathy" (▸ Fig. 2.112) describes contact of the humeral head and acromion resulting in osseous remodeling and degenerative cyst formation as well as glenohumeral osteoarthritis in long-standing, extensive rotator cuff tears.

▸ **MRI.** **Tendinopathy** displays increased signal intensity of the tendon on sequences with short echo times (T1W, PDW) and less-intense signal elevation on sequences with long echo times (▸ Fig. 2.113). The affected tendon can appear thickened but does not demonstrate any fiber discontinuity. Magic-angle artifacts may result in a similar appearance but are not usually a problem if intermediate-weighted pulse sequences (with echo times > 35 milliseconds) are used.

A **tendon tear** is diagnosed when fluidlike signal intensity is seen within the tendon on intermediate-weighted or T2W images. In a partial-thickness tear (▸ Fig. 2.114a), the alteration affects only a part of the tendon thickness, whereas the entire thickness of the tendon is involved in a full-thickness tear (▸ Fig. 2.114b). Apart from signal characteristics, attention should also be paid to tendon morphology, i.e., to evidence of interruption in the course of the tendon fibers. A limitation of conventional MRI lies in its difficulty in differentiating tendinopathy from a partial-thickness tear. While the sensitivity for detecting partial tears is therefore relatively low, the accuracy in diagnosing of full-thickness tears is high.

With the aid of **MR arthrography** the sensitivity increases to over 80% for articular-sided partial-thickness tears. An additional diagnostic criterion for diagnosing a partial-thickness tear rather than tendinopathy is the leakage of contrast into the substance of the tendon (▸ Figs. 2.115 and ▸ 2.116). With a full-thickness tear, contrast passes through the transtendinous defect into the subacromial bursa (see ▸ Fig. 2.114b).

Rotator cuff tears may result in atrophy and, over time, irreversible fatty degeneration of the affected muscles. Assessment of the rotator cuff **muscles** can be made using the semiquantitative **Goutallier classification system** (▸ Table 2.5). The most lateral image of an oblique sagittal T1W or T2W sequence (obtained without fat saturation!) where the scapula is seen to form a Y shape is used as a reference level (▸ Fig. 2.117).

> **Note**
> The amount of loss of functioning muscle in a patient with a rotator cuff tear is decisive for the prognosis of a cuff repair. Any description of a rotator cuff injury without mention of the state of the muscles is incomplete.

Table 2.4 Fox and Romeo classification of tears of the subscapularis tendon

Grade	Tear type
1	Partial-thickness tear
2	Full-thickness tear of the upper 25% of the tendon
3	Full-thickness tear of the upper 50% of the tendon
4	Full-thickness tear of all parts of the tendon

Table 2.5 Semiquantitative classification of fatty degeneration of muscles according to Goutallier

Grade	Morphology
0	Normal muscle, no fat
1	Some streaks of fat
2	Pronounced fatty infiltration, but still more muscle than fat
3	Advanced fatty infiltration; as much fat as muscle
4	Advanced fatty infiltration; more fat than muscle

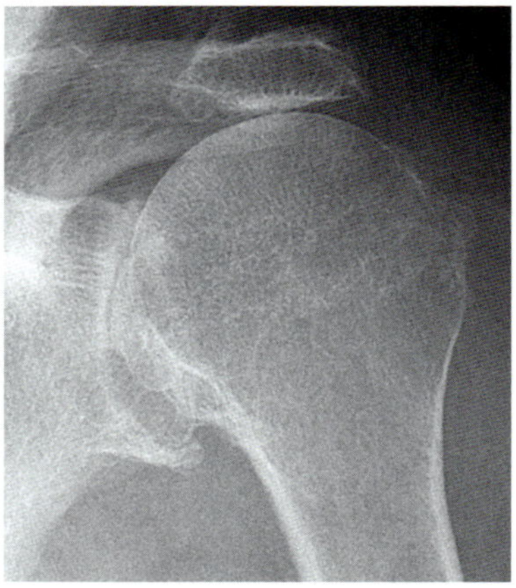

Fig. 2.112 Rotator cuff tear arthropathy.

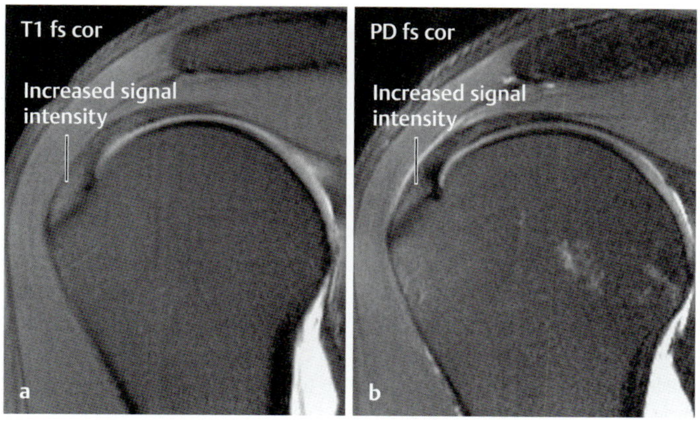

Fig. 2.113 Tendinopathy of the supraspinatus tendon. MR arthrography. **(a)** Increased intratendinous signal intensity on the FS T1W image, in part due to the magic angle effect. **(b)** Less signal increase on intermediate-weighted sequence.

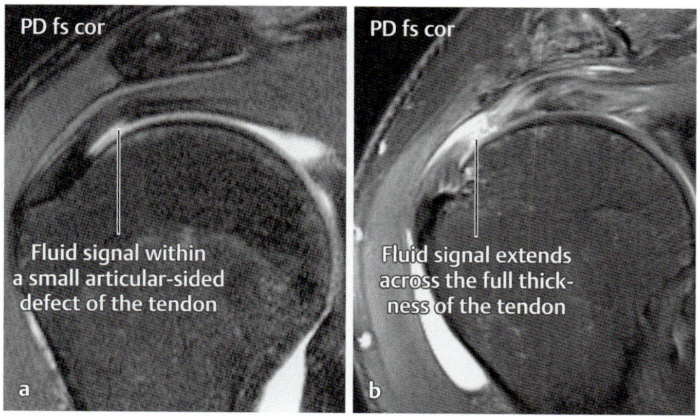

Fig. 2.114 Rotator cuff tears. Partial-thickness tear versus full-thickness tear. **(a)** Partial thickness undersurface tear of the supraspinatus tendon. **(b)** Full-thickness tear of the supraspinatus tendon.

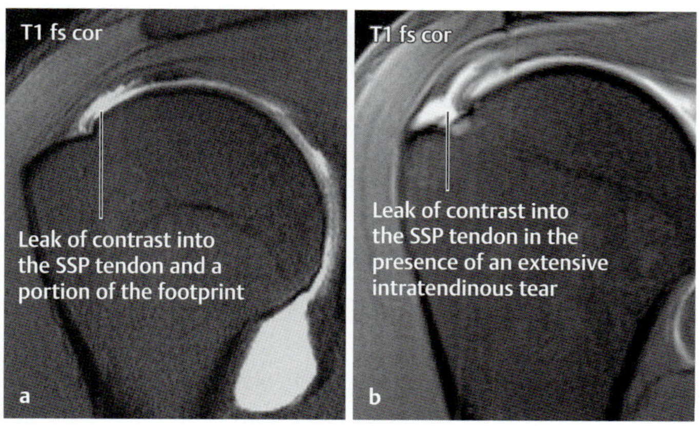

Fig. 2.115 Rotator cuff tears. MR arthrography. **(a)** PASTA lesion. **(b)** PAINT lesion. SSP = supraspinatus muscle.

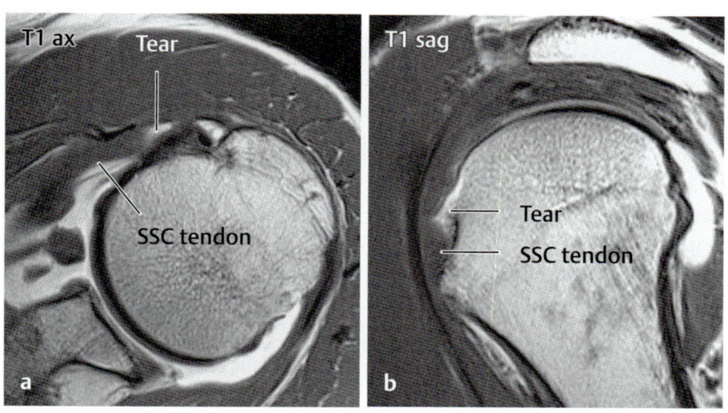

Fig. 2.116 Fox and Romeo Grade 2–3 tear of the subscapularis tendon. MR arthrography. **(a)** Leakage of contrast medium into the tendon at its insertion. **(b)** The classification according to Fox and Romeo is made using the sagittal plane. SSC, subscapularis muscle.

▸ **US.** In experienced hands, ultrasound can provide results comparable with those of conventional MRI with regard to the recognition of tendon defects. Differentiation between tendinopathy and a partial-thickness tear remains difficult, however. Furthermore, it should be borne in mind that anisotropy of tendon fibers can create the impression of a defect. To avoid this, any suspicious finding should be examined from several aspects with different probe angles. Apart from direct signs of tear, such as interruption of tendon fibers and release of fluid into the tendon or bursa (▸ Fig. 2.118a), indirect signs should also be looked for. A focal impression ("dent") in the convexity of the tendon surface or a circumscribed double contour over the surface area of the humeral head (▸ Fig. 2.118b), corresponding to hyaline articular cartilage, is encountered only with a tear, not with tendinopathy. Limitations of ultrasound include only moderate reliability in evaluating the state of muscles and its low sensitivity for concomitant pathologic states (e.g., labral pathology).

Caution

With massive full-thickness tears of the rotator cuff associated with a retracted tendon, the deltoid lies directly adjacent to the humeral head and can be confused with components of the rotator cuff.

▸ **CT.** CT arthrography using multidetector technology with image reconstructions in all three anatomical planes may be used as a "back-up procedure," for example when there are contraindications against an MRI examination. Transtendinous defects and articular surface partial tears of the supraspinatus and infraspinatus tendons are detectable with high sensitivity and specificity (▸ Fig. 2.119). This technique is limited, however, by low sensitivity for intratendinous and bursal-sided lesions and for many lesions of the subscapularis tendon. The Goutallier classification system can be used because it was originally developed for CT scanning.

▸ **DD.** There is a differential diagnosis for the clinical symptoms of a rotator cuff tear.

With the development of acute symptoms, a distinction must be made between isolated **subacromial bursitis** without rotator cuff defect, calcific tendinitis secondary to calcium hydroxyapatite deposition disease, and an **avulsion fracture** of the greater tuberosity. Suprascapular nerve palsy secondary to **entrapment neuropathy** or a **postinfectious neuritis** (Parsonage–Turner syndrome) is a relatively rare differential diagnosis. Other pathologies that can have a clinical presentation similar to that of a rotator cuff tear include **SLAP lesions** (Chapter 2.4.6) and traumatic **osteolysis of the distal clavicle** (Chapter 2.5.6).

Biceps Tendinopathy

▸ **Pathology.** Tendinopathy of the long head of the biceps tendon is often an associated condition in patients with subacromial impingement and lesions of the rotator cuff as well as secondary to instability of the tendon (pulley lesion; Chapter 2.4.4). However, biceps tendinopathy can also develop as an isolated overuse injury in athletes involved in overhead and throwing activites. Anterior shoulder pain is the cardinal clinical symptom. Partial-thickness tendon tears and eventually full-thickness tears can develop from initial tendinopathy, which typically involves the horizontal (intra-articular) part of the tendon.

▸ **MRI.** MRI signs of biceps tendinopathy are thickening and irregular contours of the tendon and increased signal intensity on sequences with short echo times. These alterations are best identified on oblique sagittal images (▸ Fig. 2.120). Partial tears can manifest as an increase in caliber and signal intensity of the tendon on T1W and T2W sequences or as attenuation of the tendon. Discontinuity or complete absence of the horizontal portion of the tendon are signs of a full-thickness tear (▸ Fig. 2.121).

▸ **US.** It is not possible to demonstrate the proximal insertion of the biceps tendon at the glenoid by ultrasound, but its more lateral intra-articular segment can be well visualized. Difficulties can arise in obese patients. Tendinopathy of the biceps tendon with thickening, heterogeneous echogenicity and increased vascularization may be detected with ultrasound, as may partial or full-thickness tears. An "empty" intertubercular groove requires differentiation between a tear and a dislocation of the long biceps tendon out of its groove (cf. ▸ Fig. 2.125). This is possible by tracing the tendon from its myotendinous junction in a cranial direction.

2.4.4 Pathology of the Rotator Interval

▸ **Pathology.** Various types of injury involving the anatomical structures of this region are subsumed under the term "rotator interval lesion." Tears of the rotator interval capsule can be found in patients with anterior shoulder instability and usually show a horizontal orientation.

Injuries of the superior glenohumeral ligament, also termed **pulley lesions**, are of more clinical significance and can occur in isolation or in combination with tears of the supraspinatus tendon and/or subscapularis tendon, resulting in instability of the long biceps tendon. Habermeyer has described four types of pulley lesions (▸ Fig. 2.122 and ▸ Table W2.2); Type 1 (frequency: 29–74%) refers to an isolated tear of the superior glenohumeral ligament.

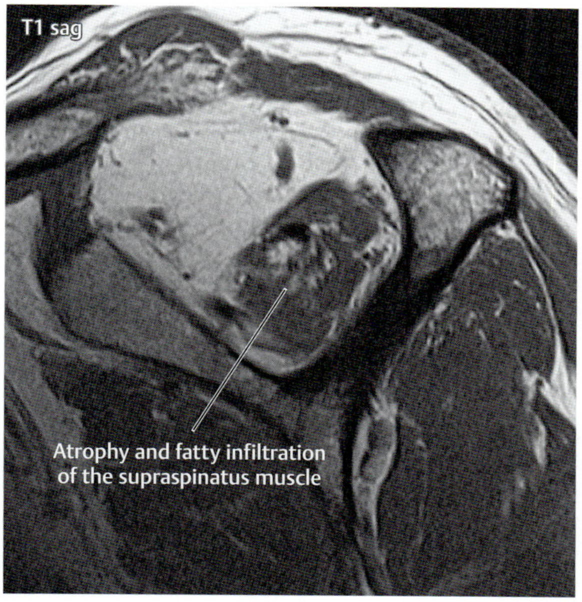

Fig. 2.117 Atrophy and fatty degeneration of the supraspinatus muscle Grade 2 to 3 according to Goutallier in a case of a full-thickness tear.

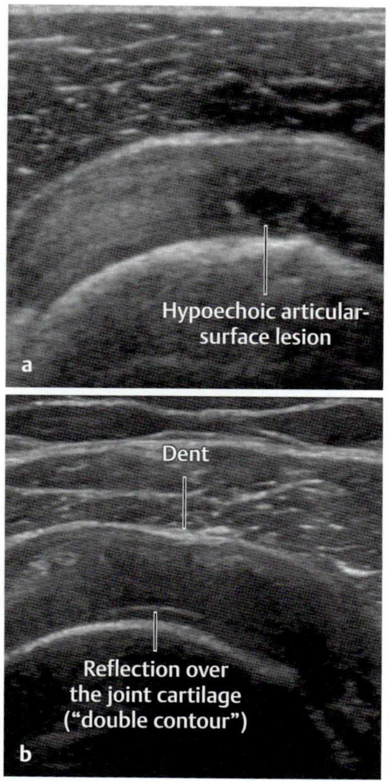

Fig. 2.118 Ultrasound of rotator cuff tears. **(a)** Partial articular-sided tear of the supraspinatus tendon (longitudinal section). **(b)** Full-thickness tear of the supraspinatus tendon (cross section).

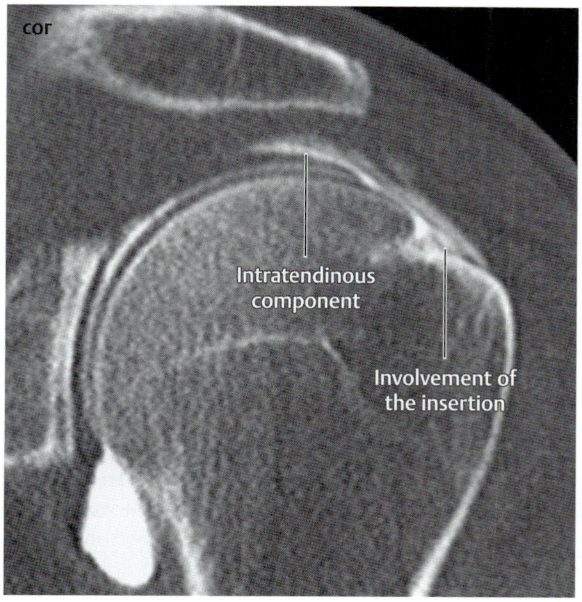

Fig. 2.119 Articular-sided partial tear of the supraspinatus tendon. CT arthrography.

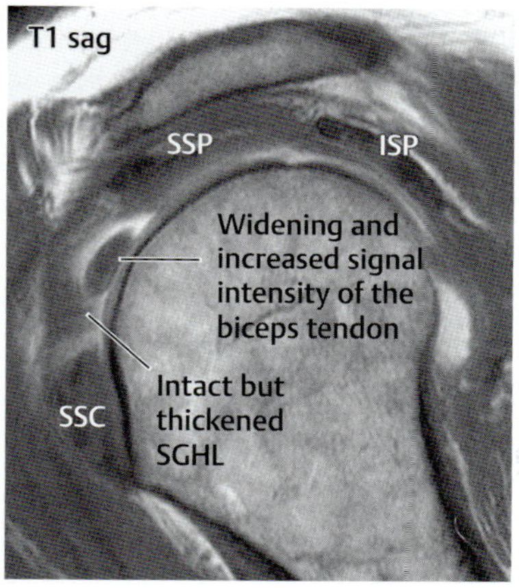

Fig. 2.120 Isolated tendinopathy of the long head of the biceps tendon. MR arthrography. ISP, infraspinatus muscle; SGHL, superior glenohumeral ligament; SSC, subscapularis muscle; SSP = supraspinatus muscle.

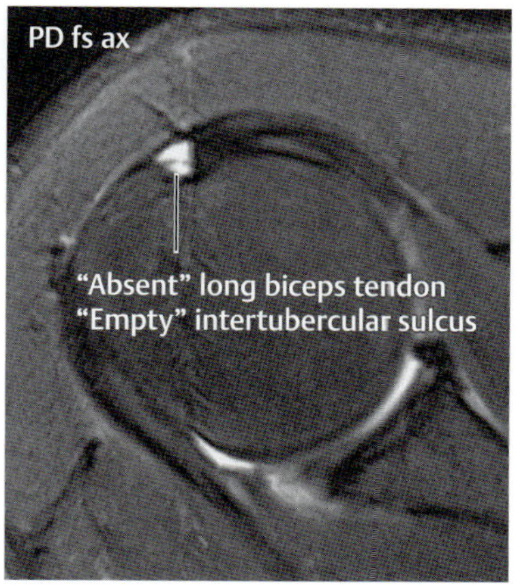

Fig. 2.121 Full-thickness tear of the long head of the biceps tendon.

▸ **MRI.** Rotator interval lesions are well demonstrated only with the aid of MR arthrography. Pulley lesions can be diagnosed on oblique sagittal MR arthrographic images with a sensitivity and specificity of more than 80%. Reliable signs are inferior displacement of the long head of the biceps tendon onto the subscapularis tendon within the rotator interval (displacement sign) and discontinuity of the superior glenohumeral ligament (▸ Fig. 2.123). This is almost always associated with tendinosis of the biceps tendon. Medial displacement of the biceps tendon, recognizable on transverse sections, is usually only encountered in conjunction with a simultaneous lesion of the subscapularis tendon, but not with an isolated tear of the superior glenohumeral ligament. With a lesion of the superior glenohumeral ligament and a partial defect of the subscapularis tendon, the biceps tendon can dislocate into the defect, i.e., deep to the coracohumeral ligament. Intra-articular dislocation can occur with a full-thickness tear of the subscapularis tendon (▸ Fig. 2.124). Extracapsular dislocations of the biceps tendon (ventral to the subscapularis tendon) associated with a tear of the coracohumeral ligament are very rare. Capsular tears can occasionally be identified as contrast leakage in the region of the interval into the subacromial/subdeltoid bursa.

▸ **US.** Instability of the long biceps tendon can be recognized using ultrasound when it is seen to subluxate or dislocate out of the intertubercular sulcus. This is best achieved with a dynamic examination during forced external rotation (▸ Fig. 2.125).

2.4.5 Shoulder Instability

Traumatic Anterior Instability

▸ **Pathology.** Anterior (anteroinferior) glenohumeral instability is the most common form of traumatic (unidirectional) shoulder instability (more than 95% of cases). Pathoanatomically there is an interruption of continuity of the anteroinferior labroligamentous complex, which results in insufficiency of the inferior glenohumeral ligament and subsequently leads to recurrent anterior dislocation or subluxation. A traumatic injury (traumatic first-time acute dislocation) results in an acute anterior shoulder dislocation in which the humeral head impacts against the anteroinferior glenoid rim; this can result in a labroligamentous injury (see following text sections) and/or a posterolateral impaction fracture of the head of the humerus (Hill–Sachs fracture).

Bankart and Perthes Lesions

Bankart lesions and Perthes lesions represent approximately 90% of the injuries that occur secondarily to traumatic anterior first-time acute dislocation. In the classic **Bankart lesion**, the anteroinferior labrum, together with the inferior glenohumeral ligament, is completely detached from osseous glenoid (▸ Fig. 2.126). Because there is also an additional disruption of the scapular periosteum, the labrum is usually displaced from its normal anatomical position, and may be "floating" freely in the anterior joint space.

A **Perthes lesion** is distinguished from a Bankart lesion by the fact that although an avulsion of the labrum off the glenoid exists, it is still attached to the glenoid via scapular periosteum, which is stripped anteromedially but not disrupted. The unstable labrum often remains in a relatively normal position and the tear can be masked by scar tissue and re-synovialization. Fluid may be seen tracking between the labrum and glenoid or beneath the periosteum and is sometimes more readily apparent in the ABER position, i.e., with the inferior glenohumeral ligament under tension (▸ Fig. 2.127).

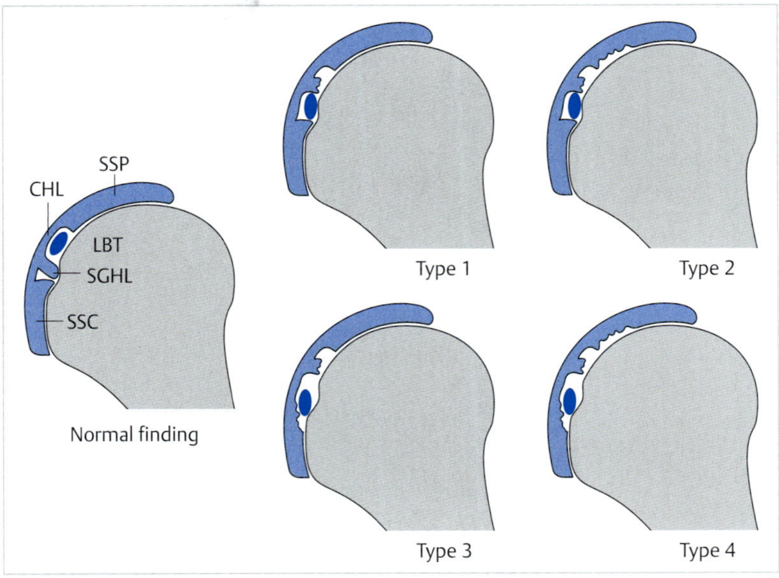

Fig. 2.122 Habermeyer classification of pulley lesions. Sagittal schematic diagrams. CHL, coracohumeral ligament; LBT, long head of the biceps tendon; SGHL, superior glenohumeral ligament; SSC, subscapularis muscle; SSP, supraspinatus muscle.

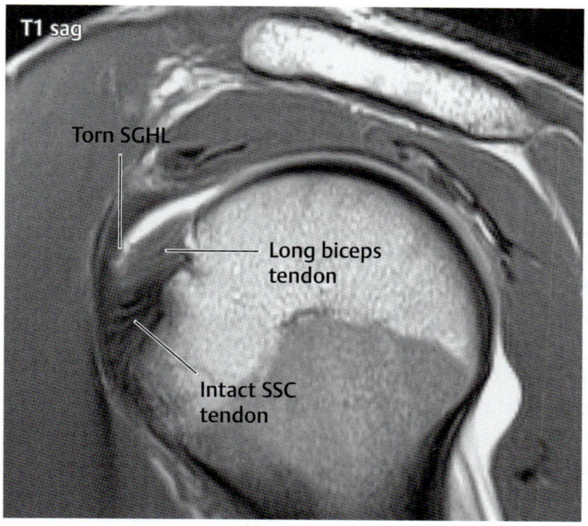

Fig. 2.123 Type 1 pulley lesion. MR arthrography. The long head of the biceps tendon shows increased signal intensity, compatible with tendinopathy, and is displaced caudally onto the subscapularis tendon (cf. ▶ Fig. 2.120). SGHL, superior glenohumeral ligament; SSC, subscapularis muscle.

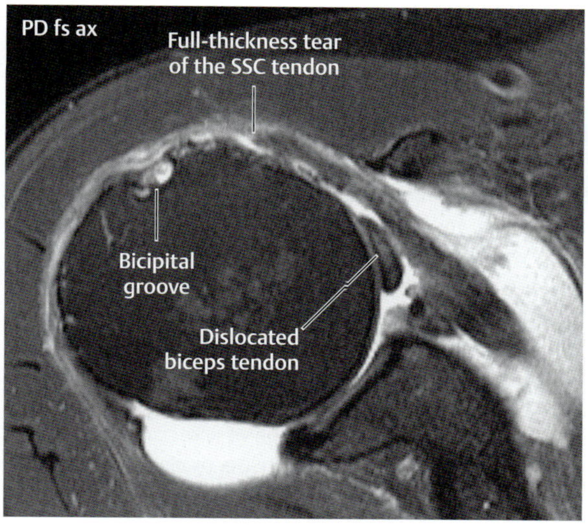

Fig. 2.124 Intra-articular dislocation of the long head of the biceps tendon. SSC, subscapularis muscle.

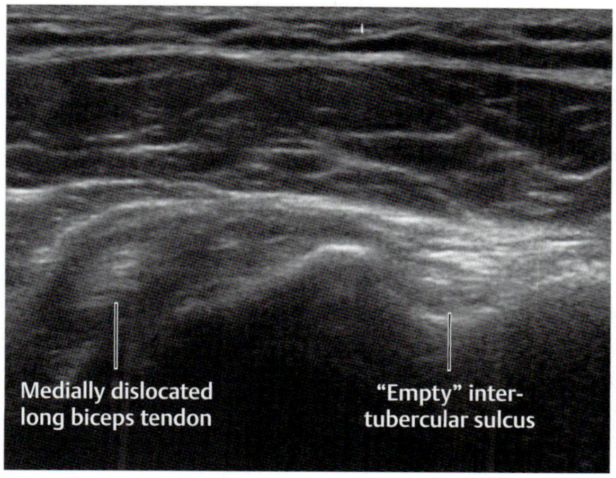

Fig. 2.125 Dislocation of the long head of the biceps tendon. Ultrasonic cross section of the proximal upper arm.

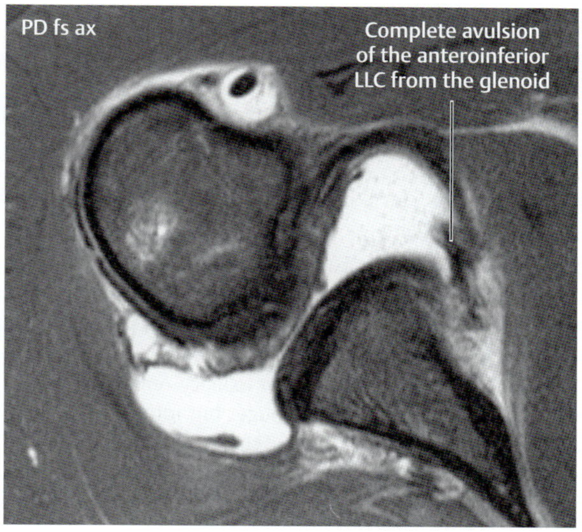

Fig. 2.126 Acute Bankart lesion. LLC, labroligamentous complex.

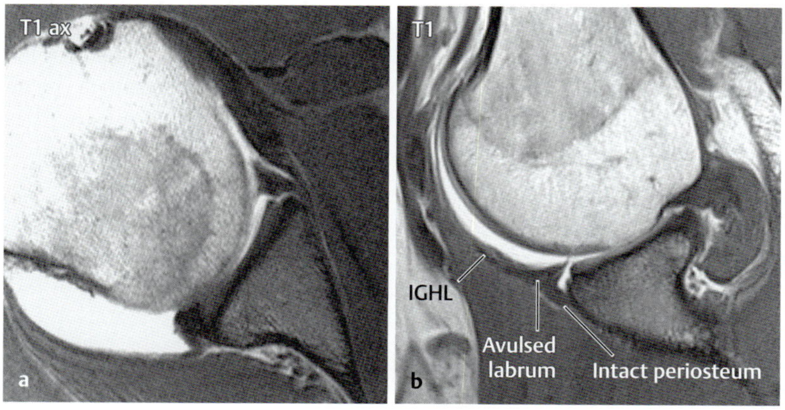

Fig. 2.127 Perthes lesion. MR arthrography. **(a)** The anteroinferior labrum is undermined by contrast medium, but remains in a normal position. **(b)** The detachment of the labrum is more clearly depicted in the ABER position. IGHL, inferior glenohumeral ligament.

ALPSA Lesion

An ALPSA lesion (anterior labroligamentous periosteal sleeve avulsion) is found as a chronic variant of a Perthes lesion, usually after multiple anterior shoulder dislocations (chronic instability). With this type of lesion, the anteroinferior labroligamentous complex becomes detached from the glenoid rim and is displaced medially, where it scars over along with its periosteal attachment to the scapular neck. Although there is no actual ligament disruption, incompetence of the inferior glenohumeral ligament develops due to the abnormal labral position. The result is shoulder instability. Characteristic signs of an ALPSA lesion are medially and caudally displaced labral tissue (▸ Fig. 2.128) which appears larger due to a proliferation of associated scar tissue along the scapular neck, and a crease, or cleft, between the glenoid and the labrum (cleft sign; see ▸ Fig. 2.128b).

Bony Bankart Lesion

The bony Bankart lesion is an avulsion fracture in which the anteroinferior labroligamentous complex is detached from the glenoid together with a bony fragment of variable size (▸ Fig. 2.129). While small bony fragments may be regarded as therapeutically and prognostically irrelevant, larger fragments require refixation or reconstruction of the glenoid.

HAGL Lesion

In the very rare HAGL lesion (humeral avulsion of glenohumeral ligament), the anteroinferior labroligamentous complex is not disrupted at its glenoid attachment but is at the humerus (▸ Fig. 2.130). The inferior glenohumeral ligament may be avulsed directly or together with a bone fragment (~20% of cases) from its insertion on the humeral neck. The anterior capsule of the axillary recess no longer appears U-shaped on coronal images but rather is J-shaped due to the lateral discontinuity of the inferior glenohumeral ligament ("J sign"). Acute HAGL lesions may be associated with fluid leakage and/or a hematoma at the insertion site of the inferior glenohumeral ligament.

Hill–Sachs Defect/Fracture

Hill–Sachs defects are detectable after traumatic first-time acute dislocations in 47 to 100% of cases. This lesion may or may not be present in patients who have sustained a significant anterior labroligamentous injury. Except for very large lesions, Hill–Sachs defects are of little clinical relevance, but detection of such a lesion indicates a previous anterior shoulder dislocation. On axial images, a Hill–Sachs defect is always located posterolaterally at or above the level of the coracoid. Acute lesions are usually surrounded by areas of bone contusion (▸ Fig. 2.131).

▸ Radiography. It is hardly possible to miss an acute anteroinferior shoulder dislocation on conventional radiographs (▸ Fig. 2.132). Follow-up films after reduction serve to exclude any associated bony injuries (osseous Bankart lesion, fracture of the greater tuberosity). Smaller bony avulsions from the anteroinferior glenoid rim are usually not visible on standard projection views. If a conventional radiological depiction is requested, then an osseous Bankart lesion is best seen on a Westpoint or axillary view, whereas a Hill–Sachs defect is best displayed on an AP radiograph in internal rotation or on a Stryker view.

▸ CT/CT arthrography. CT is the modality of choice for demonstrating the extent of an acute glenoid fracture or chronic glenoid defect resulting from progressive bone loss after multiple dislocations; quantification of the size of the bony abnormality is best accomplished on oblique sagittal image reconstructions. Hill–Sachs defects are also readily detected with CT. The results of CT arthrography are comparable to those of MR arthrography with respect to the assessment of labroligamentous injuries. The advantages of CT arthrography lie in the recognition of bony Bankart lesions and in diagnosing articular cartilage lesions. Its disadvantages include its limited ability to assess soft tissue structures and its use of ionizing radiation (especially important in young patients).

▸ MRI/MR arthrography. Conventional MRI is most suitable for demonstrating injuries immediately after the event, i.e., within a few days after the acute dislocation, since an associated joint effusion or hemarthrosis will act as a natural contrast medium and allow for more accurate assessment of the labrocapsular structures. Direct MR arthrography is the modality of choice, with a sensitivity of more than 88% and a specificity of more than 90% for the detection of labroligamentous lesions. Its accuracy in characterizing the type of injury as compared with arthroscopic findings is 84%. This technique also allows for reliable detection of associated injuries, such as SLAP lesions (Chapter 2.4.6).

▸ DD. Differentiation of a labroligamentous injury from an anatomical variant of the glenoid labrum is relatively easy. An abnormality seen exclusively within the anterosuperior quadrant of the labrum (a **sublabral foramen** or a **Buford complex**) (Chapter 2.4.1) it is always located in the anterosuperior quadrant, whereas most true labroligamentous lesions typically involve the anteroinferior quadrant, or at least begin there.

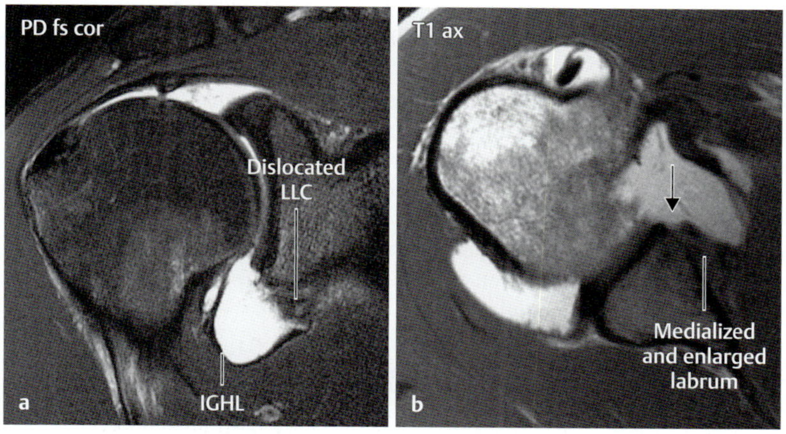

Fig. 2.128 ALPSA lesion. MR arthrography. **(a)** The labroligamentous complex is displaced medially and inferiorly. **(b)** Typical cleft sign (arrow). IGHL, inferior glenohumeral ligament; LLC, labroligamentous complex.

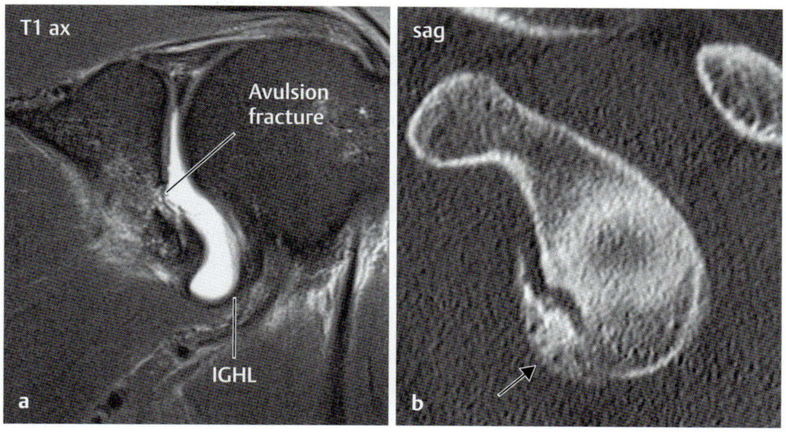

Fig. 2.129 Bony Bankart lesion. **(a)** MR arthrography. The inferior glenohumeral ligament itself is intact. **(b)** Anteroinferior bony avulsion (arrow) from the glenoid. IGHL, inferior glenohumeral ligament.

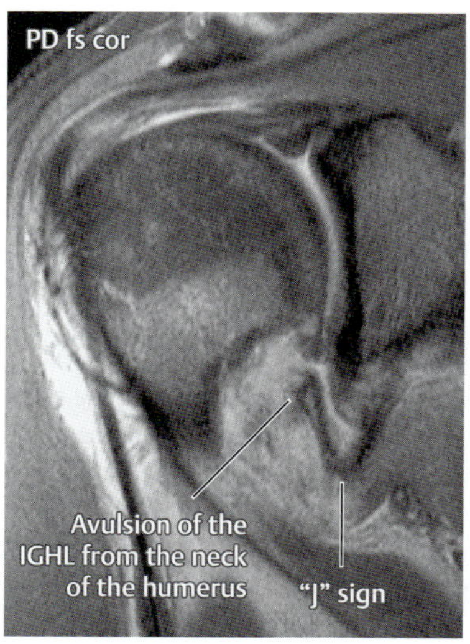

Fig. 2.130 Acute HAGL lesion. IGHL, inferior glenohumeral ligament.

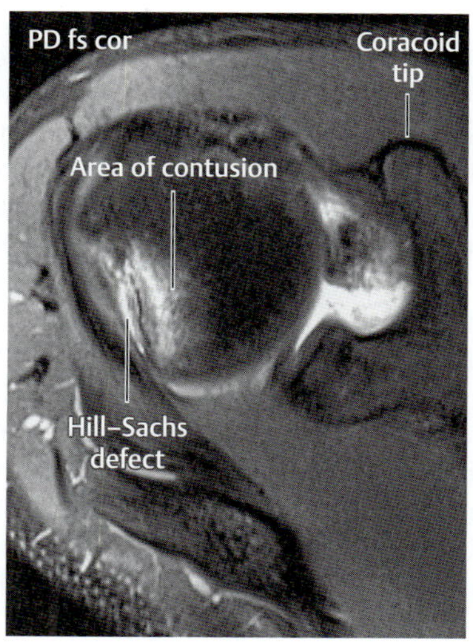

Fig. 2.131 Acute Hill–Sachs defect.

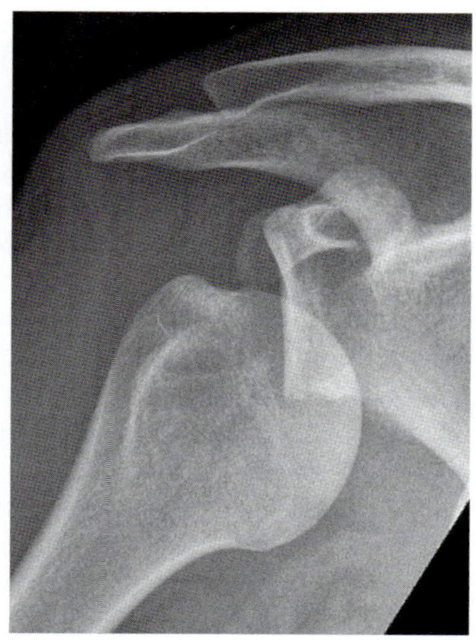

Fig. 2.132 Anteroinferior shoulder dislocation.

Traumatic Posterior Instability

▸ **Pathology.** Traumatic posterior shoulder instability is comparatively rare (2–4% of cases). In most cases, a posterior dislocation is the result of considerable muscular contraction during an epileptic seizure or an electrical accident (occasionally resulting in bilateral posterior dislocations) or during abnormal axial loading of the upper arm while it is abducted and internally rotated. The lesion pattern is a mirror image of those seen with anterior instability, including a posterior labroligamentous injury and an anteromedial "reverse" Hill–Sachs lesion of the humeral head. Classification of posterior labroligamentous lesions analogous to injuries of the anterior structures ("reverse" [bony] Bankart lesion; POLPSA [posterior labrocapsular periosteal sleeve avulsion] lesion; posterior HAGL lesion, etc.), has not become generally accepted. It is possible to miss an unreduced ("locked") posterior dislocation clinically and on standard frontal radiographs. One clue to its presence is an inability to externally rotate the arm, which is fixed in adduction and internal rotation.

▸ **Radiography.** Radiographs are diagnostic for acute or locked posterior shoulder dislocation. In a "true" AP projection, overlapping of the contours of the internally rotated head of the humerus and the joint socket is evident (▸ Fig. 2.133). There is often a line of density running parallel to the medial contour of the humeral head (trough line; see ▸ Fig. 2.133), corresponding to the lateral margin of the "reverse" Hill–Sachs defect (trough sign). In questionable cases, a radiograph in a second projection (axillary, transscapular or transthoracic) confirms the posterior dislocation of the humeral head.

▸ **CT.** CT accurately shows the size and orientation of "reverse" Hill–Sachs defects as well as additional bony injuries of the posterior glenoid rim and whether the dislocated humeral head is "locked" along the posterior glenoid rim (▸ Fig. 2.134).

▸ **MRI.** As with anterior instability, a conventional MRI examination is most useful immediately after the dislocation, whereas in the more chronic setting, MR arthrography should be considered (▸ Fig. 2.135). In addition to damage to the posterior labroligamentous complex, patients with posterior shoulder instability are not uncommonly found to have concomitant lesions of the rotator cuff.

Atraumatic Instability

▸ **Pathology.** Atraumatic shoulder instability is typically multidirectional, occurs bilaterally, and often affects patients with generalized hyperlaxity of the joints (congenital hypermobility syndrome). Multiple subluxations or dislocations are typical, and can also occasionally be produced voluntarily. Apart from a capacious joint capsule, intra-articular findings are commonly absent. However, in athletes with multidirectional shoulder instability, labral and rotator cuff lesions are not uncommonly present.

▸ **MRI.** With multidirectional shoulder instability, the primary role of MR arthrography is to exclude the presence of associated intra-articular pathology. Frequently a stretching and redundancy of the capsule can be readily recognized, especially in the region of the rotator interval. A glenohumeral ligament that does not appear to be stretched on images in the ABER position is also suggestive of capsular redundancy.

Microinstability

▸ **Pathology.** Microinstability (also known as "functional instability" or "microtraumatic instability") represents a subclinical form of shoulder instability that develops mainly in athletes secondarily to chronic overuse with repetitive injury to the capsular structures. These forms of instability are most commonly found in sports that involve abduction and external rotation of the shoulder (overhead sports). These patients typically present with pain and reduced motion of the shoulder rather than overt subluxation or dislocation events. Secondary damage to articular structures may develop, especially to the glenoid labrum and rotator cuff.

Posterosuperior glenoid impingement is a typical intrinsic form of impingement that occurs in the overhead athlete due to microinstability with abnormal anterior translation of the humeral head during the cocking phase. It most commonly manifests clinically as acute or chronic posterior shoulder pain. With posterosuperior glenoid impingement, there is repetitive pathologic contact between the joint surface of the rotator cuff (especially the posterior fibers of the supraspinatus and anterior fibers of the infraspinatus tendons) and the posterior superior glenoid rim during external rotation and abduction. These tendons may also become entrapped between the glenoid and greater tubercle, resulting in injuries to the posterior cuff and posterosuperior glenoid labrum.

Anterosuperior impingement is much less common and involves the subscapularis tendon and pulley system when the arm is brought into internal rotation and adduction (follow-through phase of throwing or striking movements) during which these structures become entrapped between the anterior superior glenoid rim and the humeral head. The most common clinical symptom is anterior shoulder pain.

▸ **MRI.** MR arthrography is the most useful imaging technique for evaluating athletes presenting with shoulder problems. A variety of often subtle articular lesions can result from microinstability: Stretching of the joint capsule, an array of labral pathology (degeneration, tear, avulsion, SLAP lesion), or rotator cuff lesions may occur in isolation or in combination (▸ Fig. 2.136).

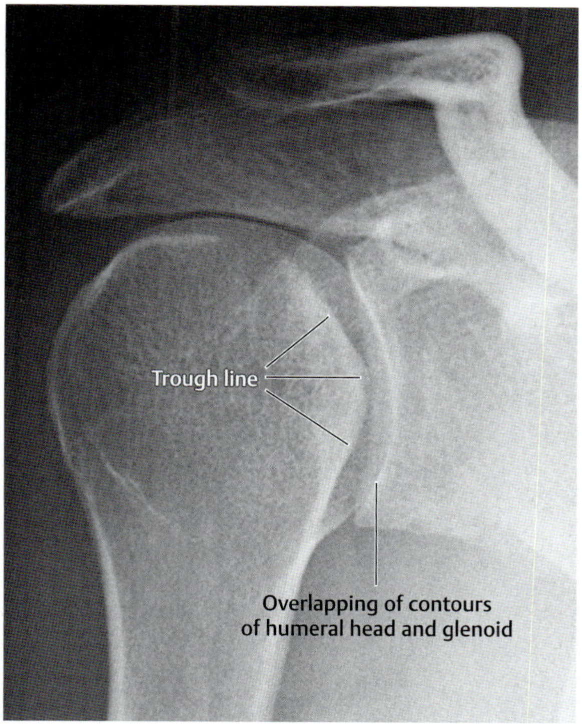

Fig. 2.133 Posterior shoulder dislocation. AP radiograph.

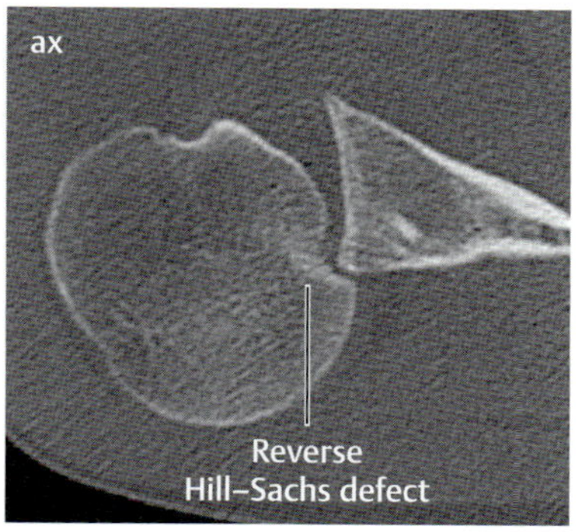

Fig. 2.134 Locked posterior shoulder dislocation.

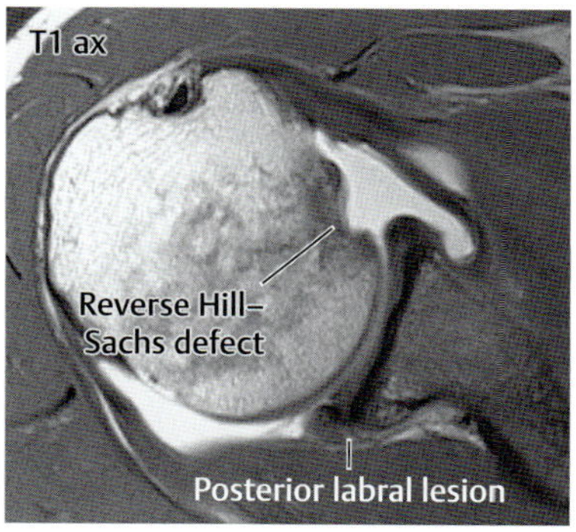

Fig. 2.135 Traumatic posterior shoulder instability. MR arthrography.

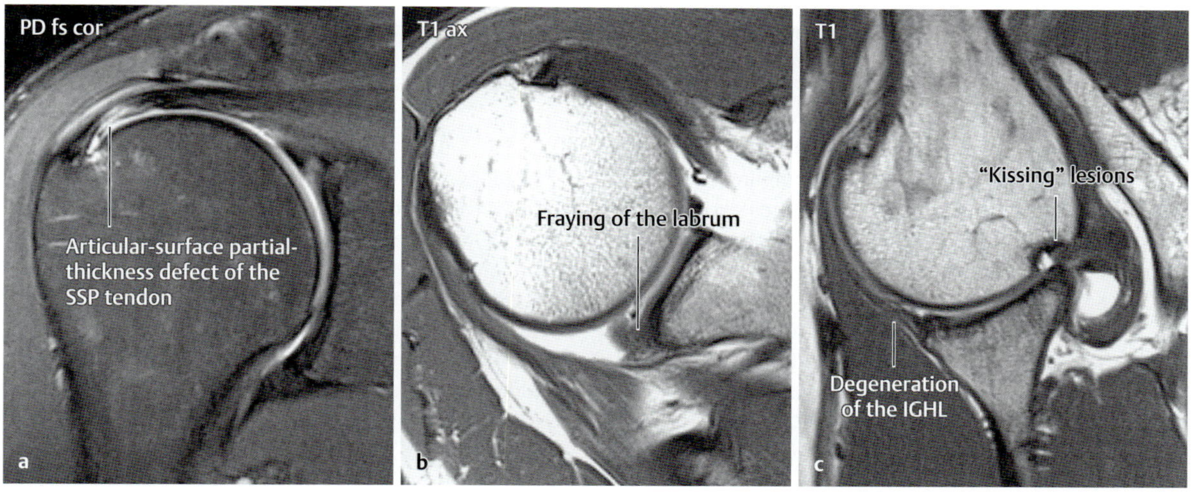

Fig. 2.136 Microinstability: posterosuperior glenoid impingement. MR arthrography. Combination of the findings from a, b, and c may be related to microinstability. The ABER position demonstrates the corresponding lesions of labrum and supraspinatus tendon. **(a)** Rotator cuff lesion. **(b)** Degenerative fraying of the posterosuperior labrum. **(c)** Degeneration of the inferior glenohumeral ligament. IGHL, inferior glenohumeral ligament; SSP, supraspinatus muscle.

A characteristic pattern of "kissing lesions" is found in patients with posterosuperior glenoid impingement (see ▶ Fig. 2.136c). MR arthrography typically demonstrates an articular-sided partial-thickness tear of the posterior fibers of the supraspinatus tendon and/or anterior fibers of the infraspinatus tendon, combined with a lesion of the posterosuperior glenoid labrum. With excessive contact, bony alterations such as bone marrow edema, cyst formation, and sclerotic changes in the greater tubercle and superior glenoid may also be seen. Lesions of the anterior joint capsule are evident on axial views and may be accentuated on views obtained in the ABER position and vary from degenerative changes to elongation and tear of the inferior glenohumeral ligament.

In cases of anterosuperior glenoid impingement, MR arthrography can demonstrate the pulley lesion with discontinuity of the superior glenohumeral ligament and the sequelae of the associated instability of the biceps tendon. Lesions of the subscapularis tendon typically start along the articular surface of the superior part of the tendon.

2.4.6 Other Labral Pathology

SLAP Lesions

▶ **Pathology.** SLAP lesions are injuries to the superior glenoid labrum and the biceps/labral anchor, extending in an anteroposterior direction. They have a frequency of 4 to 10% in arthroscopic series. Common mechanisms of injury include a fall on an outstretched hand or flexed elbow, an anterior shoulder dislocation, and chronic overuse injuries due to repetitive torsion of the biceps anchor in overhead sports (pitching and striking sports, swimming). Following a shoulder dislocation, the SLAP lesion ultimately often represents the superior extension of an anteroinferior labral lesion (e.g., Bankart lesion).

The **classification system of Snyder** distinguishes four different types of SLAP lesions (▶ Table 2.6 and ▶ Fig. 2.137). Whereas the Type 1 SLAP lesion, as a purely degenerative alteration, is of hardly any clinical relevance, Type 2 (the most common type) and Type 4 lesions often cause instability of the biceps anchor and are an indication for superior labral repair or biceps tenodesis. The biceps tendon is stable in the Type 3 SLAP lesion; treatment therefore involves only resection of the bucket-handle tear. Various other reported lesions mostly represent combination injuries of a Type 2 SLAP lesion plus damage to the labrum, the middle glenohumeral ligament or the rotator cuff. This extended classification is not typically used, however.

▶ **MRI.** Conventional MRI has only a low sensitivity for the detection of SLAP lesions and, as a result, MR arthrography is the method of choice; it exhibits high sensitivity (82–92%) and specificity (80–99%) in this regard (▶ Fig. 2.138).

Type 1 SLAP lesions manifest as contour irregularities of the superior labrum, but are only rarely detectable. With a Type 2 lesion, leakage of contrast medium into the superior labrum and the biceps/labral anchor is observed. A cleft of contrast extending laterally into the substance of the labrum is a very predictive sign of a true SLAP tear since a Type 2 SLAP tear can be very difficult to differentiate from a sublabral recess. However, the normal recess is typically oriented in a medial direction (Chapter 2.4.1). Other findings suggesting a true Type 2 SLAP lesion are irregular labral margins and a wide separation between the labrum and glenoid. Types 3 and 4 are bucket-handle tears, in which the torn fragment may be displaced caudally into the joint to a greater or lesser degree. In Type 3, the fragment typically appears triangular on coronal views and separated from the intact biceps tendon. In Type 4 the bucket-handle fragment includes both the superior labrum and parts of the biceps tendon.

▶ **CT/Arthrography.** CT arthrography is considered equivalent to MR arthrography in diagnosing SLAP lesions.

▶ **DD.** Differentiation between a Type 2 SLAP lesion and a sublabral recess (Chapter 2.4.1 and ▶ Fig. 2.137) may be difficult, if not impossible, but the orientation of the "cleft" and its morphology should provide helpful clues for accurate diagnosis.

GLAD Lesion

▶ **Pathology.** The GLAD lesion (glenolabral articular disruption) involves a combination of a focal articular cartilage defect along the anteroinferior glenoid, typically with a subtle tear of the adjacent labrum. It is not typically associated with glenohumeral instability. The cause is presumed to be an eccentric impaction of the head of the humerus against the glenoid during a fall on the outstretched arm or on the shoulder. A posterior variant of the GLAD lesion has also been reported.

▶ **MRI.** MR arthrography demonstrates a tear near the base of the nondisplaced labrum and a cartilaginous lesion involving the adjacent anteroinferior or posteroinferior quadrant of the glenoid (▶ Fig. 2.139). There is no injury to the inferior glenohumeral ligament. The extent of glenoid cartilage damage varies.

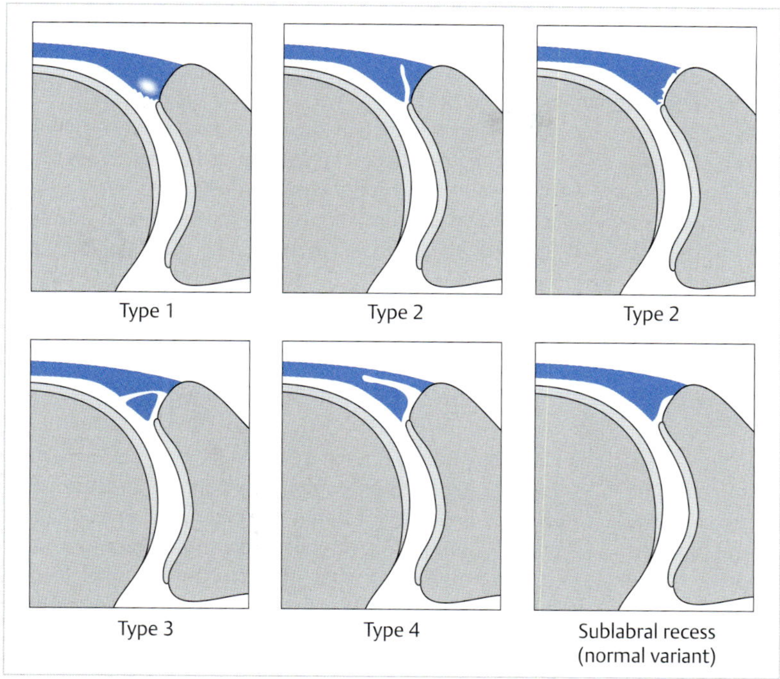

Fig. 2.137 SLAP lesions. Findings on coronal MR arthrograms.

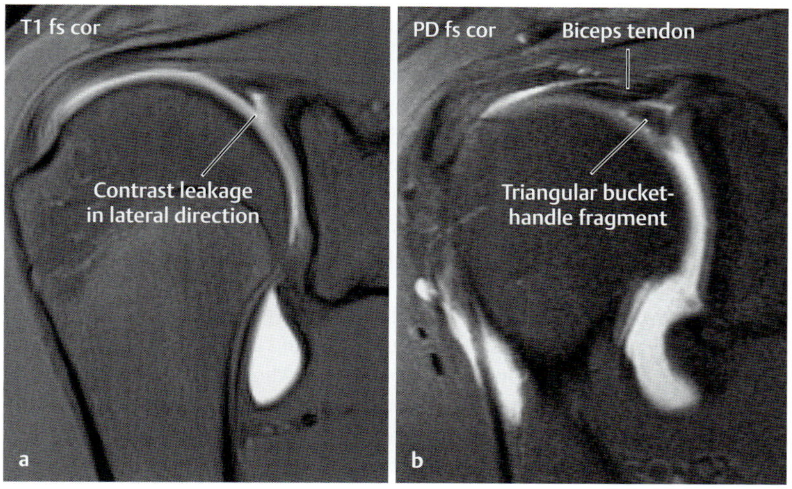

Fig. 2.138 SLAP lesions. MR arthrography. **(a)** Type 2 SLAP lesion. **(b)** Type 3 SLAP lesion.

Table 2.6 Snyder classification of SLAP lesions

Type	Lesion
1	Degenerative fraying of the superior labrum
2	Avulsion of the superior labrum and detachment of the biceps anchor from the glenoid.
3	Bucket-handle tear of the superior labrum with intact biceps anchor
4	Bucket-handle tear of the superior labrum with involvement of the biceps anchor

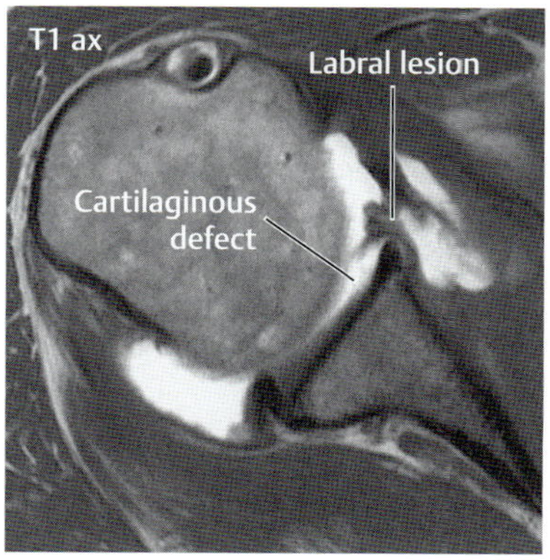

Fig. 2.139 GLAD lesion.

Ganglia

▸ **Pathology.** Ganglia are pseudocystic lesions that develop from mucoid degeneration of collagenous connective tissue and are composed of a gelatinous ground substance surrounded by a fibrous wall that lacks a true synovial lining. Since the majority of ganglia in the vicinity of the glenoid arise from labral lesions, they are often also referred to as paralabral "cysts" and are typically indicative of an injury to the adjacent labrum. Paralabral cysts most commonly originate from the posterior labrum but they can also occur in conjunction with SLAP or anteroinferior labral lesions. Dorsally situated ganglia can extend into the spinoglenoid notch, where they may cause entrapment neuropathy of the suprascapular nerve (Chapter 11.8).

▸ **MRI.** MRI demonstrates one or more rounded, often multilobulated masses which display internal fluidlike signal intensity on all pulse sequences ("cluster of grapes") (▸ Fig. 2.140a). After the intravenous administration of contrast, these demonstrate only peripheral/septal enhancement (▸ Fig. 2.140c). These are almost always in close proximity to the labrum and in some cases a "neck" of the ganglion may be seen to extend to a labral tear (▸ Fig. 2.140b). A paralabral cyst will sometimes fill with contrast medium on an MR arthrogram if it communicates with the joint space via a labral tear.

2.4.7 Postoperative Complications

Recurrences after Shoulder Stabilization

▸ **Pathology.** In the majority of cases, traumatic anterior shoulder instability is treated by an anatomical repair (known as a Bankart repair) that is usually performed arthroscopically: refixation using metallic or bioabsorbable suture anchors to reattach the labrum to the glenoid. The aim of the treatment is to restore continuity of the anteroinferior labroligamentous complex and also reduce the anterior capsular volume with a supplementary plication or a capsular shift procedure. Usually three suture anchors are used, which are inserted into the glenoid between the 2 o'clock and 5 o'clock positions. Recurrent instability after this type of repair may be due to a new traumatic shoulder dislocation or subluxation with rerupture of the labroligamentous complex. Other causes include an insufficient tightening of the anterior capsule or significant glenoid bone loss secondary to multiple dislocations.

▸ **MRI.** Imaging of the integrity of the labroligamentous complex and anterior capsular volume is best achieved by MR arthrography,

Again, images obtained in the ABER position may be helpful. Retears appear as detachment of the labrum or discontinuity of the inferior glenohumeral ligament (▸ Fig. 2.141). With a lax anterior capsule, the inferior glenohumeral ligament does not directly contact the humeral head in the ABER position.

Rerupture after Rotator Cuff Reconstruction

▸ **Pathology.** Repair of the rotator cuff can be performed arthroscopically or with an open procedure, with the choice of technique depending essentially on the size of the defect. Transosseous suture techniques or suture anchors are used to reattach the tendon to the humerus. This is almost always accompanied by subacromial decompression and removal of the subacromial/subdeltoid bursa. Postoperative retears may be due to pull-out of sutures or fixation anchors or from structural failure of the reconstructed tendon(s).

▸ **MRI.** Reconstructed tendons practically never appear homogeneously hypointense on MR images. Abnormal signal intensity, partial-thickness tears, as well as smaller full-thickness defects may be normal or irrelevant in the presence of a good functional outcome. Conventional MRI is usually sufficient for recognizing retears since clinically relevant tendon defects practically always represent transtendinous tears extending more than 1 cm in diameter (▸ Fig. 2.142).

In this context, MRI demonstrates sensitivities and specificities of approximately 85% and 90%, respectively. MR arthrography does not have any clear advantage over conventional MRI in the postoperative setting. A decisive factor for planning further treatment is the quality of and especially the degree of atrophy of the rotator cuff muscles (see Goutallier classification in Chapter 2.4.3). Fluid in the region of the former subacromial bursa usually represents a normal postoperative finding and is not, in itself, an indication of a retear or infectious process.

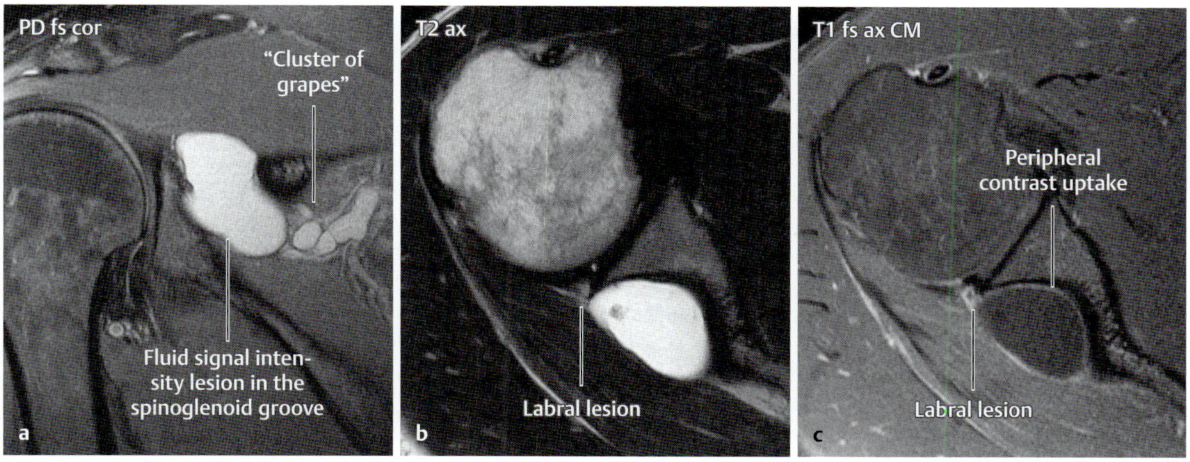

Fig. 2.140 Ganglion (paralabral "cyst"). **(a)** The lesion is isointense to water on all sequences. **(b)** Evidence of a posterior labral lesion at the level of the ganglion. **(c)** Thin peripheral contrast enhancement.

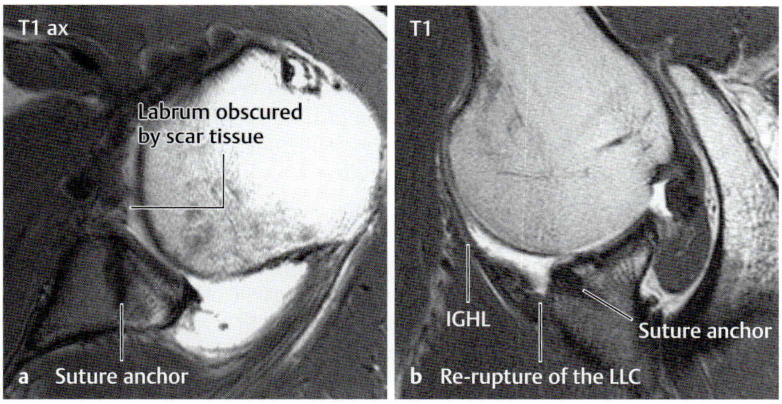

Fig. 2.141 Traumatic retear after Bankart repair (recurrent anterior instability). **(a)** Transverse MR arthrogram with the arm in neutral position. **(b)** MR arthrography in the ABER position reveals the retear. IGHL, inferior glenohumeral ligament; LLC, labroligamentous complex.

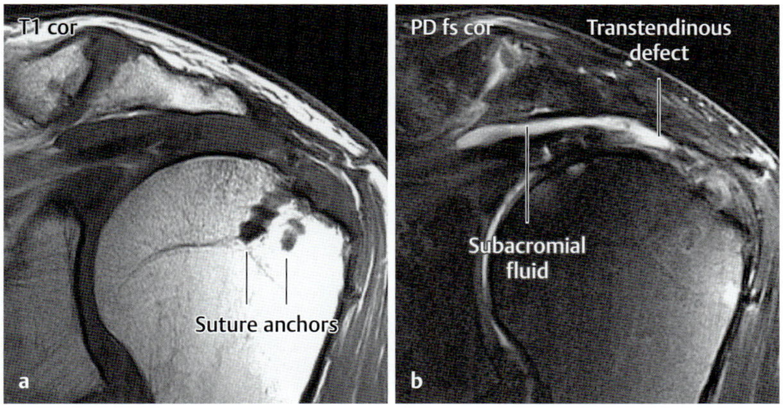

Fig. 2.142 Retear after supraspinatus tendon repair. **(a)** Increased signal intensity of the reconstructed tendon. **(b)** Evidence of a large transtendinous retear.

Implant-Associated Complications

▸ **Pathology.** Malpositioned or dislocated suture anchors and screws can cause mechanical damage to joints, and even lead to osteoarthritis. Furthermore, bioabsorbable implants can cause foreign-body reactions, which manifest as osteolysis or proliferative synovitis. Of note, osteolysis around absorbable suture anchors is not necessarily indicative of failure of the fixation device.

▸ **Radiography.** Significant malposition of metallic implants should be recognizable on radiographs (▸ Fig. 2.143). Bioabsorbable implants are not radiodense and thus are not adequately assessed on conventional films.

▸ **CT.** CT and CT arthrography are modalities of choice for the exact depiction of improper placements, loosenings, and fractures of metallic implants (▸ Fig. 2.144). Bioabsorbable implants appear as almost structureless areas in bone. If they dislocate into the joint space, they are only detectable with CT arthrography.

▸ **MRI.** Bioabsorbable materials appear as a focus of absent signal intensity on MRI and are therefore usually well demarcated in bone or the joint space. Furthermore, bioabsorbable suture anchors and interference screws often display a central cavity that is isointense to fluid (▸ Fig. 2.145). Osteolytic alterations in the vicinity of implants correspond to areas where the fatty marrow has been completely replaced by granulation tissue, and in some cases by cystic-appearing lesions as well. Foreign-body synovitis is typically proliferative and can result in extensive bone destruction.

Nerve Damage

▸ **Pathology.** Iatrogenic nerve damage is rare. In shoulder surgery it may be caused by direct nerve injury, nerve entrapment or over-aggressive intraoperative tissue retraction. The suprascapular nerve in particular may be injured during open rotator cuff repair or during tumor surgery. The axillary nerve is at risk for injury at the inferior glenoid rim, especially during shoulder stabilization surgery.

▸ **MRI.** Damage to a nerve can be indirectly diagnosed on MRI by the presence of a typical denervation pattern of the muscles innervated by that nerve.

After injury to the suprascapular nerve (▸ Fig. 2.146) there is denervation edema of the supraspinatus and infraspinatus muscles if the injury involves the nerve more proximally or only the infraspinatus muscle if the injury occurs more distally. The deltoid and/or teres minor muscles are affected by injury to the axillary nerve. Denervation edema may persist for months or even years, but over time, progressive fatty atrophy of the muscles will become evident.

Postoperative Infection

▸ **Pathology.** On the whole, postoperative infection is a rare complication of shoulder surgery, but may manifest as septic arthritis (with or without osteomyelitis), septic bursitis, or infection of the juxta-articular soft tissues. Accurate diagnosis requires joint aspiration or tissue biopsy (white cell count, pathogen identification).

▸ **US.** Ultrasound is capable of demonstrating the joint effusion, which is typically not entirely echo-free. Demonstration of hyperperfusion of the hypertrophic synovial tissue with Doppler ultrasound provides additional evidence of possible infection.

▸ **MRI.** Differentiation between septic arthritis and reactive synovitis is not possible using MRI alone (▸ Fig. 2.147). The role of MRI is to define the extent of infection, especially with regard to abscess formation in the adjacent soft tissues and any bone involvement (osteomyelitis). A standard T1W sequence is essential for detecting or excluding osteomyelitis. The most useful criterion for diagnosing osteomyelitis, as opposed to reactive (noninfectious) bone marrow alterations, is the complete replacement of the normal marrow fat by tissue that is isointense or hypointense to skeletal muscle (internal standard).

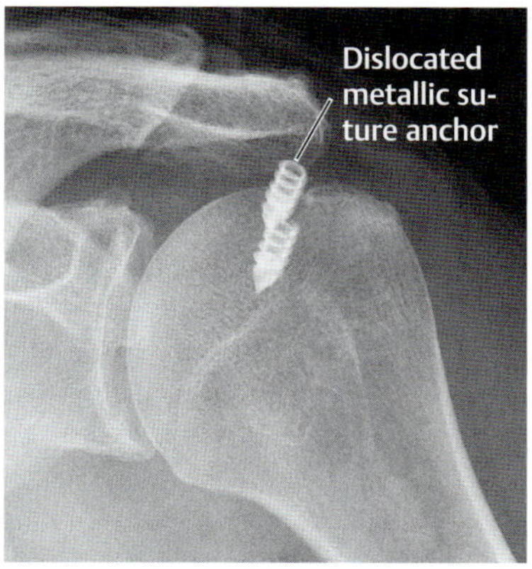

Fig. 2.143 Anchor dislocation after rotator cuff reconstruction.

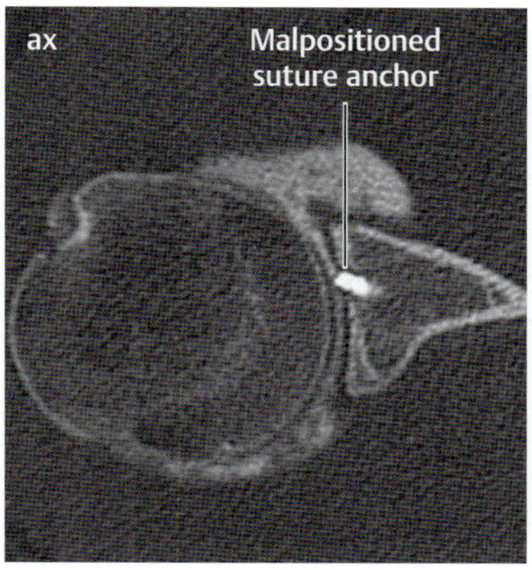

Fig. 2.144 Malpositioned suture anchor after a Bankart repair. CT arthrography.

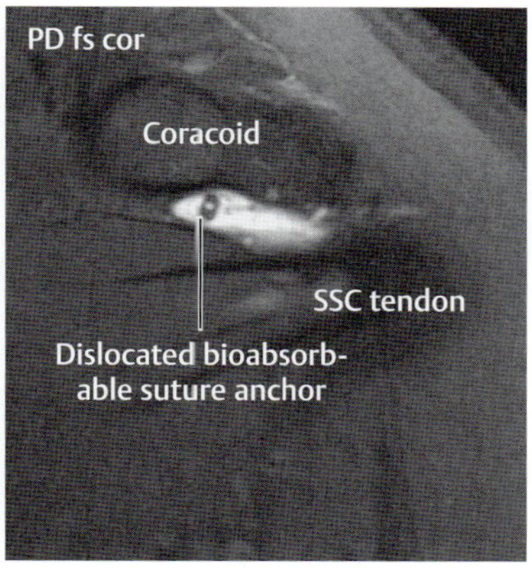

Fig. 2.145 Anchor dislocation after Bankart repair. Typical morphology of a bioabsorbable suture anchor; intra-articular position of the anchor. SSC, subscapularis tendon.

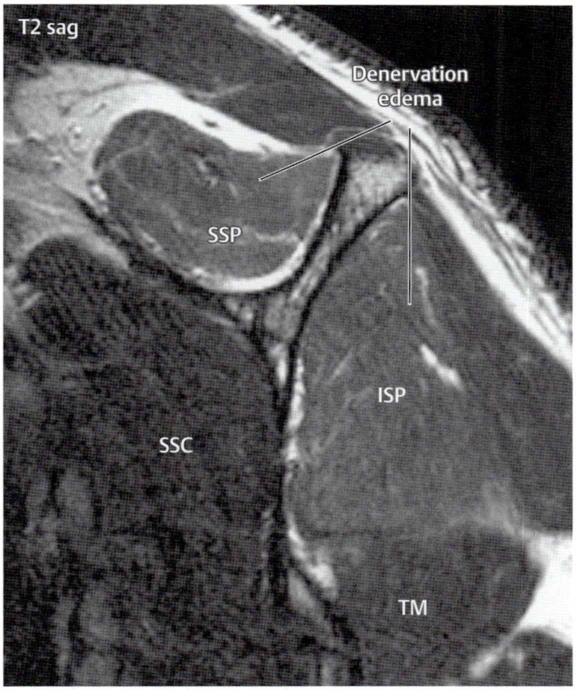

Fig. 2.146 Proximal lesion of the suprascapular nerve. ISP, infraspinatus muscle; SSC, subscapularis muscle; SSP, supraspinatus muscle; TM, teres minor muscle.

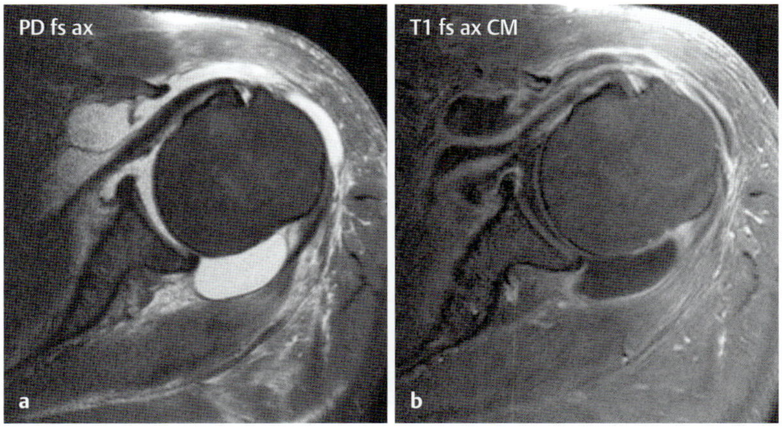

Fig. 2.147 Postoperative septic arthritis. **(a)** Significant joint distension, edematous periarticular soft tissues. **(b)** Synovitis with thickened, enhancing synovial membrane.

2.5 Shoulder Girdle and Thoracic Wall

▸ **Anatomy.** ▸ See Chapter 2.5.1 and ▸ Fig. W2.20.

2.5.1 Sternoclavicular Dislocation

In most cases **the medial clavicle is displaced** anteriorly (90% of cases), less frequently posteriorly or superiorly.

▸ **Pathology.** The degree of injury is classified according to **Allman**:

- **Grade I**: Partial-thickness tear of the joint capsule with strain of the sternoclavicular ligaments. The congruence of the articular surfaces is preserved.
- **Grade II:** Tear of the joint capsule and the sternoclavicular ligaments, with the costoclavicular ligament intact → subluxation.
- **Grade III:** Tear of the joint capsule, the sternoclavicular ligaments and the costoclavicular ligament → dislocation.

▸ **Radiography.** *Technique:* AP radiograph with the tube tilted 40° (craniocaudal or caudocranial direction). True AP views are usually nondiagnostic due to overlapping structures.

▸ **US.** In addition to demonstrating a joint effusion and soft tissue swelling, ultrasound is also able to demonstrate a sternoclavicular dislocation when compared with the contralateral side.

▸ **CT.** Depiction of the sternoclavicular joints is best achieved using CT, supplemented by coronal and 3D reconstructions (▸ Fig. 2.148).

▸ **MRI.** The MRI examination is performed in prone position, whenever possible, to reduce the risk of respiratory artifacts. It allows assessment of the disks and ligamentous and capsular structures and is used to detect Allman Grade I lesions.

▸ **Special features in children.** The medial clavicular epiphysis ossifies late (at the age of ~ 18 years) and fuses late (at the age of ~ 25 years; see ▸ Fig. 2.148). Up to the age of 18 years it is therefore difficult to distinguish epiphyseal plate injuries from a normal, unfused epiphysis.

▸ **DD.** In chronic cases of subluxation or dislocation of the medial end of the clavicle the associated swelling is most likely to be mistaken for an inflammatory or neoplastic process.

▸ **Important findings.** The extent of the dislocation of the medial end of the clavicle (subluxation versus dislocation) and the direction of the dislocation must be noted, as must any signs of possible associated injuries (tracheal indentation, vascular injury, etc.).

2.5.2 Clavicular Fracture

▸ **Pathology.** The most accepted clinical classification is that proposed by **Allman** which describes the site of the fracture:

- **Type I:** Fracture of the middle third (▸ Fig. 2.149).
- **Type II:** Fracture lateral to the coracoacromial ligaments.
- **Type III:** Fracture of the proximal segment.

▸ **Radiography.** Radiography is the modality of choice for diagnosing clavicular fractures and typically involves an AP view obtained with a 15° caudocranial tilt of the central beam. Additional imaging modalities are only required for specific indications.

▸ **CT.** CT is particularly useful for differentiating a fracture of the medial end of the clavicle from a dislocation of the sternoclavicular joint.

▸ **US.** In children with mildly displaced fractures, ultrasound may suffice as the sole modality for confirming the fracture and conducting follow-up examinations.

▸ **MRI.** MRI may be helpful in the growing skeleton to differentiate epiphyseal plate fractures from sternoclavicular dislocations; it is doubtful, however, whether this is of any therapeutic consequence. Whenever possible, acquisition is obtained with the patient in a prone position to reduce respiratory artifacts.

▸ **Special features in children.** Clavicular fractures are the most common birth injury in the newborn infant and account for 90% of all obstetrical fractures (incidence: 3–8/1000 births). Some are occult fractures and only become noticeable after callus formation. Associated neurovascular injuries should be looked for.

▸ **Important findings.** Location of the fracture, the number of fragments as well as the degree of displacement, and any overriding/foreshortening at the fracture site should be documented.

2.5.3 Acromioclavicular Dislocation

▸ **Pathology.** The most common cause of this injury is a direct blow to the shoulder. The degree of injury to the acromioclavicular joint is classified according to **Tossy** into three grades; a more comprehensive classification taking into account less common and more severe injuries has been proposed by **Rockwood** and co-workers (▸ Fig. 2.150):

- **Rockwood I (= Tossy I):** Mild sprain of the joint capsule and ligaments but no full-thickness tear.
- **Rockwood II (= Tossy II):** Ruptured joint capsule and acromioclavicular ligaments; sprain or partial-thickness tear of the coracoclavicular ligament.
- **Rockwood III (= Tossy III):** Disruption of the joint capsule, acromioclavicular and coracoclavicular ligaments.

- **Rockwood IV**: Posterior displacement of the lateral end of the clavicle into the trapezius.
- **Rockwood V**: Lateral end of the clavicle markedly displaced superiorly.
- **Rockwood VI**: Lateral end of the clavicle displaced inferiorly behind the coracoid or the acromion.

► **Radiography.** Conventional radiographs demonstrate the width of the joint space and any malalignment of the clavicle.

Technique. AP with a 3 to 5 kg weight hanging from the arm in slight external rotation with the central ray angled 10–15° caudocranially. A comparison with the contralateral side on the same radiograph is important and should be obtained unless there is an unequivocal clinical presentation (**Tossy III**). Due to differences in technical factors and patient positioning, routine films of the shoulder are not suitable for displaying the acromioclavicular joint (► Fig. 2.151).

► **US.** Ultrasound demonstrates the width of the acromioclavicular joint space in comparison with the contralateral side.

► **CT.** CT does not usually provide any additional information from that obtained with radiographs.

► **MRI.** MRI is capable of detecting capsular and ligamentous injuries (► Figs. 2.152, ► 2.153, and ► W2.21).

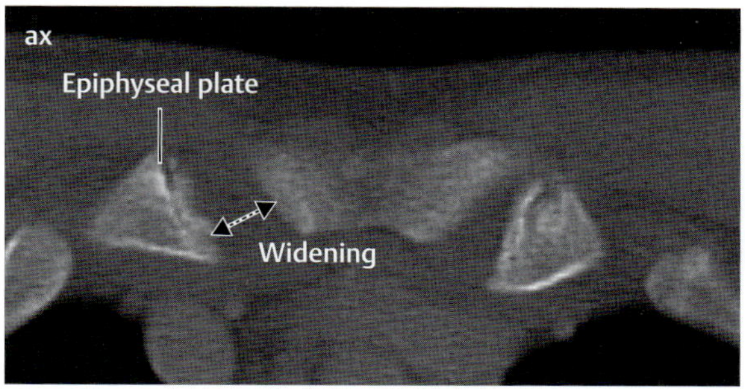

Fig. 2.148 CT of a traumatic injury to the right sternoclavicular joint in a 20-year-old man.

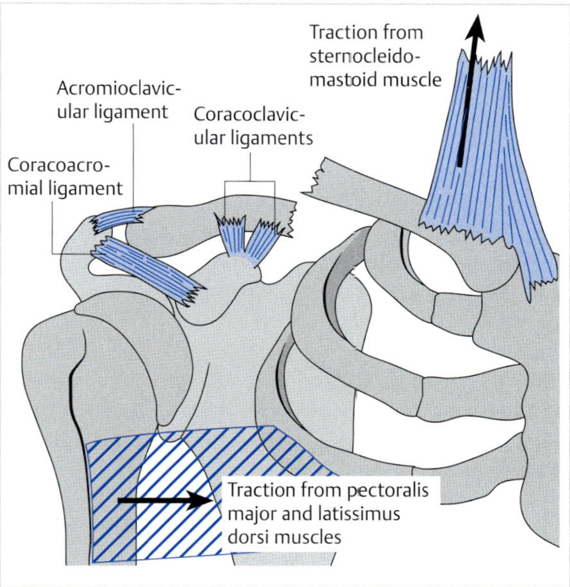

Fig. 2.149 Mechanism of displacement of clavicular fractures.

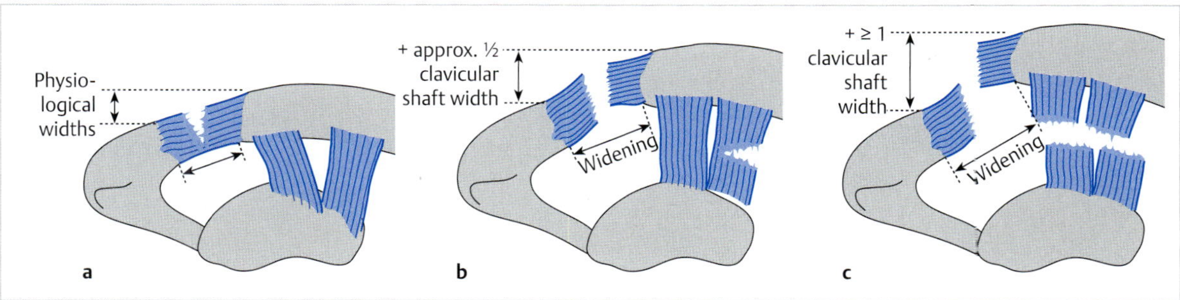

Fig. 2.150 Acromioclavicular joint dislocation. Classification according to Tossy and Rockwood. **(a)** Tossy I. **(b)** Tossy II. **(c)** Tossy III.

2.5.4 Scapular Fracture

► **Radiography.** Diagnostic radiographic examinations are of limited value due to the complexity of scapular anatomy and fracture patterns.

► **CT.** CT is the modality of choice for assessing fracture patterns and involvement of the articular surface of the glenoid (► Fig. W2.22).

► **Important findings.** With scapular fractures it is important to describe an incongruity of the articular surface of the glenoid as well as markedly angulated fractures of the scapular neck and body since these injuries are associated with increased complications and symptoms.

2.5.5 Sternal and Rib Fractures

► **Radiography.** Fractures of the ribs and sternum are insufficiently visualized on a routine chest radiographs (PA [posteroanterior] using high-kV technique). Oblique views (45°) of the affected hemithorax are obtained for the ribs, with the injured side positioned near to the film. A supplementary lateral radiograph is only rarely necessary for the sternum.

► **US.** Ultrasound is the modality of choice for confirming location, pattern, and displacement of a sternal fracture (► Fig. 2.154). It also allows exclusion of a traumatic cardiac tamponade and in some cases a larger retrosternal hematoma or an anterior pneumothorax. Ultrasound is also a substitute for radiography in localized symptoms of the ribs, especially in children.

► **CT.** CT is essential in severe thoracic trauma (e.g., in a multiple-injury setting) for detecting injuries of internal organs, in particular the heart, lungs, and major vessels, in addition to any fractures of the bony thorax.

2.5.6 Stress Phenomena of the Acromioclavicular Joint

Overuse-induced osteolysis of the lateral clavicle may manifest itself in individuals who frequently perform lifting movements (e.g., weightlifters, handball players). A reversible bone marrow edema pattern may be detected by MRI in the early phase; the edema may also involve the acromion (► Figs. 2.155 and ► W2.23).

2.5.7 Posttraumatic Conditions Secondary to Injuries of the Shoulder Girdle

Cosmetic problems secondary to displacement and/or prominent callus formation often develop after clavicular fractures. The nonunion rate is ~ 20% for conservative management and ~ 2% after surgical treatment (► Fig. W2.24).

Instability associated with secondary osteoarthritis may occur after dislocation of the sternoclavicular joint.

After disruption of the acromioclavicular joint, a residual high-riding lateral end of the clavicle is usually only a cosmetic problem.

Coracoclavicular ossification frequently appears as a late sequela of acromioclavicular joint injury—regardless of the type of treatment. In rare cases posttraumatic osteolysis of the lateral end of the clavicle is found that cannot be differentiated from the overuse-induced form with imaging.

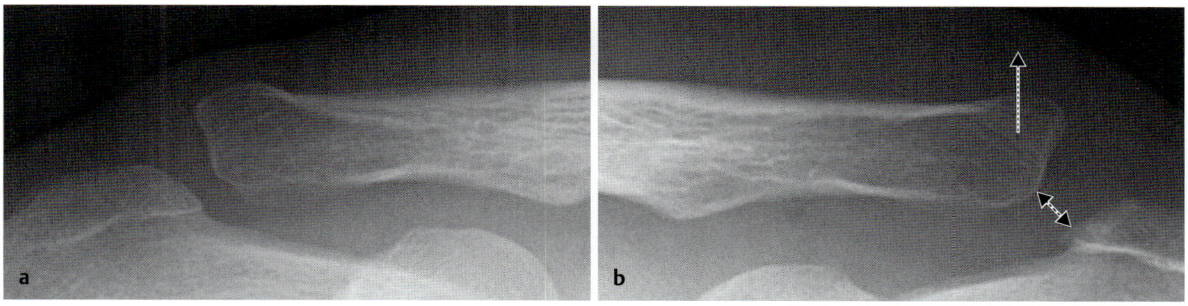

Fig. 2.151 Tossy II (arrows). Weight-bearing view. **(a)** Healthy right side. **(b)** Injured left side.

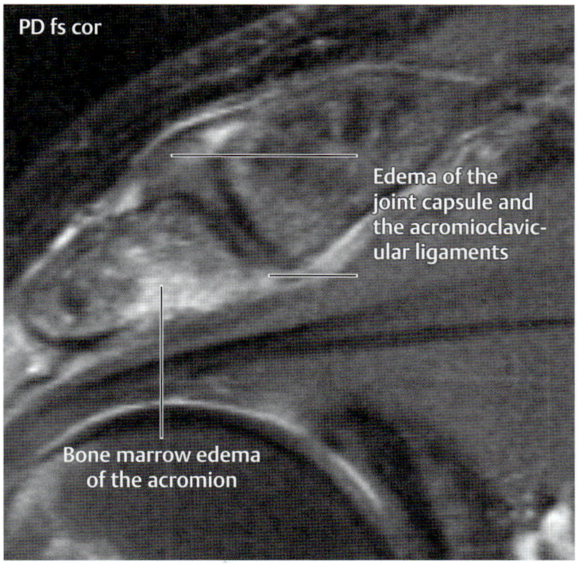

Fig. 2.152 MRI of a Tossy I injury.

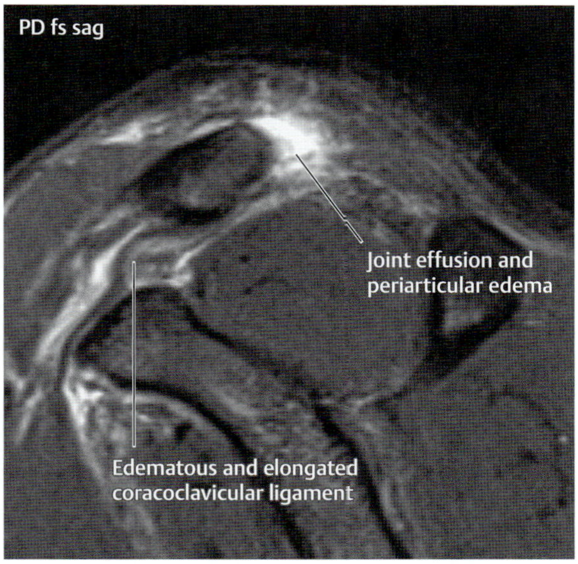

Fig. 2.153 MRI of a Tossy II injury. For additional images see ▸ Fig. W2.21.

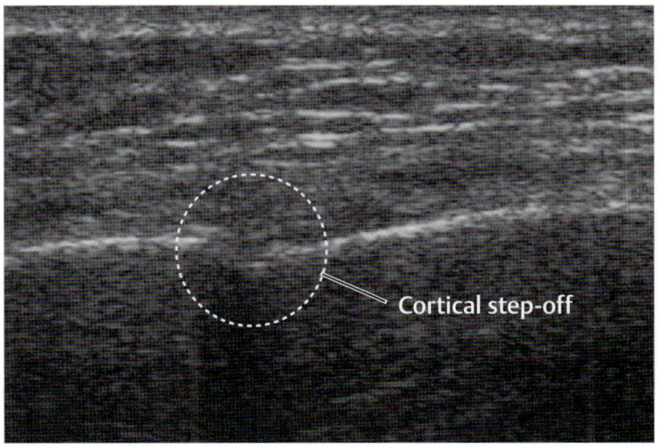

Fig. 2.154 Ultrasound of a sternal fracture. Longitudinal section.

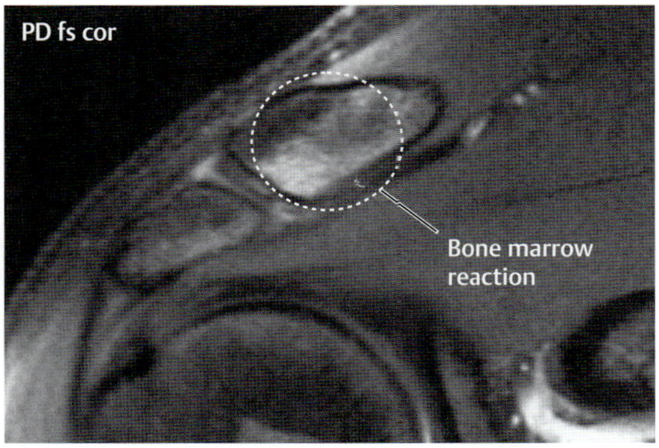

Fig. 2.155 Overuse (stress) reaction of the acromioclavicular joint in a golfer. For additional images see ▸ Fig. W2.23.

2.6 Upper Arm

2.6.1 Proximal Humeral Fractures

▸ **Anatomy.** See ▸ Figs. W2.25 and ▸ W2.26.

▸ **Pathology.** The most commonly used systems to classify humeral head fractures are the **AO and Neer classification systems** (▸ Fig. 2.156). The Neer system is based on the anatomy and prognosis of the fracture and is commonly used in clinical practice. As a rule, only segments displaced by more than 1 cm or angulated more than 45° are taken into account for classification of the fracture type (▸ Figs. 2.157 and W2.27). On the AO Foundation website (www.aofoundation.org) there is an interactive presentation of the AO classification, which is based more upon fracture management.

One variant is the head-splitting injury in which the fracture involves the cartilage-bearing portion of the humeral head. These fractures result in a step-off of the articular surface of the humeral head and may disrupt the blood supply and lead to osteonecrosis of the proximal fragment (▸ Figs. 2.158 and W2.28).

▸ **Radiography.** AP and axial views are obligatory; a supplementary transscapular or transthoracic view may also be required.

▸ **US.** Possible associated injuries, such as tears of the rotator cuff and the long biceps tendon or a hemarthrosis, may also be detected.

▸ **CT.** CT allows a confident classification of the fracture type in cases with ambiguous radiographic findings. It is also much more sensitive than radiography for displaying more subtle step-offs of the articular surface, intra-articular fragments, or associated glenoid fractures.

▸ **Special features in children.** Fractures of the proximal humerus are rare in children. They usually involve an epiphyseal separation with a metaphyseal fragment (Salter–Harris Type II) or a greenstick fracture at the level of the surgical neck (infratubercular fracture). In equivocal cases, comparison with radiographs of the contralateral side, an MRI scan, or ultrasound may help.

Stress-related changes. Widening of the proximal humeral epiphysis may develop in children and adolescents as a result of overuse (typically throwing), and is known as "little leaguer's shoulder."

▸ **Important findings.** In proximal humeral fractures, the number of fracture fragments and their degree of displacement should be described and then classified according to one of the established systems. It is important to specifically describe any head-splitting or glenoid fractures because of the risk of subsequent osteonecrosis or secondary osteoarthritis, respectively.

2.6.2 Humeral Shaft Fractures

Fractures of the humeral shaft include diaphyseal fractures with or without displacement. Displacement of the main fragment depends on the level of the fracture and the inserting muscle groups (▸ Figs. 2.159 and W2.29). There is a risk of associated injuries with humeral shaft fractures, especially when they involve its middle third. Injury of the radial nerve occurs in 18% of cases, but is reversible in more than 90% of these. Humeral shaft fractures are rarely classified and, if so, then the AO classification system may be used (see the AO website).

▸ **Radiography.** Radiographs in two projections (AP and transthoracic) are sufficient. The adjacent joints must be included on the image to exclude concomitant injuries. Important findings include the degree of distraction of the fracture fragments and any rotational malalignment.

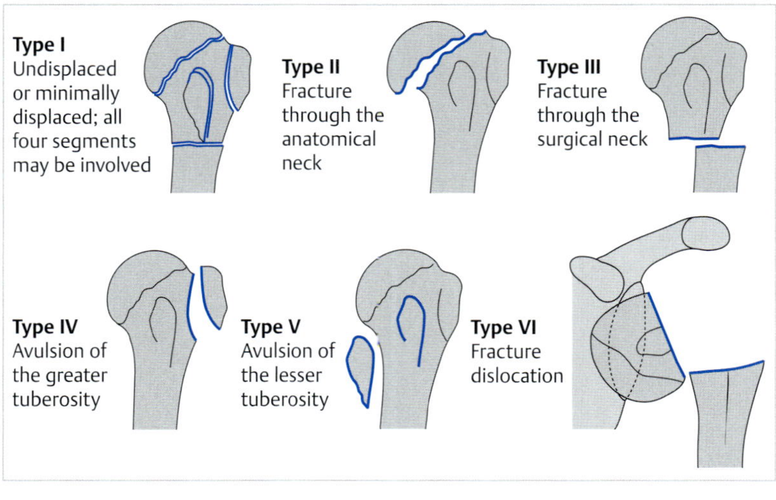

Fig. 2.156 Proximal humeral fractures: Neer classification. If several segments are displaced, then classification of the higher-grade fracture type is used.

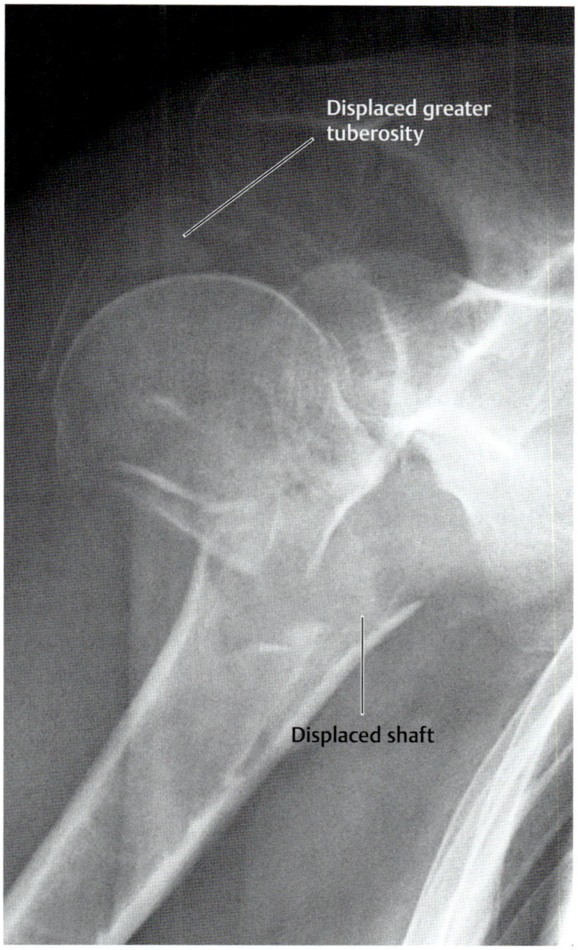

Fig. 2.157 Three-part fracture. Neer Type IV. For additional CT images see ▸ Fig. W2.27.

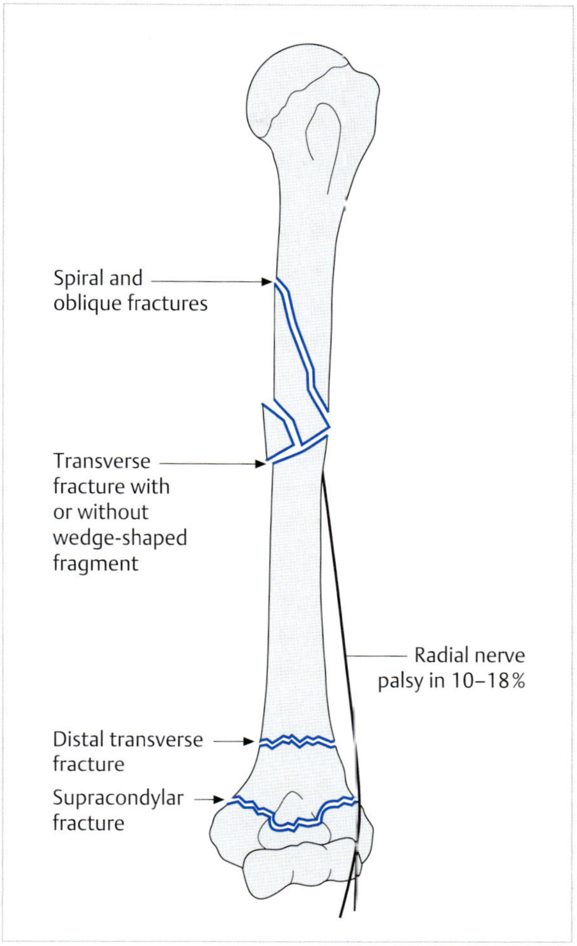

Fig. 2.159 Typical fracture patterns of the humerus.

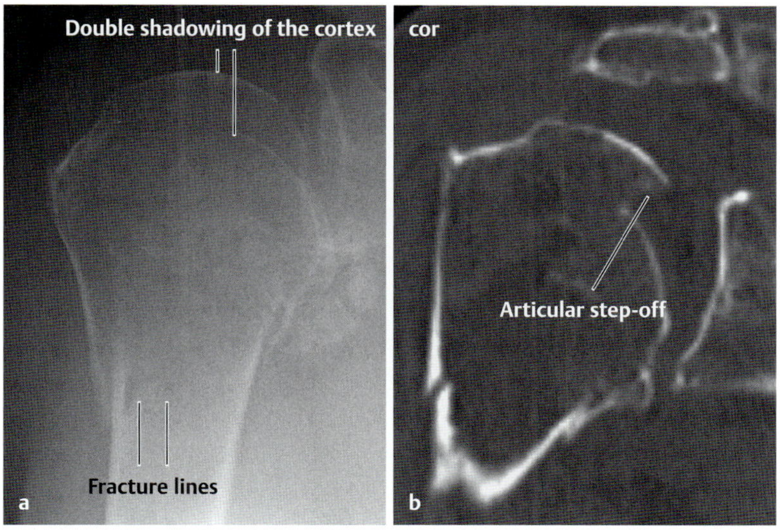

Fig. 2.158 Head-splitting fracture. **(a)** Note the double cortical shadows on the radiograph. **(b)** Assessment of the joint surfaces is best accomplished using CT (for an additional image see ▸ Fig. W2.28).

► **US.** In posttraumatic lesions of the radial nerve, ultrasound is capable of assessing whether damage to the nerve is due to focal nerve injury, fixation hardware, or callus formation.

2.6.3 Distal Humeral Fractures

► **Pathology.** In adults, 90% of distal humeral fractures involve the elbow joint. In children, by comparison, extra-articular supracondylar fractures are the most common fractures around the elbow. The fracture types are classified using the established AO systems (► Fig. 2.160).

► **Radiography.** AP and lateral radiographs with the elbow flexed at 90° should be obtained. Nondisplaced fractures may be unremarkable on AP views, and any indirect signs of a fracture, especially an elevated fat pad indicating a joint effusion, should therefore be noted (► Fig. 2.161).

► **CT.** A supplementary CT scan may help to confirm suspected joint involvement if radiographs are equivocal (► Fig. W2.30).

► **MRI.** An MRI scan is useful for suspected stress fractures, osteochondritis dissecans, and fractures in children.

► **Special features in children.** The accurate diagnosis of a distal humeral fracture in a child requires an understanding of the appearance and fusion of ossification centers. The time of appearance, however, varies considerably from one individual to another (► Fig. 2.162). The mnemonic **"CRITOL"** is helpful in listing the most common sequence of appearance of the ossification centers (**c**apitulum → **r**adial head→ **i**nternal [medial] epicondyle → **t**rochlea → **o**lecranon → external [**l**ateral] epicondyle). The absence of an expected ossification center based on this sequence should raise concern for a displaced ossification center.

These injuries are often only detectable by displacement of the ossification centers. Displacement of the capitulum secondary to a supracondylar humeral fracture or epiphyseolysis is best evaluated on a true *lateral* image with the aid of Roger's reference line (► Fig. 2.163). In equivocal cases an image comparing the contralateral side or an MRI scan may be obtained.

Rotational deformities should be especially looked for in children with a humeral fracture, often indicated by widening of the malrotated fragment (known as the rotation spur) on the lateral view (► Fig. 2.164).

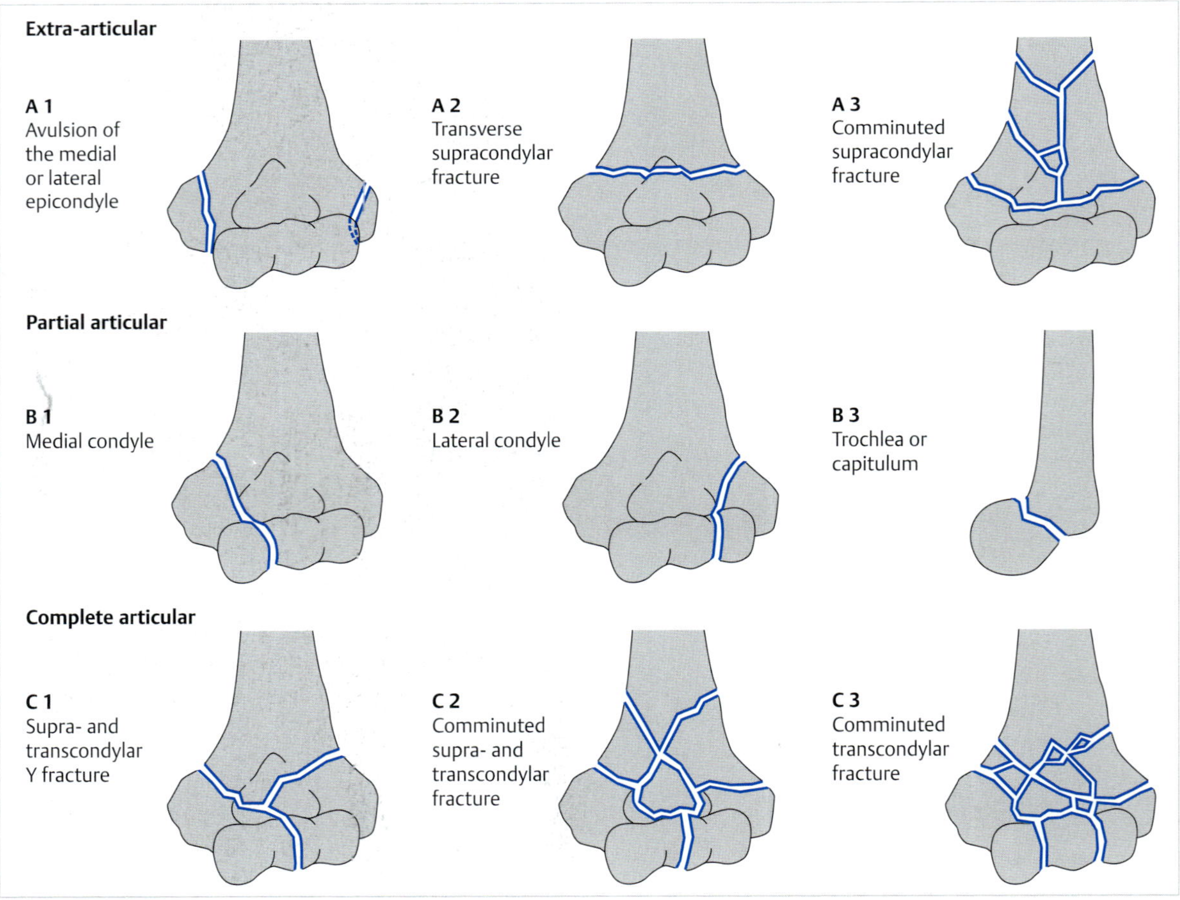

Fig. 2.160 AO classification of distal humeral fractures.

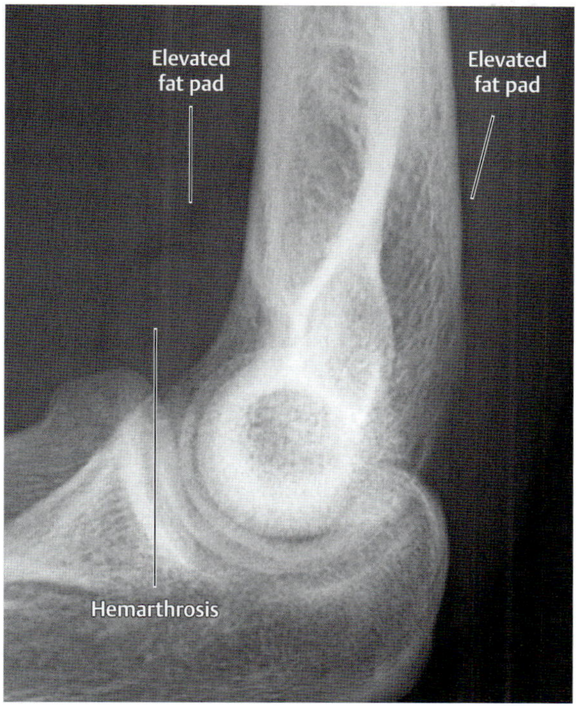

Fig. 2.161 Indirect fracture signs at the elbow.

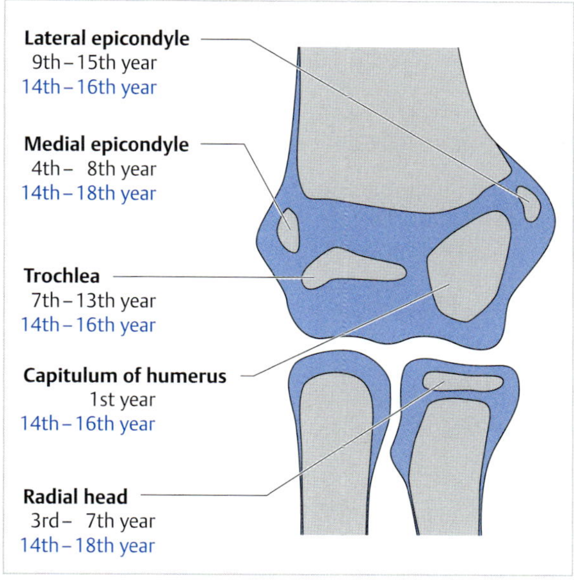

Fig. 2.162 Appearance and fusion of elbow ossification centers. Black numbers indicate age of appearance; blue numbers indicate age of fusion. Not included is the olecranon (appearance at 6th–13th year of age, fusion at 14th–18th year of age).

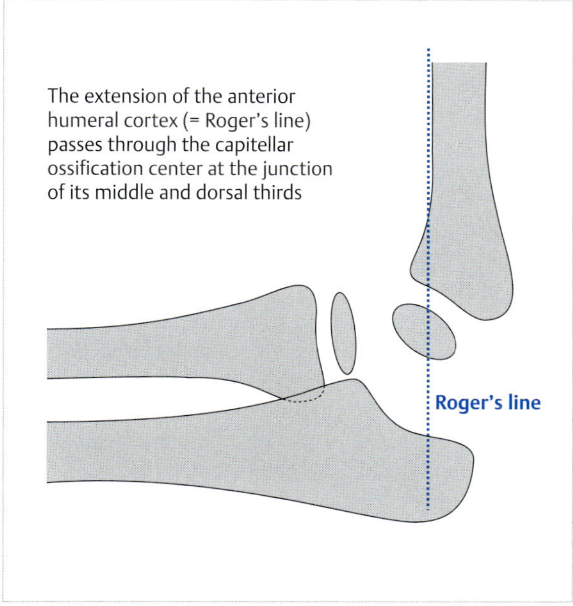

Fig. 2.163 Roger's reference line.

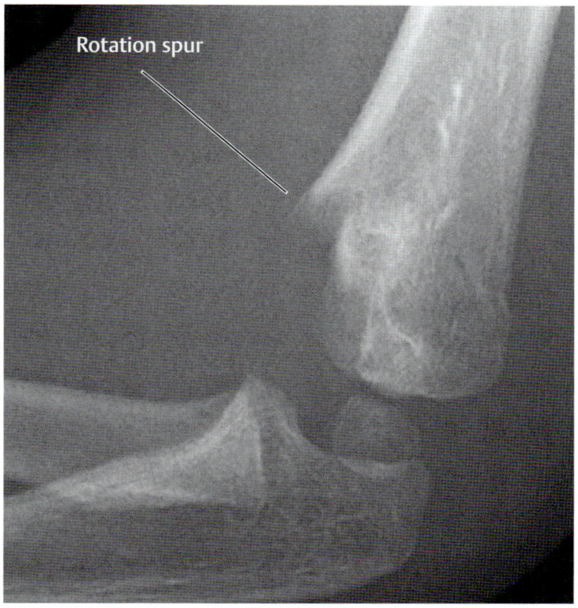

Fig. 2.164 Supracondylar humeral fracture with rotational deformity.

2.6.4 Radiological Assessment after Surgery of the Upper Arm

Proximal Humeral Fractures

There are basically three methods available for the management of proximal humeral fractures: plating, intramedullary nailing, and joint replacement.

In principle, **plate fixation** is suitable for all types of fracture of the proximal upper arm, with the angle-stable procedure being the most common. Avulsed tubercles attached to the rotator cuff tendons can be sutured to small holes in the plate, although this tension band suture is not evident on radiographs.

An intact head fragment is a prerequisite for **intramedullary nail fixation**. Tension band sutures of the tubercle can be attached to the interlocking screws. Additional stability may be achieved by a curved blade inserted from a laterocaudal direction through the nail and into the humeral head.

Joint replacement is necessary in cases of impacted four-part fractures, fractures with a severely fragmented humeral head, or severe osteoporosis. The glenoid is not usually replaced. A *reverse prosthesis* (in which the glenoid component is replaced by a head, while the head component is replaced by a corresponding socket) lends itself to cases where there is no intact glenoid or functioning rotator cuff. This results in lateralization of the pivot point of the joint, which allows the deltoid to partially replace the rotators while also reducing the risk of dislocation because of the geometry of the implant. The tendon-bearing tubercles may be secured by tension band sutures to the proximal shaft at the time the prosthesis is placed.

► Radiography.

Technique. After surgery, the majority of patients are unable to tolerate arm abduction, which is required for the axial radiograph. The scapular "Y" view is an acceptable alternative in this situation.

The **postoperative radiographic examination** must address the following questions:

- *Complete reduction?* Any angulation of the head (► Fig. 2.165) or cranial displacement of the greater tubercle (possibly resulting in impingement) should be noted.
- *Position of the screws?* The tips of the screws in the humeral head should be just a few millimeters away from the subchondral bone plate (cf. ► Fig. 1.73). Shaft screws, in contrast, must have purchase on the far cortex or project just beyond it with self-drilling screws.
- *Position of the plate?* The proximal plate end should only extend minimally beyond the circumference of the humeral head to avoid associated impingement.
- *Position of the intramedullary nail?* The proximal nail end should not project beyond the humeral head, again to avoid the risk of impingement or rotator cuff damage (see ► Fig. 2.165).
- *Alignment (instability?) and subacromial space (impingement?) after joint replacement?* Instability is recognizable by a decentralization of the humeral head replacement relative to the glenoid fossa or glenoid component (► Fig. 2.166). Scapular "Y" or axial views are also necessary for complete evaluation.

Subsequent follow-up radiographs should be scrutinized for hardware migration, loss of initial reduction (secondary fragment displacement), nonunion, avascular necrosis, heterotopic ossification, and signs of infection.

Humeral Shaft Fractures

Fractures of the humeral shaft are treated either by plating or intramedullary nailing, with a current tendency toward the latter since it is less traumatic. The nail may be inserted via the humeral head (antegrade) or through the olecranon fossa (retrograde).

► Radiography.

Technique. Technical difficulties with positioning often prevent obtaining optimal postoperative radiographs, and fluoroscopy-guided evaluation may be necessary. After surgery, complex fractures often need to be evaluated with CT if surgical revision is being considered. If extension of the elbow is inadequate, an AP projection of the distal humerus is needed. This is achieved by directing the perpendicular to the upper arm.

The **postoperative radiographic evaluation** should address the following aspects:

- *Abnormal alignment?*
- *Fragment displacement?*
- *Position of the nail?* The nail should be anchored for a sufficient length on either side of the fracture; the interlocking screws should find purchase in the far cortex. With antegrade intramedullary nailing, the proximal end of the nail should not project beyond the head. With retrograde intramedullary nailing, particular attention should be paid to the insertion site. That is where iatrogenic fractures can occur during nail insertion.

Distal Humeral Fractures

Distal humeral fractures are treated using lag screws, plates, or wire fixation.

► Radiography.

Technique. If the elbow cannot be adequately extended, then separate AP views (central ray directed first perpendicular to the upper arm and then perpendicular to the forearm) should be obtained (► Fig. 2.167). In difficult cases a CT scan will help to assess fragment reduction and restoration of the joint surfaces.

The **postoperative radiographic evaluation** should assess the following aspects:

- *Restoration of the joint surfaces?*
- *Normal joint articulation?*
- *Intra-articular fragments?*

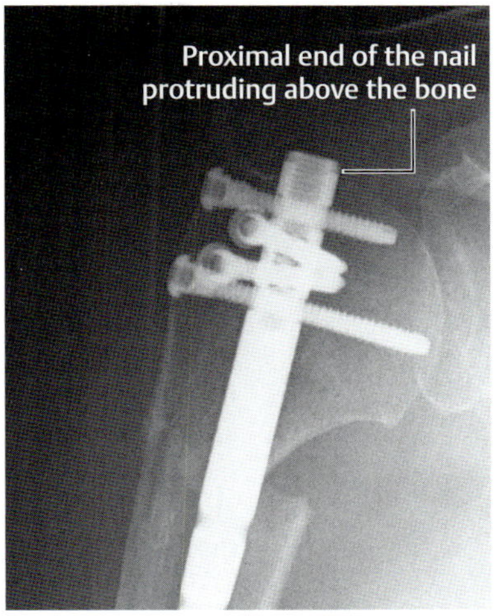

Fig. 2.165 Intramedullary nail fixation of the humeral head. The intramedullary nail projects beyond the contour of the humeral head, into the rotator cuff. Furthermore, there is varus positioning of the fracture site with angulation of the head in a medial direction.

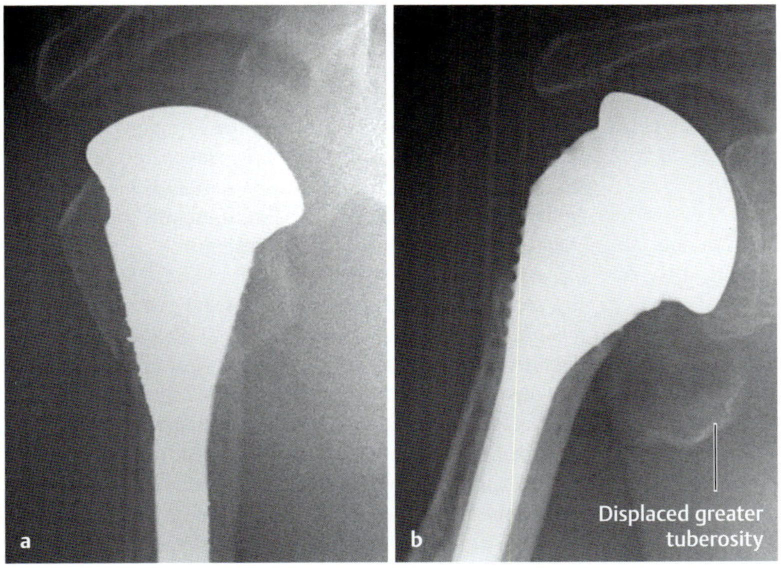

Fig. 2.166 Cemented humeral head prosthesis after a comminuted fracture dislocation. **(a)** Postoperative radiograph under suboptimal conditions: normal position. **(b)** Follow-up 6 weeks later: the greater tubercle is secondarily displaced; high-riding humeral head with loss of function of the supraspinatus tendon (superior instability).

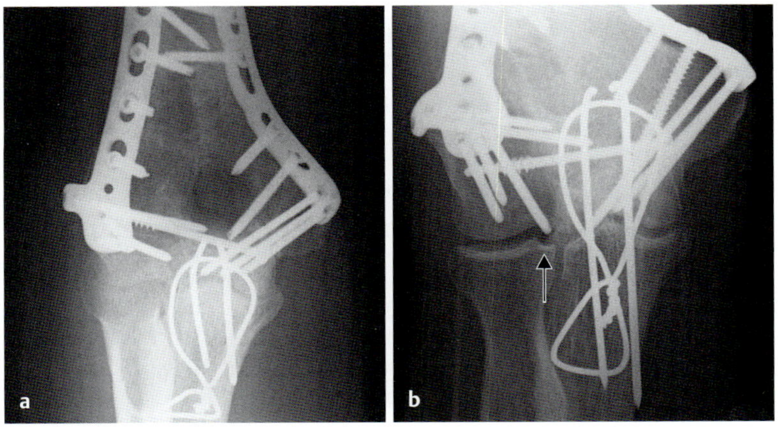

Fig. 2.167 Presentation after fixation of a comminuted transcondylar distal humerus fracture. **(a)** The distal humerus can be readily assessed with the AP view directed vertically to the upper arm. **(b)** The AP view directed vertically to the forearm also shows a defect in the radial head (arrow) caused by the protruding screw. The defect was not noticeable on image **(a)**.

2.7 Elbow Joint

▸ **Anatomy.** See Chapter 2.7 and ▸ Figs. W2.31–W2.34.

2.7.1 Medial Compartment

Medial Epicondylitis (Ulnar Epicondylitis of the Humerus)

Enthesopathy of the common flexor origin is also known as “golfer's elbow,” although this entity is seen in other sports as well.

▸ **Clinical presentation.** Physical examination reveals localized tenderness over the origin of the common flexor tendon (just proximal to the origin of the ulnar collateral ligament), which increases with resisted flexion of the wrist.

The imaging findings are analogous to those of the more common lateral epicondylitis, and for this reason reference will be made to the images presented in the following section (Chapter 2.7.2).

▸ **Radiography.** Normally there are no features of note, although soft tissue calcifications or enthesophytes may be apparent (cf. ▸ Fig. 2.174).

▸ **US.** Typical ultrasound findings include decreased echogenicity and abnormal-appearing tendon fascicles (cf. ▸ Fig. 2.175). As the disease progresses, increased vascularization develops that can be detected with Doppler ultrasound (▸ Fig. W2.35).

▸ **MRI.** The major finding is thickening of the tendon at its origin with heterogeneously increased signal intensity on fat-suppressed and T2W sequences. A heterogeneous appearance is also evident on T1W images (cf. ▸ Figs. 2.176, ▸ 2.177, and ▸ W2.36). These findings are best demonstrated in the coronal and axial planes. Concomitant bone marrow edema is often found at the tendon's origin.

The flexor muscle group may also be partially or completely avulsed from the medial epicondyle as a result of acute trauma. This may be associated with a small avulsion fracture. Such valgus injuries are often associated with chondromalacia of the radial head.

▸ **Special features in children.** **Little leaguer's elbow** is a chronic traction injury of the unfused medial epicondylar apophysis. Cumulative microtrauma from repetitive valgus stress is regarded as the cause, as occurs with repetitive throwing motions in young baseball players (see also Chapter 7.3.5).

Injuries to the Ulnar Collateral Ligament and Common Flexor Tendon Origin

▸ **Radiography.** The radiograph is unremarkable in acute injuries. A traction spur may be visible at the tip of the coronoid process in cases of chronic overuse (▸ Fig. 2.168)

▸ **US.** **Full-thickness tears** of the ulnar collateral ligament result in separation of the torn margins of the ligament (normal appearance can be seen in ▸ Fig. 2.169). Only the clinically important anterior bundle of the ulnar collateral ligament is visible on ultrasound. Joint fluid escapes from the articular space, between the torn ligament ends and into the surrounding soft tissue.

A **partial-thickness tear** is present if parts of the ligament are shown to be in continuity, or if the ligament is displayed as intact but markedly lax (wavy or undulating) during a dynamic examination or with valgus stress.

▸ **MRI.** **Full-thickness tears** are more common than partial tears. The former are usually easily delineated on coronal fat-suppressed sequences (▸ Figs. 2.170–2.172). The mechanism of injury causing the tear also commonly produces cartilage damage in the radiocapitellar joint.

By contrast, **partial-thickness tears** are often not readily visible. The deep, juxta-articular distal components of the ligament are typically involved and become separated from the ulnar attachment. These injuries are best appreciated by MR arthrography. Continuation of the contrast medium distally beyond the tip of the coronoid beneath the distal fibers of the ligament is indicative of an articular-surface partial-thickness tear. In these cases the distribution of the contrast medium resembles the form of horizontal “T,” for which reason it is referred to as the “T” sign (▸ Fig. 2.173). In addition, widening of the overlying common flexor tendon is often found in cases of chronic ligament tears.

2.7.2 Lateral Compartment

Lateral Epicondylitis (Radial Epicondylitis of the Humerus)

Chronic pathology of the common extensor tendon at its origin is also known as “tennis elbow,” although this pathology is not confined to that particular sport. It is 10 times more common than medial epicondylitis. Histologically, mucoid degeneration in the region of the origin of extensor carpi radialis brevis develops; in about one-third of cases the extensor digitorum is also involved.

▸ **Clinical presentation.** The clinical appearance is similar to that of medial epicondylitis, only on the lateral aspect.

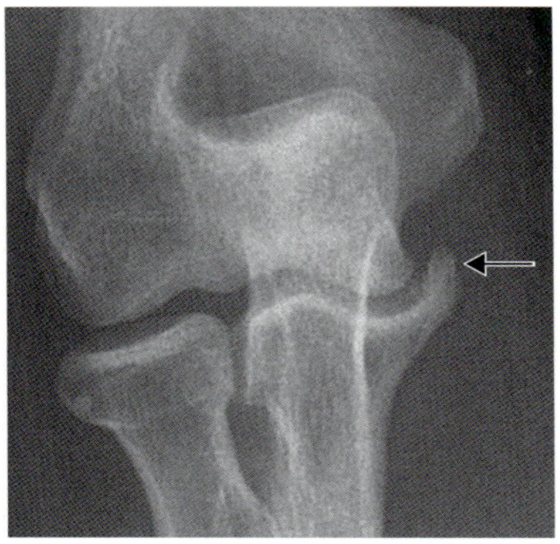

Fig. 2.168 Bone spur on the ulnar surface of the coronoid process (arrow). The bone spur is consistent with a traction osteophyte.

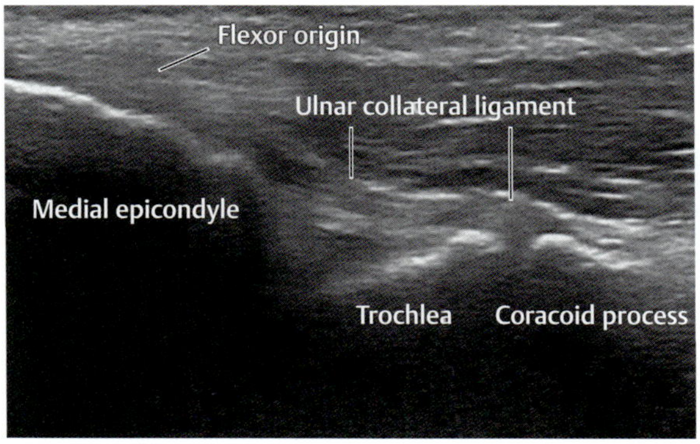

Fig. 2.169 Normal ulnar collateral ligament under ultrasound. Longitudinal section.

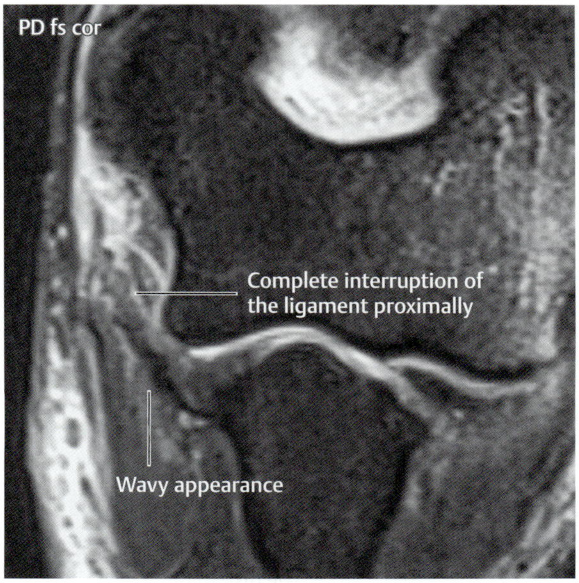

Fig. 2.170 Full-thickness tear of the ulnar collateral ligament.

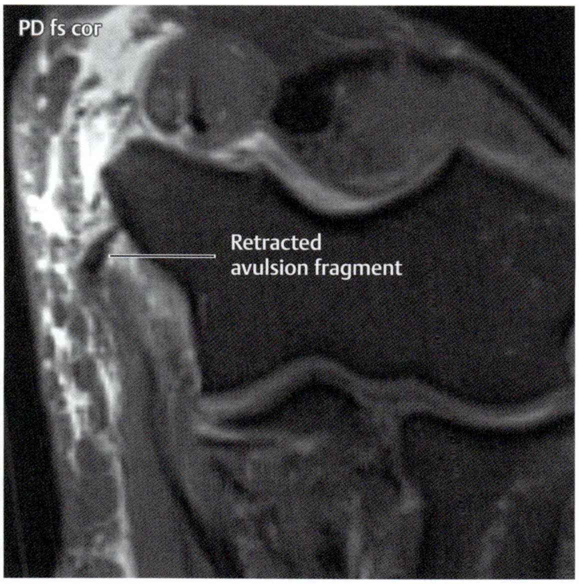

Fig. 2.171 Bony avulsion of the flexor origin on the medial epicondyle in an adolescent.

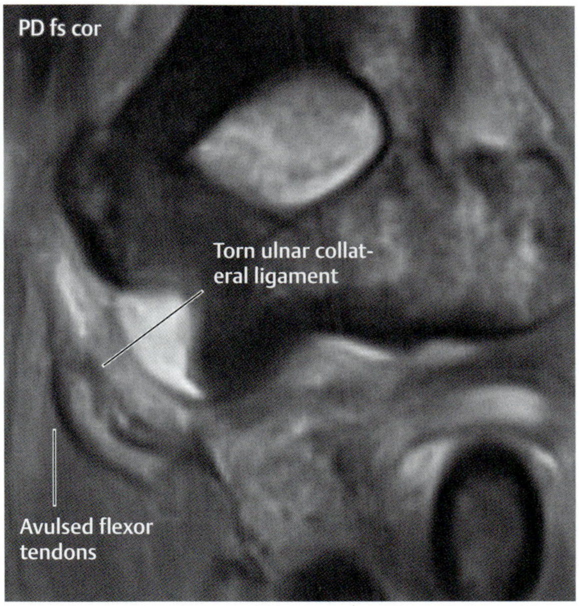

Fig. 2.172 Avulsion of the flexor tendons from the medial epicondyle associated with a collateral ligament avulsion.

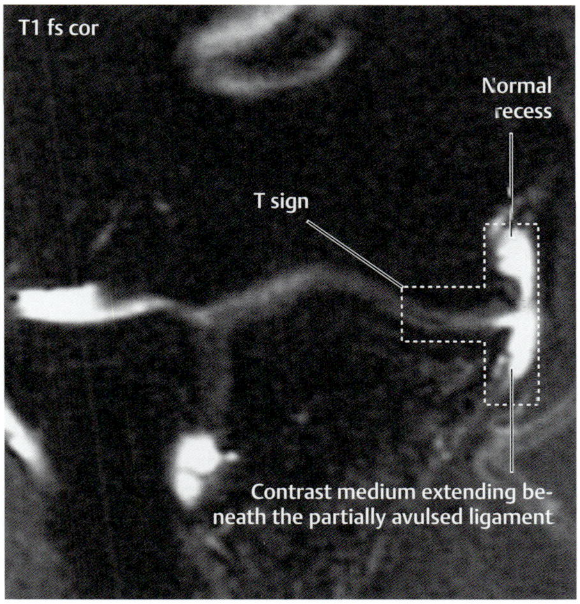

Fig. 2.173 Articular-surface partial tear of the ulnar collateral ligament. MR arthrography.

▶ **Radiography.** Radiographs are generally unremarkable in a case of lateral epicondylitis; occasionally intratendinous calcifications or enthesophytes are evident near the tendon origin (▶ Fig. 2.174).

▶ **US.** Similarly to its use in medial epicondylitis, ultrasound displays a thickened and hypoechoic proximal common extensor tendon at its origin (▶ Fig. 2.175). The anterior and deeper fibers of the tendon are more affected than the posterior and more superficial fibers, corresponding to the position of extensor carpi radialis brevis within the common extensor tendon origin.

As the disease progresses, there is an increase in vascularity with increased flow signal on Doppler ultrasound (▶ see ▶ Fig. W2.35).

▶ **MRI.** Coronal fat-suppressed sequences are best suited for reaching a diagnosis; the changes are also well defined on axial slices (▶ Figs. 2.176 and ▶ 2.177; also ▶ Fig. W2.36). Corresponding signal changes may also occur on T1W sequences, but these are less specific than the increase in signal intensity on T2W sequences.

Injuries of the Radial (Lateral) Collateral Ligaments, the Extensor Origin, and the Annular Ligament

▶ **Pathology.** Both the radial collateral ligament and the lateral ulnar collateral ligament are important dorsolateral stabilizers of the elbow joint. A fall on the outstretched hand results in an axial compression of the radius (with or without a fracture of the radial head) with displacement of the radius in a dorsal direction. The result is a partial- or full-thickness tear of these ligaments, even to the extent of a complete avulsion of the radial ligamentous system, together with the common extensor tendon origin at the lateral epicondyle.

With even more severe trauma, the tear progresses beyond the anterior and posterior parts of the capsule until it finally reaches the medial collateral ligament. Here, the posterior components of the medial collateral ligament rupture before the anterior components tear. Along with the rupture of the annular ligament and subsequent displacement of the radius, this results in a circumferential capsuloligamentous disruption (known as the circle of Horii).

A fracture of the coronoid process, another important stabilizer of the elbow joint, is often found in these cases as an indication of the prior (and commonly spontaneously reduced) dorsal displacement of the ulna. Typically there is also a partial tear of the dorsal fibers of the brachialis muscle and those parts of the flexor digitorum superficialis muscle close to its origin.

▶ **Radiography.** Incongruence between radial head and capitellum on survey views suggests injury to the radial (lateral) collateral ligament.

▶ **US.** The radial collateral ligament appears on ultrasound as a delicate fascicular structure that is somewhat thickened proximally. A synovial plica (meniscal homologue of the elbow) can be well demonstrated along its articular surface. Tears of the radial collateral ligament result in abnormal contour of the ligament and/or disruption of fibers along its course. Involvement of the lateral ulnar collateral ligament may be detected by ultrasound in cases of a tear of the common extensor origin. Widening is an indication of an old injury. Subluxation of the radial head can be visualized by ultrasound.

▶ **MRI.** Pathologies of the common extensor tendon origin are often associated with a tear of the radial collateral ligament, which should be specifically looked for. Increased intrasubstance signal intensity or tear of the ligament are well demonstrated on MRI.

An elbow dislocation can result in simultaneous avulsions of both the radial collateral ligament and the lateral ulnar collateral ligament. The ruptured ligament may be detected along with fluid leaking into the soft tissues (▶ Fig. 2.178). Injury to the annular ligament can also be demonstrated. There is often joint incongruence between the radial head and capitellum (▶ Fig. 2.179).

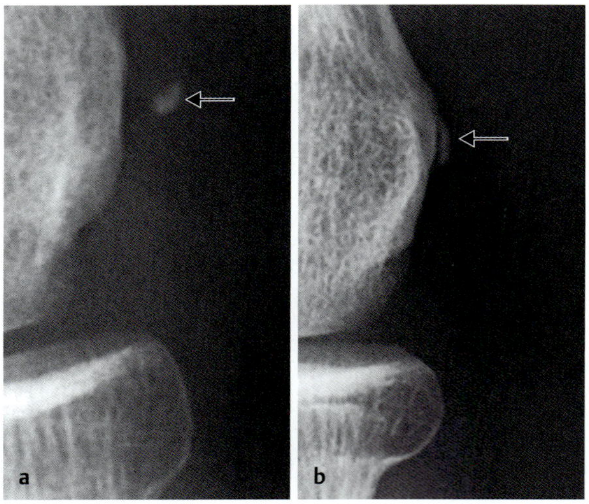

Fig. 2.174 Radiological signs of chronic lateral epicondylitis. **(a)** Small intratendinous calcifications (arrow). **(b)** Enthesophyte (arrow).

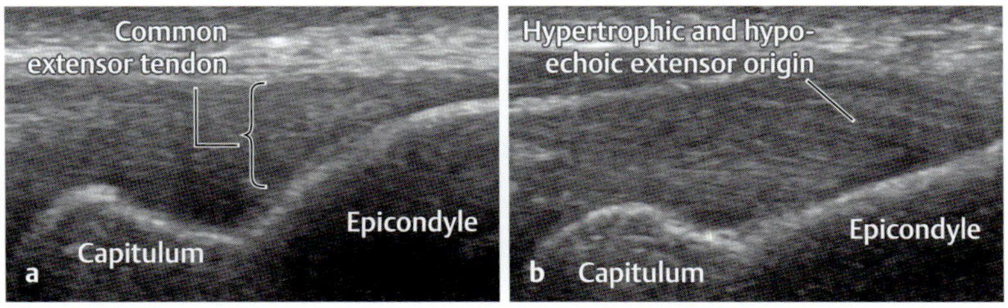

Fig. 2.175 Ultrasound of the common extensor origin on the lateral epicondyle. Longitudinal section. **(a)** Normal finding. **(b)** Chronic epicondylitis.

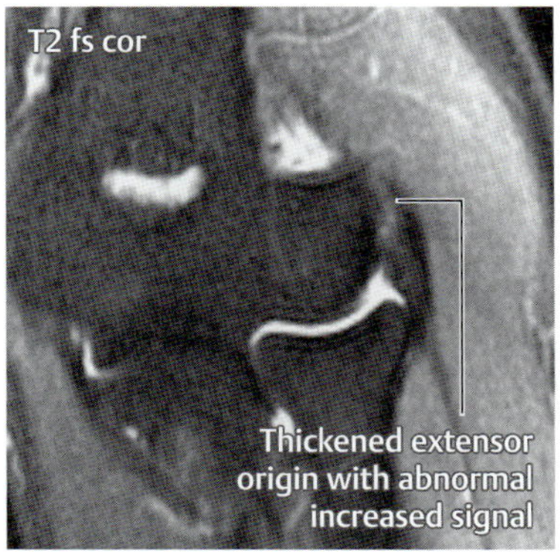

Fig. 2.176

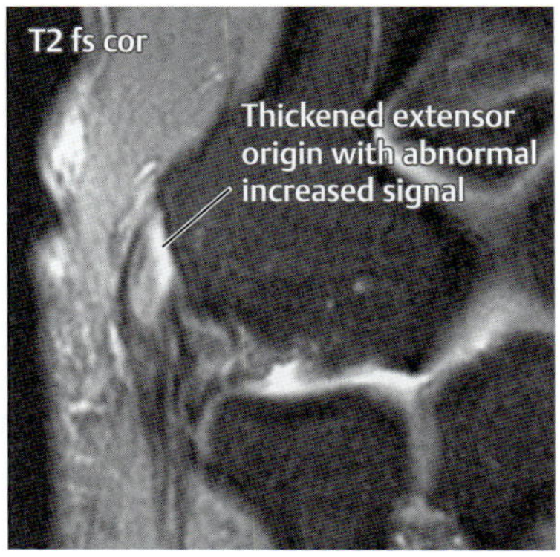

Fig. 2.177

Fig. 2.176 Lateral epicondylitis of the humerus.

Fig. 2.177 Lateral epicondylitis of the humerus. Different patient from ▶ Fig. 2.176.

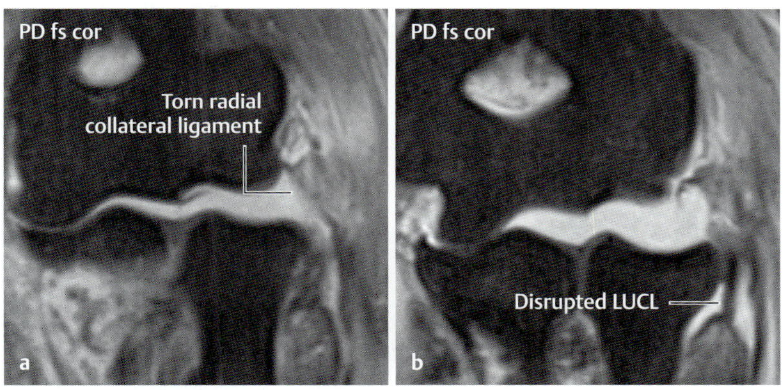

Fig. 2.178 Injury to the radial ligamentous system secondary to a varus injury. **(a)** Lateral collateral ligament tear and extensive avulsion of the extensor origin. **(b)** Somewhat further dorsally, the torn lateral ulnar collateral ligament is visible. LUCL, lateral ulnar collateral ligament.

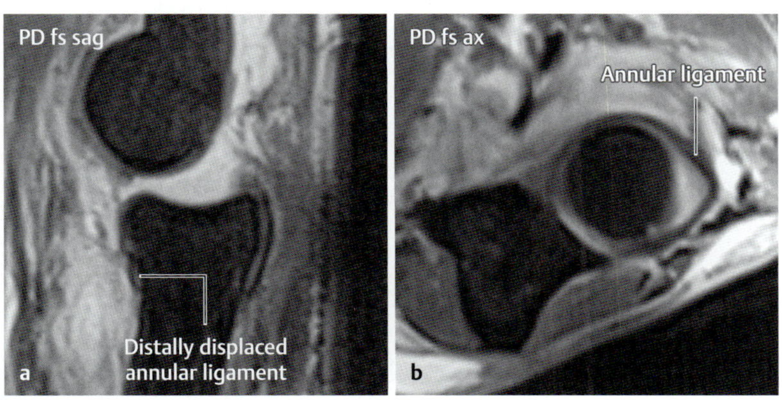

Fig. 2.179 Presentation after elbow dislocation. **(a)** Posterior subluxation of the radial head, which is also displaced proximally relative to the annular ligament. **(b)** The annular ligament appears "too loose" on this axial slice.

2

2.7.3 Anterior Compartment

Biceps Tendon Disorders

▸ **Pathology.** The most important pathologic entities of the anterior compartment include tears and tendinopathy of the distal biceps tendon. The bicipital aponeurosis often sustains a tear at the same time. In this case the tendon retracts proximal to the elbow. Clinically detectable retraction may be absent if the aponeurosis is intact, with the torn tendon margin remaining close to the radial tuberosity.

▸ **US.** Ultrasound can demonstrate tendon pathology and/or associated bursitis. Tendinosis appears as a hypoechoic, thickened tendon; Doppler ultrasound may show increased vascularity. With full-thickness tears, the proximal stump may appear retracted with the distal tendon bed empty or merely filled with fluid. A dynamic ultrasound examination in flexion and extension will help in equivocal cases to distinguish between partial- and full-thickness tears.

▸ **MRI.** Using conventional positioning and imaging techniques, axial slices are best suited for assessing the biceps tendon. If there is strong clinical suspicion of pathology of the distal biceps tendon, the patient may be placed in the FABS position (prone, arm overhead, flexed, abducted, and supinated). It is possible to visualize the entire distal biceps tendon on a single slice with the patient in this position (▸ Fig. 2.180).

Tendinosis demonstrates mildly increased signal intensity within a thickened tendon on T1W and PDW sequences that does not increase significantly on T2W images. Partial- or full-thickness tears of the tendon may develop. Splitting of the tendon is characterized by evidence of multiple smaller tendinous structures (▸ Fig. 2.181). Enthesopathy may be differentiated from tendinosis at the insertion site of the tendon (▸ Fig. 2.182). Tendon continuity is disrupted in acute full-thickness tears, accompanied by edema or hemorrhage in the adjacent soft tissues (▸ Fig. 2.183). Distal biceps tendinopathy is often associated with a bicipitoradial bursitis (▸ Fig. 2.184), which may lead to nerve compression syndrome and may create the clinical impression of a possible tumor (▸ Fig. 2.185).

2.7.4 Posterior Compartment

Olecranon Bursitis

The olecranon bursa is found within the dorsal subcutaneous tissues overlying the olecranon. Common causes of bursitis are chronic mechanical irritation and rheumatic disorders. Direct trauma can lead to hemorrhage into the bursa with a subsequent inflammatory reaction.

▸ **Radiography.** Survey views demonstrate soft tissue swelling over the olecranon and other potential causes, such as rheumatoid arthritis of the elbow joint.

▸ **US.** Olecranon bursitis appears as a fluid-filled structure with a thin or thickened wall, depending on its chronicity. Doppler ultrasound demonstrates increased flow signal in the adjacent inflamed soft tissues. Chronic bursitis (e.g., in association with a rheumatic disorder) may present clinically as a mass in this region.

▸ **MRI.** Rarely is there a need to resort to MRI to reach a diagnosis. However, the scan will demonstrate a high-signal intensity, fluid-filled structure on fluid-sensitive, fat-saturated sequences.

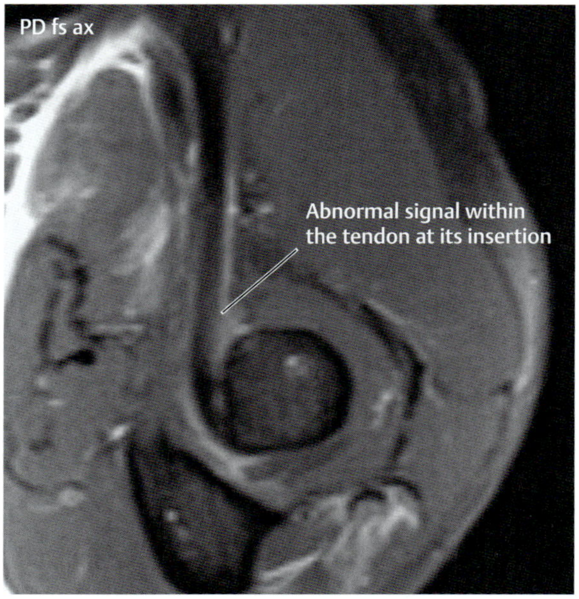

Fig. 2.180 Mild injury to the insertion of the distal biceps tendon secondary to trauma (MRI obtained in the FABS position).

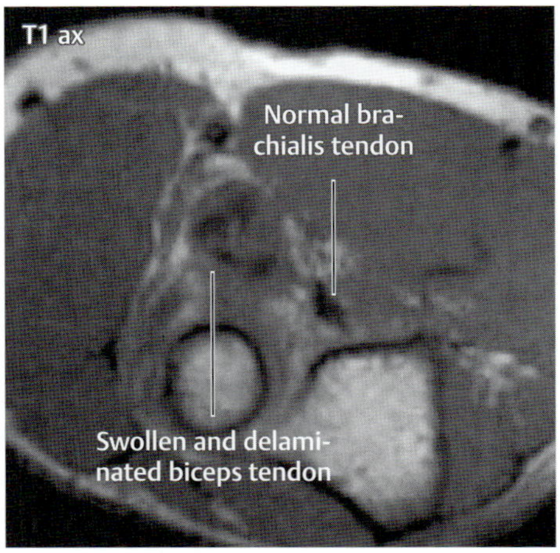

Fig. 2.181 Advanced tendinosis of the distal biceps tendon.

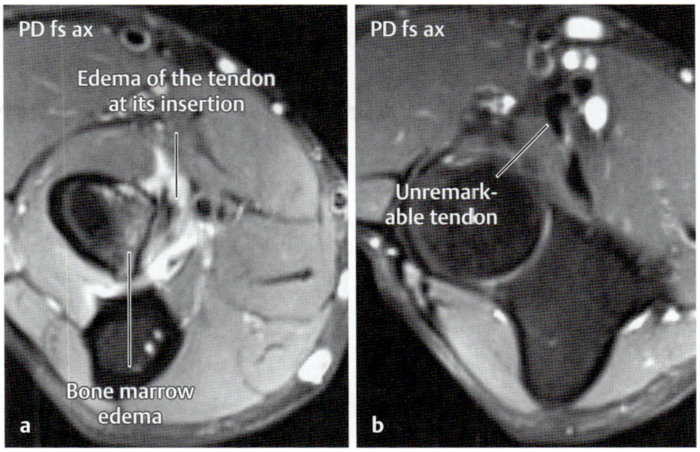

Fig. 2.182 Enthesopathy of the insertion of the distal biceps tendon. **(a)** Inflammatory changes of the tendon insertion. **(b)** The tendon is unremarkable 2.5 cm proximally; there is no tendinosis at this level.

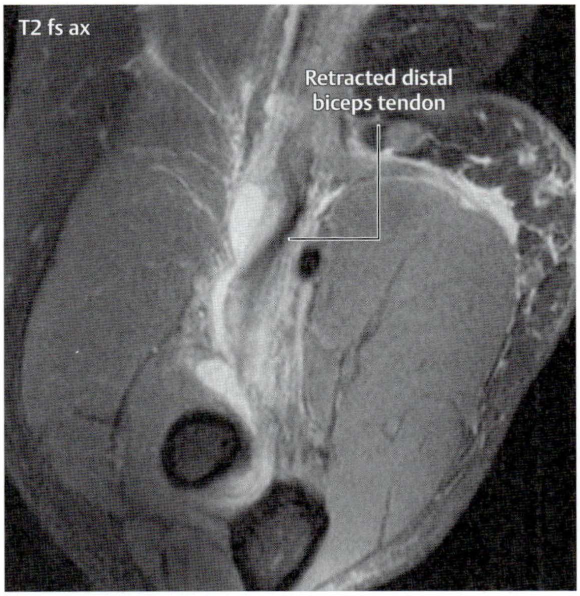

Fig. 2.183 Full-thickness tear of the distal biceps tendon (FABS position).

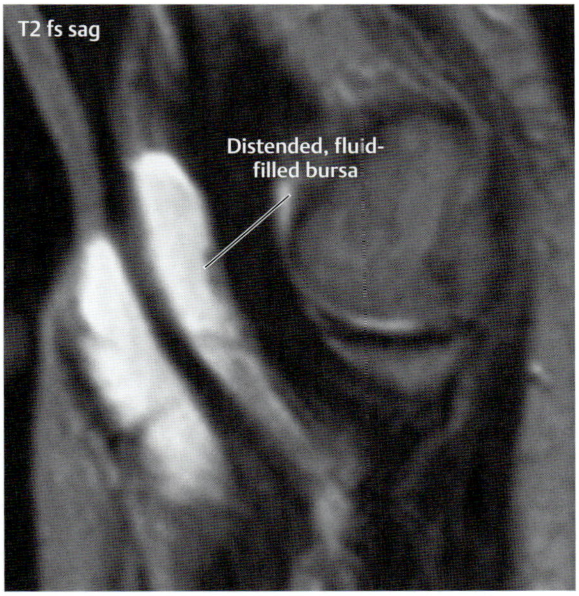

Fig. 2.184 Marked bursitis of the distal biceps tendon. Sharply demarcated fluid accumulation.

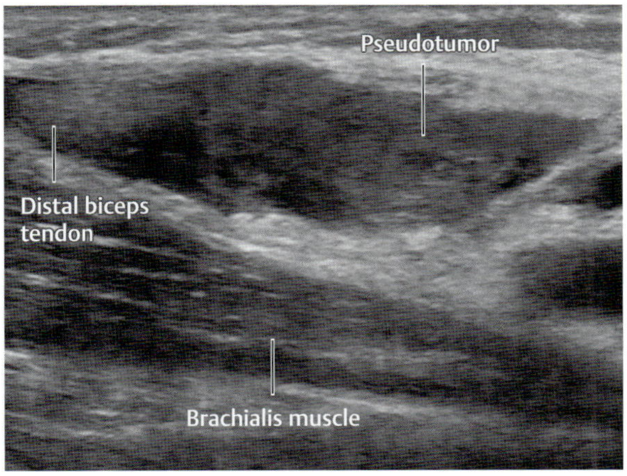

Fig. 2.185 Pseudotumor secondary to tear of the distal biceps tendon. Ultrasound, longitudinal section.

Triceps Tendon Disorders

▸ Pathology. The triceps tendon is much less commonly involved with pathology than is the biceps tendon. Tears are encountered most commonly at its insertion on the olecranon and are usually caused by a fall or a direct blow. Occasionally there is a concomitant fracture of the radial head. Tears of the triceps tendon occur in diabetics and rheumatic patients, as well as in weightlifters, often in association with the misuse of anabolic steroids.

▸ Radiography. Bony avulsions in the region of the olecranon and associated radial head fractures may be demonstrated by conventional radiography. Spur formation is seen in the case of chronic enthesopathy (▸ Fig. 2.186).

▸ US. Ultrasound provides an excellent depiction of all types of triceps tendon pathology. For findings see biceps tendon disorders in Chapter 2.7.3.

▸ MRI. An MRI scan is rarely required, although it does provide unequivocal findings.

2.7.5 Osteochondral Lesions: Traumatic Lesions, Panner's Disease, and Osteochondritis Dissecans

▸ Pathology. **Acute or chronic trauma** to the cartilage and subchondral bone is the most common cause of osteochondral pathology. Involvement of the joint surface is regularly encountered, especially after an elbow dislocation.

Panner's disease is a benign, self-limiting epiphyseal osteochondrosis (a developmental disorder of the growing cartilage) that occurs in childhood and adolescence, most commonly in prepubertal boys (age 5–10 years). This entity usually goes on to develop normal ossification.

True **osteochondritis dissecans** occurs most commonly in the second decade of life, but before skeletal maturity (Chapter 7.2.5). As a result, an unstable osteochondral fragment may develop and result in an osteochondral defect and associated loose body.

Both Panner's disease and osteochondritis dissecans typically involve the capitellum.

▸ Radiography. Particular attention should be paid to subtle irregularities of the bone on survey views. Flattening, subchondral sclerosis and lucencies may be apparent in the capitulum. Sclerotic changes around the contour irregularity suggest a chronic process. Often only a joint effusion is detected in the acute phase. Special attention must be directed toward any free fragments (▸ Fig. 2.187).

▸ US. Ultrasound may demonstrate irregularity or a step-off in the joint surface (▸ Fig. 2.188) or a defect in later stages. Corresponding loose joint bodies are commonly found in the coronoid and/or olecranon recesses. Particular attention should therefore be directed toward these regions during the ultrasound examination.

▸ CT. Loose bodies are better displayed on a CT scan than on routine radiographs. CT arthrography provides excellent spatial resolution which can be helpful for identifying even small cartilage lesions (▸ Fig. 2.189).

▸ MRI. With acute lesions, abnormal signal intensity may be present within cartilage as well as the underlying cancellous bone (▸ Figs. 2.190 and ▸ 2.191). Unstable lesions demonstrate fluid surrounding the subchondral fragment or larger cystic foci along the fragment/bone interface. Defects of the overlying cartilage are best demonstrated with MR or CT arthrography.

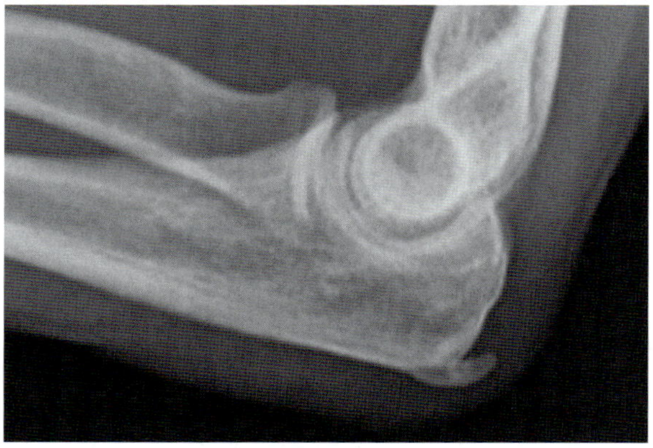

Fig. 2.186 Olecranon traction osteophyte.

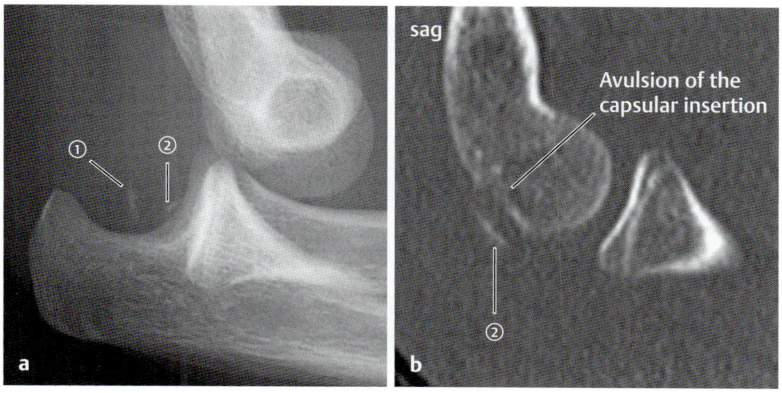

Fig. 2.187 Posterior dislocation of the elbow. **(a)** The radiograph demonstrates two small, flakelike fragments (circled numbers). **(b)** CT after reduction.

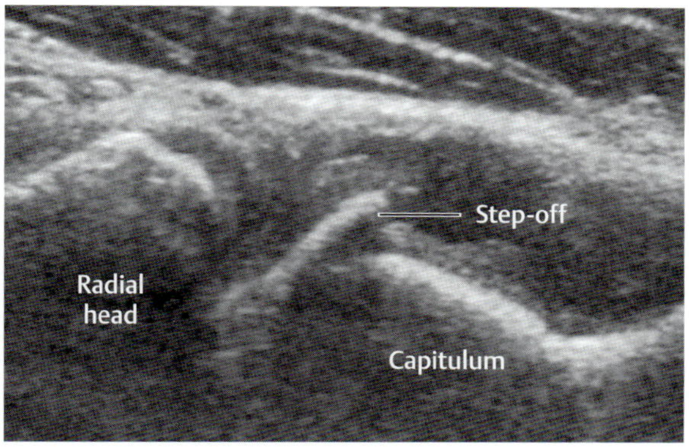

Fig. 2.188 Osteochondral lesion of the capitulum with clear step-off. Longitudinal section.

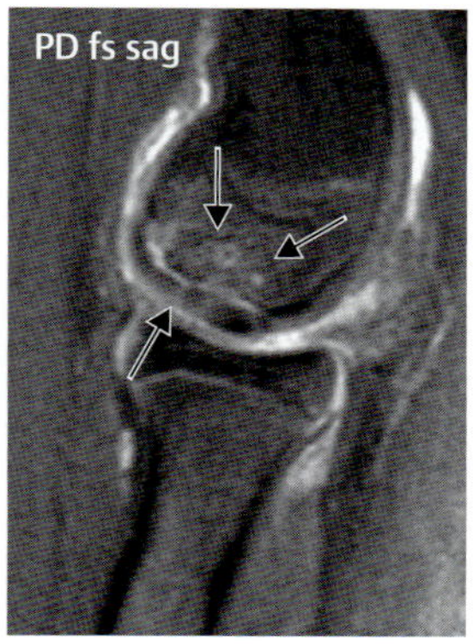

Fig. 2.190 Osteochondral lesion of the capitulum. Note the fracture lines (arrows) near the subchondral bone and the overlying cartilage.

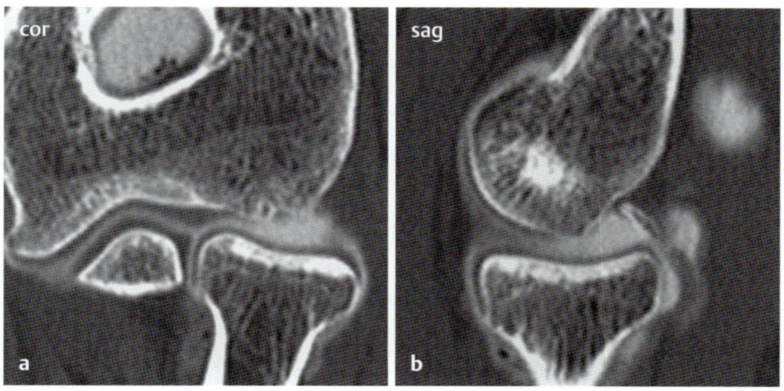

Fig. 2.189 Older osteochondral avulsion from the capitulum. CT arthrography. **(a)** Absent cartilage at the site of the defect. **(b)** The fragment lies in the dorsal recess and is attached to the capsule.

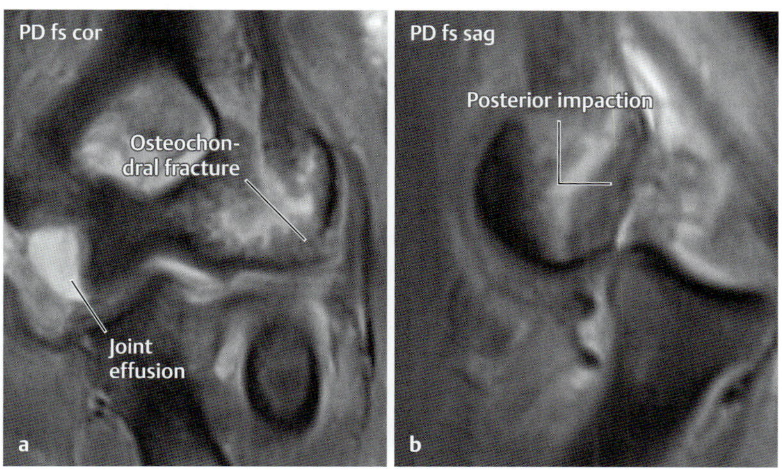

Fig. 2.191 Osteochondral impaction fracture secondary to an elbow dislocation. **(a)** Disruption of the cortex and edema of the capitulum. **(b)** Humeroradial dislocation.

Caution

There are anatomical variants that should not be confused with osteochondral lesions. These include a posterior pseudodefect of the capitellum, a physiological dorsal bony groove between capitellum and lateral epicondyle (▶ Fig. 2.192), and the so-called trochlear groove, an apparent cartilage defect along the articular surface of the ulna between the olecranon and coronoid process (▶ Fig. 2.193).

2.7.6 Neuropathies

Ulnar Nerve

Compression of the ulnar nerve causes pain in the region of the medial elbow and sensory disturbances of the ring and little fingers. There is an association with medial epicondylitis.

▶ **Radiography.** Occasionally bony irregularities are found in the region of the groove for the ulnar nerve and may be well displayed by radiography or CT (▶ Fig. 2.194).

▶ **US.** On a transverse section the normal ulnar nerve displays an oval shape with a "speckled" internal structure. When the nerve is compressed, it appears narrowed at the level of the cubital tunnel, proximal to which there is edematous swelling with loss of the normal fascicular structure (▶ Fig. 2.195a).

A cause of nerve compression may also be visible and may include a thickened retinaculum, ganglion, aberrant anconeus muscle spanning the cubital tunnel (anconeus epitrochlearis), or a bony spur. Medial subluxation of the nerve when the elbow is flexed occurs in 15% of the general population and may be demonstrated with a dynamic US examination. Chronic friction or dislocation may be another cause of neuritis.

▶ **CT.** Bony irregularities and osteophytes are more easily distinguished by CT than with conventional radiography or MR imaging. A bony narrowing of the cubital tunnel is also a relevant finding.

▶ **MRI.** The relationship of the ulnar nerve to the cubital tunnel may be demonstrated on axial T1W sequences. Axial fat-suppressed T2W sequences are well suited for detecting pathologic signal alterations. Compression of the nerve at the level of the groove and thickening proximal to this site may be demonstrated by MRI, as can abnormally increased signal intensity on PDW or T2W sequences (▶ Fig. 2.195b). Subluxation or dislocation of the nerve, or surgical transposition will produce an "empty groove." Ulnar neuropathy may also result from chronic traction, in which case abnormal internal signal intensity is evident without signs of nerve compression.

Median Nerve

▶ **Pathology.** The median nerve may be compromised at various levels. This happens most commonly in the region of the distal humerus as it passes beneath the bicipital aponeurosis and between the two heads of pronator teres, especially when accessory muscle bands are present.

A supracondylar process (spurlike bony projection arising from the anteromedial surface of the distal humerus) is found in ~ 0.7% of the general population and is connected to the medial epicondyle via the ligament of Struthers, and compression of the median nerve may also develop within this osteofibrous tunnel.

▶ **Radiography.** The presence of a supracondylar process may be related to pathology of the median nerve (▶ Fig. 2.196).

▶ **US.** The normal median nerve demonstrates an oval shape in cross section and a "patchy" internal reflection pattern. Nerve compression results in narrowing of the nerve with swelling proximal to the site of compression. It is usually possible to demonstrate the causes of the compression (see "Ulnar Nerve" above).

Compression of the anterior interosseous nerve, one of the two major distal branches of the median nerve, is most commonly caused by a hematoma of the forearm.

▶ **MRI.** Apart from demonstrating the compressed nerve (or the lesion causing the compression), an MRI scan can also detect denervation changes (edema and/or atrophy) within the affected muscle groups. The pattern of involvement allows conclusions to be made regarding the level of the lesion. For example, compression of the median nerve above the elbow joint results in edema and atrophy of the pronator muscle, while compression of the nerve by the muscle itself does not lead to atrophy because those parts of the nerve supplying the muscle are not directly affected.

Radial Nerve

▶ **Radiography.** Lesions of the radial nerve are not usually identified on routine radiographs. It may be possible in some cases to demonstrate a space-occupying soft tissue mass or abnormal soft tissue calcifications.

▶ **US.** The fascicles of the radial nerve course in a more loosely arranged pattern and are spread farther apart than those of the median or ulnar nerves. Narrowing of the nerve is visible at the site of compression, with swelling proximal to it. Possible causes of compression may be detected with ultrasound, such as fractures of the humeral shaft, fibrous cords, vascular aberrations, and compression of the deep branch of the radial nerve (posterior interosseous nerve) as it emerges from the two heads of the supinator (arcade of Frohse).

► **MRI.** In addition to swelling of the nerve or demonstration of the actual cause of the nerve compression, MRI is able to demonstrate denervation edema of the affected muscles at an early stage, and the distribution pattern allows conclusions to be drawn regarding the level of the nerve damage. Thus, nerve compression above the elbow joint, for example, results in edema (► Fig. 2.197) and later in atrophy of the supinator muscle (► Fig. W2.37); if these changes are found in the extensor muscles of the forearm the nerve lesion is located more distally.

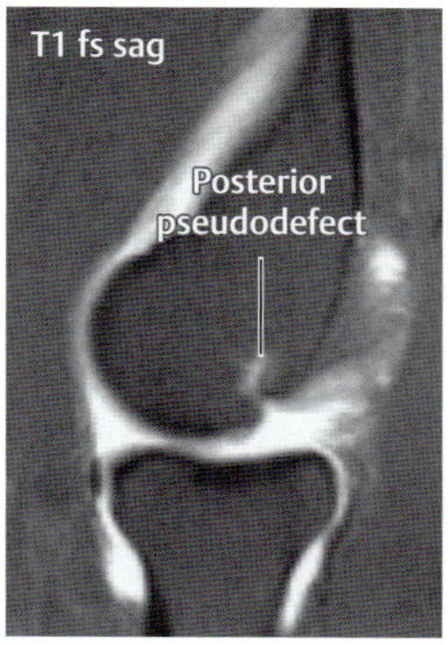

Fig. 2.192 Normal variant: posterior pseudodefect. Sagittal MR arthrography displays a small focus of contrast within the epimetaphyseal region. Cartilage intact, no edema.

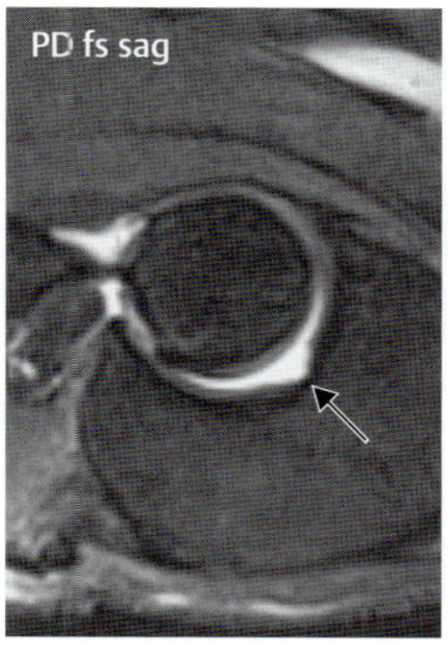

Fig. 2.193 Normal variant: Trochlear groove (arrow).

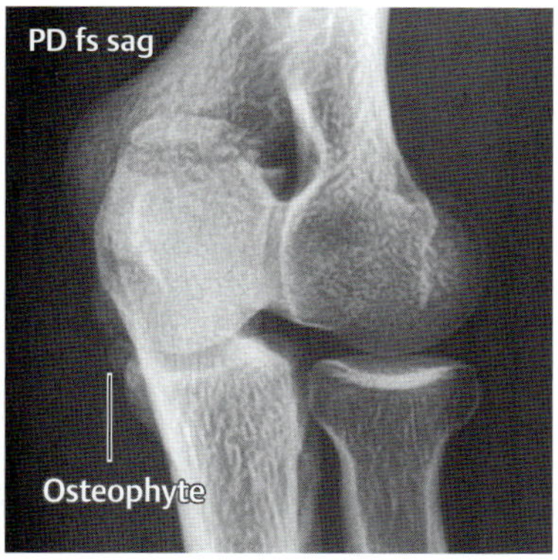

Fig. 2.194 Osteophyte formation at the cubital tunnel.

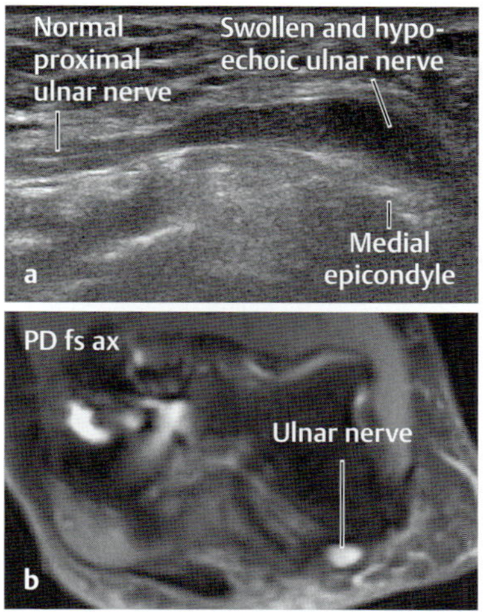

Fig. 2.195 Ulnar neuropathy. (Images courtesy of K. Scheglmann, Augsburg, Germany.) **(a)** Depiction of the ulnar nerve by ultrasound (longitudinal section). **(b)** Significantly increased signal intensity of the nerve on this axial fat-saturated PDW image.

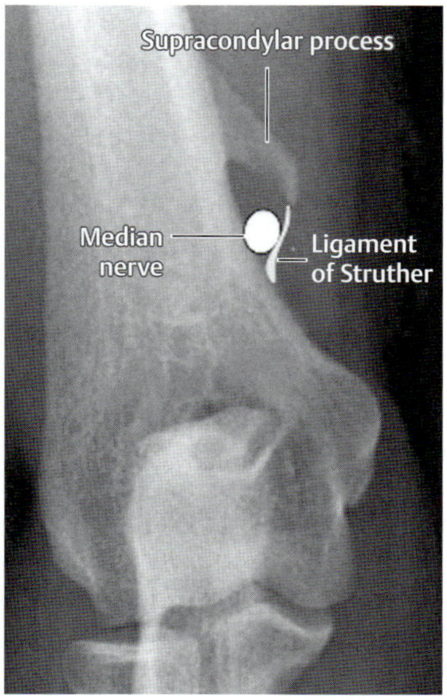

Fig. 2.196 Supracondylar process with schematic representation of Struther's ligaments and the median nerve.

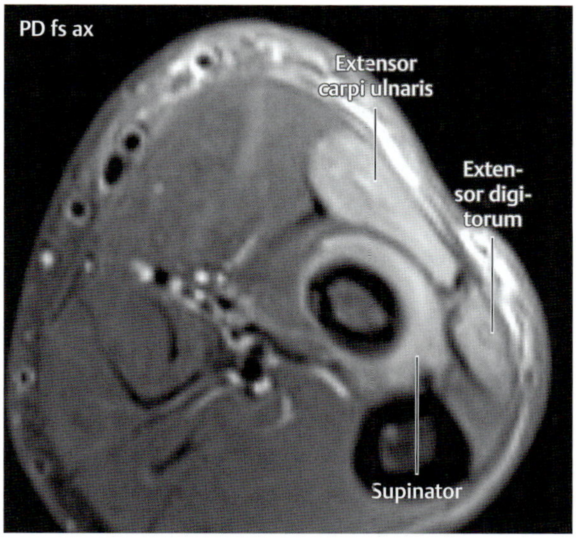

Fig. 2.197 Acute denervation edema secondary to injury of the deep branch of the radial nerve that occurred during surgical management of a radial head fracture.

2.8 Forearm

▶ **Anatomy.** See Fig. W2.38.

2.8.1 Proximal Fractures of the Forearm

Olecranon Fractures

▶ **Pathology.** Olecranon fractures account for more than one-third of elbow fractures. They are usually the result of a direct blow and are usually intra-articular transverse fractures; the less common extra-articular fractures are predominantly oblique. Traction from the triceps brachii muscle commonly results in distraction of the proximal fragment with an associated high risk of nonunion.

A clinically practical **classification of olecranon fractures** proposed by **Weigel** (▶ Figs. 2.198 and ▶ 2.199) is based, from a therapeutic standpoint, on the established classifications of Schatzker and Morrey (▶ Figs. W2.39 and ▶ W2.40).

> **Caution**
> The patella cubiti, an accessory sesamoid bone within the triceps tendon, and/or the dorsal supratrochlear bone, an accessory ossicle located in the olecranon fossa, can both mimic an olecranon fracture fragment.

Fractures of the Ulnar Coronoid Process

Fractures of the coronoid process of the ulna are usually associated with a posterior dislocation of the elbow. Given the importance of the coronoid process of the ulna for dorsal stability and the tendency for recurrent dislocation, it is important to exclude a corresponding injury after reduction of the elbow such as medial and lateral ligament tears or injuries of the anterior capsule or brachialis muscle.

The **classification system of Regan and Morrey** takes into account the size of the fragment, which in turn is an indirect assessment of humeroulnar instability (▶ Figs. 2.200–2.202).

▶ **Radiography.** Screening radiographs should consist of AP and lateral views (if at all possible with the elbow in 90° of flexion). It is sometimes only possible to recognize a nondisplaced fracture with the aid of supplementary 45° oblique views.

▶ **CT.** CT is the modality of choice for equivocal or complex fracture patterns in order to assess articular incongruity and any intra-articular fragments.

▶ **MRI.** MRI serves to demonstrate tendon and ligament injuries as well as chondromalacia. It should be considered in the presence of avulsion fractures and in cases where there is clinical evidence of instability and a tendency for redislocation after reduction.

With a tear of the common flexor tendon or avulsion of the medial epicondyle secondary to a posterior dislocation of the elbow joint, the median nerve should be carefully evaluated for possible entrapment.

2.8.2 Radial Head and Neck Fractures

▶ **Pathology.** Fractures of the radial head and radial neck are the most common elbow fractures in the adult, accounting for 20 to 30% of these injuries. Usually they result from an axial force sustained during a fall on the outstretched hand with compression of the radial head on the capitellum. Capitellar avulsion fractures and collateral ligament tears are commonly associated injuries which also increase the degree of elbow instability.

The most commonly used **classification** of **radial head fractures** is that proposed by **Mason**; it includes the number of fragments and their degree of displacement (▶ Figs. 2.203–Fig. 2.205).

Fractures of the radial neck are most common in children, in whom the degree of displacement and angulation is of importance (▶ Figs. 2.206 and ▶ 2.207).

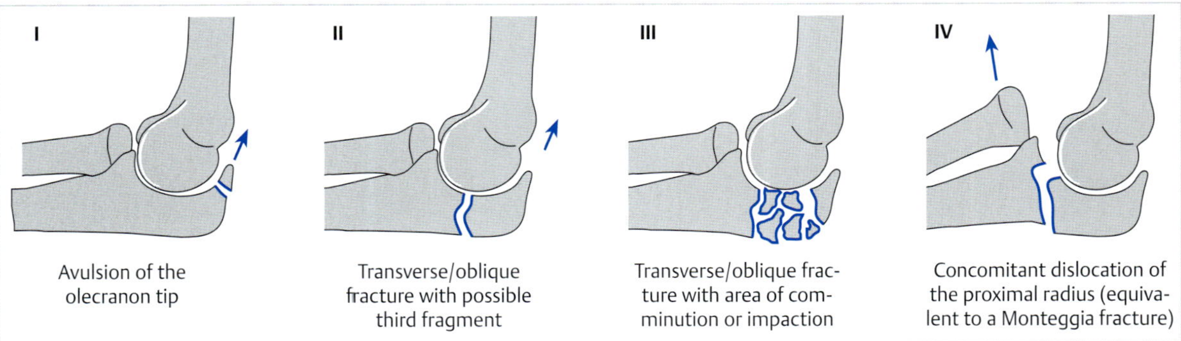

Fig. 2.198 Classification of olecranon fractures according to Weigel.

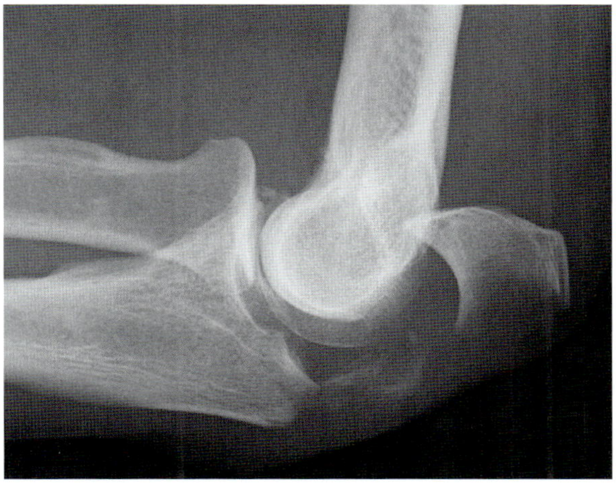

Fig. 2.199 Olecranon fracture with central area of comminution and dislocation of the proximal radius. Weigel Type IV.

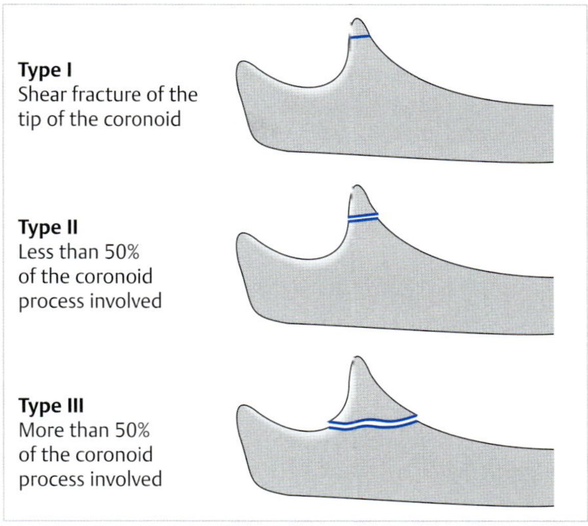

Fig. 2.200 Classification of coronoid fractures according to Regan and Morrey.

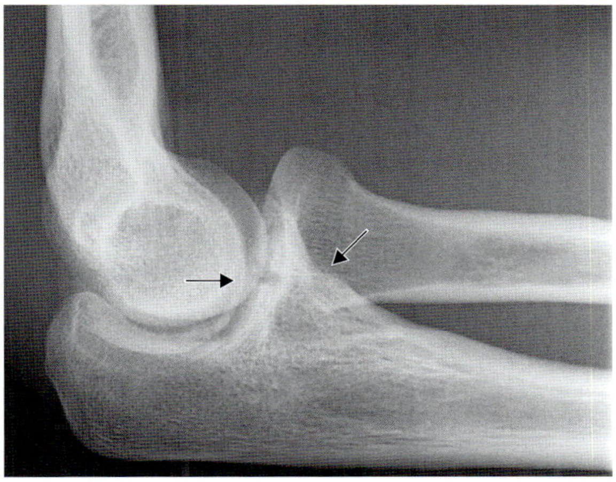

Fig. 2.201 Fracture of the coronoid process (arrows). Regan and Morrey Type II.

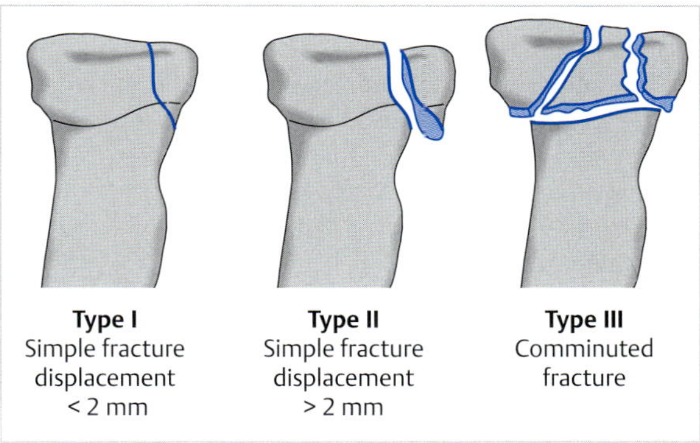

Fig. 2.203 Classification of radial head fractures according to Mason.

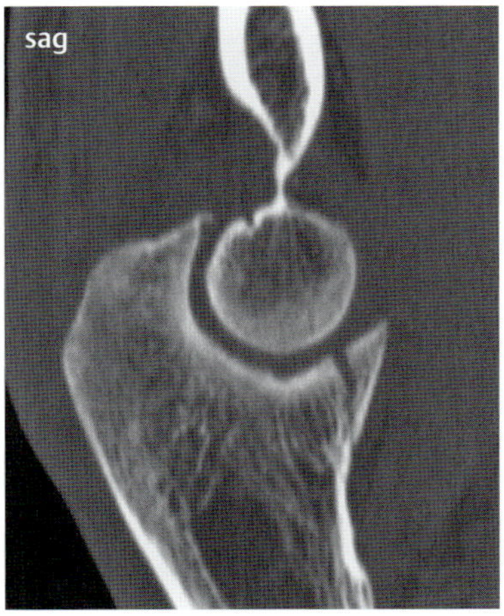

Fig. 2.202 Fracture of the coronoid process. Regan and Morrey Type II.

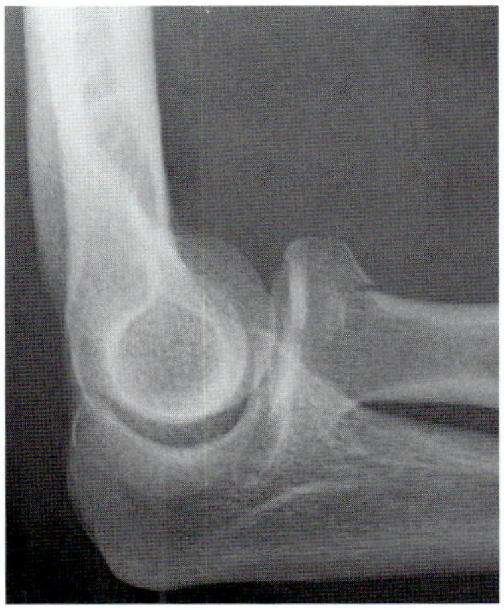

Fig. 2.204 Chisel-type fracture of the radial head. Mason Type I.

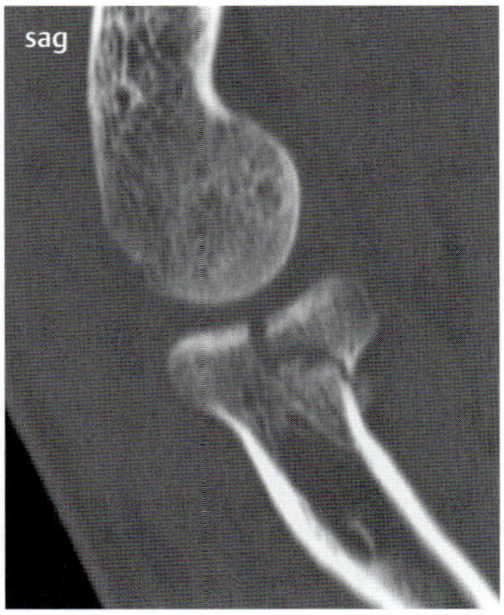

Fig. 2.205 Chisel-type fracture of the radial head. Mason Type I (different patient from ▶ Fig. 2.204).

An **Essex-Lopresti fracture** involves either a comminuted fracture of the radial head or a severely displaced proximal radius fragment, combined with disruption of the interosseous membrane and dislocation of the distal radioulnar joint, resulting in relative shortening of the radius. After extreme axial loading (high-velocity injuries), therefore, a complete radiological evaluation of the entire forearm and the adjacent joints should be undertaken.

The so-called **terrible triad of the elbow** refers to a severe, unstable injury with a combination of radial head fracture, fracture of the coronoid process, and disruption of the ulnar collateral ligament typically associated with a posterior dislocation of the humeroulnar joint.

► **Radiography.** Radiographs are obtained primarily in two projections, AP and lateral (with the elbow joint flexed at 90°). Since nondisplaced radial head fractures (present in up to 50% of cases) are difficult to detect on survey views, it is important to look for indirect signs, such as a hemarthrosis with elevation of the periarticular fat pads (**fat pad sign**; ► Figs. 2.207a and ► 2.208). An additional 45° oblique view should be obtained in cases with suspicious soft tissue signs but no demonstrable fracture. The forearm and the wrist in two projections should also be included in cases of comminuted radial head fractures to exclude an Essex–Lopresti fracture. Focal impaction fractures may simply produce a focus of increased subchondral density together with indirect soft tissue signs.

► **CT.** CT allows for detection of fractures and intra-articular fragments as well as the evaluation of complex fracture patterns that would otherwise go unnoticed using standard radiographs (► Fig. 2.209).

► **MRI.** Soft tissue injuries of the capsuloligamentous and myotendinous structures with or without involvement of the bone (avulsion fracture) may be seen using MRI (Chapter 2.7). MRI is also able to demonstrate radiographically occult bone contusions and osteochondral lesions, and to reveal epiphyseal plate injury in children.

► **US.** Ultrasound is used in children for diagnosing fractures that are difficult to detect on radiographs (see ► Fig. 2.207). The contralateral extremity should be scanned to detect epiphyseal plate injuries (epiphyseolysis).

► **Special features in children.** In children and adolescents, proximal radius fractures present in one-third of cases as Salter–Harris Type I or II epiphyseal plate injuries and in two-thirds as metaphyseal/radial neck fractures. Articular fractures are rare when the growth plates are still open. The degree of angulation of proximal radius fractures is important for treatment, although there is a potential for spontaneous correction of up to 50° until the age of 10 years and of up to 20° even after the age of 10 years.

Displaced olecranon fractures have hardly any potential for correction with conservative treatment.

As a general principle, a gap of up to 2 mm is regarded as the maximal amount of displacement allowed for the conservative treatment of an intra-articular fracture.

Given the variations of skeletal maturity, radiographs of the contralateral side should be obtained for comparison in cases of diagnostic uncertainty in order to differentiate between normal ossification nuclei and fracture fragments.

In mildly angulated fractures of the proximal radius, which are otherwise difficult to detect, a sclerotic metaphyseal compression zone, typically located on its radial aspect, will indicate the presence of the lesion.

2.8.3 Shaft Fractures of the Forearm

► **Pathology.** Forearm shaft fractures usually involve both forearm bones. Fracture dislocations of the distal forearm are less common than classic shaft fractures (only 10% of cases), but deserve particular attention due to the possible functional impairment of rotation in the distal radioulnar joint (an indication for immediate surgery!).

AO classification of fractures of the forearm

- **Type A fractures:** Two-fragment fractures of ulna (A1), radius (A2), or both bones (A3).
- **Type B fractures:** Wedge fractures of ulna (B1), radius (B2), or both bones (B3).
- **Type C fractures:** Complex comminuted fractures of ulna (C1), radius (C2), or both bones (C3).

Fracture Dislocations

Monteggia Fracture

This fracture is usually sustained with the forearm in pronation in defense against a direct blow and involves a combination of proximal fracture of the ulnar shaft or olecranon and dislocation of the radial head in the proximal radioulnar joint (► Fig. 2.210).

Note should be made of possible associated injuries to the annular ligament of the radius and the coronoid process.

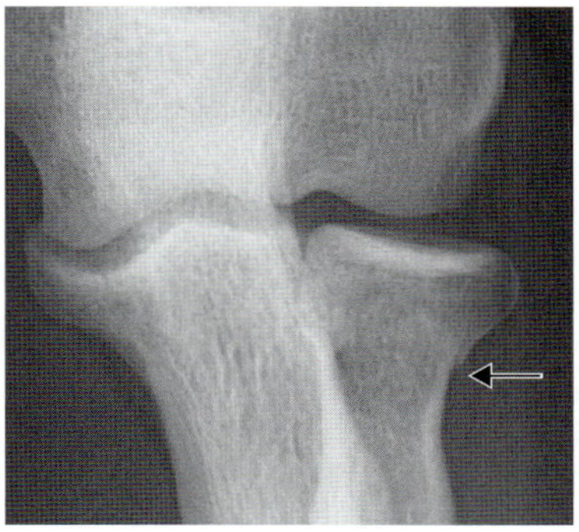

Fig. 2.206

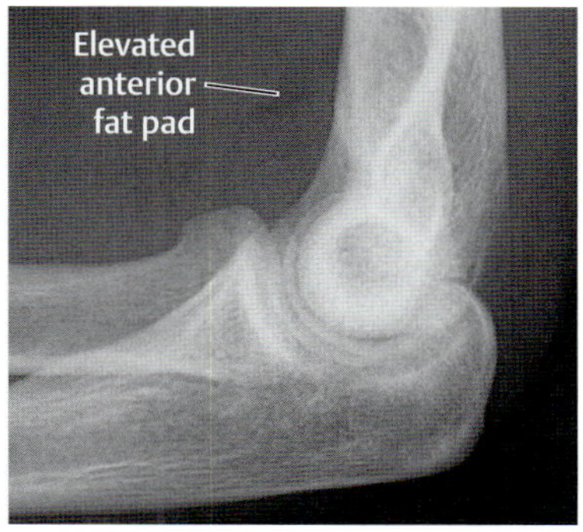

Fig. 2.208

Fig. 2.206 Mildly impacted fracture of the radial neck (arrow).

Fig. 2.208 Positive fat pad sign as an indirect sign of a fracture.

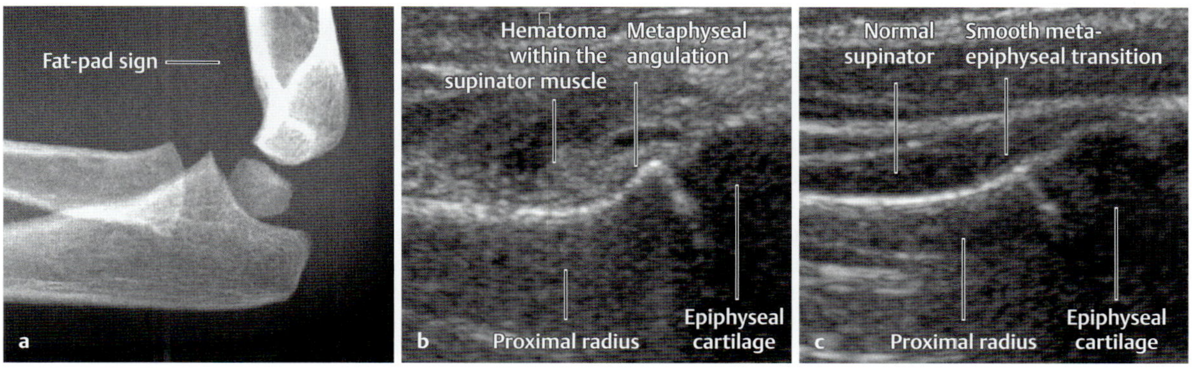

Fig. 2.207 Fracture of the radial neck in a 4-year-old child that was only diagnosed unequivocally by ultrasound. Hemorrhage in the soft tissues ventral to the radius. **(a)** No unequivocal sign of a fracture on the radiograph, but fat pad sign as an indirect fracture sign. **(b)** Metaphyseal angulation and hematoma within the supinator muscle. **(c)** Healthy contralateral side.

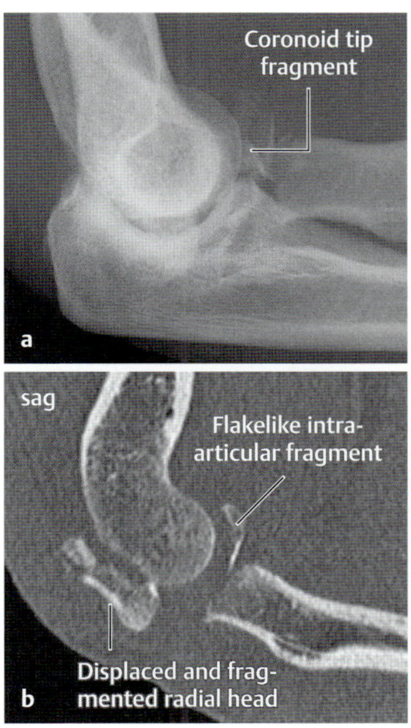

Fig. 2.209

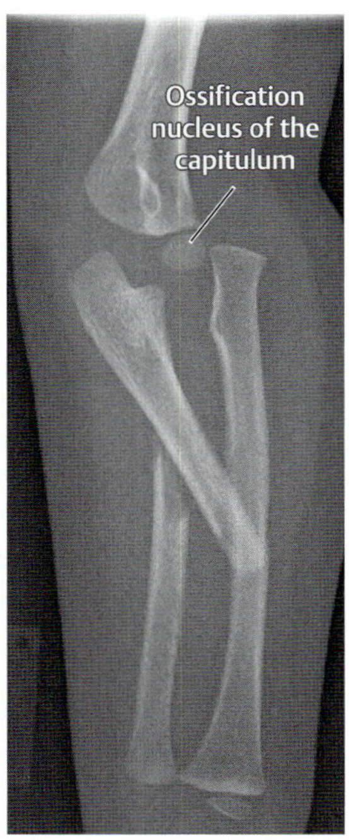

Fig. 2.210

Fig. 2.209 Complex proximal radius fracture with associated shearing fracture of the tip of the coronoid. **(a)** Lateral radiograph: unclear presentation of the fracture pattern. **(b)** On the CT image the extent of the injury is evident.

Fig. 2.210 Monteggia fracture. Fracture of the ulnar shaft with dislocation of the radial head.

Galeazzi Fracture (Also Known as Reverse Monteggia Fracture)

This fracture usually occurs when warding off a blow with the arm in supination and refers to a combination of distal radial shaft fracture and dorsal dislocation of the ulnar head in the distal radioulnar joint (▸ Fig. 2.211). The dislocation is associated with disruption of the triangular fibrocartilage complex.

Divergent Radioulnar Dislocation

This involves disruption of the interosseous membrane with interposition of the carpus between the distal radius and ulna with associated dissociation at the distal radioulnar joint (very rare).

Essex–Lopresti Fracture

See Chapter 2.8.2.

▸ **Radiography.** Radiographs are obtained in two projections, centered on the hand or elbow joint, with exact lateral views to exclude fracture dislocations. The entire forearm including both joints should be visualized, especially after high-velocity injuries. The images should overlap.

▸ **MRI.** In fracture dislocations, MRI allows assessment of capsular and ligamentous structures of the proximal and distal joints, including the status of the triangular fibrocartilage complex, which is often injured with a Galeazzi fracture.

▸ **Special features in children.** Fractures of the forearm in children are usually the result of a fall on the outstretched hand. Apart from complete fractures (complete disruption of the cortex), incomplete fractures are commonly encountered here: greenstick, buckle, and compression fractures (▸ Fig. 2.212; Chapter 1.3.1). There is a potential for correction of axial malalignment by up to as much as 20° up to the age of 5 years, and up to 10° beyond that age; rotational deformities on the other hand are not acceptable.

2.8.4 Distal Forearm Fractures

▸ **Anatomy.** ▶ See ▸ Fig. W2.41.

▸ **Pathology.** Distal radius fractures, with or without involvement of the ulna, are the most common fractures in adults, representing 20% of all fractures; isolated epiphyseal fractures of the ulna are rare. They are usually due to an impaction mechanism following a fall on the outstretched hand, either with the wrist extended (Colles' extension fracture, 90% of cases) or flexed (Smith's flexion fracture, 10% of cases).

As a rule, with a distal forearm fracture, a distinction should be made between intra-articular fractures involving the radiocarpal and/or radioulnar joint surfaces and extra-articular fractures without joint involvement. However, with higher-grade dislocations, even an extra-articular fracture can result in disruption of the capsule and ligaments of the involved joint.

The indication for surgery is based upon the fracture pattern, joint alignment and associated injuries (as covered by the various fracture classifications), and a number of radiological criteria for instability:

- Avulsion fracture of the base of the ulnar styloid process.
- Dislocation or fracture involvement of the distal radioulnar joint.
- Comminution of the metaphysis (more than 50% of the dorsopalmar diameter).
- Shearing or dislocation fractures.
- Positive ulnar variance (or radial shortening) by more than 3 mm.
- Dorsal angulation of the distal radial fragment by more than 20°.

Additional injuries commonly associated with distal radius fractures include scaphoid fracture, scapholunate ligament injury with subsequent scapholunate dissociation, tears of the triangular fibrocartilage complex, and injuries with instability of the distal radioulnar joint.

Possible **posttraumatic complications** include carpal tunnel syndrome (Chapter 11.8), compartment syndrome (Chapter 11.6) and CRPS (Chapter 1.7.4).

Rupture of the extensor pollicis longus tendon in Lister's canal weeks or even months after injury is also possible, even in nondisplaced or only mildly displaced fractures.

Classifications (the agony of choice!). There are numerous classification systems for distal radial fractures, each with its own significance for fracture-specific treatment strategies as well as for prognostic value with regard to anticipated treatment results. However, describing the fragments and their position is ultimately more important than being able to assign the fracture to a particular classification.

The **AO classification** (▸ Fig. 2.213) is often used, but the **Fernandez classification system** (▶ Fig. W2.42) has also proven itself useful for therapeutic planning. Less often applied are the **Melone** and **Frykman classification systems** (▶ Chapter 2.8.4 and ▶ Fig. W2.43).

The old classifications with their respective eponyms and synonyms for characterizing fractures of the distal radius (Colles, Smith, Barton, reversed Barton, Hutchinson/Chauffeur, die punch; ▸ Fig. 2.214) describe primarily the type of force involved and the direction of displacement, but refer only in part to joint involvement or other prognostic criteria, such as the involvement of the styloid process of the ulna.

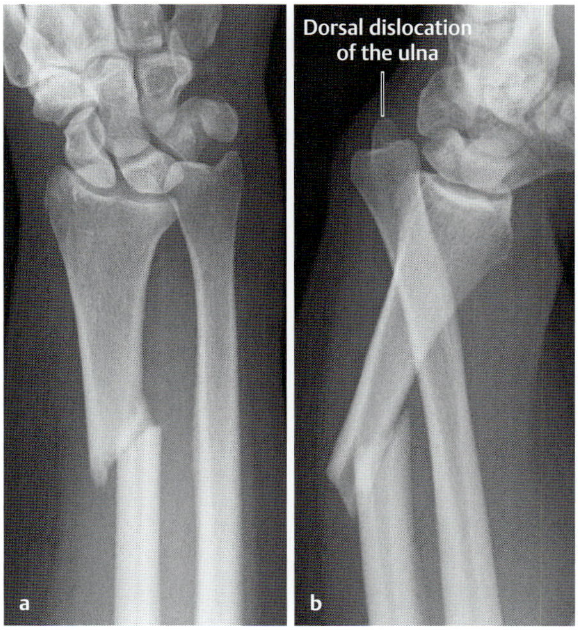

Fig. 2.211 Galeazzi fracture. Radial shaft fracture with dislocation of the ulnar head at the distal radioulnar joint. **(a)** PA view: positive ulnar variance with fracture-related radial shortening. **(b)** Lateral.

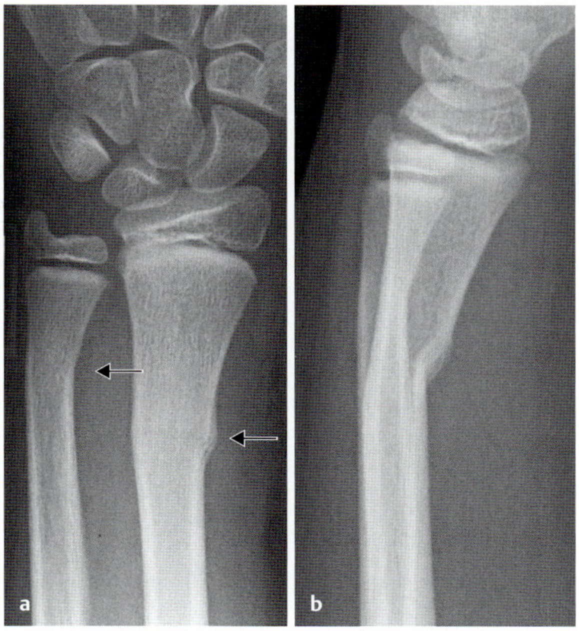

Fig. 2.212 Buckle/compression fractures of radius and ulna (arrows). **(a)** Mild radial angulation of the distal radius. **(b)** Mild palmar angulation.

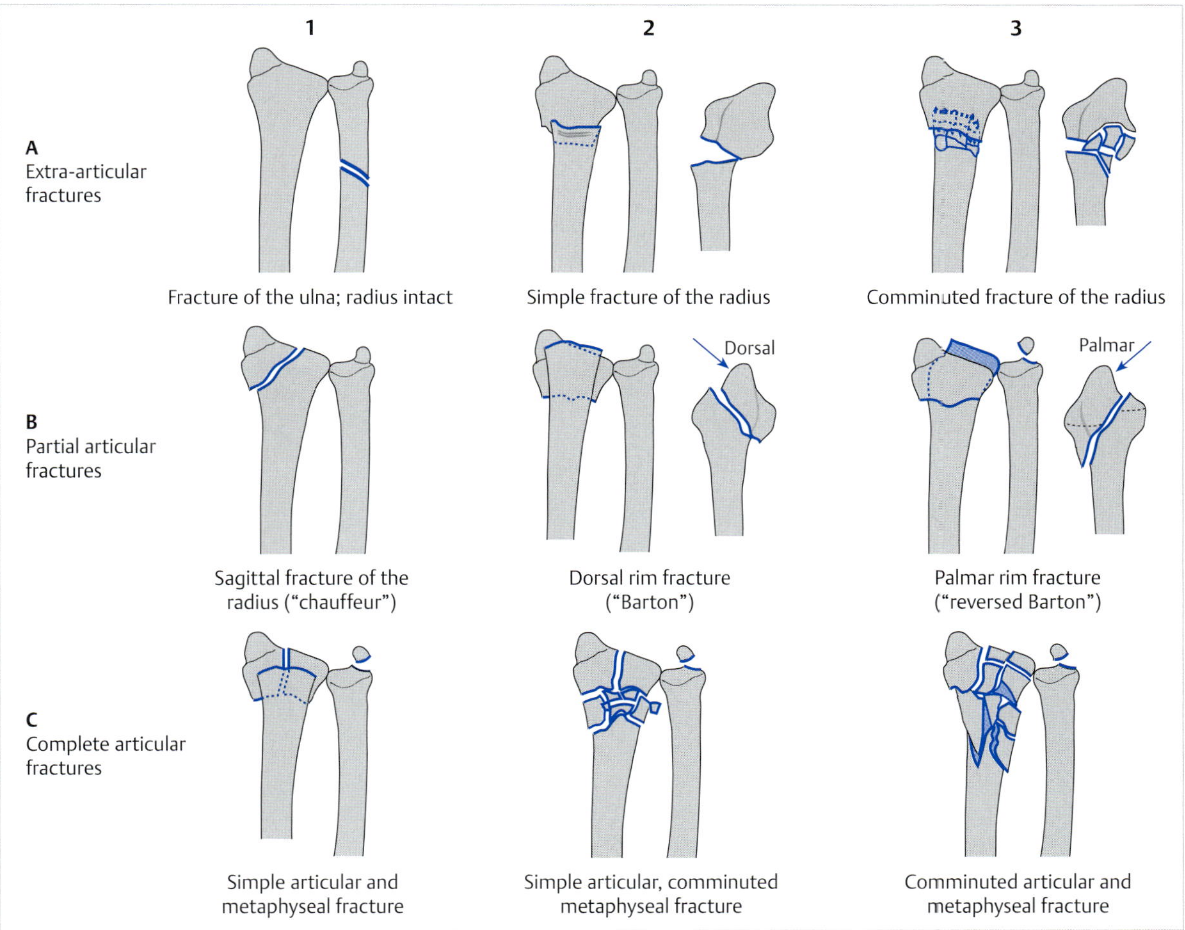

Fig. 2.213 AO classification of distal forearm fractures.

Concomitant injuries of the distal radioulnar joint are assessed with regard to stability of the joint after primary reduction and fixation of the radius. Disruption of the triangular fibrocartilage complex or an avulsion fracture of the base of the ulnar styloid process are regarded as unstable injuries (▶ Fig. 2.215).

▶ Radiography. Initial radiographs should be obtained in two planes (dorsopalmar and lateral) and, if necessary, supplemented by additional oblique views in 45° of pronation or supination for better assessment of the lunate and scaphoid fossae if joint involvement is suspected. An exact view of the distal radioulnar joint is particularly important. There are a number of criteria for assessing whether or not a projection obtained in the neutral position is adequate (▶ Fig. W2.44). Various morphological criteria (▶ Fig. 2.216) allow for quantitative assessment of posttraumatic deformities of the wrist and of articular congruity after reduction.

The term **"radius shift"** refers to the dorsopalmar or radioulnar offset of the distal radial fragment. When judging distal radioulnar alignment, attention should be paid to obtaining an exact neutral position when taking the radiographs as ulnar variance is dependent upon positioning (ulnar shortening in supination, ulnar lengthening in pronation) (▶ Fig. W2.45).

In order to distinguish between **pathologic ulnar lengthening** secondary to impaction of the distal radius and **inherent ulna-plus** or **ulna-minus variance**, comparison with the contralateral side, or even better an MRI scan, provides additional information in uncertain cases.

When examining radiographs of a distal forearm fracture, associated carpal injuries should be assessed by evaluating the carpal joint lines and alignment, especially of the scaphoid and lunate (Chapter 2.9.3). Furthermore, attention should also be paid to any indirect signs of fracture, such as obliteration or palmar displacement of the pronator fat pad (which lies between the pronator quadratus and the deep flexor tendons) by hemorrhage (**pronator quadratus sign**; ▶ Fig. 2.217).

▶ US. Ultrasound is especially useful for examining children after trauma. It is able to demonstrate cortical step-offs as well as trauma-associated soft tissue injuries. Ultrasound is also able to assess tendon injury and tendon function. For less experienced investigators, comparison with the normal contralateral side is useful for identifying true abnormalities.

▶ CT. With the use of high-resolution imaging and triplanar reconstructions, CT allows exact assessment of the radiocarpal and radioulnar joint surfaces in complex fracture dislocations and any incongruity of the joint surfaces. Questionable fractures on conventional radiographs, joint incongruity, and intra-articular fragments can be best depicted by CT. 3D reconstructions (volume rendering technique, surface shaded display) may provide a clearer presentation of a complex fracture, especially when planning fracture fixation (▶ Fig. 2.218).

Axial CT projections in comparison with the contralateral side allow an exact assessment of the degree and direction of the axial malrotations of a distal radial fragment versus the proximal shaft.

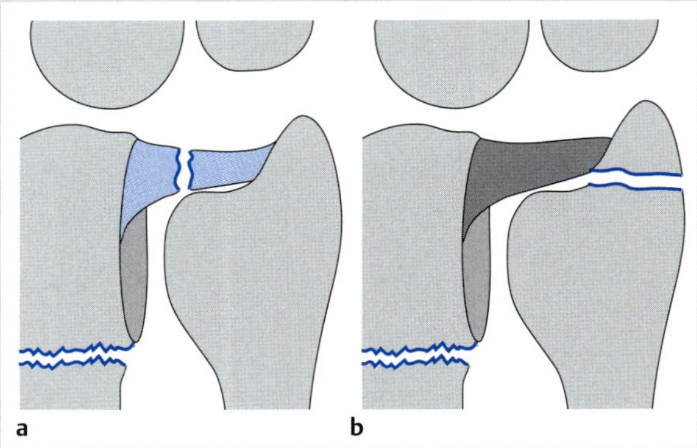

Fig. 2.215 Unstable associated injuries of the distal radioulnar joint. **(a)** Disruption of the triangular fibrocartilage complex. **(b)** Avulsion fracture of the base of the ulnar styloid process.

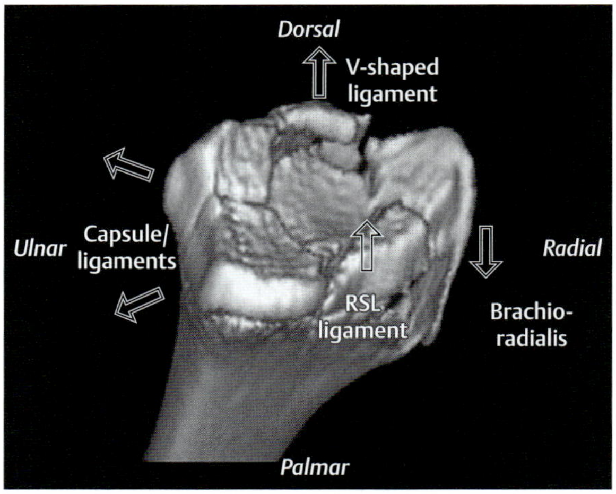

Fig. 2.218 3D reconstruction from a thin-slice CT dataset of a compression fracture of the distal radius with typical fragment distribution and direction of the traction forces on the fragments (arrows). RSL, radioscapholunate ligament.

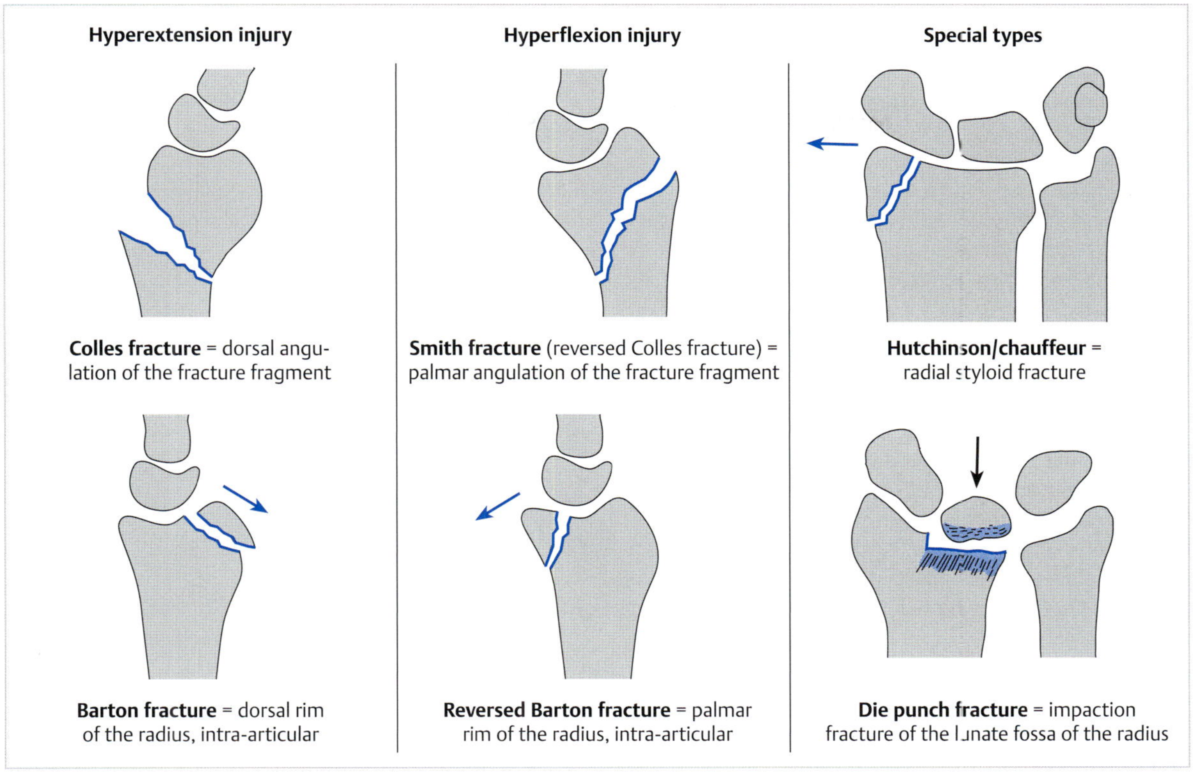

Fig. 2.214 Diagram representing the classic eponyms and synonyms for characterizing distal radius fractures. Blue arrow indicates the direction of displacement; black arrow indicates the direction of force.

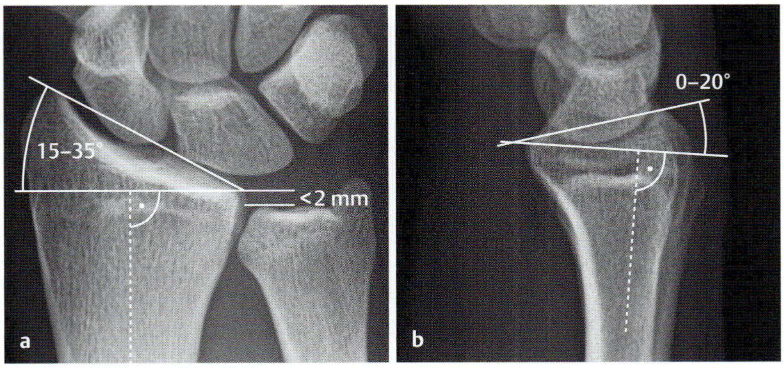

Fig. 2.216 Morphometric assessment of the distal radius. **(a)** Radial angle in the frontal view (radial inclination), 15 to 35°; ulnar variance (the relative length of ulna in relation to the radius) in neutral position, < 2 mm. **(b)** Sagittal radial angle (palmar inclination or volar tilt), 0 to 20°.

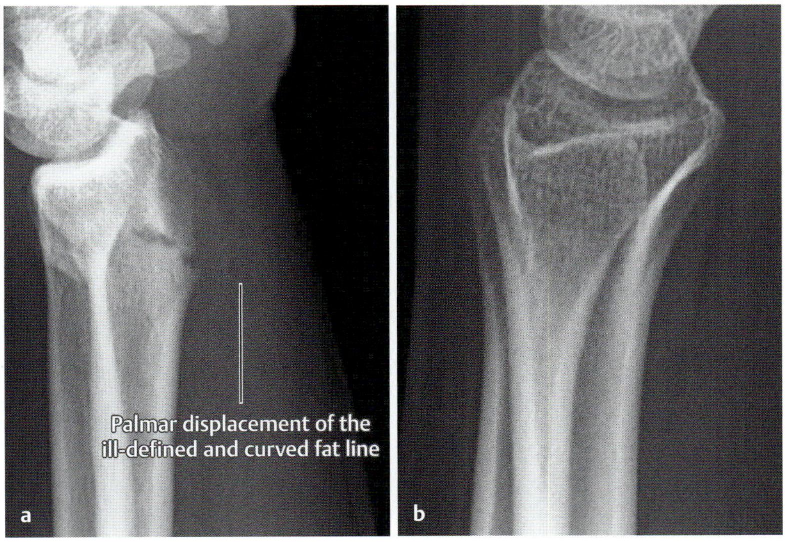

Fig. 2.217 Pronator quadratus sign. **(a)** Metaphyseal distal radius fractures. **(b)** Normal finding for comparison.

▸ **MRI.** MRI is particularly helpful for detecting occult fractures and osteochondral injuries. Edemalike signal within the bone marrow on T2W fat-suppressed sequences is extremely sensitive for detecting acute fractures. The fracture line is evident as a linear area of signal abnormality (on T1W or T2W sequences).

Furthermore, MRI or MR arthrography allows for detection of associated ligament (▸ Fig. 2.219) and triangular fibrocartilage complex injuries (see also Chapter 2.9.4).

▸ **Special features in children.** In children, distal radial fractures generally present as Salter–Harris type I and II physeal injuries or as buckle or greenstick fractures suitable for conservative management. Given the high contribution of the distal forearm growth plates to longitudinal growth (80% distal as opposed to 20% proximal), there is here a high potential for spontaneous correction. Malalignment of as much as 40° can be corrected spontaneously up to 10 to 12 years of age; larger angular deformities and degree of shortening should be reduced and, if necessary, stabilized.

2.8.5 Instability of the Distal Radioulnar Joint

▸ **Pathology.** Instability of the distal radioulnar joint may result from fracture dislocations of the distal forearm or from isolated ligament damage secondary to hyperpronation (palmar ligament disruption) or, less often, to hypersupination (dorsal ligament disruption) with or without involvement of the triangular fibrocartilage complex. During rotational movements at the distal radioulnar joint, the ulna represents the fixed point around which the radius physiologically rotates (by about 150°).

Subluxation is diagnosed on the axial images if 25 to 50% of the ulnar head is lying beyond the radius tangent (referred to as Mino's lines; ▸ Fig. 2.220). If more than 50% of the ulnar head lies beyond Mino's lines, then dislocation is present.

Palmar subluxation/dislocation of the radius (or dorsal subluxation of the ulna) occurs in the presence of a disruption of the palmar radioulnar ligament; dorsal subluxation/dislocation of the radius (or palmar subluxation of the ulna) results from disruption of the dorsal radioulnar ligament.

> **Caution**
> True subluxation of the ulna in the distal radioulnar joint must be distinguished from a functional positional variant where pseudo-subluxation of the ulnar head occurs in a dorsal direction in pronation and in a palmar direction in supination.

▸ **Clinical presentation.** Dorsal dislocation of the ulna at the distal radioulnar joint presents clinically with restricted rotation and a painful dorsal prominence of the ulnar head with a springing resistance (so-called piano-key sign or spring test).

▸ **Radiography.** These are the radiological signs of radioulnar dislocation (view taken in neutral position):

- Palmar or dorsal axial malalignment of the distal ulna on the lateral view.
- Widening of the distal radioulnar joint space on the AP projection to over 3 mm.
- Fracture-related radial shortening by more than 5 mm.

> **Note**
> Views in neutral position are not usually possible because of the fixed malalignment in cases of hyperpronation dislocation or hypersupination dislocation.

▸ **CT.** Subluxations and dislocations can be easily recognized on axial CT sections with the help of Mino's lines (▸ Fig. 2.220).

Whereas dislocations are largely independent of standard positioning, an axial CT scan in maximal pronation and supination in comparison with the contralateral side may be required for exact grading of the degree of subluxation. In this way, purely functional instabilities can also be detected.

A CT scan also allows for accurate diagnosis of associated osseous injuries and intra-articular fragments, unobscured by overlying structures.

▸ **MRI.** Malalignment may also be demonstrated on axial MR images.

Furthermore, MRI allows for direct demonstration of associated injuries to the radioulnar ligaments, the triangular fibrocartilage complex, and the interosseous membrane, which provides static stabilization. MRI also allows evaluation of the myotendinous structures, such as the pronator quadratus muscle and flexor and extensor carpi ulnaris tendons, which provide dynamic stabilization.

2.8.6 Ulnar Impingement Syndrome

▶ **Pathology.** Ulnar impingement syndrome results from posttraumatic or postoperative ulnar shortening.

> **Caution**
> Ulnar impingement syndrome should not be confused with ulnocarpal impingement (= ulnocarpal impaction syndrome) (Chapter 2.9.5).

▶ **Radiography.** Ulnar shortening, radioulnar deviation, and, in advanced stages, sclerosis and erosive changes are well demonstrated on in this schematic based on a PA radiograph (▶ Fig. 2.221).

▶ **MRI.** MRI provides a high degree of sensitivity in the early stages of this process because of its ability to demonstrate subchondral edema.

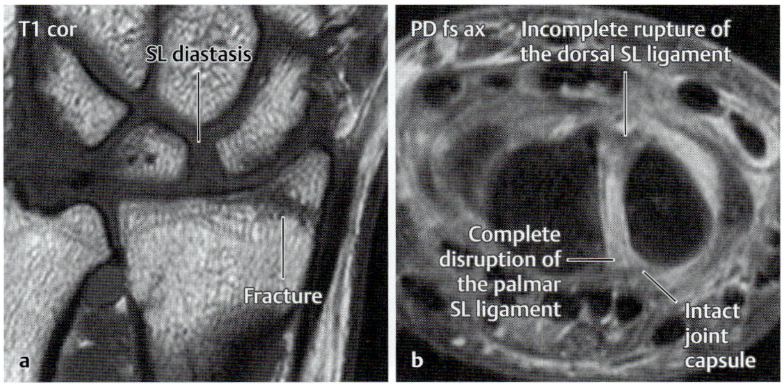

Fig. 2.219 MRI scan of an intra-articular distal radius fracture (AO Type B1, chauffeur's fracture) with associated disruption of the palmar and dorsal portions of the scapholunate ligament. SL ligament = scapholunate ligament. **(a)** Linear hypointensity of the fracture gap; scapholunate dissociation. **(b)** Complete disruption of the palmar and subtotal partial tear of the dorsal component of the scapholunate ligament.

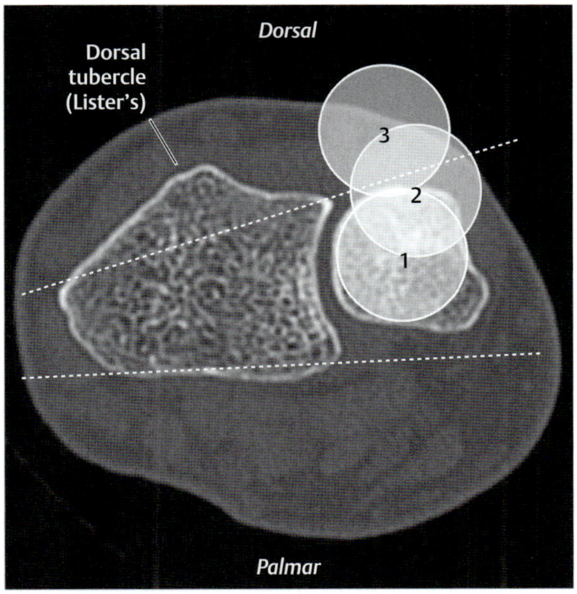

Fig. 2.220 Assessment of the position of the articular surface of the distal radioulnar joint with the aid of Mino's lines (tangents through the dorsal and palmar radius contour). 1, Normal finding; 2, subluxation; 3, dislocation.

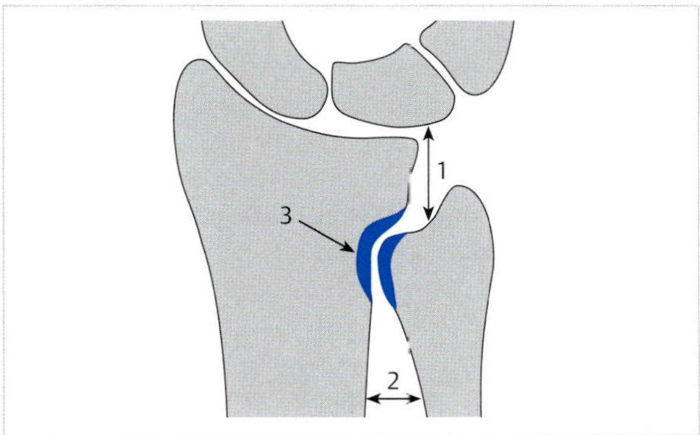

Fig. 2.221 Ulnar impingement syndrome with ulnar shortening (1): approximation of the radius to the ulna (2), and scalloping (3) of the distal radius.

2.8.7 Radiological Assessment after Surgery of the Forearm

Proximal Forearm

Classic management of olecranon fractures involves the use of tension band wiring (▶ Fig. 2.222). Plate fixation and external fixator application, in contrast, are generally used for complex fractures of the proximal forearm. Management of a radial head fracture is usually done using screws.

▶ Radiography.
Technique. If extension of the elbow is inadequate, then the central beam must be placed vertical to the forearm for the AP view (Chapter 2.6.4). In difficult cases a CT scan will help in assessing fragment reduction and restoration of the joint surfaces as well as in detecting small intra-articular loose bodies.

The **postoperative radiographic evaluation** should assess the following questions:

- *Are the joint surfaces restored* (▶ Fig. 2.223)?
- *Is there a malpositioned intra-articular screw?*
- *Is the position of the joint correct (including the position of the proximal radioulnar joint)?*
- *Are there any intra-articular fragments?*

Forearm Shaft

Fractures of the forearm are preferentially treated by plate fixation (compression or neutralization plate) or intramedullary nailing (especially in children). It is important when using elastic nails (known as Prevot nails) that the nails are advanced along almost the full length of the shaft, reaching but not penetrating the epiphyseal plate to avoid interference with growth.

▶ Radiography. The **postoperative radiographic evaluation** must assess the following:

- *Is there any angulation of the shaft?*
- *What is the alignment of the proximal and distal radioulnar joints?*

Distal Forearm

A large number of internal fixation techniques may be used for fractures of the distal forearm, depending on which fracture classification system is used. Over time, plate fixation (usually palmar and preferably angular-stable) has gained acceptance as the standard procedure for fractures with joint involvement and for complex extra-articular fractures.

▶ Radiography.
Technique. A 15°-inclined PA view parallel to the joint surface will help exclude screw penetration into the radiocarpal joint. Complex fractures usually require additional CT scanning for better assessment of the joint surfaces.

The **postoperative radiographic evaluation** should assess the following aspects:

- *Are the joint surfaces restored?*
- *Is the position of the joint correct?* Attention should also be paid to the position of the proximal radioulnar joint.
- *Is there a malpositioned intra-articular screw* (▶ Fig. 2.224)?
- *Are there any signs of associated injuries that were not apparent before surgery?* It is essential to thoroughly assess the carpus for structural disruption (most frequent: scapholunate dissociation) or other fractures (most frequent: scaphoid fracture).

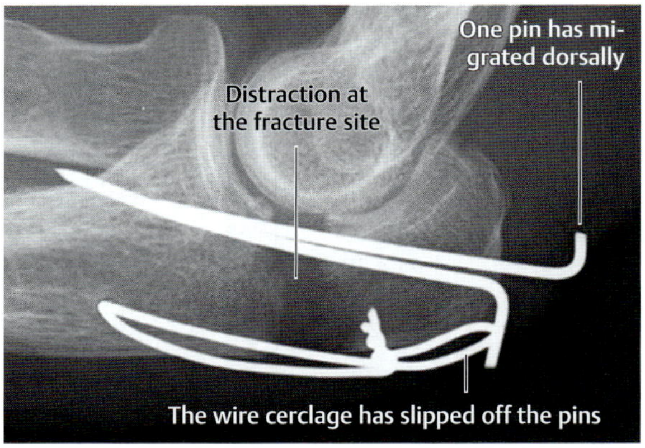

Fig. 2.222 Failure of tension band wiring of the olecranon.

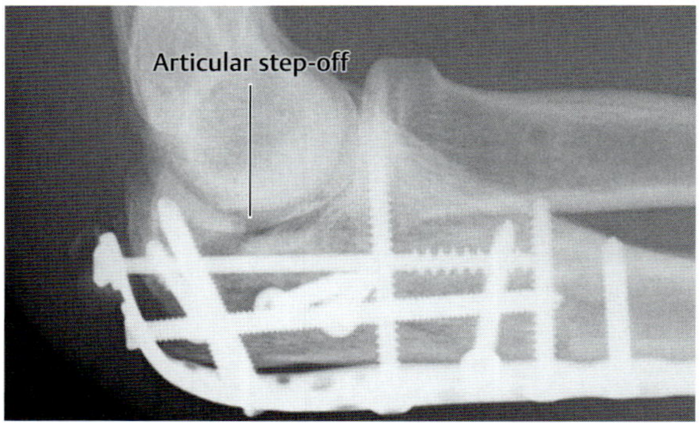

Fig. 2.223 Obvious articular step-off (2 mm) in the trochlear notch after fixation of a complex fracture of the proximal ulna.

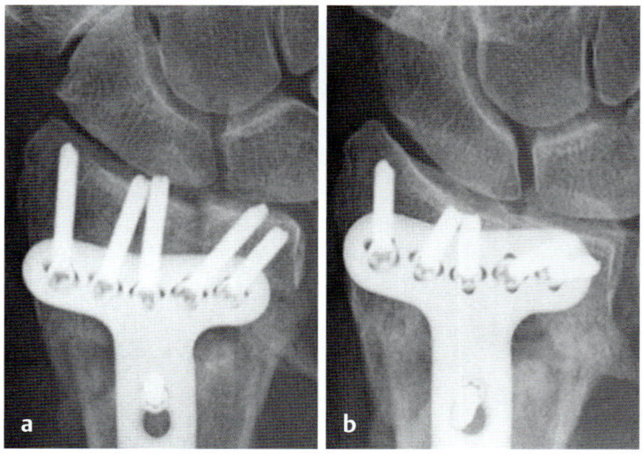

Fig. 2.224 Plate fixation of a distal radius fracture. **(a)** The dorsopalmar view does not provide unequivocal evidence of whether or not screws are penetrating the radiocarpal joint. **(b)** The 15°-inclined dorsopalmar view shows the correct extra-articular position of the screws.

2.9 The Wrist

2.9.1 Anatomy, Variants, Technique, and Indications

▸ Anatomy. ▸ See Chapter 2.9.1 and ▸ Figs. W2.46–W2.48).

Technique and Indications

▸ Radiography. Basic diagnostic examinations of the wrist include radiographs in PA and lateral projections. It is important to ensure correct positioning (PA view with the shoulder in 90° abduction and the forearm at the same level; lateral view with the shoulder joint in abduction and the elbow joint in 90° flexion). Assessment of the proximal and distal carpal rows is based on Gilula's three carpal arcs, which normally demonstrate smooth continuous contours (▸ Fig. 2.225). The M line, as it is known, serves to assess alignment of the carpometacarpal joints (▸ Fig. 2.226).

For quality criteria regarding properly positioned views see ▸ Fig. W2.44.

Stecher's PA projection with the fist clenched in ulnar deviation is taken as a **special view** for suspected scaphoid fracture (▸ Fig. 2.227). The image is centered on the radial side of the wrist.

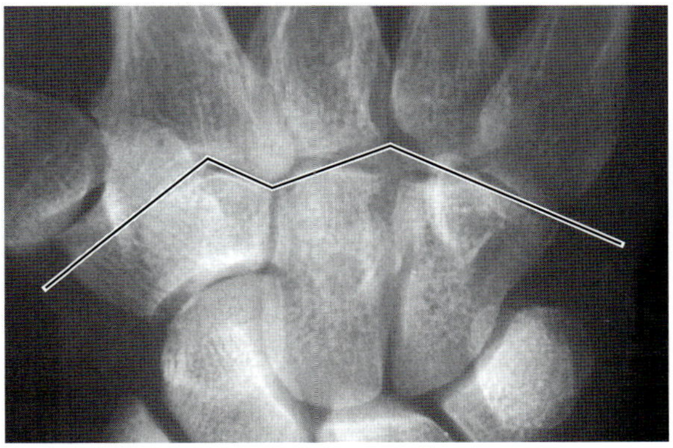

Fig. 2.226 M line. This line helps in assessing alignment of the carpometacarpal joints.

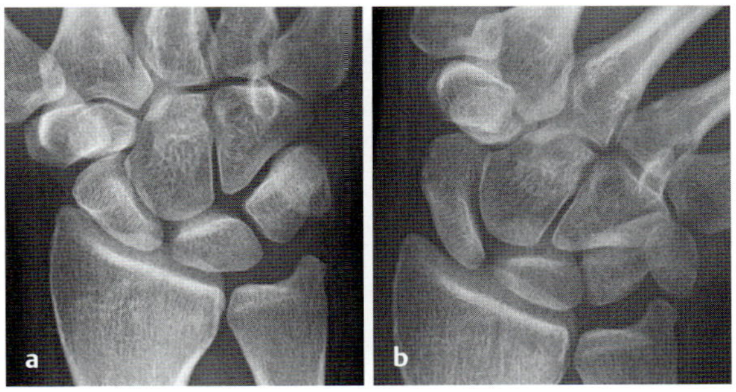

Fig. 2.227 Comparison of the dorsopalmar radiograph using the Stecher view. Normal finding. **(a)** Dorsopalmar view. **(b)** Stecher view of the scaphoid.

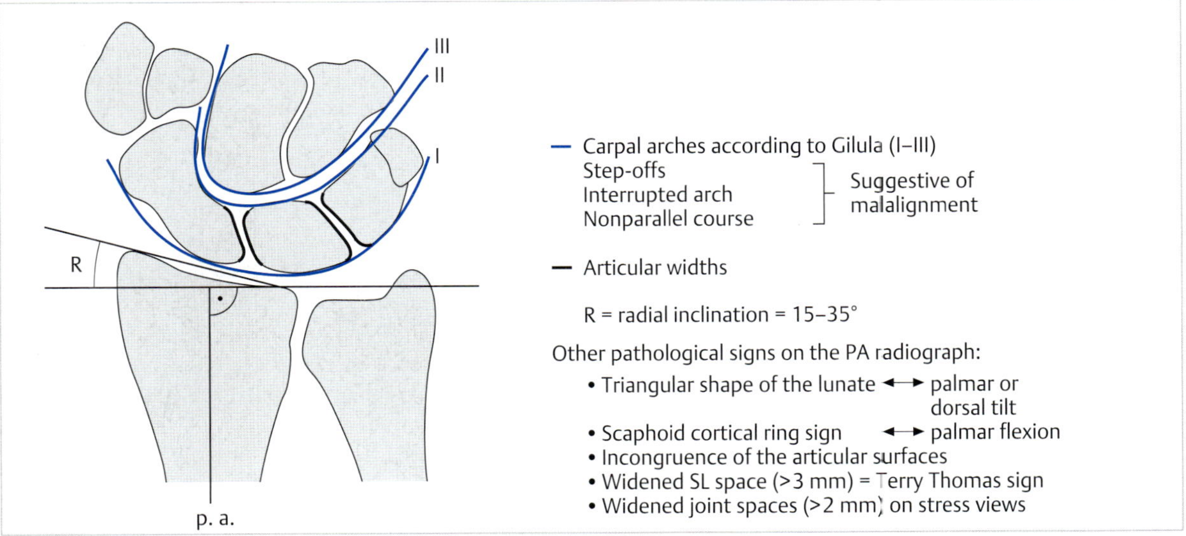

Fig. 2.225 The most important reference lines for assessing the dorsopalmar radiograph of the wrist. SL, scapholunate.

When looking for scapholunate dissociation, a grip-loaded PA view with the fist clenched over an object (e.g., a tennis ball) is helpful as stress is transferred to the scapholunate ligament via flexor tendon contraction (▶ Fig. 2.228).

▶ **US.** Ultrasound, with its ability to provide a dynamic examination, is an excellent tool for investigating tendon pathology and for confirming the presence of joint effusions and ganglia. Ultrasound guidance also allows for accurate therapeutic injections for various painful and inflammatory conditions.

▶ **CT.** Thin-slice CT scans with triplanar reconstructions are performed for investigating complex fractures. Additional indications include evaluation of possible scaphoid nonunion, avascular necrosis of the lunate, and, less often, distal radioulnar joint instability in which the affected wrist is compared with the contralateral side in pronation and supination.

▶ **MRI.** MRI plays an important role in evaluating a patient with wrist pain of unknown origin, avascular necrosis of the scaphoid and lunate, and in the investigation of inflammatory conditions and tumors.

▶ **Cinefluoroscopy/Arthrography.** Cinefluoroscopy together with appropriate stress maneuvers may be undertaken to clarify ligamentous damage and dynamic joint instability. Furthermore, it is possible to perform arthrography in the same session that is typically combined with CT or MRI. The injection site is chosen according to the issue in question. A unicompartmental, radiocarpal injection is usually sufficient to evaluate the common problem of intrinsic ligament disruption (▶ Fig. W2.49a). For investigation of a tear in the triangular fibrocartilage complex, a bicompartmental injection is more appropriate (first into the radiocarpal joint and then, if there is no leakage of contrast, into the distal radioulnar joint; ▶ Fig. W2.49b). CT or MR arthrography (▶ Fig. W2.50) allows for the evaluation of ligaments and the triangular fibrocartilage complex, as well as chondral pathology.

2.9.2 Fractures and Dislocations and Their Complications

The most common carpal fractures are scaphoid fractures (more than 70% of cases) and triquetral fractures (approximately 25% of cases). Dislocations and fracture dislocations of the carpal region must be accurately diagnosed since perilunate dislocations or fracture dislocations may result in avascular necrosis of the lunate.

Scaphoid Fracture

Ten percent of scaphoid fractures involve the distal third of the scaphoid, 70% the middle third, and 20% the proximal third of the bone.

The **Krimmer, Schmitt, and Herbert classification** (▶ Fig. 2.229) distinguishes between stable (Type A) and unstable fractures (Type B). The majority of fractures fall into the unstable (Type B) group by virtue of an oblique fracture line, fracture separation greater than 1 mm, or fracture displacement.

▶ **Radiography/CT.** A Stecher view often confirms the presence of a fracture (▶ Fig. 2.230). However, in 15 to 30% of cases the results are uncertain, and an early CT scan is indicated. CT scanning is less sensitive but more specific than MRI for fracture detection. CT is also superior to MRI scanning for fracture staging and treatment planning. Furthermore, CT is often required to assess fracture healing (▶ Fig. 2.231).

▶ **MRI.** An MRI scan is usually able to detect a fracture line (either hyper- or hypointense) on fluid-sensitive sequences. In the absence of a fracture line, diffuse edema does not indicate a fracture worthy of treatment but rather only trabecular microfractures (▶ Fig. 2.232).

▶ **Important findings.** Accurate classification of a scaphoid fracture is decisive for primary diagnostic assessment (see ▶ Fig. 2.229). A humpback deformity (dorsal rotation of the proximal fragment combined with palmar rotation of the distal fragment) is regarded as an unequivocal sign of instability. Accordingly, the majority of fresh scaphoid fractures, with the exception of A1 fractures, are typically stabilized using a Herbert screw. During follow-up CT examinations, fine bony bridges may become visible from the sixth week onward (see ▶ Fig. 2.231). Bony union is considered to have been achieved when central consolidation of the fracture gap is detected.

> **Caution**
> Important complications of a scaphoid fracture include partial avascular necrosis of the scaphoid (up to 13% of cases) and scaphoid nonunion which may occur if a fracture has been missed, healing has not occurred, or treatment was inadequate (up to 18% of cases). Early and definitive recognition of the fracture is therefore essential.

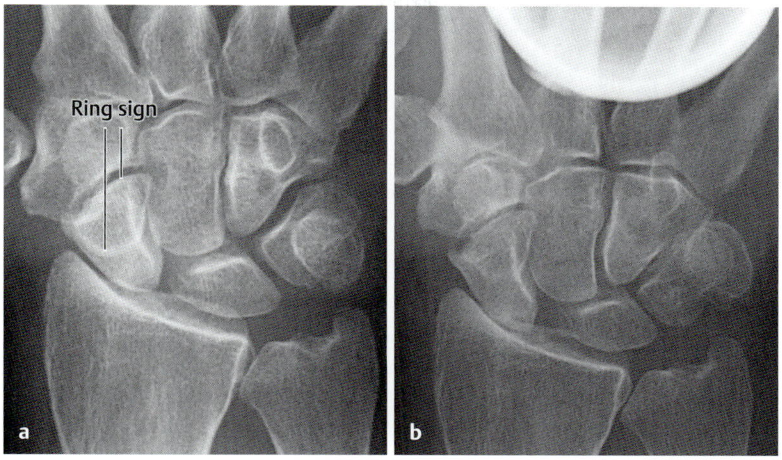

Fig. 2.228 The significance of the grip-loaded view in scapholunate dissociation. (a) In the normal dorsopalmar view there is an accentuated scapholunate space and a pathologic ring sign of the distal scaphoid. (b) Clear widening of the scapholunate space with the fist gripped over a ball.

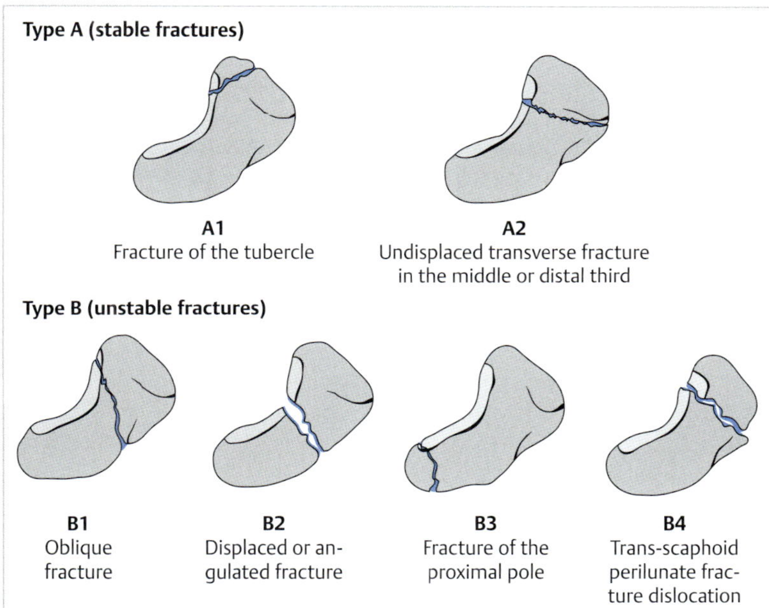

Fig. 2.229 Classification of scaphoid fractures according to Krimmer, Schmitt, and Herbert.

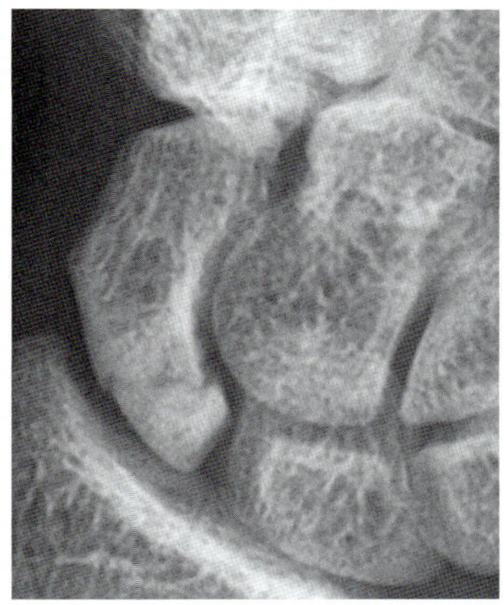

Fig. 2.230 Proximal pole fracture of the scaphoid. Type B3 according to Krimmer et al (unstable fracture). Stecher view.

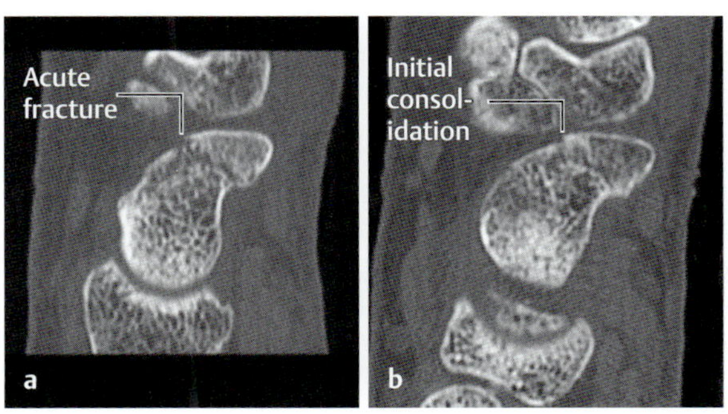

Fig. 2.231 Progressive healing of scaphoid fracture. **(a)** One week after injury. **(b)** Six weeks after injury.

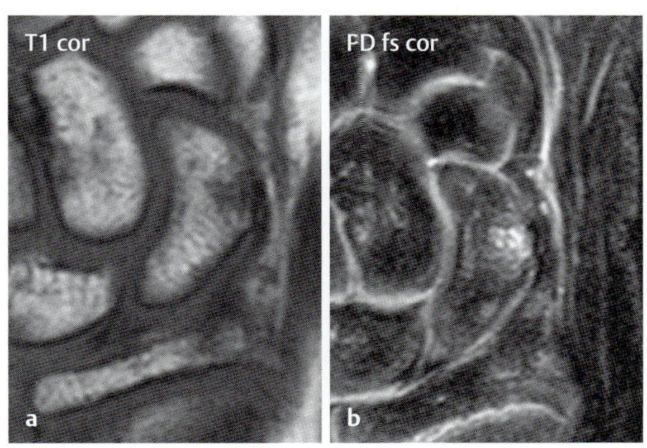

Fig. 2.232 Posttraumatic trabecular microfractures in the scaphoid. **(a)** No clear fracture line definable; cortex intact. **(b)** Focal bone marrow edema at the scaphoid waist.

Scaphoid Nonunion

> **Note**
> A scaphoid fracture normally heals within 8 weeks. Scaphoid nonunion is diagnosed when bone resorption and cyst formation are detected by CT and/or when no bony healing has occurred by 6 months after the injury.

▸ **Radiography/CT.** Nonunion stage is diagnosed when bone resorption and cyst formation are detected at the fracture margins (▸ Fig. 2.233) and should not be confused with the normal bone resorption and widening of the fracture gap in the early stage of fracture healing. Over time, nonunion progressive sclerosis of the fracture margins occurs and carpal collapse develops with subsequent osteoarthritis (SNAC wrist, see immediately below).

SNAC Wrist

The SNAC wrist (SNAC = scaphoid nonunion advanced collapse) is regarded as the final stage of an untreated scaphoid nonunion. SNAC wrist is classified into three stages (▸ Figs. 2.234–2.236).

Avascular Necrosis of the Scaphoid

> **Note**
> In contrast to secondary osteonecrosis after a scaphoid fracture, the rare "primary" osteonecrosis of the scaphoid (Preiser's disease) is of unknown etiology.

The site of predilection for posttraumatic avascular necrosis is the proximal pole of the scaphoid (secondary to interruption of the normal distal to proximal blood supply).

▸ **Radiography/CT.** Depending on the stage of the disease, subchondral sclerosis and cyst formation may be seen (▸ Fig. 2.237), followed by collapse (see ▸ Fig. 2.235) and, ultimately secondary osteoarthritis.

▸ **MRI.** MRI with intravenous contrast is used in the early diagnostic work-up to investigate viability of the proximal fragment. It is regarded as nonviable if there is diffuse hypointense signal within the affected area on conventional T1W sequences and absence of enhancement after gadolinium administration (▸ Fig. 2.238). T2W image signal is irrelevant for diagnosing viability.

Fracture of the Triquetrum

▸ **Radiography.** Usually dorsal flakelike cortical avulsion fractures are found that are recognizable on the lateral view (▸ Fig. 2.239).

▸ **CT.** CT is the best modality for determining the size and degree of displacement of the avulsed fragment, which will influence whether a conservative or surgical approach is used.

▸ **Important findings.** With fractures of the triquetrum, the description of an avulsion fragment, even if it is small, is of therapeutic relevance because the associated ligament avulsion may result in instability.

Other Carpal Fractures

Less common fractures, in descending order, include those involving the hamate, capitate, lunate, pisiform, trapezium, and trapezoid. These fractures are easily overlooked on conventional radiographs. A CT scan is indispensable in the case of a clinically suspected fracture but negative radiographs.

Avascular Necrosis of the Lunate (Kienbock's Disease)

Avascular necrosis of the lunate as a result of an acute injury is rare. See Chapter 6.3.2 for "primary," idiopathic avascular necrosis of the lunate (Kienbock's disease).

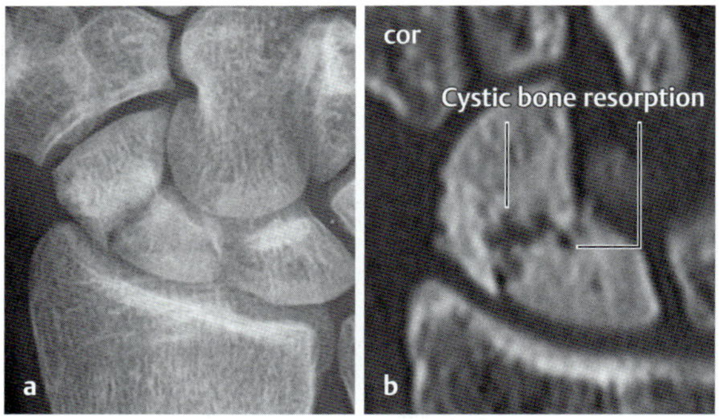

Fig. 2.233 Scaphoid nonunion. **(a)** Initial finding: 2-week-old scaphoid fracture, Type B2 according to Krimmer et al. **(b)** After 3 months, evidence of bone resorption and cyst formation on CT.

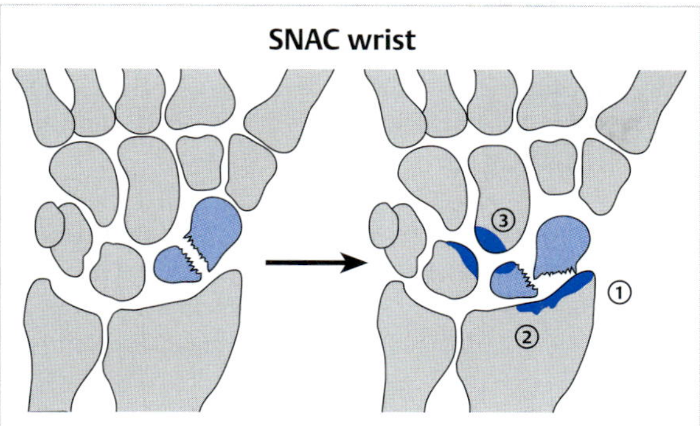

Stage 1: Osteoarthritis of the radial styloid process ①
Stage 2: Plus radioscaphoid osteoarthritis ②
Stage 3: Plus midcarpal osteoarthritis between the lunate and capitate with proximal migration of the capitate ③

Fig. 2.234 Watson's staging system for SNAC wrist.

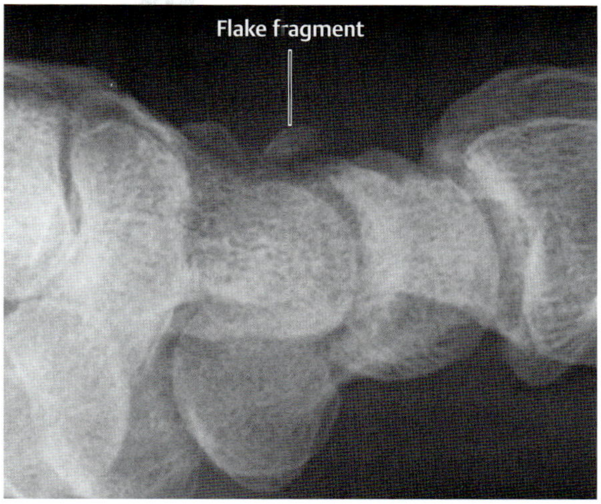

Fig. 2.239 Typical dorsal avulsion fracture of the triquetrum. Lateral radiograph.

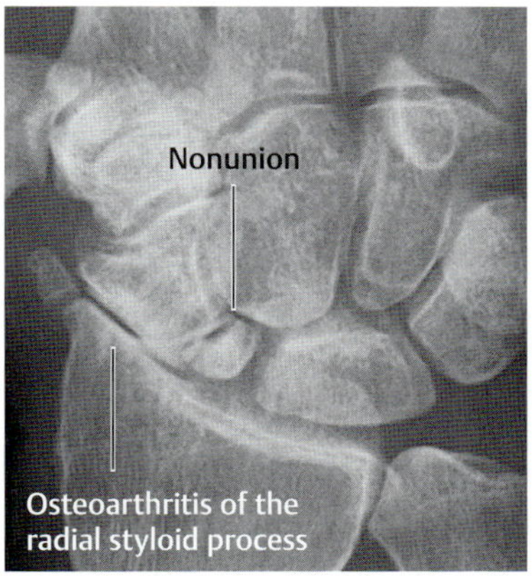

Fig. 2.235 SNAC wrist. Watson Stage I.

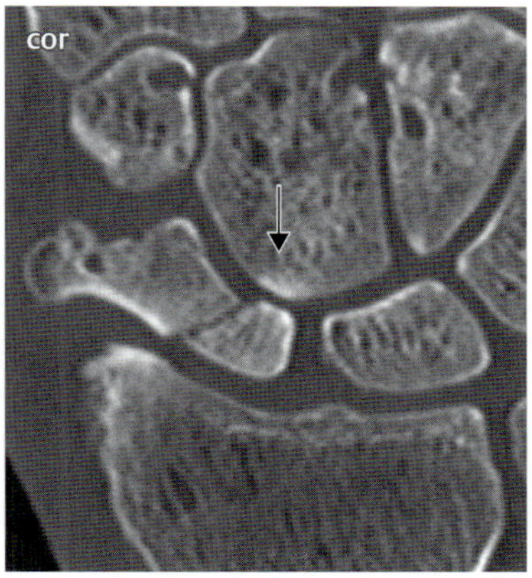

Fig. 2.236 SNAC wrist. Watson Stage III, as midcarpal osteoarthritis is already present (arrow).

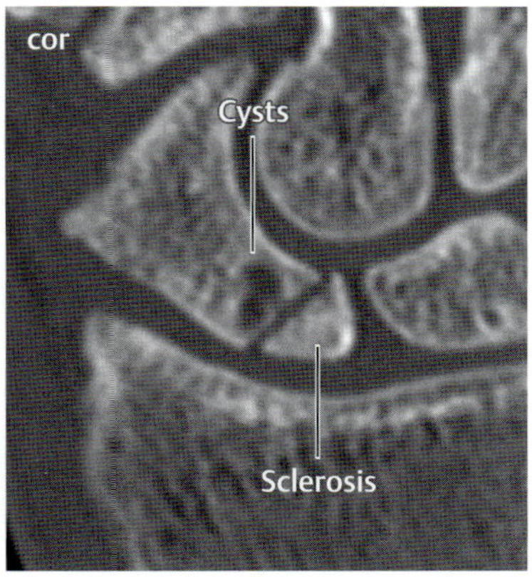

Fig. 2.237 Avascular necrosis of the proximal pole of the scaphoid.

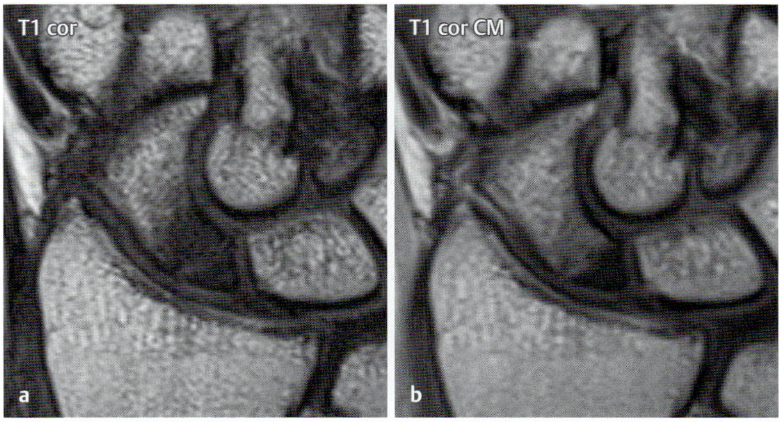

Fig. 2.238 Posttraumatic avascular necrosis of the proximal pole of the scaphoid. **(a)** In the plain T1W view differentiation between necrosis and edema is not certain. **(b)** After IV administration of contrast, nonenhancement is seen in the proximal pole, indicating that it is nonviable.

Perilunate Dislocation and Fracture Dislocations

A **perilunate dislocation** refers to dislocation (most commonly dorsal) of the carpus relative to the lunate due to a combination of intrinsic and extrinsic ligament disruption. If the carpus is subsequently reduced by traction of the forearm muscles, the lunate is rotated in a palmar direction (resulting in the image of the tipped-out tea cup; see ▶ Fig. 2.243b) and manifests itself as a palmar **dislocation of the lunate.** In fact, this should be regarded pathophysiologically as the ultimate stage of a perilunate dislocation and indicates disruption of all ligamentous support of the lunate.

Perilunate fracture dislocations are also associated with fractures of the adjacent carpal bones or radius and/or ulna. A careful search must therefore always be made for associated fractures when a perilunate dislocation is diagnosed; these are classified by Johnson according to which carpal injury arcs are injured (▶ Fig. 2.240):

- The greater arc with perilunate carpal fracture/dislocation (▶ Fig. 2.241).
- The lesser arc without carpal but with radial and/or ulnar fractures (▶ Fig. 2.242).

The most common fracture patterns are transradial, transscaphoid (= de Quervain's fracture dislocation), and transtriquetral.

▶ **Radiography.** Interruption of the Gilula lines along with a triangular form of the lunate is seen on the PA view (▶ Fig. 2.243a). Interruption of alignment of the radius, lunate, capitate, and third metacarpal as well as a pathologic angle between the individual carpal bones (▶ Fig. 2.243b) may be detected on the lateral view.

▶ **CT.** A CT scan is obligatory for assessing the full extent of the osseous injuries. It must be obtained urgently because of the risk of avascular necrosis of the lunate.

Axial Dislocation and Fracture Dislocations

This injury occurs as a result of axial compression. A distinction is made between ulnar and radial dissociation (▶ Fig. 2.244).

Ulnar-sided dissociation passes between the bases of the third and fourth metacarpals as well as through the hamate and capitate to extend proximally through the lunotriquetral ligament or the lunate (▶ Fig. 2.245). Associated fractures of the metacarpal bases are possible.

The less common **radial dissociation** passes between the bases of the second and third metacarpals with disruption of the STT joint (articulation formed between the scaphoid, trapezium and trapezoideum) and in some cases with associated fractures of the metacarpal bases.

▶ **Radiography.** This injury pattern may be underestimated due to projection-related superimposition at the carpometacarpal junction. An essential criterion is interruption of the M-shaped line formed by the carpometacarpal joints on the PA view (cf. ▶ Fig. 2.226).

▶ **CT.** An absolute indication for a CT scan is a suspected complex injury pattern and evaluation of its severity (▶ Fig. 2.245).

2.9.3 Carpal Instabilities and Malalignments

Carpal instability is defined as the inability to maintain normal carpal alignment during physiological loads. The causes of carpal instability are either traumatic, constitutional, degenerative or osteoarthritic. Classification is undertaken according to anatomical aspects:

- **CID (carpal instability dissociative):** This is a structural disruption within the proximal carpal row (scapholunate and lunotriquetral ligament tear).
- **CIND (carpal instability nondissociative):** This is a structural disruption of the entire proximal carpal row in relation to the forearm or the distal carpal row.
- **CIC (carpal instability complex):** This includes perilunate dislocations and fracture dislocations (Chapter 2.9.2).
- **Axial carpal instability:** Axial dislocations and fracture dislocations are included in this category (Chapter 2.9.2).

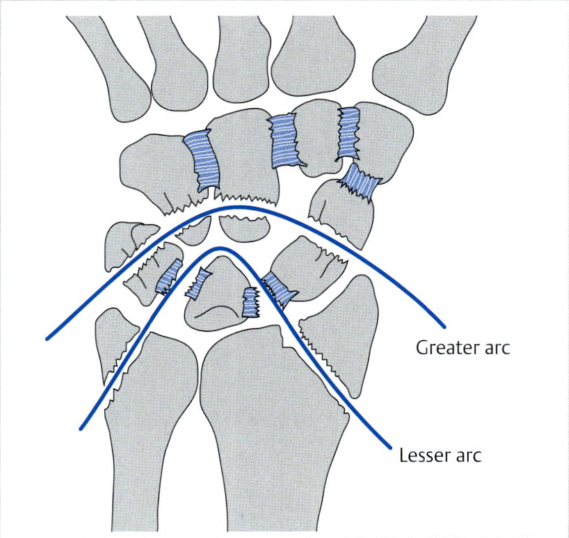

Fig. 2.240 Common injury patterns of perilunate fracture dislocations according to Johnson.

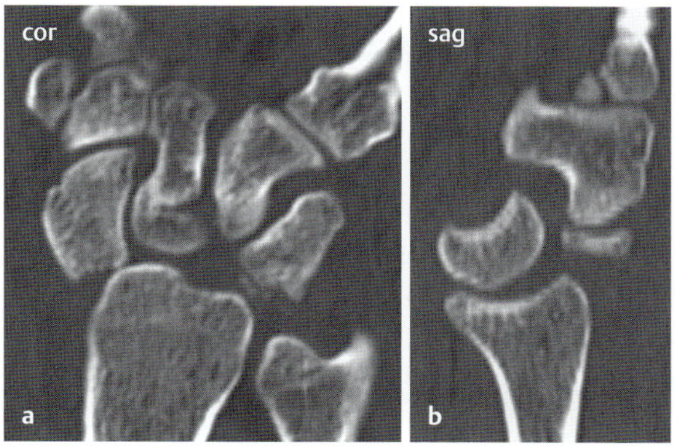

Fig. 2.241 Perilunate fracture dislocation. Greater arc injury. **(a)** Scaphoid fracture; this is therefore a De Quervain's fracture-dislocation. **(b)** The distal carpus is dislocated dorsally.

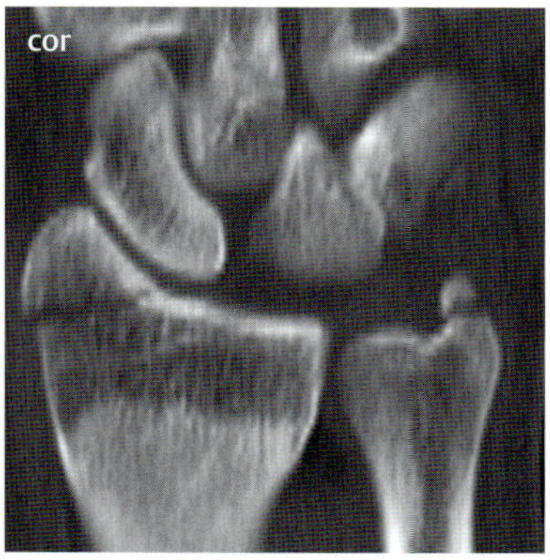

Fig. 2.242 Lesser arc injury. Lunate dislocation, fracture of the radial styloid process and the ulnar styloid process. Thick-slice MPR (4 mm).

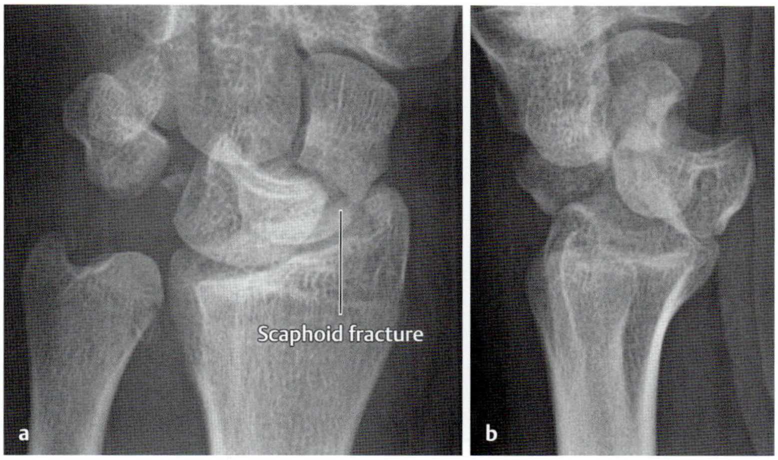

Fig. 2.243 Transscaphoid fracture dislocation. **(a)** Note the triangular shape of the lunate on the dorsopalmar projection, which is indicative of the dislocation. **(b)** The lateral view confirms the palmar dislocation of the lunate.

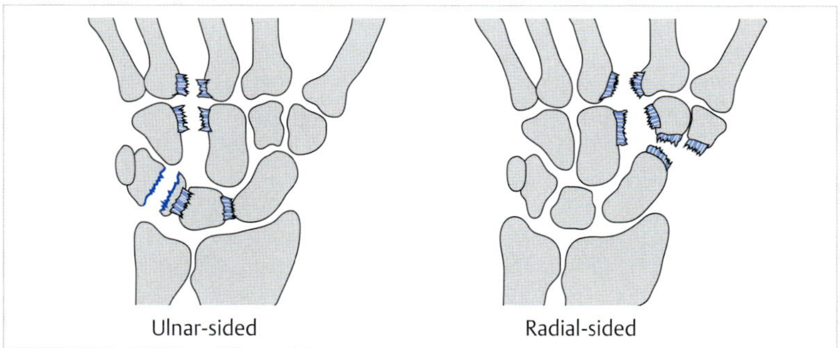

Fig. 2.244 Axial dislocation injuries of the carpus.

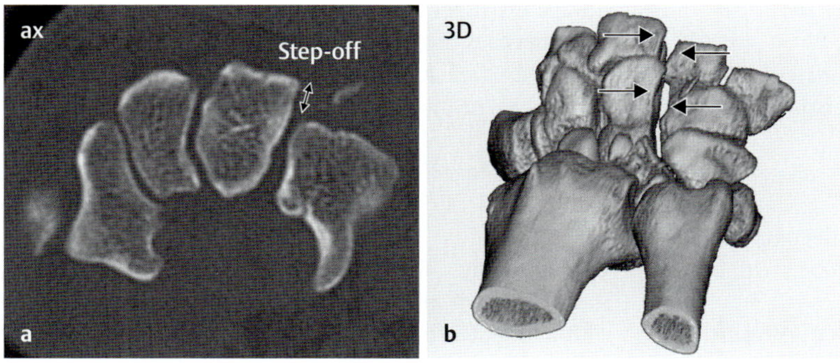

Fig. 2.245 Complex carpal injury as a result of an axial force. **(a)** Step-off between the articular surfaces of capitate and hamate. **(b)** 3D reconstruction (proximal–dorsal view) reveals the step-off (arrows) between the radial and ulnar carpal pillars; concomitant fracture of the lunate.

The terms "DISI" (dorsal intercalated segment instability deformity) and "VISI" (volar intercalated segmental instability) are important when dealing with carpal instability (► Fig. 2.246). **DISI deformity** refers to a rotation of the lunate dorsally in the sagittal plane; the radiolunate angle then amounts to more than 15°. In contrast, a **VISI deformity** refers to a palmar rotation of the lunate.

Furthermore, severity distinguishes between dynamic and static instability. With **dynamic instability**, pathologic alignment is evident only at dynamic clinical examination or on stress radiographs; in contrast, with **static instability** the structural disruption is consistently evident on conventional radiographs.

► Radiography/CT. A radiograph of the wrist will provide initial diagnostic imaging information. A stress view with the fist clenched may demonstrate evidence of dynamic scapholunate dissociation. A CT scan is capable of clearly depicting any malalignment (► Fig. 2.247).

► MRI. MRI (with or without MR arthrography), allows the direct identification of ligament injuries.

► Cinematography/Arthrography. Dynamic instability may be verified using cinefluoroscopy. It also allows for correlation of any clinical signs, such as a click or "clunk," with the actual structures involved during motion studies under fluoroscopy. Arthrography (with subsequent CT or MR arthrography) may be performed to achieve improved diagnostic confidence.

Dissociative Instability

Scapholunate Dissociation (Scapholunate Ligament Lesion)

► Pathology. This commonly occurs after hyperextension injuries or may be related to an intra-articular distal radial fracture extending to the scapholunate joint. Differentiation between acute-traumatic and chronic-degenerative lesions of the scapholunate ligament is not entirely possible using imaging. If the strong dorsal fibers of the ligament are disrupted in a young patient, this would indicate a traumatic origin.

A distinction is made between four stages:
- **Stage I:** Partial rupture of the scapholunate ligament in which at least one component (e.g., the palmar segment) is still intact.
- **Stage II:** Dynamic full-thickness tear, i.e., all components of the ligament are involved.
- **Stage III:** Static full-thickness tear, i.e., all components of the scapholunate ligament are involved along with the extrinsic radioscaphocapitate ligament.
- **Stage IV:** Collapse with varying degrees of osteoarthritis ("SLAC wrist"; see below).

► Radiography. No abnormalities are evident in Stage I. A Stage II injury can be diagnosed using a stress view and/or cinefluoroscopy.

Stage III:
- Diastasis of the scapholunate joint space of more than 3 mm (known as the Terry Thomas sign; ► Fig. 2.248).
- Ring sign of the distal scaphoid pole (see ► Figs. 2.228 and ► 2.248) due to rotatory subluxation of the scaphoid.
- DISI position of the lunate (see ► Figs. 2.246 and ► 2.247).

Stage IV is consistent with a SLAC wrist (► Fig. 2.249).

SLAC Wrist

The SLAC (scapholunate advanced collapse) wrist is regarded as the final stage of an untreated scapholunate dissociation. SLAC wrist is classified into three stages (see ► Fig. 2.249).

► CT/MR arthrography. CT arthrography and MR arthrography are the most accurate imaging modalities for determining the extent of ligament disruption and the exact stage of injury (► Figs. 2.250 and ► 2.251).

> **Note**
> The scapholunate ligament is comprised of dorsal, palmar, and central components. The dorsal component is decisive for stability and therefore must be carefully evaluated on CT and MRI studies. The central component is a thin membrane in which age-related perforations are common in older patients. Therefore, leakage of contrast medium through the scapholunate interval during arthrography is not necessarily clinically important.

Lunotriquetral Dissociation (Rupture of the Lunotriquetral Ligament)

► Pathology. This form of dissociation is much less common. It is usually secondary to an acute hyerpronation injury or chronic process, often associated with lesions of the triangular fibrocartilage complex.

A distinction is made between three stages:
- **Stage I:** Dynamic full-thickness tear with disruption of all ligamentous components.
- **Stage II:** Static full-thickness tear, in which extrinsic ligaments are involved in addition to the entire lunotriquetral ligament.
- **Stage III:** Stage II findings as well as midcarpal osteoarthritis.

► Radiography. The radiograph is often unremarkable in Stage I. There is interruption of the arcs of Gilula in Stage II with a VISI deformity of the lunate, which is palmar-flexed

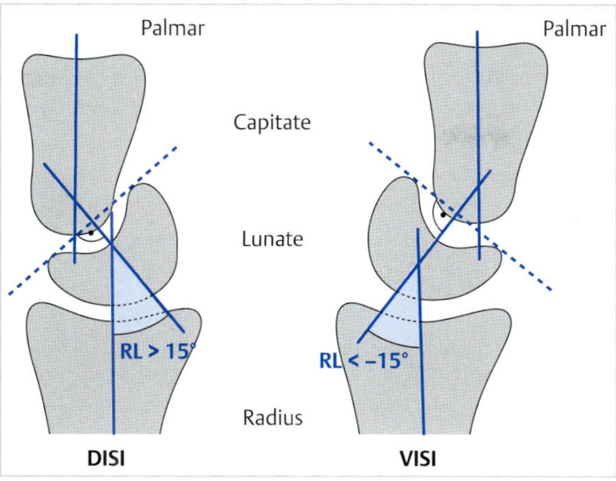

Fig. 2.246 Determination of the instability direction and angle on the lateral radiograph. RL = radiolunate angle.

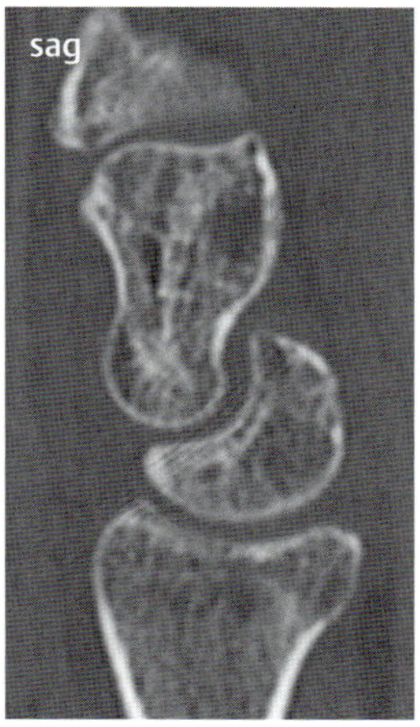

Fig. 2.247 DISI deformity. Obvious malrotation of the lunate relative to the radius and the capitate.

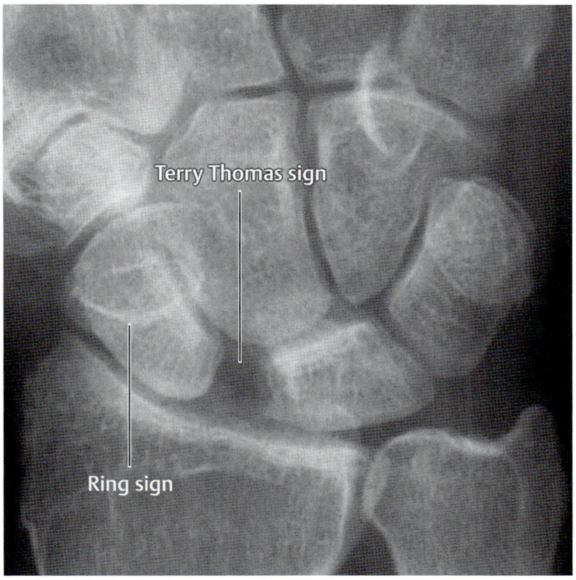

Fig. 2.248 Grade III scapholunate dissociation. No SLAC wrist as yet.

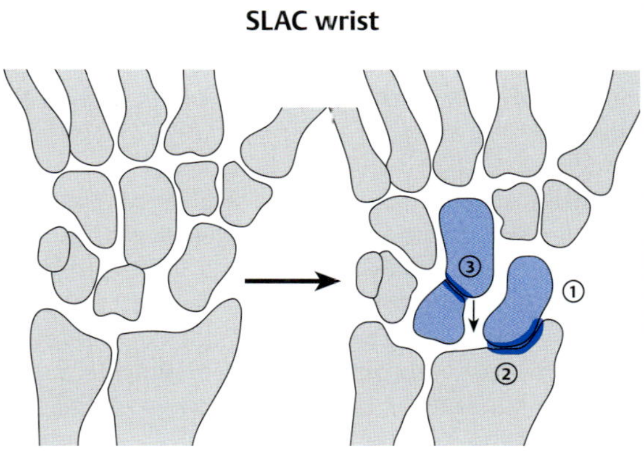

Stage 1: Osteoarthritis of the radial styloid process ①
Stage 2: Additional radioscaphoid osteoarthritis ②
Stage 3: Additional midcarpal osteoarthritis between lunate and capitate with proximal migration of the capitate ③

Fig. 2.249 Staging system of the SLAC wrist according to Watson.

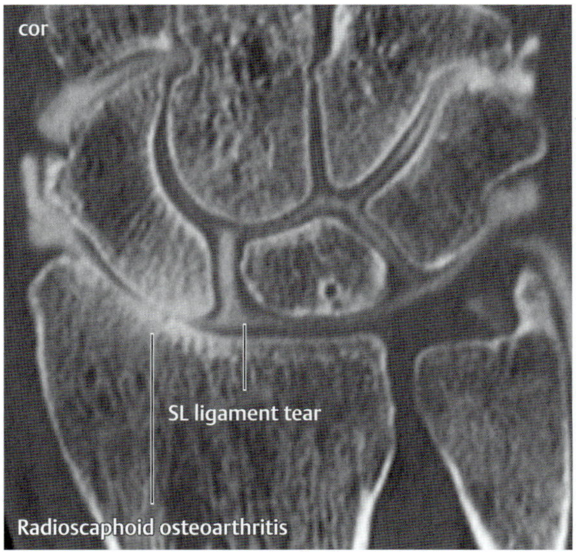

Fig. 2.250 Grade II SLAC wrist. SL, scapholunate.

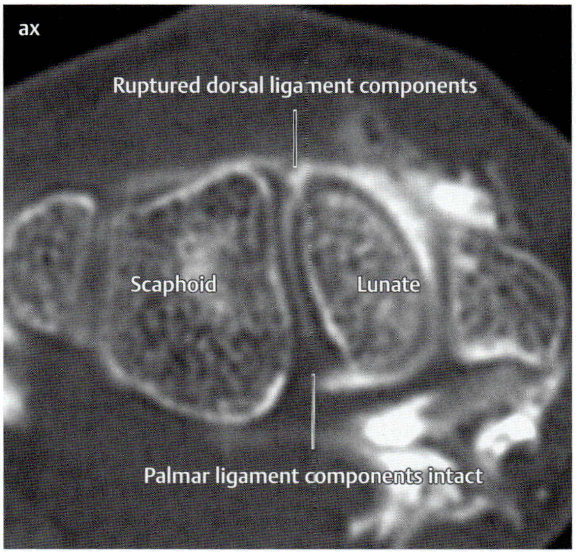

Fig. 2.251 Scapholunate dissociation, Stage I.

on a lateral radiograph; diastasis of the lunotriquetral joint space is less commonly seen.

▸ **CT/MR arthrography).** The same findings as for a lesion of the scapholunate ligament are seen. Here too, CT arthrography and/or MR arthrography provide the highest diagnostic accuracy (▸ Fig. 2.252).

Nondissociative Instability

A distinction is made between radiocarpal instability, carpal translocation, midcarpal instability, and capitatolunate instability. The scope of this book only allows a detailed account of the two most important forms; the specialized literature should be referred to for further information.

Carpal translocation. This may occur in all four directions and does not occur only after trauma but may also result from ligament disruption secondary to rheumatoid arthritis or CPPD arthropathy. This is related to lesions of the extrinsic ligaments. Ulnar carpal translocation (▸ Fig. 2.253) is common and is often found in patients with rheumatoid arthritis.

Midcarpal instability. This results from either congenital or posttraumatic insufficiency of the dorsal V-shaped ligament and intrinsic ligaments. With the dynamic form, the triquetrum is seen to jump within the spiral-shaped hamatotriquetral joint during cinefluoroscopy ("click phenomenon"). Ligamentous laxity is sometimes evident on an MRI scan, especially an MR arthrogram after a midcarpal injection of contrast medium.

2.9.4 Triangular Fibrocartilage Complex

▸ **Anatomy.** See Chapter 2.9.4 and ▸ Fig. W2.51.

▸ **Pathology.** The **classification system according to Palmer** is commonly used in daily clinical practice to describe lesions of the triangular fibrocartilage complex; it distinguishes between *traumatic* (Types Ia–d; ▸ Figs. 2.254–2.256) and *degenerative alterations* (Types IIa–e; ▸ Figs. 2.257 and ▸ 2.258). In practice, however, this distinction is often difficult, since a combination of the two is often present, given that degeneration of the triangular fibrocartilage itself may begin between 20 and 30 years of age.

▸ **MRI.** Routine high-resolution (noncontrast) MRI is accurate for diagnosing TFC pathology. Intravenous administration of contrast medium allows identification of vascularized components of triangular disk defects.

▸ **MR arthrography.** Unicompartmental or bicompartmental MR arthrography may also be used to increase diagnostic confidence. Clarification of the state of the undersurface of its ulnar attachment is paramount after injury (▸ Fig. 2.255) as it is often symptomatic but not usually amenable to direct inspection using standard arthroscopic portals. Another advantage of MR arthrography lies in its ability to better demonstrate chondropathy associated with degenerative (Palmer II) changes (see ▸ Fig. 2.258).

> **Note**
> If the distal radioulnar joint fills after a radiocarpal injection, then an additional injection may be dispensed with. Otherwise, the distal radioulnar joint will also require injecting in order to clarify the status of the undersurface of its ulnar attachment after a traumatic injury (▸ Fig. W2.49).

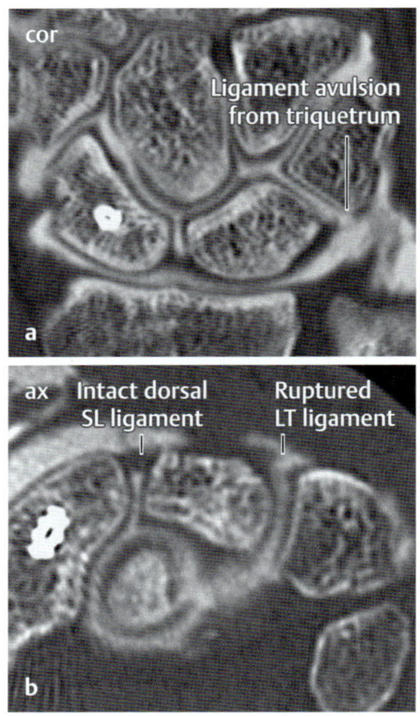

Fig. 2.252 Full-thickness lunotriquetral ligament tear. CT arthrography. LT, lunotriquetral; SL, scapholunate. **(a)** Mild lunotriquetral step-off in the proximal and middle Gilula arcs. **(b)** Contrast medium present over the entire lunotriquetral space, extending from dorsal to palmar.

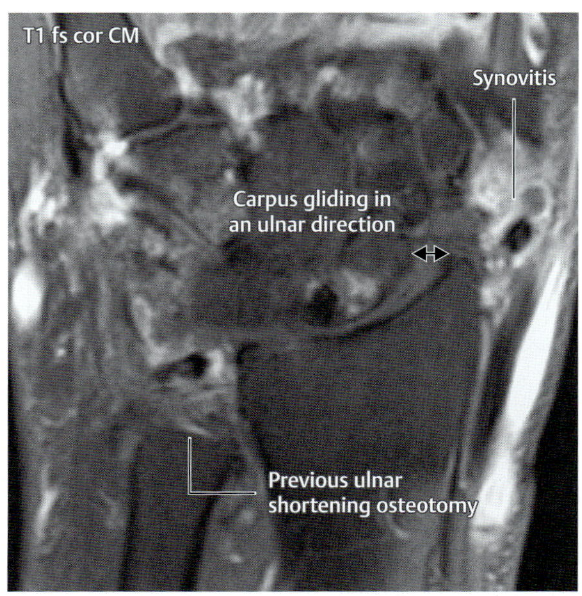

Fig. 2.253 Ulnar carpal translocation in rheumatoid arthritis.

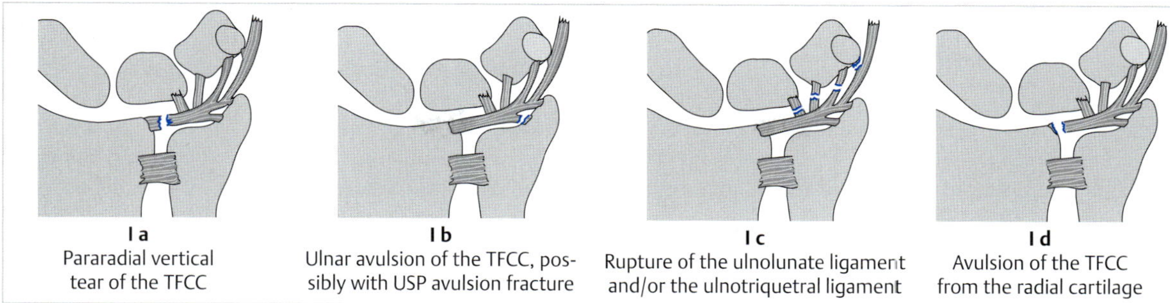

Fig. 2.254 Palmer classification of **traumatic lesions** of the triangular fibrocartilage complex. USP, ulnar styloid process; TFCC, triangular fibrocartilage complex.

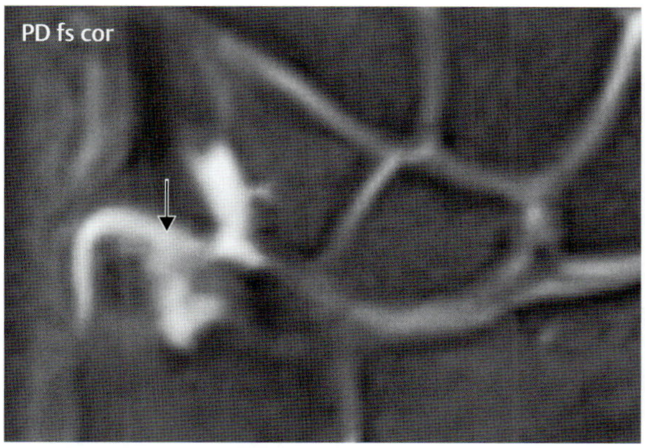

Fig. 2.255 Palmer Ib lesion (arrow).

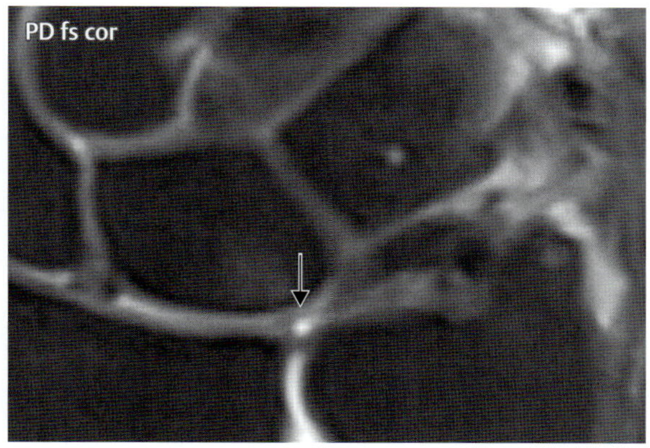

Fig. 2.256 Palmer Id lesion (arrow).

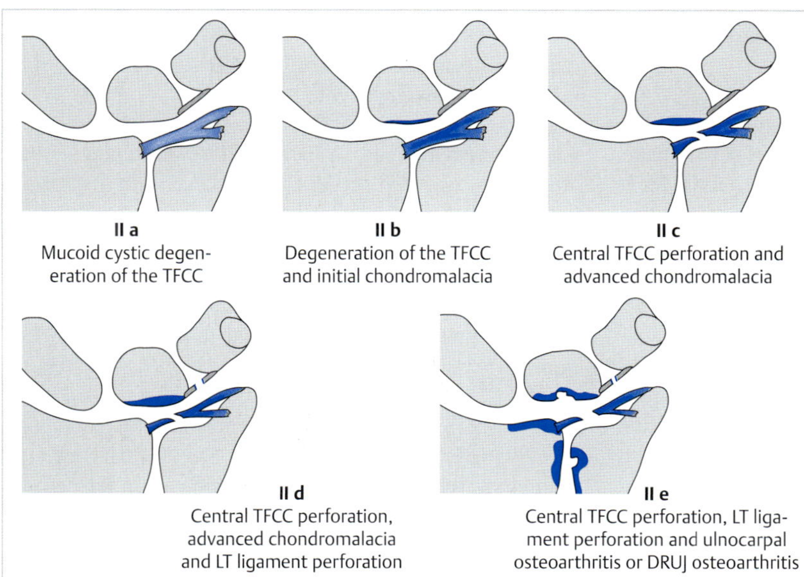

Fig. 2.257 Palmer classification of **degenerative lesions** of the triangular fibrocartilage complex. DRUJ, distal radioulnar joint; LT, lunotriquetral; TFCC, triangular fibrocartilage complex.

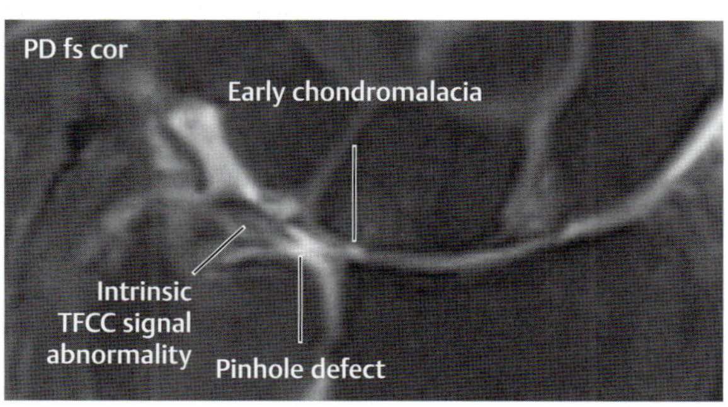

Fig. 2.258 Degenerative TFCC lesion, intermediate finding between Palmer Stages II b and II c.

2.9.5 Ulnocarpal Impaction Syndrome

Ulnocarpal impaction syndrome is a broad term representing varying forms:

- **Ulnolunate impaction:** Force transmission onto the lunate (▶ Figs. 2.259–2.261).
- **Ulnotriquetral impingement:** Force transmission onto the triquetrum with impaction of an elongated ulnar styloid process.
- **TILT (triquetral impingement ligament tear):** Ligamentous tissue becomes trapped between the ulnar styloid process and triquetrum after disruption of ulnar-sided capsuloligamentous structures.

Hamate-tip syndrome (hamatolunate impaction syndrome; ▶ Fig. 2.259) may also be considered an ulnocarpal impaction syndrome. This occurs with a type II lunate that has a medial articular facet on its distal surface which articulates with the hamate bone. It leads to chondral defects of the proximal pole of the hamate and consequent subchondral bone remodeling.

An **ulnar plus variant** is often present, in the setting of ulnocarpal impaction; however, this syndrome may also develop in the presence of ulnar-neutral variance, for example, when an increased ulnar force component is transmitted via a hypertrophic triangular fibrocartilage disk (▶ Fig. 2.262). Furthermore, there is not only a static, but also a dynamic form of impaction, which in turn can be identified by cinefluoroscopy

▶ **Radiography/CT.** Patchy sclerosis of the proximal lunate should be looked for; unlike avascular necrosis of the lunate, however, these changes are localized to its proximal ulnar aspect. Sometimes a small amount of osteolysis is the prominent finding, along with subchondral lucencies surrounding sclerosis of varying degrees (see ▶ Fig. 2.260a). Sclerosis of the ulnar head and/or the triquetrum and possibly the tip of the hamate may be identified.

▶ **MRI.** Ulnar impaction syndrome is often combined with a wide central perforation of the triangular fibrocartilage disk. In some cases this is also associated with a lunotriquetral ligament tear. Localized chondropathy, together with focal osseous abnormalities ranging from edemalike signal intensity to sclerotic changes (▶ Fig. 2.260b), allows a differentiation from avascular necrosis of the lunate.

▶ **Important findings.** Avascular necrosis of the lunate should be differentiated from ulnocarpal impaction syndrome because they require different therapeutic approaches. An ulnar shortening osteotomy can reduce the ulnar force transmission in ulnocarpal impaction syndrome. This procedure would be contraindicated for necrosis of the lunate as it would increase the abnormal forces upon the lunate even more.

2.9.6 Tendons of the Wrist

▶ **Anatomy.** ▶ See Chapter 2.9.6 and ▶ Fig. W2.52.

▶ **Pathology.** At the level of the wrist, chronic overuse-related degeneration of the tendons (tendinosis) and their surrounding structures are common, as are friction syndromes. Less frequently, acute damage to the extensor pollicis longus tendon occurs secondarily to an angulated distal radial fracture or as a result of irritation by screws after the placement of a palmar plate. Alterations to tendons and tendon sheaths secondary to inflammatory disorders are dealt with in Chapter 10.

Tendinoses

Tendinoses most commonly involve the flexor carpi radialis, flexor carpi ulnaris, and extensor carpi ulnaris tendons.

Osteoarthritic changes of the STT joint are often the cause of tendinosis in the case of the **flexor carpi radialis tendon.**

The **flexor carpi ulnaris tendon** is the most common site of a calcific tendinosis of the wrist.

The **extensor carpi ulnaris tendon** can suffer chronic damage as a result of friction in its osteofibrotic tunnel over the sulcus of the ulnar styloid process. Rupture of its overlying retinaculum, in comparison, may result in palmar subluxation of the tendon (corresponding clinically to a painful snapping when moving from supination to pronation), with secondary tendinopathy of the tendon, an injury that is commonly associated with tennis.

▶ **US.** Ultrasound is an excellent modality for tendon evaluation because of their superficial position. In addition, US allows a dynamic examination of the tendons. Tendinosis is associated with localized thickening of the tendon (▶ Fig. 2.263). Tenosynovitis involves thickening of the tendon sheath and fluid within it. Ultrasound is also ideal for providing guidance during targeted tendon sheath injections.

▶ **MRI.** MRI is equally capable of demonstrating tendon pathology (▶ Fig. 2.264). The administration of IV contrast medium may provide improved visualization of tendon pathology.

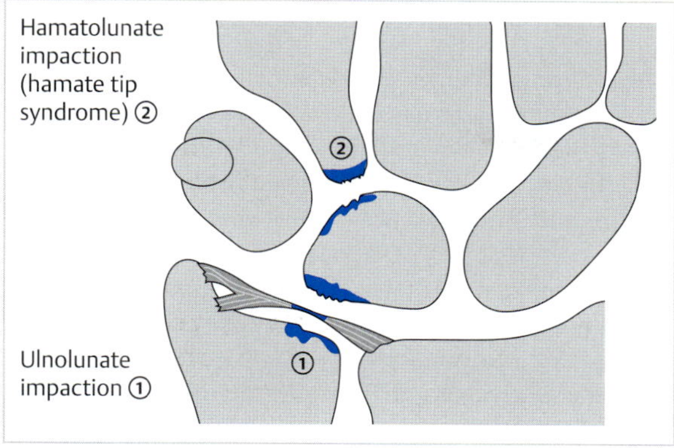

Fig. 2.259 Common manifestations of ulnar-sided impaction syndromes.

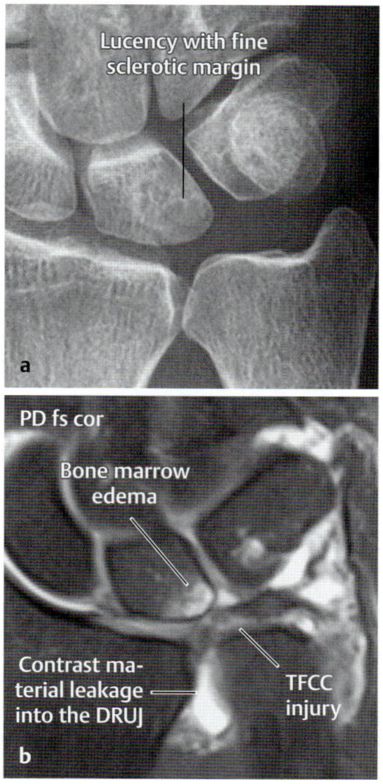

Fig. 2.260 Ulnolunate impaction. DRUJ, distal radioulnar joint; TFCC, triangular fibrocartilage complex. **(a)** Mild ulnar plus variance. Typical location of lunate abnormality. **(b)** MR arthrography: three pathologic findings.

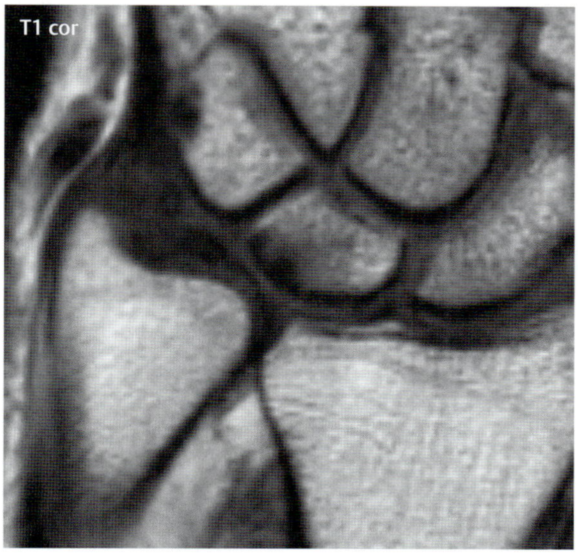

Fig. 2.261 Ulnolunate impaction. Different patient from ▶ Fig. 2.260.

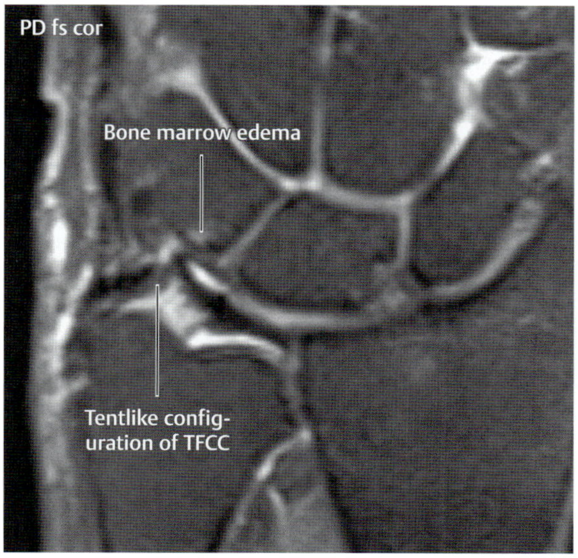

Fig. 2.262 Triquetral impingement with a variant of the triangular fibrocartilage complex.

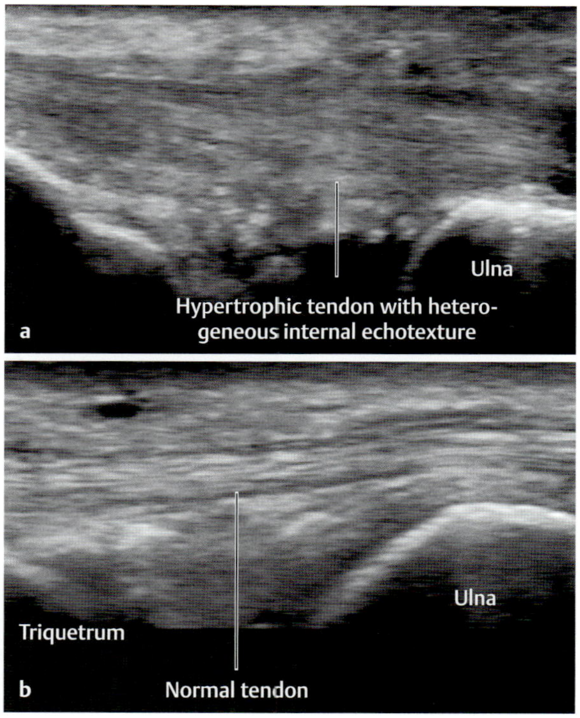

Fig. 2.263 Ultrasound of the extensor carpi ulnaris tendon. Longitudinal section. **(a)** Tendinosis of the extensor carpi ulnaris tendon. **(b)** Normal finding for comparison.

Friction Syndromes

De Quervain's stenosing tenosynovitis involves the tendons of the first extensor compartment at the radial styloid process (▶ Fig. 2.265). It is important to be aware of any normal variants preoperatively, such as a vertical septum within the tunnel or the occurrence of accessory tendons, which is by no means rare.

This should be distinguished from **distal intersection syndrome** in which the extensor pollicis longus tendon within the third extensor compartment crosses over the second extensor compartment at the level of the proximal scaphoid pole.

Proximal intersection syndrome, however, is located approximately 5 cm proximal to the wrist where the first extensor tendons cross over those of the second.

▶ **US.** Ultrasound is the primary imaging technique for evaluating these syndromes. Apart from thickening of the tendon or tendon sheath proximal to the friction site, a concomitant effusion within the tendon sheath is often seen on static images. The sheath is compressed at the level of the friction (▶ Fig. 2.265a). The major advantage of this modality is the ability of perform a dynamic examination, which may demonstrate restricted gliding of tendons and allow for targeted therapeutic injections.

▶ **MRI.** MRI is also an excellent modality for evaluating these friction syndromes (▶ Fig. 2.265b).

2.10 Metacarpals and Fingers

2.10.1 Anatomy, Technique, and Indications

▶ **Anatomy.** ▶ See Chapter 2.10.1 and ▶ Figs. W2.53–W2.56.

Technique and Indications

▶ **Radiography.** Conventional radiographs, typically in two projections, are an excellent screening modality.

▶ **US.** As with the wrist, ultrasound is the primary modality for assessing the soft tissues. In particular, tendon pathology and collateral ligament injuries (especially of the ulnar collateral ligament of the thumb MCP joint—skier's thumb) are well evaluated with ultrasound.

▶ **MRI.** MRI scanning plays a supplementary role in the diagnostic work-up of traumatic or overuse-related injuries.

2.10.2 Fractures

The following findings are of particular importance when evaluating metacarpal and phalangeal fractures:

- Fractures with joint involvement.
- Extra-articular fractures, but near the base.
- Shaft fractures and subcapital fractures.

Apart from indicating the site of the fracture, description of the direction and degree of displacement is important.

Fractures of the basal joint of the thumb (▶ Fig. 2.266) include the Bennett (▶ Fig. 2.267) and Rolando fractures, both of which are intra-articular, as well as the Winterstein fracture, which is extra-articular.

Attention should also be paid to avulsion fractures sustained during tendon and ligament injuries, in particular bony avulsions related to the extensor tendons and the ulnar collateral ligament of the thumb MCP joint (see next subsection).

2.10.3 Tendon and Ligament Lesions

Extensor Tendon Injury

Various finger deformities may arise as a result of an extension tendon injury, depending on the site of the lesion:

- **Mallet finger** with a dorsal avulsion of the base of the distal phalanx.
- **Boutoniere deformity** due to rupture of the central slip and palmar subluxation of the lateral slips at the level of the proximal interphalangeal joint.
- **Malalignment of the metacarpophalangeal joint** (boxer knuckle) due to a rupture of the sagittal band (usually along its radial aspect) with either partial or complete dislocation of the extensor tendon into the intermetacarpal space.

▶ **Radiography.** Radiological diagnostic examination is suitable for excluding or confirming an avulsion fracture (▶ Fig. 2.268).

▶ **US/MRI.** Dynamic ultrasound is superb for demonstrating extensor tendon injuries and injuries to the extensor hood over the metacarpophalangeal joint and any associated subluxation of the extensor tendon with finger flexion. MRI may be indicated in questionable cases.

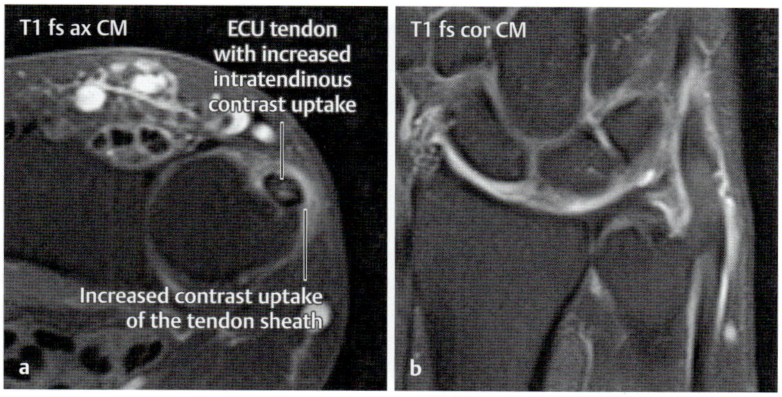

Fig. 2.264 Tendinosis and tenosynovitis of the extensor carpi ulnaris tendon. ECU, extensor carpi ulnaris. **(a)** Thickened extensor carpi ulnaris tendon with increased contrast enhancement of tendon and synovial sheath. **(b)** Demonstration in the coronal plane.

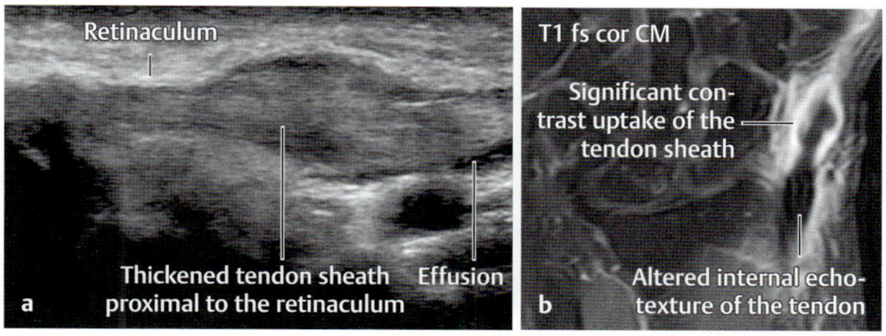

Fig. 2.265 Stenosing tenosynovitis (de Quervain). **(a)** Typical ultrasound finding (longitudinal section). **(b)** Tendinosis and tenosynovitis of the first extensor compartment on an MRI scan.

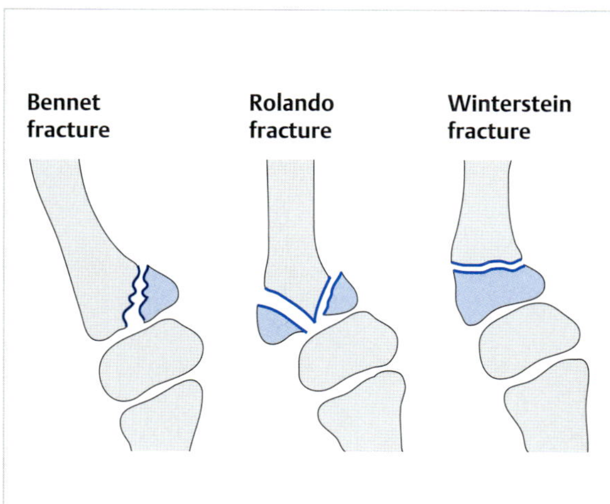

Fig. 2.266 Typical appearance of a fracture at the base of the first metacarpal.

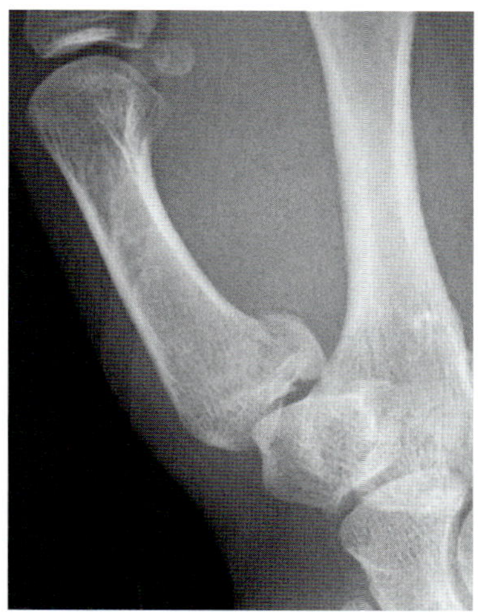

Fig. 2.267 Bennett fracture.

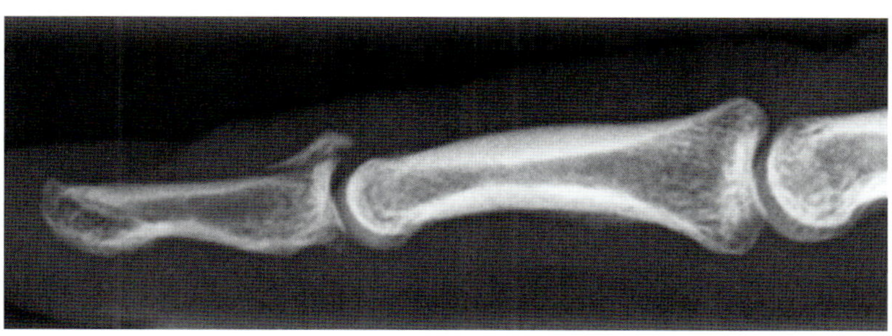

Fig. 2.268 Bony avulsion of the extensor tendon from the distal phalanx.

Flexor Tendon and Pulley Injuries

Flexor tendon injuries are assessed for the extent of tendon retraction and the presence of a bony avulsion fragment.

An avulsion injury of the flexor digitorum profundus (FDP) tendon from its insertion on the distal phalanx can occur when the FDP muscle is maximally contracted while the distal interphalangeal (DIP) joint is forcefully hyperextended. This may happen, for example, when a player of American football or rugby grabs an opponent's jersey while the latter pulls away (jersey finger injury). This may rupture the flexor tendon or even avulse the palmar base of the distal phalanx with the FDP tendon attached. The bony fragment is usually evident on a lateral radiograph of the involved finger, which in 75% of cases is the ring finger due to its anatomically weaker insertion.

Pulley injuries must be considered in the presence of a flexion deficit.

▶ **Radiography.** Radiographs allow for evaluation of an avulsion fracture.

▶ **US/MRI.** Ultrasound can display the extent of tendon retraction after a flexor tendon injury (▶ Fig. 2.269). US is also employed for a suspected pulley injury (climber's finger) and has the advantage of allowing a dynamic assessment. In this case, displacement of the tendon away from the bone (normal: 1 mm or less) increases significantly during flexion against resistance (bowstringing). Supplemental MRI is not usually necessary.

Stenosing Tenosynovitis

"Trigger finger" refers to degeneration of the flexor tendon at the level of the A1 pulley over the metacarpal head.

▶ **US.** The stenosing alterations can be exactly located by a dynamic examination. In addition to increased thickness of the A1 pulley (normal: up to 1.5 mm), tendinosis, and tenosynovitic changes, Doppler US may demonstrate the presence of increased vascularization.

Collateral Ligament Injuries

▶ **Radiography.** Radiography allows evaluation of the presence of an avulsion fracture (▶ Fig. 2.270).

▶ **US/MRI.** A diagnostic ultrasound examination allows assessment of the extent of the collateral ligament tear.

Skier's thumb requires differentiation between a nondisplaced ligament stump and one where the aponeurosis of the adductor pollicis is interposed between the stump and the torn ligament (**Stener lesion**), which is important for treatment (▶ Fig. 2.271). A supplementary MRI scan may be obtained in equivocal cases (▶ Fig. 2.272).

> **Note** !
> Stress radiographs are no longer used to evaluate skier's thumb.

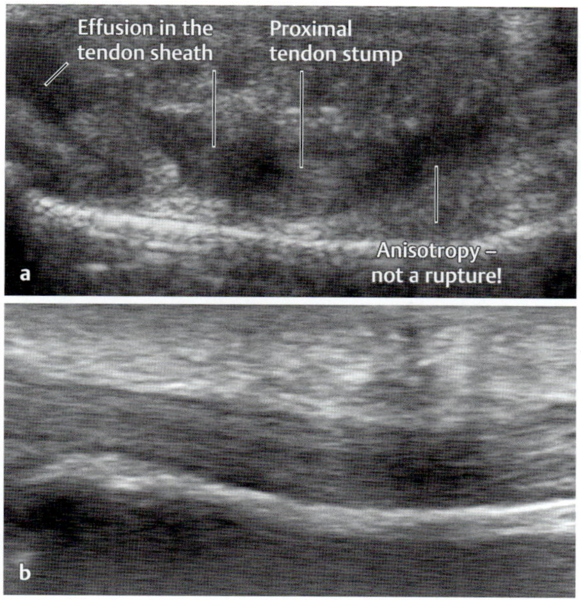

Fig. 2.269 Ultrasound of the flexor tendon of a finger. Longitudinal section. **(a)** Full-thickness traumatic tear of the tendon. **(b)** Normal finding.

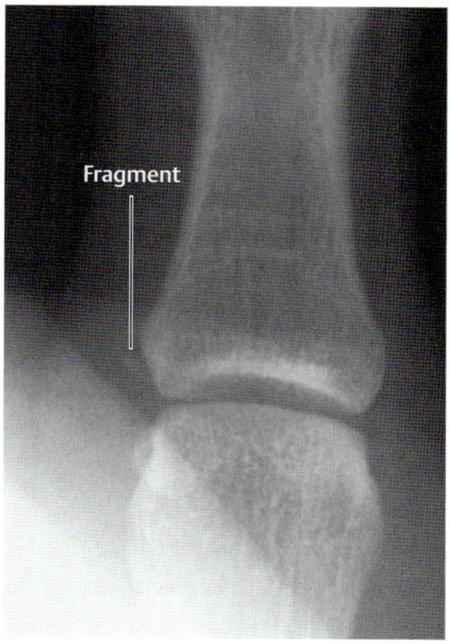

Fig. 2.270 Skier's thumb with a small bony avulsion.

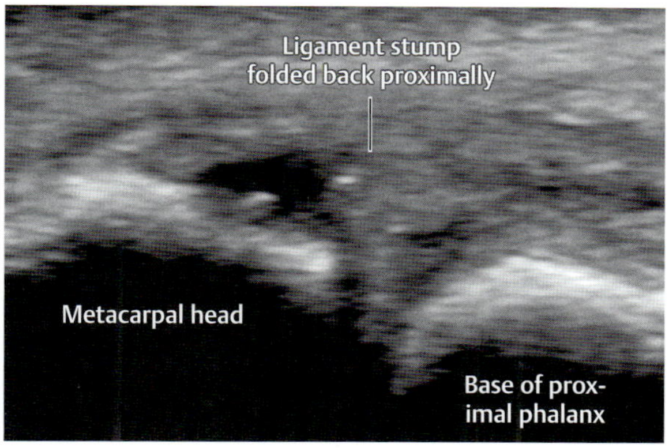

Fig. 2.271 Skier's thumb with a displaced ligament stump. Stener lesion.

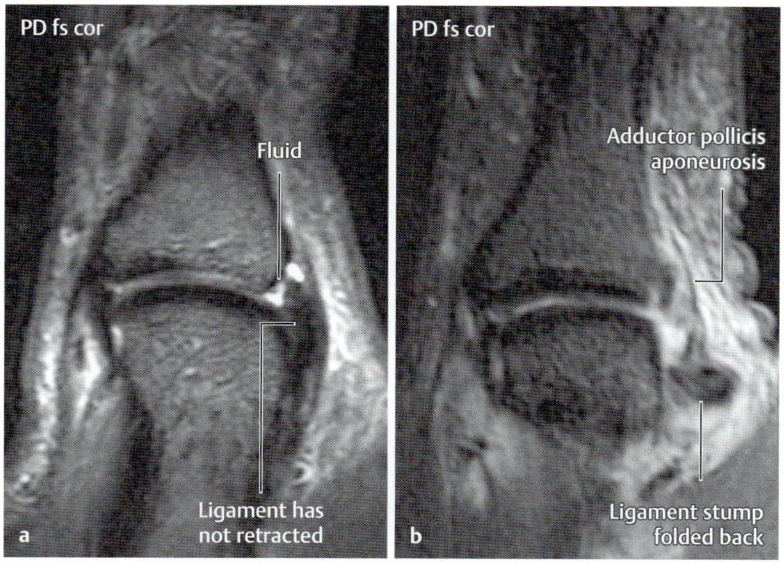

Fig. 2.272 Two patients with skier's thumb. **(a)** Distal ligament tear; conservative treatment is possible. **(b)** Displaced ligament stump; surgical treatment is indicated.

2.11 Hip Joint

2.11.1 Anatomy, Variants, and Techniques

▸ **Anatomy.** See Chapter 2.11.1 and ▸ Fig. W2.57.

Variants

There are several synovial folds or plicae within the hip joint which, in part, carry blood vessels from the hip joint capsule to the bone. The most significant synovial fold can be recognized in 95% of cases by MR arthrography: It courses from the medial border of the femoral neck to the hip joint capsule and is referred to as the "pectineofoveal fold" (or **medial synovial plica**) (▸ Fig. 2.273).

At the femoral head–neck junction there is often a cystic structure known as a **"herniation pit,"** which corresponds to a synovial fold. Whereas this alteration has previously been regarded as a normal variant, individual studies have identified an increased occurrence of herniation pits in patients with femoroacetabular impingement (FAI) (▸ Fig. 2.274). However, since a herniation pit also occurs in one-fourth of the general population, the diagnosis of FAI cannot be assumed from the presence of a herniation pit.

Bursae may be present at several sites, directly adjacent to the hip joint. An **iliopectineal bursa** is the most common finding. It is located between the musculotendinous junction of the iliopsoas muscle and the hip joint capsule and communicates in 15% of cases with the hip joint (▸ Fig. 2.275).

Indications

▸ **Radiography.** Initially, the pelvis should be assessed by a well-positioned AP radiograph. Apart from any possible fracture or joint-space narrowing, this will allow evaluation of the roof and orientation of the acetabulum, which is important for assessing FAI or dysplasia of the hip.

▸ **CT.** CT is employed for assessing fractures or tumors of the pelvis and for the diagnostic work-up of unclear radiological findings. The labrum and articular cartilage can also be evaluated by CT arthrography in patients with contraindications to MRI.

▸ **US.** The presence of an effusion of the hip joint may be assessed by ultrasound; US is also used for evaluation of soft tissues (muscles, tendons) or for possible abscess. Ultrasound is of particular importance in pediatric cases especially for the evaluation of developmental dysplasia of the hip.

▸ **MRI.** MRI of the pelvis and hips is commonly performed and is useful for fracture detection, tumor staging, the diagnostic work-up of inflammatory processes of bone and soft tissue, and for the assessment of muscles, tendons, the acetabular labrum, and articular cartilage of the hip. Oblique axial and/or radial slices are useful for evaluating the proximal femur in cases of suspected FAI. MRI of the whole pelvis is usually obtained without the administration of contrast; direct MR arthrography may be used when the focus is directed to the hip joint. During MR arthrography, needle position is confirmed with the injection of a small amount of iodine-containing contrast, followed by 8 to 12 mL of dilute gadolinium-based contrast under fluoroscopic guidance (an "off label" use in several countries) (Fig. W2.58). Alternatively, the injection may be performed under ultrasound guidance.

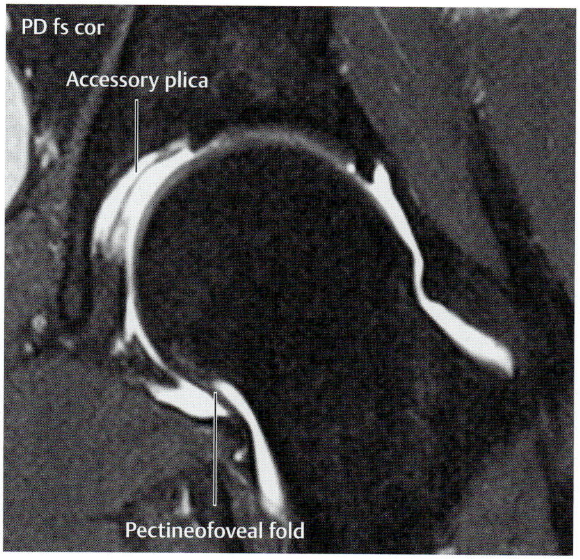

Fig. 2.273 Medial synovial plica as a normal variant. MR arthrography.

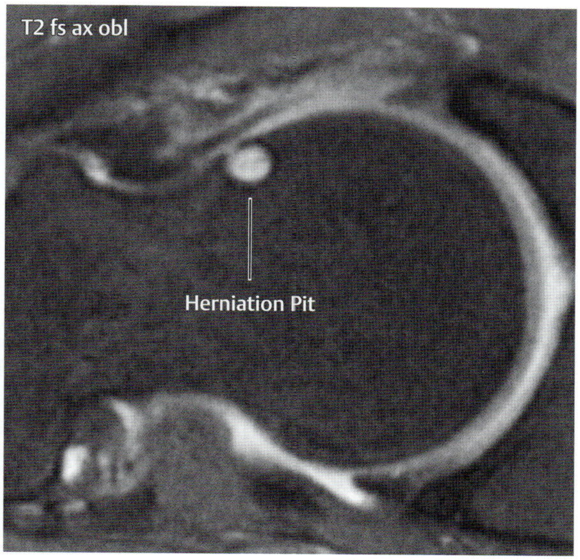

Fig. 2.274 Herniation pit in a female patient with FAI. MR arthrography.

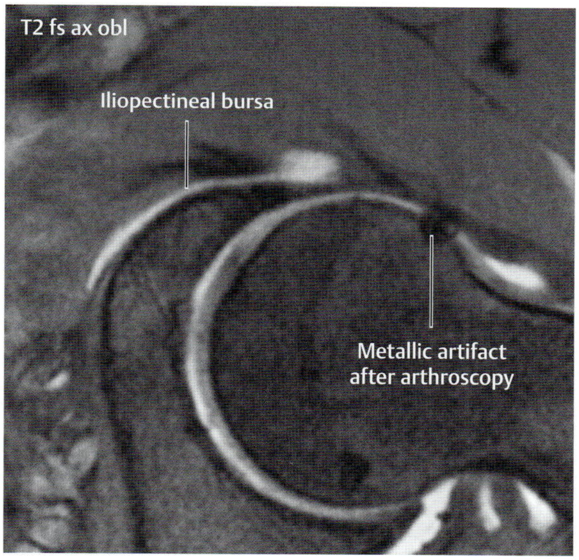

Fig. 2.275 Iliopectineal (iliopsoas) bursa. MR arthrography. The bursa is fluid-filled due to communication with the hip joint.

2

2.11.2 Fractures

Fractures of the acetabulum are dealt with in Chapter 2.3.2, fractures of the femoral head in Chapter 2.3.4 and Chapter 2.12.2. Insufficiency fractures of the hip are described in Chapter 1.5.1.

2.11.3 Femoroacetabular Impingement

▸ **Pathology.** There are two basic forms of FAI (▸ Fig. 2.276), **cam impingement** (in which the shape of the aspherical femoral head and neck resembles a camshaft and involves a **reduced femoral-neck offset** at the femoral head–neck junction) and **pincer impingement** (in which there is acetabular overcoverage). There is also a mixed form of FAI. The common factor in all forms of FAI is that an abnormal contact occurs between the proximal femur and the acetabulum that results in abnormal bony abutment and secondary damage to the labrum and articular cartilage.

With cam type FAI, the alpha angle is increased (▸ Fig. 2.277). The pincer form of FAI occurs when the acetabulum is too deep or retroverted, resulting in acetabular overcoverage (▸ Figs. 2.278 and ▸ 2.279).

▸ **Clinical presentation.** Patients with FAI often experience pain in the hip or groin, especially with adduction or internal rotation. Commonly young active individuals between the ages of 20 and 50 years who participate in sports are affected. As a rule of thumb, symptoms of the cam form of FAI tend to develop in males between the ages of 20 and 40 years, while the pincer form is more likely to affect females between 30 and 50 years of age.

In the presence of clinical symptoms, FAI is treated by femoral head–neck junction osteochondroplasty and trimming of the acetabular rim. Given that long-term results are lacking, it is not clear which clinical and radiological findings represent clear indications for surgery.

▸ **Radiography/CT.** In a patient with suspected FAI, a technically well-positioned pelvic radiograph should be obtained initially in order to determine the depth and orientation of the acetabulum (see ▸ Fig. 2.279). An abnormal head–neck offset of the proximal femur (cam FAI) is sometimes recognizable on this radiograph. However, an abnormal offset is sometimes underestimated on radiographs, especially if it involves the anterosuperior portion of the femur. CT can demonstrate retroversion of the acetabulum, but it is preferable to assess this on a well-positioned radiograph since the method for measuring acetabular version described in ▸ Fig. 2.278 can only quantify the mean version. Pincer FAI is frequently associated with a **cranial** retroversion, which cannot be assessed using the method described in ▸ Fig. 2.278.

▸ **MRI.** MR arthrography is obtained as a second step in suspected FAI. An abnormal offset at the head–neck junction may be identified with standard imaging planes or using special radial images (▸ Fig. 2.280). This technique is also able to demonstrate associated damage to the labrum and articular cartilage. This is most important because surgical management is associated with a significantly poorer prognosis in the presence of substantial labral or cartilage damage.

▸ **DD.** A mildly abnormal offset or a mild coxa profunda is not necessarily an indication of an FAI as these are often present in asymptomatic individuals. The correlation of radiological and clinical findings is mandatory.

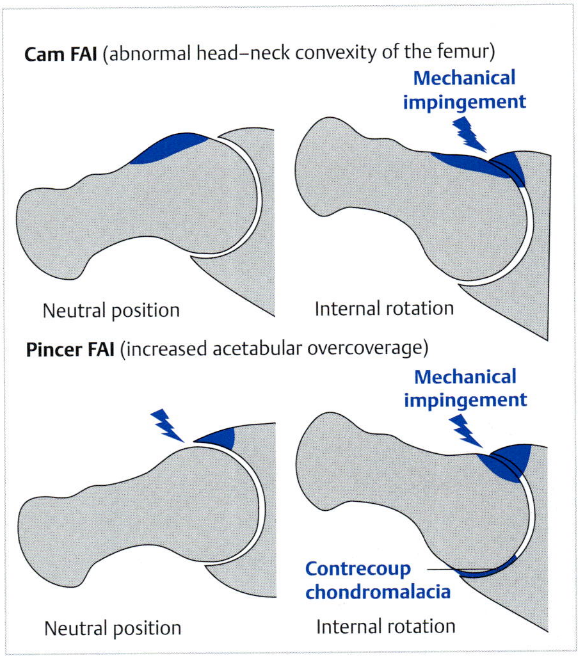

Fig. 2.276 Basic forms of femoroacetabular impingement (FAI).

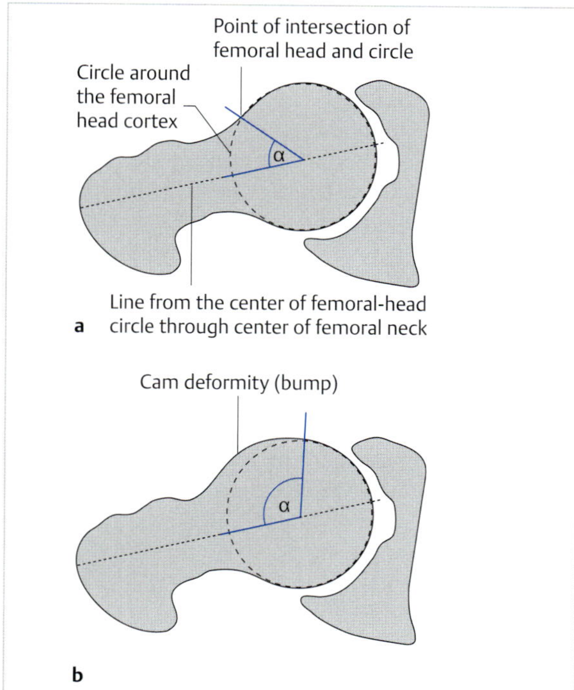

Fig. 2.277 Alpha angle of the proximal femur. Normal value < 55°. Measurement on a para-axial section (plane along the femoral neck). **(a)** Determination of the alpha angle (normal finding). **(b)** Pathologically enlarged alpha angle in cam deformity.

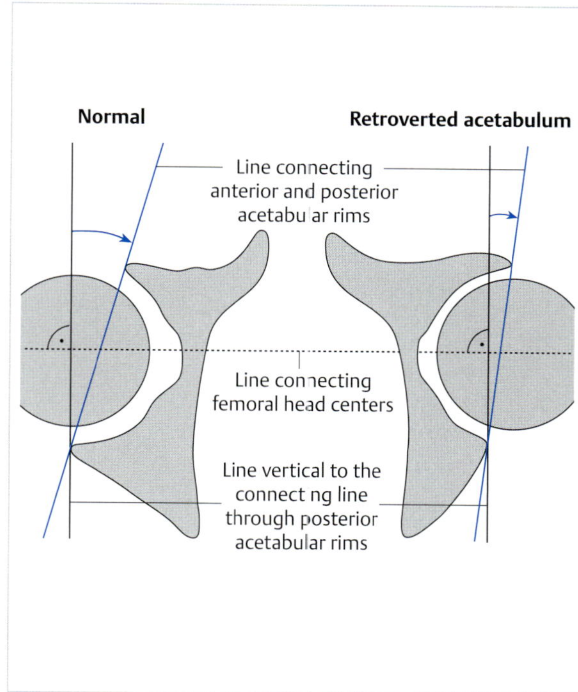

Fig. 2.278 Measurement of acetabular inclination on the axial CT image. Normal value ~ 15 to 25° anteversion.

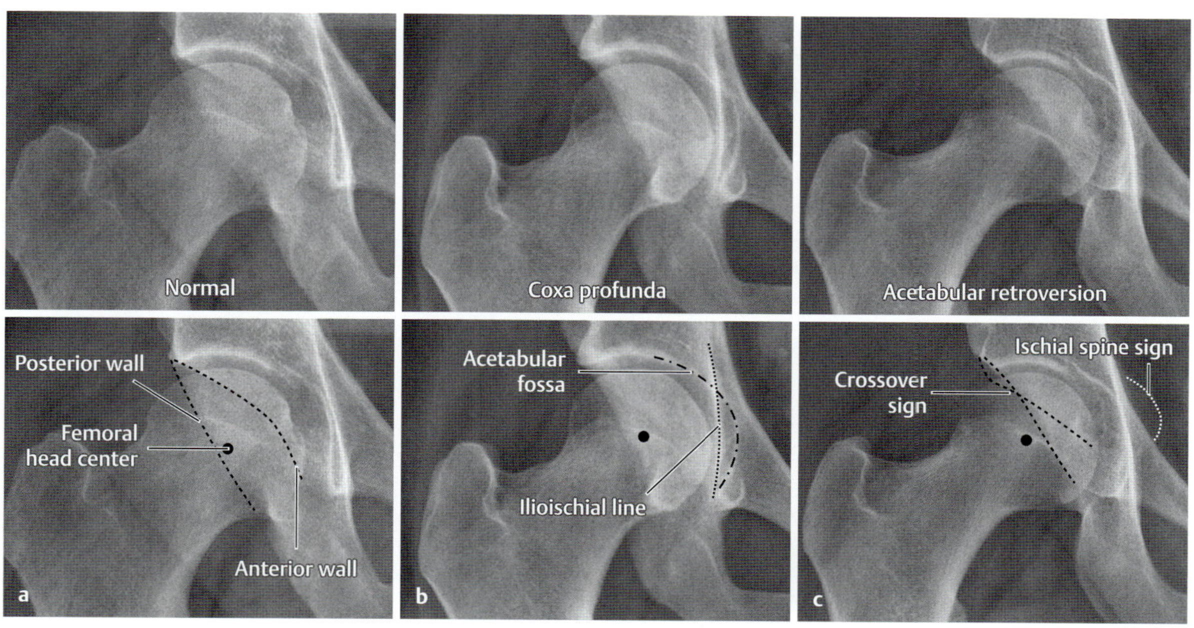

Fig. 2.279 Radiographic findings of pincer FAI. **(a)** Normal finding. **(b)** Coxa profunda: the acetabular fossa overlaps the ilioischial line. **(c)** Acetabular retroversion: the center of the femoral head is projected lateral to the posterior rim of the acetabulum (posterior wall sign); the ischial spine is brought into profile. The anterior wall overlaps the posterior wall, corresponding to a positive crossover sign.

2.11.4 Labral Lesions

▶ **Pathology.** Labral tears may present as pain in the hip or groin, but may also be asymptomatic. Labral damage commonly results from chronic overload, e.g., secondary to acetabular dysplasia or FAI; acute traumatic tears are less frequent. Labral injury is often associated with damage to the articular cartilage, with the labral pathology usually developing first. Progressive labral degeneration is also seen with advancing age. In 10 to 14% of the general population, the labrum is absent in its anterior segment; this is to be regarded as a normal variant. In 20% of individuals a sublabral sulcus is found in the anterior to anteroinferior labrum (▶ Fig. 2.281). A posteroinferior sublabral groove is found in about 25% of individuals (▶ Fig. 2.282).

▶ **Radiography.** In some cases it is possible to distinguish an os acetabuli lateral to the acetabular rim, corresponding to an unfused secondary ossification center (▶ Fig. 2.283). However, the ossification of the labrum can also occur after a tear; it is not possible to differentiate these two entities with certainty radiographically.

▶ **MRI.** A labral tear most commonly occurs at its base (in over 50% of cases); the labrum is then detached both from the acetabulum and from the articular cartilage (▶ Fig. 2.284). An intralabral tear is less frequently encountered. The labrum must be assessed in several different planes because it lies in an oblique orientation to the standard imaging planes. MR arthrography should also be considered on account of its ability to identify small labral tears.

▶ **DD.** A labral tear must be differentiated from known normal variants of the labrum. A **sublabral sulcus** is most often encountered posteroinferiorly, anteroinferiorly, or anteriorly, whereas in the anterosuperior quadrant labral tears are much more common than a sulcus. A labral tear is sometimes associated with a **paralabral cyst**, which may become quite large. In general, paralabral cysts are an indication of underlying labral pathology (▶ Fig. 2.285).

2.11.5 Chondromalacia and Synovitis

Chondromalacia

▶ **Pathology.** Defects of the joint cartilage are often found near the acetabular rim. Initially, the anterior segment of the acetabular cartilage is usually affected. In addition to focal defects, delamination of the acetabular cartilage is also possible and is often found in patients with FAI. Edema or cysts may develop in the subcortical bone in advanced cases (▶ Fig. W2.59).

▶ **Radiography.** The severity of osteoarthritis of the hip is determined using a radiograph; attention is drawn to osteophyte formation, joint space narrowing, and subchondral sclerosis as well as malalignment and deformity (Chapter 10.2).

▶ **CT.** CT arthrography is a very sensitive method for demonstrating articular cartilage defects.

▶ **MRI.** Defects of the articular cartilage may be quite small, so the cartilage must be carefully examined using several different imaging planes. MR arthrography is especially useful for evaluating the articular cartilage (▶ Fig. 2.286). It should be noted that the cartilage is not equally thick at all points—for example, the femoral cartilage appears thicker in the central part while acetabular cartilage is more prominent laterally.

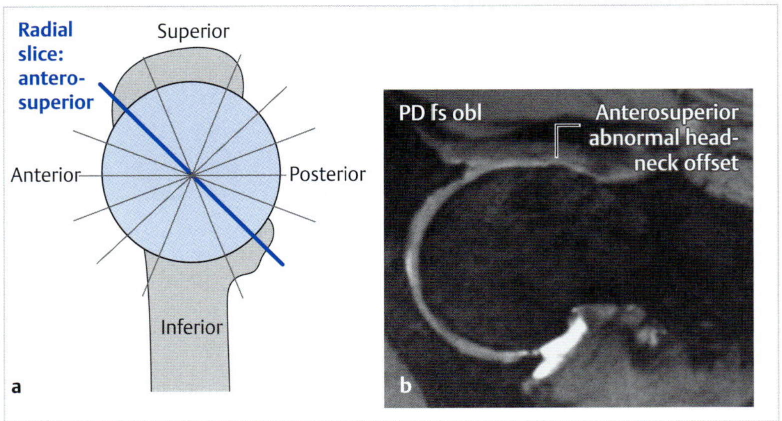

Fig. 2.280 Assessment of the femoral head–neck offset using radial MRI slices in a patient with a cam form of FAI. **(a)** Schematic diagram of radial slices (drawn on a sagittal projection). **(b)** MR arthrography in radial slice orientation (see panel **a**).

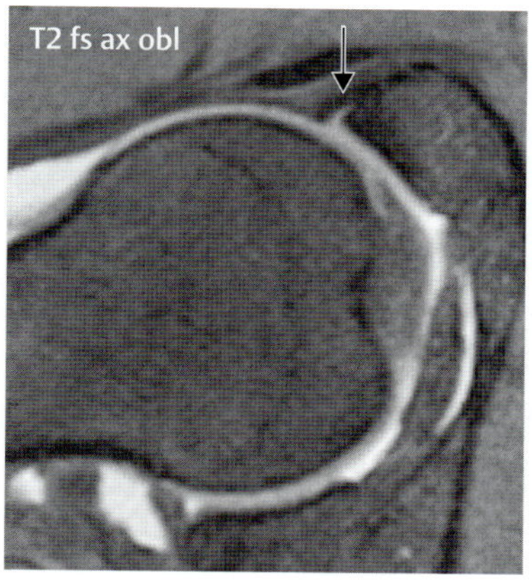

Fig. 2.281 Anteroinferior sublabral sulcus (arrow) as a normal variant of the labrum. MR arthrography.

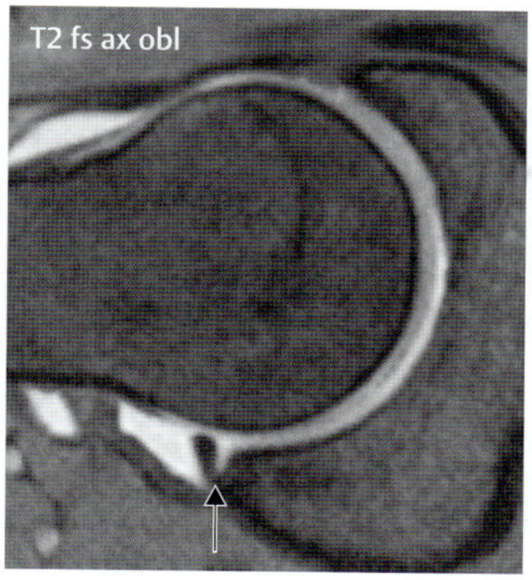

Fig. 2.282 Posteroinferior sublabral groove (arrow) as a normal variant of the labrum. MR arthrography.

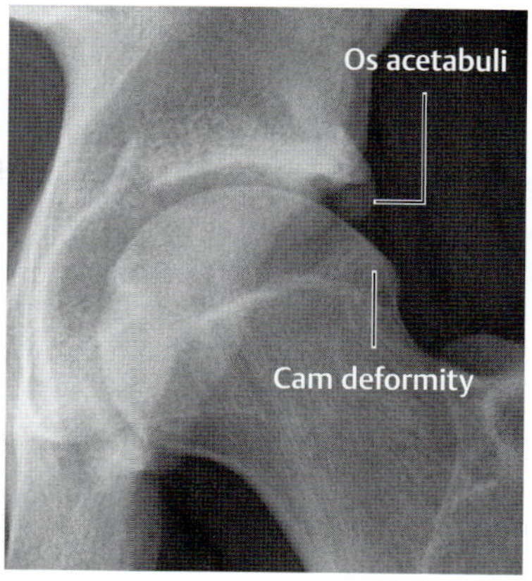

Fig. 2.283 FAI and os acetabuli.

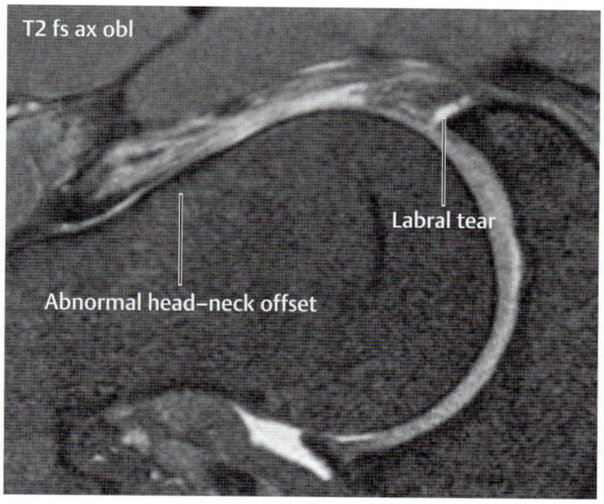

Fig. 2.284 Tear at the base of the labrum in a patient with FAI. MR arthrography.

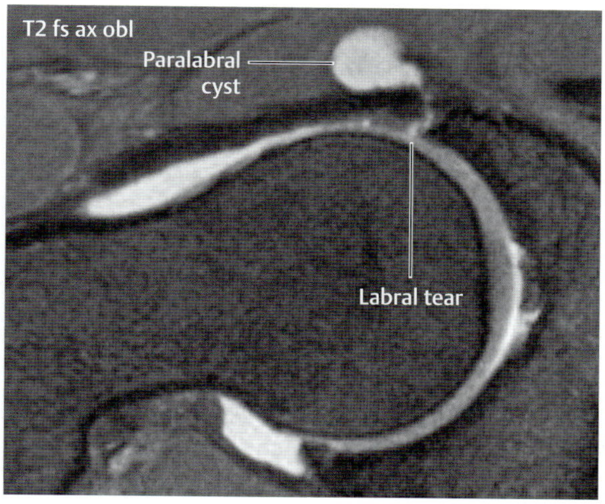

Fig. 2.285 Labral tear with associated paralabral cyst. MR arthrography.

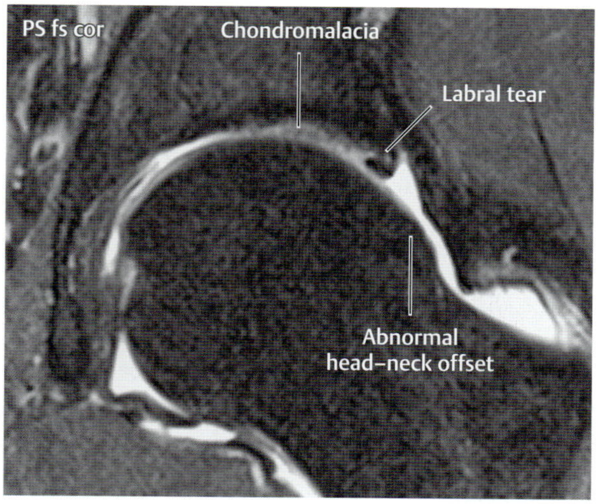

Fig. 2.286 Chondromalacia in a case of FAI. MR arthrography.

Synovitis

▸ **Pathology.** Acute synovitis along with a joint effusion may result from inflammatory disease, from osteonecrosis, and after trauma. Chronic irritation of the hip joint or involvement of the joint in rheumatoid arthritis results in hypertrophy of the synovial membrane and joint effusion. Furthermore, PVNS (pigmented villonodular synovitis; Chapter 4.6.5) can also occur in the hip joint.

▸ **US.** Joint effusion and thickening of the synovial membrane can be well visualized by ultrasound (▸ Fig. 2.287). The effusion may also be aspirated under ultrasound guidance.

▸ **MRI.** Synovitis manifests itself as hypertrophy of the synovial villi associated with a joint effusion (▸ Fig. 2.288). Prominent enhancement of the hypertrophied synovial membrane is evident after administration of IV contrast.

2.11.6 Muscle and Tendon Injuries

Abductor Muscles

▸ **Anatomy.** ▸ See Chapter 2.11.6 and ▸ Fig. W2.60.

▸ **Clinical presentation.** Pathological findings of the abductor tendons are found in elderly women and in patients with total hip replacement. Disruption of the gluteal tendon insertions on the greater trochanter occurs most commonly at an anterolateral location. Tendinopathy or tear of the gluteal tendons or a trochanteric bursitis can result in symptoms known as the greater trochanteric pain syndrome, which manifests as chronic pain and tenderness over the lateral part of the hip joint. Insufficiency of the hip abductors may also result in a limited range of motion and a Trendelenburg gait pattern.

▸ **US.** Ultrasound is capable of diagnosing a trochanteric bursitis quickly and reliably (▸ Fig. W2.61). Ultrasound-guided injection of the bursa is commonly used for pain management.

▸ **MRI.** The abductor tendons are normally dark on all sequences. Tendon degeneration (tendinopathy) results in increased signal intensity within an often thickened tendon and surrounding tissues on water-sensitive sequences and after the administration of intravenous contrast medium (▸ Fig. 2.289). It is sometimes difficult to differentiate between tendinopathy and a partial-thickness tear. Full-thickness tears may also occur but are less common (▸ Fig. 2.290). Fatty atrophy of the gluteal muscles may develop in cases of chronic abductor tendon pathology and is well demonstrated with MRI (▸ Fig. 2.291).

> **Caution**
>
> Edematous changes around the insertions of the abductor muscles are also seen in patients without any clinical signs or symptoms. The diagnosis of greater trochanter pain syndrome is not possible based on imaging findings alone without correlation with the clinical presentation.

Hamstring Muscles

▸ **Anatomy.** ▸ See Chapter 2.11.6 and ▸ Fig. W2.62.

▸ **Pathology.** The hamstring muscles provide for hip extension and knee flexion during walking and are the most commonly injured muscles. This type of injury often presents with tenderness over the ischial tuberosity and pain, particularly on flexion of the hip. Hamstring injuries can become very recalcitrant to therapy, especially in athletes. Tendon avulsions most commonly occur proximally; bony avulsions are a rarity in adults.

▸ **Radiography.** Bony avulsions and fractures may be detected with radiographs. Chronic hamstring injuries may ossify.

▸ **US.** Sonographic assessment of hamstring injuries is possible, although it does require a good understanding of the complex anatomy on the part of the investigator. Hypoechoic edema, combined with partial or complete interruption of tendon continuity is characteristic.

▸ **MRI.** MRI is the most reliable modality for investigating a suspected hamstring injury. It adequately demonstrates tendon avulsions and the gap between the margins of the torn tendon (▸ Fig. 2.292).

Rectus Femoris Muscle

▸ **Anatomy.** ▸ See Chapter 2.11.6 and ▸ Fig. W2.63.

▸ **Pathology.** Injuries of the proximal component of the rectus femoris muscle are common in soccer players and sprinters. Patients with an injury to the proximal part of the rectus femoris muscle may complain of stabbing inguinal pain. The central part of the rectus femoris tendon is most commonly injured. As with hamstring injuries, full-thickness tears of the rectus femoris are managed surgically. Tears of the muscle itself are often the result of a direct blow and are located more distally, where they may be associated with large hematomas (pseudotumor).

▸ **Radiography.** Bony avulsions may be demonstrated on radiographs and are particularly common in adolescents. An old partial-thickness tear or an apophyseal injury may ossify and appear as small ossicles or, in an extreme case, as a bony spur on the anterior inferior iliac spine (▸ Fig. 2.293).

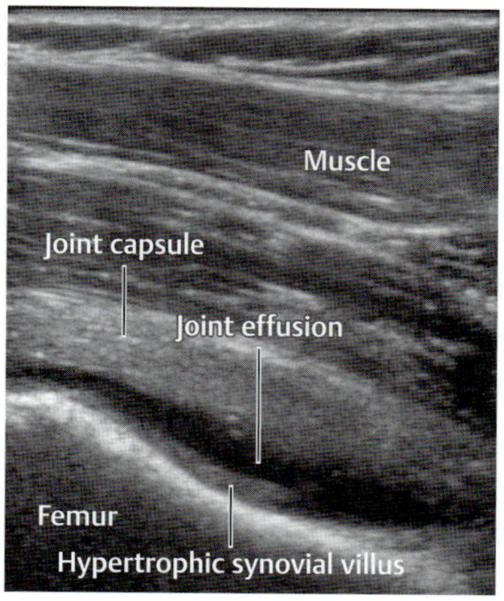

Fig. 2.287

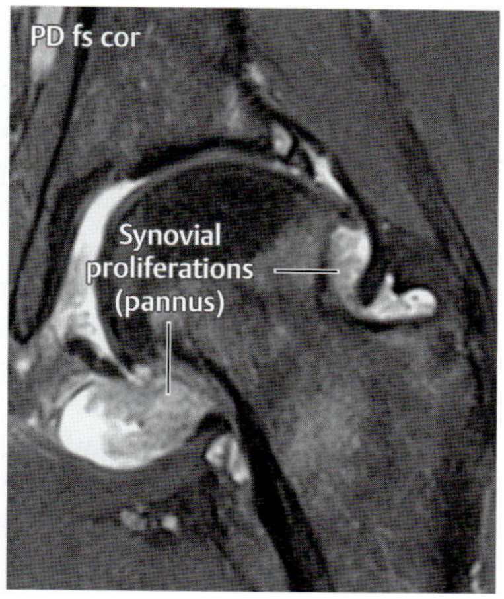

Fig. 2.288

Fig. 2.287 Ultrasound of a hip joint with synovitis. Mild joint effusion.

Fig. 2.288 Severe synovitis in a case of rheumatoid arthritis with secondary osteoarthritis of the hip. MR arthrography.

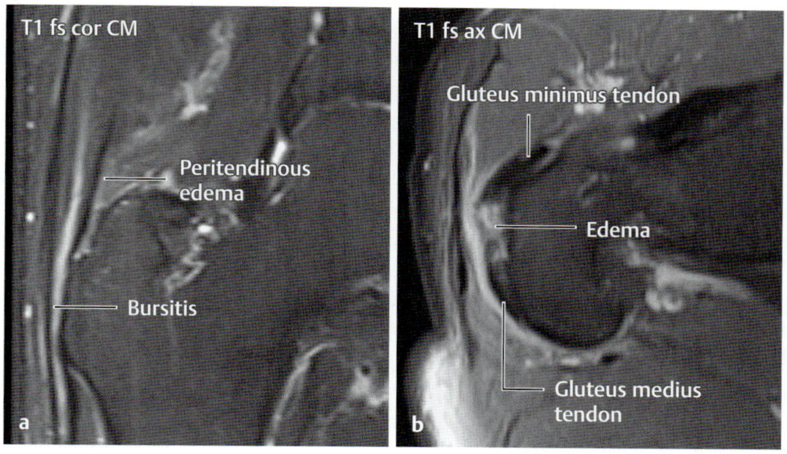

Fig. 2.289 Trochanteric pain syndrome. **(a)** Increased contrast uptake within the bursa. **(b)** Peritendinous edema and increased contrast medium uptake.

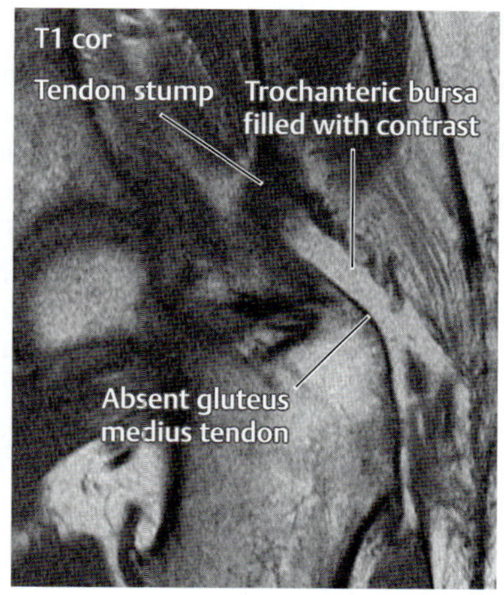

Fig. 2.290 Avulsion of the gluteus medius tendon.

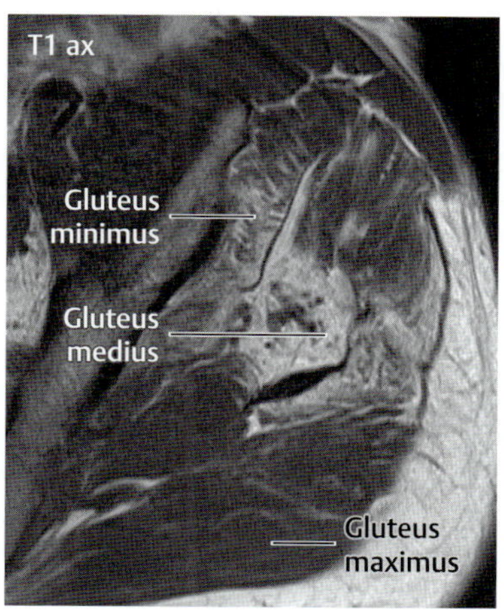

Fig. 2.291 Fatty atrophy of the abductor muscles secondary to gluteal tendon disruption.

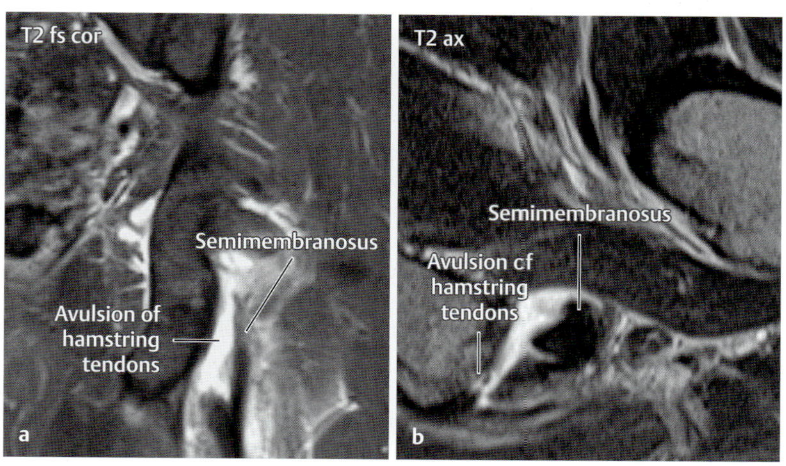

Fig. 2.292 Avulsion of the hamstring tendons with retraction of ~ 1 cm. **(a)** Coronal slice. **(b)** Axial slice.

▸ **US.** The rectus femoris muscle and tendon are well visualized by ultrasound, as are injuries to these structures. Ultrasound can also identify an associated intramuscular hematoma and provide guidance for its aspiration.

▸ **MRI.** The extent and type of injury are well displayed with MRI, which can demonstrate the location of the margins of the torn tendon and size of any associated hematoma.

Adductors

The adductors are most commonly affected by insertional tendinopathies and muscle avulsions (▸ Fig. 2.294) resulting from acute trauma or chronic overuse (Chapter 1.8 and Chapter 2.12.3).

Snapping Hip

This syndrome is defined clinically by pain in and around the hip, accompanied by an audible and/or palpable "snap" during hip motion (especially when running). Intra-articular causes (labral pathology, synovial osteochondromatosis) are rare. It is more commonly related to the iliopsoas tendon "snaps" across a prominent iliopectineal eminence. Similarly the iliotibial tract may not glide smoothly over the greater trochanter, resulting in a snapping sensation laterally.

2.11.7 Slipped Capital Femoral Epiphysis

This disorder is also known as epiphysiolysis capitis femoris (adolescent coxa vara). The slipped capital femoral epiphysis is an epiphysiolysis of the proximal femoral growth plate resulting in separation of the epiphysis. It occurs in adolescents between the ages of 10 and 14 years in whom the epiphyseal plate is still open. Boys are more commonly affected than girls. Both hips are affected in 20 to 40% of cases, often at different times.

▸ **Pathology.** The exact etiology is unknown. Since slipped capital femoral epiphysis occurs during puberty, hormonal influences have been suggested. Most affected patients are overweight and this likely is a factor as well. The disorder may occur in the absence of trauma. Slipped capital femoral epiphysis is divided into an acute ("acuta") and an insidious ("lenta") form, depending on the duration of development and its extent.

Acute epiphysiolysis (less than 3 weeks) usually results in a complete dislocation of the epiphysis. The risk of avascular necrosis of the femoral head and thus the probability of early hip replacement is clearly increased if treatment is delayed or inappropriate.

With the **insidious form** (over 3 weeks to months) the degree of dislocation is variable, with complete epiphysiolysis being rare. The epiphysis remains in its socket. Dislocation ceases once ossification of the epiphyseal plate has occurred. A so-called femoral bump often remains as a residual appearance (similar to the bumps associated with cam impingement; Chapter 2.11.3); this is regarded as a preosteoarthritic condition.

▸ **Clinical presentation.** The clinical presentation varies from rather mild symptoms with a protective limp and pain on weight-bearing, to immobilizing pain.

▸ **Radiography.** Basic diagnostic examinations include AP and lateral Lauenstein views of both hips. Widening of the epiphyseal plate and an irregularity of the metaphyseal plate are found on the AP view (▸ Fig. 2.295a) in the **initial stage**. It is not possible to detect dislocation of the epiphysis on this projection. If **dislocation** has already occurred, then the reference line drawn along the lateral border of the femoral neck misses the femoral epiphysis, which is normally transected at its lateral margin. Additionally, because of the displacement, the epiphysis appears shorter. Signs of metaphyseal cystic regeneration and repair become apparent with longer-standing slipped capital femoral epiphysis, with callus dorsomedially between the slipped epiphysis and the femoral neck. Dislocation of the femoral head in a dorsal and caudal direction can be detected early on a lateral projection (▸ Fig. 2.295b).

> **Note**
> Radiological confirmation of the diagnosis of slipped capital femoral epiphysis may be difficult during the early stage, in which the radiographs may appear normal.

▸ **CT.** Performed as low-dose CT, this allows for early diagnosis and accurate determination of the slip angle.

▸ **US.** The diagnosis is usually easily made with ultrasound (▸ Fig. 2.295c).

▸ **MRI.** MRI is capable of detecting the earliest diagnostic signs of incipient slipped capital femoral epiphysis. Hyperintense signal within the bone marrow along the epiphyseal growth plate on fat-saturated T2W sequences is an indication of stress and incipient slipped capital femoral epiphysis. Axial and sagittal slices reveal the extent of any dislocation. Standard imaging of the pelvis includes both hips, which is important given the high prevalence of bilateral involvement. Serial MR imaging studies allow for early recognition of delayed involvement of the contralateral side.

2.11.8 Radiological Assessment after Fracture Fixation and Joint Replacement of the Hip

See Chapters 1.6.3 and 1.6.4.

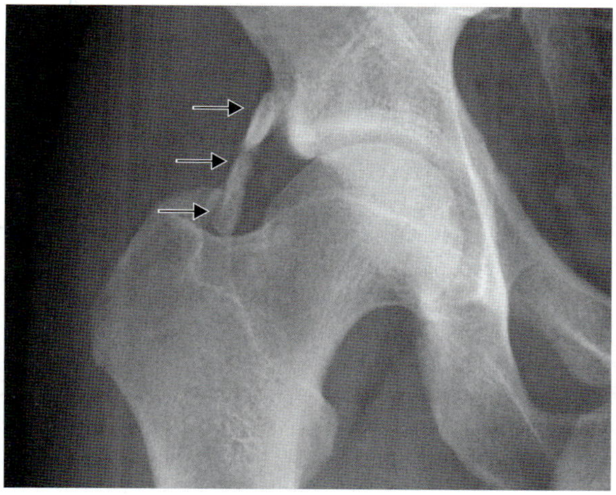

Fig. 2.293 Posttraumatic bony spur (arrows). Three years after a partial-thickness tear of the rectus femoris tendon.

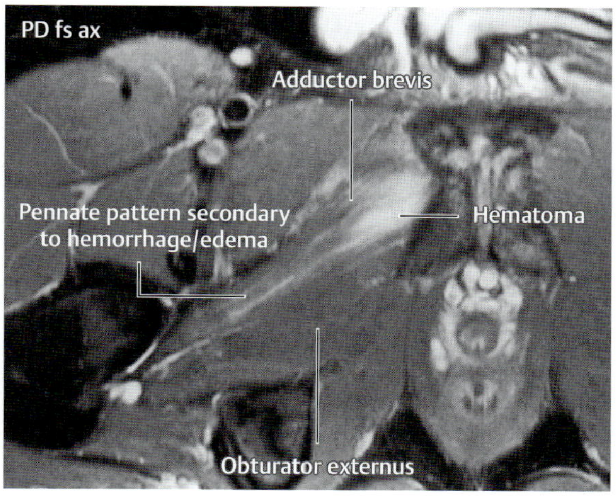

Fig. 2.294 Partial-thickness tear of the adductor brevis at its origin on the pubic bone.

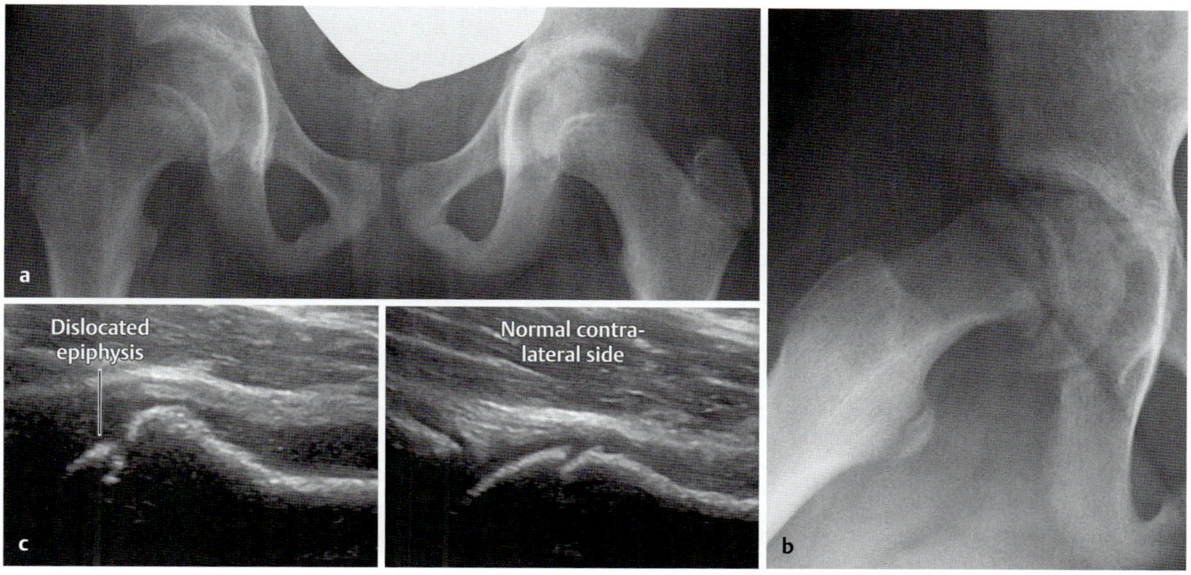

Fig. 2.295 Right chronic slipped capital femoral epiphysis in an obese 10-year-old girl. **(a)** Epiphyseal dislocation is recognizable on the AP radiograph only by widening of the epiphyseal plate. The metaphysis has already undergone remodeling (sclerosis). **(b)** The Lauenstein view shows the slipping of the epiphysis in a dorsocaudal direction. **(c)** Well demonstrated by ultrasound.

2.12 Femur and Soft Tissues of the Thigh

2.12.1 Anatomy and Technique

▶ **Anatomy.** ▶ See Chapter 2.12.1.

Technique

▶ **Radiography.** For cases of trauma involving the proximal femur, routine radiographs should include AP and lateral views of the hip. On the AP view the lesser trochanter should just about overlie the medial cortex of the femur. If the leg is externally rotated too much, the lesser trochanter will appear too prominent and the femoral neck will appear shortened. The Lauenstein view is used for special indications (such as slipped capital femoral epiphysis, etc.).

▶ **CT.** CT provides a better depiction of unclear radiographic findings and is also particularly useful for assessing the position and origin of fragments in cases of complex fractures.

▶ **MRI.** The main strengths of MRI in this setting include its ability to display radiographically occult fractures, trauma-related soft tissue injuries (e.g., muscle fiber tears), and complications of fractures such as aseptic necrosis of the femoral head or osteomyelitis.

▶ **US.** Ultrasound is useful for diagnosing epiphysiolysis in children and for assessing soft tissue lesions.

2.12.2 Fractures

Fractures of the Proximal Femur

▶ **Pathology.** Fractures of the proximal femur include fractures of the femoral head related to hip dislocations (Chapter 2.3.4) and the femoral neck as well as the intertrochanteric and subtrochanteric regions.

Proximal femoral fractures are typical injuries of the elderly. Even relatively minor trauma (such as a fall on the hip) can result in a fracture in the presence of osteoporosis. On the other hand, proximal femoral fractures in younger patients are most often the result of high-velocity injuries. Less common causes are stress fractures in athletes and pathologic fractures associated with focal bone lesions.

A distinction is made between intracapsular (and therefore intra-articular) femoral neck fractures and those that are extracapsular, the former having a higher risk of developing complications. Femoral neck fractures are intra-articular and are subdivided into **subcapital, transcervical, and basicervical** fractures. Inter- and subtrochanteric fractures are extracapsular. An intact femoral calcar, a dense plate of cortical bone projecting from the medial cortex into the trabecular bone (▶ Fig. 2.296), is important for stability of proximal femoral fractures.

Classification of proximal femoral fractures is usually descriptive and takes into account location and fracture pattern (see ▶ Fig. 2.296). The AO classification (▶ Chapter 2.12.2) is less important for daily clinical practice, see ▶ Fig. W2.64.

Subcapital Femoral Neck Fractures

A subcapital femoral is the most proximal form of a femoral neck fracture, is still located within the capsule, and is the most common proximal femoral fracture. Due to its location, this fracture places at risk the lateral epiphyseal vessels that arise from the deep branch of the medial circumflex femoral artery and enter the femoral neck dorsally in the region of the fracture. In adults these vessels supply the major part of the femoral head. As a result, avascular necrosis of the femoral head develops in 10 to 20% of all cases of subcapital fractures (depending on the morphology of the fracture). Other complications include delayed fracture healing or nonunion (5–25% of cases) and the development of secondary osteoarthritis of the hip.

Abduction fractures with lateral impaction can be mechanically stable; adduction fractures and shear fractures, in contrast, are always unstable.

The **classification according to Pauwels** takes into account the obliquity of the fracture line with regard to the horizontal plane (▶ Fig. 2.297). The risks of the femoral head slipping, of developing nonunion, and of necrosis of the femoral head increase with more vertically oriented fractures.

The Garden classification system works for all intra-articular femoral neck fractures and emphasizes the degree of fragment displacement (▶ Fig. 2.298). With increasing fragment displacement, the risk of injury to the epiphyseal vessels and subsequent avascular necrosis of the femoral head rises. In Stages III and IV the risk of developing avascular necrosis is up to 50%.

▶ **Radiography.** Diagnosis and classification of a fracture are not difficult when it is displaced (▶ Fig. 2.299). However, with nondisplaced fractures or fatigue fractures of the femoral neck, radiographic findings are often very subtle, with trabecular discontinuity or a vague linear density being the only clues.

▶ **CT.** CT may be helpful for confirming a fracture in equivocal cases.

▶ **MRI.** MRI is the most sensitive method for demonstrating fractures, even those that are radiographically occult. Early diagnosis of avascular necrosis of the femoral head can be

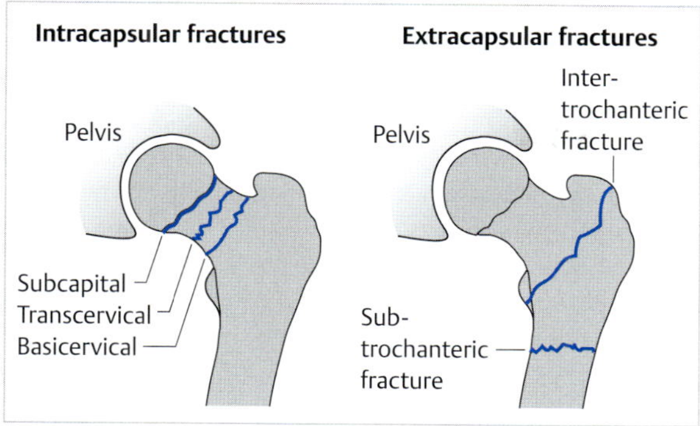

Fig. 2.296 Description of intra- and extracapsular fractures of the proximal femur.

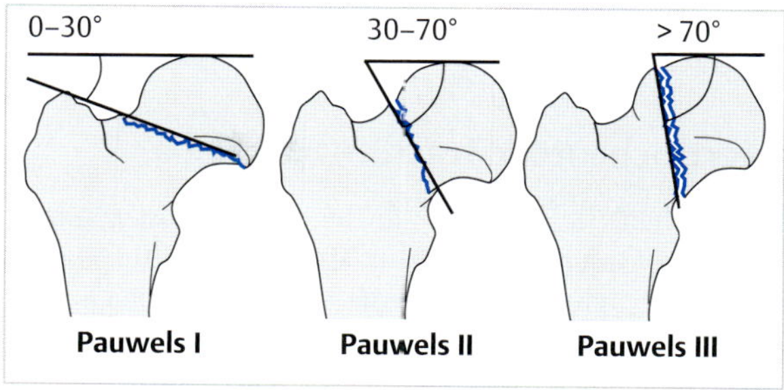

Fig. 2.297 Classification of subcapital femoral neck fractures according to Pauwels.

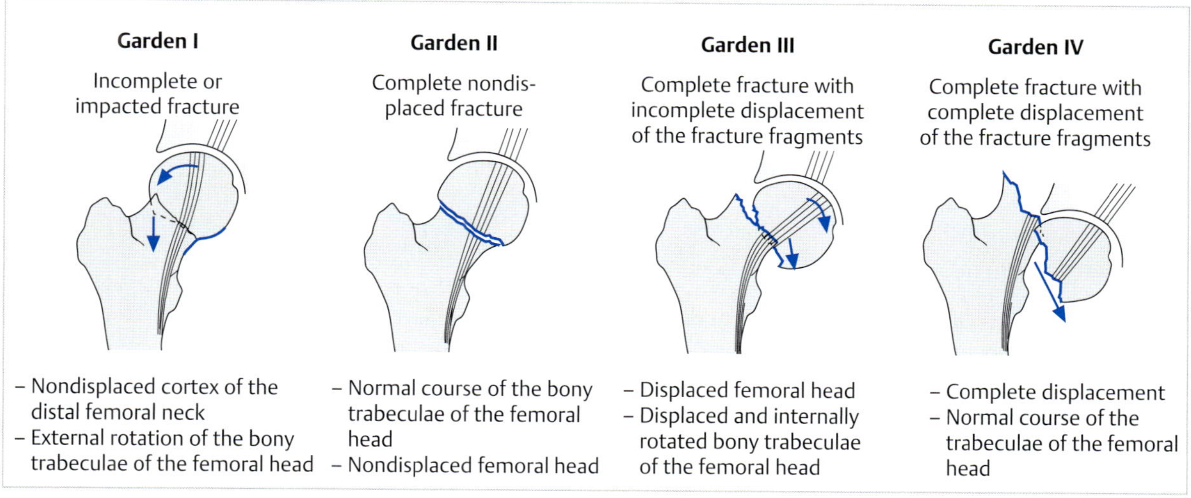

Fig. 2.298 Classification of fractures of the medial femoral neck according to Garden.

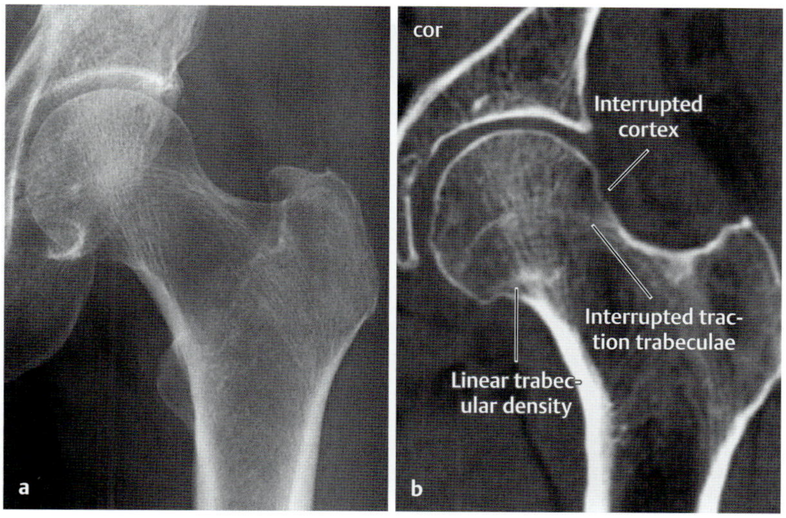

Fig. 2.299 Female patient with acute hip pain after an accident. **(a)** Initial radiograph reveals no signs of a fracture. No further diagnostic investigations followed. **(b)** On CT imaging 10 days later there is evidence of a nondisplaced femoral neck fracture.

achieved with MRI; but it is not able to predict the risk of developing avascular necrosis after a fracture of the femoral neck.

Intertrochanteric Fractures

Intertrochanteric fractures are the second most common fractures of the proximal femur. They run from the greater trochanter obliquely in a medial–caudal direction to the lesser trochanter. Less frequently there is an inverse fracture pattern in a medial–cranial direction (reverse oblique intertrochanteric fracture; ▶ Fig. 2.296). In addition, the trochanters and/or other fragments may be avulsed, resulting in a comminuted fracture.

Subtrochanteric Fractures

The subtrochanteric femoral segment extends from the lower portion of the intertrochanteric region to the junction of the proximal and middle thirds of the femoral shaft. Fractures of this region are comparatively rare and, like other proximal femoral fractures, occur more commonly in elderly patients or in others who also suffer from osteoporosis. Classification is done using the AO classification system for femoral shaft fractures (see below).

“Occult” Fractures of the Femoral Neck

The radiograph of the femoral neck—especially in the presence of osteoporosis—does not always allow the diagnosis of a nondisplaced fracture of the femoral neck. The fracture is then radiologically “occult” (▶ Fig. 2.299). With an appropriate history of trauma and severe pain, the radiological report must recommend that further diagnostic imaging be performed (CT or, especially, MRI).

Insufficiency Fractures of the Femoral Head and Neck

The femoral head and neck are classic sites of insufficiency fractures (▶ Fig. 2.301; see also ▶ Fig. 2.300). See also Chapter 1.5.1.

Fractures of the Femoral Shaft

▶ **Pathology.** Considerable force is required to fracture the femoral shaft. The most common cause is traffic accidents that typically involve multiple injuries. Muscle traction from the adductors, which originate medially on the distal fragment, results in a typical varus malalignment of this fragment with leg-length shortening, while the proximal fragment assumes an adducted, externally rotated and flexed position as a result of the combined traction of the pelvic muscles.

Classification of fractures of the femoral shaft according to AO

- **Type A fracture:** Simple spiral, oblique or transverse fracture.
- **Type B fracture:** Additional avulsion of a single or multifragmentary wedge (▶ Fig. 2.302).
- **Type C fracture:** Complex multisegmental or comminuted fracture.

> **Caution**
> Femoral shaft fractures are commonly associated with considerable **soft tissue damage** and proximal femoral fractures. These should not be overlooked.

Fractures of the Distal Femur

▶ **Pathology.** Distal femoral fractures result from axial loading, combined with valgus stress and rotation.

The most common classification is that of the **AO system** (▶ Fig. 2.303). Sectional imaging is indicated for partial or complete intra-articular fractures.

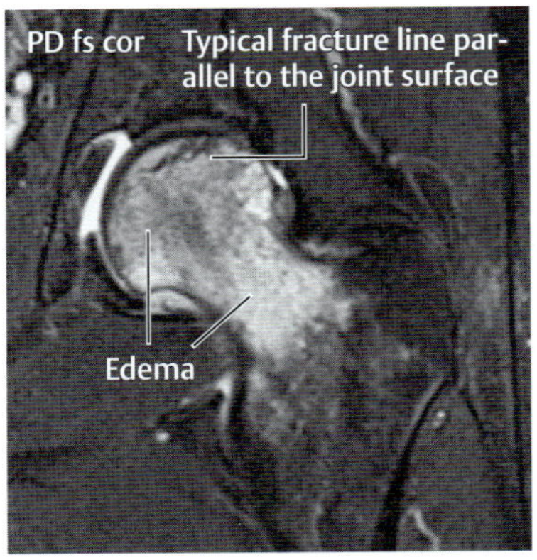

Fig. 2.300 Insufficiency fracture of the femoral head in a case of severe obesity.

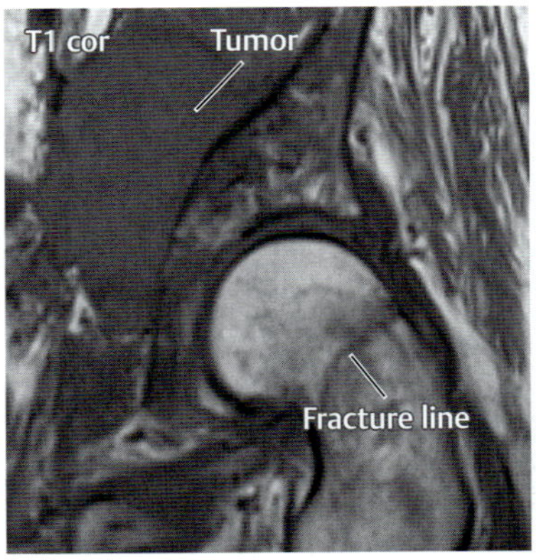

Fig. 2.301 Insufficiency fracture of the neck of the femur in a patient with recurrent carcinoma of the bladder and osteoporosis. This patient’s pain was not entirely due to the tumor.

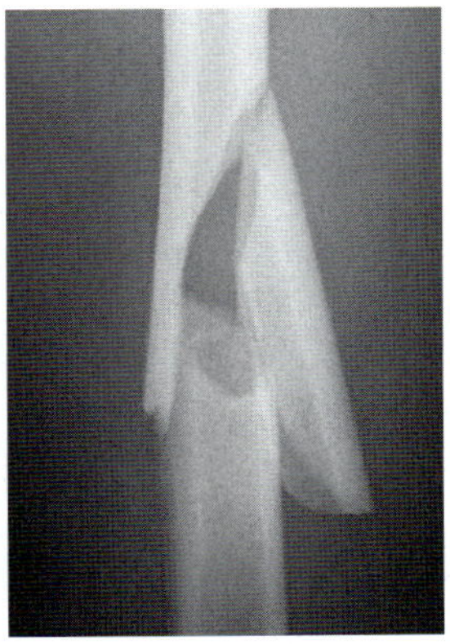

Fig. 2.302 Femoral shaft fracture with avulsion of a monofragmentary wedge. AO Type 32-B1.

2.12.3 Muscle Injuries of the Thigh

Muscle injuries of the thigh often result from sports injuries (▶ Fig. 2.304). Other, accident-related injuries of the thigh muscles without bone involvement are rare.

Thigh muscle injuries are subdivided into three groups according to anatomy (▶ Fig. 2.305). The injuries are assessed by applying general rules (see Chapter 1.8.1).

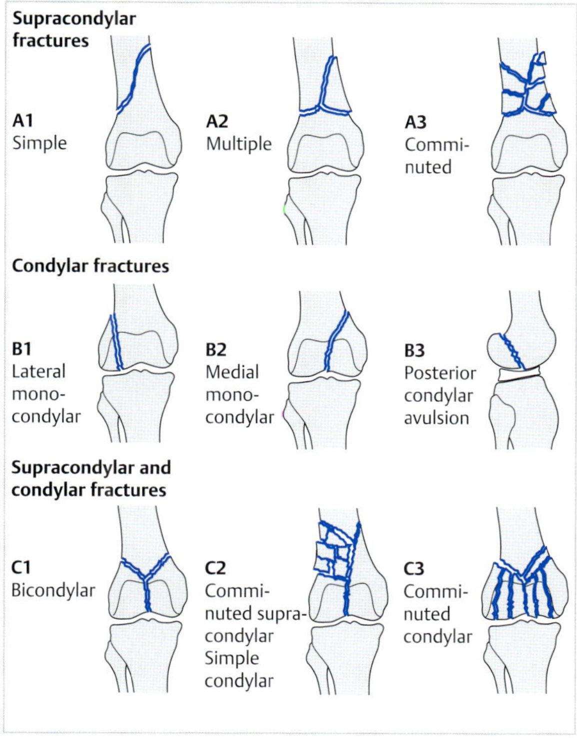

Fig. 2.303 AO classification of distal femoral fractures.

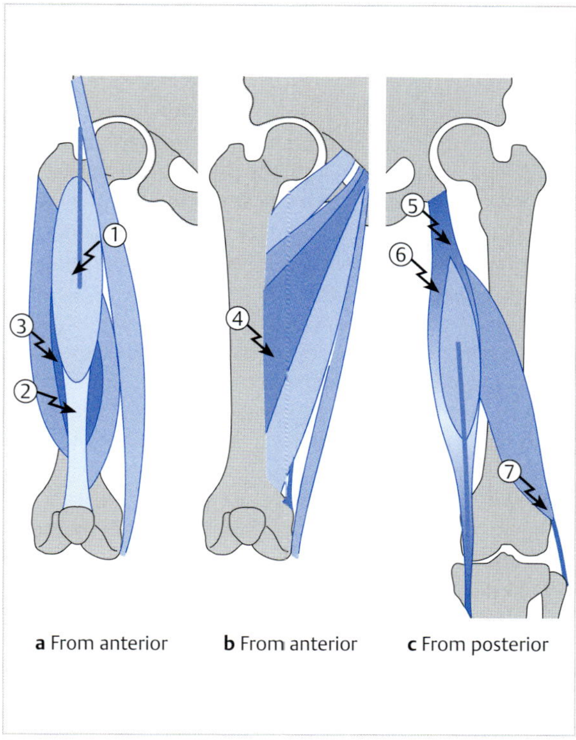

Fig. 2.305 Common sites of muscle injuries of the thigh. **(a)** Extensors: central (1) and distal aponeurosis (2) of rectus femoris; muscle belly of vastus intermedius (3). **(b)** Adductor: distal attachment of adductor longus (4). **(c)** Flexors: proximal myotendinous junction of semitendinosus (5) and semimembranosus (6); distal myotendinous junction of biceps femoris (7).

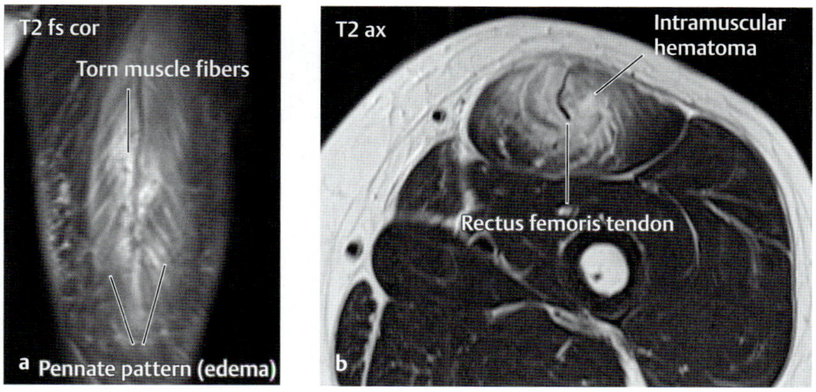

Fig. 2.304 Central muscle tear within the rectus femoris muscle associated with an intramuscular hematoma. Edematous pennate appearance of the muscle secondary to a muscle strain. **(a)** Coronal slice level. **(b)** Axial slice level.

2.12.4 Radiological Assessment after Surgery of the Thigh

Proximal Femur

Lag screw fixation, intramedullary nailing (proximal femoral nail), or dynamic hip screw fixation are primarily available for fractures of the proximal femur, in addition to hip replacement. An avulsed lesser trochanter is usually not reattached.

Radiological assessment of hip implants is dealt with in Chapter 1.6.4.

In addition to general postoperative findings (fragment adaptation, axial and length discrepancy, hardware failure, iatrogenic fracture, etc.) **postoperative radiographic evaluation** of the hip should also assess the following issues:

- *Position of the fracture fixation hardware?* When using dynamic hip screws or proximal femoral nails for fracture fixation, the screw shaft should be placed near the medial cortex of the femoral neck and the thread in the posteroinferior quadrant of the femoral head (▸ Fig. 2.306). This position ensures the best mechanical stability, yet at the same time protects the vascular supply and cartilage covering of the main weight-bearing area. The screw head or the gliding nail should be at least 5 mm away from the joint and lie somewhat posteroinferiorly within the femoral head (see ▸ Fig. 2.306).
- *Screw migration?* Subsidence of the femoral neck over time is not pathologic but rather due to the sliding capabilities of the screws within the shaft; similarly, lateral migration of a screw is also normal (▸ Fig. 2.307).
- *Penetration of the screw into the joint?* (▸ Fig. 2.306b).
- *Evidence of avascular necrosis of the femoral head?* Compare Chapter 6.3.1.
- *Posttraumatic heterotopic ossification?* This occurs relatively commonly in the hip.

Femoral Shaft

Fractures of the femoral shaft are usually treated by intramedullary nailing. Alternative options are plate and external fixation. Intramedullary nails may be inserted via an antegrade approach (through the greater trochanter) or a retrograde approach (through the intercondylar notch). Static or dynamic locking of the nail is possible. Plates are always placed laterally.

Postoperative radiographic evaluation should assess the following aspects:

- *Is there a rotational deformity?* The position of the femoral condyles is assessed in relation to the femoral neck.
- *Position and integrity of the screws and interlocking screws* (▸ Fig. 2.308)? Bending or breaking of the interlocking screws is a sign that fracture stability has not yet been achieved.

Distal Femur

The majority of distal femoral fractures are currently treated by plate fixation (preferably angle-stable), and less commonly with retrograde intramedullary nailing or external fixation.

Postoperative radiographic evaluation should assess the following aspects:

- *Fragment adaptation and restoration of the joint surface?*
- *Position of the end of the nail?* With retrograde femoral nails it should be ensured that the distal end of the nail is countersunk below the level of the femoral condyles (▸ Fig. 2.309).

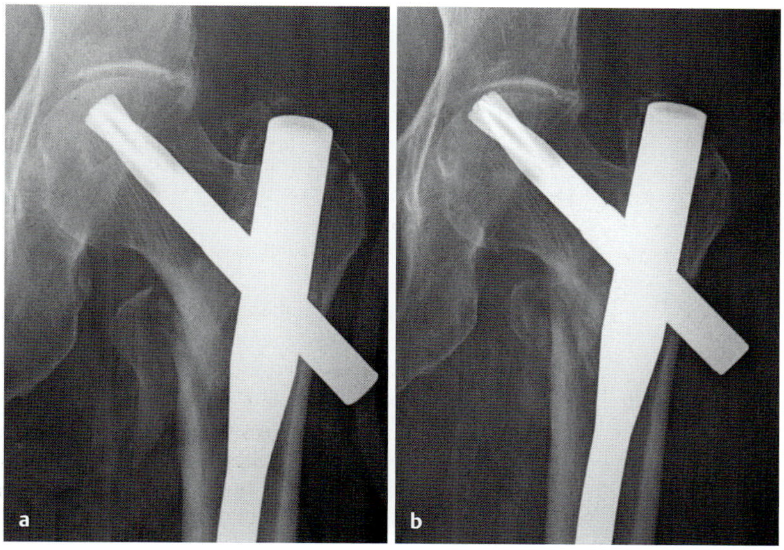

Fig. 2.306 Intramedullary nail fixation of an intertrochanteric femoral fracture. The type of nail used (Type A proximal femoral nail) can obviate the need for an antirotation screw. **(a)** Suboptimal position of the blade, which is situated too far cranially. **(b)** Later in the postoperative course the blade penetrated into the joint ("cutting out").

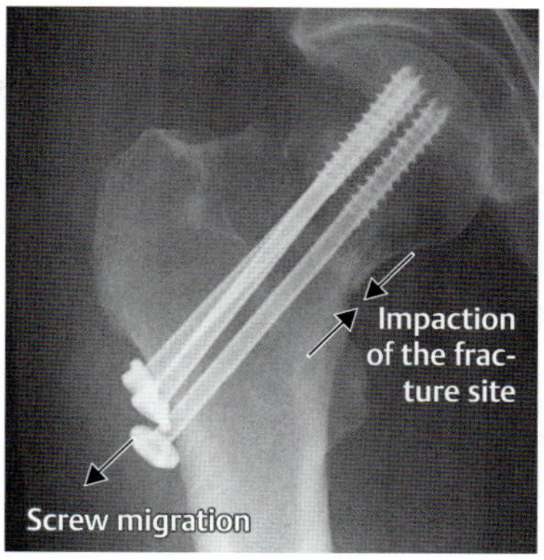

Fig. 2.307 Subcapital femoral neck fracture, treated with three cannulated cancellous screws. Migration of the screws is not pathologic but is the result of (tolerable and desired) compression of the fracture.

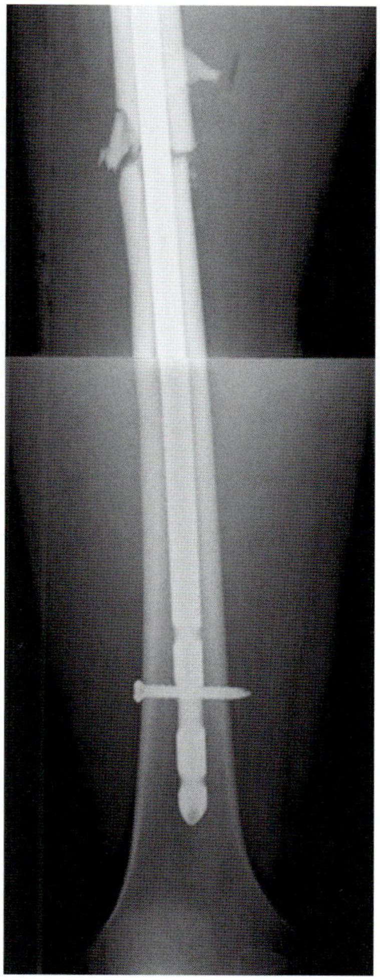

Fig. 2.308 Transverse fracture of the femoral shaft. Antegrade intramedullary nail with planned dynamic distal locking. The screw was mistakenly inserted into the proximal end of the slit instead of distally, which is why the nail is preventing any (desired) compression with weight bearing.

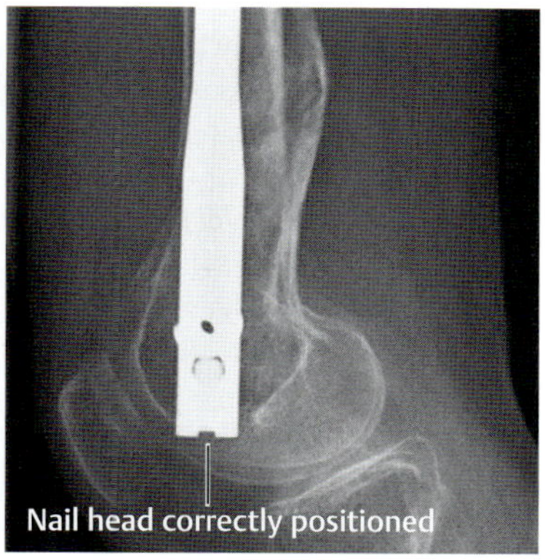

Fig. 2.309 Distal femoral fracture, treated with a retrograde femoral nail.

2.13 Knee Joint

2.13.1 Indications and Technique

▶ See Chapter 2.13.1.

2.13.2 Cruciate Ligaments

Anterior Cruciate Ligament

▶ **Anatomy.** ▶ See Chapter 2.13.2.

▶ **Pathology.** The anterior cruciate ligament (ACL) is the most commonly injured ligament of the knee joint. The proximal attachment is most often involved; avulsion at its tibial insertion is rare (and more common in children).

▶ **MRI.** Fat as well as some fluid is interspersed in and between the anteromedial and posterolateral bundles. That part of the anterior cruciate ligament near the tibia therefore appears somewhat striated and typically contains some degree of increased signal intensity (▶ Fig. 2.310).

Mucoid degeneration of the anterior cruciate ligament is not uncommon. It manifests itself as loss of detail with a masslike configuration of the ligament that has preserved continuity and normal orientation of the fibers (▶ Fig. 2.311).

Direct signs of a full-thickness tear of the anterior cruciate ligament

- **Interruption of continuity:** There is complete interruption of continuity (▶ Fig. 2.312).
- **Abnormal course:** Distal fibers assume an abnormally flat course or are folded over (▶ Fig. 2.314); proximal fibers are "hanging down" (no longer parallel to the roof of the intercondylar notch; ▶ Fig. 2.313).
- **Increased signal intensity along the course of the anterior cruciate ligament:** Localized increase in signal intensity of the ligament on non–fat-saturated T2W images has a positive predictive value for rupture of about 90%. Fat-saturated intermediate sequences are less specific in their predictive value, making a—supplementary—T2W sequence worthwhile for this type of indication.
- **Thickening and "blurring" of the ligament:** These findings are often seen, but are nonspecific.

> **Note**
> The knee joint should be examined in extension to best assess the integrity of the ACL

Secondary signs of a full-thickness tear of the anterior cruciate ligament

- Areas of **bone marrow edema** at the posterolateral tibial plateau and the lateral femoral condyle (▶ Fig. 2.315), with the latter possibly also associated with an impaction fracture (known as a "deep notch sign") at the site of the terminal sulcus, a normal physiologic depression of the lateral femoral condyle (▶ Fig. 2.316). **Note:** These distribution patterns involving bone marrow edema can also occur in children, even without a tear of the anterior cruciate ligament, due to the elasticity of their ligaments.
- Capsular avulsion of the lateral tibial plateau (**Segond fracture**).
- Combination of bone marrow edema of the anterior tibia and the anterior femur secondary to a hyperextension injury; in this case the anterior or posterior cruciate ligament may be injured individually or in combination.
- Increased curvature ("buckling") of the posterior cruciate ligament.
- Anterior subluxation of the tibia of more than 7 mm beyond the posterior contour of the lateral femoral condyle (anterior drawer sign; ▶ Fig. 2.317).
- Associated meniscal tears (approximately 50% of cases).

Criteria for a partial-thickness tear of the anterior cruciate ligament

- Signal isointense to fluid between the ligament fibers (▶ Fig. 2.318).
- Some of the fibers are intact along their entire course, some are interrupted.

> **Note**
> It is particularly helpful to carefully follow the ligament on the axial slices when diagnosing a partial-thickness tear of the ACL.

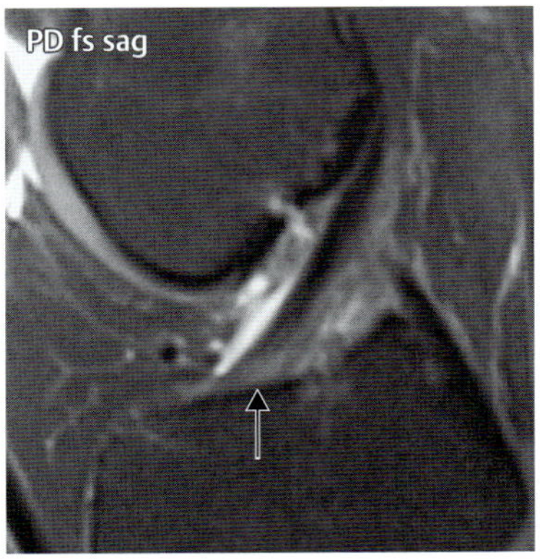

Fig. 2.310

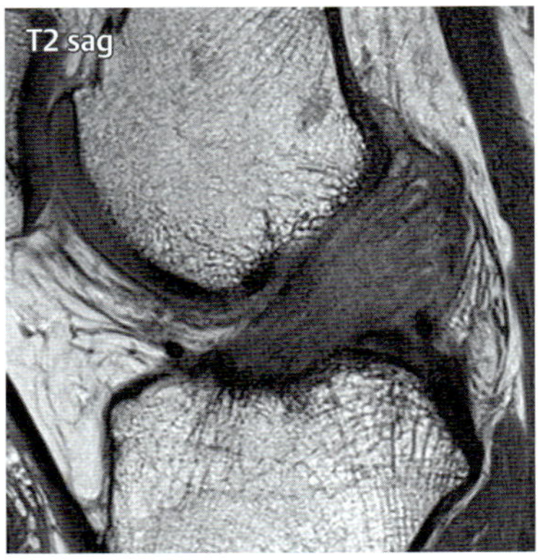

Fig. 2.311

Fig. 2.310 Normal anterior cruciate ligament. The ligament commonly demonstrates intermediate signal intensity stripes (arrow).

Fig. 2.311 Mucoid degeneration of the anterior cruciate ligament.

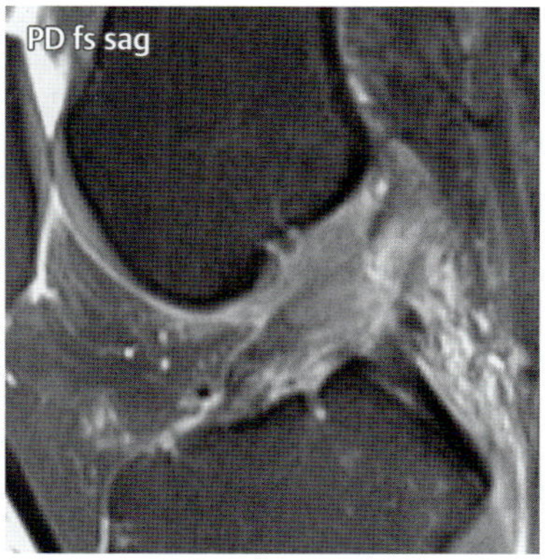

Fig. 2.312 Tear of the anterior cruciate ligament. Complete discontinuity of the ligament.

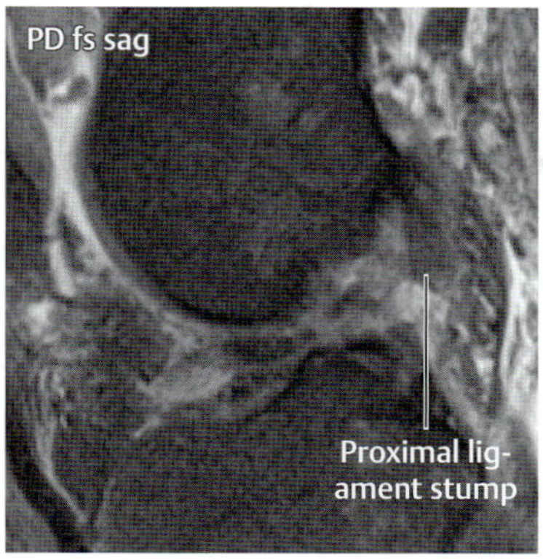

Fig. 2.313 Tear of the anterior cruciate ligament. The proximal fibers no longer run parallel to the roof of the intercondylar notch, but "hang down."

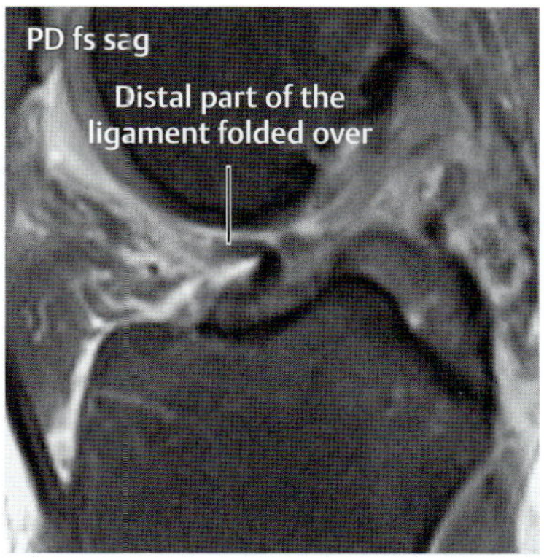

Fig. 2.314 Tear of the anterior cruciate ligament. The distal ligament stump is folded over anteriorly.

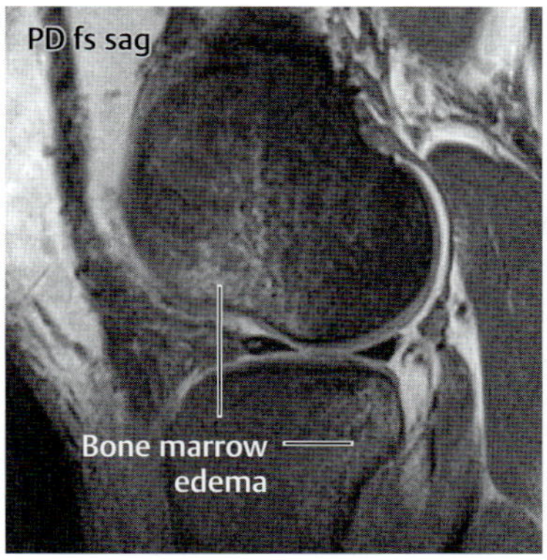

Fig. 2.315 Typical bone marrow edema of the lateral femoral condyle and posterolateral tibial plateau.

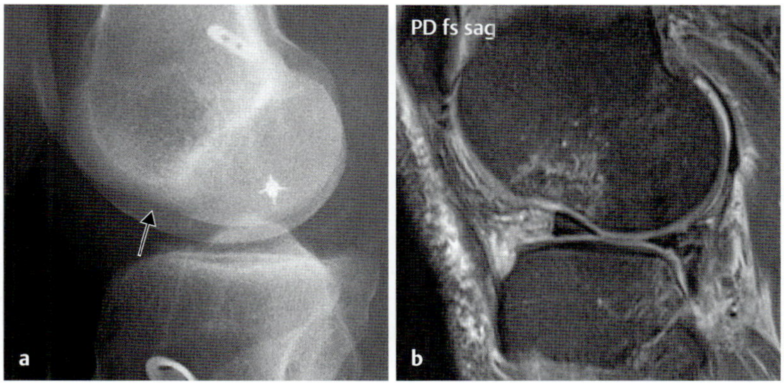

Fig. 2.316 "Deep notch" sign. (a) Trough-shaped depression (arrow) at the junction of the patellofemoral and tibiofemoral articular surfaces (terminal sulcus) on the lateral radiograph. Surgical implants are from prior ACL reconstruction. (b) An osteochondral impaction fracture is evident on MRI after the accident, corresponding to the radiographic sign.

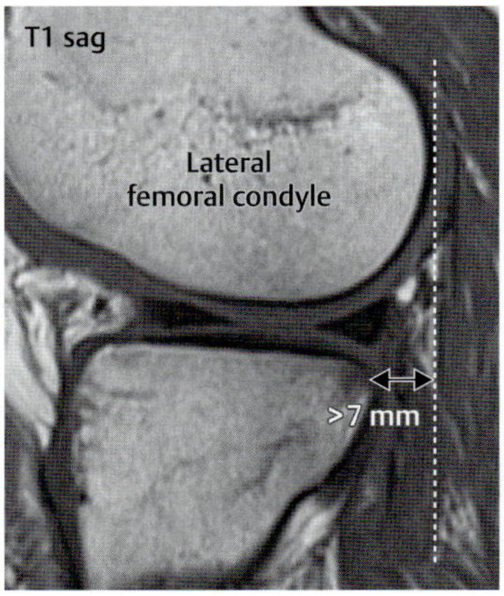

Fig. 2.317 Anterior subluxation of the tibia as a secondary sign of insufficiency of the anterior cruciate ligament.

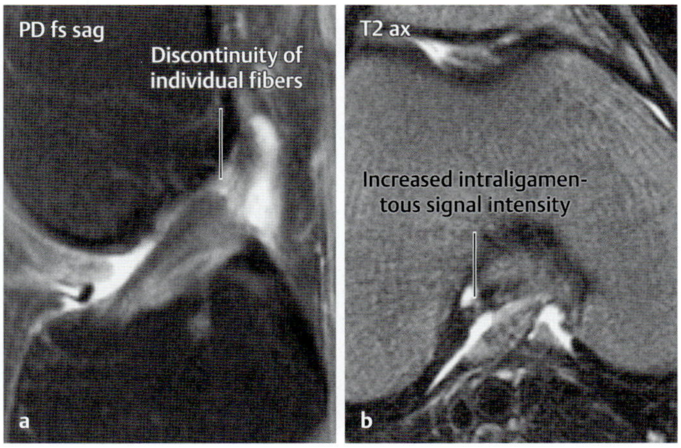

Fig. 2.318 Partial-thickness tear of the anterior cruciate ligament.
(a) Partial interruption of continuity near the femoral attachment.
(b) Intraligamentous increased signal intensity is evident on the T2W axial slice.

Criteria for an old tear of the anterior cruciate ligament

- Thinning or complete "absence" of the anterior cruciate ligament (▶ Fig. 2.319).
- Abnormal course.
- "Deep" notch sign (▶ Fig. 2.316) without bone marrow edema.
- Clinical evidence of a positive drawer sign.

Posterior Cruciate Ligament

▶ **Anatomy.** ▶ See Chapter 2.13.2.

▶ **Pathology.** Injuries to the posterior cruciate ligament are clearly less common than those of the anterior cruciate ligament, and they often only tear partially.

▶ **MRI.** The posterior cruciate ligament is primarily assessed on sagittal slices and appears uniformly hypointense on all sequences. The normal course of the posterior cruciate ligament is curved when the knee is fully extended.

Direct signs of a tear of the posterior cruciate ligament

- **Full-thickness tear:** discontinuity of all fibers with hyperintense signal extending across the entire ligament on fluid-sensitive sequences in the acute phase (▶ Fig. 2.320).
- **Partial-thickness tear:** some intact fibers with localized areas of increased signal intensity involving other portions of the ligament.

Indirect signs of a tear of the posterior cruciate ligament

- There is isolated bone marrow edema in the anterior aspect of the proximal tibia (dashboard injury).
- Bone marrow edema is located on opposing sites of the anterior femur and tibia (less specific).
- Avulsion injuries of the posterior cruciate ligament are usually on the tibial aspect and often have a large, nondisplaced fragment of the posterior tibial plateau (▶ Fig. 2.321).
- There are avulsion fractures of the fibular head, Gerdy's tubercle, and the medial capsule.

Assessment of Anterior Cruciate Ligament Reconstruction

Caution
Examination in extension is essential for a proper assessment of ACL reconstruction.

Anterior cruciate ligament reconstruction using a **patellar tendon graft** should appear homogeneously hypointense on all sequences.

In contrast, **hamstring tendon grafts** (gracilis and semitendinosus) display a characteristic streak of increased signal intensity (because they are doubled up ▶ Fig. 2.322) and demonstrate changes in their signal intensity during the postoperative healing phase: During the first 3 months they remain hypointense; 4 to 8 months after the procedure they usually demonstrate an intermediate intrinsic signal and then finally, 12 months after surgery, return to the signal intensity of the original anterior cruciate ligament.

Symptoms after anterior cruciate ligament reconstruction (most characteristically, a feeling of instability) may be due to the following causes:

- **Tear of the graft:** On MRI, complete interruption of the ligament fibers, severe attenuation, or even "absence" of the graft (▶ Fig. 2.323).
- **Stretching of the graft:** MRI shows a normal course of the graft with increased signal intensity. **Caution:** Consider the time interval after surgery.

Limitation of the range of motion following anterior cruciate ligament reconstruction may be related to:

- Impingement of the graft (▶ Fig. 2.324).
- Improper placement of the tibial or femoral tunnel.
- Increased signal intensity in the intercondylar part of the graft.
- Osteophytes at the roof of the intercondylar notch.
- Loose intra-articular bodies, e.g., cartilage fragments.
- Postoperative scar formation: focal (known as cyclops lesion = scar tissue immediately anterior to the intra-articular segment of the graft; ▶ Fig. 2.325) or diffuse (hypointense synovial thickening on T2W sequences).

The development of a ganglion in the drill hole may be associated with degenerative alterations of cruciate ligament reconstruction and may be an indication of an incipient tear of the graft. However, small fluid collections in the osseous tunnels are a common finding on MRI within the *first* year after ACL repair with an autologous hamstring graft. The fluid collections usually resolve over time and do not progress to ganglion formation or lead to tunnel expansion. They are not associated with clinical instability.

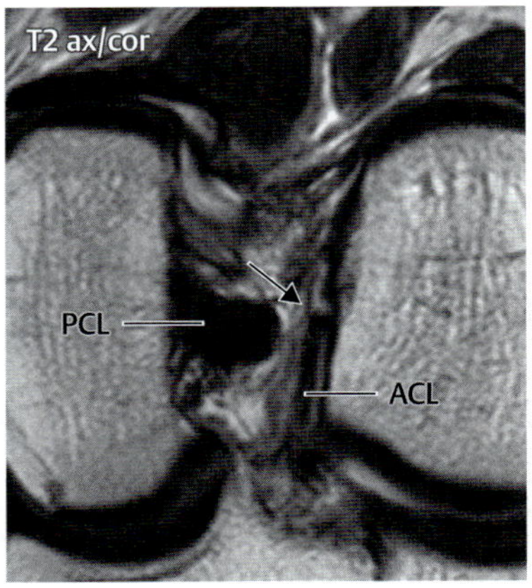

Fig. 2.319 Chronic tear of the anterior cruciate ligament. The ligament is attenuated; there is an extensive partial-thickness tear of the femoral insertion (arrow).
PCL, posterior cruciate ligament;
ACL, anterior cruciate ligament.

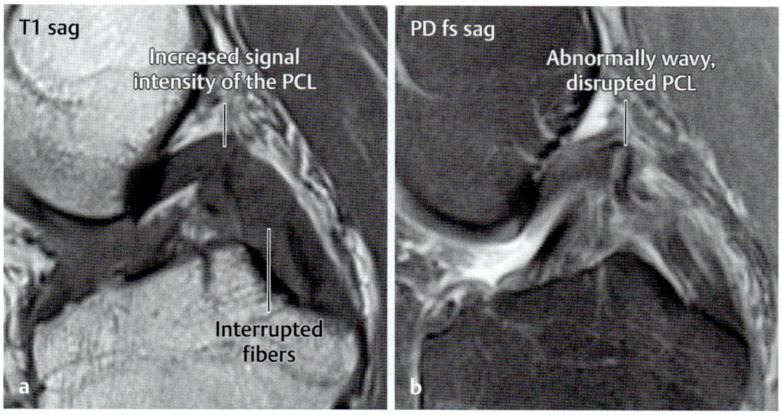

Fig. 2.320 Full-thickness tear of the posterior cruciate ligament. **(a)** The posterior cruciate ligament displays increased signal intensity and complete fiber disruption. **(b)** Elongated, wavy course of the torn ligament. PCL, posterior cruciate ligament.

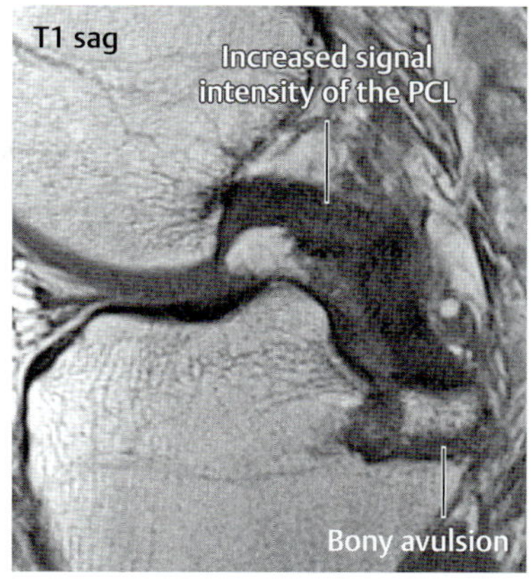

Fig. 2.321 Bony avulsion of the posterior cruciate ligament. There is no marked bone marrow edema. PCL, posterior cruciate ligament.

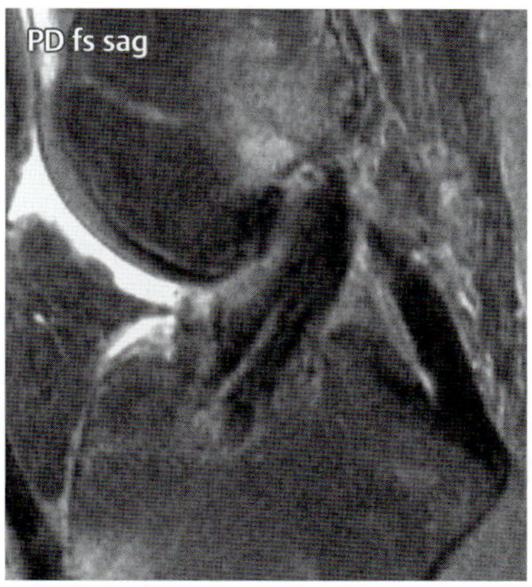

Fig. 2.322 Semitendinosus graft of the anterior cruciate ligament, 3 months after surgery. Typical streaks are due to folding of the graft.

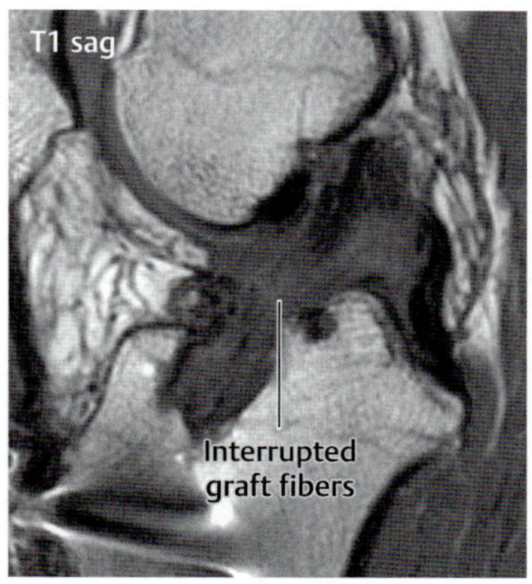

Fig. 2.323 Tear of anterior cruciate ligament graft after reconstruction.

Fig. 2.325 Localized arthrofibrosis (cyclops lesion) after anterior cruciate ligament reconstruction. ▶

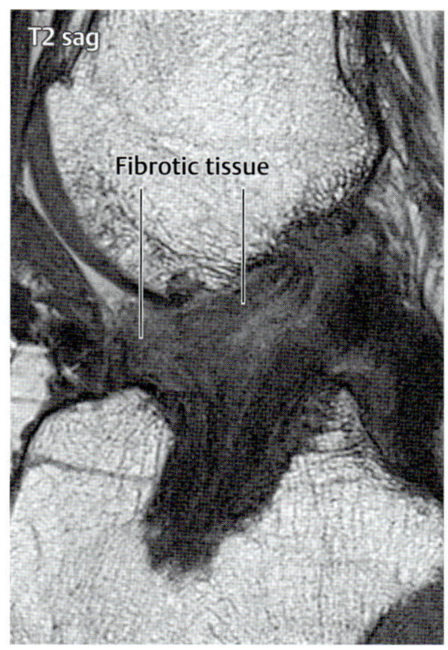

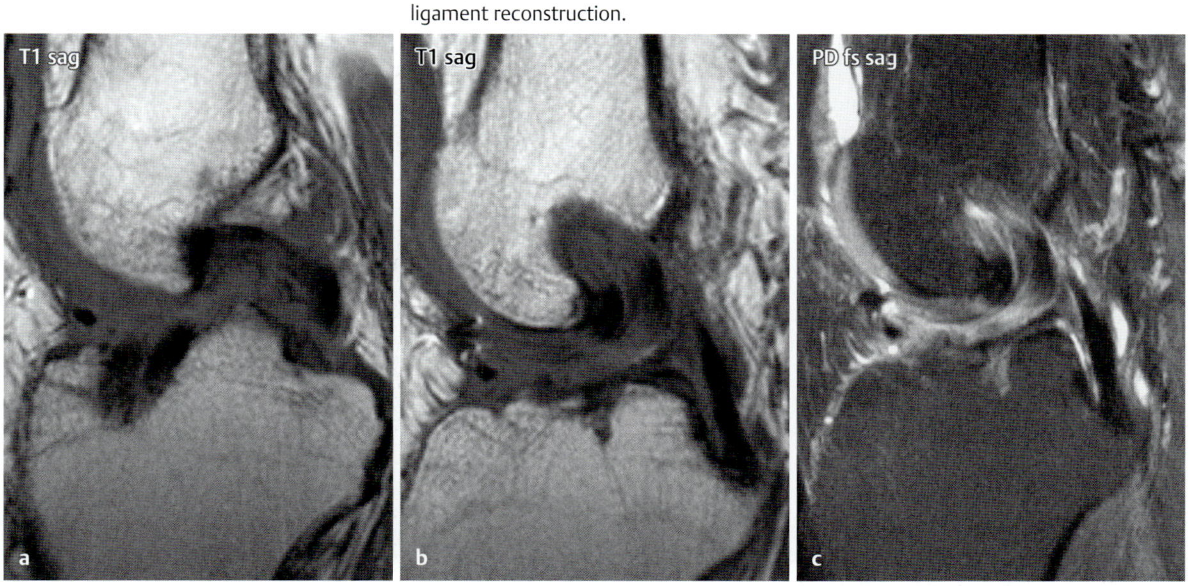

Fig. 2.324 Impingement of the anterior cruciate ligament graft. **(a)** The tibial tunnel has been placed too far anteriorly. **(b)** The femoral tunnel should be located farther dorsocranially. **(c)** The result is graft impingement with intrasubstance edema.

Complications may also arise at the donor site of the material used for the reconstruction. These include, for example, tendinopathy or tear of the remaining portions of the patellar tendon and patellar fractures.

> **Caution**
> Signal intensity changes and thickening of the patellar tendon are normal during the first 2 years after graft harvesting cruciate ligament reconstruction; therefore the patient's clinical symptoms are crucial in this phase.

2.13.3 Medial Supporting Structures

▸ **Anatomy.** See Chapter 2.13.3.

▸ **Pathology.** Injuries to the medial supporting structures are more frequent than those to the lateral. Various mechanisms, such as patellar dislocation, valgus stress, or rotational injury, result in injury to the structures along the medial joint.

Medial Patellofemoral Ligament and Medial Patellar Retinaculum

These structures are best assessed with MRI using axial slices. Although contiguous with the retinaculum, the medial patellofemoral ligament is situated proximally (▸ Fig. 2.326) at the level where the vastus medialis obliquus is also be visualized; here the ligament lies immediately deep to the muscle. Injuries to the medial patellofemoral ligament most commonly occur at the femoral insertion site but may involve its patellar attachment or midportion. A typical contusion pattern involving the lateral femoral condyle and medial patellar facet after lateral patellar dislocation indicates the mechanism of injury (Chapter 2.13.5).

Medial Collateral Ligament

Injuries of the medial collateral ligament (MCL) are classified into three grades (the same applies to the lateral collateral ligament):

- **Grade 1:** Soft tissue edema along an intact ligament.
- **Grade 2:** Partial-thickness tear, evident as increased intraligamentous signal intensity (without complete discontinuity) or thickening of the ligament (▸ Fig. 2.327).
- **Grade 3:** Full-thickness tear, complete disruption of the substance of the ligament or at its femoral or, less commonly, tibial attachment (▸ Fig. 2.328).

A **Stieda fracture** refers to an avulsion of a femoral bony fragment; bony avulsions of the medial collateral ligament at the tibia are rare.

> **Note**
> A tibial avulsion of the medial collateral ligament and a tear of the ligament (Grade 3 lesion) at the level of the meniscus in particular should be repaired if the meniscocapsular attachment is also involved (▸ Fig. 2.329). It is therefore important that the MRI report contains exact details about the location of the tear.

Chronic injury to the tibial collateral ligament is visualized as thickening of the ligament without edema, possibly also associated with calcifications (▸ Fig. 2.330).

> **Caution**
> With chronic **meniscal lesions of the intermediate zone**, increased signal intensity in and around the medial collateral ligament is commonly found. This finding most likely reflects an "irritation" of the medial collateral ligament by the pathologic meniscus (▸ Fig. 2.331). The finding is nonspecific and is also found in the presence of a chronic effusion.

▸ **US.** The medial collateral ligament can be well visualized by ultrasound. Thickening, tears, and calcifications may be identified, as may bony avulsions of the femoral and tibial insertion sites.

The (**superficial**) **pes anserinus** is the common insertion of the gracilis, sartorius, and semitendinosus tendons along the medial aspect of the tibial tuberosity. The bursa deep to this insertion site may become inflamed due to repetitive overload and is well delineated with MRI or ultrasound (▸ Fig. 2.332).

Injury to the distal insertion of the semimembranosus tendon is also commonly referred to as posteromedial corner injury; this may involve tears of the distal tendon or avulsion of a small bony fragment of the posteromedial tibial plateau.

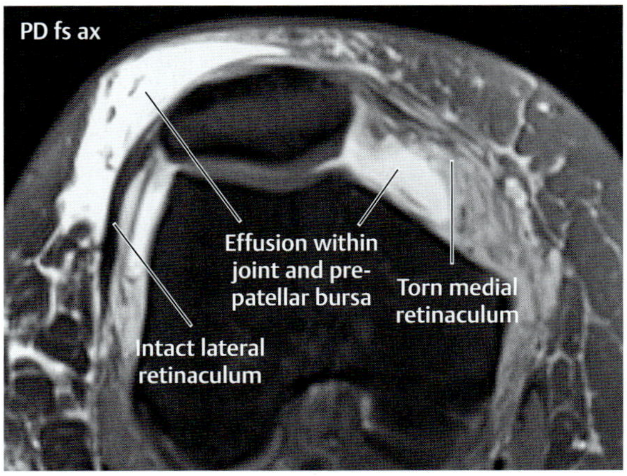

Fig. 2.326 Tear of the medial patellar retinaculum at the level of the medial patellofemoral ligament (MPFL).

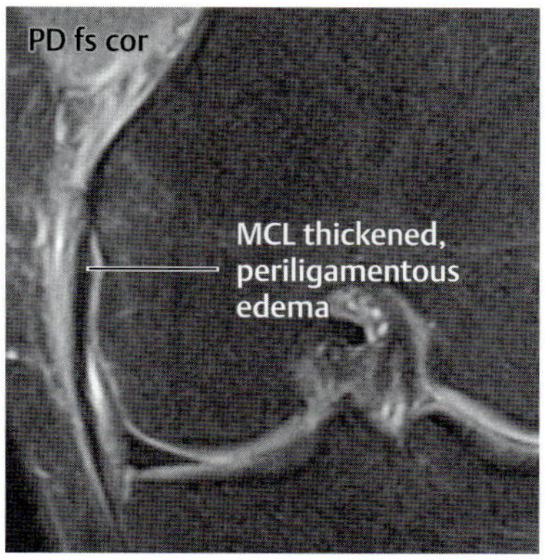

Fig. 2.327 Injury to the medial collateral ligament. Periligamentous edema and thickening of the ligament with a normal intraligamentous signal. MCL, medial collateral ligament.

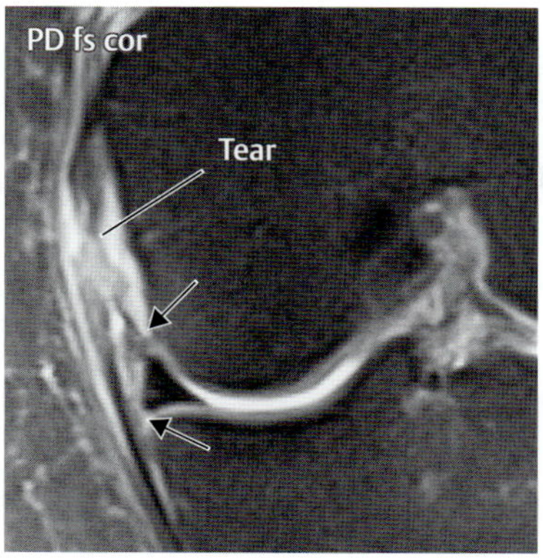

Fig. 2.328 Full-thickness tear of the medial collateral ligament (superficial layer) with associated tears of its deep fibers leading to meniscocapsular separation (arrows).

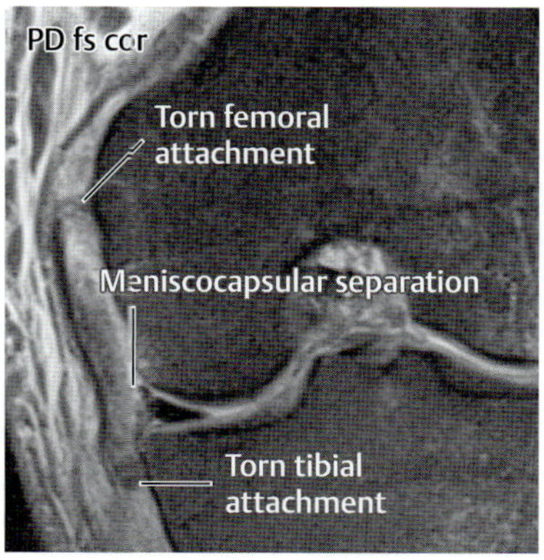

Fig. 2.329 Grade 3 injury of the medial collateral ligament.

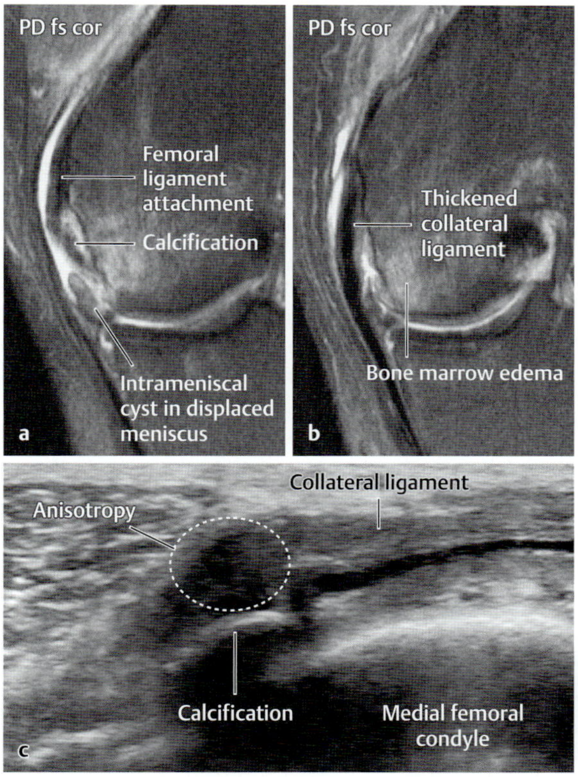

Fig. 2.330 Calcification deep to the femoral attachment of the medial collateral ligament. **(a)** There is additional evidence of an adjacent perimeniscal cyst. **(b)** The collateral ligament is irregularly thickened as a sign of chronic alteration. **(c)** Ultrasound also demonstrates the thickening just above the calcification within the ligament. The hypoechoic focus within the proximal tendon is artificial (anisotropy).

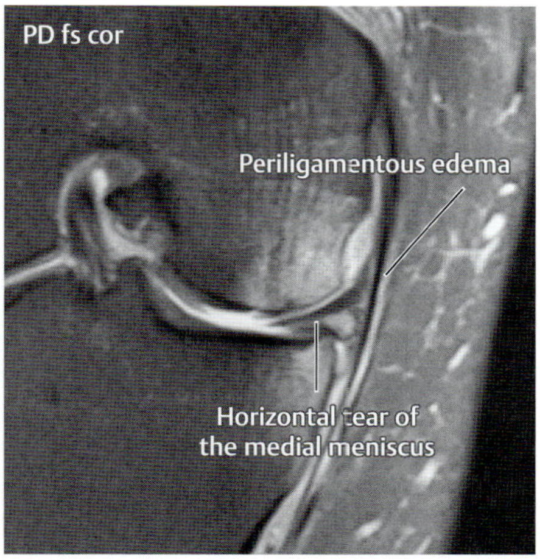

Fig. 2.331 Concomitant edema around the medial collateral ligament with a horizontal tear of the medial meniscus (no history of trauma).

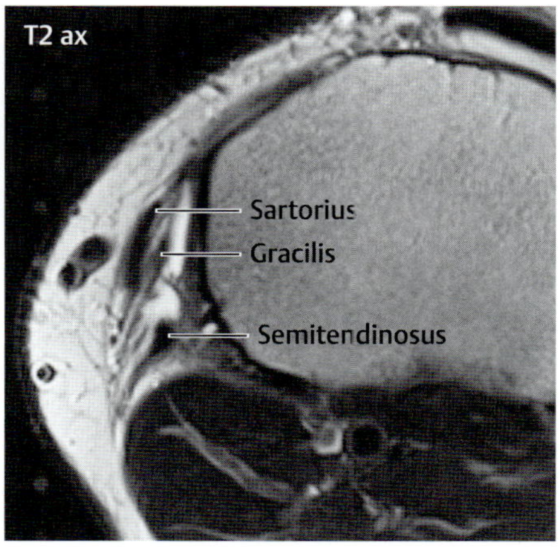

Fig. 2.332 Pes anserine bursitis.

2

2.13.4 Lateral Supporting Structures

▸ **Anatomy.** See Chapter 2.13.4 and ▸ Fig. W2.65.

▸ **Pathology.** Injuries to the lateral collateral ligament are significantly less common than those to the medial. The injury mechanisms are manifold and are often combined with cruciate ligament injuries. Iliotibial band syndrome (synonym: **runner's knee**) develops from continual friction of the iliotibial band on the lateral femoral condyle, in particular in long-distance runners.

▸ **MRI.** The signs of a sprain or tear of the lateral collateral ligament correspond to those of the medial collateral ligament and are graded into three groups (▸ Fig. 2.333). If a bony avulsion of the lateral collateral ligament or the biceps tendon (▸ Fig. 2.334) from the fibular head is observed (arcuate sign), it may be assumed that one of the cruciate ligaments is injured.

A **Segond fracture** is an avulsion of the mid-lateral joint capsule at its tibial attachment (▸ Fig. 2.335).

Posttraumatic lesions of the **popliteus** tendon are assessed like those of the collateral ligaments (▸ Fig. 2.336). About 95% of the tears occur at the myotendinous junction (▸ Fig. 2.337).

> **Caution**
> Mild increase in signal intensity at the femoral attachment of the popliteus tendon is normal.

Of the reinforcing ligaments of the posterolateral knee, the popliteofibular ligament (which anchors the lateral part of the myotendinous junction of the popliteus muscle to the tip of the fibular head; ▸ Fig. 2.338) should be known. Meniscopopliteal fascicles are located dorsolaterally and dorsally and are identifiable in the presence of a significant joint effusion.

The **iliotibial band syndrome** appears on MRI as soft tissue edema between the lateral femoral condyle and the band itself (▸ Fig. 2.339). In addition, adjacent bone marrow edema and thickening of the band may also be observed. Ultrasound reveals longitudinal hypoechoic areas between the band and the femur.

2.13.5 Patella, Quadriceps Muscle, and Anterior Ligaments

▸ **Anatomy.** See Chapter 2.13.5.

Variants

A bipartite patella results when two ossification nuclei of the patella have not fused together. It is a normal variant and is usually of no clinical significance. This should not be confused with a fracture. However, marrow edema may be evident along the synchondrosis of the bipartite patella on MRI in patients with anterior knee pain resulting from trauma or overuse. A distinguishing feature of a bipartite patella from a fracture is that the cartilage of a bipartite patella is continuous (▸ Fig. 2.340), and analysis of the ("fracture") margin on the radiograph or CT slice will also allow differentiation (▸ Fig. 2.341).

Patellar Fractures and Dislocations

▸ **Pathology.** **Patellar fractures** are usually the result of a direct blow; only rarely does massive traction of the muscle indirectly cause a fracture. The fracture lines can run in any direction through the body of the patella. A transverse fracture is the commonest form. Possible complications after fracture are fragment necrosis and early osteoarthritis of the patellofemoral joint.

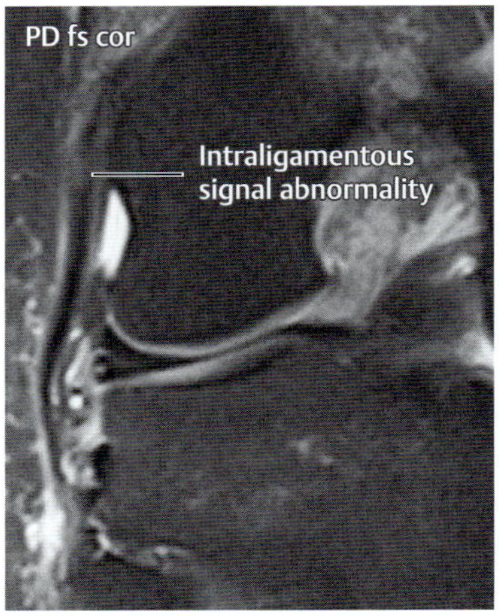

Fig. 2.333 Grade 2 lesion of the lateral collateral ligament.

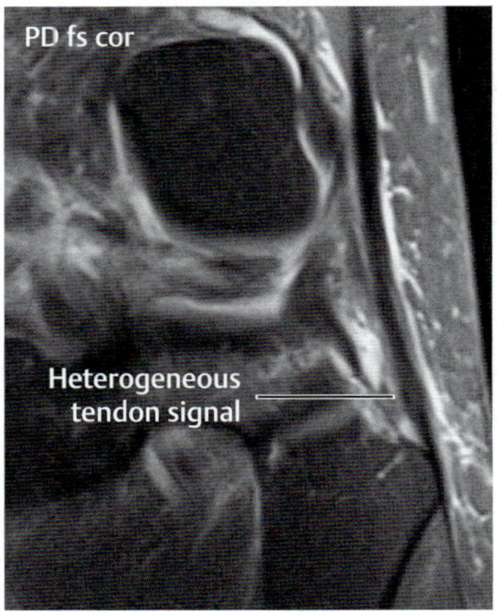

Fig. 2.334 Tear of the biceps femoris tendon with surrounding edema. Grade 2 injury.

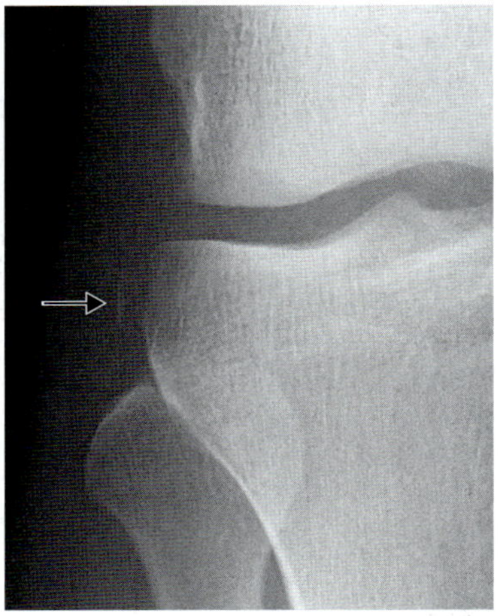

Fig. 2.335 Segond fracture. Bony avulsion (arrow) from the mid-lateral tibial plateau.

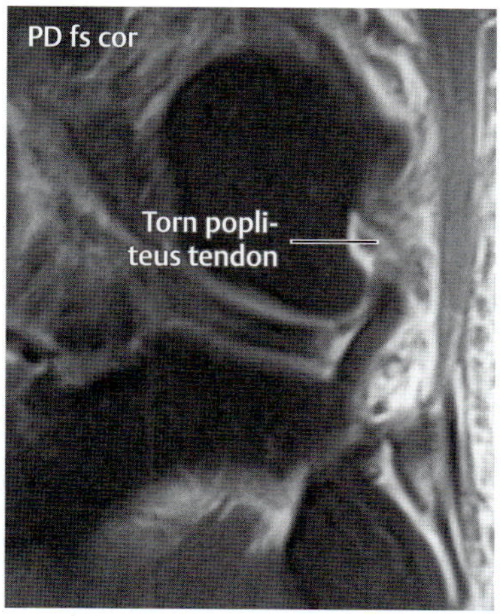

Fig. 2.336 Grade 3 lesion (full-thickness tear) popliteus tendon at its femoral attachment.

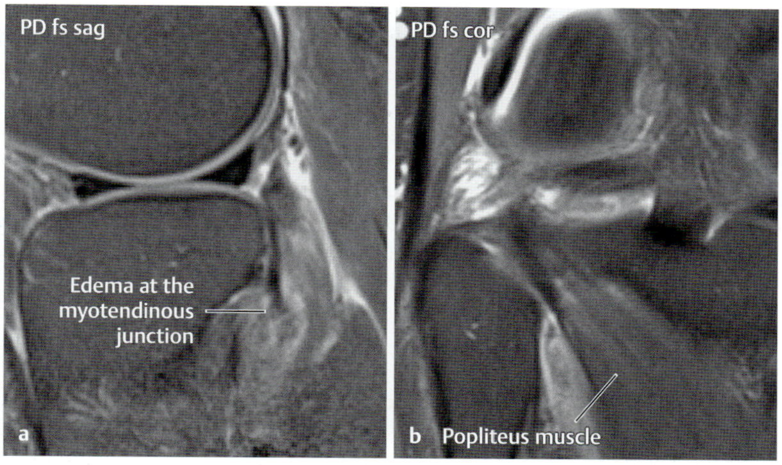

Fig. 2.337 Partial-thickness tear of the popliteus muscle at the myotendinous junction (most common site). **(a)** Edema, hemorrhage, and partial interruption of muscle fibers. **(b)** The muscle displays a pennate appearance with intrasubstance edema.

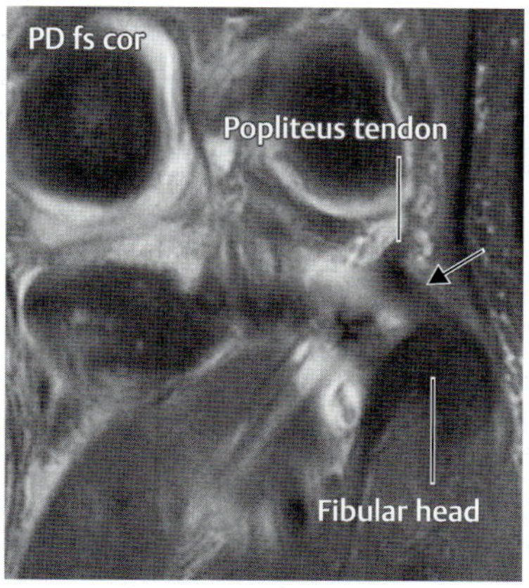

Fig. 2.338 Intact popliteofibular ligament (arrow).

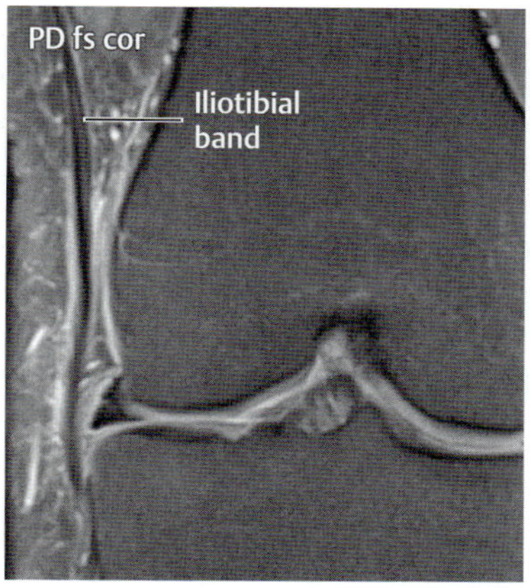

Fig. 2.339 Iliotibial band syndrome with adjacent soft tissue edema.

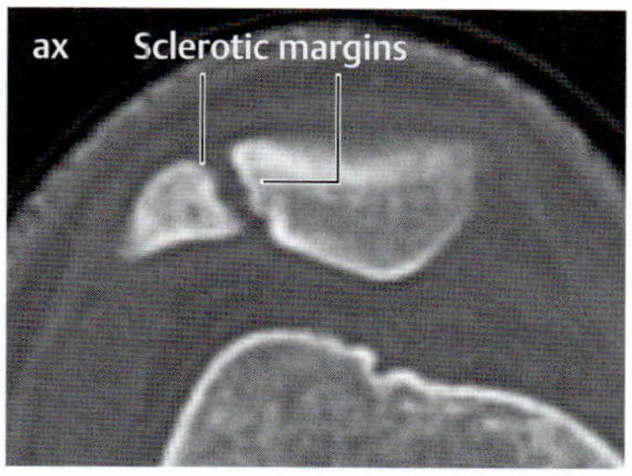

Fig. 2.341 Bipartite patella. The sclerotic margins mitigate against a fresh fracture.

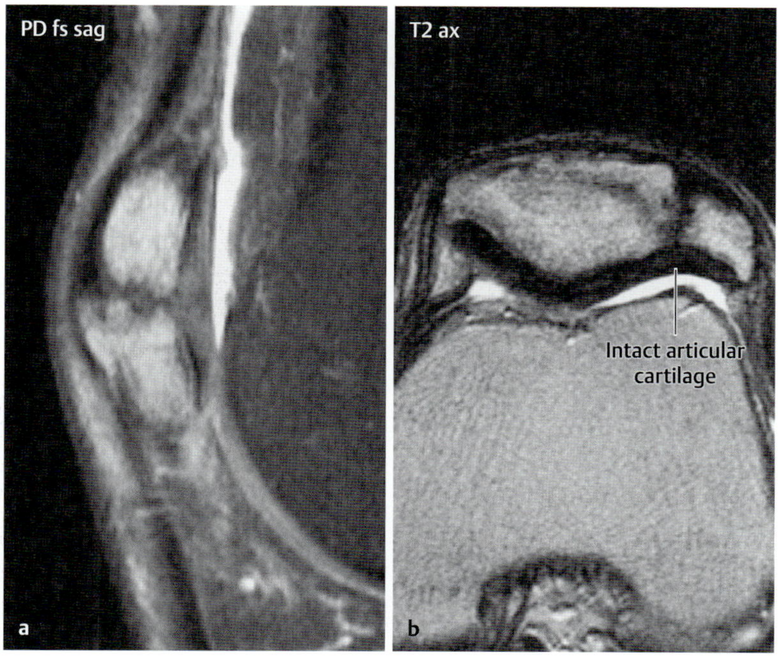

Fig. 2.340 Bipartite patella. **(a)** Marked edema of the nonfused ossification nuclei related to a stress reaction. **(b)** The continuous cartilage allows differential diagnosis from an (older) patellar fracture.

Traumatic tears and stress-related alterations of the extensor mechanism are common. Patellar dislocation can also occur as result of biomechanical instability or trauma.

Unilateral loading of the articular cartilage can develop from axial malalignment or decentralization of the patella. After other factors have been excluded (especially pathologic conditions of the tendons and cartilage), there are a number of measurement techniques (angles, distances, displacements) to help evaluate the patient's complaints, which are often very nonspecific. Please refer to the specific literature for more details (Chapter 9.4).

▸ **MRI.** The typical constellation of findings after patellar dislocation include:

- Increased signal intensity anteriorly within the marrow of the lateral femoral condyle and also in the medial portion of the patella (▸ Fig. 2.342).
- Soft tissue edema.
- Joint effusion.
- Possible tear of the medial retinaculum, the medial patellofemoral ligament, and the joint capsule.
- Possible injury to the patellar cartilage.
- Possible avulsion fracture of the medial margin of the patella.
- Possible osteochondral injury of the lateral femoral condyle (▸ Fig. 2.343).

Quadriceps Tendon and Patellar Tendon

▸ **MRI/US.** A traumatic tear of the patellar tendon typically results in a transversely oriented disruption of its fibers and is easily distinguished from degenerative tendinosis. Indirect signs are also evident, such as a wavy or undulating pattern of the tendon fibers plus surrounding soft tissue edema. In these cases, the patellar tendon often demonstrates a lax, undulating appearance. Partial tears (usually the superficial layers of the tendon) can be distinguished from full-thickness disruptions by MRI as well as by ultrasound (▸ Figs. 2.344 and ▸ 2.345).

A patella baja is found in the presence of a disruption of the **quadriceps tendon**. Otherwise the same criteria apply as for the patellar tendon.

Jumper's knee is an overuse-related tendinopathy of the patellar tendon *and* the quadriceps tendon. In 65% of cases the tendon insertion at the lower pole of the patella is affected, in ~ 25% the patellar insertion of the quadriceps tendon, and in 10% the tibial insertion of the patellar tendon. Chronic tendinopathy appears on MRI as thickening with increased intrasubstance signal; on ultrasound it demonstrates decreased echogenicity, and color Doppler ultrasound reveals hypervascularization (comparison with the contralateral side, ▶ Fig. W2.66).

During adolescence, overuse of the knee joint can result in enthesitis and disturbance of development of the apophysis at the inferior pole of the patella (**Sinding–Larsen–Johansson syndrome**).

> **Caution**
>
> A jumper's knee should not be diagnosed if there is only increased intrasubstance signal intensity within the proximal patellar tendon. This is very common and of no significance. Thickening of the proximal tendon and increased signal intensity in the surrounding soft tissues are also required (▸ Fig. 2.346). Strong contrast enhancement is also a helpful sign.

"Irritation" of **Hoffa's fat pad** presents as edematous swelling of the fatty tissue and less prominent edema within the surrounding tissues (▸ Fig. 2.347). A similar finding following trauma is not unusual.

2.13.6 Menisci

▸ **Anatomy.** The menisci of the knee are divided anatomically into an anterior horn, an intermediate part (or body) and a posterior horn. A particularly important clinical aspect regarding menisci is their vascularization, which may be divided into a vascular "red zone" (involving approximately its peripheral third), an avascular "white" zone, and variable "red/white" intermediate zone (▸ Fig. 2.348). The attachments of the meniscus to the tibia (especially dorsal) are also of great clinical significance (▸ Fig. 2.349). ▶ For further information on anatomy, see Chapter 2.13.6 and ▸ Fig. W2.67.

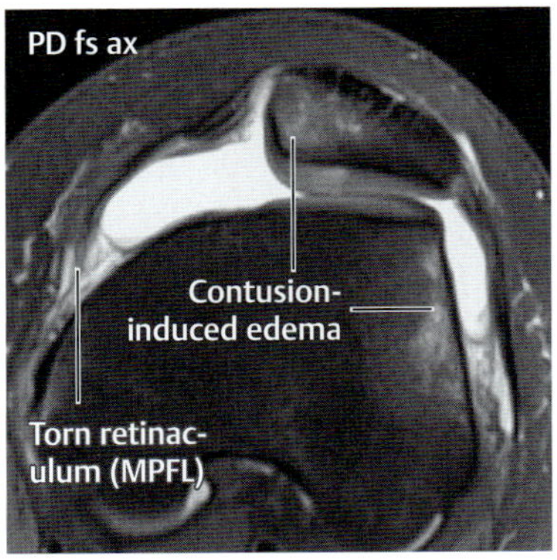

Fig. 2.342 Typical injury pattern after lateral patellar dislocation. MPFL, medial patellofemoral ligament.

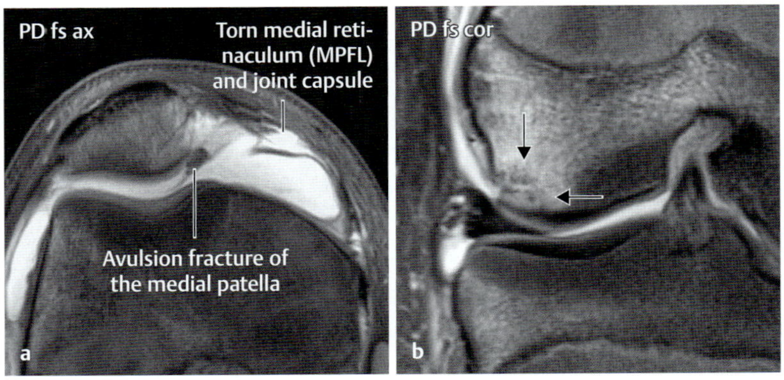

Fig. 2.343 Concomitant injuries of patellar dislocation. **(a)** Disruption of the medial supporting structures and avulsion fracture of the patella. **(b)** Osteochondral fracture of the lateral femoral condyle (arrows). MPFL, medial patellofemoral ligament.

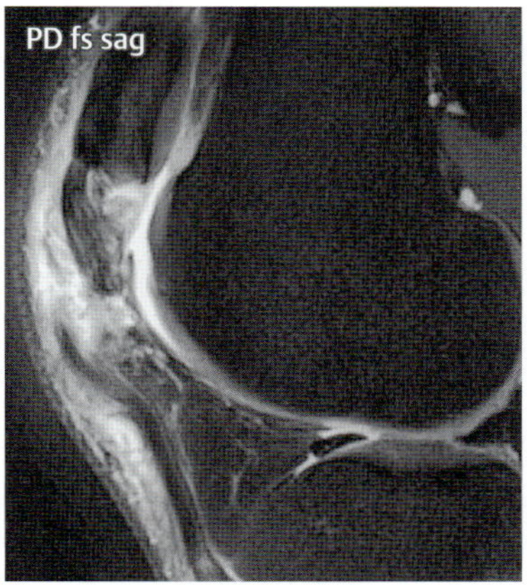

Fig. 2.345 Patellar tendon tear.

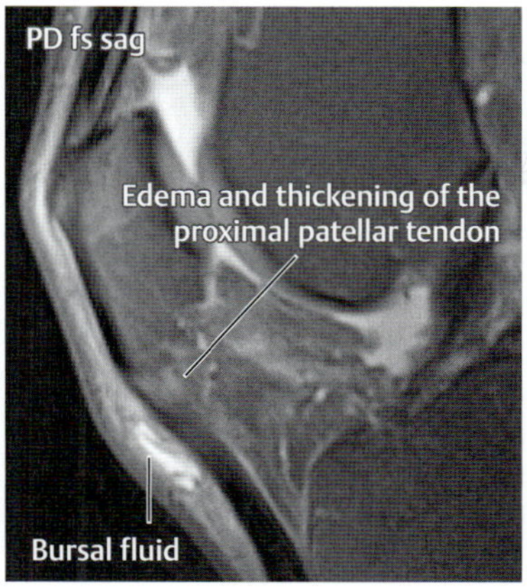

Fig. 2.346 Jumper's knee. Overuse-related tendinosis of the proximal patellar tendon. Associated prepatellar bursitis.

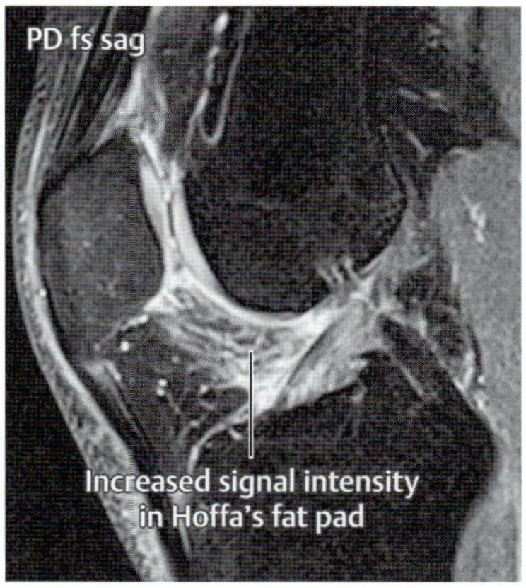

Fig. 2.347 Overuse-related irritation of Hoffa's fat pad ("Hoffaitis").

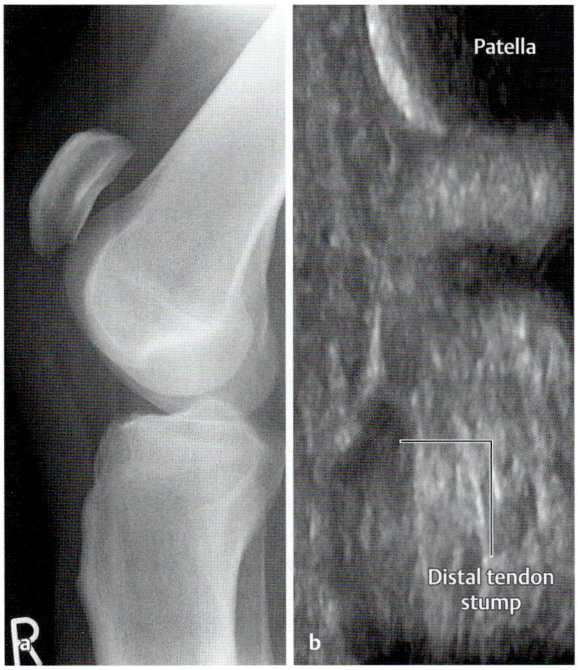

Fig. 2.344 Patellar tendon tear. **(a)** Patella alta is evident. **(b)** Ultrasound (longitudinal section) demonstrates tendon dehiscence at the inferior patellar pole.

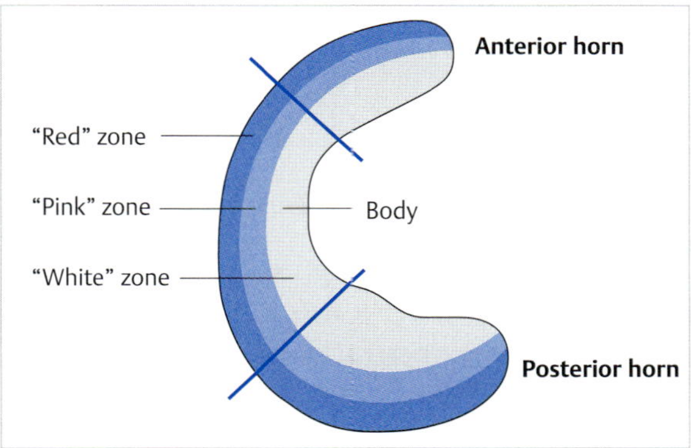

Fig. 2.348 Zones used for the classification of the meniscal tears according to Stoller.

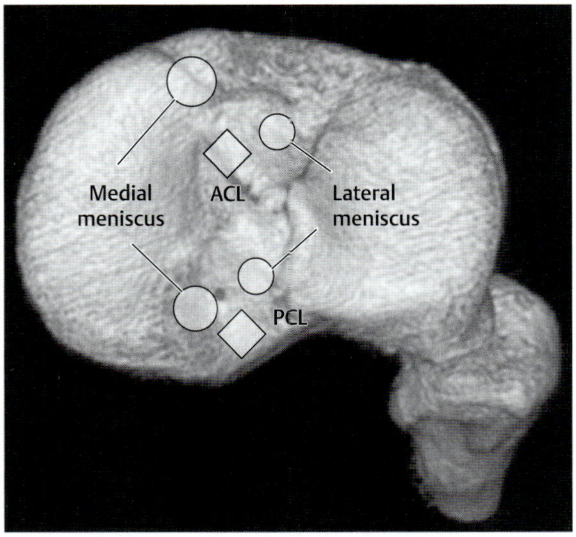

Fig. 2.349 Attachment sites of the menisci and cruciate ligaments. Superior view of the tibial plateau (3D model). ACL, anterior cruciate ligament. PCL, posterior cruciate ligament.

2

Some "golden rules" for assessing menisci

- A normal meniscus is always wider than it is thick (in the sagittal plane).
- The posterior horn of the medial meniscus is always wider than the anterior horn. They are equally wide in the lateral meniscus.
- The posterior horns of the menisci should cover the entire tibial plateau in the coronal plane.
- The connection between the medial meniscus and its capsular attachment is firm. Fluidlike signal intensity at the menisco-capsular junction is a sign of pathology.
- The transverse ligament of the knee connects the anterior horns of the menisci. Both structures are visible in the sagittal plane where the ligament attaches to each anterior horn (▶ Fig. 2.350). Correlation with the coronal plane helps avoid a false-positive diagnosis of a "tear."
- The popliteus tendon passes dorsolaterally, between the lateral meniscus and joint capsule (take care when diagnosing a tear at this site!).

Variants

A **discoid meniscus** (usually lateral) demonstrates a more circular shape in the transverse projection instead of the usual C shape; it can be closed like a disk or open in the middle (▶ Fig. 2.351). On MRI, therefore, the body of the meniscus is visible on more than three sagittal slices (when 3 mm thick slices are obtained). Another variant is the **"flounce" meniscus**, i.e., the inner part of the meniscus seemingly creates a fold or wave (especially with the knee slightly flexed). One should avoid considering this fold to be an indirect sign of a meniscal tear. If a tear is not evident, then this should be considered a normal variant.

> **Caution**
> In children, the vascularized part of the meniscus normally has a very high signal on water-sensitive sequences. Do not interpret this as "degeneration."

▶ **MRI.** Healthy menisci of adults are hypoechoic on all sequences. Areas of increased signal intensity within the meniscus are an indication of (mucoid) degeneration. Linear, increased intrameniscal signal intensity, on the other hand, should be considered a tear if it contacts with the joint space (▶ Fig. 2.352).

> **Note**
> **Rule of thumb:** A meniscal tear should only be diagnosed if an alteration of signal intensity is visible within the meniscus on two consecutive slices or on two slices in different planes and extends through an articular surface (**two-slice-touch rule**). If this contact is not present or is at best equivocal, then a tear is not usually detectable at arthroscopy. The meniscus should be examined in every plane using this rule as meniscal tears are variable in their form.

Morphology of Meniscal Tears

▶ Fig. 2.353 demonstrates the morphology of classic types of meniscal tears.

- **Longitudinal tears** (▶ Fig. 2.354) tend to be trauma-related. The inner fragment resulting from the tear can become displaced within the joint.
- **Horizontal tears** are usually of degenerative origin and are most often situated in the posterior horn. Occasionally they demonstrate a "frayed" appearance with multiple tears (▶ Figs. 2.355 and ▶ 2.356). **Caution:** Meniscal fragments originating from the undersurface can become displaced to lie adjacent to the tibia along the medial or lateral joint lines.
- **Radial tears** are more difficult to detect because they may be visualized on only a few slices (▶ Fig. 2.357). They are usually of traumatic origin. These tears are often unrepairable since they always involve the avascular, "white" zone and cut transversely across the all-important longitudinal collagen bundles.

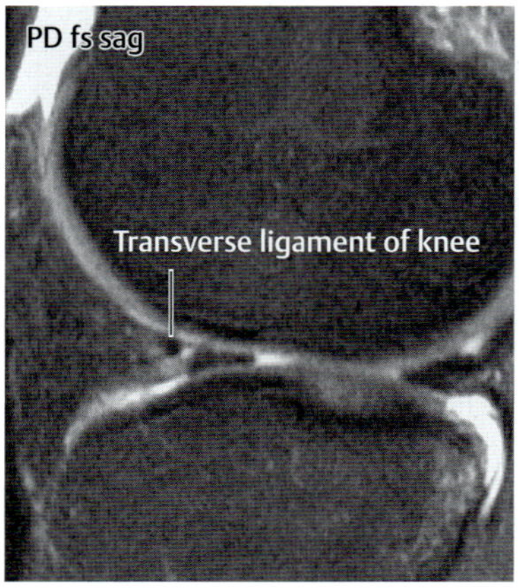

Fig. 2.350

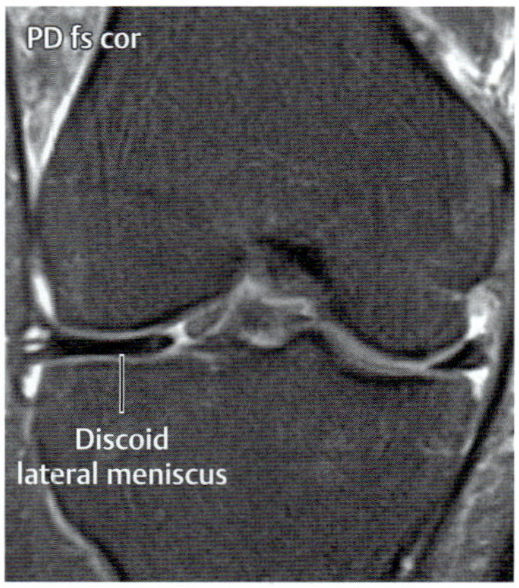

Fig. 2.351

Fig. 2.350 The transverse ligament of the knee must not be mistaken for a tear or avulsed portion of the anterior horn of the meniscus.

Fig. 2.351 Discoid meniscus.

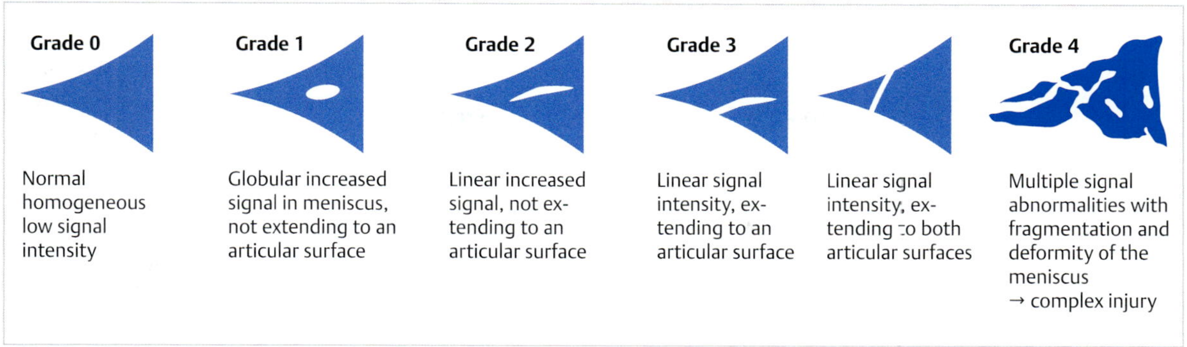

Fig. 2.352 Grading system of meniscal signal intensity (according to Stoller).

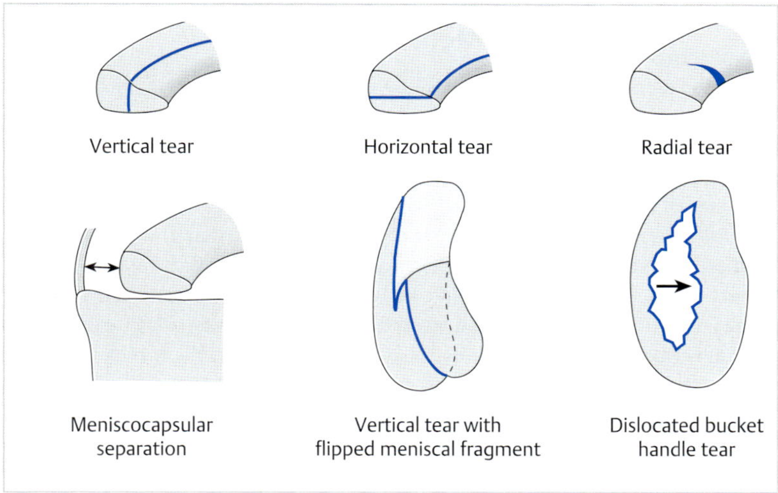

Fig. 2.353 Morphology of meniscal tears.

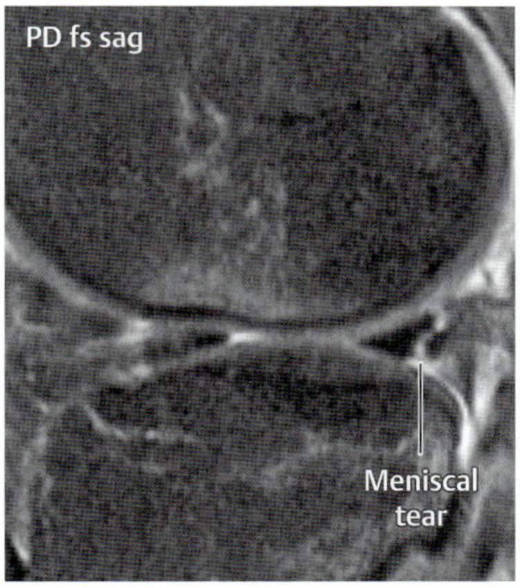

Fig. 2.354 Vertical tear of the posterior horn in the red zone.

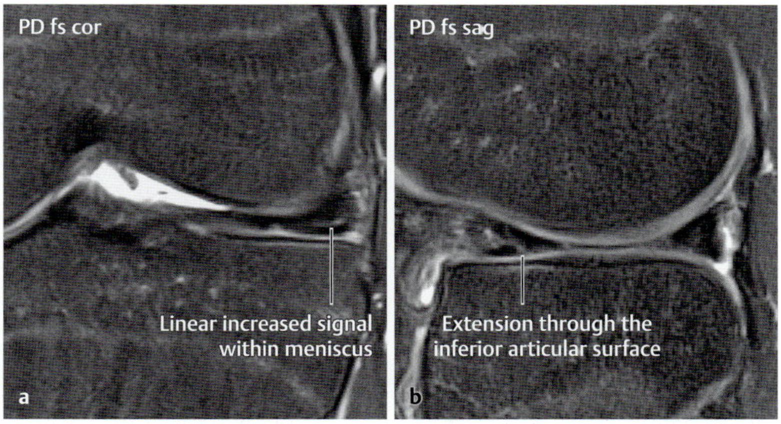

Fig. 2.355 Horizontal tear of the anterior horn of the lateral meniscus. **(a)** Horizontal line, isointense to fluid, within the meniscus. **(b)** The sagittal plane confirms extension through the inferior articular surface.

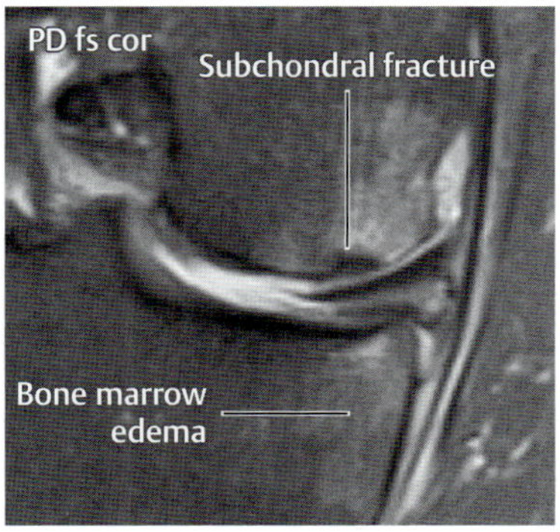

Fig. 2.356

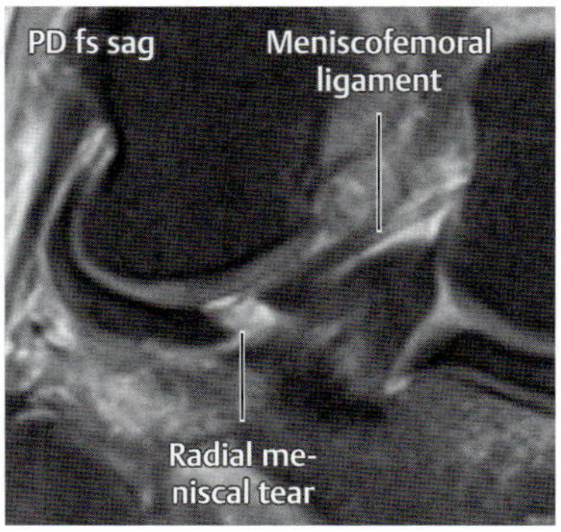

Fig. 2.357

Fig. 2.356 Posttraumatic subchondral fracture of the medial femoral condyle. It is not certain whether the horizontal tear of the posterior body of the medial meniscus was already present. Mild meniscal extrusion.

Fig. 2.357 Radial tear posterior horn lateral meniscus near posterior root attachment.

- **Bucket-handle tears** are longitudinal tears that have extended far enough to result in the inner fragment becoming unstable and displacing into the intercondylar notch. They look like the handle of a bucket and come to lie adjacent to the posterior cruciate ligament. In the sagittal plane it then looks as if there are two posterior cruciate ligaments (the **double posterior cruciate ligament sign;** ▸ Fig. 2.358).

Displaced meniscal fragments can result from all types of tears. The **flipped meniscus sign** (▸ Fig. 2.359) almost exclusively involves the lateral meniscus and typically represents a tear of the meniscal attachment of the posterior horn with subsequent displacement of part of the meniscus.

If a part of the meniscus becomes completely separated, then this is known as an **amputated meniscus.** If the meniscus is avulsed from the capsule, then this is referred to as a **meniscocapsular separation.**

▸ **Important findings.** The radiological report should indicate whether there is in fact a meniscal tear or whether degenerative signal intensity ("mucoid degeneration") is present. The location, pattern, and type of tear must be described. The zonal classifications of menisci described above are useful here. Tears in the red zone have a better prognosis after suture repair, whereas torn tissue in the white zone is usually removed.

Meniscocapsular Separation

A diagnosis of meniscocapsular separation cannot usually be made with any degree of certainty by MRI. The suspected diagnosis should not be expressed unless certain signs are present (▸ Figs. 2.360–2.362).

Tears of the **meniscal root attachments to the tibia** are often underestimated on MRI. A systematic search for the root attachments should be made. In many cases, these tears provide an explanation for meniscal extrusion.

The term **meniscal extrusion** should be used with care as it is merely descriptive. Strictly speaking, meniscal extrusion refers to a situation in which the meniscus projects beyond the tibial plateau by 3 mm (which is not uncommon). It is essential to look for a potential cause—meniscal tear? Tear at the meniscal root attachment?

Intrameniscal or parameniscal cysts are fluidlike structures that are typically associated with a torn or degenerated meniscus. If the meniscus appears normal, then it should be considered whether it is actually a normal joint recess, bursitis, or para-articular ganglion.

Postoperative Assessment of the Meniscus

Both postoperative alterations and posttraumatic healing processes, such as granulation tissue formation, can demonstrate a similar degree of signal intensity as a meniscal tear. This signal may remain visible for a long time after surgery or after a tear has healed. Furthermore, normal criteria for evaluating menisci cannot be applied after a partial meniscal resection because preexisting intrasubstance degeneration may gain contact with the surface as a result of the resection and give the false impression of a tear. So if a recurrent tear is suspected (▸ Fig. 2.363) it is necessary to look for a displaced fragment or a tear at a site which was previously intact (prior studies for comparison are indispensable here!). Many authors therefore also recommend MR arthrography for this indication.

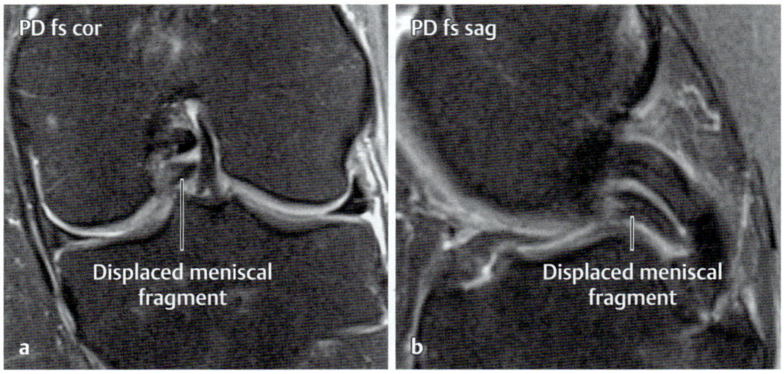

Fig. 2.358 Bucket-handle tear of the medial meniscus. **(a)** The rest of the medial meniscus is attenuated and demonstrates abnormal signal intensity. **(b)** The bucket-handle fragment is located in the intercondylar area, deep to the posterior cruciate ligament (double PCL sign).

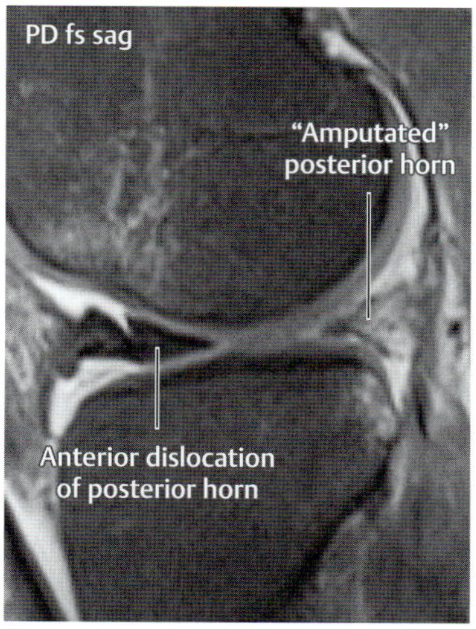

Fig. 2.359 Lateral meniscal tear with flipped-meniscus sign. The posterior horn is avulsed and displaced anteriorly. As a result the anterior horn appears larger than the posterior horn ("double anterior horn" sign).

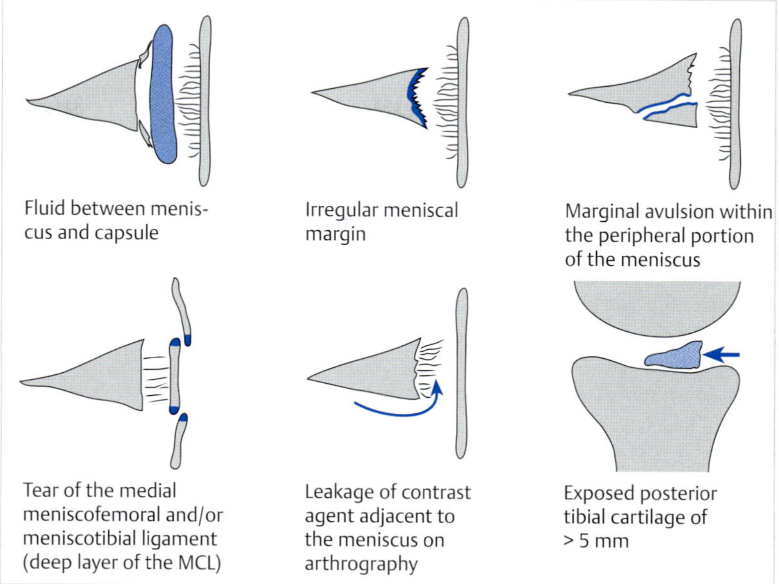

Fig. 2.360 Signs of meniscocapsular separation (according to Fischer). MCL, medial collateral ligament.

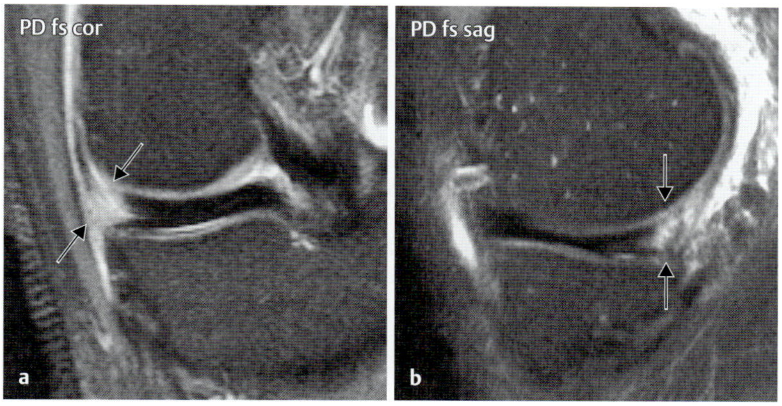

Fig. 2.361 Meniscocapsular separation. **(a)** Disruption of the meniscal attachment (arrows). **(b)** Disruption of the meniscal attachment (arrows; different slice level).

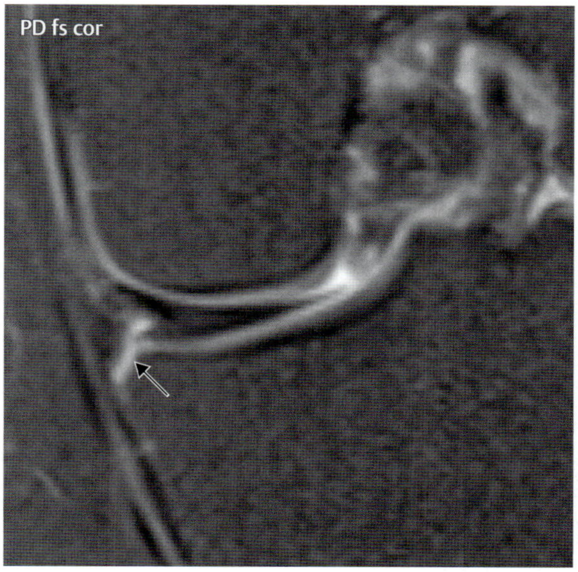

Fig. 2.362 Partial meniscocapsular separation (arrow) of the medial meniscus on the tibial side.

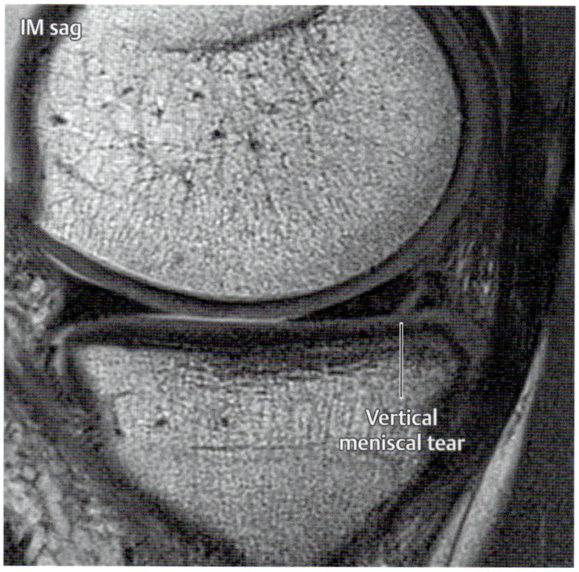

Fig. 2.363 Retear of the medial meniscus posterior horn after previous suture repair.

2.13.7 Cartilage

Compare also Chapter 1.4 (Fractures of the Articular Surface), Chapter 7.2.5 (Osteochondritis Dissecans), and Chapter 10.2 (Osteoarthritis of the Peripheral Joints).

▶ Anatomy/Pathology. ▶ See Chapter 2.13.7.

Of the proposed grading scales for cartilaginous lesions, the **modified Outerbridge classification** is the best established. This classification system was originally developed for arthroscopy, but has been modified for MRI as follows:

- **Grade 0:** Normal cartilage.
- **Grade 1:** Superficial roughness, abnormal intrachondral signal intensity.
- **Grade 2:** Superficial cartilage defects involving less than 50% of the cartilage thickness.
- **Grade 3:** Cartilage defects involving more than 50% of the cartilage thickness.
- **Grade 4:** Full thickness chondral defect; exposed subchondral bone.

▶ MRI. Apart from this grading system there should follow a measurement of the chondral defect in at least two planes It is also essential to assess any concomitant involvement of the bones or intra-articular structures of the knee.

2.13.8 Bursae and Plicae

Bursae

▶ Anatomy. There are a number of different bursae that can become filled with fluid, either as a result of overuse-related inflammation or due to communication with the knee joint. Particular mention should be made of the popliteal cyst (Baker's cyst), the prepatellar bursa, and bursae at the insertion of the pes anserinus and the semimembranosus tendons. There are others, however (see the specialized literature).

▶ MRI/US. Bursitis is characterized on MRI by increased signal intensity on water-sensitive sequences and peripheral gadolinium uptake. On ultrasound, it appears as a hypoechoic area with hyperperfusion of the adjacent soft tissue observed with color Doppler imaging.

Plicae

Plicae are synovial folds that are usually asymptomatic. These lie:

- In front of the anterior cruciate ligament: infrapatellar plica (▶ Fig. 2.364).
- Above the patella, dorsal to the quadriceps tendon: suprapatellar plica.
- Medial to the patella: mediopatellar plica (▶ Fig. 2.365).
- Lateral to the patella: lateral patellar plica.

Pain at the medial patellar margin, especially in young patients, is commonly assigned to plica syndrome, with the mediopatellar plica cited as the cause. It is purely a clinical diagnosis, although, if suspected clinically, a well-developed plica should be evident on MRI.

2.13.9 Findings after Cartilage Replacement Therapy

Given the frequency of cartilage lesions and the only slight chance of their spontaneous healing, modern cartilage replacement therapy is the treatment of choice for permanent restoration of a healthy and functional cartilage.

Arthroscopic and open surgical procedures may be summarized as follows:

- Bone marrow–stimulating procedures, such as drilling and microfracture.
- OATS (osteochondral autograft transfer system) using autografts or allografts.
- Autologous chondrocyte implantation.
- MACT (matrix-associated autologous chondrocyte implantation).

▶ MRI. MRI serves as a noninvasive technique for monitoring these surgical procedures with regard to ingrowth of the bone–cartilage cylinders placed during an OATS procedure (▶ Fig. 2.366), filling of a defect, and morphology of various types of replacement tissue. It can identify complications, such as articular incongruity, incomplete filling, progressive enlargement of filling defects, and hypertrophy of the cartilage-repair tissue relative to the original defect (▶ Fig. 2.367).

The **MOCART classification** (Magnetic Resonance Observation of Cartilage Repair Tissue) was introduced for monitoring the postoperative course of cartilage replacement therapy. This classification system evaluates morphology and signal intensity of the repair tissue using a number of variables.

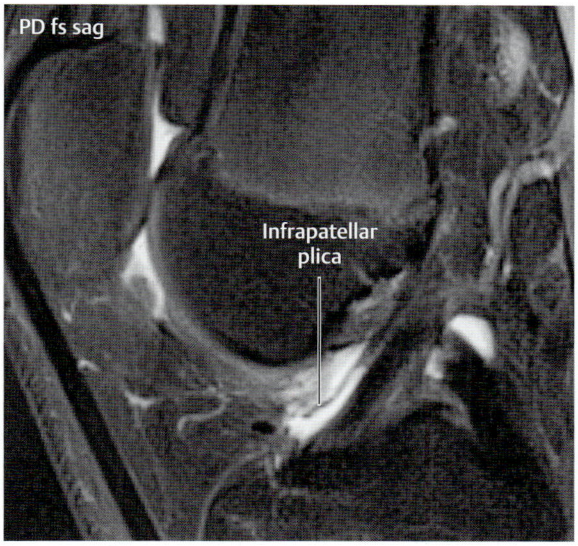

Fig. 2.364 Infrapatellar plica.

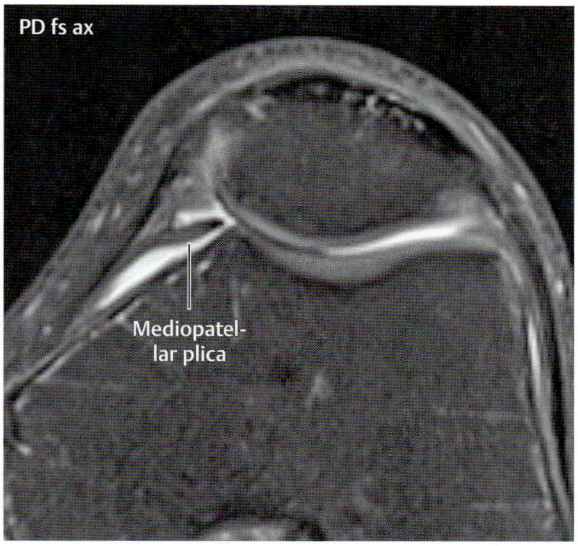

Fig. 2.365 Mediopatellar plica. Clinically the patient did not present with symptoms of plica syndrome. There is also chondral injury to the medial patellar facet.

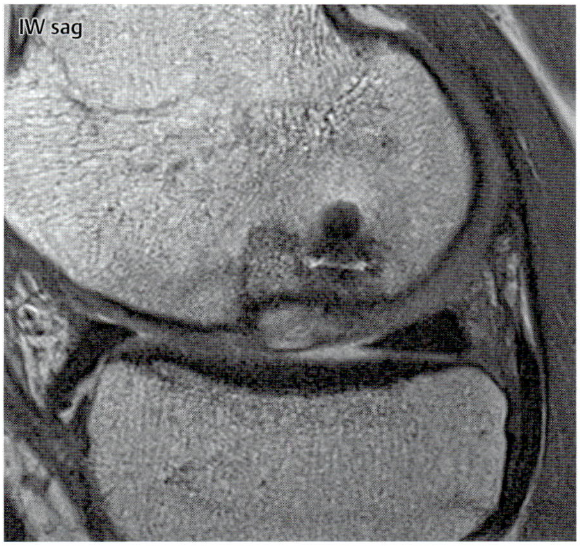

Fig. 2.366 Previous OATS. The cartilage of the transplanted cylinder displays higher signal than the original cartilage but the cartilage surface appears intact.

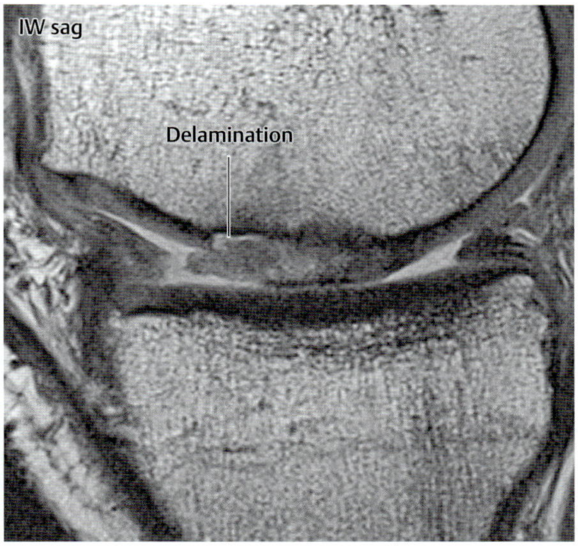

Fig. 2.367 Previous matrix-associated autologous chondrocyte transplantation (MACT) with evidence of chondral delamination as a complication.

2

2.13.10 Radiological Assessment of Knee Replacement Surgery

Knee joint replacements may be classified according to the extent of the repaired joint surface (ranging from total joint replacement of the patellar, tibial, and femoral joint surfaces to unicondylar prostheses), according to the type of joint stabilization (ligament-retaining, constrained, or fixed-bearing prosthesis), and according to their fixation (cemented or uncemented).

Postoperative Assessment

The surfaces of the joint prosthesis should be perpendicular to the weight-bearing axis; this corresponds on the AP view to a femoral shaft–tibial shaft angle of 5 to 9°. A dorsal inclination of the tibial joint surface up to 5° on the lateral projection is tolerable. The patella should be orthotopic. If subluxation is suspected (usually laterally) then a tangential view of the patella usually helps.

Exactly positioned radiographs are essential for recognizing postoperative axial malalignment on the survey view. If the femoral *or* the tibial component of the joint implant is positioned exactly but the corresponding part is not, then this may be regarded as an indication of rotational deformity.

Complications

Instabilities: The extent of implant dislocation may be identified on radiographs by a gaping or narrowing of the "joint space" or incongruence between the implant surfaces. The radiographic markings of the polyethylene inlay should be noted to assess possible dislocation of this component.

Foreign body granulomas, as a response to debris from prosthetic wear, manifest as honeycomb-like periprosthetic osteolysis (cf. Chapter 1.6.4).

Periprosthetic lucent zones of more than 2 mm and their progression are an indication of **loosening of the implant**, especially if the metaphyseal pedestal is involved. Subsidence of the tibial (rarely the femoral) component in its bed is considered pathologic.

The diagnosis of **periprosthetic infection** is made based on clinical, laboratory and imaging findings. Specific radiological signs include gas formation and periosteal reaction; less specific findings include soft tissue swelling and lucent zones at implant interfaces (▶ Fig. 2.368). In individual cases, other imaging modalities (CT, MRI, ultrasound, nuclear medicine) or ultrasound-guided aspiration of fluid collections will be of assistance.

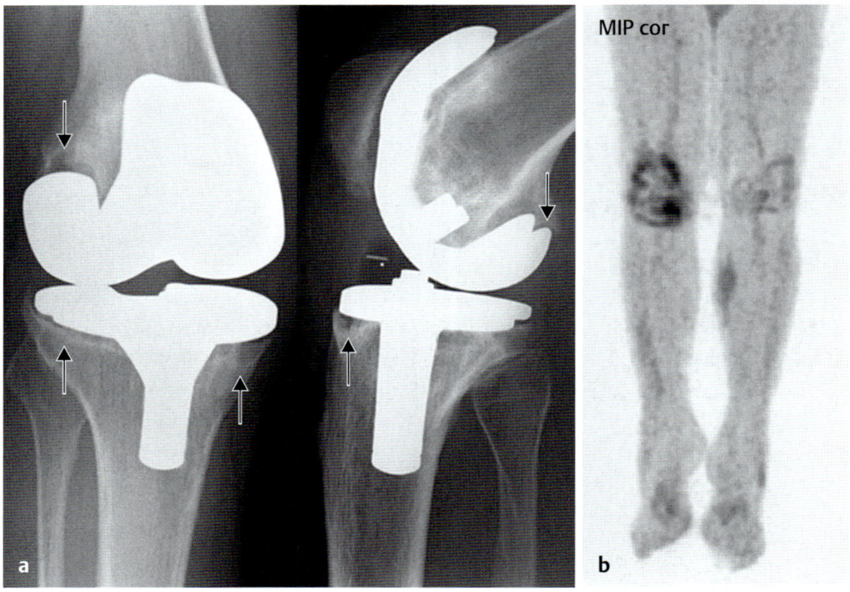

Fig. 2.368 TJR 3 years previously. Increasing pain. **(a)** Lucent zones (arrows) around the femoral and tibial components. **(b)** Increased accumulation on the ^{18}F-FDG PET image is nonspecific and cannot differentiate between aseptic and infectious loosening. A swab finally confirmed septic loosening.

2.14 Lower Leg

▸ **Anatomy.** See Chapter 2.14.

2.14.1 Fractures

Fractures of the Tibial Plateau

On the whole, a distinction is made between depression, dislocation, and comminuted fractures, with dislocations usually having already been reduced spontaneously by the time of any diagnostic imaging. The lateral tibial plateau is more frequently fractured than is the medial.

There are a large number of fracture classification systems, of which the AO Classification is the best established (▸ Figs. 2.369 and ▸ 2.370). The **Schatzker classification** is also popular in North America (▸ Fig. W2.68). Comminuted fractures of the tibial plateau after high-velocity injuries, however, are often difficult to classify exactly using radiographs alone, and CT provides an exact assessment of the fracture morphology.

Tibial margin fracture (shearing fracture). This type of fracture is not represented in the established classification systems. It involves the posterior margin of the tibial plateau (uni- or bicondylar) and has a transverse fracture pattern.

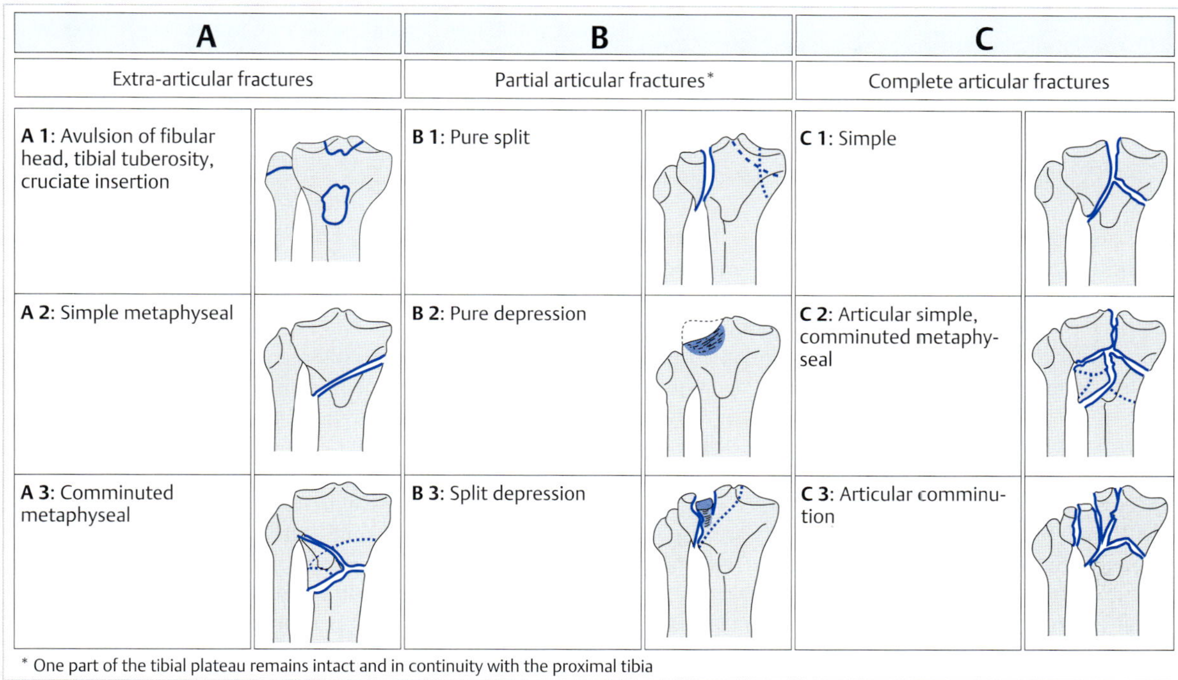

Fig. 2.369 AO classification of fractures of the tibial plateau.

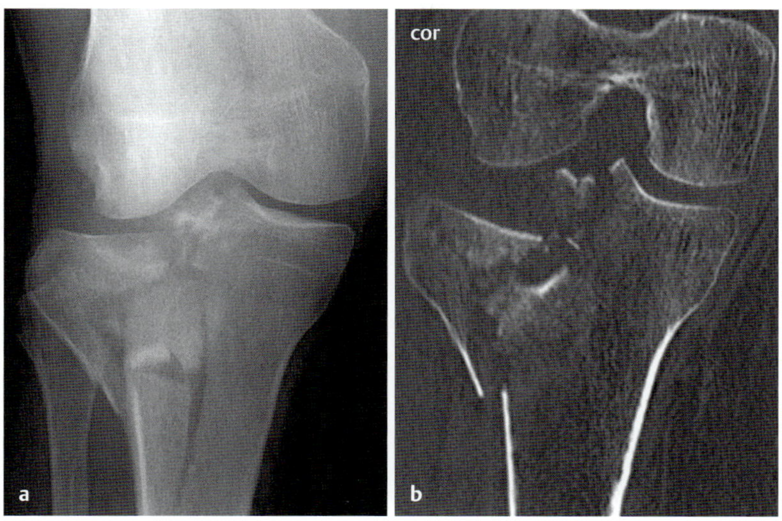

Fig. 2.370 Fracture of the tibial plateau. Type B3 according to the AO classification or Type II according to Schatzker (see ▸ Fig. W2.68). **(a)** Comminuted and depressed lateral tibial plateau. **(b)** The central depression and involvement of the intercondylar eminence are better visualized on CT.

The cause is subluxation of the anterior part of the plateau and tibial shaft; the posterior part of the plateau and the distal femur remain intact.

Avulsion fractures of the proximal lower leg. If the injury results in joint distraction or twisting, then often a ligamentous or tendinous avulsion is the result.

- **Segond fracture:** This is a bony avulsion of the lateral capsule–ligament complex (▶ Fig. 2.371).
- **Arcuate sign:** This refers to a bony avulsion of the arcuate complex from the fibular head. It commonly demonstrates a curved contour, giving it its name (▶ Fig. 2.371).
- Bony **avulsion of the iliotibial band** from the tibial plateau (avulsion of Gerdy's tubercle).

> **Caution**
> If this type of bony avulsion occurs at the proximal lower leg secondary to trauma, then a supplementary MR image should always be obtained because usually there is additional, often extensive, intra-articular damage to the knee not evident on the radiographs.

Other avulsion fractures

- **Avulsion fractures of the intercondylar eminence** are most common during adolescence. They result from a bony avulsion at the insertion of the anterior cruciate ligament with the tibial eminence being partially or completely avulsed (▶ Fig. 2.372). The isolated avulsion fracture of the intercondylar eminence is a Type A fracture according to the AO classification of tibial plateau fractures. Avulsion of the posterior cruciate ligament attachment is rare.
- **Avulsion fractures of the tibial tuberosity** are also more common during adolescence (▶ Fig. 2.373). They must be differentiated from a secondary ossification center of the tibial tuberosity and from Osgood–Schlatter disease (cf. Chapter 7.3.2); the history and clinical presentation are very helpful in this scenario.

▶ **Special features in children.** Epiphyseal fractures and epiphyseal separation of the tibial plateau are indeed rare, but they may escape detection on diagnostic imaging, especially if the clinical presentation is not available during image interpretation. An isolated fracture of the fibular head may also occur. MRI is useful in equivocal cases.

Fractures of the Tibial and Fibular Shafts

Fractures of the tibial shaft are the most common diaphyseal fractures in the body and are associated with a fibular fracture in 80% of cases.

> **Caution**
> Concomitant injury of the neurovascular structures of the lower leg is not rare in fractures of the tibial shaft. The same holds true for acute compartment syndromes.

The **AO classification** (for precise illustrations and examples: http://www.aofoundation.org) is the overall accepted fracture classification system:

- **Type A:** Simple fracture.
- **Type B:** Wedge fracture.
- **Type C:** Complex fracture.

A modified **classification according to Ellis and Edwards** is favored in American textbooks. This incorporates the degree of associated soft tissue damage and severity of injury, both of which have a major impact on prognosis (▶ Table W2.3 in Chapter 2.14.1).

> **Caution**
> Distal fibular fractures are not classified with shaft fractures but with ankle fractures, since these are usually related to a completely different injury mechanism and not uncommonly occur in combination with a syndesmotic injury.

▶ **Special features in children.** The term **"toddler's fracture"** covers stress-induced fissures and infractions of the lower extremity between the ages of approximately 1 and 3 years. The majority of cases are isolated, nondisplaced tibial shaft fractures, usually with an oblique fracture line (▶ Fig. 2.374). These children draw attention to themselves by their limp. Sometimes the diagnosis is only made on MRI or on follow-up radiography in which callus formation has become evident. Ultrasound may allow visualization of periosteal elevation by an associated hematoma.

The **metaphyseal compression fracture** in childhood is a variant of the shaft fracture in which trabecular and cortical bone are impacted proximally or distally at the metaphysis secondarily to an axial load. It is often difficult to make the diagnosis and the fracture is commonly recognizable only by bandlike densities within the cancellous bone or a concomitant buckle fracture of the cortex (▶ Fig. 2.375). MRI or ultrasound is indicated in equivocal cases (to detect the cortical buckle fracture) (▶ Fig. 2.376).

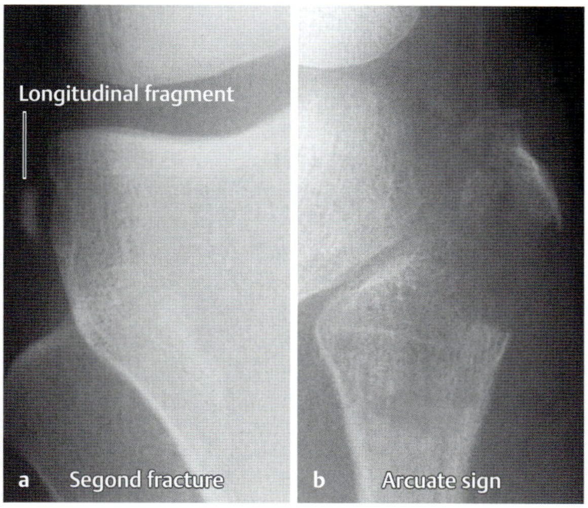

Fig. 2.371 Lateral avulsions. **(a)** Avulsion of the lateral capsular ligament (Segond fracture). **(b)** Biceps tendon avulsion of the fibular head (arcuate sign).

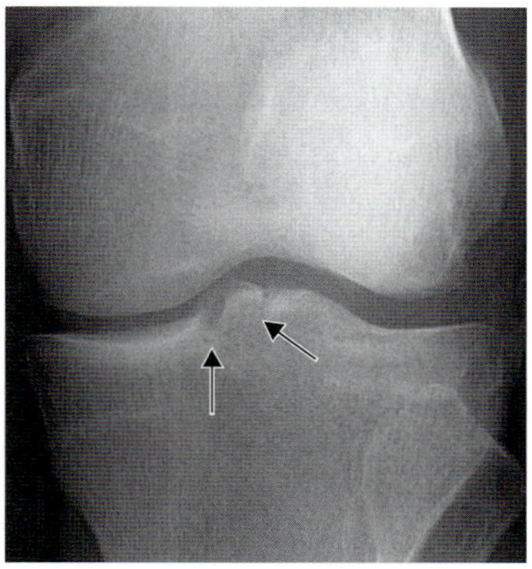

Fig. 2.372 Avulsion (arrows) of the intercondylar eminence.

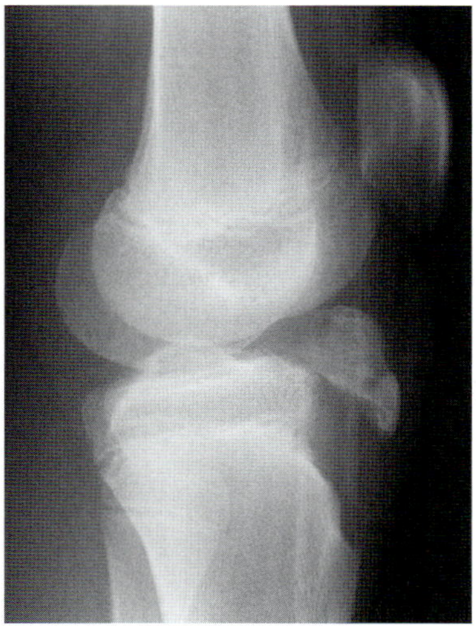

Fig. 2.373 Avulsion of the tibial tuberosity in a 17-year-old boy. Secondary patella alta.

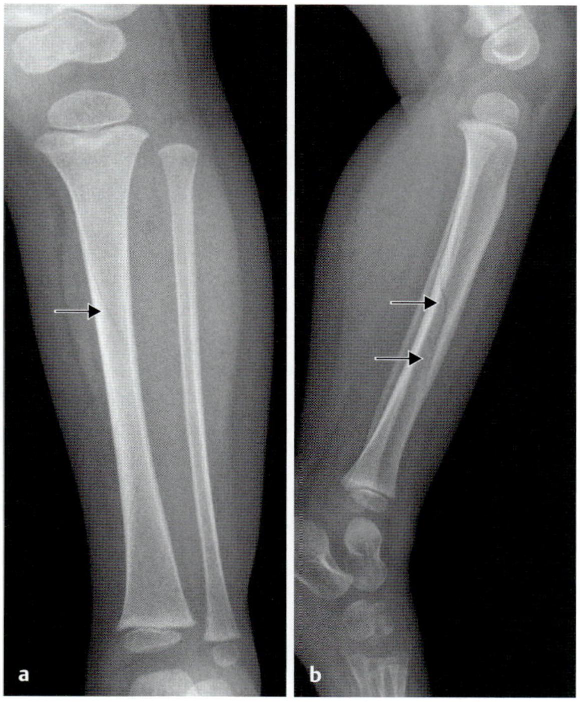

Fig. 2.374 Toddler's fracture (arrows). **(a)** Oblique fracture line on the AP view. **(b)** Typical oblique-spiral pattern on the lateral view.

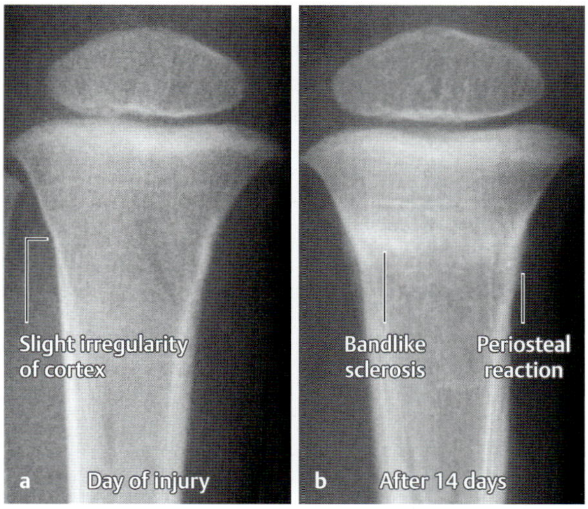

Fig. 2.375 Metaphyseal compression fracture of the proximal tibia in a 1-year-old girl. **(a)** On the day of injury. **(b)** After 14 days.

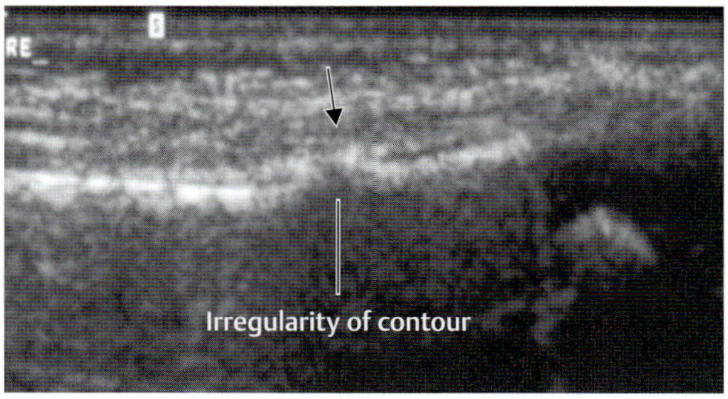

Fig. 2.376 Ultrasound of a diametaphyseal compression fracture in a child.

Distal Tibial Fractures and Tibial Plafond or Pilon Fractures

The most important feature of a distal tibial fracture is involvement of the articular surface resulting from an axial loading injury in which the talus is driven into the distal tibial surface (French *pilon* = pestle).

Here too, **classification** is done **according to the AO system** (▸ Fig. 2.377), which also includes extra-articular fractures of the distal tibial metaphysis. Tibial pilon fractures themselves are Types B and C fractures (▸ Fig. 2.378). Although, strictly speaking, pilon fractures are tibial fractures, the fibula is also commonly involved. Distinction from **malleolar fractures** (Chapter 2.15.2) is therefore sometimes only possible based on the mechanism of injury, and sometimes not even then.

> **Caution**
> Radiological classification of distal tibial fractures is usually quite difficult; intra-observer and, above all, inter-observer variability are moderate. This is why CT should be strongly considered, especially for Type B and Type C fractures.

▸ **Special features in children.** **Epiphyseal separations** of the distal tibia are among the most common anywhere in the body. Distal tibial epiphyseal fractures commonly involve the medial malleolus. They are situated along the medial tibial margin and may occur with or without a metaphyseal wedge. If the fracture is displaced, there is the risk of premature partial or complete epiphyseal closure.

Transition fractures are another type of fracture occurring in adolescence. They usually occur in children between the ages of 12 and 15 years, at the "transition" from youth to adulthood, usually involving the distal tibia when the epiphyseal plate is just *partially* closed. The shearing forces do not completely disrupt the growth plate but affect only that lateral part of the plate that has not undergone bony closure (▸ Fig. 2.379). The fracture line extends to the medial epiphysis, which has already ossified and which remains intact (**two-plane fracture**). If there is an additional bending component, then a metaphyseal fragment is also sheared off (**triplane fracture**; ▸ Figs. 2.379 and ▸ 2.380).

> **Note**
> The term "transition fracture" is not used in some countries or continents (e.g., the United States). It is considered a subtype of a Salter–Harris fracture and, rather than using this term, usually the fracture morphology is just described.

2.14.2 Radiological Assessment of Surgery of the Lower Leg

Tibial Plateau

Fractures of the tibial plateau are usually treated by plate fixation, less commonly with a supplemental lag screw. Sometimes augmentation with cancellous bone or bone replacement is performed.

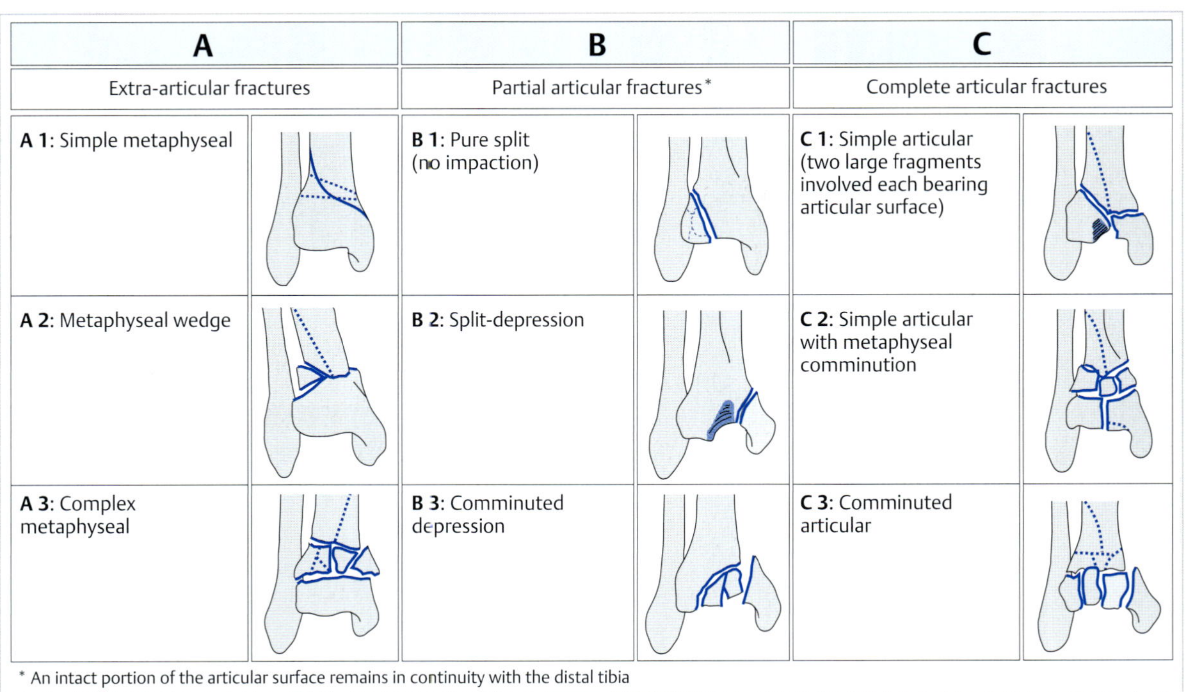

Fig. 2.377 AO classification of distal fractures of the tibia. Each type of fracture can occur with or without an associated fibular fracture.

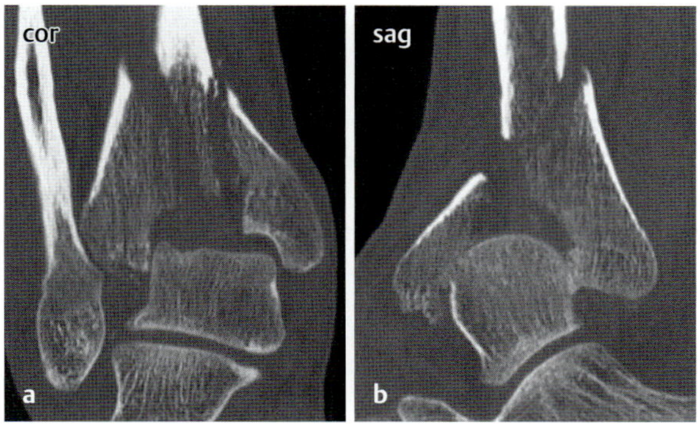

Fig. 2.378 Tibial pilon fracture secondary to an axial loading injury. Type C3 according to the AO classification. **(a)** Coronal reconstruction. **(b)** Sagittal reconstruction.

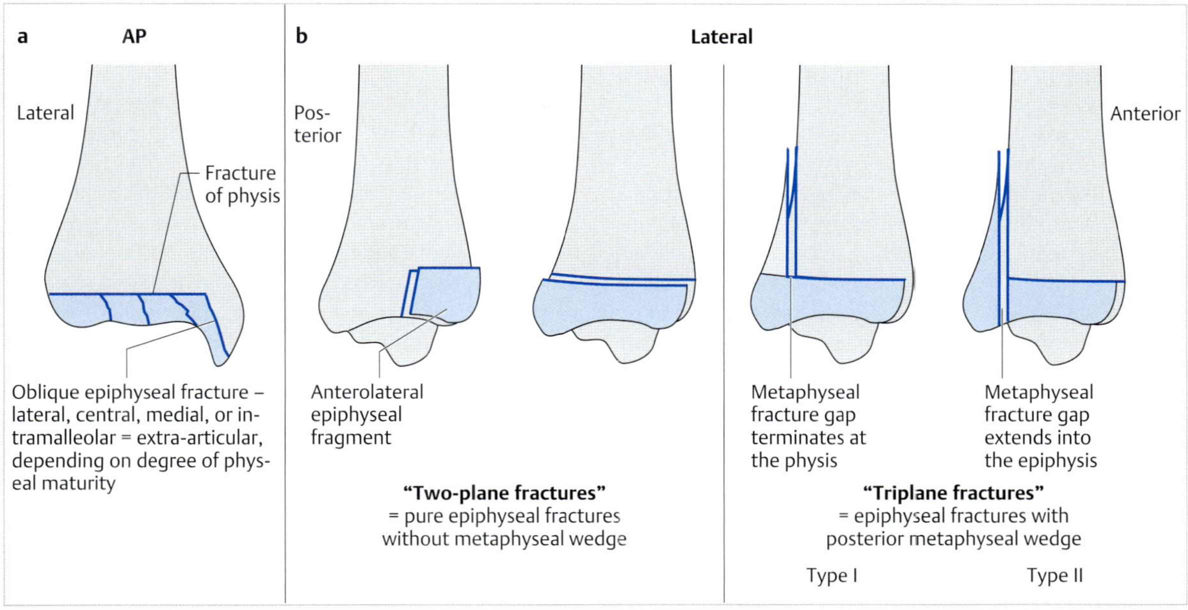

Fig. 2.379 Transitional fractures of the distal tibial epiphysis. **(a)** Possible fracture patterns on an AP radiograph or a coronal image. **(b)** Classification of transitional fractures using the lateral view.

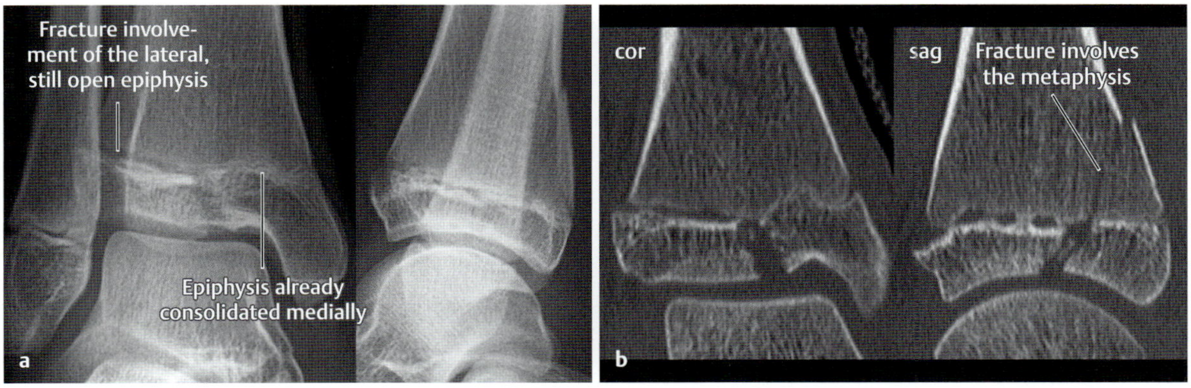

Fig. 2.380 Transitional fracture (triplane fracture) of the distal lower leg. **(a)** Radiographs: the line of fracture is anterolaterally through the growth plate. **(b)** CT: unlike with a two-plane fracture, there is additional fracture involvement of the metaphysis.

Here, the main objective of fracture fixation is restoration of the tibial joint surface. For this reason the postoperative radiograph should be evaluated for any step-offs, defects, or dehiscences of the articular surface (▶ Fig. 2.381). Special attention should be directed toward any intra-articular fragments as well as axial alignment. A supplementary CT scan is often beneficial.

Lower Leg Shaft

Currently, fractures of the lower leg are usually managed by intramedullary nailing, or plate fixation. Combined procedures are also employed (e.g., intramedullary nail of the tibia with plating of the fibula).

▶ Radiography. **Postoperative radiographic evaluation** must assess the following features:

- *Abnormal axial alignment, fragment dislocation or leg-length discrepancy?*
- *Stability of the intramedullary nailing?* There should be a gap of a few millimeters between the fracture line and interlocking screw (stability). The nail must occasionally be advanced until just proximal to the ankle joint. It should neither split the distal fragment nor penetrate the joint. The interlocking screws must find purchase in the far cortex to obtain sufficient hold.
- *Hardware failure?* If the proximal static interlocking screw goes on to bend or break, this may achieve a desired "autodynamization" (▶ Fig. 2.382). However, the fracture zone should be examined for development of malalignment. A problem may arise if the distal interlocking screw breaks and the nail migrates distally toward the ankle.

Tibial Pilon (Plafond)

Tibial pilon fractures are usually managed with an angular-stable screw plate after the obligatory interim stabilization with an external fixator.

▶ Radiography. Radiographs centered exactly on the ankle joint are required for correct evaluation of the operative repair. About one-half of the lower leg should also be displayed to completely image the fixation hardware.

Postoperative radiographic evaluation must assess the following features:

- *Axial alignment* (▶ Fig. 2.383)?
- *Restoration of the joint surface?* Any step-off, defect or dehiscence should be identified.
- *Intra-articular fragments?*
- *Position of the screws relative to the joint?*
- *Width of the ankle mortise?* A (persistent) widening of the ankle mortise after surgery is an indication of instability of the tibiofibular syndesmosis and must be mentioned in the radiological report.

2.14.3 Soft Tissue Injuries and Stress Reactions of the Lower Leg

Compartment syndromes (Chapter 11.6) most commonly involve the lower leg, especially its anterior compartment (▶ see Chapter 2.14 for anatomy). In addition to trauma, heavy strain of the muscles can also result in symptoms of compartment syndrome. The diagnosis is primarily reached by clinical examination. Ultrasound and MRI demonstrate respectively decreased echogenicity and increased signal intensity on water-sensitive sequences. The compartment involved is swollen and the normal architecture of the muscles is disrupted. If compromise of perfusion has been present for a longer period, then necrotic tissue may be demonstrated within the affected muscles using IV contrast medium.

Fractures of the lower leg may be associated with **muscle injuries** and hemorrhage, with subsequent vascular and nerve damage being relatively common. Competitive athletes can sustain tears of the gastrocnemius/soleus muscles, especially at their musculotendinous junctions (▶ Fig. 2.384).

The term **"shin splints" (runner's leg)** usually refers to an activity-related pain syndrome of the lower leg of an athlete that is associated with a nonspecific (noninfectious) inflammatory reaction of the soft tissue and bone. Four important causes are recognized:

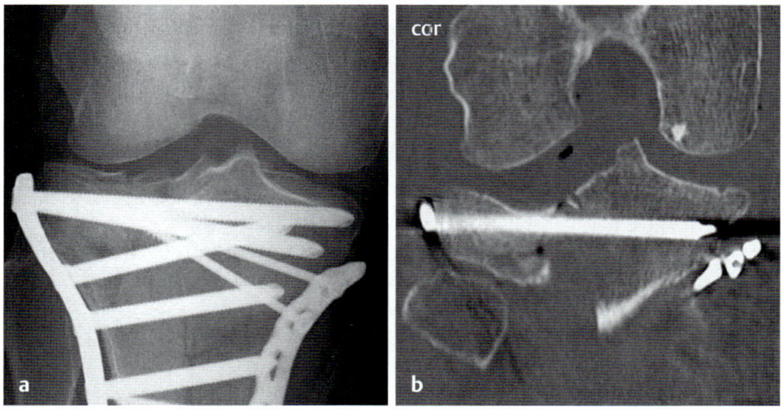

Fig. 2.381 Bilateral plating of a comminuted fracture of the tibial plateau. **(a)** Marked articular step-offs are still evident at the lateral tibial plateau. **(b)** There is a posterior trough-shaped impression of the plateau.

- Tibial stress fractures (▶ Fig. 2.385).
- Tibialis posterior syndrome (myositis, fasciitis).
- Overuse-related anterior compartment syndrome.
- Periostitis of the (anterior margin of the) tibia.

These causes may be differentiated using MRI.

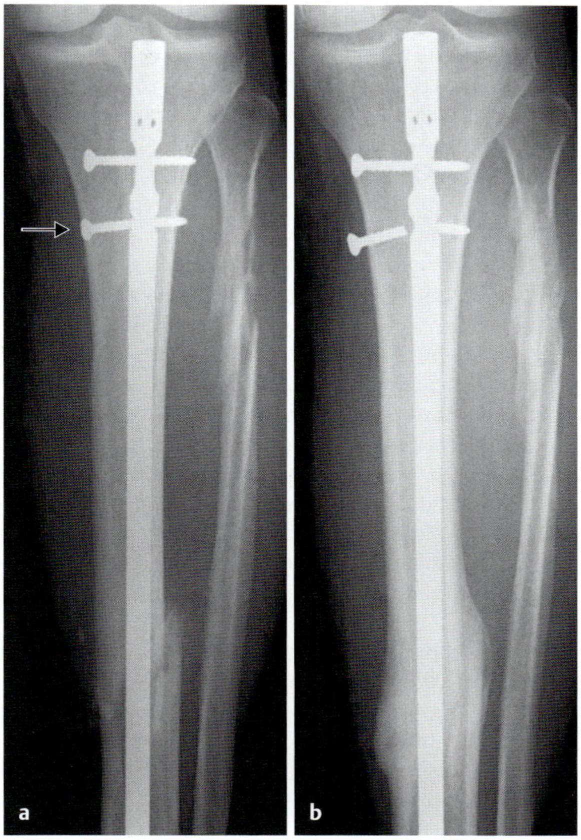

Fig. 2.382 Intramedullary nailing of a lower leg fracture. **(a)** Bending of the proximal static interlocking screw (arrow) is apparent 6 weeks after surgery. **(b)** Six months later: spontaneous dynamization secondary to breakage of the screw. This resulted in complete consolidation of the fracture.

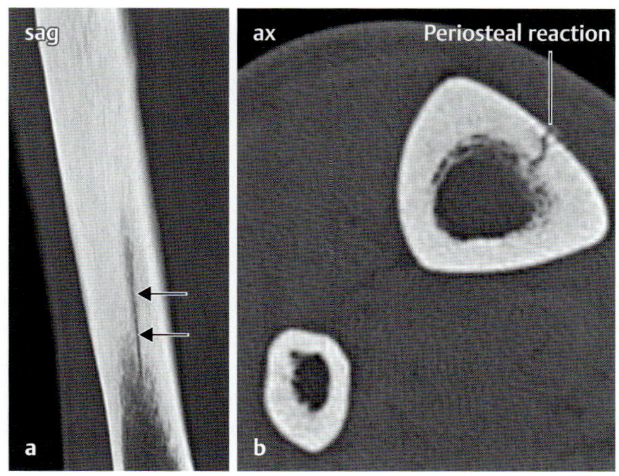

Fig. 2.385 Stress-related fracture of the tibia (shin splint). **(a)** Longitudinal fracture (arrows). **(b)** Early periosteal reaction.

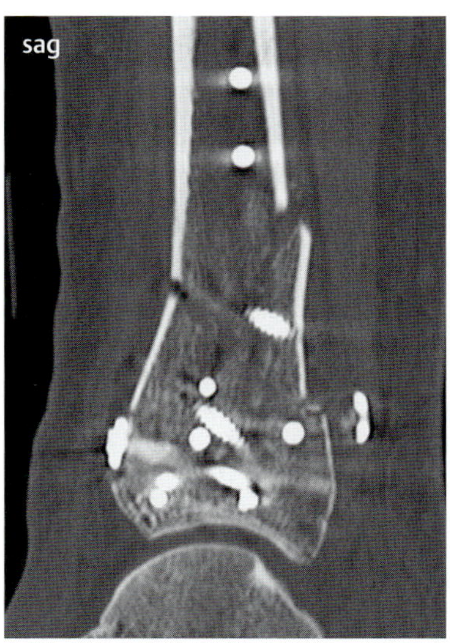

Fig. 2.383 Excellent restoration of the distal tibial joint surface after a tibial pilon fracture. Nevertheless, there is residual apex posterior angulation at the diametaphyseal transition.

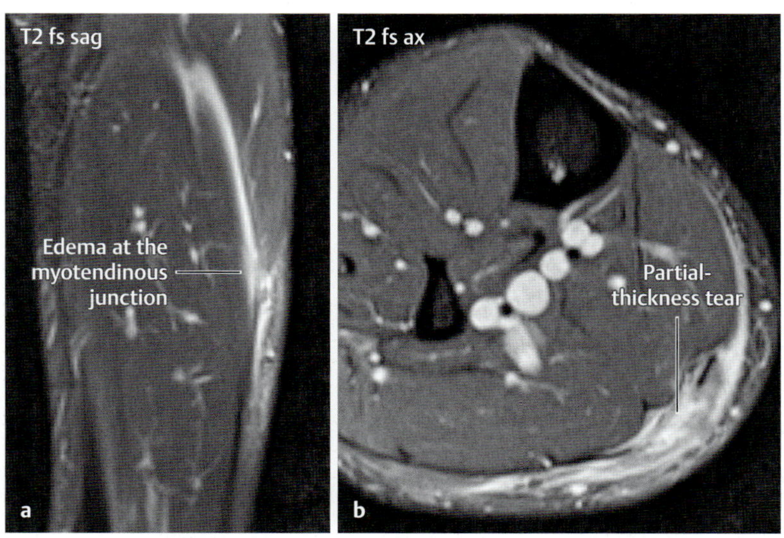

Fig. 2.384 Partial-thickness tear of the gastrocnemius muscle in a competitive athlete. **(a)** This injury typically involves the myotendinous junction. **(b)** Edema and partial discontinuity of the fibers.

2.15 Ankle Joint and Foot

2.15.1 Anatomy, Variants, and Technique

▸ Anatomy. ▸ See Chapter 2.15.1 and ▸ Figs. W2.69–W2.71.

Variants

There is a large number of possible **accessory bones** around the ankle and foot that are of no clinical significance (▸ Fig. 2.386). It is sometimes difficult to distinguish these from small avulsed fragments using diagnostic imaging. An os naviculare accessorium and an os trigonum may become symptomatic secondary to an impingement syndrome (Chapter 2.15.11).

Normal variants that occur during adolescence can pose further diagnostic difficulties, e.g., multiple secondary nuclei of the calcaneal attachment of the Achilles tendon (▸ Fig. 2.387).

A **tarsal coalition** is found in 1 to 2% of the general population and refers to an abnormal congenital connection between tarsal bones that can be either bony, cartilaginous, or fibrous. **Talocalcaneal and calcaneonavicular coalitions** are the two most common types, and occur bilaterally in 50% of cases. They do not usually become symptomatic until the second decade of life when they present with pain in the tarsal region. The lateral radiograph of a talocalcaneal coalition typically displays what is known as the **C sign** (▸ Fig. 2.388) (a continuous line from the dorsal cortex of the talus to the inferior border of the sustentaculum tali) and the **talar beak sign**, which is not to be confused with the talar nose, a fibro-ostosis of the capsular insertion of the ankle at the talar neck (▸ Fig. 2.388). A calcaneonavicular coalition typically appears as an elongation of the anterior calcaneal process, known as **"anteater nose sign"** (▸ Fig. 2.389).

Technique

▸ Radiography. Basic radiographs for almost all acute and chronic indications involving the ankle joint require the collection of images in two projections. The *leg* must be internally rotated by 15° for the AP view. A common mistake during positioning is supination of the subtalar joint, which mimics internal rotation. When obtaining a lateral view, care should be taken that the foot, together with the lower leg, is placed laterally and completely on the cassette, otherwise the talus will demonstrate a double contour and the lateral malleolus will simulate an anterior dislocation. Features of a good AP radiograph positioning include a clear space between the medial malleolus and the talus and the calcaneal tuberosity not being projected lateral to the tip of the fibula. A tangential view into the lateral (fibulotalar) joint space is not compulsory because the medial and lateral contours of the talus do not run parallel but converge posteriorly.

In order to exclude a proximal fibular fracture, which may occur with fractures of the ankle, the entire lower leg, including the knee, must be visualized. Stress views to exclude a collateral ligament tear or to test the syndesmosis are often inconclusive. Direct imaging of the ligaments is often obtained using MRI and/or ultrasound. If anatomical anomalies are detected, then a comparison radiograph of the contralateral side is advisable.

There are important **radiographic findings** for assessing normal articulation of the ankle joint (▸ Fig. 2.390):

- Regular joint space width.
- Correct length of the fibula.
- The position of the fibulotalar joint surface at the level of the tibiotalar joint surface (recognizable by Weber's nose, a small bony extension on the medial side of the distal fibula).
- Tibiofibular overlap of at least 1 mm with 20° internal rotation and of 10 mm on the strict AP projection.
- Distance between tibia and fibula 1 cm cranial to the joint plateau of less than 5 mm (widening of more than 5 mm suggests syndesmotic injury).

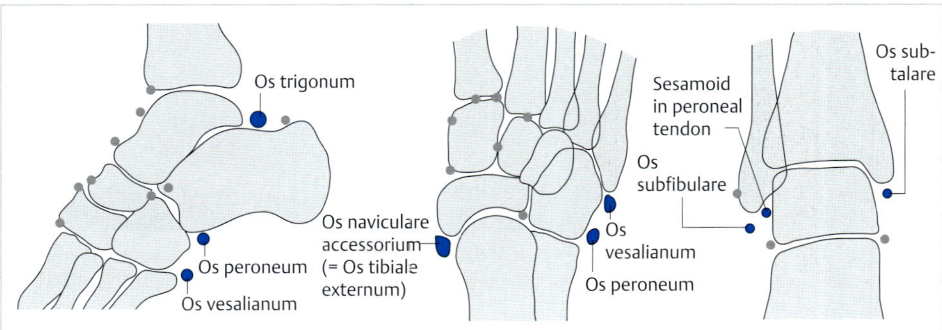

Fig. 2.386 Accessory bones of the ankle and tarsus.

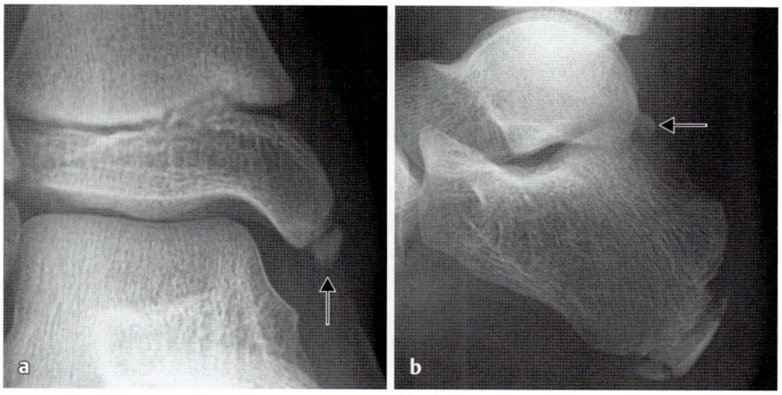

Fig. 2.387 Anatomical variants that could be mistaken for sequelae of trauma. **(a)** Separate ossification nucleus of the medial malleolus (arrow). **(b)** Multiple nuclei of the apophysis of the calcaneus and os trigonum (arrow).

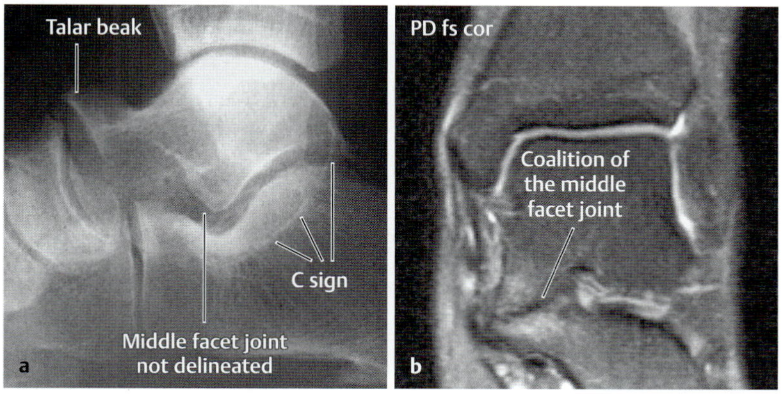

Fig. 2.388 Talocalcaneal coalition. **(a)** Typical radiographic signs on the lateral image. **(b)** Discrete bone marrow edema at the site of the coalition (middle subtalar facet).

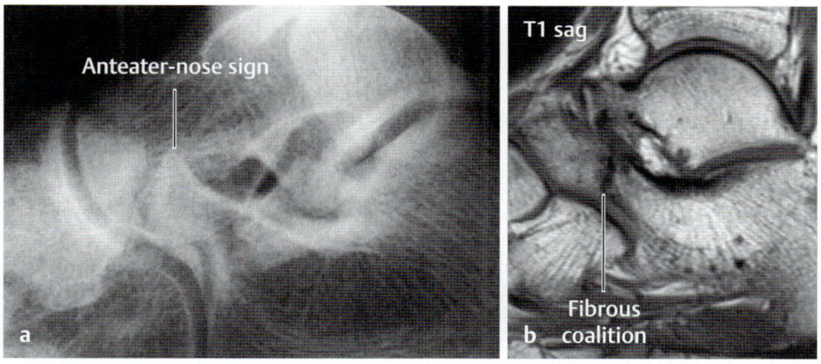

Fig. 2.389 Calcaneonavicular coalition. **(a)** Anteater nose sign on the lateral radiograph. **(b)** Sagittal MRI demonstrates a fibrous coalition.

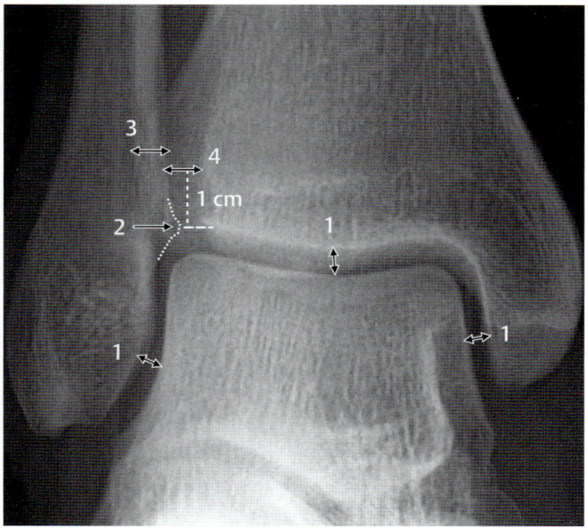

Fig. 2.390 Radiological parameters for assessing the correct positioning of the tibiotalar joint. Radiograph with 15° internal rotation. 1, regular joint space width; 2, Weber's nose; 3, tibiofibular overlap; 4, tibiofibular clear space.

▸ **US.** Assessment of the lateral ligament structures, the anterior syndesmosis, and tendons is possible using ultrasound, which has the advantage of allowing a dynamic examination. An effusion within the ankle joint is easily detected.

▸ **CT.** CT is used for equivocal radiological findings or for complex fractures.

▸ **MRI.** MRI is indicated for suspected ligament or tendon injuries, as well as for assessing the cartilage and occult osseous pathology.

2.15.2 Fractures of the (True) Ankle Joint

These are caused by a (transient) dislocation of the ankle (talocrural) joint, which is often associated with injuries to the collateral ligaments and the tibiofibular syndesmosis (Chapter 2.15.9).

Fractures of the ankle joint are classified according to the **AO system** (http://www.aofoundation.org). The AO classification system combines the **classification system proposed by Danis and Weber**, which assesses fractures of the distal fibula with respect to the syndesmosis, and the **Lauge-Hansen classification system,** which combines fracture morphology with the pathomechanism. For daily clinical use, the classification according to Danis and Weber is still commonly used internationally and is supplemented with descriptive subdivisions into uni-, bi-, and trimalleolar fractures, allowing conclusions to be drawn regarding possible associated injuries (▸ Fig. 2.391 and ▸ Table 2.7). The posterior tibial margin is regarded as a third malleolus and, when avulsed, is known as **"Volkmann's triangle."** ▶ Images illustrating the various fracture types can be found in ▸ Figs. W2.72–W2.75.

Variants of fractures of the ankle joint

- **Tillaux–Chaput fracture:** Bony avulsion of the anterior tibiofibular ligament at the anterolateral tibial margin (▸ Fig. 2.392).

Table 2.7 Concomitant injuries associated with fractures of the lateral malleolus

Danis/Weber	Type A	Type B	Type C
Syndesmotic injury	Never	Possible	Always
Injury to the interosseous membrane	Never	Never	Common, up to the fracture level
Fracture of the medial malleolus or medial ligament tear	Possible	Possible	Always

- **Wagstaffe facture**: Bony avulsion of the anterior talofibular syndesmosis from the fibula.
- **Maisonneuve fracture:** Combination of a proximal fibular shaft fracture with a tear of the anterior syndesmosis and disruption of the interosseous membrane (▶ Fig. W2.76).

In **children**, fractures of the ankle joint are usually classified with reference to the epiphysis according to Aitken or Salter–Harris (Chapter 1.3.1).

2.15.3 Osteochondral Lesions of the Talus

Note

- Osteochondral lesions are not rare, occurring in 1 to 5% of all ankle injuries.
- The majority of acute osteochondral lesions are radiologically occult.

Acute Articular Fractures of the Talar Shoulder

▸ **Pathology.** These are impaction or shear fractures of the lateral or medial shoulders of the talar dome. The articular cartilage and subchondral bone are involved. There is a clear association with trauma.

▸ **XR/CT.** Elongated, oval-shaped, or triangular fragments are observed running parallel, or slightly oblique, to the joint surface (▸ Fig. 2.393). These may come to lie "upside down" within the fragment bed and may rarely be displaced. In some cases, only a mild depression of the joint surface may be present without a fragment.

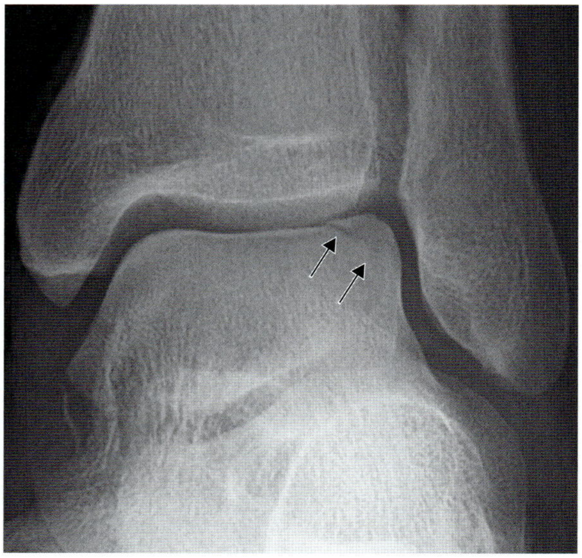

Fig. 2.393 Acute shear fracture (arrows) of the lateral talar shoulder.

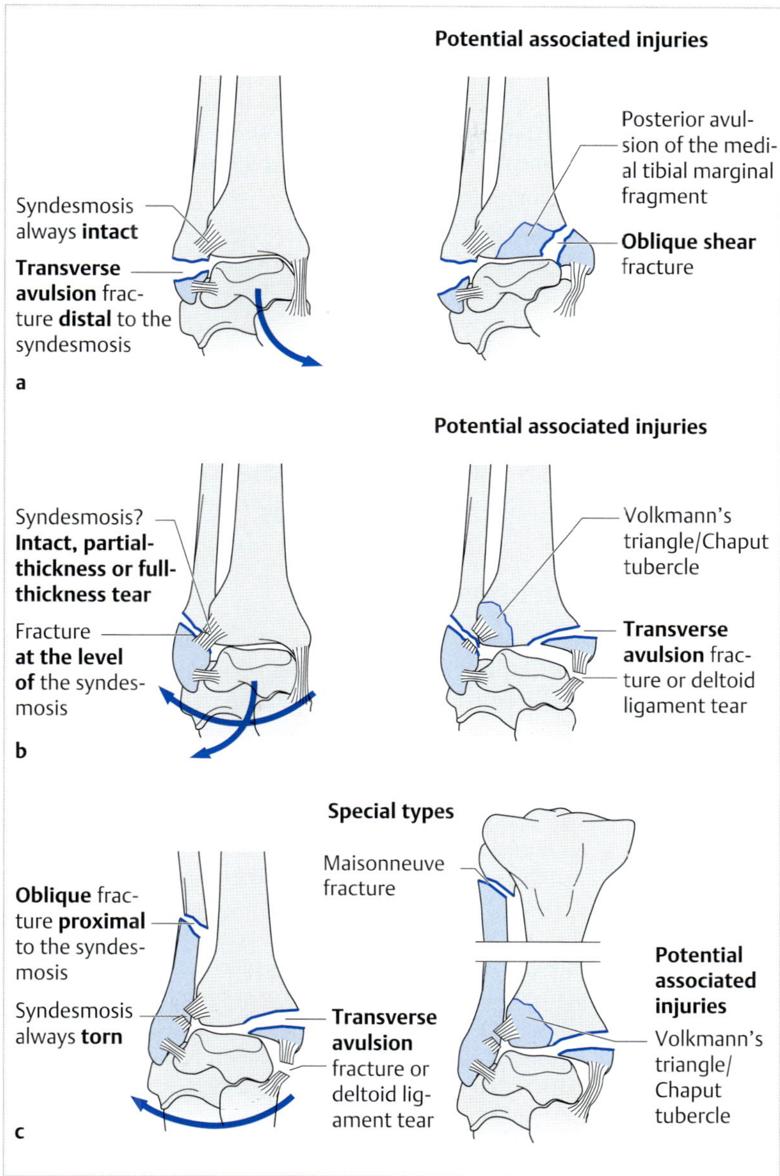

Fig. 2.391 Schematic diagram of ankle fractures according to Danis and Weber, including common associated injuries. **(a)** Type A: adduction of the talus with the foot supinated. **(b)** Type B: external rotation of the talus with the foot supinated or abduction of the talus with the foot pronated. **(c)** Type C: external rotation of the talus with the foot pronated.

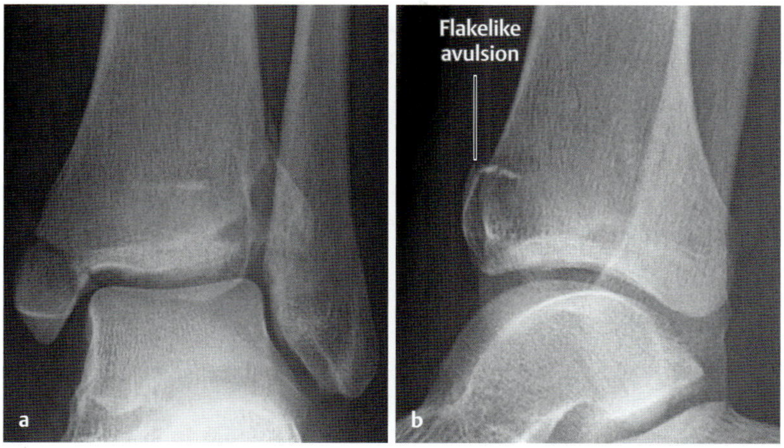

Fig. 2.392 Tillaux–Chaput fracture. Bony tibial avulsion of the anterior syndesmosis. **(a)** Fracture of the lateral tibia at the level of the syndesmosis. There is an additional fracture of the medial malleolus. **(b)** The lateral view confirms the anterior position and morphology of the avulsion fracture.

▸ **MRI.** On the whole, only subchondral signal alterations (typically increased signal intensity on fluid-sensitive sequences) are evident directly beneath the joint surface. The thin articular cartilage is often difficult to evaluate because of the limited resolution obtained with the majority of MRI scanners Larger cartilage defects are usually evident (▸ Fig. 2.394). As with radiography or CT, it should be possible to distinguish corresponding fragments or osteochondral impaction of the talus with MRI.

▸ **Important findings.** If an osteochondral lesion is identified after an acute injury (e.g., fracture of the talus), then the age of the lesion should be estimated (acute or chronic). This will affect treatment decisions since an acute lesion will usually be addressed more quickly, while a chronic osteochondral lesion might not be addressed until after the talar fracture heals (see the next subsection).

Chronic Osteochondral Lesions of the Talar Dome

▸ **Pathology.** Many of these patients do not recall a specific traumatic event. Nevertheless, thickening/scarring of the ankle ligaments suggests an old ankle injury. The medial talar dome is more commonly involved. These lesions indicate an incomplete posttraumatic recovery, and these may be associated with small necrotic fragments. The term "osteonecrosis" is *not* appropriate for bony remodeling and defects in these cases; it should be reserved for complications of talar neck and body fractures.

▸ **Radiography/CT.** The following features are found in traumatic osteochondral lesions:

- Mild depression of the subchondral bone plate.
- Craterlike defect of the joint surface with sclerotic margin.
- Diffuse sclerosis of the subchondral bone along the margin of the talar dome (▸ Fig. 2.395).
- Juxta-articular radiolucencies ("cysts"; see ▸ Fig. 2.395).

With **osteochondritis dissecans**, on the other hand, a rounded osteochondral fragment with an opposing fragment bed is seen, surrounded by a sclerotic margin (▸ Fig. 2.396).

▸ **MRI.** With posttraumatic lesions, MRI may reveal regions of cartilage damage (provided the spatial resolution is high), hypointense fragments, and a varied picture of diffuse sclerotic changes and subchondral cystic foci on fluid-sensitive sequences (▸ Fig. 2.397).

With **osteochondritis dissecans,** the osteochondral fragment is fat-containing or hypointense on T1W sequences (sclerotic). Increased signal intensity may be present on T2W images, and fluid or contrast (in the case of an MR arthrogram) may extend between an unstable osteochondral fragment and fragment bed (▸ Fig. 2.398).

> **Note**
> Arthrography combined with CT (CT arthrography) is currently the gold standard for assessing the articular surface of the talus in the presence of chronic osteochondral lesions (▸ Fig. 2.399).

2.15.4 Fractures of the Talus and Calcaneus

Fractures of the Talus

▸ **Pathology.** Fractures of the talus usually result from an axial loading injury. A shearing component is usually the cause of osteochondral fractures of the talar dome.

The talus has a precarious vascular supply, for which reason posttraumatic osteonecrosis is a common complication of a talar fracture. The probability of developing avascular necrosis is directly related to the degree of fracture displacement and this is taken into account in all fracture classifications.

A distinction is made between fractures of the talar neck (about 50% of fractures) and body (about 25%) and peripheral fractures involving the lateral or posterior processes of the talus or the talar dome (in total about 25%). The ICI (Integral Classification of Injuries) classification is a comprehensive classification system, but is impractical for daily clinical practice. On the other hand, the classification of vertical **talar neck fractures** according to **Hawkins** is clinically useful and commonly employed (▸ Figs. 2.400–2.402).

Using this system, the fracture type is strongly correlated with the risk of developing **posttraumatic osteonecrosis:** 10% for Type I, 40% for Type II, 90% for Type III, and 100% for Type IV.

> **Note**
> **Fractures of the talar body** always involve the tibiotalar and/or subtalar joint surfaces, but are not easily differentiated from talar neck fractures, which are, by definition, extra-articular and are located anterior to the lateral process of the talus. This is especially true for comminuted fractures. A fracture of the talus is (with the exception of Type 1; ▸ Fig. 2.402) an emergency requiring immediate surgical management.

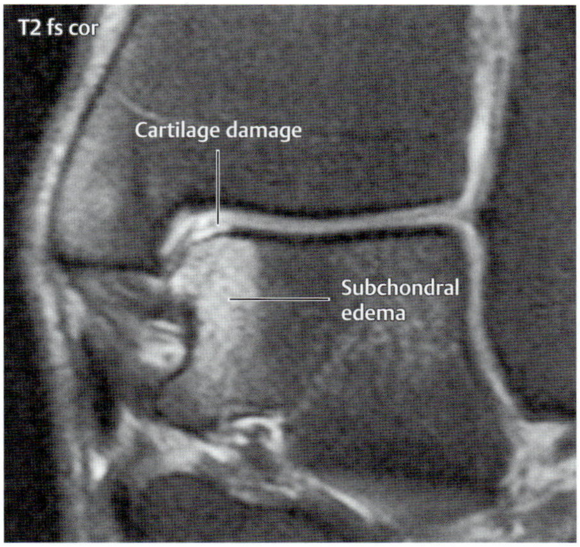

Fig. 2.394 Acute osteochondral lesion with cartilage damage, minimal impaction and subchondral edema.

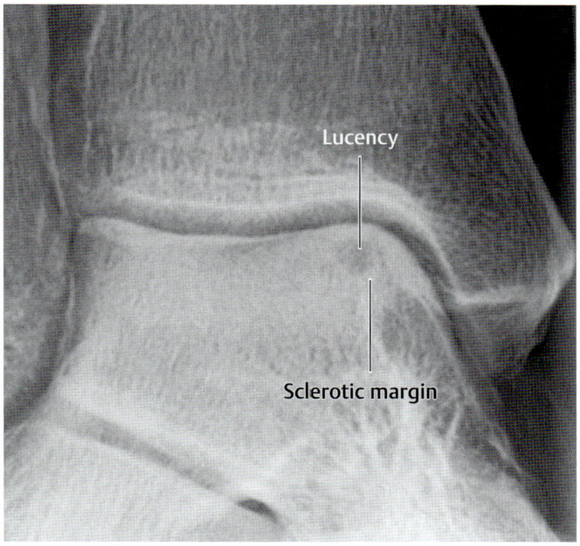

Fig. 2.395 Rounded subchondral lucency at the medial talar shoulder with sclerotic margin. Classic chronic posttraumatic appearance.

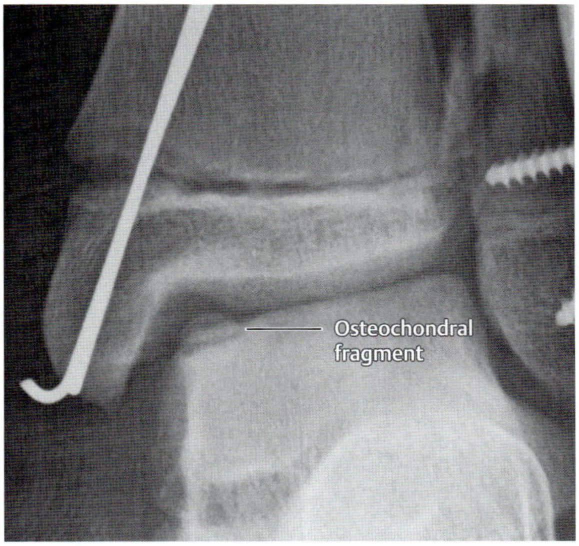

Fig. 2.396 Appearance after reduction and fixation of fractures of the distal tibial epiphysis and lateral malleolus. The osteochondrosis dissecans at the medial talar shoulder is not related to the acute fractures.

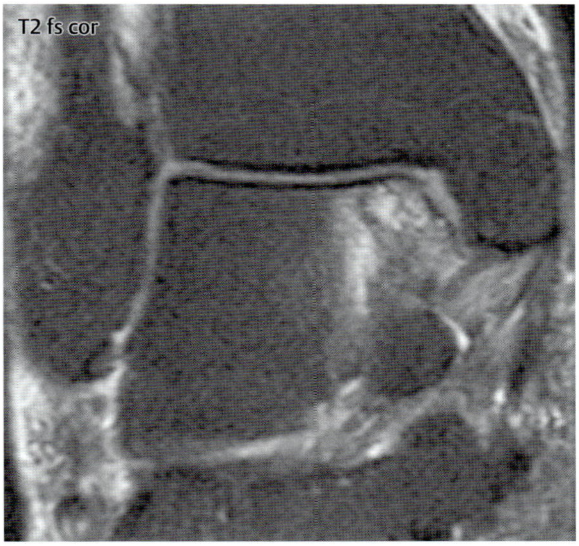

Fig. 2.397 Subchondral cystic foci in the medial talar shoulder. There had been pain for the previous 2 years, with no recollection of injury, but this is most likely posttraumatic in origin.

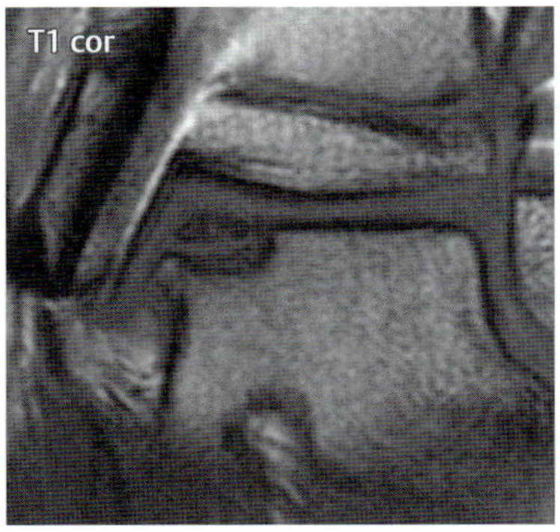

Fig. 2.398

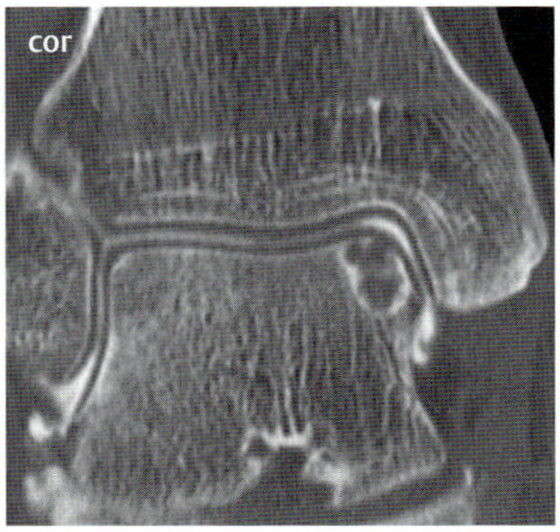

Fig. 2.399

Fig. 2.398 Osteochondritis dissecans of the medial talar shoulder. The osteochondral fragment is hypointense as a sign of osteosclerosis. The same patient as in ► Fig. 2.396.

Fig. 2.399 Osteochondral lesion before treatment. CT arthrography. The cartilage is completely intact.

▸ **Radiography/CT/MRT.** For suspected talar fractures, the conventional radiographic examination should include imaging of the ankle joint in two projections and of the foot in three (dorsoplantar, oblique, and strict lateral). CT imaging should also be obtained in every case of proven (or even strongly suspected) talar fracture. MR imaging may be useful in the case of an older fracture (older than 4–6 weeks) to assess osseous viability.

Talar head fractures usually occur with complex talar fractures.

Fractures of the **posterior talus** and the **lateral process of the talus** (▸ Fig. 2.403) are distinguished from fractures of the talar body. For example, **snowboarder fracture** refers to a nondisplaced fracture of the lateral process of the talus, and a **shepherd fracture** is a fracture of the lateral tubercle of the posterior process of the talus, which should not be confused with an os trigonum. CT should be used for optimal fracture assessment since surgical management is pursued with fracture displacement of as little as 1 to 2 mm in adults and 5 mm in children.

Fractures of the Calcaneus

▸ **Pathology.** A distinction is made between extra- and intra-articular fractures of the calcaneus. **Extra-articular fractures** (~ 30% of cases) can occur at the anterior process, the posterior tuberosity, in the body below the posterior articular facet, and at the medial sustentaculum (▸ Fig. 2.404). A **duck-bill fracture** occurs when the Achilles tendon removes the superior part of the posterior tuberosity (▸ Fig. 2.405).

> **Note**
>
> A duckbill fracture of the calcaneus is an emergency because of the associated soft tissue compression (▸ Fig. 2.405) which, without immediate surgical intervention, may lead to soft tissue necrosis.

Intra-articular fractures of the calcaneus (▸ Fig. 2.406) occur as a result of a vertical impact on the foot, which thrusts the middle part of the talus, including its lateral process, like a wedge onto the calcaneus.

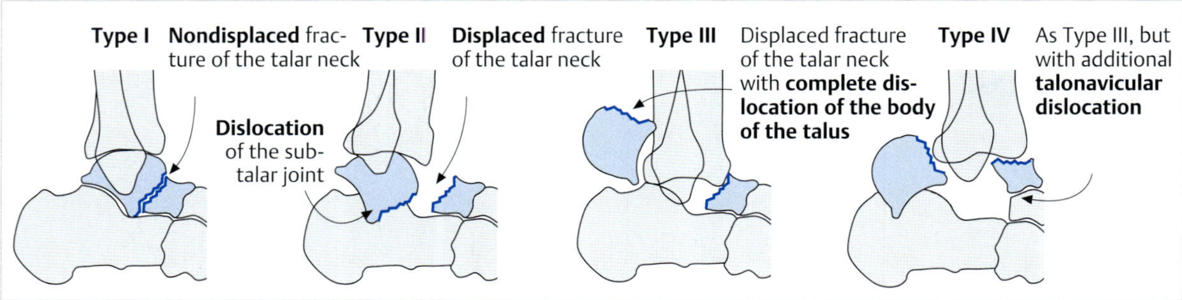

Fig. 2.400 The Hawkins classification of fractures of the talar neck. STJ, subtalar joint.

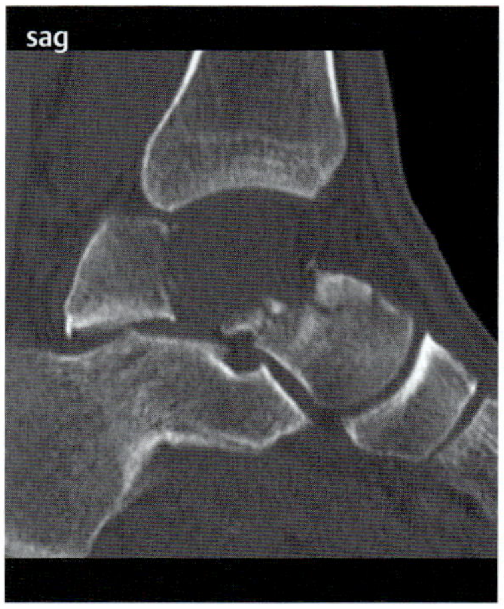

Fig. 2.401 Talar fracture, Hawkins Type III. Displacement of the posterior talar fragment relative to the ankle and subtalar joints.

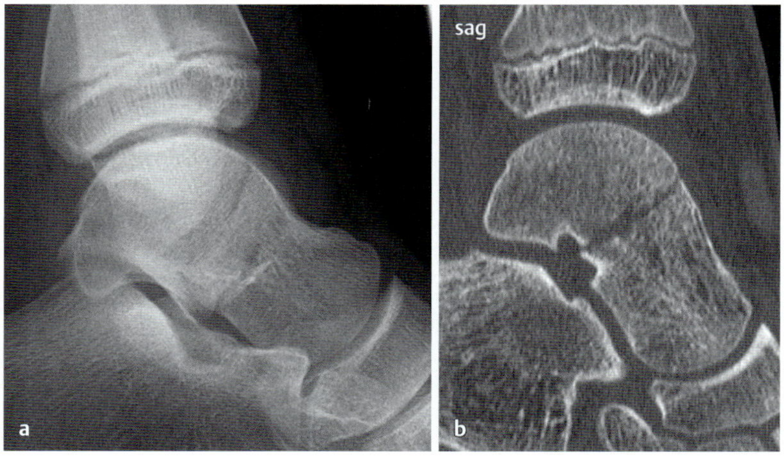

Fig. 2.402 Nondisplaced fracture of the talar body. The fracture line lies dorsal to the lateral process of the talus; it is therefore not a fracture of the talar neck. **(a)** Radiolucent line through the anterior talar body. **(b)** No dislocation of the ankle and subtalar joint.

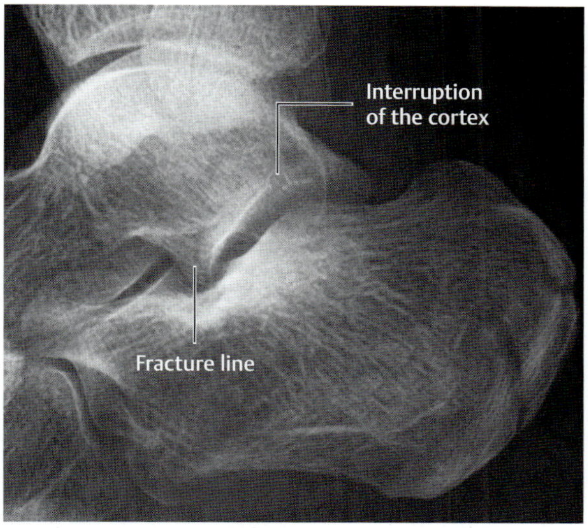

Fig. 2.403 Fracture of the lateral process of the talus and posterior part of the calcaneus.

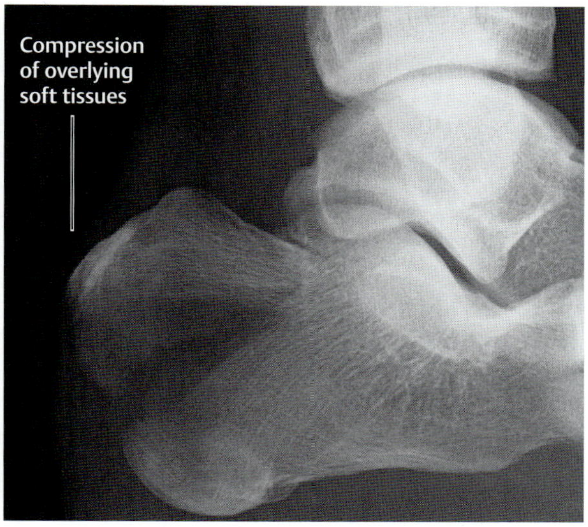

Fig. 2.405 Duck-bill fracture of the calcaneus.

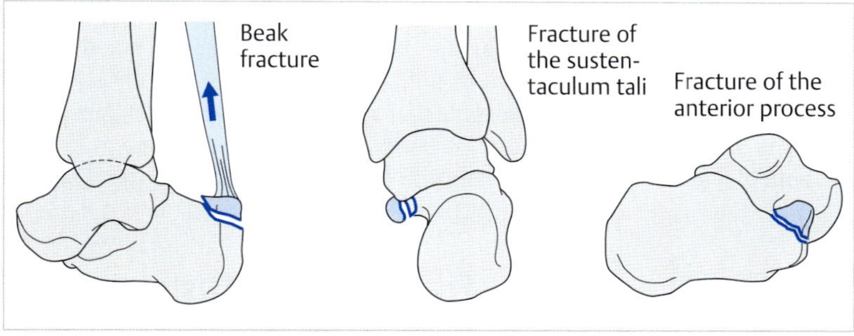

◀ **Fig. 2.404** Extra-articular calcaneus fractures (without involvement of the subtalar joint surface).

Fig. 2.406 (a–c) Intra-articular calcaneus fracture with involvement of the subtalar joint surface (according to Essex-Lopresti). Major fragments: 1, posterior facet fragment; 2, tuberal fragment; 3, sustentacular fragment; 4, anterior process fragment. ▼

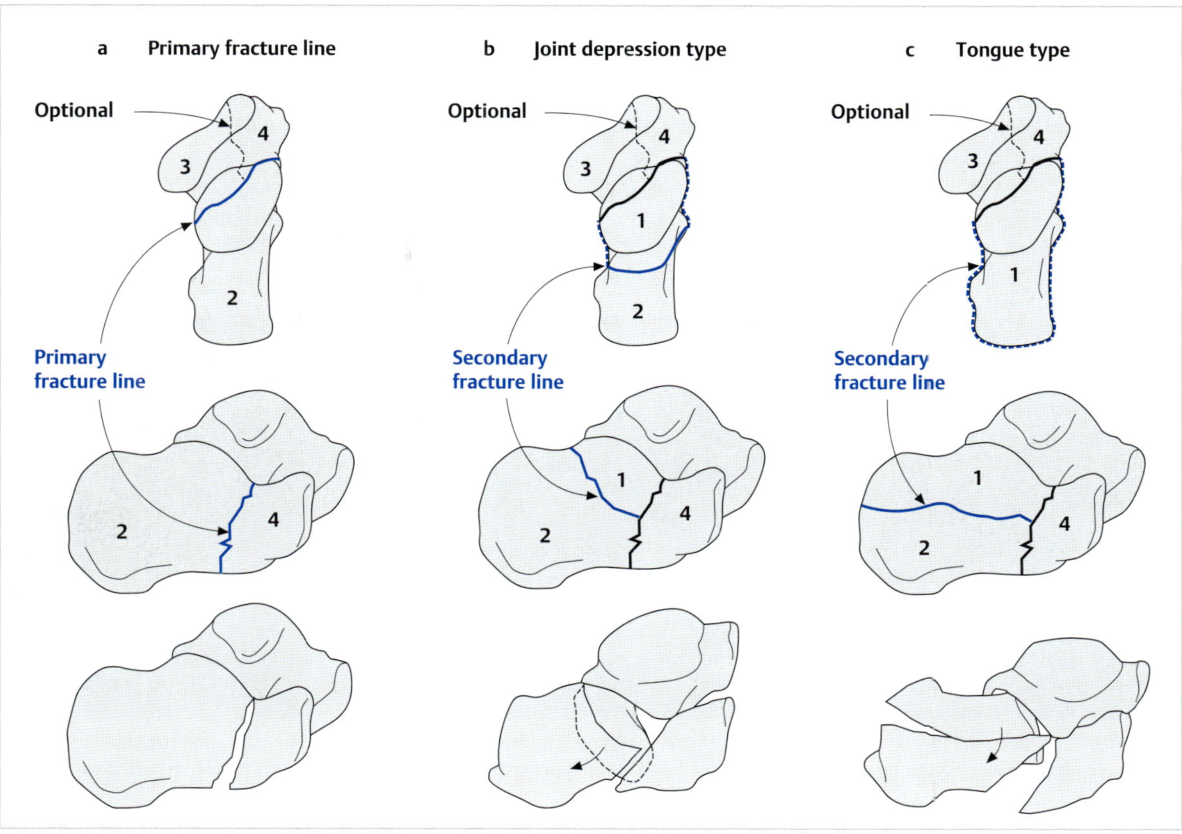

This results in a shear fracture because the weight-bearing axis is always somewhat medially displaced and never centrally. As a result, the medial part of the calcaneus (major sustentacular fragment) remains practically undisplaced beneath the talus, while the lateral part of the calcaneus is displaced cranially past the talus and is compressed along with the joint surface. Secondary and tertiary fracture lines form if the compression energy is not exhausted at the time of the initial shear fracture. If the secondary fracture line runs superiorly around the subtalar joint surface, then (according to Essex-Lopresti) it is a **joint-depression type fracture** (▶ Fig. 2.407). In this case the superolateral fragment and the posterior facet remain attached to the tuberosity posteriorly. If the fracture line runs posteriorly and exits posteriorly to the cortex of the posterior tuberosity, then it is a **tongue-type fracture** (▶ Fig. 2.408), producing a tongue-shaped posterior facet fragment. In both cases, the posterior facet fragment is impacted and rotated into the tuberosity fragment and may also be fractured within itself. This results in widening of the talus with loss of height and rotation of the tuberosity out of the weight-bearing axis of tibia and talus (Saltzmann view, see ▶ Fig. 2.410).

Apart from the classification according to Essex-Lopresti, which is still clinically in use, there is also the complex ICI classification and the CT-based system according to Sanders (▶ see references to Chapters 2.15.1–2.15.4), both of which are utilized in certain centers.

▶ **Radiography.** Radiographs are obtained in three views (calcaneus lateral, axial, and foot dorsoplantar to depict the calcaneocuboid joint). An important parameter for assessing the fracture position of the subtalar joint is **Boehler's angle** (**"tuber angle"**) (▶ Fig. 2.409), which should also be determined for the contralateral side since it is subject to significant variability between individuals. The Saltzmann view allows for assessment of the axial alignment of the tibia, talus and calcaneus (▶ Fig. 2.410).

▶ **CT.** CT, with triplanar reconstructions, is essential for precise evaluation of the fracture, given that an articular step-off of as little as 1 mm is considered an indication for surgical management.

▶ **Important findings.** Assessment of the subtalar joint surface (step-offs as well as the size, number, and position of fragments) after fracture of the calcaneus is of paramount significance for preoperative planning. Furthermore, alignment of the calcaneus relative to the weight-bearing axis must be documented.

Calcaneal Stress Fractures

A calcaneal stress fracture is a hairline crack or fracture in the calcaneus. The cause may be overuse injury ("fatigue fracture"), which was originally seen mostly in soldiers marching long distances carrying heavy weights. However, these fractures are also seen in long distance runners, ballet dancers, and sports involving jumping. They are the second most common stress fracture of the foot after navicular stress fractures. Insufficiency fractures are seen in the elderly (see Chapter 1.5).

Often a radiograph of the injured bone will not show any sign of fracture until the fracture has actually started to heal. It is possible that a stress fracture will not appear on a radiograph at all. Bone scans and MRI scans are more likely to be of assistance in diagnosing a calcaneal stress fracture (see Chapter 1.5).

2.15.5 Fractures and Dislocations of the Tarsal Bones

Technique

Conventional radiographic evaluation of fractures and dislocations of the tarsal bones should include plain views of the foot in three projections (dorsoplantar, oblique, and strict lateral), possibly supplemented by radiographs of the ankle in two planes. Supplementary diagnostic CT imaging is usually indicated to better assess complex injuries and for preoperative planning.

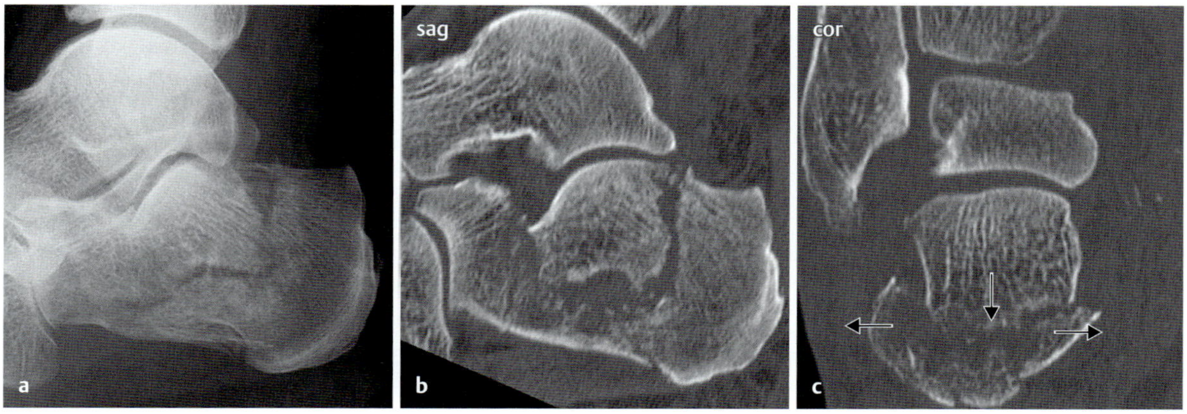

Fig. 2.407 Calcaneus fracture of the joint depression type. **(a)** Fragment involving the posterior facet of the joint. **(b)** The fragment is clearly compressed in a plantar direction. **(c)** The coronal projection demonstrates the resulting impaction and bursting (arrows) of the calcaneus.

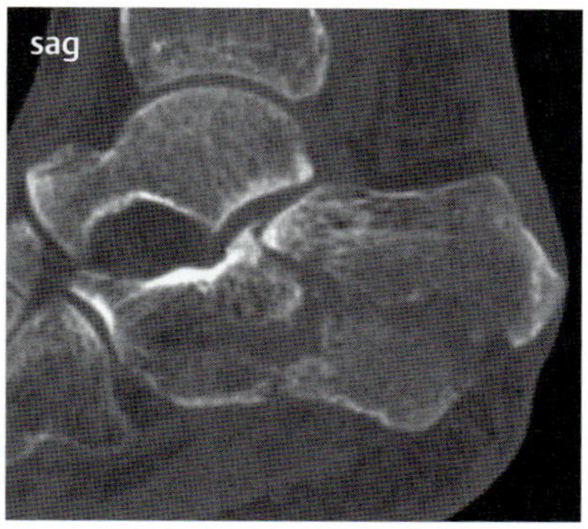

Fig. 2.408 Calcaneal tongue-type fracture.

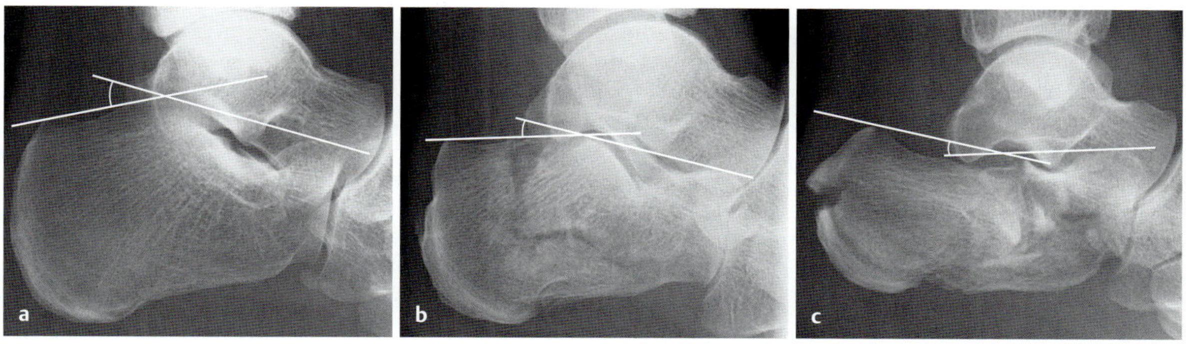

Fig. 2.409 Boehler angle. The angle formed between a line connecting the highest point of the calcaneal tuberosity and the posterior margin of the subtalar joint surface with a line from there to the highest point of the anterior process should be between +20° and +40°. **(a)** Normal finding (here +26°). **(b)** Joint-depression calcaneal fracture. Decreased Boehler angle (here +16°). **(c)** Calcaneal tongue-type fracture. Pathologic negative Boehler angle (here −15°).

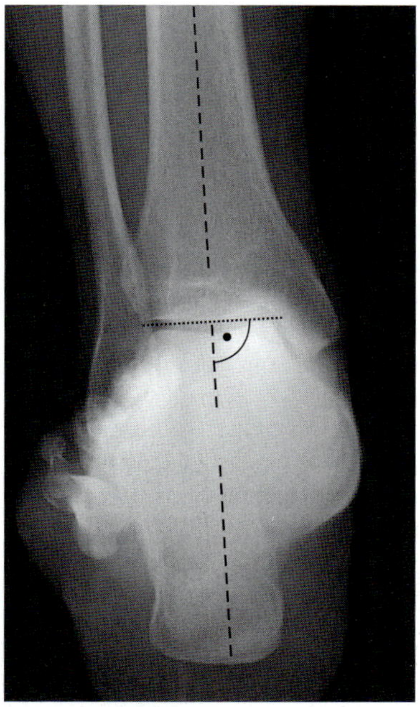

Fig. 2.410 Saltzmann view to assess axial alignment between tibia, talus, and calcaneus demonstrates normal relationships.

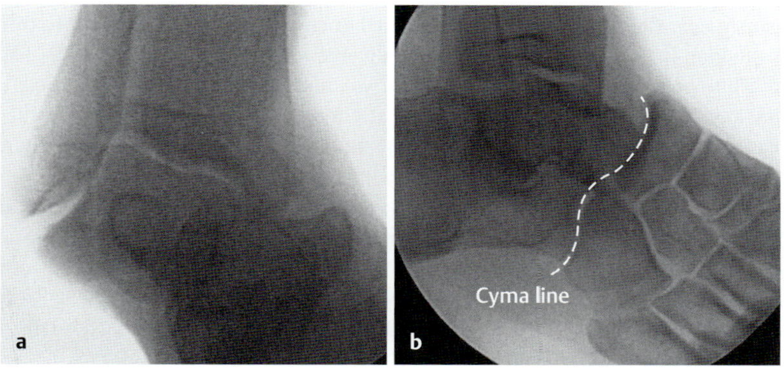

Fig. 2.411 Subtalar dislocation of the foot. Fluoroscopic images. **(a)** AP view: medial dislocation of the subtalar joint. **(b)** Lateral view (slightly tilted): talonavicular dislocation. The Cyma line (between talonavicular and calcaneocuboid bones) shows the normal calcaneocuboid articulation.

Total dislocation of the talus. In this rare injury, the entire capsule–ligament complex is disrupted at the ankle joint, taking with it the dislocated tendons. These dislocations are usually open and associated with a significant degree of soft tissue damage. Unlike a fracture-dislocation of the ankle, the ankle mortise is intact or there are only smaller bony avulsions present.

Subtalar dislocation. Unlike total talar dislocation, the talus remains in the ankle mortise with this type of talar dislocation. After disruption of the strong talocalcaneal ligament and the joint capsule of the subtalar joint, the calcaneus dislocates medially at the subtalar joint. An important distinguishing feature in comparison with Chopart's fracture-dislocation, however, is the fact that the calcaneus remains in contact with the anterior portion of the foot. The cyma line is preserved on the lateral radiograph in a case of a talonavicular dislocation (▶ Fig. 2.411).

Chopart's fracture-dislocation. Compared with a subtalar dislocation of the foot, Chopart's fracture-dislocation is a dislocation of the talus from the talonavicular joint with a concomitant dislocation of the calcaneocuboid joint (▶ Fig. 2.412). These injuries commonly demonstrate spontaneous reduction, often resulting in only minimal radiographic findings, best detected by CT (widened or eccentric joint space, bony avulsions of the ligament; ▶ Fig. 2.413).

Lisfranc fracture-dislocation. Lisfranc injuries are usually fractures/dislocations of varying degrees, with fractures usually near the base of the second to fourth metatarsals. A distinction is made between convergent, divergent (relative to a line between the first and second rays), and isolated first-ray dislocations. The main focus of attention must be placed on the Lisfranc ligament. In a large number of cases this ligament is avulsed along with a bony fragment, usually from the base of the second metatarsal (▶ Fig. 2.414), less commonly from the base of the first. Unless proven otherwise, fractures of the base of the second to fourth metatarsals are strongly suspicious for a prior Lisfranc fracture-dislocation. Here too, the radiographic findings can be very subtle and easily overlooked, which is why CT is often indicated in this scenario.

Isolated tarsal dislocations. Unlike Chopart and Lisfranc injuries, these unusual injuries are the result not of a distortion mechanism but of direct force. They are often combined with severe soft tissue damage; a secondary compartment syndrome is not uncommon.

Fractures of the tarsus. Isolated tarsal fractures are rare, so a search should always be made for associated injuries or dislocations. *Navicular fractures* are usually bony avulsions. Fractures of the navicular body are usually the result of high-velocity injuries and they may severely affect the biomechanics of the foot. For this reason even mild axial shortening (> 2 mm) and articular incongruity of > 1 mm are of clinical importance. Posttraumatic osteonecrosis is common.

Stress fractures of the tarsus. These are not uncommon in athletes and most often involve the navicular at the junction between its middle and lateral thirds, where significant force from the head of the talus is applied to this area of relatively poor bone perfusion. Patients present nonspecific pain in the midfoot. These fractures are difficult to detect on conventional radiographs and MRI is the modality of choice if one is clinically suspected.

▶ **Important findings.** It is important to carefully evaluate the appearance and alignment of the tarsal bones at the Chopart and Lisfranc joints, which are essential for maintaining an even load distribution.

2.15.6 Fractures and Dislocations of the Forefoot

Fractures of the second to fourth metatarsals are treated conservatively in the absence of any rotational deformity of the toes. On the other hand, surgical repair of the first and fifth metatarsals is indicated to prevent transfer pain in the forefoot.

Fractures of the metatarsal bones. Metatarsal fractures are the most common factures of the foot. Traumatic fractures most commonly involve the first and fifth metatarsals. A common injury is *bony avulsion of the peroneus tendon* from the tuberosity of the proximal fifth metatarsal, often involving the fifth tarsometatarsal joint. The *Jones fracture* is adjacent to this, at the base of the fifth metatarsal at the metaphyseal–diaphyseal junction. Also known as "dancer's fracture," it does not involve the tarsometatarsal joint; however, this fracture is prone to nonunion—particularly after conservative therapy (▶ Fig. 2.415).

Stress fractures in the region of the metatarsus and forefoot. These are among the most common stress fractures and primarily involve the shafts of the second to fourth metatarsals. Patients often present later when radiographs already demonstrate callus formation (▶ Fig. 1.43).

Dislocations of the metatarsophalangeal joints and interdigital dislocations. These can be usually treated with closed reduction under local anesthesia, but entrapment of a palmar plate, or an extensor or flexor tendon, may inhibit reduction of a metatarsophalangeal joint. A sign of inadequate reduction is a widened joint space with dislocation of the toes.

Sesamoids. Sesamoids can fracture as a result of trauma; they are also a common site for fatigue fractures. A bipartite sesamoid is a common congenital variant (especially of the medial sesamoid) that may mimic a fracture. A tangential view of the foot is helpful for assessing sesamoids on a radiograph; if radiographic findings are equivocal, sectional imaging (CT or MRI) may be helpful (▶ Fig. 1.50).

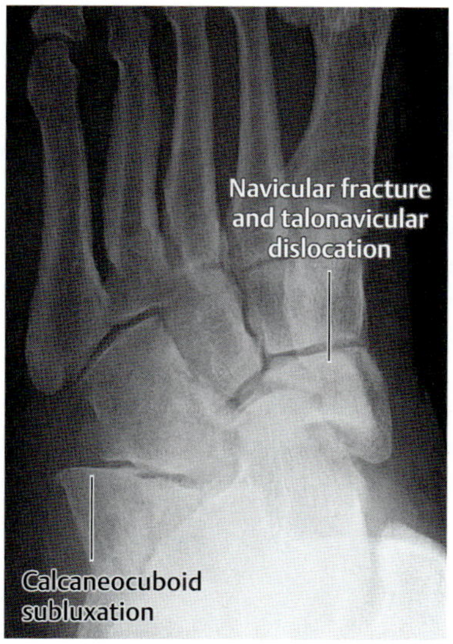

Fig. 2.412 Chopart's fracture-dislocation.

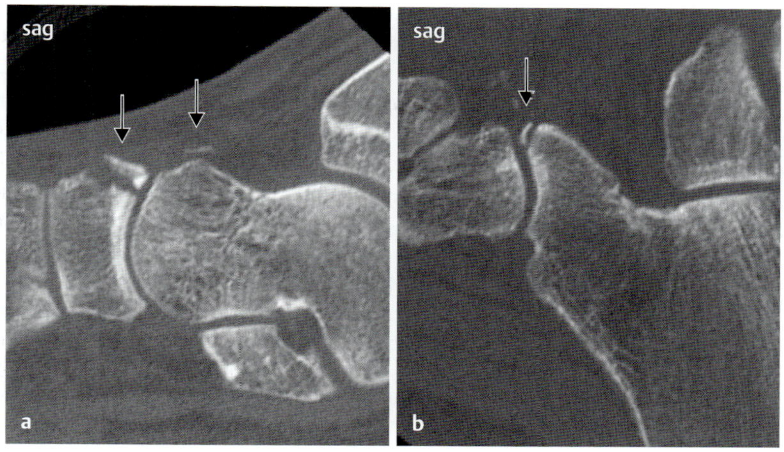

Fig. 2.413 Signs of prior Chopart fracture-dislocation following spontaneous reduction. **(a)** Talonavicular ligament avulsion fractures (arrows). **(b)** Bony avulsion (arrow) of the anterior process of the calcaneus.

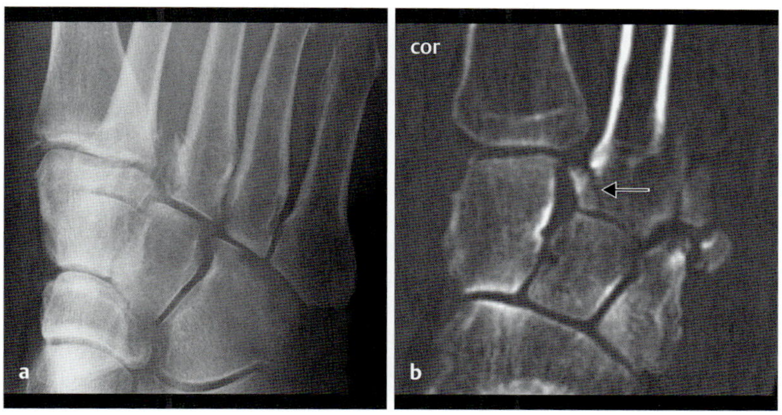

Fig. 2.414 Lisfranc fracture-dislocation. **(a)** Multiple small fracture fragments of the first to fifth rays with offset of the third tarsometatarsal joint. **(b)** CT confirms the bony avulsion of the Lisfranc ligament from the base of the second metatarsal (arrow).

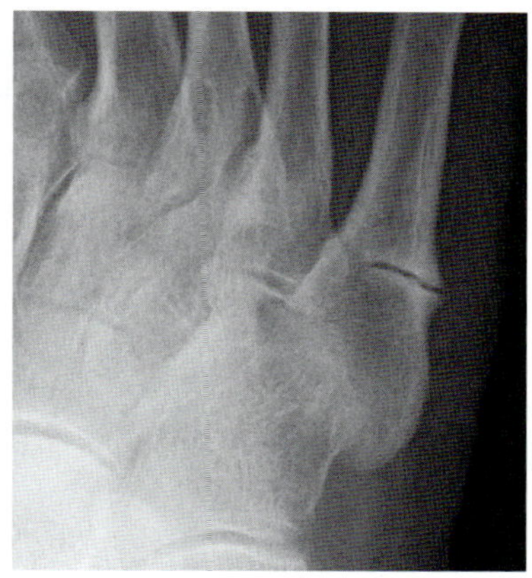

Fig. 2.415 An ununited fifth metatarsal (Jones) fracture that had occurred 2 years previously.

▶ **Important findings.** With fractures and dislocations of the forefoot, the integrity of the first and fifth rays is critical as they are the main weight-bearers in the foot. Any length or rotational deformity of these metatarsals should be reported.

2.15.7 Radiological Assessment after Surgery of the Ankle and Foot

Ankle

▶ **Radiography.** Well-positioned views are essential for proper evaluation (Chapter 2.15.1).

Postoperative radiographic evaluation must address the following:

- *Position of the malleoli* (▶ Fig. 2.416)? The medial and lateral malleoli must be superimposed on the lateral view.
- *Width of the ankle mortise?* Evaluate the distance between fibula and tibial tubercle, posterior to the fibular notch (< 6 mm) and the distance between the malleoli and talus (▶ Fig. 2.417).
- *Screw position* (▶ Figs. 2.418 and ▶ 2.419)? The proximal screws of a plated lateral malleolus must reach and extend slightly beyond the far cortex. The screws at the level of the talus and syndesmosis should be positioned within the bone.
- *Articular incongruity, loose bodies within the joint, any separate fragments* (▶ Fig. 2.420)?

Foot

Tarsal bones. Management of *calcaneal fractures* includes anatomical reduction of fragments, restoring the position of the tuberosity with regard to the mechanical axis, and the Boehlert angle (tuber angle). Posttraumatic osteoarthritis of the subtalar joint is a common complication. *Anatomical reduction of tarsal fractures* is critical because of their important role in supporting the longitudinal and transverse arches of the foot. Even a small degree of shortening (impaction) should be mentioned in the radiological report.

Forefoot. In the forefoot, it is important to document that length has been maintained after reconstruction of the first and fifth rays and to assess any rotational deformities of the metatarsals (▶ Fig. 2.421).

2.15.8 Acquired Malalignments

Splay foot. Splay foot (pes transvers planus), involves loss of the normal transverse arch at the level of the ball of the foot that results in spreading of the metatarsals. Clinical presentation includes plantar calluses beneath the second and third metatarsophalangeal joints. The main cause is certain types of shoes—pumps (i.e., court shoes) in particular. Loading of the forefoot increases to five times normal in high-heeled shoes as the transverse arch of the forefoot is pressed down into the shoe. Splay foot is also a risk factor for developing a hallux valgus deformity. A complication of chronic splay foot is irritation of the plantar nerves, which may result in the development of metatarsal neuralgia (Morton's neuralgia; see Chapter 2.15.16).

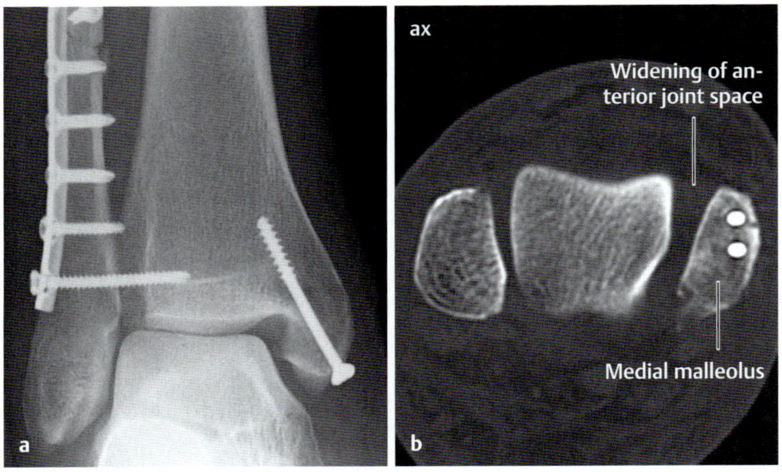

Fig. 2.416 Presentation after fixation of a bimalleolar fracture. **(a)** Incongruence of the articular surface of the medial malleolus. **(b)** The medial malleolus has been stabilized in an externally rotated position.

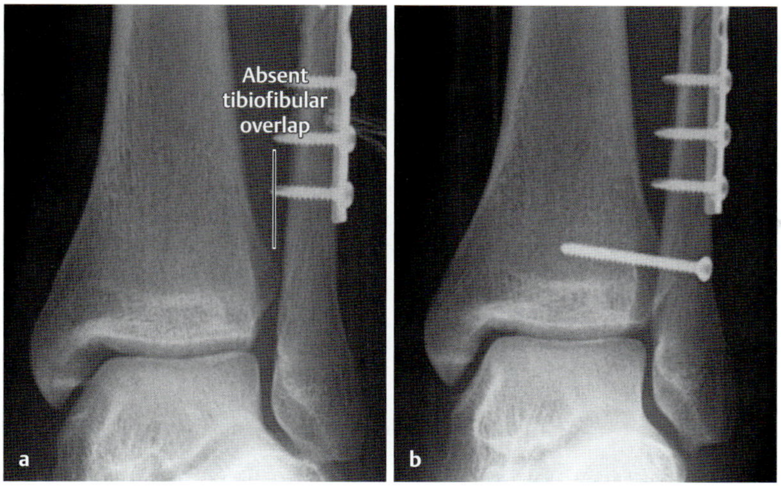

Fig. 2.417 Weber C fracture of the lateral malleolus. **(a)** The postoperative radiograph displays widening of the syndesmosis. Widening of the space between the medial malleolus and talus is an additional sign of disruption of the syndesmosis but remains concealed because the leg is excessively internally rotated. **(b)** The radiographic evaluation after insertion of an additional syndesmotic screw is ideal.

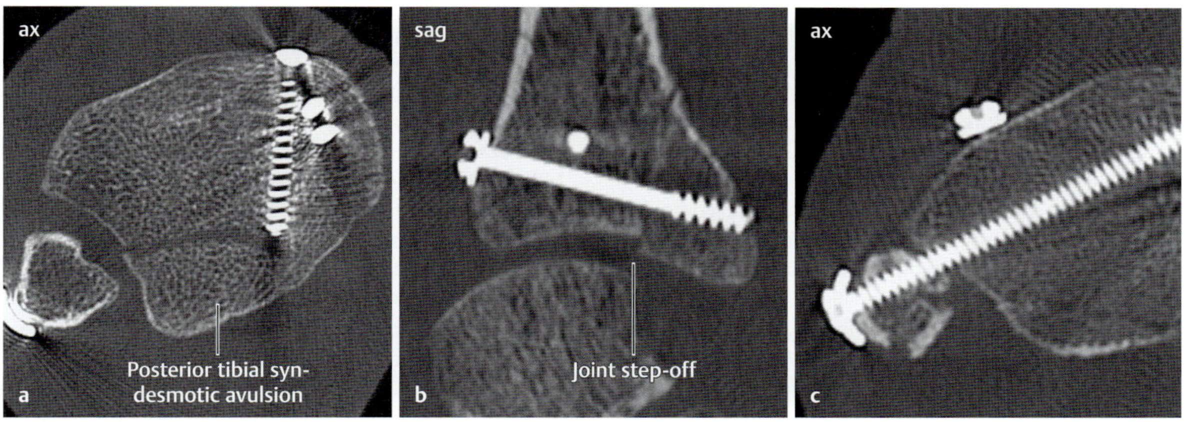

Fig. 2.418 Ankle fracture with an avulsion of the posterior malleolus. **(a)** The posterior tibial fragment was not engaged anteriorly by the screw during the primary procedure. **(b)** The fragment was fully engaged during the revision procedure, but this resulted in an articular step-off. **(c)** During revision surgery, the syndesmotic screw has stabilized the fibula too far anteriorly.

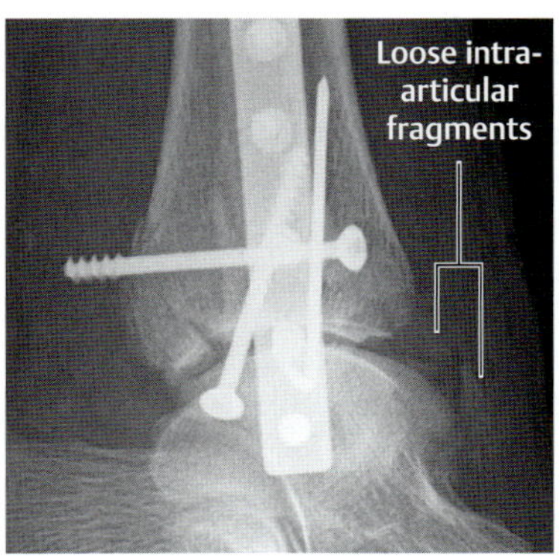

Fig. 2.419 Malplaced positioning screw with significant dorsal protrusion. Anterior loose bodies.

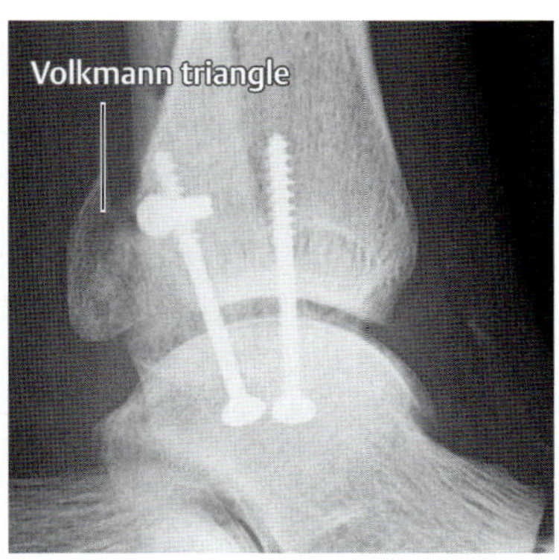

Fig. 2.420 The posterior malleolus avulsion fracture has not been stabilized. This would be tolerable with a fragment size of up to ~ 25% of the joint surface, but in this case it appears to be slightly greater than that.

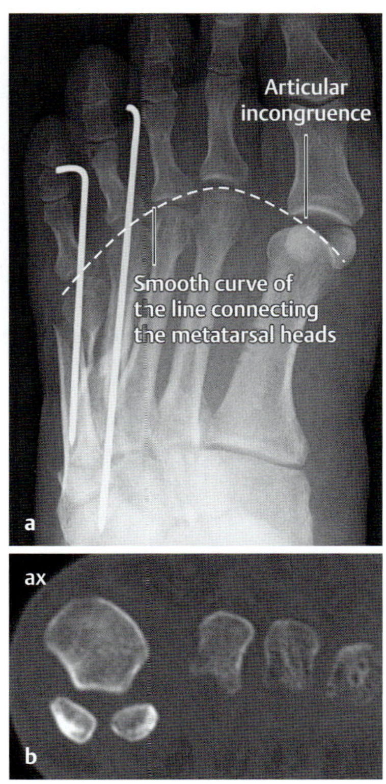

Fig. 2.421 Postoperative appearance after complex Lisfranc fracture-dislocation with metatarsal shaft fractures. **(a)** Correct restoration of the metatarsal length. **(b)** There is a rotational deformity of the first metatarsal in a medial direction, with resulting severe subluxation of the sesamoids.

Hallux valgus. Hallux valgus refers to lateral deviation of the great toe at the metatarsophalangeal joint (▸ Fig. 2.422). The angle between the axes of the first metatarsal and the proximal phalanx is increased (normal: 10°) and the angle between the first and second metatarsals may also be increased (normal: 10–12°), termed metatarsus primus varus. The combination of hallux valgus and metatarsus primus varus results in increased prominence of the first metatarsal head along the medial border of the foot. Additionally, the hallux tendons no longer run centrally across the joint, but further laterally, thereby pulling the toe into an increasingly deviated position along with lateral subluxation of the sesamoid bones, which are embedded in the flexor tendons. In addition, hammer and claw toe deformities of the adjacent toes are common (▸ Fig. 2.422). Apart from a hereditary disposition, the cause of a hallux valgus deformity is most often the development of a splay foot related to footwear.

Hallux rigidus. "Hallux rigidus" refers to stiffness of the first metatarsophalangeal joint secondary to osteoarthritic changes. The diagnosis is primarily made on clinical grounds. Typical signs of osteoarthritis are present on radiographs.

Hammer toe and claw toe. *Hammer toe* is the commonest toe deformity. It consists of a flexion deformity of the proximal interphalangeal (PIP) joint and less commonly the distal interphalangeal (DIP) joint (see ▸ Fig. 2.422). In contrast to hammer toe, *claw toe* is characterized by dislocation or subluxation of the metatarsophalangeal (MTP) joint, resulting in its hyperextension with concomitant flexion of the PIP and DIP joints. Hammer toe is most commonly caused by inappropriate footwear, and less often by neuromuscular disorders, high-arch foot (pes cavus), splay foot, compartment syndrome, poliomyelitis, or rheumatic disorders.

2.15.9 Ligaments

The ligaments of the ankle joint are made up of the distal tibiofibular syndesmosis along with the lateral and the medial collateral complexes. ▶ See ▸ Figs. W2.70 and W2.71.

▸ **MRI.** MRI is the gold standard for evaluating these ligaments and images are best obtained with the foot in the neutral position. Undamaged ligaments are hypointense on all sequences. Sometimes a longitudinal stripe of increased signal intensity is also visualized, especially in the posterior tibiofibular ligament.

▸ **US.** With the exception of the posterolateral ligaments (posterior tibiofibular and posterior talofibular ligaments), the ligaments of the ankle joint are usually well demonstrated by ultrasound. The ligaments normally demonstrate a sharply delineated fibrillar structure and a thickness of up to 2 mm. Injuries result in thickening of the ligament, which also becomes hypoechoic and loses its fibrillar appearance. A dynamic examination, with stretching of the affected ligaments, can assist in differentiating between partial- and full-thickness tears.

Distal Tibiofibular Syndesmosis

Syndesmotic injuries are commonly combined with fibular fractures or are part of complex ligament injuries secondary to severe ankle trauma. These are often difficult to detect clinically, resulting in a delayed or missed diagnosis.

If there is malalignment of the talus within the ankle mortise on radiographs, the diagnosis of a syndesmotic injury can be made (▸ Fig. 2.423). MRI is usually required for accurate assessment of the syndesmosis. Given its low sensitivity, ultrasound (▸ Fig. 2.424) should not be used in place of MRI. The following points should be borne in mind:

- The thinner anterior tibiofibular ligament consists of several oblique fascicles, which can mimic a tear on axial slices. Coronal and obliquely oriented images are more reliable (▸ Figs. 2.425 and ▸ 2.426).
- The posterior tibiofibular ligament may be torn and avulse a flake of bone from the posterior tibia.
- A tear of the caudal parts of the interosseous membrane produces proximal extension of the tibiofibular recess of the ankle; this may be regarded as an indirect MRI sign. If the fascicles of the distal interosseous membrane are well developed, their integrity can be assessed directly.

Lateral Collateral Ligaments

Disruption of the lateral ligaments secondary to a supination injury (plantar flexion, inversion, internal rotation) is by far the most common ligament injury of the ankle. Depending on the severity of the injury, the three ligamentous components (anterior talofibular [ATAF]; calcaneofibular [CF]; posterior talofibular [PTAF]) tear from anterior to posterior almost without exception, with the PTAF ligament tearing only rarely.

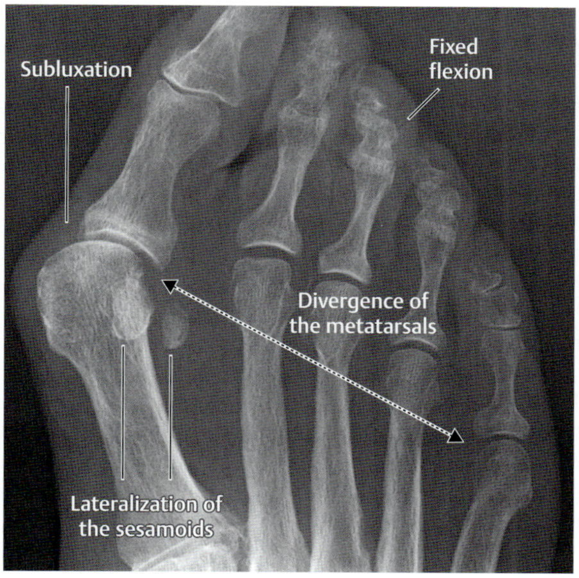

Fig. 2.422 Splay foot with typical sequelae: hallux valgus, hammer toes.

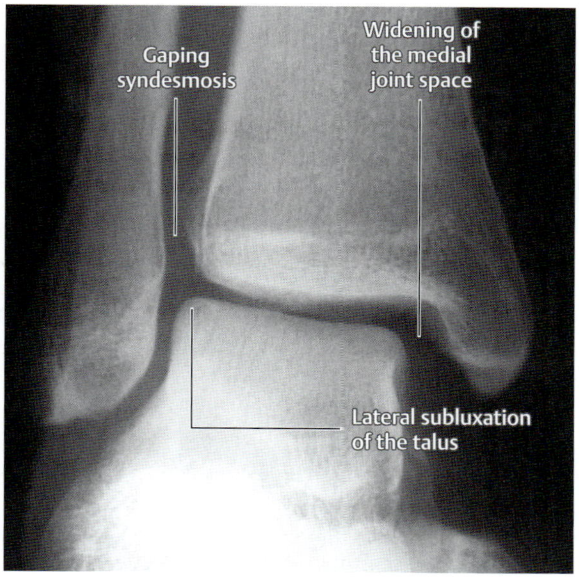

Fig. 2.423 Signs of a syndesmotic injury seen on the radiograph. AP view in 20° internal rotation.

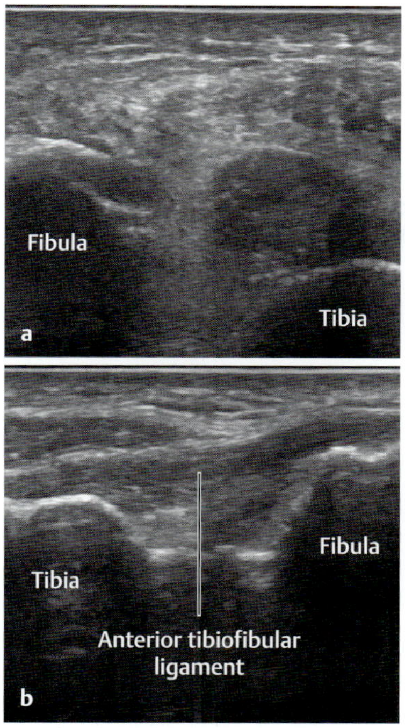

Fig. 2.424 Disruption of the anterior tibiofibular ligament visualized on ultrasound. Longitudinal section. **(a)** Interruption of continuity with thickened and retracted ligament ends. **(b)** Healthy contralateral side for comparison.

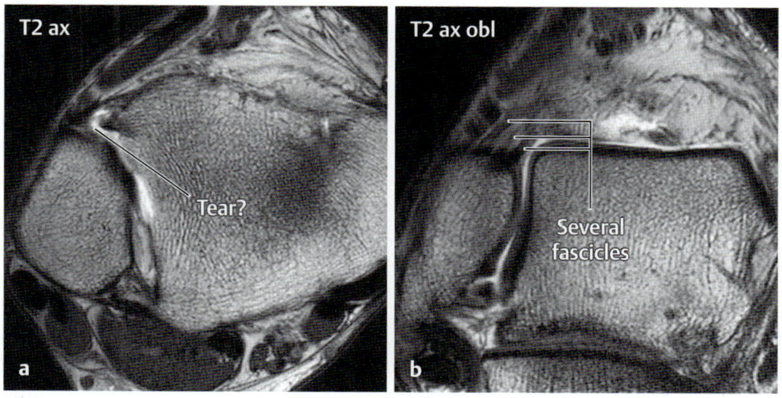

Fig. 2.425 Assessment of the anterior tibiofibular ligament. **(a)** The individual fascicles of the anterior tibiofibular ligament can mimic a tear on the axial slice. **(b)** The oblique axial plane confirms continuity of the ligament.

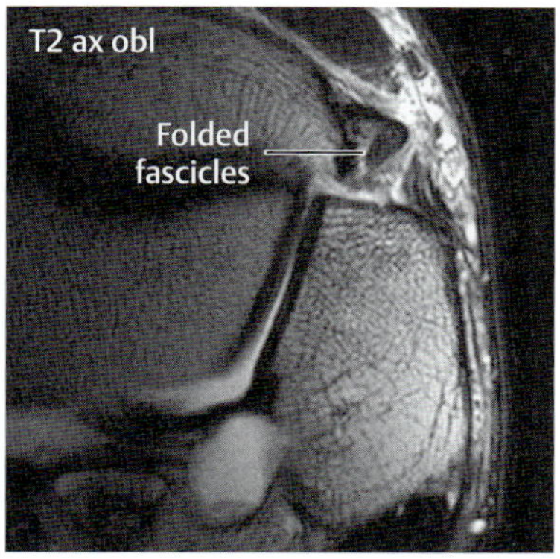

Fig. 2.426 Tear of the anterior tibiofibular ligament on the oblique axial slice.

Full-thickness tears of the **ATAF ligament** at the level of the tip of the lateral malleolus are usually easy to diagnose on axial slices. Partial-thickness tears may simply manifest as thickening of the ligament with slightly increased signal intensity on T2W sequences (▶ Fig. 2.427).

Due to its oblique course, the **CF ligament** is most easily assessed on an oblique axial slice orientation obtained at an angle of approximately 45° (▶ Fig. 2.428).

The **PTAF ligament** takes origin on the concave inner side of the lateral malleolus and tapers as it courses toward the talus. On non-fat-suppressed sequences, it often demonstrates some intrasubstance signal intensity (▶ Fig. 2.429).

> **Note**
>
> Routine MRI for a simple supination injury in a patient presenting with isolated lateral ankle pain is usually not indicated. Imaging evaluation is often indicated in cases in which there is clinical suspicion of more severe injury or for persistent symptoms. It is important to evaluate other ligamentous structures, tendons, and joint surfaces along with the damaged lateral ligaments (▶ Fig. 2.430).

Medial Collateral Ligaments (Deltoid Ligament)

Sprains of the medial collateral ligaments are much less frequent than those on the lateral side and are therefore more often missed. The strong **posterior tibiotalar component** may normally demonstrate some increased, streaklike signal intensity. For this reason, discontinuity of the ligament should be observed in order to diagnose a tear, especially at its talar insertion (▶ Fig. 2.431). With injury of the superficial layers of the deltoid ligament, an avulsion of the tip of the medial malleolus may occur (▶ Fig. 2.432).

The **tibiocalcaneal component** merges continuously into the **tibiospring ligament,** located somewhat farther anteriorly and radiating into the superomedial portion of the spring ligament along the medial aspect of the head of the talus (▶ Figs. 2.433 and ▶ W2.71).

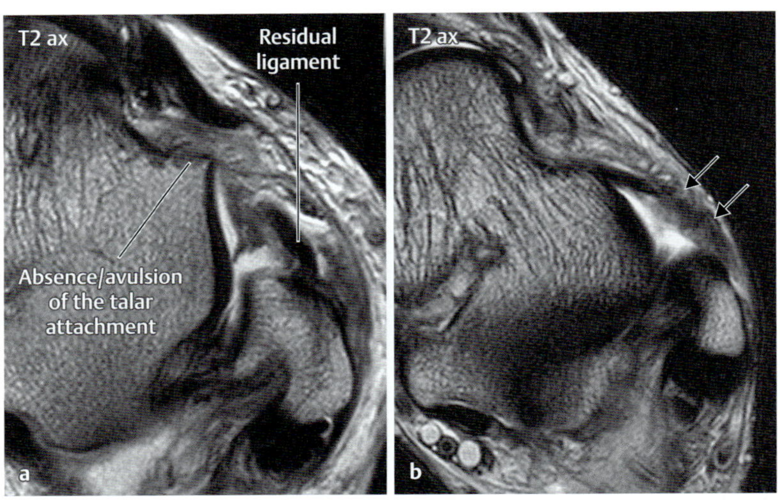

Fig. 2.427 Anterior talofibular ligament. **(a)** Full-thickness tear of the ligament. **(b)** Significant partial-thickness tear (arrows). There is no discontinuity, but there is increased signal intensity and thickening of the ligament.

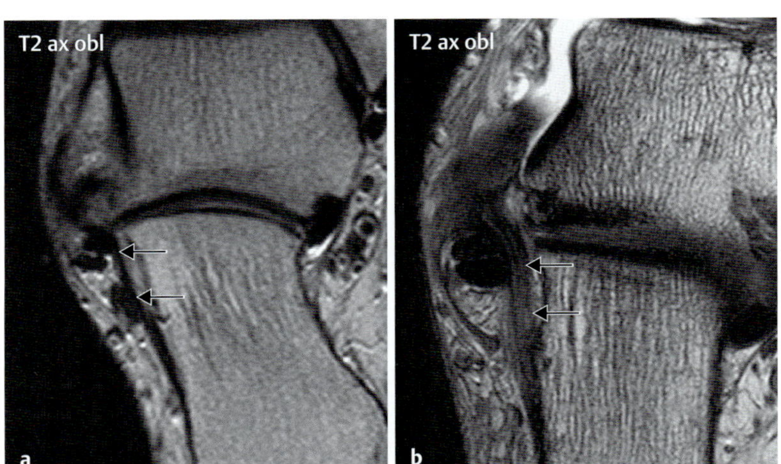

Fig. 2.428 Calcaneofibular ligament. The calcaneofibular ligament is displayed longitudinally using a transverse oblique imaging plane angulated ~ 45° dorsocaudally. **(a)** Normal finding. The ligament is visualized between the peroneal tendons and calcaneus as a delicate dark stripe (arrows). **(b)** There is a partial-thickness tear of the calcaneofibular ligament (arrows) with thickening and increased signal intensity, yet continuity is preserved.

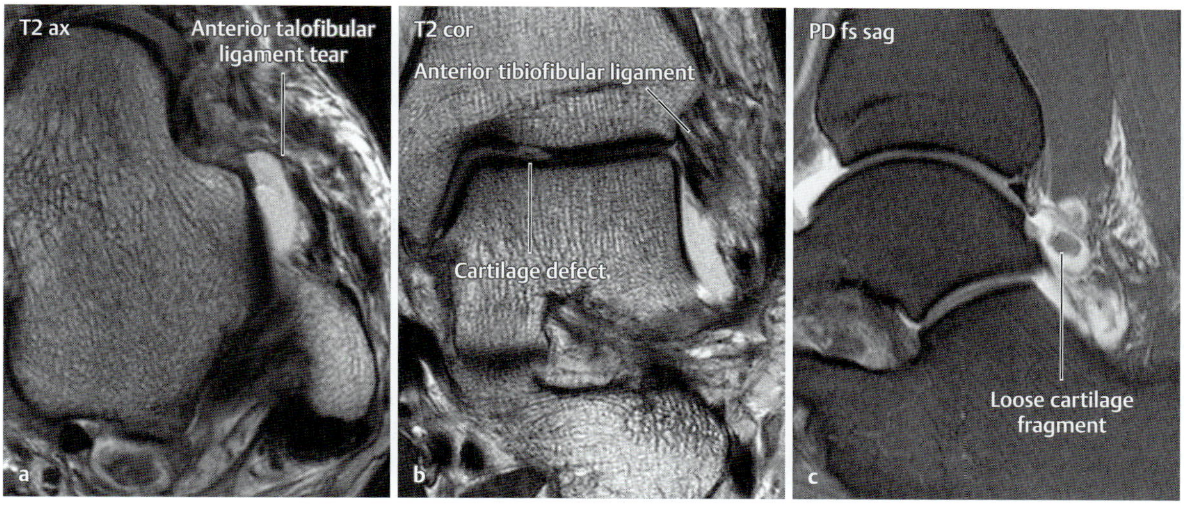

Fig. 2.430 A patient after supination injury. **(a)** The lateral ligament tear is evident. **(b)** Circumscribed cartilage lesion of the anterior distal tibia. **(c)** The loose fragment of cartilage is identifiable in the posterior joint recess [the fragment is also evident in image **(a)**].

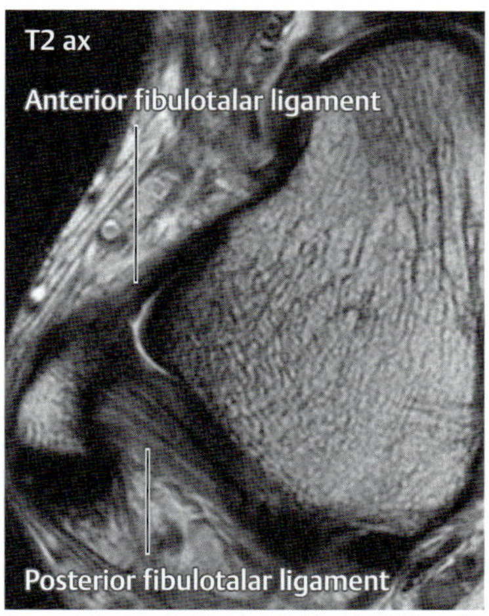

Fig. 2.429 Normal posterior talofibular ligament. The normal posterior talofibular ligament commonly has a striped appearance.

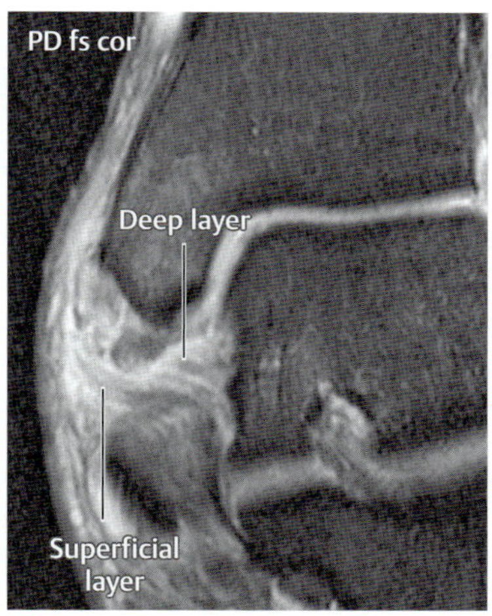

Fig. 2.431 Full-thickness tear of the deltoid ligament. The deep layers are disrupted in the middle of the ligament; the superficial layers are torn near their tibial attachment.

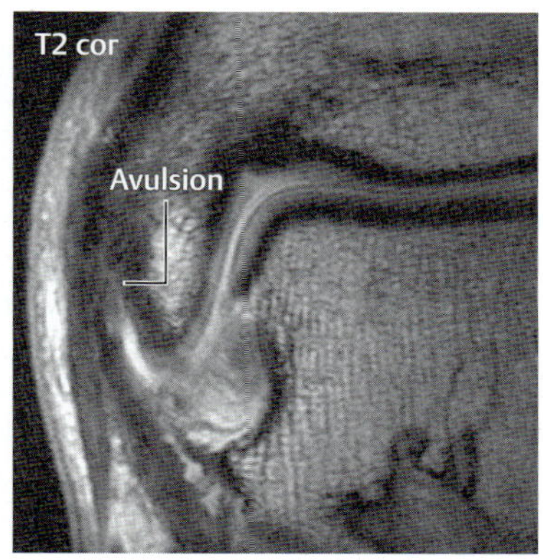

Fig. 2.432 Deltoid ligament injury in a professional footballer. The superficial layers are not torn but are avulsed from the tip of the medial malleolus.

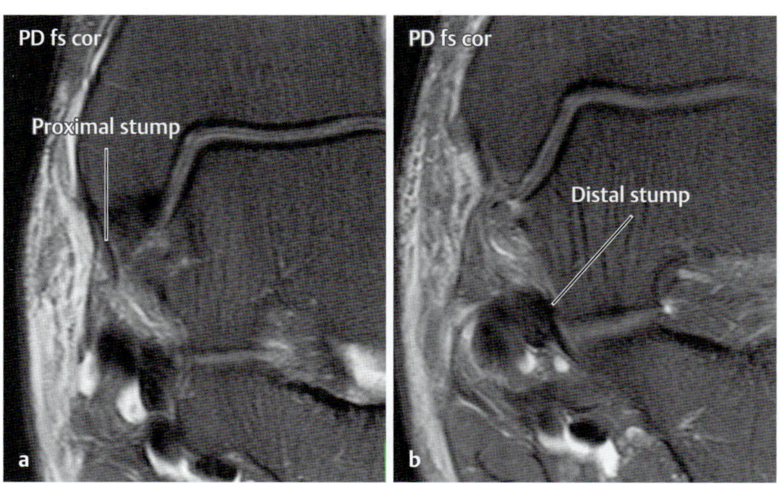

Fig. 2.433 Tibiospring ligament tear. **(a)** The proximal stump appears attached to the tip of the medial malleolus. **(b)** Two slices farther anteriorly, the superomedial fascicles of the spring ligament are visualized as a hypoechoic structure beneath the tibialis posterior tendon.

Plantar Calcaneonavicular Ligament

The plantar calcaneonavicular ligament, also known as the spring ligament, is an important stabilizer of the arch of the foot. Tears of this ligament occur in conjunction with complex ankle injuries; however, chronic degenerative alterations are more common and may result in insufficiency of the ligament and ultimately degenerative tearing (▶ Fig. 2.434). The adjacent tibialis posterior tendon merges into the superomedial portion of the tibiospring ligament. The inferoplantar and medioplantar portions of the ligament are often difficult to identify even in healthy individuals.

2.15.10 Tendons

Full-thickness tendon tears commonly retract, resulting in a gap between the torn ends of the tendon. With **partial-thickness tears**, the tendon may appear attenuated or even thickened with loss of the normal fibrillar tendon architecture. Differentiation from **tendinopathy** may be difficult in the presence of a thickened tendon. Apart from surrounding soft tissue swelling, an indirect, though nonspecific, sign of a tear is fluid in the tendon sheath. Ultrasound allows comparison with the contralateral side to help in differentiating a pathologic amount of fluid from a physiologic amount.

▶ US. One advantage of US over MRI is the fact that changes in direction of the tendons as they pass around the malleoli do not present any diagnostic difficulties (such as occurs with the magic angle artifact on MRI), although it must always be remembered that anisotropy of the tendons may result in a diagnostic error. Again, comparison with the contralateral side is helpful in equivocal cases.

Achilles Tendon

Achilles tendon tears usually occur on the basis of a preexisting, often asymptomatic tendinopathy. The most common site of tearing is an avascular zone 4 to 6 cm above its calcaneal insertion (▶ Figs. 2.435 and ▶ 2.436).

Tendinopathy of the Achilles tendon results in tendon thickening and, over time, internal signal intensity related to myxoid degeneration. Advanced tendinopathy can result in intratendinous calcifications and small intratendinous partial-thickness tears. The Achilles tendon does not have a tendon sheath so you will not see well defined peritendinous fluid such as is seen with tenosynovitis involving other tendons.

Following an Achilles tear, the tendon often heals with considerable thickening, regardless of the type of treatment. The scarred tendon can show significantly high signal over a long period of time (12 months and in rare cases even longer); this should be kept in mind, particularly with the question of a retear.

▶ US. A healthy Achilles tendon appears as a homogeneously hypoechoic, fibrillar structure, usually with a thickness of less than 6 mm.

Dynamic examination facilitates differentiation between partial-thickness and full-thickness tears; this is easier with fresh disruptions than with older tears, in which it is more difficult to distinguish a hematoma from the torn edges of the tendon. Myxoid degeneration is hypoechoic and differentiation of tendinopathy from partial-thickness tears is difficult using ultrasound. Another typical feature of tendinopathy is neovascularization, which can be visualized by Doppler ultrasound. Doppler ultrasound is also of help in diagnosing peritendinitis.

▶ MRI. A normal Achilles tendon appears as a low-signal intensity structure with a concave or flat ventral margin, though small punctate or linear foci of increased signal intensity may be present normally.

Tendinopathy is associated with thickening, increased signal intensity, and hypervascularity of the tendon and, in advanced cases, necrotic areas can develop within its substance (▶ Fig. 2.437). The abnormalities usually extend over a long segment, with maximal tendon thickening occurring 4 to 5 cm above its calcaneal insertion. Distal tendinopathy near the superior margin of the calcaneus may be associated with a Haglund deformity of the calcaneal tuberosity (▶ Fig. 2.438).

T2W sequences are most reliable for assessing the tendon.

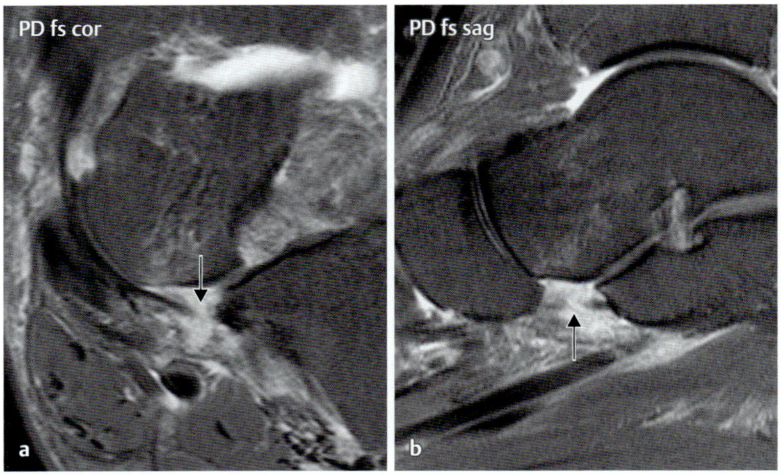

Fig. 2.434 Tear of the spring ligament. **(a)** The avulsion (arrow) of the calcaneal insertion of the superomedial limb is well visualized in the coronal projection. **(b)** The sagittal plane displays the stump of the oblique inferior limb (arrow). Inspection of the adjacent slices will allow clarification as to whether a "tear" is only being simulated by the oblique course of the ligament.

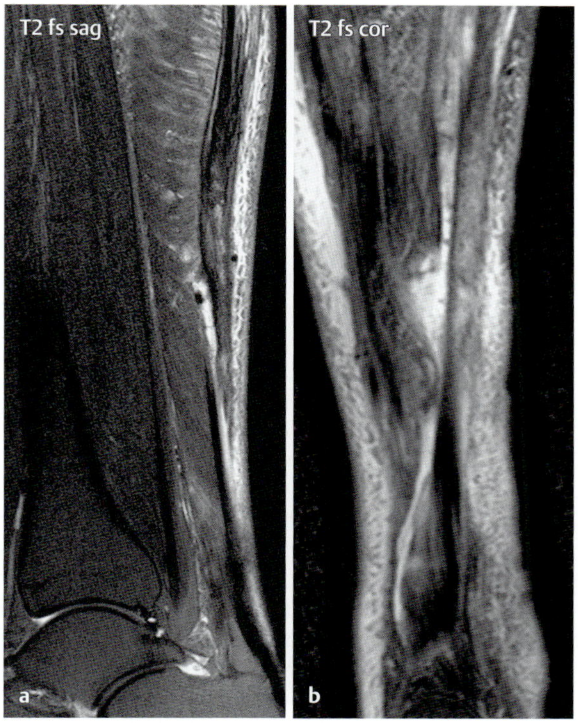

Fig. 2.435 Long-segment longitudinal disruption between the fascicles of the Achilles tendon as a variant of a tendon rupture. Since the tear exits proximally and distally to the longitudinal tear in a posterior and anterior direction, it is confirmed as a full-thickness tear. **(a)** Sagittal slice level. **(b)** Coronal slice level.

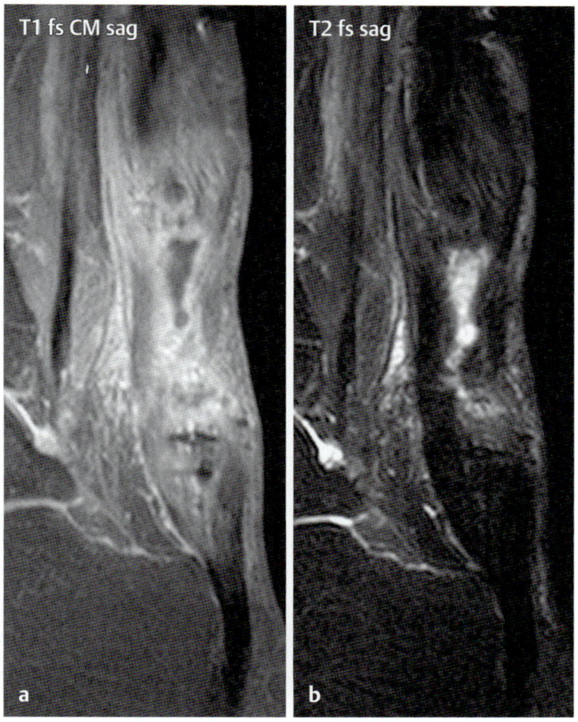

Fig. 2.436 Appearance of a full-thickness tear of the Achilles tendon 4 months after the tear and conservative treatment. **(a)** Contrast administration reveals the considerable degree of hypervascularization. **(b)** A T2W sagittal image obtained at the same time demonstrates relatively low signal intensity of a large proportion of the tendon.

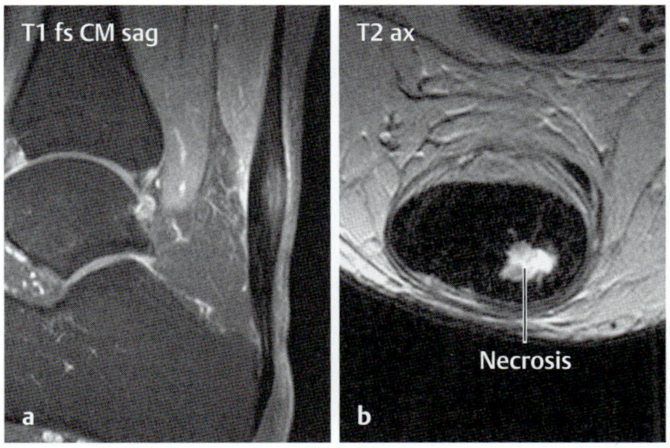

Fig. 2.437 Typical spindle-shaped thickening of the Achilles tendon secondary to chronic tendinopathy. **(a)** Hypervascularity is evident within parts of the tendon after administration of contrast. **(b)** Within this area there is a focus that is isointense to fluid on the T2W image, corresponding to necrosis.

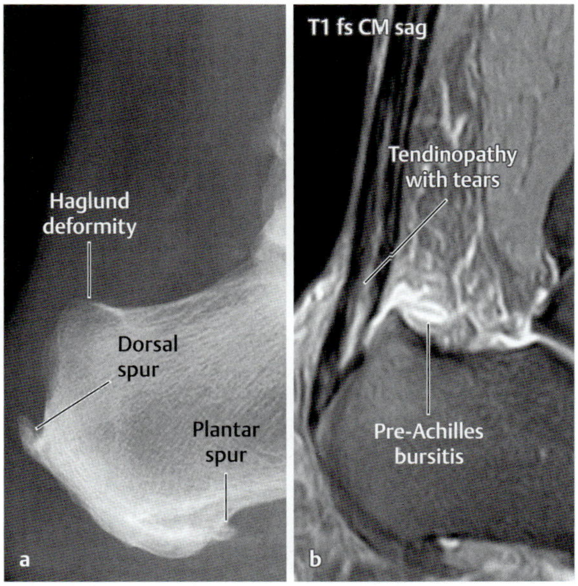

Fig. 2.438 Insertional tendinopathy of the Achilles tendon with a heel spur (Haglund deformity). **(a)** Plantar and dorsal heel spurs. A slightly obliquely positioned lateral view has not fully projected the Haglund deformity at the superior margin of the calcaneal tuberosity. **(b)** MRI demonstrates the true extent of the bony spur and displays significant insertion tendinopathy with an interstitial tearing of the distal tendon and concomitant pre-Achilles bursitis.

Flexor Group

Of the flexor tendons, the posterior tibial (PT) is most commonly affected by pathology. Full-thickness **tears** are rare, however. **Chronic tendinopathy** is most common with thickening, progressive degeneration, and ultimately attenuation of the (likely insufficient) tendon (▶ Fig. 2.439). Because it is the primary arch support in the foot, progressive PT tendon insufficiency leads to increased stress upon the spring ligament and ultimately the development of pes planus deformity.

Peroneal Tendons

Injuries to the peroneal tendons are often associated with pathology of the lateral ligaments. The peroneus brevis tendon commonly tears longitudinally, resulting in two separate tendon segments lying either anterior to or on each side of the peroneus longus tendon (▶ Fig. 2.440).

▶ **US.** Ultrasound is particularly important for assessing **dislocation of the peroneal tendons** secondary to injury to the superior peroneal retinaculum, which can be provoked by a dynamic examination.

▶ **MRI.** The extent of tendon damage and condition of the superior peroneal retinaculum can be accurately assessed with MRI (▶ Fig. 2.441). It should also be noted whether a retromalleolar groove is present just above the tip of the lateral malleolus since absence of this groove predisposes to tendon dislocation.

Extensor Group

Pathologic alterations of the extensor group are much less common and almost always involve the tibialis anterior tendon. Tears are usually the result of direct injuries to the tendons that lie superficially along the dorsum of the foot; these often occur between the superior and inferior extensor retinacula and result in retraction of the margins of the torn tendon. Chronic tendinopathy typically involves the distal parts of the tendons near their insertions (▶ Fig. 2.442).

▶ **Important findings.** It is important to provide information on the location and extent of a tendon tear and, with full-thickness disruptions, the position of the retracted tendon margins, since these factors will directly influence therapy.

2.15.11 Impingement Syndromes

Entrapment phenomena at various sites are referred to as "impingement syndromes." Posttraumatic capsular thickening is usually the cause. Anterolateral impingement following injury to the lateral collateral ligaments is by far the most common (▶ Fig. 2.443). This is followed by anteromedial and posteromedial impingement syndromes and those located in the region of the syndesmosis (▶ Fig. 2.444). Unlike these soft tissue entrapment phenomena, impingement of the anterosuperior ankle is the result of anterior osteophyte development along the distal tibia and opposing talus (▶ Fig. 2.445). These impingement syndromes lead to localized synovitis, secondary cartilage lesions, and—in some cases—a mechanical restriction of motion.

Posterior impingement can result from entrapment of soft tissue near the posterior talar process. One variant is the **os trigonum syndrome**: this results from impingement of the os trigonum and is suggested when marrow edema is seen within the ossicle and adjacent talus along with reaction within the surrounding tissues, often including tenosynovitis of the flexor hallucis tendon (▶ Fig. 2.446).

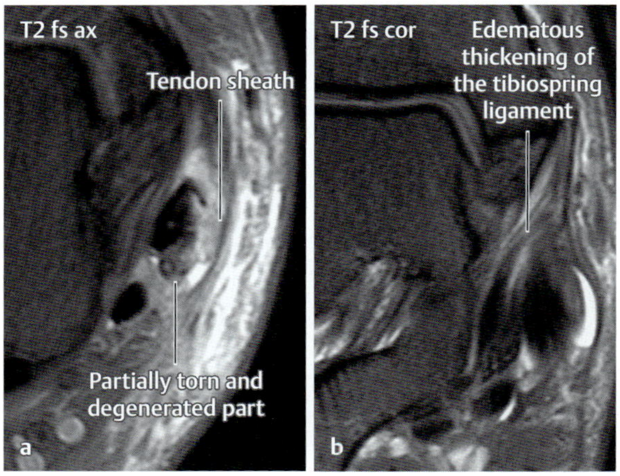

Fig. 2.439 Degeneration of the tibialis posterior tendon. Degeneration of the tibialis posterior tendon is often associated with tendinopathy, tenosynovitis, and peritendinitis. **(a)** Note the abnormally small cross section of the tendon that contains abnormal signal intensity, the fluid in the tendon sheath, and also the edema in the surrounding tissues. **(b)** Insufficiency of the tendon often leads to failure of other structures that support the arch of the foot, in this case the tibiospring ligament.

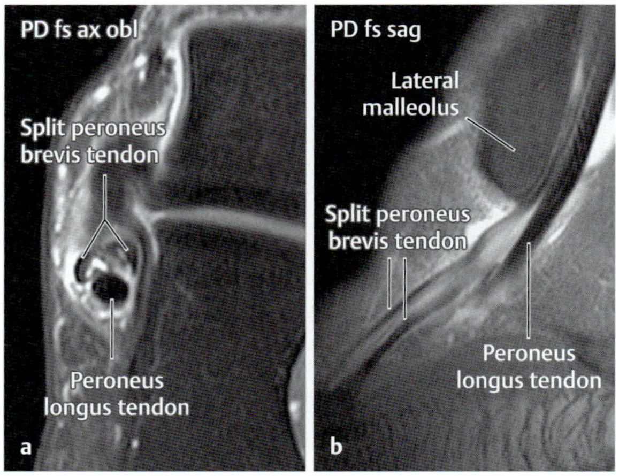

Fig. 2.440 Long-segment longitudinal tear of the peroneus brevis tendon with significant tenosynovitis. **(a)** Oblique transverse plane. **(b)** Sagittal.

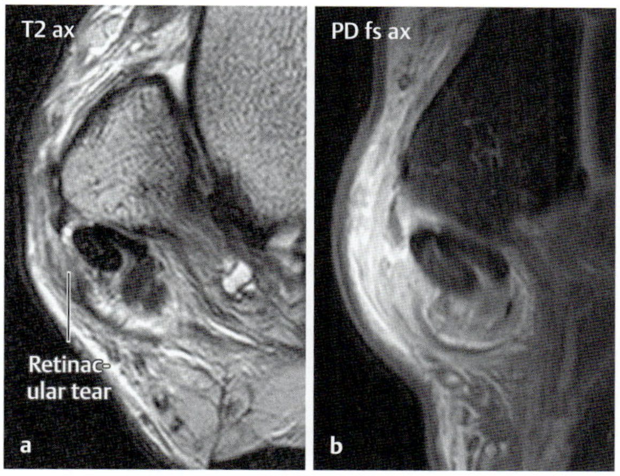

Fig. 2.441 Peritendinitis around the peroneal tendons with a clinically confirmed tendon dislocation secondary to a supination injury. **(a)** Tear of the retinaculum. **(b)** Edematous tissue in the region of the retinacular tear and around the tendon. The tendons themselves are still intact.

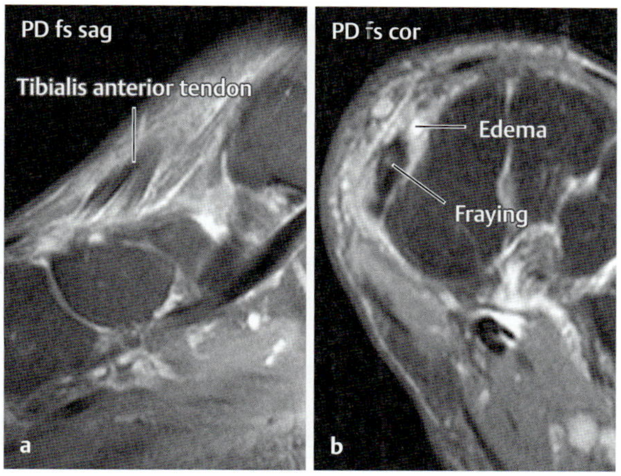

Fig. 2.442 Insertional tendinopathy of the tibialis anterior tendon. **(a)** Increased fraying of the tendon fascicles. **(b)** Peritendinous edema.

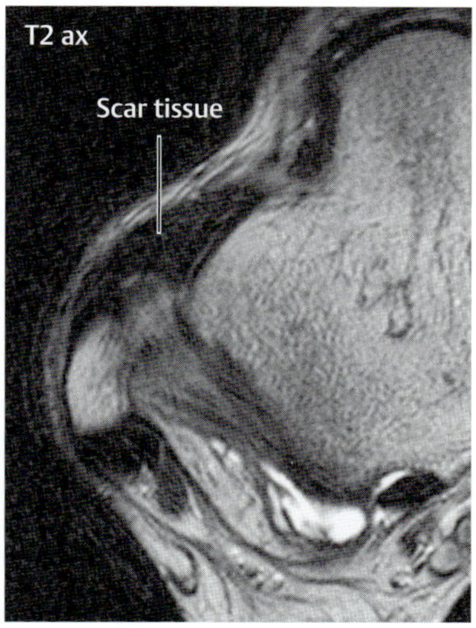

Fig. 2.443 Anterolateral impingement syndrome. The syndrome developed as a result of excess scar formation along the anterior fibulotalar ligament after disruption of the ligament 8 months previously.

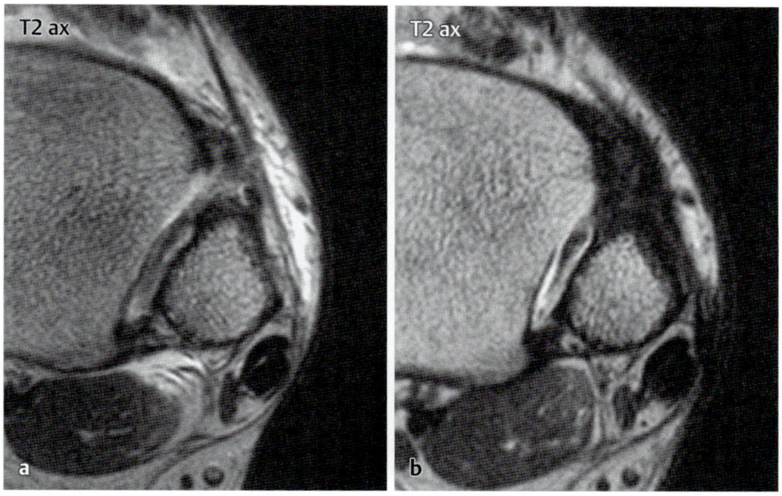

Fig. 2.444 Impingement of the anterior syndesmosis. **(a)** The cause was a tear of the anterior tibiofibular ligament. **(b)** Excess scar formation with a space-occupying tendency is evident about 1 year after the tear.

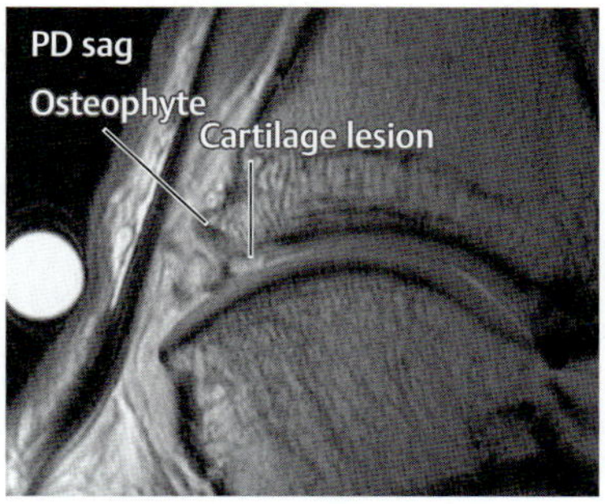

Fig. 2.445 Anterior osteophyte formation of the distal tibia with clinical signs of anterior impingement. Note the presence of an associated cartilage lesion.

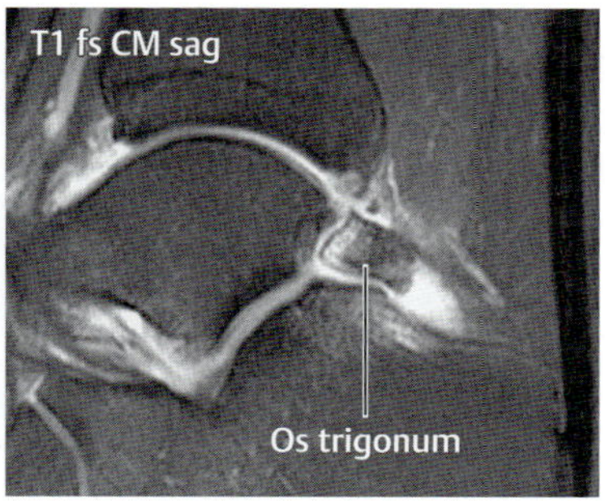

Fig. 2.446 Posterior impingement, here in the form of an os trigonum syndrome. The clinical presentation was posterior ankle pain for some months.

2.15.12 Tarsal Tunnel Syndrome

Tarsal tunnel syndrome refers to a neuropathy of the branches of the tibial nerve (the medial plantar and the lateral plantar nerves) secondary to pathology within the tarsal tunnel. In many cases, MRI can demonstrate the cause of the nerve compression, such as a ganglion, tumor, accessory muscle, or scar (▶ Fig. 2.447). It is not uncommon, however, for the MRI to be unrevealing in electrophysiologically confirmed cases.

2.15.13 Sinus Tarsi

The interosseous talocalcaneal ligament runs posteriorly as a wide, sail-like ligament through the sinus tarsi. The cervical ligament runs anteriorly. Although rare, injuries to these ligaments can result from trauma to the ankle and hindfoot, often in conjunction with injuries to the medial and lateral collateral ligaments.

The **sinus tarsi syndrome** is a painful condition of uncertain etiology. Posttraumatic instability of the subtalar joint, along with associated synovitis and scar formation within the sinus tarsi is thought to be a cause due to impingement of the scar upon the numerous sensory nerve endings in this region (▶ Fig. 2.448). In some cases, MRI demonstrates diffusely abnormal signal intensity within the sinus tarsi and can also exclude a space-occupying lesion or inflammatory process as a cause. Evaluation of the lateral ligamentous complex, the spring ligament, and the tibialis posterior tendon is important in these cases since these structures may be affected as well.

2.15.14 Plantar Fascia

The plantar fascia is functionally composed of two components: a thicker medial band and a somewhat thinner lateral band. **Plantar fasciitis** arises at its calcaneal origin, usually as a chronic degenerative process brought on by overuse, and may occur along with a plantar heel spur (▶ Fig. 2.438a). The medial component is more commonly involved and more significantly affected. In advanced cases, partial—or even complete—fascial tears may occur.

▶ **US.** On ultrasound the plantar fascia appears as a well-defined fibrillar structure. Fusiform thickening (> 4 mm) is seen with plantar fasciitis and Doppler ultrasound often displays neovascularization of the fascia and hyperemia of the surrounding tissues.

▶ **MRI.** MRI may demonstrate fascial thickening alone, but increased signal intensity and contrast enhancement of the affected portion of the fascia are often observed as well (▶ Fig. 2.449).

▶ **DD.** **Plantar vein thrombosis** is a rare, but important, condition that may mimic plantar fasciitis. It is most easily recognized on MRI after contrast administration; the hypointense thrombus appears surrounded by a strongly enhanced venous wall.

2.15.15 Plantar Plate and Turf Toe

The joint capsule of a metatarsophalangeal joint is most prominent along the plantar aspect of the joint. This structure is known as the plantar plate. Chronic overuse can lead to degeneration and eventual rupture of the plate (▶ Fig. 2.450).

Acute disruption of the plantar plate of the great toe secondary to a hyperextension injury is known as "turf toe." Differential diagnostic considerations include sesamoid pathology (fracture, stress reaction, necrosis), insertion tendinopathy, or bursitis.

2.15.16 Morton's Neuroma

"Morton's neuroma" is a misnomer since it is not a true tumor but rather a proliferation of fibrous tissue around a plantar digital nerve. These lesions are common in healthy, asymptomatic individuals but are usually smaller than 5 mm in those cases. Symptomatic lesions most commonly affect the second or third interdigital spaces and present a typical teardrop-shaped configuration on sectional imaging (▶ Fig. 2.451). They appear more prominent with the patient in a prone position.

▶ **US.** A Morton's neuroma is best assessed on ultrasound by applying digital pressure to the dorsal soft tissues between the metatarsal heads in a plantar direction, thus pushing the Morton's neuroma against the probe, which is placed on the plantar aspect of the foot. A hypoechoic structure may then be delineated within the plantar fatty tissue. An alternative technique in which scanning is performed dorsally is also possible.

▶ **MRI.** The fibrous tissue of Morton's neuroma results in a very hypointense appearance on both T1W and T2W sequences (▶ Fig. 2.451) but the neuromas typically demonstrate avid enhancement after contrast administration.

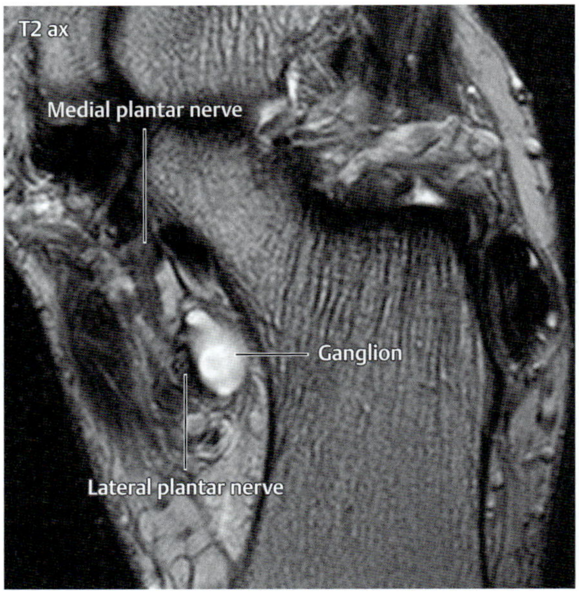

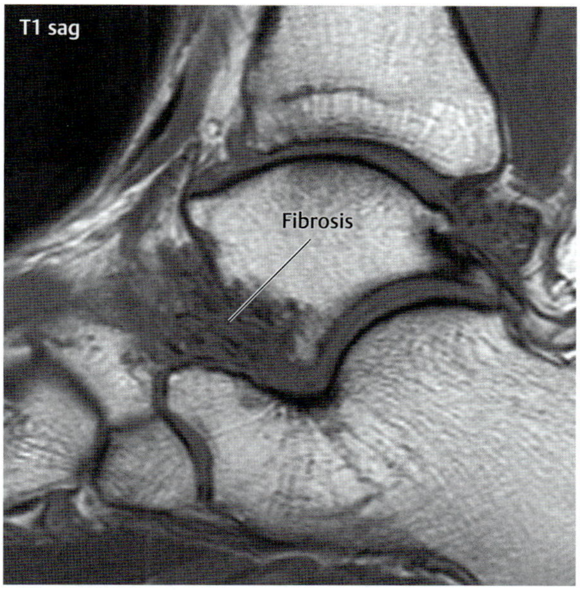

Fig. 2.448 A fibrotic sinus tarsi in a 48-year-old man. It remains unclear in this case whether or not there was an association with an injury that had occurred 3 months previously.

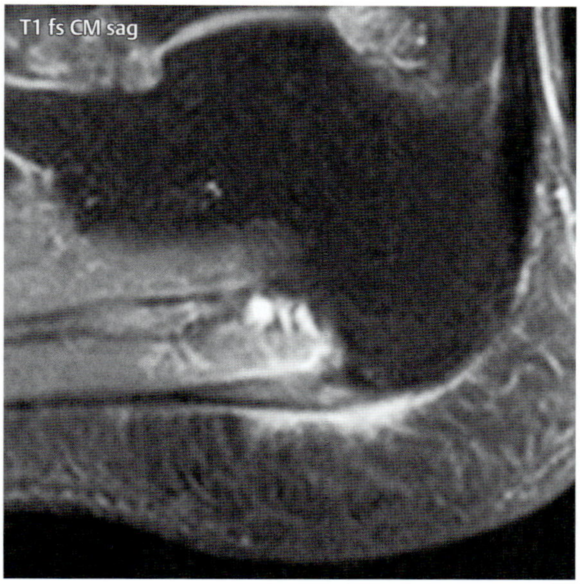

Fig. 2.449 Plantar fasciitis with edematous thickening and markedly increased contrast enhancement. The medial band is typically more affected than the lateral.

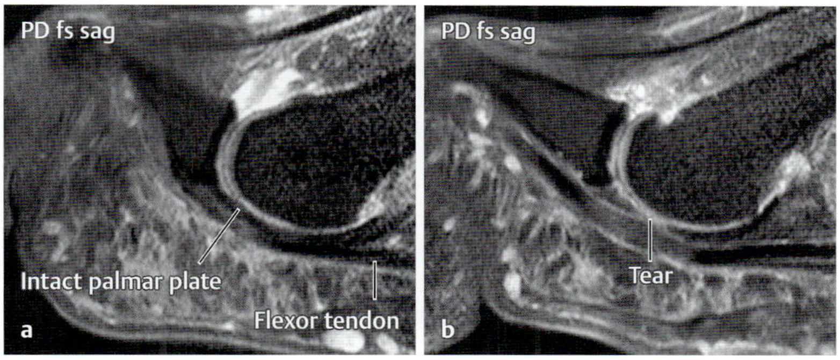

Fig. 2.450 Plantar plate. **(a)** The plantar plate consists of fibrocartilage; when intact it appears as plantar capsular thickening with absent signal intensity, in this case at the metatarsophalangeal joint of the third ray. **(b)** A torn plantar plate is evident at the metatarsophalangeal joint of the second ray.

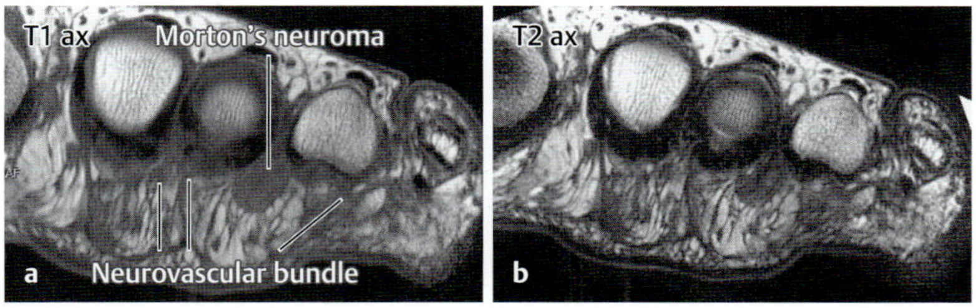

Fig. 2.451 Morton's neuroma. **(a)** The bulbous teardrop shape and its location along the interdigital neurovascular bundle are characteristic features. **(b)** Typical low signal intensity on the T2W scan due to fibrosis.

◀ **Fig. 2.447** Clinically suspected tarsal tunnel syndrome. The cause was found to be a ganglion that was stretching the lateral plantar nerve. The medial plantar nerve was not involved.

3 Infections of the Bones, Joints, and Soft tissues

3.1 Osteomyelitis and Osteitis

Osteomyelitis is defined as an inflammation of the bone marrow and/or bone due to an infection. The term "osteitis" (also ostitis) is a more general term indicating an inflammation of bone.

In Europe and North America, the majority of bone infections (~ 70%) occur after trauma and operations or secondary to the underlying condition "diabetic foot."

3.1.1 Terminology, Classification, and Infection Routes

Osteomyelitis. Infection of the bone initially arising in the bone marrow and/or cortex.

Osteitis (exogenous). Bone infection with an infection route from the outside (e.g., after trauma or surgery).

Periostitis. An inflammatory response (degenerative or rheumatological) of the periosteum. A primary infection of the subperiosteal space is very rare. Periostitis commonly appears as a noninfectious finding secondary to rheumatological disorders or chronic trauma/overuse.

Soft tissue infection. Infection of the soft tissue surrounding the bone and the joints.

(Septic) arthritis. Infection of the synovial membrane with identification of the causative pathogen in the joint fluid. Invasion of the contiguous bone is often seen.

Sequestrum. This term refers to a fragment of nonviable bone surrounded by granulation tissue and fluid. Other foreign bodies, such as antibiotic-impregnated beads or residual screw material, are also potential sequestrum-like structures.

Involucrum. A thick sheath of periosteal new bone surrounding a sequestrum.

Classification of osteomyelitis differs **according to**

- **The portal of entry** (endogenous/hematogenous versus exogenous/posttraumatic) or according to the **direction of spread** (centripetal/centrifugal): With primary hematogenous infection located in the bone marrow, the infection spreads from the center to the periphery (centrifugal route). With exogenous osteomyelitis, the pathogen makes its way from the outside into the bone marrow (centripetal route).
- **The time course** (acute/primary versus chronic/secondary): Acute osteomyelitis is commonest in infants and children. The chronic form of the disease clearly predominates in adults. The dividing line between acute and chronic bone infection is defined arbitrarily. Depending on the author, a chronic course is considered to have established itself any time between 4 and 8 weeks. Two different variations should be noted: a form in which continuous symptoms present for more than 8 weeks and a phasic form with asymptomatic intervals. It should be noted with posttraumatic and postoperative infections that within just hours of the infection irreversible alterations can develop in the bone. This places strict time limits on the acute phase within which there is still a chance of complete healing with adequate treatment.
- **The type of causative pathogen:** Almost every human-pathogenic bacterium, fungus, virus, or helminth can, albeit some very rarely, manifest itself at osteoarticular sites and in the peripheral soft tissues:
  - Gram-positive bacteria, above all *Staphylococcus aureus*, are the most common pathogens.
  - Gram-negative bacteria (e.g., *Escherichia coli, Klebsiella, Pseudomonas*) are more commonly seen in posttraumatic infections and in immunocompromised patients.
  - *Salmonella* infections classically occur in patients with sickle cell anemia—although *Staphylococcus* is still the commonest pathogen.
  - Mycobacteria are—even in Europe and the United States —important pathogens for spondylitis (Chapter 3.1.5), osteomyelitis, and septic arthritis.
- **The patient's age:** With osteomyelitis presenting an acute clinical course, a distinction is made between neonatal, pediatric, and (less common) adult forms.

3.1.2 Hematogenous Osteomyelitis

About 95% of cases of hematogenous osteomyelitis assume an acute course. It is divided according to age into neonatal, pediatric, and adult osteomyelitis, with the latter more frequently seen in patients over the age of 50 years (see spondylitis and spondylodiskitis in Chapter 3.1.5).

Brodie abscess is the predominant manifestation of the chronic hematogenous forms of osteomyelitis. If primarily acute hematogenous osteomyelitis assumes a chronic course, due to inadequate therapy, then this is also referred to as chronic hematogenous osteomyelitis. This applies, for example, to patients with a mixed spectrum of pathogens that has not been fully covered by antibiotics. Abscesses inadequately treated surgically are possible causes. It almost exclusively affects adults. The bacteria present in bone that has undergone reactive change and is commonly sclerotic are capable of triggering a renewed inflammatory episode at some future time. A reduced immune response, e.g., due to HIV infection or during chemotherapy and/or steroid therapy, is a possible contributory factor to reactivation.

▸ **Pathology.** The medullary cavity is saturated with edema and filled with granulocytes. Osteocytes are hardly, or no longer, detectable. The associated ischemia can lead to sequestrum formation. Liquefaction of necrotic tissue results in the development of an abscess within the bone. Healing commences with the proliferation of connective tissue and capillary ingrowth.

Neonatal osteomyelitis. This is a highly acute disease with a predilection for the femoral metaphysis. Organisms are predominantly streptococci. If the infection spreads via the haversian canals into the subperiosteal space and/or via the still patent metaphyseal–epiphyseal vascular connections, the infection will involve the epiphysis.

Pediatric osteomyelitis. The metaphyseal–epiphyseal vessels occlude with increasing age. Dilated vascular loops are present in the metaphysis, favoring pathogen colonization. This is the reason why the focus of inflammation initially develops in the metaphysis. Rapid penetration of the thin cortical bone ensues, with subsequent subperiosteal spread of the infection. The periosteum is elevated. The infection can then spread to the adjacent joint, especially if the metaphysis is located within the joint capsule, as with the hip and knee joints.

Acute osteomyelitis of adulthood. Acute osteomyelitis at this age is being increasingly diagnosed, affecting primarily the vertebrae (Chapter 3.1.5).

▸ **Clinical presentation.** Acute hematogenous osteomyelitis is a systemic disorder. Early symptoms include fever, chills and localized pain with focal swelling, erythema, and increased skin temperature. CRP and white blood cell count are elevated. In ~50% of cases it is possible to identify the pathogen in blood cultures.

▸ **Radiography.** A number of findings should be looked for on the radiographs:

- The type and degree of bone destruction vary. A wide spectrum is possible, ranging from diffuse reduction of density, via solitary radiolucency, irregular multiple radiolucencies (moth-eaten or mottled pattern) to an extensive permeative pattern.
- The margins of the lesions are usually ill-defined and irregular (▸ Fig. 3.1) so that it is not possible to determine the exact extent of the infection.
- Uni- to multilaminated (onion skin) periosteal reactions are invariably found (▸ Fig. 3.2).
- The reparative phase during treatment and neglected chronic forms of osteomyelitis are characterized by endosteal and periosteal new bone formation, development of marginal sclerosis around the lesion and, in part, extensive areas of osteosclerosis.

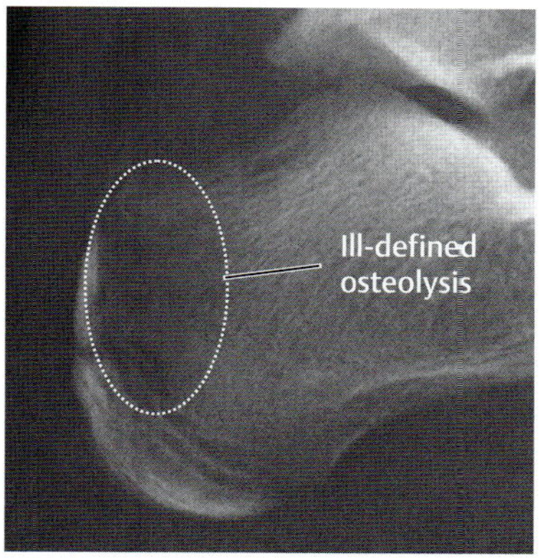

Fig. 3.1 Acute hematogenous osteomyelitis. The dense calcaneal apophysis is normal.

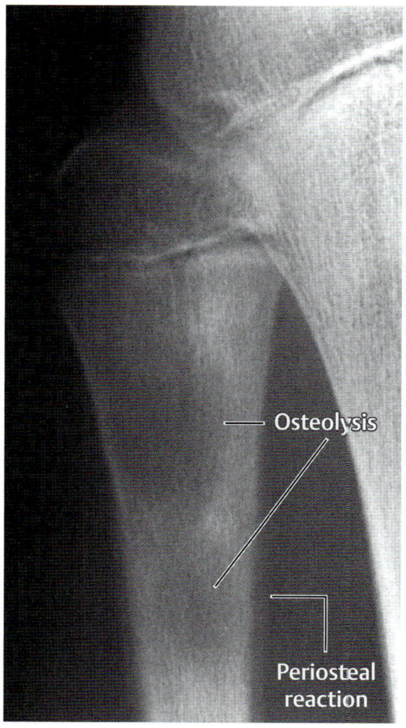

Fig. 3.2 Acute hematogenous osteomyelitis.

- In neonatals and small children, radiographs already allow an early (within the first days after onset of symptoms) presumptive diagnosis of soft tissue swelling based on the obliteration of fat lines. The skeletal alterations require at least 7 to 10 days before they become radiographically evident. The laminated periosteal reactions are sometimes recognized before bone destruction. A late sign in this age group is swelling of the metaphysis, sometimes also involving the epiphysis. During the late phase of the disease, the extensive periosteal reaction can appear as periosteal ossification.

Caution

Nowadays, patients with acute osteomyelitis during the neonatal period, and above all in childhood, commonly present at such an early stage of the disease that only subtle radiographic findings, or even none at all, are present (cf. section on "Recommendations for an Examination Strategy" at the end of the general part of Chapter 3.1.2).

▶ **US.** Imaging conditions are particularly favorable during the neonatal period. The first sign, evident even before any periosteal reaction, is the hypoechoic, or even hyperechoic, edematous soft tissue swelling. Then a thin, hypoechoic fluid layer develops, elevating the periosteum (▶ Fig. 3.3). This can go on to form a space-occupying abscess with an anechoic to hypoechoic intralesional structure and hyperechoic wall (▶ Fig. 3.4). With good imaging conditions, destruction of the cortex can be well visualized as disruption or distortion of the contour (▶ Fig. 3.5).

The diagnostic value of ultrasound decreases with increasing age of the patient. In osteomyelitis, its indication is essentially restricted to providing additional diagnostic soft tissue information. Abscesses, cysts, and hematomas are excellently visualized as anechoic or hypoechoic lesions and are therefore amenable to ultrasound-guided aspiration.

▶ **MRI. Examination technique.** Fluid-sensitive fat saturated sequences (STIR, PDW or T2W) serve as sequences for screening; the T1W sequence demonstrates the anatomy and provides characteristic findings within the bone marrow, while the T1W sequence with fat saturation after administration of contrast agent is of help with reliably diagnosing abscesses and sequestrum formation, although it is not generally required for routine diagnostics.

Morphology and signal behavior. This usually involves circumscribed, very signal-intense areas on fluid-sensitive sequences. Intramedullary lesions are hypointense on T1W images (▶ Figs. 3.6a and ▶ 3.8b). An edematous halo forms around the focal lesion, extending as an irregular and ill-defined manifestation of normal bone marrow. Instead of small circumscribed lesions, large diffuse areas of increased signal intensity are also possible (▶ Fig. 3.8).

Note

With hematogenous osteomyelitis, an area of low signal intensity is always evident in the bone marrow on the T1W image, clearly marking the extent of the inflammatory lesion (▶ Fig. 3.6a). Care should be taken before establishing the diagnosis "acute osteomyelitis" when there is no clear area of low signal intensity on the T1W images. The rule is that periosteal edema should always be identifiable (▶ Figs. 3.6b and ▶ 3.7). The periosteal areas of edema can be very subtle in early cases.

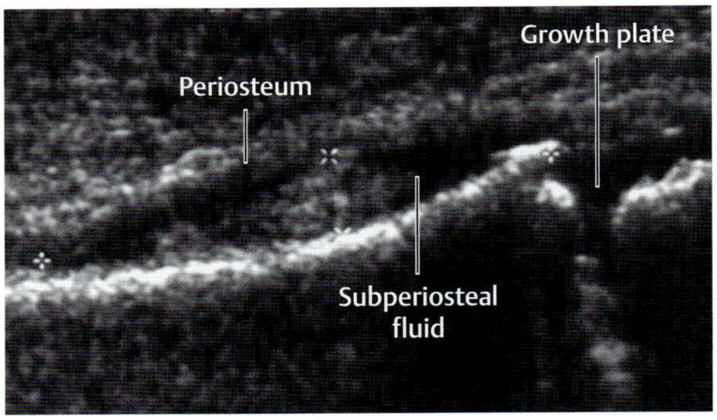

Fig. 3.3 Acute osteomyelitis of the distal fibula on ultrasound. Longitudinal section.

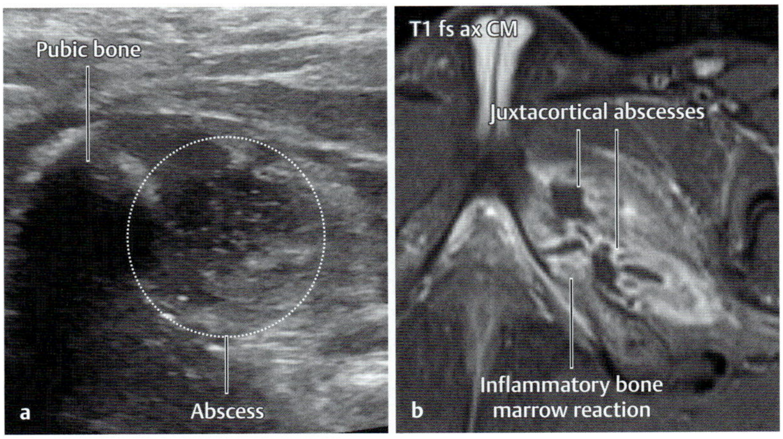

Fig. 3.4 Periosteal abscesses in osteomyelitis of the coccyx. **(a)** Ultrasound, transverse section. **(b)** Correlation with MRI after IV contrast administration.

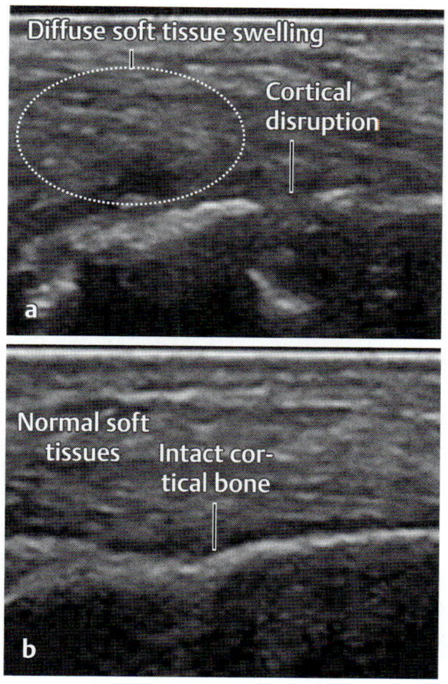

Fig. 3.5 Acute osteomyelitis with cortical bone destruction. **(a)** Ultrasound finding, longitudinal section. **(b)** Healthy contralateral side for comparison.

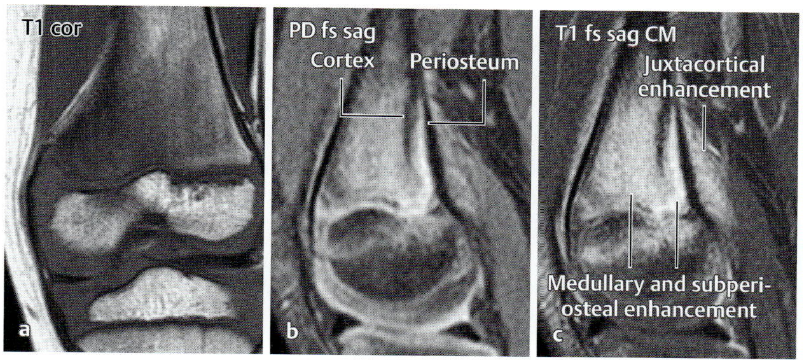

Fig. 3.6 Acute osteomyelitis. **(a)** Hypointense bone marrow edema on the T1W image. **(b)** Medullary, subperiosteal, and periosteal edema. **(c)** No abscess.

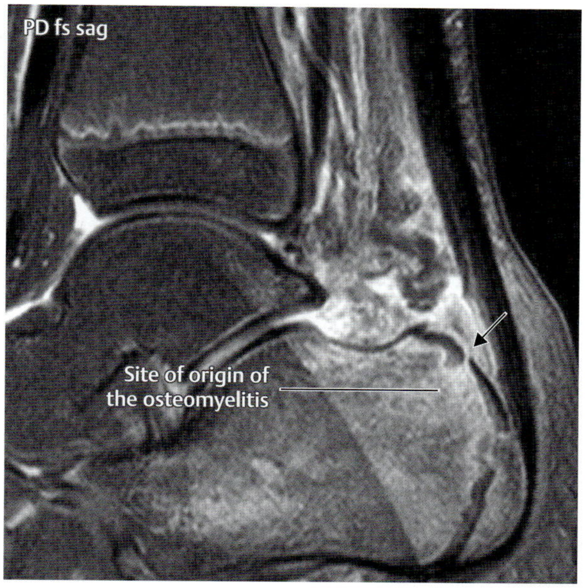

Fig. 3.7 Acute hematogenous osteomyelitis. Cortical penetration (arrow) and concomitant involvement of the soft tissue deep to the Achilles tendon, especially the bursa.

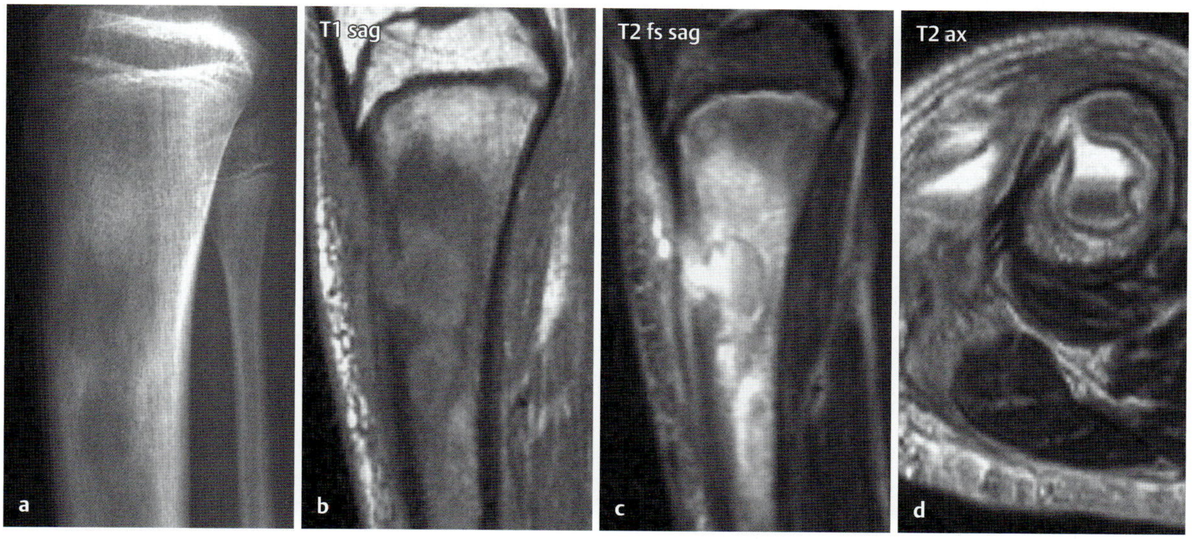

Fig. 3.8 Acute osteomyelitis of the proximal tibia. **(a)** Ill-defined margin of the osteolytic area. **(b)** Disruption of the anterior cortical bone. **(c)** Extensive perifocal bone marrow edema and abscess cavity. **(d)** Intraosseous abscess with sedimentation.

Differentiation between osteomyelitis and arthritis can be problematic. Septic arthritis may result in concomitant (completely unspecific) edematous involvement of the epiphysis and metaphysis, without any pathogen-induced osteomyelitis having to be present. On the other hand, juxta-articular osteomyelitis often results in a reactive joint effusion (▶ Figs. 3.9 and ▶ 3.10; cf. Chapter 3.3). The diagnosis of (concomitant) osteomyelitis in association with septic arthritis should only be made if the cortical bone is clearly disrupted (clarification is best obtained on T1W or T2W sequences without fat saturation).

Intraosseous abscesses tend to be small in size in acute osteomyelitis (0.5–3 cm); commonly they are relatively sharply delineated and occasionally display a hypointense cuff of normal tissue on fluid-sensitive sequences. Additional confirmation of an abscess is the marked marginal enhancement with no, or distinctly less, contrast enhancement in the center of the lesion corresponding to the abscess (▶ Fig. 3.10).

▶ **NUC MED.** Bone-seeking tracers are used for acute osteomyelitis. Multiphase bone scintigraphy using technetium (^{99m}Tc)-labeled diphosphonates is primarily used. Here, fully developed osteomyelitis will display a marked focal accumulation of the radionuclide in all three phases. Increased uptake in the blood-pool phase, without accumulation in the bone phase, is regarded as being indicative of an inflammation of only the soft tissue. Because of its radiation exposure, the use of multiphase bone scintigraphy has been reduced in favor of ultrasound and MRI, especially in children. Nor have other nuclear medicine imaging procedures (leukocyte scintigraphy, PET, and hybrid procedures such as PET-CT) been able to assert themselves as diagnostic modalities of choice for acute osteomyelitis.

Signs of healing of acute osteomyelitis. The first sign of healing to appear on the radiograph is progressive sclerosis, beginning at the periphery. The bone scan displays a reduction in activity, the MRI scan a resolution of the edematous changes and the soft tissue swelling with the development of contrast-enhanced (fibrovascular) granulation tissue. Contrast agent uptake becomes less and less over the course of time (months). In the ideal case, complete resolution occurs (▶ Fig. 3.11). Many cases, however, end up with an incomplete recovery. Increased sclerosis or fibrosis with periosteal thickening or even fatty marrow conversion can remain on MRI as a "scar."

Recommendations for an examination strategy

- Where there is clinical suspicion of **acute osteomyelitis**, radiography is the primary modality of choice, supplemented routinely by ultrasound in the neonatal period and early childhood. MRI should be used to confirm the diagnosis.
- When there is justified suspicion of **multifocal involvement** (particularly in the neonatal period), then a bone scan or whole-body MRI scan is useful. CT and nuclear medicine imaging modalities are reserved for special cases. Confirmation of the diagnosis "acute osteomyelitis" by biopsy is only rarely necessary, given that the combination of clinical presentation, laboratory results, and imagery is confirmation enough. Biopsy/aspiration is required for identification of the pathogen prior to commencement of appropriate antibiotic therapy.

▶ **DD.** **Primary and secondary bone tumors.** *Ewing's sarcoma* and, less frequently, *osteosarcoma*, are important differential diagnoses in children and adolescents, given that their clinical presentation and laboratory findings often resemble an inflammatory process. Radiography and bone scan may not allow for differentiation. MRI is a great help here. The solid tumor has space-occupying character and has often already breached the cortex. The peritumoral edema is often well defined from the tumor. *Osteoid osteoma* may resemble a focal lesion of osteomyelitis on MRI. Characteristic for an osteoid osteoma, however, is the surrounding sclerotic margin, which is absent in acute osteomyelitis (a radiograph or CT image must be available when assessing the MRI findings; ▶ Fig. W3.1). In adults, the differential diagnosis "tumor versus inflammation" rarely arises as a clinical issue. The same criteria for differentiation apply as for children and adolescents.

Cysts and other lesions. Marginal enhancement around fluid-filled cavities is also found on MRI around cysts, necrotic tumors, and posttraumatic seromas (see also chronic osteomyelitis in Chapter 3.1.3). In these cases, differentiation is only possible from the thickness of the marginal enhancement and identification of an associated edema. An abscess typically displays the latter.

Brodie Abscess

▶ **Pathology.** A pus-filled cavity measuring 1 to 5 cm is present within the cancellous bone. This is surrounded by marked sclerosis of the cancellous bone. *Staphylococcus aureus* can be grown from the abscess aspirate in one half of cases.

▶ **Clinical presentation.** The clinical findings are relatively limited. Some patients do not consult a physician until late. The disorder has its peak incidence in the second decade of life. The findings are primarily located in the metaphyseal part of the distal femur or at the proximal tibia.

▶ **Radiography.** Brodie abscesses cause osteolysis in the metaphysis or diametaphysis. Round, oval, and polymorphic forms are possible (▶ Fig. 3.12). The margin is characteristic, always being sharply delineated and demonstrating signs of surrounding sclerosis.

The osteosclerosis starts to fade toward the periphery so that the transition from sclerosis to normal bone is often ill-defined. Solid periosteal reactions are possible

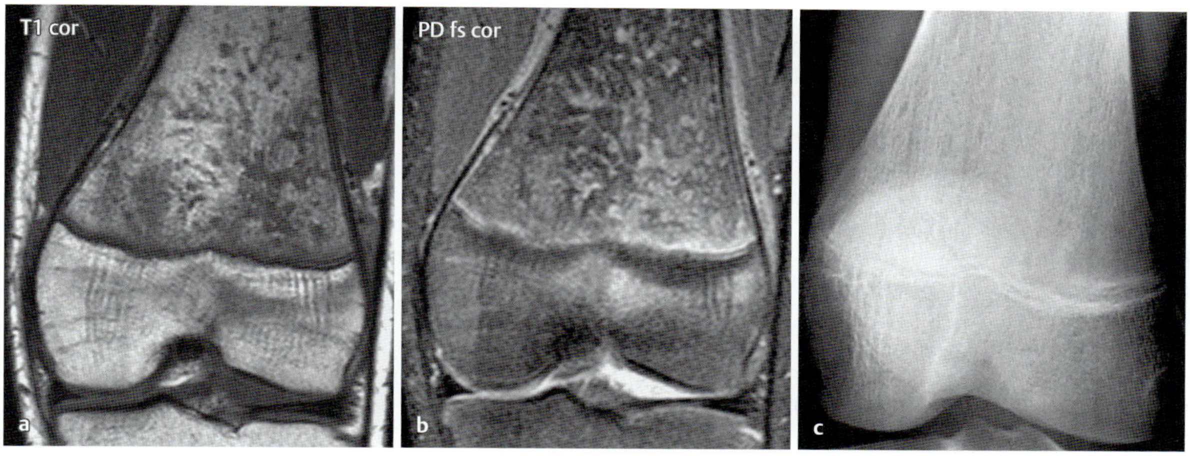

Fig. 3.9 Acute osteomyelitis. **(a)** Confluent small areas of low signal intensity in the metaphysis. **(b)** Incipient epiphyseal involvement. **(c)** The radiograph shows subtle osteolysis that could be overlooked were it not for knowledge of the MRI report.

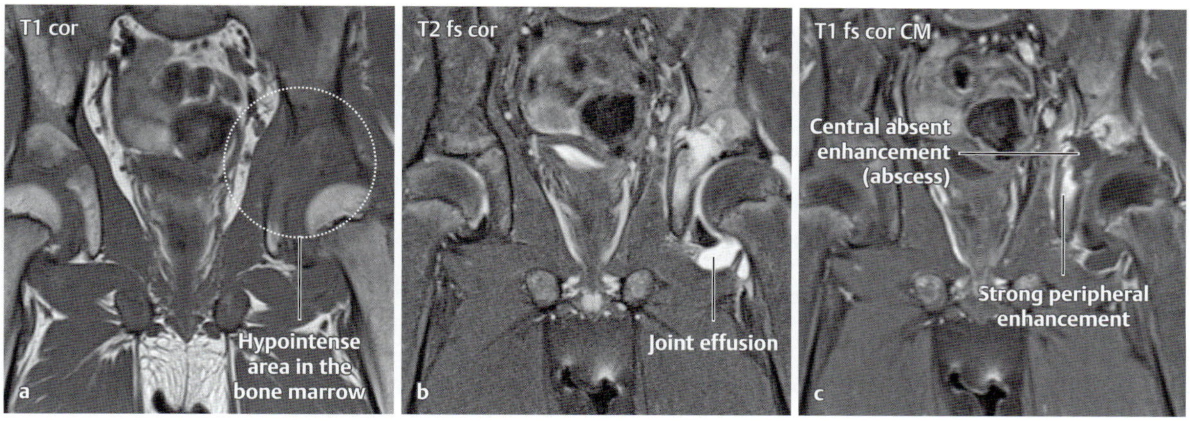

Fig. 3.10 Acute hematogenous osteomyelitis with abscess formation. **(a)** Loss of signal in the iliac bone on the T1W image. Cortical bone destruction. **(b)** Strong signal in the abscess with perifocal edema. **(c)** Contrast administration confirms the diagnosis of an abscess.

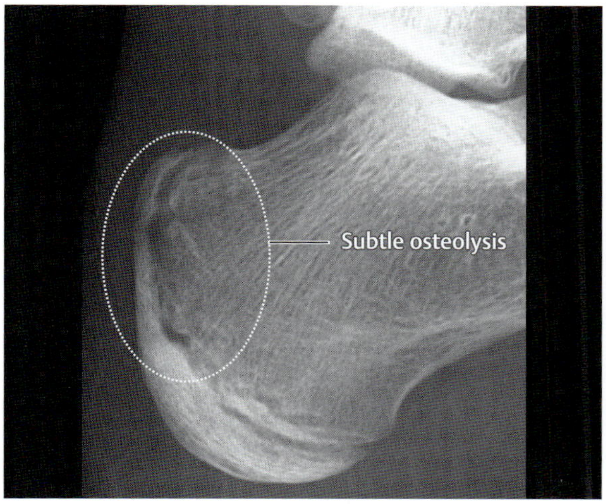

Fig. 3.11 Appearance after healing of an osteomyelitis. Compare with the original finding in ▶ Fig. 3.1.

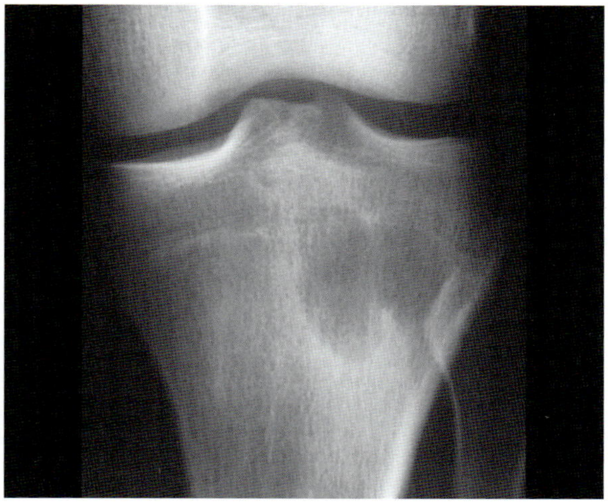

Fig. 3.12 Brodie abscess. Osteolysis associated with a rim of surrounding sclerosis.

(▶ Fig. 3.13a). Brodie abscesses may be located in the cortex, where they are then associated with strong, solid periosteal reactions that cause the bone to appear "distended."

▶ **MRI.** The typical appearance of an abscess is a strongly contrast-enhanced margin around a fluid, nonenhancing center (▶ Fig. 3.14). However, weak contrast filling of the center can result from a rapid diffusion of contrast medium. A signal-intense edema is always recognizable around the abscess (on water-sensitive sequences and after contrast administration).

The "**Penumbra sign**" refers to the mildly hyperintense rim lining the abscess that is already evident on the unenhanced T1W image, especially in the case of a Brodie abscess (▶ Fig. 3.13b). This lining enhances readily.

▶ **DD.** The radiological differential diagnosis includes osteoblastoma, chondroblastoma, nonossifying fibroma, giant cell tumor, eosinophilic granuloma, aneurysmal bone cyst, and fibrous dysplasia. It is possible to shorten this comprehensive list using MRI because tumors and tumorlike lesions usually enhance with contrast more clearly in their center when MRI is used. The differentiation between a simple cyst and a Brodie abscess is usually possible by a combined assessment of radiographs and MRI scans. A cyst displays only a narrow sclerotic margin on the radiograph and lacks perifocal edema on MRI—provided there are no fractures. Septations and fluid levels, as with an aneurysmal bone cyst, are not seen on MRI of a Brodie abscess.

3.1.3 Chronic Exogenous Osteomyelitis

Chronic exogenous osteomyelitis is an infection of the bone that is not induced hematogenously and demonstrates a chronic recurrent course (cf. Chapter 3.1.1).

▶ **Pathology.** The disorder can be initiated by the migration of pathogens through natural barriers such as skin, teeth, or paranasal sinuses. Another route of spread results from injury to natural barriers, such as after cuts and lacerations, or secondarily to burns and bed sores.

The **direct inoculation** of pathogens into the bone due to trauma or iatrogenically is the most common form of exogenous osteomyelitis. The spread of the infection in posttraumatic osteomyelitis depends not only on the number and virulence of the pathogens and the resistance of the patient, but also, and above all, on local conditions such as the degree of soft tissue damage, disruption of vascularization of the bone, the stage of fracture healing, and the type of foreign material introduced. Poor vascularization and altered stability of the traumatized soft tissue and bone are cofactors, or even the cause, of the insidious development of chronic osteomyelitis.

▶ **Clinical presentation.** The majority of cases of posttraumatic and postoperative forms of osteomyelitis begin acutely. As a rule, this is what is known as a "full-blown infection." Cardinal symptoms are erythema, increased skin temperature and swelling of the surgical site, associated with abnormal wound healing. Fistula formation with purulent discharge or serous fluid is possible. Inflammatory parameters (white blood cell count, ESR and CRP) of laboratory tests are elevated. After these signs of early infection, the further course of such exogenous infections is chronic-recurrent. Even after several years of a clinically inapparent chronic infection, acute flares can recur (also known as the reactivation of chronic osteomyelitis).

▶ **Radiography.** The radiological findings differ clearly depending on the route of infection. With posttraumatic, direct inoculation of the pathogen, the radiograph depends strongly on the presence of fractures and their healing and transformation processes. In some cases the infectious process is difficult to recognize. After surgery, especially after the introduction of fracture fixation hardware, screws, plates, and nails can superimpose and obscure the picture (▶ Fig. 3.16). If a soft tissue infection results in osteomyelitis, then the periosteum will react very early. Depending on the route of infection usually to be expected from the clinical presentation, the various imaging modalities will be accorded different degrees of importance.

In cases of pathogen migration or injury to the skin

- Consolidation of the soft tissue, disappearance of the fat lines.
- Periosteal reaction of varying degrees of expression and form.
- Mixed appearance combining destruction (small lytic areas) and consolidation.
- Lytic destruction of larger parts of the bone, particularly in the fingers and toes (▶ Fig. 3.15).

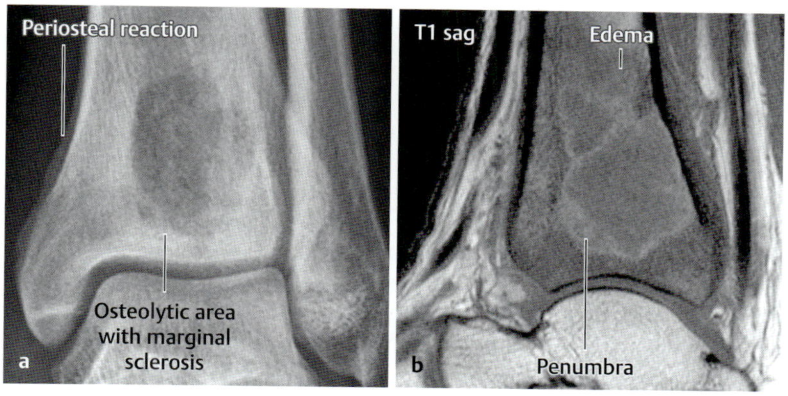

Fig. 3.13 Brodie abscess. **(a)** Solid periosteal reaction indicating a chronic process. **(b)** The margin of the abscess on the unenhanced T1W image appears slightly hyperintense to the abscess contents (known as penumbra, see text).

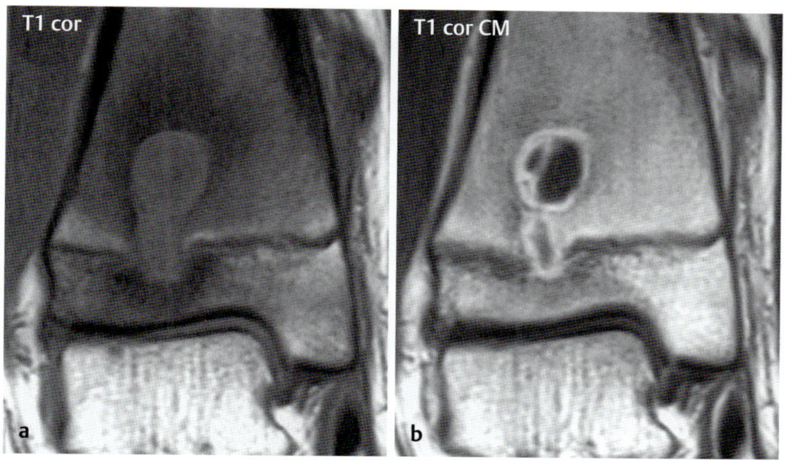

Fig. 3.14 Classic Brodie abscess on MRI. **(a)** Extensive perifocal edema (hypointense). **(b)** Strong enhancement of the lining of the abscess.

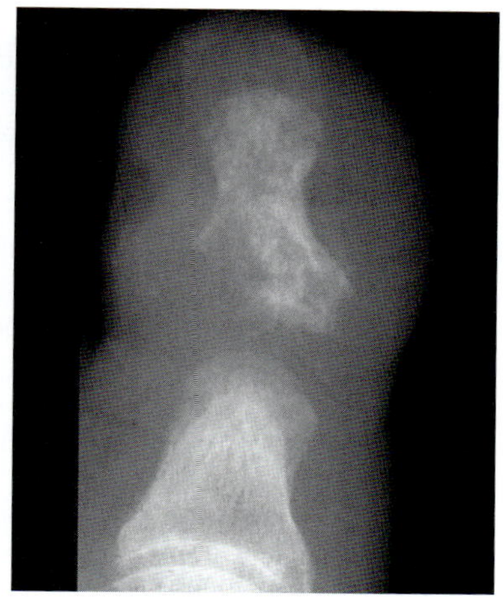

Fig. 3.15 Exogenous osteomyelitis and arthritis secondary to soft tissue infection. Ill-defined bone destruction of the terminal phalanx.

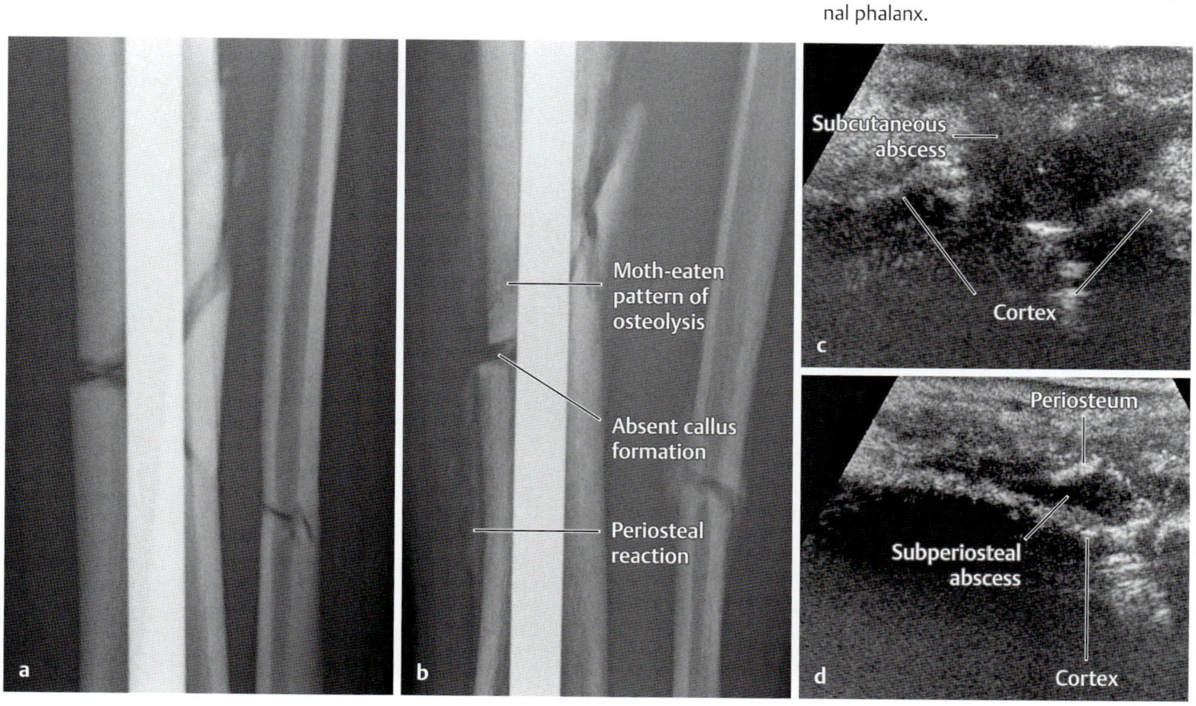

Fig. 3.16 Exogenous osteomyelitis. **(a)** Initial postoperative radiograph. **(b)** Radiograph 2 months later. **(c)** Subcutaneous abscess originating from the fracture line. **(d)** Subperiosteal abscess and periosteal reaction, correlating with the radiograph.

Posttraumatic, postoperative

- Mixed lytic and sclerotic appearance of the bone (▶ Figs. 3.17–3.19).
- Typically solid periosteal reaction with consecutive widening of the cortical bone (sclerosis of the internal table, even to the extent of eburnization of the entire bone marrow, can also result in increased thickness of the cortical bone [▶ Fig. 3.17]; *caution*—likelihood of confusion with cortical thickening secondary to callus formation!).
- Bony sequestrum formation (irregular, circumscribed zone of marked consolidation) or involucrum (▶ Fig. 3.18).
- Apparent "widening" of the fracture gap (▶ Fig. 3.18).
- Circumferential radiolucent lines without sclerotic margin around screws.
- Lucent zones with ill-defined margin around implants of more than 1.5 mm in size (cf. ▶ Fig. 2.358; *caution*—artifactual lucent zones at the high-contrast metal–bone interface on digital radiography).

▶ US. Soft tissue abscesses around bones are well demarcated. Diffuse phlegmons may be seen as hypoechoic ill-defined areas. Cortical destruction and periosteal reaction can be detected (▶ Fig. 3.15).

▶ CT. CT is ideally suited for the detection of a nonviable sequestrum, involucrum, and osseous fistulas. The sequestration is of high density and surrounded by a cuff of fluid and soft tissue.

▶ MRI. The examination technique in cases of posttraumatic exogenous osteomyelitis is similar to that of the acute form (Chapter 3.1.1). Metal artifacts can restrict the diagnostic value of MRI due to local field inhomogeneities. The same also applies after removal of implants because troublesome metal debris remains. Even radiologically invisible abrasion artifacts can produce circumscribed signal distortions up to 1 cm in size: an area of complete signal loss is surrounded by a very hyperintense (semi-)circle. This ring is larger with fat-suppressed sequences than with normal SE sequences.

Findings

- Extensive bony remodeling, with hypointense sclerosis, fibrosis, and cortical thickening found on all sequences, determines the overall picture.
- Nevertheless, the principal rules applied for diagnosing inflammation, as described for acute osteomyelitis (Chapter 3.1.2), remain valid.
- On T1W sequences, bone marrow alterations are hypointense to fatty marrow (▶ Fig. 3.20a).
- The inflammed areas are hyperintense on fat-saturated fluid-sensitive sequences; abscesses are practically fluid-equivalent with a somewhat less signal-intense halo (▶ Fig. 3.19c).
- After injection of contrast, variable but increased signal intensity is seen in the abscess membrane and granulation tissue. The abscess cavity takes up no contrast, or takes it up only in a delayed manner (▶ Figs. 3.20b and ▶ 3.21). After contrast administration, at least a mild signal enhancement should be evident in the presence of an active process (▶ Fig. 3.21); otherwise, the diagnosis of an abscess should be challenged or only a very mildly active process should be assumed.
- Fistula tracts usually appear as contrast enhancements with a meandering pattern (see ▶ Fig. 3.25). They present as linear hyperintensities on fluid-sensitive sequences.

During the initial weeks after injury or a surgical intervention it is often not possible to diagnose an infection with any degree of confidence because edema, granulation tissue, fibrosis, and callus formation produce signal intensity changes that strongly resemble those of an infection. Only the positive identification of abscesses and fistulas should give cause for the unequivocal diagnosis of posttraumatic or postsurgical bacterial inflammation.

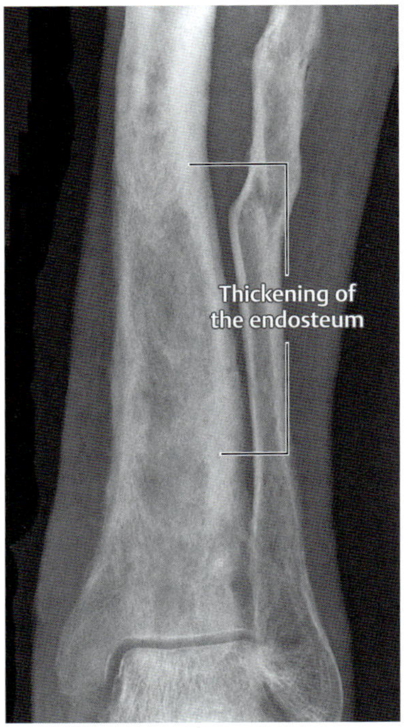

Fig. 3.17 Posttraumatic osteomyelitis. Mixed lytic and sclerotic appearance of the bone.

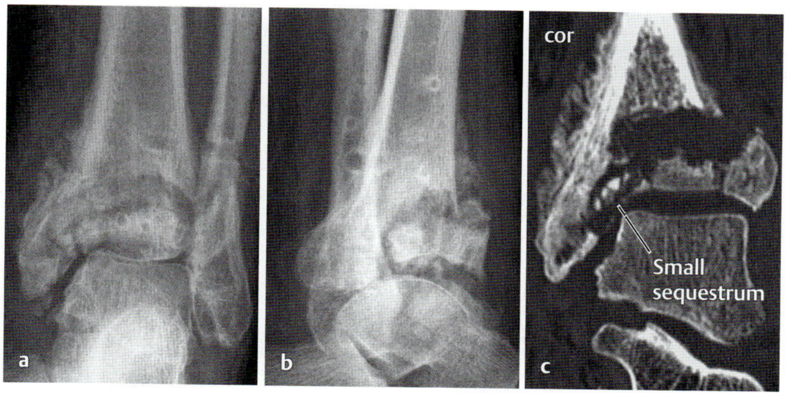

Fig. 3.18 Posttraumatic osteomyelitis following a pilon fracture of the tibia. **(a)** Mixed lytic and sclerotic appearance of the bone with marked periosteal reaction. **(b)** Apparent widening of the former fracture gap. **(c)** Knowing the CT finding, the small sequestrations are identifiable on the radiograph (**a**).

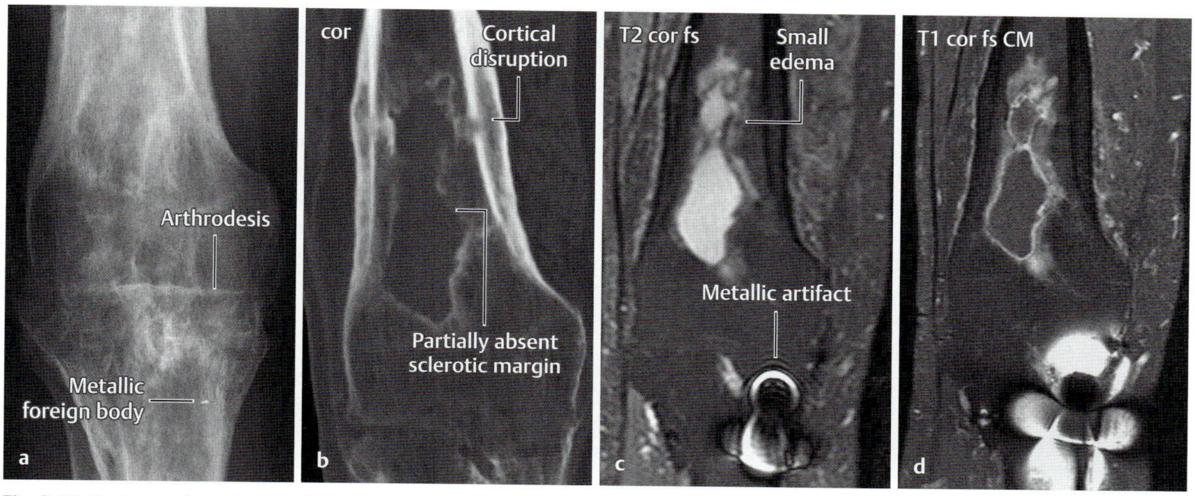

Fig. 3.19 Postoperative osteomyelitis after knee joint fusion. **(a)** Nonspecific, mixed lytic and sclerotic appearance of the distal femur. **(b)** Large area of osteolysis with partial, fine sclerotic margin as a sign of a slowly progressive process. **(c)** A subtle cuff of edema is an indication of mild activity. **(d)** The metal artifact is larger on the fat-saturated T1W sequence than on the T2W sequence (**c**).

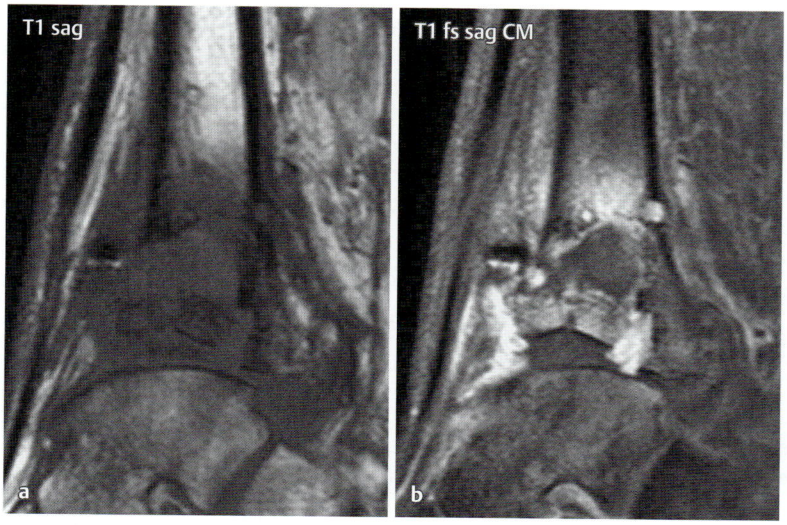

Fig. 3.20 Posttraumatic osteomyelitis. Same patient as in ▶ Fig. 3.18. **(a)** Hypointense bone marrow reaction around the enhanced abscess of intermediate signal intensity. **(b)** Those parts of the bone around the abscess that are still perfused show enhancement.

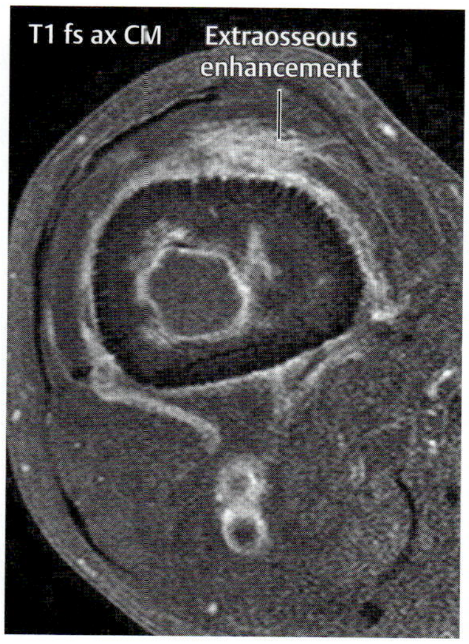

Fig. 3.21 Exogenous osteomyelitis. Same patient as in ▶ Fig. 3.19.

▶ NUC MED. The classic nuclear medicine imaging procedure for diagnosing osteomyelitis is **three-phase bone scintigraphy.** The technique has high sensitivity, but its specificity is low. Increased tracer uptake following fractures and surgical procedures, in particular, produces differential diagnostic problems. Bone scintigraphy alone may not be sufficient. When it is combined with leukocyte scintigraphy (▶ Fig. 3.22), a chronic osseous inflammatory lesion may at least be excluded in all probability.

There are two types of procedures used for **leukocyte scintigraphy**:

- The patient's own leukocyte suspensions are isolated, marked with indium 111 (^{111}In) compounds or technetium Tc 99 m-HMPAO (hexamethylpropyleneamine oxime), and reinjected.
- Alternatively there is the in-vivo marking of granulocytes with technetium 99 m- or iodine 123-labeled fragments of murine monoclonal antibodies. The antibody can bind with circulating granulocytes as well as diffuse through the capillary wall of inflamed tissue.

Any tracer accumulation that differs from the physiological distribution pattern is indicative of an infection. An increase in the activity accumulation during the course of the examination procedure (early image, 4-hour image, 24-hour image) reinforces the diagnosis of "infection."

On fluorine-18 fluorodeoxyglucose PET (**^{18}F-FDG-PET**), infections produce intensive, circumscribed activity accumulations. This modality can be used regardless of metal implants. PET is a highly sensitive method for diagnosing an exogenous osteomyelitis (▶ Fig. 3.23). This procedure has often been combined with CT and more recently also with MRI. Initial experience has shown that use of the hybrid modality can increase the specificity of these examinations.

Recommendations for an examination strategy. The initial examination for chronic osteomyelitis is projection radiography in two planes. The second step is MRI to provide supplementary diagnostic information. A radiograph in two projections should be available when the MRI is performed. Given the high specificity of radiographs and the excellent sensitivity of MRI, the combination of both procedures can generally achieve an accurate diagnosis. This is true for initial diagnosis and for a reactivated chronic osteomyelitis or osteitis. PET should be preferentially used particularly when metal implants are in situ. When combined with sectional imaging in the form of PET-CT or PET-MRI, this method ensures an increase in specificity. PET is also an option for the identification of residual activity after surgery for abscesses or sequestrations. The classic three-phase bone scan is only useful in combination with leukocyte scintigraphy.

Variant: Infected Diabetic Foot

"Diabetic foot" is the condition of the foot of a person with diabetes associated with characteristic soft tissue, joint, and bone alterations (Chapter 11.9.2). Exogenous infections are common concomitant phenomena during the course of chronic progressive disease particularly if poorly controlled. Imaging does not always allow distinction between a diabetic (Charcot/neuropathic) foot with and one without infection.

▶ Radiography. Signs found on projection radiography:

- Reactive erosions and lytic areas, even to the extent of a "melting away" of the bone, which is superimposed on the sclerosis of the Charcot foot (▶ Fig. 3.24a).
- Laminated periosteal reactions.
- Loculi of gas in the soft tissue.

▶ MRI. Confirmation is obtained by the identification of an abscess in the soft tissue and/or joint and/or bones (▶ Figs. 3.24b and ▶ 3.25). The direct comparison of the very bright structures on fluid-sensitive sequences and absent enhancement after administration of gadolinium confirms the presence of an abscess or—as is common—diffuse phlegmons in the soft tissues.

A connection with a **cutaneous fistula** supports the diagnosis of an abscess-related or phlegmonous infection (▶ Fig. 3.25). Diffuse increased signal intensity in the soft tissues and the bone is nonspecific, especially in the case of a diabetic foot, and should in no way be interpreted as the sign of an infection in isolation. Here too the rule applies: if the medullary cavity is not really hypointense on T1W images, then the diagnosis "osteomyelitis" should not be made.

▶ NUC MED. Only leukocyte scintigraphy is suitable for increasing specificity. It is, however, not a routine modality for confirming or excluding infection because this method is not specific enough. Nor is ^{18}F-FDG-PET an established method for diagnosing an infection because it is not capable of distinguishing with certainty between an infection and a nonspecific inflammatory response found during the course of the continual repair and remodeling processes of the diabetic foot.

3.1.4 Forms of Osteomyelitis (Specific Pathogens)

Tuberculosis

Tuberculosis is an infection caused by *Mycobacterium tuberculosis*, rarely by *Mycobacterium bovis*. An osteoarticular manifestation develops in about 1 to 2% of all tuberculosis patients. This is almost always preceded by a primary infection in other organs. The spine is most commonly involved (more than 50% of cases) (Chapter 3.1.5). Primary or secondary joint involvement is not uncommon.

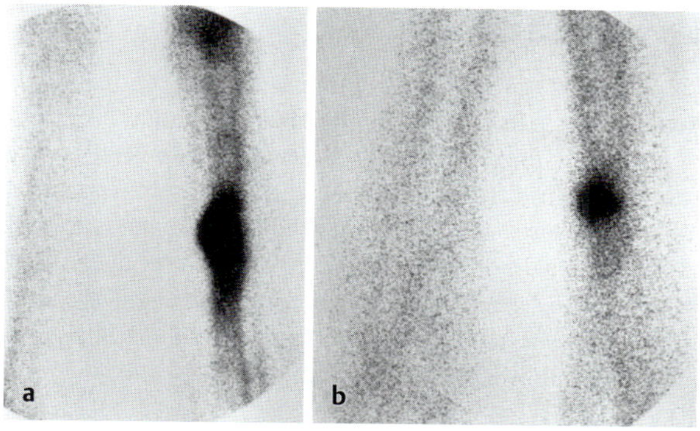

Fig. 3.22 Posttraumatic chronic osteomyelitis of the tibia. (Image courtesy of J. Sciuk, Augsburg, Germany.) **(a)** Marked activity in the static phase of the bone scan. **(b)** Leukocyte scintigraphy results in tracer accumulation in the infected part of the bone.

Fig. 3.23 Infected sequestration of the tibia. (Image courtesy of J. Sciuk, Augsburg, Germany.) **(a)** The sequestration is hardly demarcated in the thickened bone. **(b)** An ^{18}F-FDG-PET confirms the infectious focus by the increased carbohydrate metabolism.

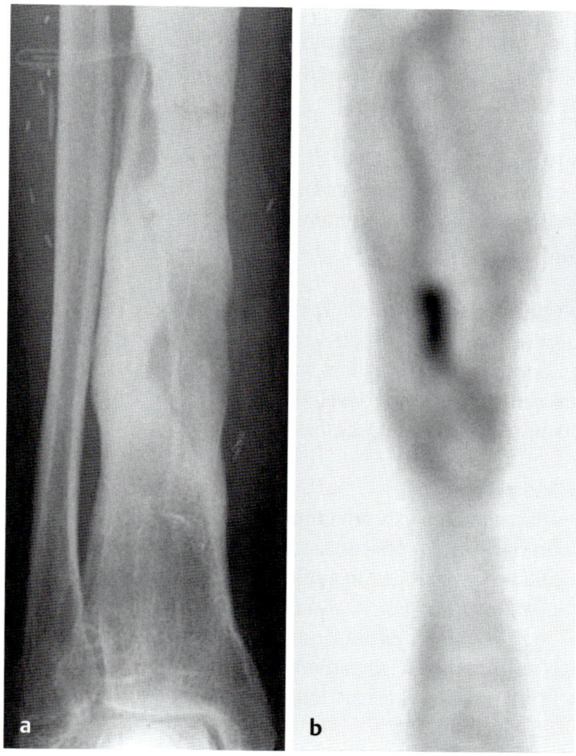

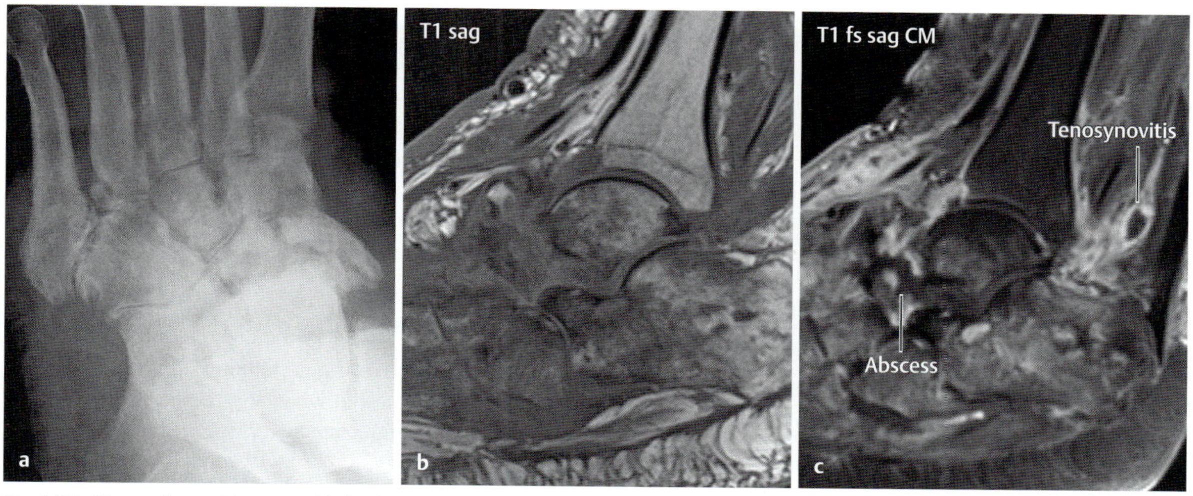

Fig. 3.24 Charcot foot with superadded infection. **(a)** Fragmentation of the navicular bone and osteolysis of the other tarsal bones; the infection is not evident on the radiograph. **(b)** Hypointense bone marrow reaction in the tarsal bones. **(c)** Acministration of contrast agent allows differentiation between abscesses and granulation tissue/edema.

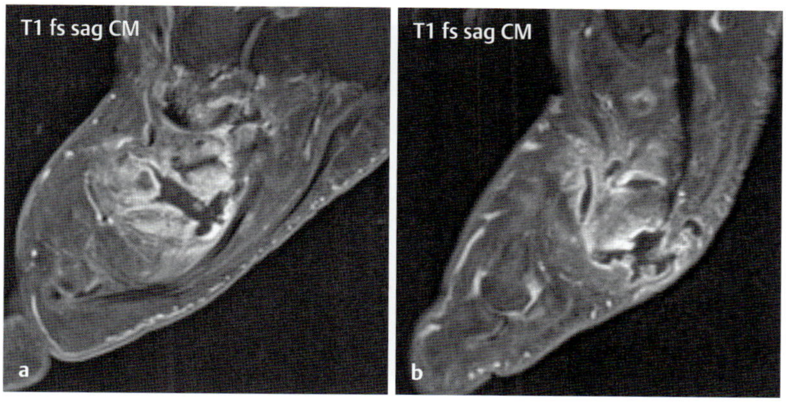

Fig. 3.25 Fistula formation in an infected Charcot foot. **(a)** Abscess of the midfoot. **(b)** Fistula formation extending to the sole of the foot.

The worldwide increasing prevalence of tuberculosis affects above all immune-compromised and immune-suppressed patients (those with HIV, alcoholism, malignancies, or undergoing chemotherapy).

▸ **Pathology.** Large parts of the bone marrow become necrotic in the exudative caseous form (unlike the productive form of tuberculosis); granulation tissue develops at the margin.

▸ **Clinical presentation.** The disease is characterized by its insidious course. The patient's general condition is affected, associated with weight loss and subfebrile temperatures. Local pain and swelling develop, but there is no erythema. Inflammatory parameters are elevated.

▸ **Radiography/CT.**

- Reactive osteolysis predominates (▸ Figs. 3.26 and ▸ 3.27). Primary diffuse sclerosis is found only in rare cases (above all in the spine) and in adults. A sclerotic margin, as a sign of a slow progression, also develops (▸ Fig. 3.28).
- The periosteal reaction can differ considerably in its extent from patient to patient (▸ Fig. 3.29).
- "Punched-out" destruction patterns are possible in children (▸ Fig. 3.26).
- Dactylitis in the phalanges of hands and feet of neonates and small children is a rarity these days. This involves a periosteal reaction and diffuse fusiform expansion of the phalanx (known as spina ventosa; ▸ Fig. 3.30).
- A permeative or "moth-eaten" pattern is rare (▸ Fig. 3.31a).

▸ **MRI.** The granulomatous inflammation often creates the impression of a multicentric "tumor" with corresponding signal intensity (hypointense on T1W sequences, hyperintense on fluid-sensitive sequences). A specific diagnosis should only be attempted together with the radiograph (▸ Fig. 3.31b, c).

▸ **NUC MED.** Tuberculous nodules are detected using ^{18}F-FDG-PET. The activity of the nodules during treatment can be assessed. This method does not differentiate between infectious and malignant disorders.

▸ **DD.** Any distinction from other, more chronic, forms of nonspecific osteomyelitis can be difficult or even impossible in some cases. Biopsy is mandatory in the majority of cases.

Brucellosis

Brucellosis is transmitted to humans via milk products; it is nowadays rare in Europe and the United States. In 30 to 40% of cases the clinically acute form results in arthritis that may primarily be regarded as reactive. A radiograph is obtained for the purposes of exclusion and for basic diagnostics but is usually negative. In chronic clinical forms, spondylitis predominates in cases of osteoarticular involvement. The radiological and MR images are reminiscent of tuberculosis and only really allow a presumptive diagnosis.

Leprosy

Osseous and articular affection with *Mycobacterium leprae* is uncommon in Europe and the United States but not in parts of Asia and Africa. Bone invasion by the pathogen—usually per continuitatem—results in significant osteodestruction. A secondary, neurogenic osteoarthropathy is typical of leprosy. Arthritis of the major and minor joints, primarily and most likely of a reactive nature, is commonly a concomitant symptom of leprosy.

Salmonella infection

A salmonella infection of the bone manifests itself as subacute to chronic osteomyelitis or spondylitis. The pathogens do not produce any specific radiological findings. It is, however, characteristic for the organisms to colonize the bone within areas of bone infarction, where they cause an infection. In patients with sickle cell anemia this poses the problem of differentiating a sickle cell crisis (infarction) from a superadded infection. Imaging techniques, even MRI, are not always capable of making this differentiation with absolute confidence

Fungal diseases

Humans have a high resistance to fungal infections. They are therefore to be expected when the health of the "host" is compromised (immunodeficiency, malignant disease, specific medication). *Cryptococcus, Aspergillus fumigatus*, histoplasmae, *Coccidioides immitis, Candida* spp., and *Bastomyces dermatides* are, amongst others, pathogens that can exhibit osteoarticular involvement. Radiographic, CT, and MRI findings are nonspecific: Osteodestruction and sharp borders with healthy bone predominate (▸ Figs. 3.32 and ▸ 3.33).

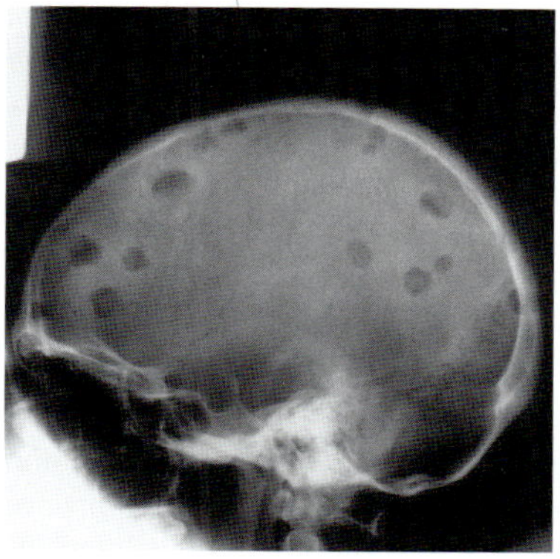

Fig. 3.26 Skeletal tuberculosis of the skull. "Punched out" osteolytic lesions with minimal sclerotic reaction.

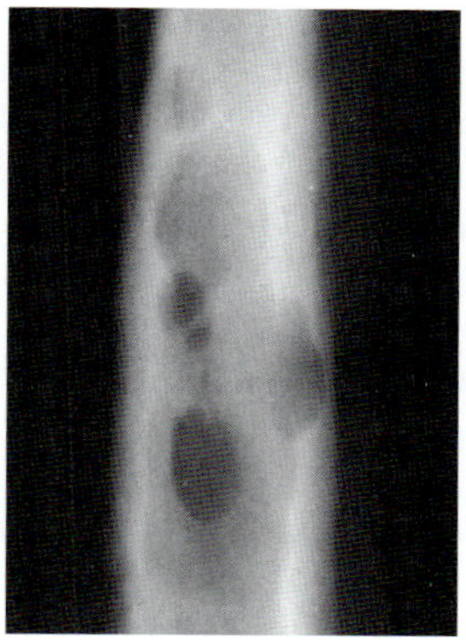

Fig. 3.27 Skeletal tuberculosis of the femur.

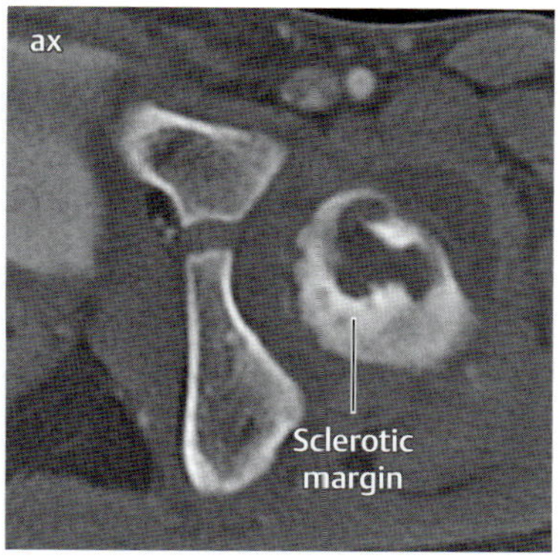

Fig. 3.28 Osseous tuberculosis of the proximal femur. The sclerotic margin indicates a slowly progressive process.

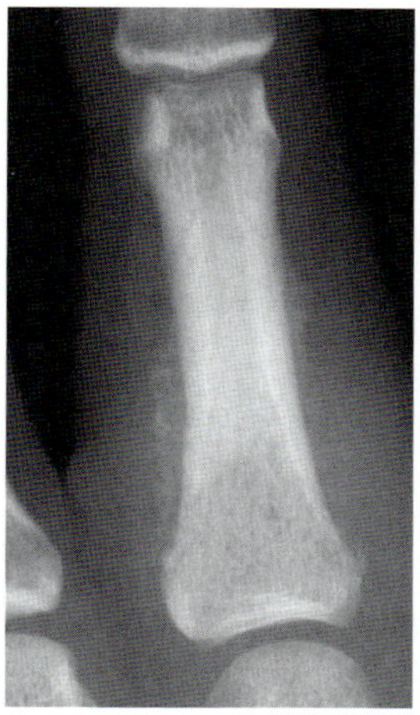

Fig. 3.29 Skeletal tuberculosis. Irregular periosteal reaction.

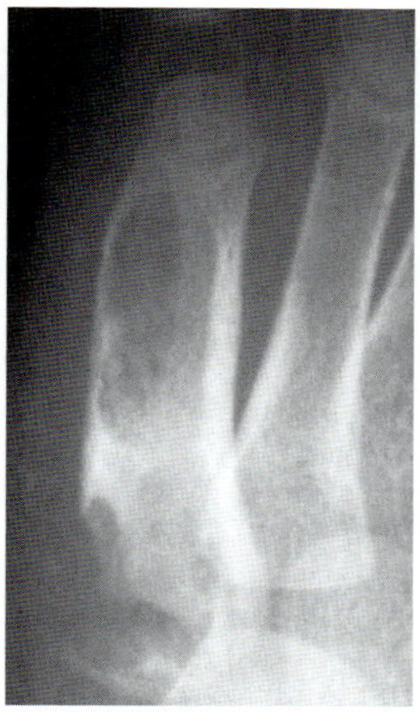

Fig. 3.30 Spina ventosa with typical fusiform swelling of the phalanx.

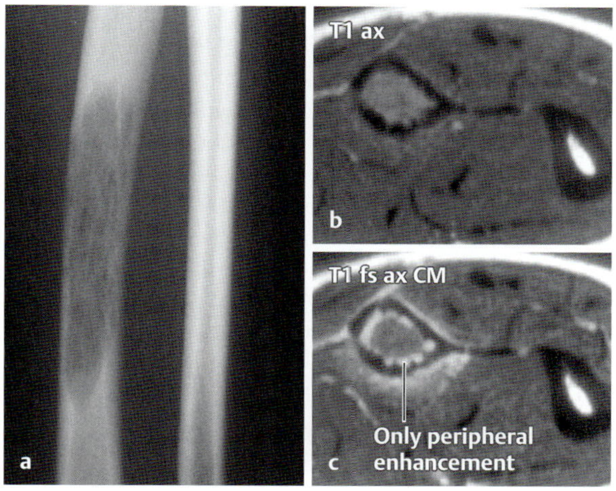

Fig. 3.31 Tuberculosis of the radius. **(a)** "Moth-eaten" pattern of osteolysis. **(b)** Loss of fat marrow signal in the medullary cavity on the plain T1W image. **(c)** Contrast enhancement only in the periphery as a sign of caseation (necrosis) of the center.

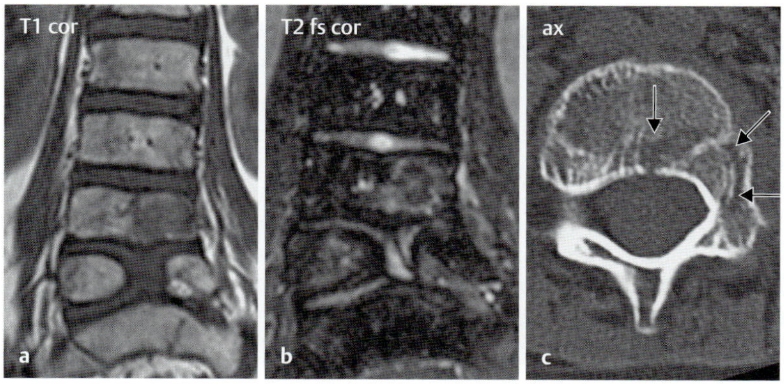

Fig. 3.32 Early finding of *Aspergillus* osteomyelitis in L4. Additional finding of a congenital butterfly vertebra at L5. **(a)** A nonspecific area of low signal intensity on the T1W image. **(b)** Mildly increased signal intensity, mainly in the periphery, on the T2W sequence. **(c)** The CT shows that the central portion of the bone is preserved. Fine lytic margin (arrows).

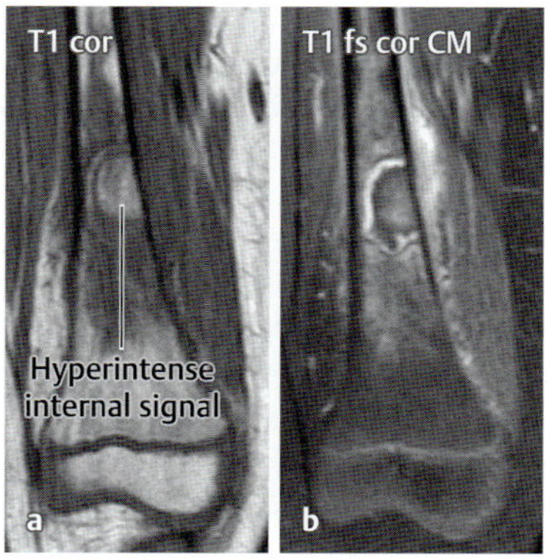

Fig. 3.33 *Aspergillus* osteomyelitis of the femur. **(a)** The very bright internal signal found in the lesion on the T1W image has been reported in aspergillosis and must not be mistaken for an infarction. **(b)** Very peripheral, less so central, contrast enhancement and perifocal edema.

Mycetoma

Mycetomas are classic forms of exogenous osteomyelitis secondary to fungal infection, commonly mixed with bacteria, which result in a chronic, granulomatous infection of the soft tissues and, subsequently, in an infection of the bone. The main site is the foot. Reference is widely made to the term Madura foot following its first description from the Indian region of Madura (▶ Fig. 3.34).

Echinococcosis

The most common pathogen is the parasite *Echinococcus granulosus* (giving hydatid disease). In about 2% of cases, the skeleton becomes involved as a result of seeding of pathogens via the blood circulation. Main sites are the pelvic bones and the sacrum. Multiloculated, expansile, "cystic" areas of osteolysis, occasionally traversed by trabeculae, are characteristic on radiographs. Cortical destruction may also be evident (▶ Fig. 3.35). Fluid-equivalent areas are found on MRI on T2W sequences. Radiologically there is a similarity with fibrous dysplasia, giant cell tumor, aneurysmal bone cyst, enchondromas, skeletal metastases, brown tumors, and angiosarcomas. A chordoma of the sacrum should be considered as a special differential diagnosis at that site. MRI is particularly helpful in distinguishing echinococcosis from a cystic tumor presenting on the radiograph. A diagnostic biopsy with aspiration of cystic contents is important in equivocal cases.

3.1.5 Infections of the Spine

▶ **Pathology.** Unlike with osteomyelitis, the route of infection is usually hematogenous via the arteries or the epidural venous plexus from the pelvis. Iatrogenic, i.e., exogenous, cases of spondylodiskitis are nevertheless not uncommon (postoperative or postinterventional complication). Staphylococci are also the most common pathogens in the spine. Another important disorder is spinal tuberculosis. *Salmonella* as a responsible pathogen should be considered in patients with sickle cell anemia and in diabetics. Fungi are very rare as potential pathogens. Brucellosis should be considered in endemic areas.

In a classic case, the infection takes origin at the anterior and lateral parts of a **vertebra**, adjacent to the intervertebral disk. At this very early stage (**spondylitis**) the avascular disk is excluded from the inflammatory process. The inflammation makes its way to the disk via the bony and cartilaginous end plates. This is particularly the case when the disko-vertebral transition zone has degenerated. We see the infection starting in the paravertebral soft tissue (epidural and paravertebral abscesses) and proceeding to invade in a **secondary stage** the vertebral body and intervertebral disk.

Because the vascular supply is different in children, a primary site of infection is also possible in the disk (**diskitis**).

▶ **Clinical presentation.** Apart from a general feeling of malaise and fever, patients present localized pain in the spine (often of a dull character, mainly at night) with a reactive protective posture. These cases are often diagnosed late because the clinician must consider the whole differential diagnostic spectrum of spinal pain. In severe cases patients may present with spinal cord compression. Tuberculous spondylitis typically develops over a period of weeks to months and is therefore often not detected until very late.

Distribution pattern. Although the entire spinal column may be affected, ***pyogenic spondylodiskitis*** tends to involve the lumbar spine (~ 70% of cases) and tuberculous spondylitis the thoracic spine and the thoracolumbar junction.

> **Note**
>
> CT-guided biopsy has an important role in classifying the pathogen causing infections of the spine and—to a lesser extent—for distinguishing between infection, degeneration, and tumor. However, a positive pathogen result is achieved in only 30 to 50% of cases with spondylodiskitis. The most common reason for these disappointing results is the fact that broad-spectrum antibiotic therapy will already have been commenced prior to biopsy. Some of the biopsy material should also always be sent for histological assessment as it may show chronic inflammation, in the absence of a positive culture, thereby confirming the diagnosis of infection.

▶ **Radiography.** In the early stage only soft tissue signs will point to the inflammation; attention should therefore be directed toward the paravertebral lines and, above all, the psoas shadow (▶ Fig. 3.36).

> **Caution**
>
> Early spondylodiskitis is to be suspected with any nonreactive (i.e., osteophytes and irregular end plates being absent) monosegmental reduction of disk height. This applies particularly in children and adolescents as other causes, such as degeneration, are highly unusual.

The first radiologically visible bony alterations are not detectable until **3 to 8 weeks** after the onset of clinical symptoms, and display various findings depending on the time lapse between onset of symptoms and imaging as well as during the further clinical course under (antimicrobial) treatment (▶ Figs. 3.37 and ▶ 3.38):

- Indistinct vertebral end plates.
- Reduction of the intervertebral disk space.
- Contour defects of the superior and/or inferior end plates.
- Vertebral body destruction, followed later by collapse.
- Reactive sclerosis.
- Gibbus deformity.

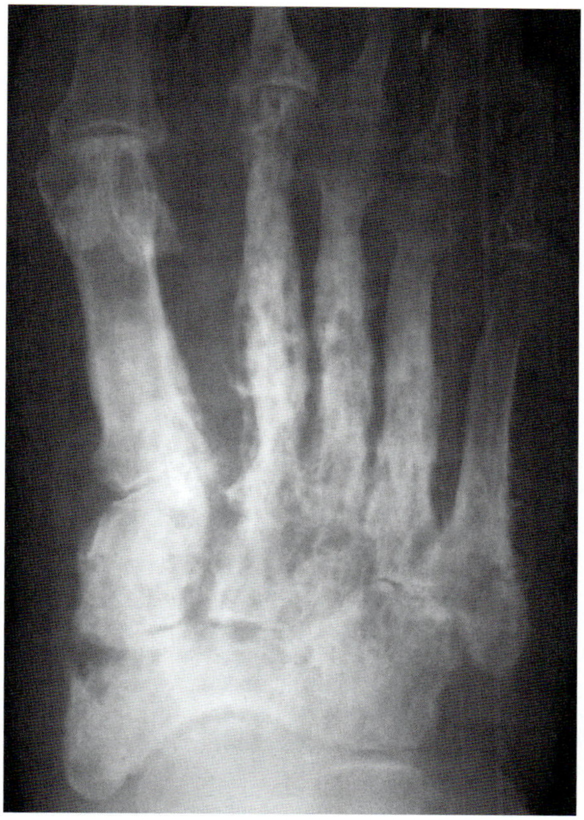

Fig. 3.34 Madura foot. Diffuse mixed sclerotic and lytic destructive process.

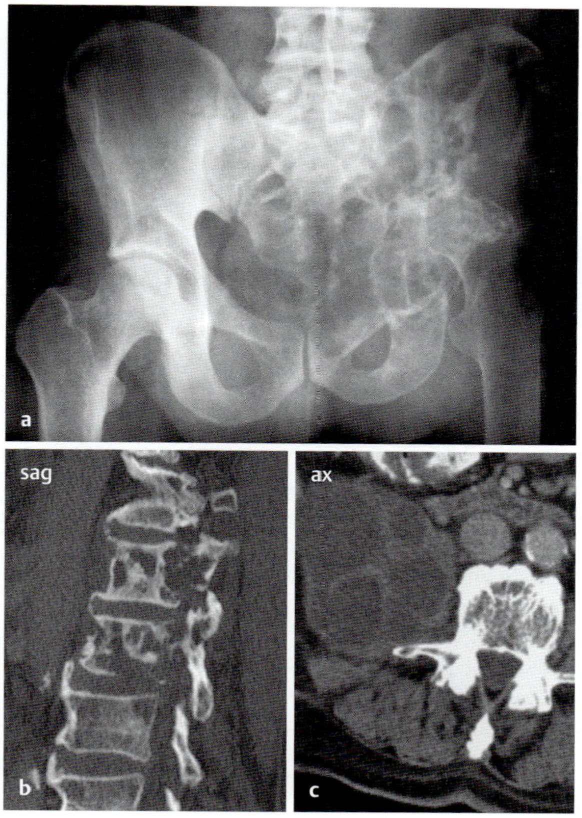

Fig. 3.35 Echinococcosis (hydatid disease). **(a)** Honeycomb, "multicystic" areas of osteolysis in the left pelvis. **(b)** The lumbar spine is also involved. **(c)** Lobulated hypodense soft tissue masses in the right psoas muscle.

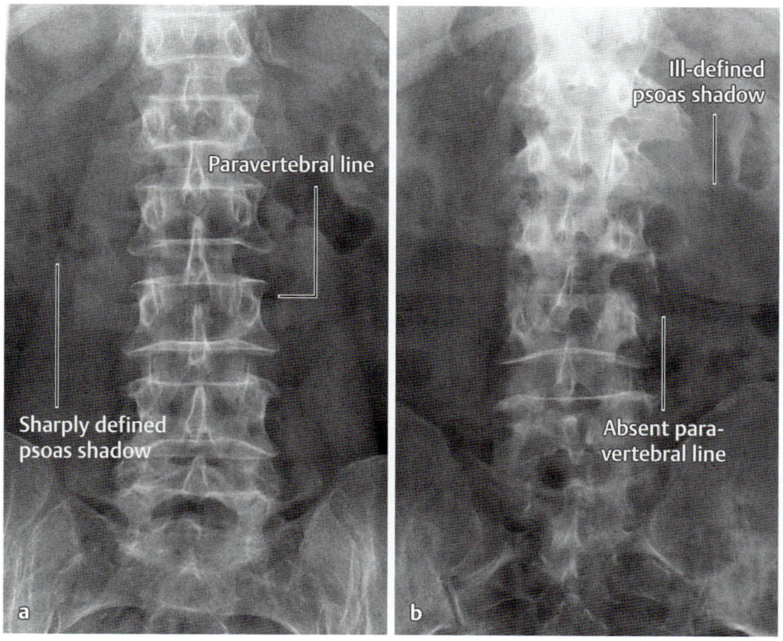

Fig. 3.36 Paravertebral soft tissue shadow. **(a)** Normal. **(b)** Pathologic finding in the presence of spondylodiskitis L3–L4.

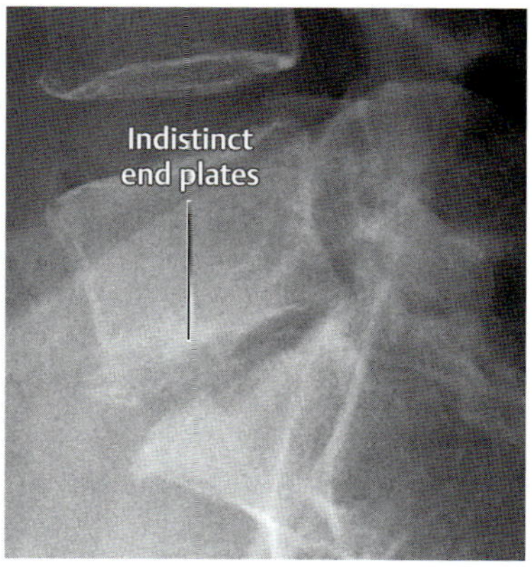

Fig. 3.37 Spondylodiskitis of L5–S1.

Fig. 3.38 Spondylodiskitis of L4–L5.

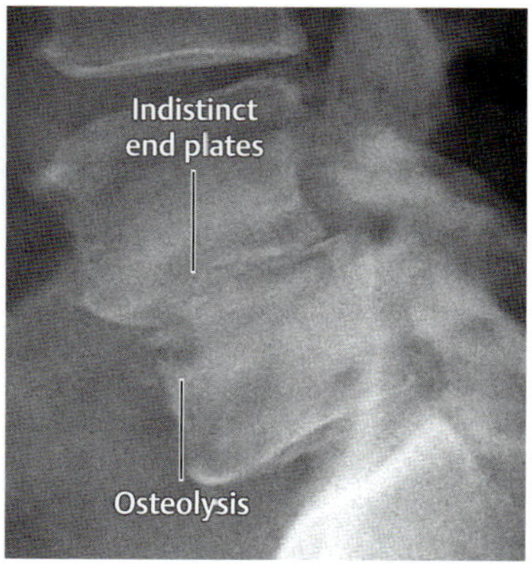

▸ **CT.** CT is superior to radiography in detecting the findings listed above under "Radiography." CT is most useful for the important practical differentiation between "degeneration" and infectious disease (▸ Fig. 3.39; also ▸ Table 3.1). For CT-guided biopsy, see Chapter 12.2.

▸ **NUC MED.** Nuclear medicine imaging procedures are employed when there are contraindications for MRI. Advantages over radiographic examination are the early detection and the ability to examine the whole body. A massively increased accumulation in all phases is seen in the two- or three-phase technetium Tc 99 m diphosphonate bone scan (▸ Fig. 3.40). This may well be nonspecific in itself but very worthwhile in correlation with a radiograph. Especially when the radiograph is (still) negative and *without* any sign of degeneration, the suspicion of an infection will be reinforced. ^{18}F-FDG-PET is also helpful for diagnosing and monitoring vertebral inflammations and paravertebral soft tissue involvement on the grounds of its high spatial resolution, especially when implants create artifacts and so restrict the informative value of MRI (▸ Fig. 3.41).

▸ **MRI.** Today, MRI is the modality of choice for early diagnosis, for differentiation from other pathologies (osteochondrosis, tumor), and in particular for clarifying the therapeutic approach (conservative, interventional, surgical). It allows the detection of the following findings:

- It shows low signal intensity on T1W sequences and increased signal intensity on fluid-sensitive sequences in one or both vertebrae as well as in the intervertebral disk (▸ Figs. 3.42 and ▸ 3.43). Depending on the point in time when the diagnosis is established, the entire vertebra or only parts of it may be involved. It should be borne in mind that, with paraspinal origin of the inflammation (soft tissue or epidural abscesses; ▸ Fig. 3.44), the finding in the bone and disk is not very pronounced and only develops secondarily.
- The inflammatory tissue enhances with contrast (▸ Figs. 3.44–3.46).
- Intervertebral disk height is usually reduced.
- The "black" bony-hyaline end plate is (partially) no longer visible (T1W and T2W images without fat saturation; ▸ Fig. 3.42).
- Abscesses (epidural, paravertebral, intradiskal) are hyperintense or even demonstrate a fluid-equivalent signal on fluid-sensitive sequences and do not enhance with contrast other than at the margins (▸ Figs. W3.2 and ▸ W3.3; see also ▸ Figs. 3.45 and ▸ 3.46).

Note

- Confirmation (or exclusion) of an epidural or paravertebral **abscess** is highly important as it is an indication for interventional drainage or surgical procedure in the presence of appropriate signs and symptoms.
- Establishing the diagnosis of a spondylodiskitis on MRI is not easy in the early stage because the "classic" signs have yet to develop. A **fat-saturated sequence** (T2W or STIR/T1 W sequences after contrast administration) should be obtained in any case. This allows increased signal intensities to be detected more sensitively.

Clinical course. There is almost always a discrepancy between the clinical course and laboratory results on the one hand and imaging on the other. In follow-up reviews 3 to 6 weeks after starting treatment, the finding in the vertebral body and the intervertebral disk is often more marked than in the initial examination. For this reason "follow-up review" using MRI is rarely of any use where there is evidence of a clinical improvement.

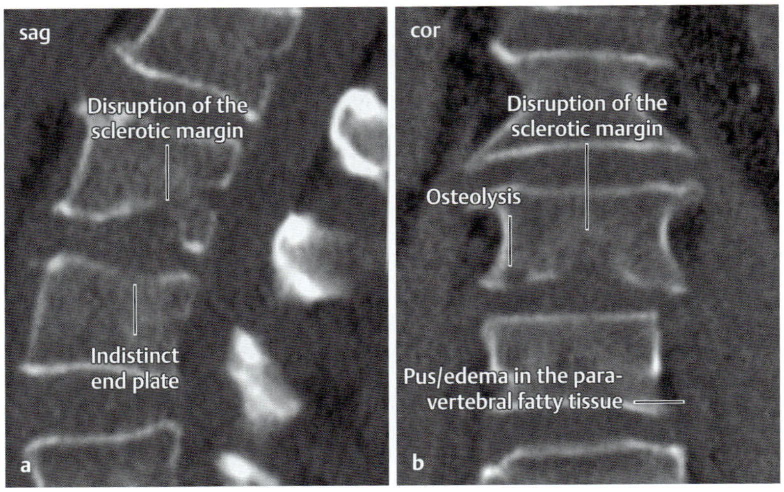

Fig. 3.39 Spondylodiskitis with a preexisting Schmorl's node. **(a)** Loss of definition of the sclerotic margin around the Schmorl's node and opposing superior end plate as a very early sign of spondylodiskitis. **(b)** Furthermore, there is a small area of osteolysis in the inferior end plate.

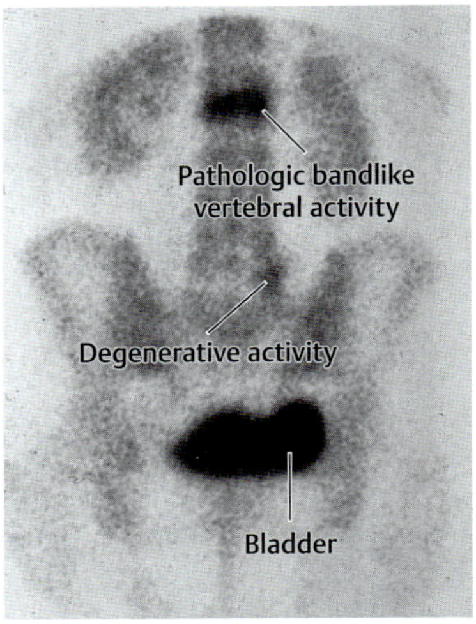

Fig. 3.40 Technetium Tc99m methylene diphosphonate (^{99m}Tc-MDP) bone scan in a case of spondylodiskitis. Late phase.

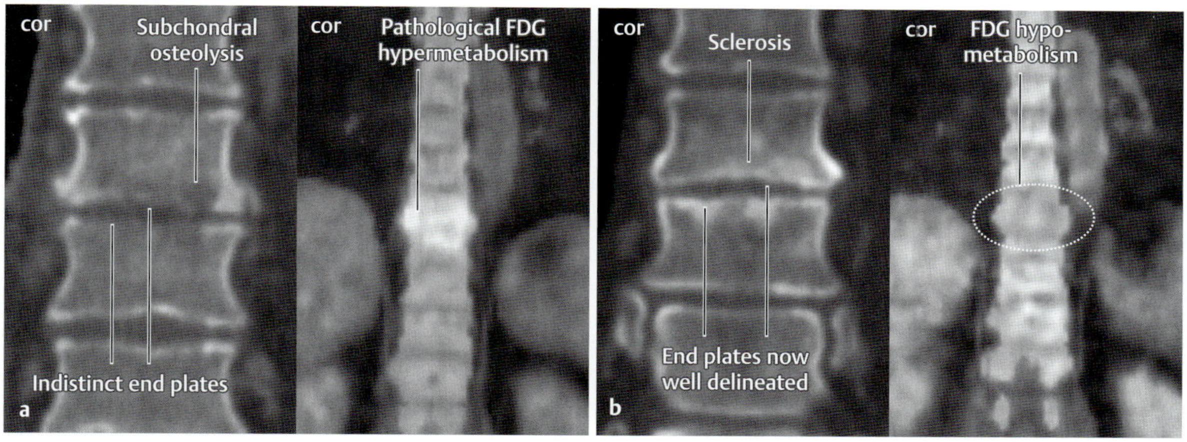

Fig. 3.41 Clinical course of a spondylodiskitis on antibiotic therapy. CT and corresponding ^{18}F-FDG-PET images. (Images courtesy of J. Sciuk, Augsburg, Germany.) **(a)** Fully developed spondylodiskitis with typical morphological changes and focal FDG-accumulation. **(b)** Healed spondylodiskitis 9 months later. The increased sclerosis is causing a reduction of physiological bone marrow metabolism in comparison with the surrounding vertebrae.

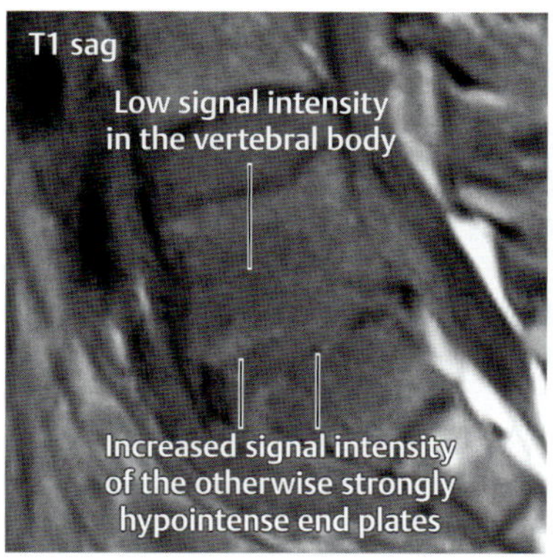

Fig. 3.42 Spondylodiskitis.

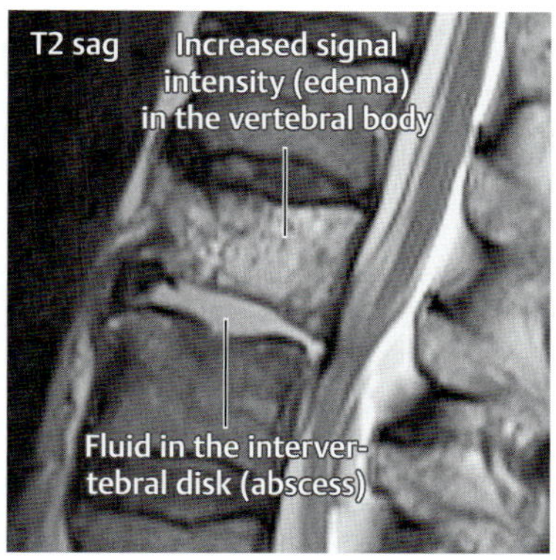

Fig. 3.43 Spondylodiskitis. Different patient from ▸ Fig. 3.42.

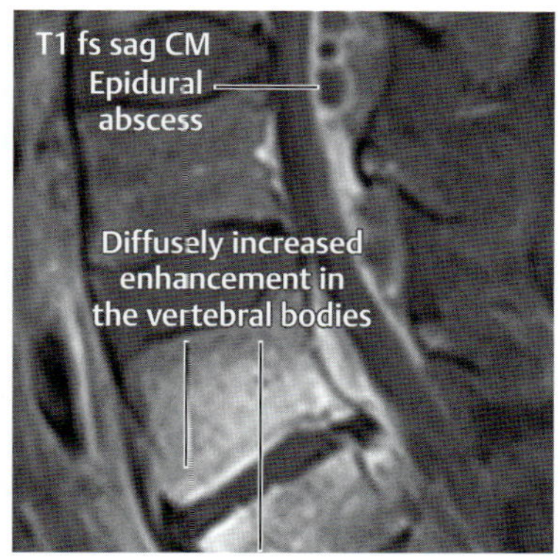

Fig. 3.45 Spondylodiskitis with epidural abscesses.

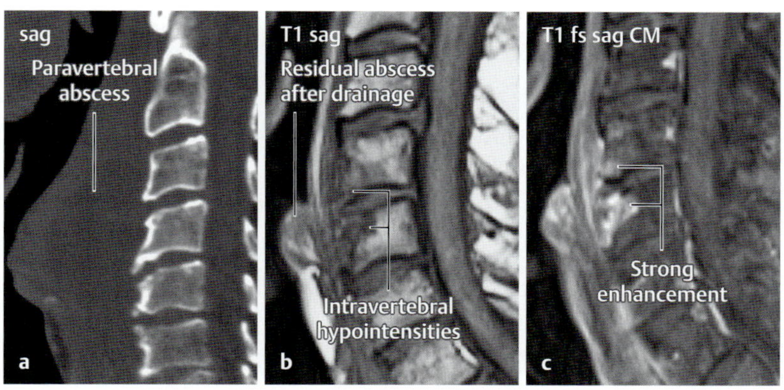

Fig. 3.44 Prevertebral abscess. Despite surgery, the abscess is affecting the vertebrae secondarily from the anterior aspect (secondary spondylitis). **(a)** The postoperative CT demonstrates a large abscess anterior to C3–C5. **(b)** Hypointense areas on the postoperative plain MR image confirm concomitant involvement of the vertebrae. **(c)** The MR image after IV contrast administration displays intervertebral enhancement.

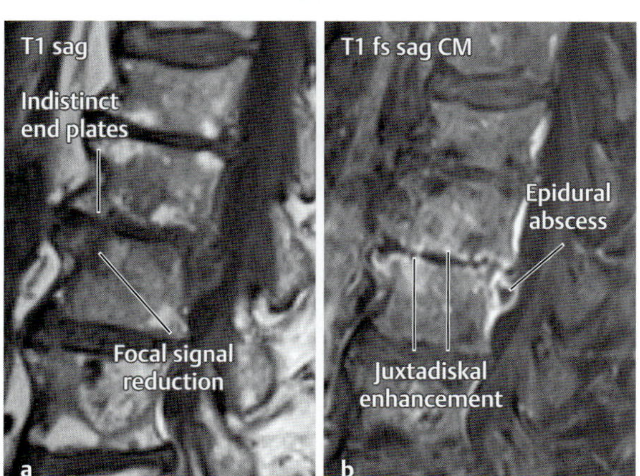

Fig. 3.46 Spondylodiskitis. Different patient from ▸ Fig. 3.45. **(a)** Heterogeneous bone marrow signal, not inappropriate in a 75-year-old patient. **(b)** Low contrast enhancement along the end plates, which is actually nonspecific. Concomitant evidence of a small epidural abscess that indicates the diagnosis of infection.

Initial signs of healing on MRI are reduction of inflammatory signs in the paraspinal soft tissues, with conversion of the vertebral signal into a normal fat signal (i.e., sclerosis) being a later-stage sign. Incomplete recovery of the involved vertebrae (collapse, deformation) is usually found.

▸ **DD.** Herniations of disk material into the superior and inferior end plates (**Schmorl's nodes**) are commonly associated with impressive perifocal increased signal intensities on fluid-sensitive sequences or after contrast administration. These findings are easily mistaken for spondylodiskitis or spondylitis (▸ Fig. 3.47). Exact analysis of the findings will usually lead to a correct diagnosis (▸ Table 3.1).

The differentiation between **pyogenic and tuberculous spondylodiskitis** (▸ Figs. 3.48–3.50 and ▶ Fig. W3.4) is not usually possible on the basis of imaging alone. Details are provided in ▸ Table 3.2. Clarification requires a CT-guided needle biopsy from the bone or soft tissue.

In some cases, differentiation from **erosive osteochondrosis** (▸ Figs. 3.51 and ▶ W3.5) is very difficult, not only on plain radiographs but also on MRI. Details are provided in ▸ Table 3.1.

The distinction from metastasis is only rarely a practical problem (Chapter 4.4). **Modic Type 1** changes are also hypointense on T1W and hyperintense on T2W images. In spondylodiskitis these appearances are more extensive in the majority of cases. An important distinguishing feature is that the vertebral end plates are intact in Modic Type 1 changes in the majority of cases, but one or both end plates is eroded/destroyed in spondylodiskitis.

In **children**, an **acute calcifying diskitis** should be considered. The etiology is not clear; this is not an infection. With the presence of calcification of the intervertebral disk, the diagnosis is not difficult from a radiograph or CT. The cervical spine is primarily affected (▸ Fig. 3.52).

3.2 Soft Tissue Infections

As with bones, soft tissue infections can develop from hematogenous seeding during bacteremia. However, the cause is far more commonly a wound infection. Here, the infection can spread per continuitatem from the site of entry of the pathogen to the surrounding soft tissue or result in extension of the infection along the lymphatic channels. A distinction is made between the following patterns of infection:

Panniculitis (cellulitis). Generally speaking, this is an exogenous infection of the subcutaneous tissue without involvement of muscle or fascia.

Pyomyositis. Infectious pyomyositis is classified according to the pathogen and has its origin in the muscle. It manifests itself as a diffuse or abscess-forming inflammation. Tuberculosis also commonly presents more granulomatous clinical forms. However, pyomyositis only rarely develops via a primarily hematogenous route.

Erysipelas. Bacterial infection of the superficial layers of the skin and the lymphatic channels, usually originating from minor skin injuries (see ▸ Fig. 3.56).

Table 3.1 Distinguishing spondylodiskitis from erosive osteochondrosis based on MRI findings

Feature	Spondylodiskitis	Erosive osteochondrosis
End plates	Partially ill-defined	Usually definable throughout, CT analysis of the end plates is very helpful in some cases
Vertebral body edema	Major parts of the vertebra	Tend to be near the end plates, bandlike (exceptions possible)
Intervertebral disk	Very variable findings	Very variable findings
Vacuum phenomenon	Unusual	Sometimes present, then very specific
Abscess formation/phlegmon	Common	None
Soft tissues	Often extensive soft tissue involvement	Usually no, or only mild, concomitant reaction of the soft tissues

Table 3.2 Details of the differential diagnosis between pyogenic and tuberculous spondylodiskitis

Feature	Pyogenic spondylodiskitis	Tuberculous spondylodiskitis
Clinical presentation	Acute, high inflammatory parameters	Chronic, few inflammatory parameters
Segments	Usually monosegmental	More commonly oligosegmental
Disk involvement	Early	Late
Soft tissues	Mostly small epidural abscesses	Large paraspinal abscesses, possibly with calcification

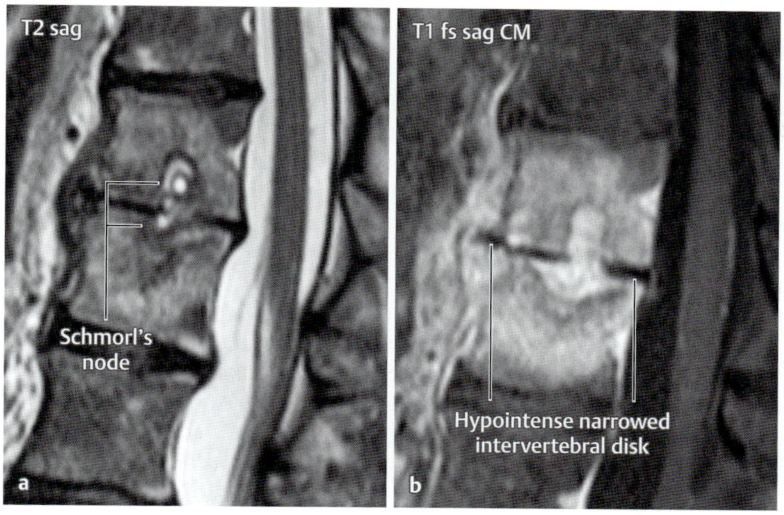

Fig. 3.47 Two "confluent" Schmorl's nodes with massive edema. No spondylodiskitis. Note the "black" intervertebral disk outside the Schmorl's node as an important indication of osteochondrosis. **(a)** Diffuse edema in both vertebrae. **(b)** Diffuse contrast enhancement of the vertebrae.

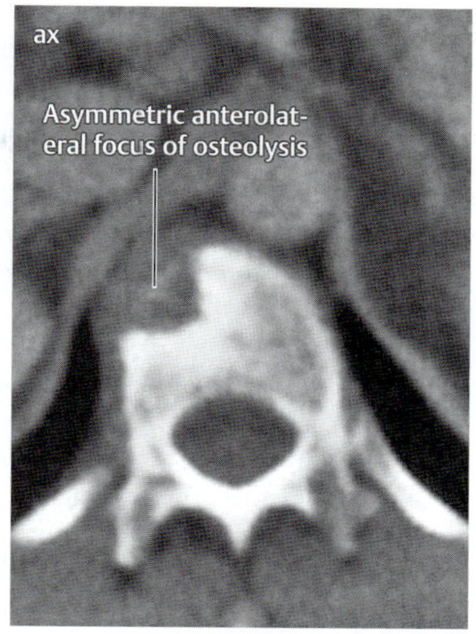

Fig. 3.48 Tuberculous spondylodiskitis. The CT image displays asymmetrical lysis of the vertebrae ("nibbled"); this is indicative of tuberculosis.

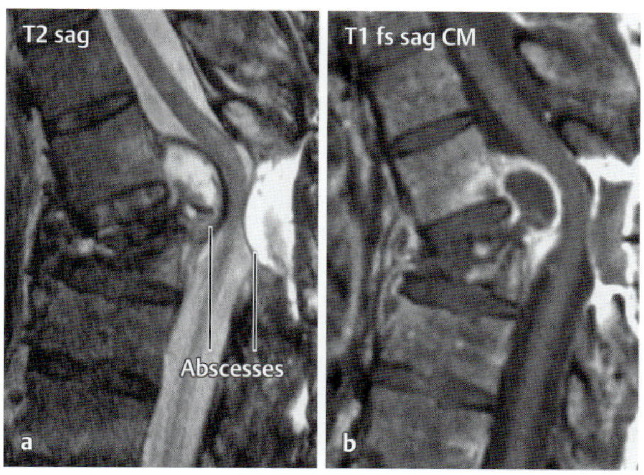

Fig. 3.49 Tuberculous spondylodiskitis. Destruction of the vertebra with wedging (gibbus). **(a)** Additionally, the spinal cord is displaced and compressed by large abscesses. **(b)** Strong contrast enhancement of the abscess capsule; the abscesses themselves remain hypointense on T1W sequences.

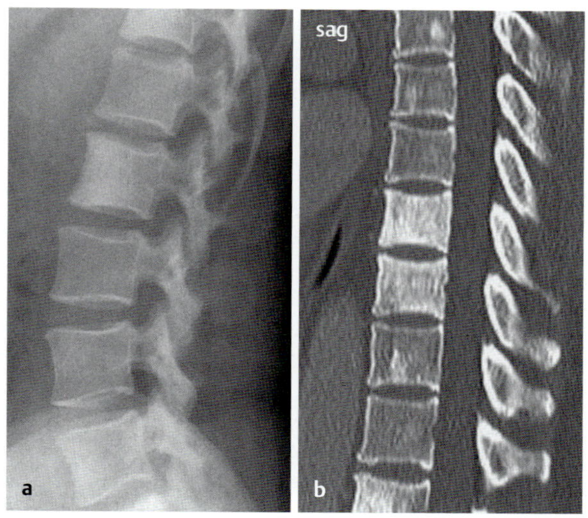

Fig. 3.50 Sclerotic, multifocal spondylitis secondary to infection with *Mycobacterium avium*. ▶ For supplementary MRI images see ▸ Fig. W3.4 (images courtesy of H. Rosenthal, Hannover, Germany). **(a)** Extensive sclerotic areas on the radiograph of the lumbar spine. **(b)** Multisegmental involvement of the thoracic spine on CT.

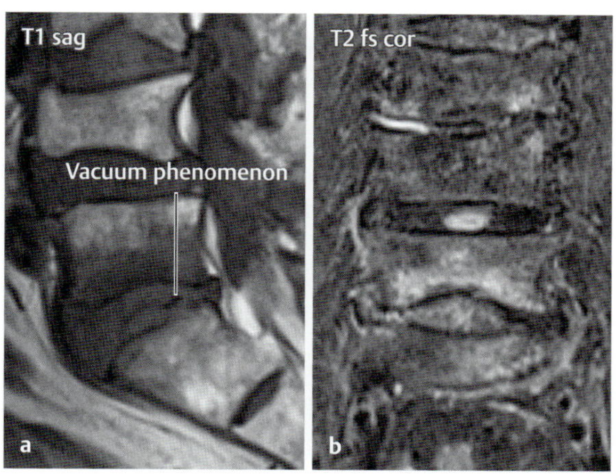

◀ **Fig. 3.51** Erosive lumbosacral osteochondrosis as a differential diagnosis of spondylodiskitis. Bandlike, "classic" distribution of edema. **(a)** Bandlike hypointensities along the normal configuration of the end plates. **(b)** The bandlike edema patterns are also evident near the end plates on the fat-suppressed T2W sequence.

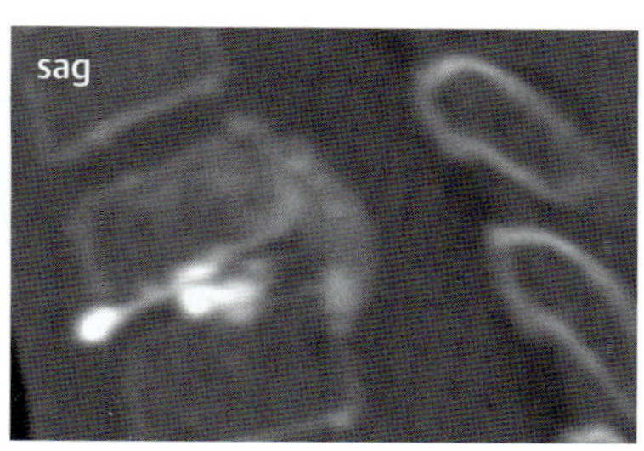

Fig. 3.52 Low-dose CT showing calcifying spondylodiskitis of the cervical spine in a 12-year-old boy.

Phlegmon. This is diffuse form of inflammation, involving the subcutaneous tissue and also muscle, fascia, and tendon sheath. The individual soft tissue regions are affected in different ways. The "fox's den-like" spread of the inflammation is characteristic, even without the presence of any relevant abscesses. A *palmar abscess* is a variant that can spread from beneath the palmar aponeurosis in the region of the flexor tendons and progress up the forearm.

Abscess. As in other organs, an abscess is a circumscribed, encapsulated collection of pus. *Staphylococcus* is usually the causative organism.

Necrotizing fasciitis. This is a highly acute disorder of the periosseous soft tissue, in particular the fascia (see Chapter 3.2.1).

> **Caution**
> It should be recognized that the route of spread of the soft tissue infection cannot always be distinguished. With myositis and fasciitis in particular, the subcutaneous tissue is also commonly involved.

Infections of the **tendon compartments and the bursae** should be distinguished from diffuse soft tissue infections (▶ Figs. 3.53, ▶ W3.6, and ▶ 3.54).

Nowadays, examination of the soft tissues is performed using ultrasound; further diagnostic investigations using MRI are required in equivocal cases or for more exact localization.

▶ **Radiography.** A number of soft tissue infections develop radiologically evident calcifications, e.g., cysticercosis (▶ Fig. 3.55). Gas formation is also well recognizable.

▶ **US.** The sonographic findings of soft tissue infections can be divided into three categories:

- **Diffuse increase in echogenicity of the tissue:** this reflects the soft tissue edema (▶ Fig. 3.56). However, it is not possible to make any statement about its origin with the aid of ultrasound (e.g., erysipelas versus congestion).
- **Circumscribed hypoechoic to anechoic areas:** this is advanced tissue liquefaction of varying degrees (▶ Fig. 3.57). It is only possible to decide with certainty by ultrasound whether a circumscribed abscess is present once an abscess capsule has been clearly demarcated. This is also only possible in some of the cases.
- **Linear or circumscribed hypoechoic to anechoic "fox's den-like" areas:** these correspond to collections of pus in the presence of a phlegmon (▶ Fig. 3.58).

> **Caution**
> Venous congestion-related water retention can produce linear or fox's den–like, hypoechoic to anechoic images similar to soft tissue infection (e.g., lymphedema). Identification or exclusion of inflammatory hyperperfusion by Doppler ultrasound aids the differentiation.

Gas collections appear as hyperechoic tissue alterations with signal loss.

▶ **CT.** Diffuse inflammations are recognizable, if at all, by an edematous infiltration of the fatty tissue (increased density). Abscesses appear as ringlike contrast enhancements around a hypodense center (▶ Fig. 3.59a). Gas collections are very well defined and are an important sign for urgent therapeutic intervention.

▶ **MRI.** The inflammatory edema is easily recognizable in all soft tissue areas as increased signal intensity on fluid-sensitive sequences with fat suppression. On these sequences an abscess presents as a very signal-intense lesion with a hypointense margin. However, abscesses only rarely display a truly water-equivalent signal, but show a more inhomogeneous signal intensity (▶ Fig. 3.60a). After administration of contrast, a characteristic enhancement of varying width is found around the abscess (▶ Fig. 3.60). Especially in the case of panniculitis, the fat signal is also reduced or lost in advanced stages; this should be verified on T1W images. In the case of inflammation of the fatty tissue, enhancement with contrast allows differentiation from lymphedema that does not take up contrast.

▶ **NUC MED.** Abscesses and other soft tissue inflammations are sensitively demonstrated on ^{18}F-FDG-PET (▶ Fig. 3.59b). The activity of the nodules during treatment can be assessed. This method does not differentiate between infectious and malignant disorders.

3.2.1 Necrotizing Fasciitis

Necrotizing fasciitis is a potentially **life-threatening soft tissue infection**, prompting immediate surgical intervention to curb the fulminant progressive infection associated with signs of systemic toxicity. The speed with which the clinical picture develops and the high mortality of 30 to 80% of cases explains why diagnostic imaging only plays a secondary role. The diagnosis of necrotizing fasciitis is essentially based on the clinical presentation and just a few laboratory tests.

▶ **Pathology.** Necrotizing fasciitis is an **infection of the deep fascial layers** caused by mixed bacterial flora that leads to rapidly progressive **necrosis of the affected tissue layers** associated with massive release of toxins. Apart from immune-compromised patients (e.g., transplant patients, HIV sufferers), diabetic patients, alcohol abusers, patients with peripheral arterial occlusive disease, and cancer patients, as well as intravenous drug users are particularly susceptible. The extremities and the perineum (Fournier's gangrene) are most commonly affected, less often the trunk.

▶ **Radiography.** Radiographs do not have a role in the diagnosis of necrotizing fasciitis. Only the demonstration of gas in the soft tissues can indicate the disease, though it is absent in two-thirds of cases.

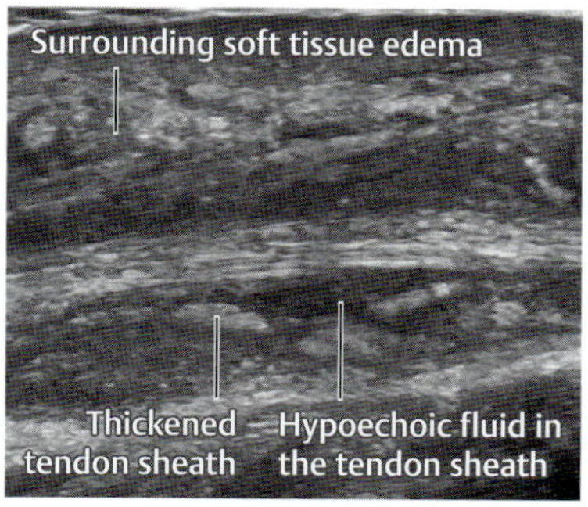

Fig. 3.53 Purulent tendinopathy on ultrasound. Longitudinal section. For a supplementary Doppler image see ▶ Fig. W3.6.

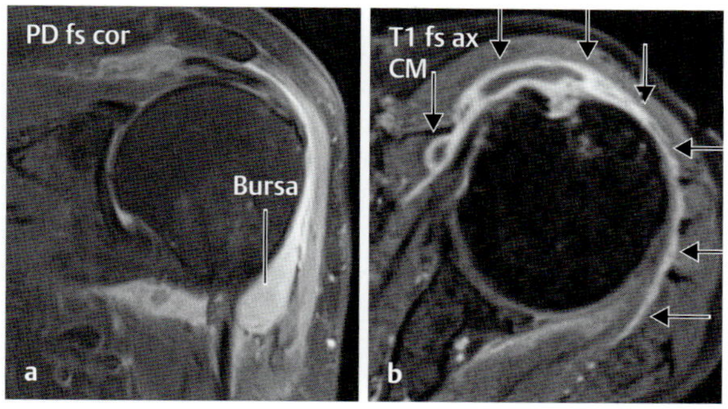

Fig. 3.54 Purulent subdeltoid bursitis. **(a)** Fluid collection in the bursa and edema of the surrounding soft tissue. **(b)** Increased contrast enhancement of the bursa (arrows). The joint cavity, however, is spared.

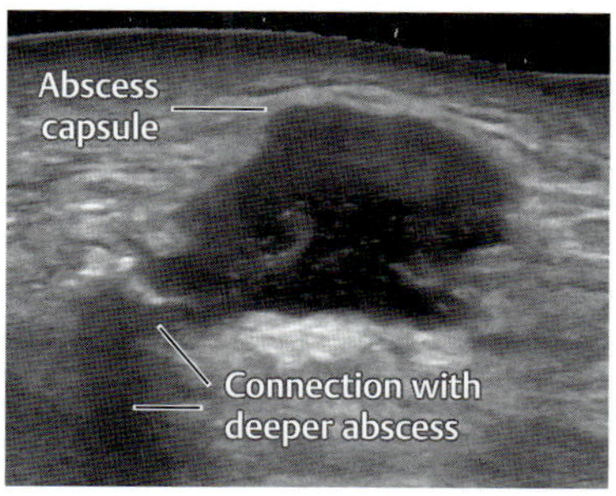

Fig. 3.57 Typical ultrasound appearance of a soft tissue abscess.

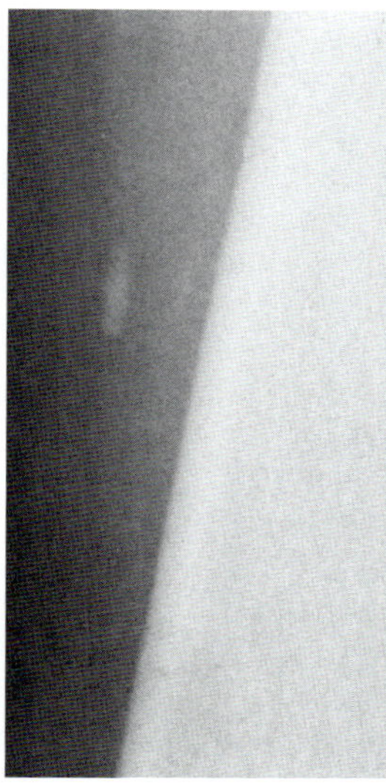

Fig. 3.55 Cysticercosis with calcified larva in the muscles.

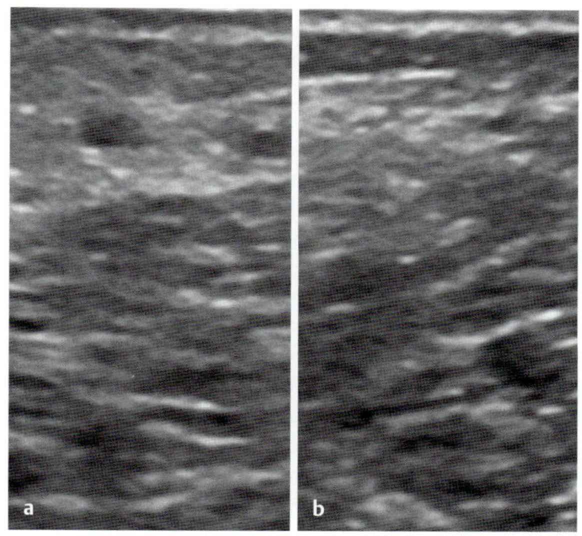

Fig. 3.56 Erysipelas. Diffuse increased echogenicity of the superficial tissue. **(a)** Erysipelas. **(b)** Healthy contralateral side for comparison.

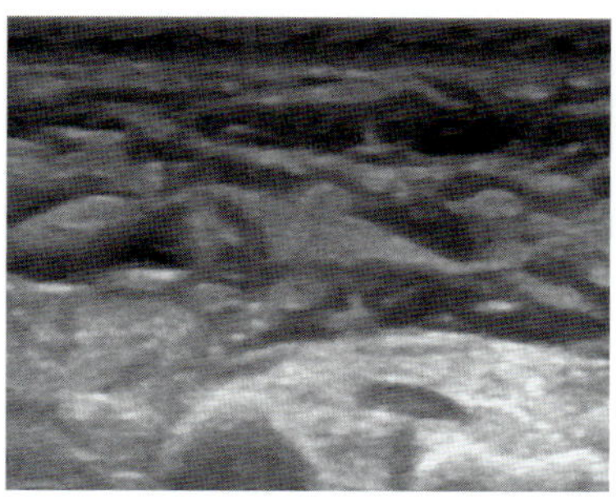

Fig. 3.58 Ultrasound appearance of a phlegmon. The tissue is interspersed with hypoechogenic streaks of fluid.

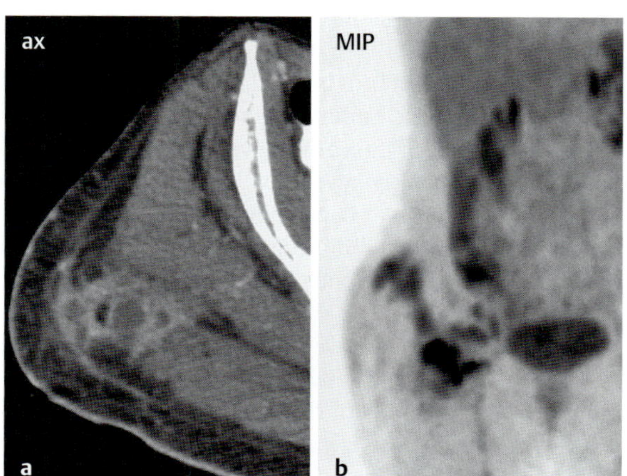

Fig. 3.59 Gluteal soft tissue abscess. (Images courtesy of J. Sciuk, Augsburg, Germany.) **(a)** Typical CT appearance after IV administration of contrast agent. **(b)** Correlation of the soft tissue inflammation with the ^{18}F-FDG-PET image. There is also concomitant involvement of the right total hip replacement.

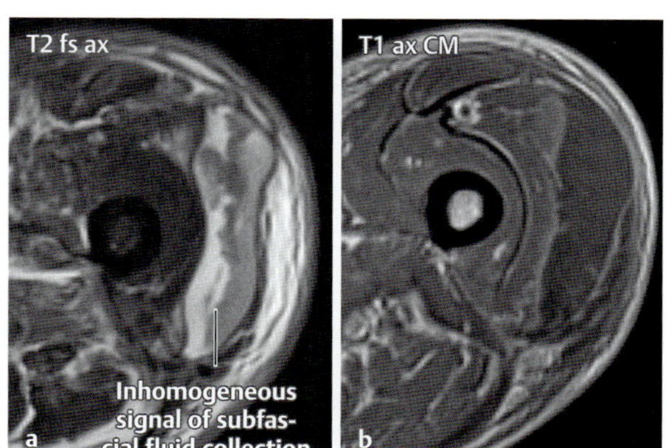

Fig. 3.60 Multifocal subfascial abscess formation. **(a)** Signal inhomogeneity due to hemorrhage and debris. **(b)** Marginal contrast enhancement around the abscess.

▸ **CT.** CT is capable of demonstrating the smallest of gas collections along the saturated and widened fascial planes. It is also possible to determine the extent of pathological spread throughout the fascia and the degree of subcutaneous involvement. Muscle compartments are excluded from assessment due to the low soft tissue contrast; complications such as muscle abscesses and hematomas, on the other hand, are recognizable. Enhancement with contrast is inconstant and is of diagnostic assistance only when the deep fascial layer is involved.

▸ **MRI.** Fluid-sensitive, fat-saturated sequences display a hyperintense signal both for the subcutaneous fat and for the fascial spaces. Whereas the former does not allow any differentiation from soft tissue phlegmon, involvement of the deep muscle fascia is regarded as typical for necrotizing fasciitis. Assessment of the **deep fascial layers** is therefore decisive: A hyperintense thickness of the fascia of 3 mm and more is considered pathological (▸ Figs. 3.61 and ▸ W3.7). Intrafascial hypointense areas and areas absent of signal on T2W sequences, corresponding to **gas bubbles**, have been reported as another, very specific pattern. If fascial enhancement with contrast is identifiable in the early infection phase, it becomes less and less conspicuous as the necrosis progresses. An unequivocal distinction between necrotizing fasciitis and other soft tissue infections can be made by identifying nonenhancing, **necrotic areas of the thickened fascia.** Other pathomorphological criteria of necrotizing fasciitis include extensive involvement of the deep fascia and the involvement of at least three compartments. Concomitant involvement of juxta-fascial areas of muscle in the edema is common for necrotizing fasciitis, albeit nonspecific. Increased contrast enhancement of muscle may be regarded as a sign of an aggressive disease course. Muscular necroses and abscesses tend to be encountered less often in cases of necrotizing fasciitis.

3.3 Septic Arthritis

Pathogens include *Staphylococcus* (more than 60% of patients), followed by *Pseudomonas* (15%), *Streptococcus, Enterococcus, Salmonella*, and *Haemophilus influenzae*. Arthritis secondary to fungi and viruses is very uncommon.

3.3.1 Nonspecific Pathogens

▸ **Pathology.** The inflammation is caused directly by colonization of the joint. Pathogens can enter the joint by various routes:

- Penetration (injection, surgery, injury).
- Per continuitatem in cases of soft tissue infection or osteomyelitis.
- Hematogenous seeding in bacteremia.

With metaphyseal osteomyelitis, a route of infection per continuitatem is extremely uncommon during the growth phase because the cartilaginous growth plate acts as an effective barrier and prevents the spread of pathogens. In infancy and after completion of skeletal maturity, on the other hand, there are metaphyseal and epiphyseal vascular connections that facilitate the spread of the infection to the joint.

> **Note** !
> Intra-articular injection or aspiration is the most common cause of bacterial arthritis.

▸ **Clinical presentation.** Apart from general signs of sepsis (poor general condition, episodes of high fever), the typical local appearance is that of an acute arthritis with erythema, increased skin temperature, swelling, pain, and limitation of motion. When several joints are involved, the signs and symptoms usually appear sequentially; this is of particular relevance for differential diagnosis.

Distribution pattern. This disorder is usually monoarticular, less commonly oligoarticular. Any joint can be affected.

> **Note** !
> Septic arthritis is a surgical emergency. Untreated, it can result in irreversible cartilage destruction within 24 to 48 hours.

▸ **Radiography/CT.** *Bony alterations are not to be expected in the early stage of acute arthritis.* Recognizable radiographic signs are restricted to soft tissue swelling and possibly joint-space widening (effusion). Juxta-articular osteoporosis is evident a few days after onset of symptoms, followed by joint-space narrowing secondary to destruction of articular cartilage. Erosions then appear over the further clinical course (▸ Fig. 3.62). Repair is indicated by the appearance of sclerotic changes (▸ Fig. 3.63). Nowadays, the final stage in the form of ankylosis is rare.

▸ **US.** The early use of US is beneficial in any case of suspected joint infection. The cardinal finding is an effusion. It may be anechoic; in the presence of empyema, however, it is typically inhomogeneously hypoechoic. Gas inclusions may be evident (▸ Fig. 3.64b). Depending on the degree of echogenicity, it may be difficult to differentiate effusion and thickened synovial membrane.

▸ **MRI.** MRI is an alternative modality in areas of complex anatomy that are sonographically difficult to access (e.g., sacroiliac joints and joints of the foot). Cardinal findings include effusion and a strongly enhancing synovial membrane (▸ Figs. 3.64 and ▸ 3.65).

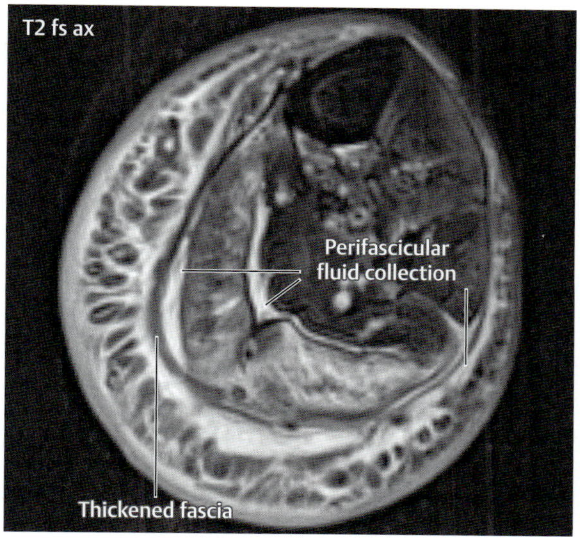

Fig. 3.61 Fasciitis of the lower leg. Contrast agent could not be administered because of renal failure; the identification of necrotic components of the fascia is therefore not possible.

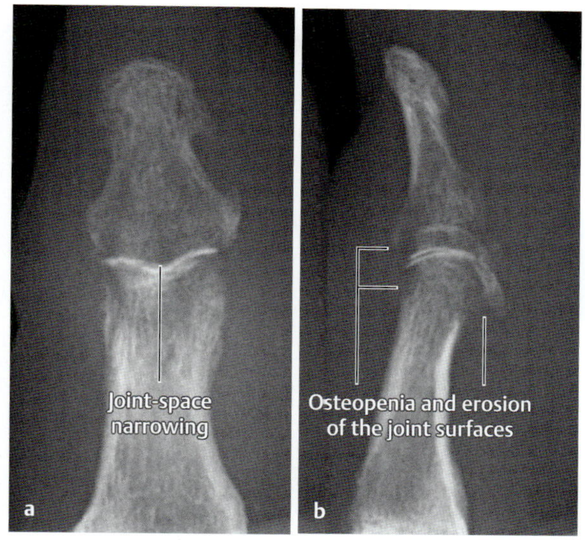

Fig. 3.62 Exogenous septic arthritis with osteomyelitis. **(a)** Joint-space narrowing secondary to arthritis-related loss of cartilage. **(b)** Juxta-articular osteopenia.

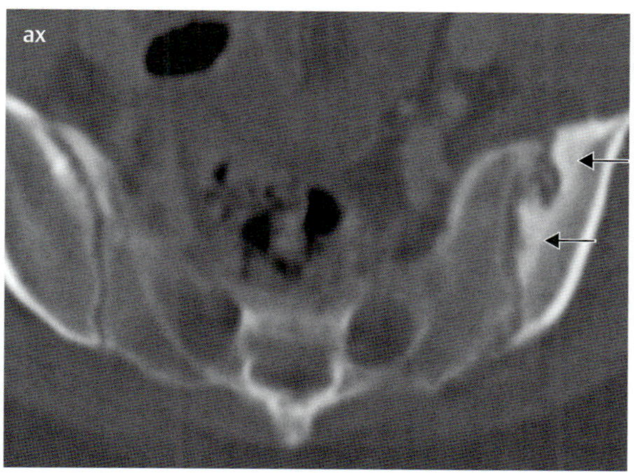

Fig. 3.63 Appearance after septic arthritis of the sacroiliac joint with areas of reparative sclerosis (arrows).

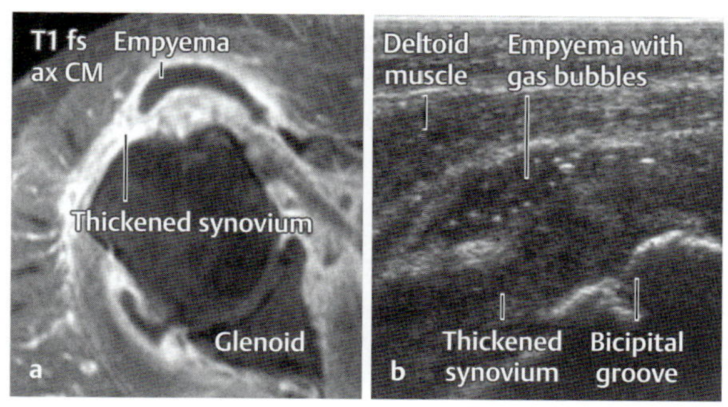

Fig. 3.64 Septic arthritis of the shoulder joint. **(a)** Empyema, significant synovitis. **(b)** Ultrasound demonstrates gas bubbles in the joint.

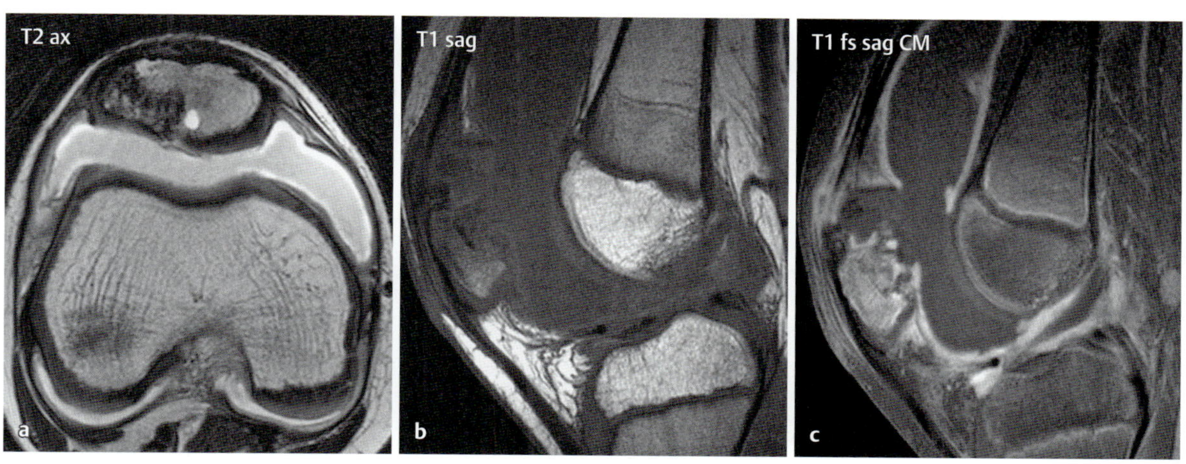

Fig. 3.65 Knee joint empyema secondary to osteomyelitis of the patella. **(a)** Postoperative osteomyelitis and concurrent septic arthritis developed after surgical management of a patellar fracture. Nonspecific effusion on the T2W image. **(b)** The T1W scan demonstrates the origin at the superior pole of the patella. **(c)** Massively increased signal intensity in the patella after administration of contrast agent. Marked synovitis, which should prompt early aspiration.

The adjacent subchondral bone marrow is signal-enhanced at a very early stage on fluid-sensitive sequences and following the administration of contrast medium; here the edema should be regarded as a reactive phenomenon (▶ Fig. 3.66). Hyperintense edema is no proof of (concomitant) osteomyelitis. If a triad of effusion, significant synovitis, and edema is present in the articular bones on both sides of the joint, then generally infectious arthritis should be assumed (▶ Figs. 3.67 and ▶ 3.68).

▶ **NUC MED.** ^{18}F-FDG-PET can detect septic arthritides very sensitively.

▶ **DD.**

> **Note**
>
> Any acute monoarthritis should initially be expected to be of bacterial origin. Given that no imaging modality is capable of confirming or excluding the infectious origin of arthritis, a diagnostic joint aspiration should be performed without delay in *any suspicious joint.*

Especially in a male subject, an acute monoarthritis is also commonly the initial manifestation of gout. The typical location of gout plus laboratory findings usually allows a distinction to be made.

Bacterial arthritis as a complication of a preexisting arthropathy poses particular diagnostic problems, especially in **rheumatoid arthritis.** Suspicion should arise as soon as there is a disproportionately rapid destruction of the joint or the clinical and radiological alterations are confined to one joint and do not match the overall pattern of the disorder (▶ Table 3.3).

The question often arises whether osteomyelitis or septic arthritis is present (or even whether both are). Osteomyelitis takes origin from a single bone. Thus if one joint-supporting bone is significantly destroyed but its counterpart is still unremarkable, then osteomyelitis is probable. Septic arthritis, on the other hand, affects both articulating bones more or less simultaneously (▶ Fig. 3.68).

The differential diagnosis of **pediatric or juvenile hip** includes above all transient synovitis of the hip (coxitis fugax/irritable hip syndrome). The clinical finding and the aspirate differ from those of bacterial arthritis.

3.3.2 Tuberculous Arthritis

Tuberculous arthritis predominantly affects the major joints (knee, hip, and sacroiliac), less commonly the carpal and tarsal joints. The clinical course is protracted in comparison with nonspecific cases of arthritis; the radiological changes are slow to develop over a period of months.

The differentiation from pyogenic arthritis is difficult based on radiomorphological findings. Occasionally extensive "cyst formation" is found in the juxta-articular parts of the bone (▶ Fig. 3.69). In the hand, the radiological features may resemble those of the cystic form of sarcoidosis.

3.4 Musculoskeletal Inflammations associated with HIV Infections

Involvement of the skeletal system and the joints in HIV patients is influenced by geographical considerations and therapeutic options with regard to frequency, manifestation, and spectrum of pathogens. Osteoarticular involvement in Asia and Africa differs entirely from the situation in Europe and North America.

Infections secondary to a wide range of bacteria pathological to humans are to be distinguished from autoimmune reactions in joints and bones. During the course of their disease, HIV patients can suffer from the following infections:

- Septic arthritis (broad pathogen spectrum, including tuberculosis).
- Osteomyelitis (commonly multifocal; in 50% of cases *Staphylococcus aureus*, otherwise mixed flora; tuberculosis is also possible, especially in the spinal column; tuberculosis develops in HIV patients 500 times more commonly than in the general population).

Table 3.3 Infectious versus noninfectious arthritis: Aspiration is highly diagnostic

Diagnostic measure	Infectious arthritis	Noninfectious arthritis
Case history	Previous joint injection or aspiration?	Known oligo- or polyarthritis?
Clinical presentation	Painful, warm monoarthritis; rapid course	Less rapid course; pain and increased skin temperature less marked in rheumatoid arthritis; but very similar in CPPD
Ultrasound, MRI	Possible concomitant abscess and osteomyelitis	
Aspiration	Empyema	Serous, fibrinous

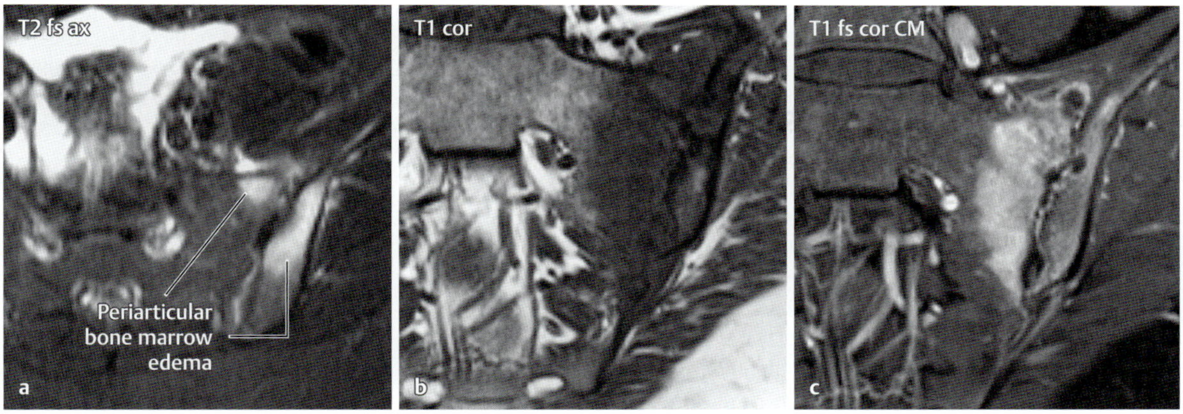

Fig. 3.66 Septic arthritis of the sacroiliac joint. Same patient as in ▶ Fig. 3.63. **(a)** Early stage: increased signal intensity, not only in the articular bones but also in the cranial joint space and the joint capsule (markings). **(b)** Four months later, after inadequate treatment: increased involvement of the bone. The erosions are new. **(c)** The corresponding slice after administration of contrast displays the new finding of a distended capsule. Aspiration confirmed purulent material.

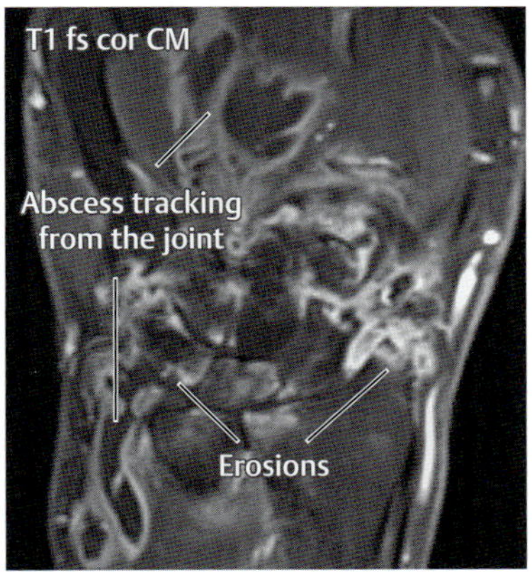

Fig. 3.67 Septic arthritis of the wrist.

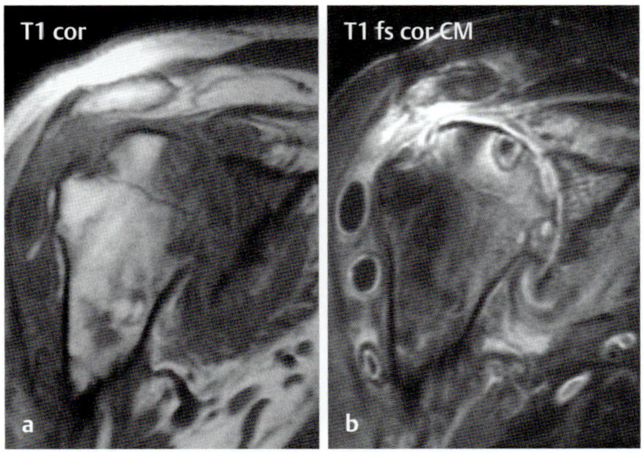

Fig. 3.68 Empyema of the shoulder joint. **(a)** Hypointense bone marrow reaction in the humeral head and in the glenoid. **(b)** Extension into the soft tissue, accompanied by multiple abscesses.

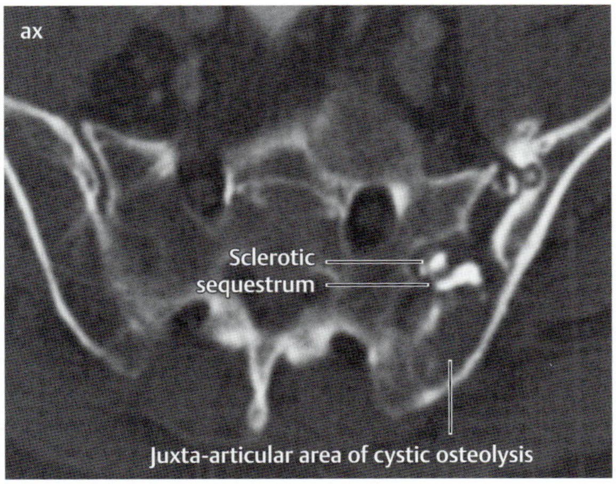

Fig. 3.69 Tuberculous arthritis of the sacroiliac joint.

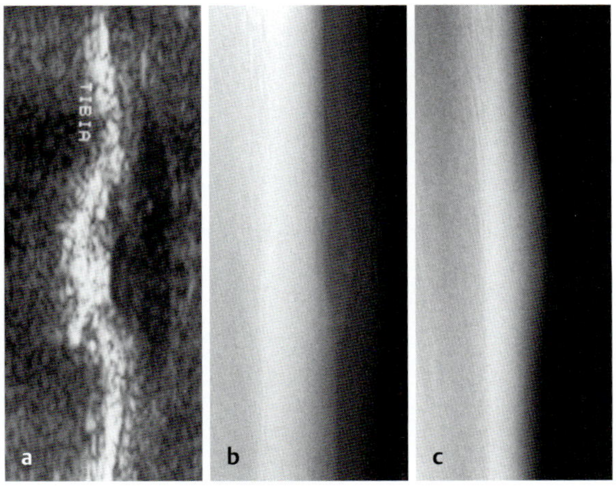

Fig. 3.70 Clinical course of periosteal abscess in an HIV-related infection. **(a)** Primary finding on ultrasound. **(b)** Primary finding of the radiograph. **(c)** Healed solid periosteal reaction 6 months later.

- Periostitis (also in association with abscess formations; ▶ Fig. 3.70).
- Pyomyositis (bacterial infection of the muscles).
- Polymyositis (rheumatoid, reactive inflammation of the muscles).
- Nonseptic arthritis (clinical presentation and radiographs as in rheumatoid arthritis; so-called HIV arthritis [virus-related]; in the shorter term, painful monoarthritides without pathologic radiograph; Reiterlike arthropathy of the spine).
- Bacillary angiomatosis (vascular proliferation involving the skin, but also, less commonly, the bone; pathogens are *Bartonella henselae* and *Bartonella quintana*).

From a differential diagnostic perspective, it should not be forgotten that HIV patients also have an increased susceptibility to bone infarctions and osteonecroses (especially of the hip) and to hypertrophic osteoarthropathy (secondary to infection with *Pneumocystis carinii*).

Chapter 4

Tumors and Tumorlike Lesions of Bone, Joints, and the Soft Tissues

4 Tumors and Tumorlike Lesions of Bone, Joints, and the Soft Tissues

4.1 General Aspects of Diagnostic Imaging of Skeletal Tumors

4

Primary bone tumors are very rare (1% of all neoplasms) unlike metastases or hematologic malignancies. Plasmacytomas and malignant lymphomas belong to this latter group (see Chapter 5.5). **Tumorlike lesions** are invariably covered with primary bone tumors, as in this book, but differ fundamentally from primary bone tumors. They are a heterogeneous group of benign lesions with the possibility of spontaneous cessation of growth or even regression. In addition, these lesions do not have the potential to metastasize. Even inflammatory (e.g., osteomyelitis, enthesopathies) or degenerative conditions (e.g., intraosseous ganglia) are capable of mimicking tumors. Important criteria for the evaluation and differential diagnosis of bone tumors are **location** in the skeleton (e.g., appendicular versus axial skeleton) and in the bone (epiphyseal, metaphyseal, diaphyseal; central, eccentric; intracortical or juxtacortical) as well as the **patient's age** (peak age in childhood and adolescence and in late adulthood). There is rarely a significant gender prevalence. Most entities can also arise as rare variants located at intracortical, periosteal, parosteal, or extraosseous sites (▶ Fig. 4.1). A distinction is made between bone tumors and soft tissue tumors (see Chapter 4.5).

Overview of tumorlike lesions

- Bone island/osteoma.
- Nonossifying fibroma (fibrous metaphyseal cortical defect).
- Periosteal desmoid.
- Simple ("juvenile/unicameral") bone cyst.
- Aneurysmal bone cyst (primary aneurysmal bone cysts are nowadays considered to be benign bone tumors).
- Eosinophilic granuloma (solitary form of Langerhans cell histiocytosis).
- Fibrous and osteofibrous dysplasia.
- Heterotopic ossification (see Chapter 11.5.2).
- Intraosseous ganglion.
- Epidermoid.
- Giant-cell reparative granuloma.
- Brown tumor (of hyperparathyroidism).

> **Note** !
>
> Tumorlike lesions, unlike primary bone tumors, are relatively common. The majority are incidental findings of the 1st to 3rd decades of life. Often tumorlike lesions do not require treatment ("leave-me-alone" or "do-not-touch" lesions) and should be confidently diagnosed radiographically. Here the radiologist has a decisive contribution to make toward avoiding unnecessary biopsy/surgery.

The overview presented in ▶ Table 4.1 is based on the **WHO Classification** and deliberately omits rare conditions (for which the reader is referred to the specialized literature). The basic principle of the classification of primary bone tumors is based on the type of **matrix production**. However, this principle is not applicable to a large number of tumors, so the tumor origin should also be included. The matrix is the intercellular substance produced by mesenchymal cells and includes osteoid (osteogenic), chondroid (chondrogenic), and myxoid ground substance, and (fibrous) collagen fibers.

4.1.1 The Role of the Radiologist in Assessing a Suspected Bone Tumor

1. Once a lesion has been recognized as being pathological and has been distinguished from a normal variant, an attempt should be made to **interpret** and correctly diagnose it. A reasonable differential diagnosis should be proposed comprising, where possible, a maximum of three diagnoses. In some cases it will only be realistic to make a distinction between "probably benign" and "probably malignant." Providing a **synopsis** of the results of all the imaging techniques (scintigraphy, PET, MRI, etc.) lies in the hands (and eyes!) of the radiologist.
2. The site for a **biopsy** should be indicated that ensures the most representative tissue is obtained. The radiologist must be familiar with the principles of staging primary bone tumors to be able to recommend the **appropriate imaging modalities**. In particular, it should be ensured that a biopsy is not taken until all the imaging studies have been performed. The trauma from a needle or open biopsy will alter signal intensity on MRI, which can distort the apparent size of the lesion.
3. The radiologist must know which imaging modalities should be appropriately utilized for **monitoring treatment and subsequent follow-up**. Matrix components

should be taken into consideration (e.g., calcium or bone: radiography and CT; cysts or fluid levels: MRI).

4. With close **cooperation**, only the trio of surgeon/pathologist/radiologist is capable of establishing the correct diagnosis and drawing up a rational therapeutic strategy for primary bone tumors. **Regular multidisciplinary team (MDT) conferences** are an absolute prerequisite.

4.1.2 General Approach to a Suspected Bone Tumor

In many cases it will already be possible to deduce the (differential) diagnosis, speed of growth of a lesion (growth rate) and benign or malignant nature of the tumor, as well as the nature of a disorder (systemic disease, circumscribed lesion) from the radiographs.

The "Five Ds"

The basic steps of radiological assessment of a bony abnormality are encompassed by the "five Ds":

- Detect.
- Describe.
- Discuss.
- Differential diagnosis.
- Diagnosis.

Based on the "five Ds," basic questions should be addressed after taking the radiographic, CT, MRI, scintigraphic, etc. findings into consideration.

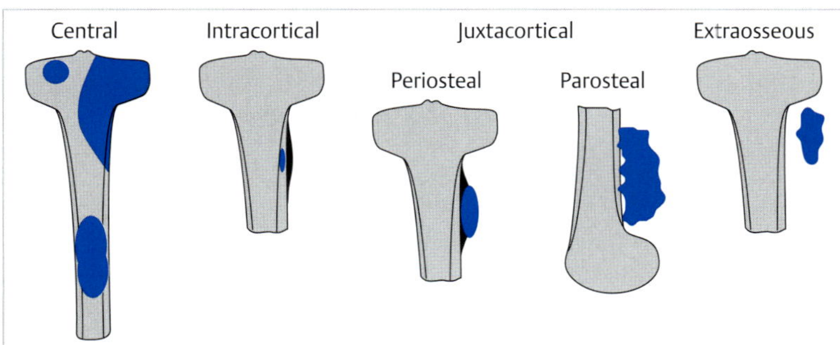

Fig. 4.1 Depiction of the location of tumors.

Table 4.1 Summary of primary bone tumors (according to WHO)

Tumor groups	Benign tumors	Malignant tumors
Chondrogenic tumors	• Osteochondroma • Chondroma • Chondroblastoma • Chondromyxoid fibroma	• Chondrosarcoma (note subclassifications)
Osteogenic tumors	• Osteoid osteoma • Osteoblastoma	• Osteosarcoma (note subclassification)
Fibrogenic and fibrohistiocytic tumors	• Desmoplastic fibroma • Benign fibrous histiocytoma	• Fibrosarcoma • Malignant fibrous histiocytoma
Ewing's sarcoma/primitive neuroectodermal tumor		• Ewing's sarcoma/primitive neuroectodermal tumor
Giant cell tumor	• Giant cell tumor	
Vascular tumors	• Hemangioma	• Angiosarcoma
Lipogenic tumors	• Lipoma	• Liposarcoma
Other tumors		• Adamantinoma • Chordoma

Detect. Is this a pathologic bony abnormality? In many cases this may be obvious; however, the initial detection of the lesion is often a difficult task. Detecting pathologic structures is ultimately a matter of experience as, over time, the spectrum of what is normal versus abnormal will develop in the radiologist's mind. At present, this conscious and subconscious ability is still based on conventional radiomorphology in two planes. These always (!) form a mandatory part of primary imaging work-up. Bone lesions involving the cortex are more readily recognized on radiographs than lesions confined to cancellous bone. Loss of bone substance (e.g., osteoporosis) will make detection of subtle osteolytic lesions difficult.

Describe. Any description involves first determining whether the lesion arises in bone, soft tissues, or joints. Where is the finding located with respect to the skeletal system? In a tubular bone? If yes, where exactly (epiphyseal, metaphyseal, diaphyseal; central or eccentric)? Is it a solitary lesion or are there multiple lesions? Focal bone lesions pose their own specific questions: What type of bone lesion is it (lytic, sclerotic, or a mixed lesion)? Are there cortical changes or periosteal new bone formation? Can matrix production be deduced from the radiograph, the CT, or the MRI? Is the surrounding soft tissue involved? A correct answer to these questions is a prerequisite for the other three "D's."

Discuss. This step involves the initial evaluation of the questions addressed above. The speed of growth of a lesion (*growth rate*) may be inferred from the apparent reaction of the host bone to the pathologic lesion as seen on the radiograph. This is an important factor in differentiating between a benign and a malignant lesion.

Differential diagnosis. In order to develop a differential diagnosis, the radiological findings have to be taken into account together with the clinical findings and laboratory results.

> **Note**
>
> The differential diagnosis of a focal bone lesion is based on the overall assessment of the following parameters:
>
> - Tumor matrix (cf. Chapter 4.1.3).
> - Growth rate (cf. Chapter 4.1.4).
> - Exact location of the lesion (▸ Fig. 4.1).
> - Patient's age.
> - History and clinical findings (above all pain and its duration).
> - Laboratory parameters (ESR, CRP, alkaline phosphatase).

Diagnosis. A diagnosis should only be made if either the radiograph is unequivocal or the combination of radiograph, case history, and clinical findings gives grounds for a clear diagnosis (e.g., the diagnosis of a metastasis based on osteolysis in the presence of the simultaneous identification of multiple lesions and a known primary tumor).

> **Note**
>
> The correlation between the histological biopsy result and the radiograph (*validity check*), in the broadest sense, is part of establishing and signing off the diagnosis before a treatment plan is implemented. If there is a discrepancy between the proposed radiological differential diagnosis and the histological diagnosis, then the case must be reviewed with regard to all the imaging, the histology and the biopsy site. Radiologists and pathologists should not be reluctant to request a second opinion. The histological differentiation of primary bone tumors is often challenging and belongs in the hands of experts and their multidisciplinary colleagues.

4.1.3 Description of a Focal Bone Lesion

Type of Bone Lesion

The radiomorphological description of bone lesions continues to rely primarily on conventional radiographs in two projections. The following patterns are common:

- Solitary radiolucency (▸ Fig. 4.2a).
- Solitary radiodensity (▸ Fig. 4.2b).
- Solitary, mixed lesion (▸ Fig. 4.2c).
- Irregular multiple radiolucencies (moth-eaten pattern; ▸ Fig. 4.3a).
- Homogeneous, multiple radiolucencies ("permeative" pattern; ▸ Fig. 4.3b).

Border of a Bone Lesion

The border or margin of a lesion within the host bone reflects the relation between destruction and repair in the bone and is an important indicator of growth rate:

- The border of the lesion is **sharp** or well-defined if the transition between normal and pathologic bone follows a clearly recognizable line (i.e., can be traced with a pencil without hesitation; ▸ Fig. 4.4a). A sharply marginated lesion can be partially or completely surrounded by a sclerotic margin.
- The border of the lesion is **ill-defined** if the zone of transition between normal and pathologic bone is wide and the margin of the lesion is barely recognizable (▸ Fig. 4.4b). An **irregular** (jagged, wavy, ridged) border does not indicate that one is dealing with an ill-defined border.
- A bone lesion may, on occasion, show a mixed pattern margin with both well- and ill-defined sections.

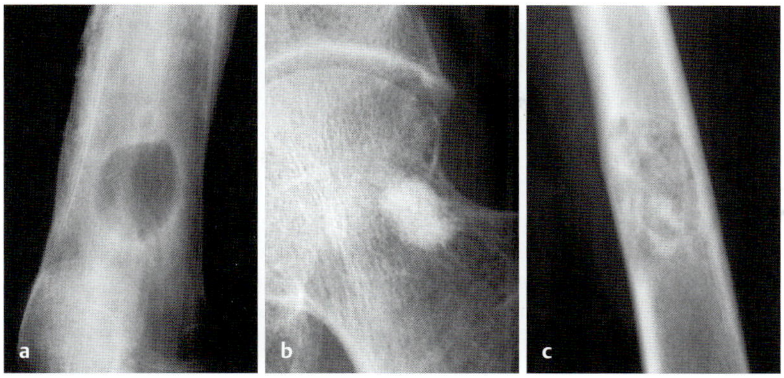

Fig. 4.2 Solitary bone lesions. **(a)** Solitary radiolucency. **(b)** Solitary radiodensity. **(c)** Mixed lesion.

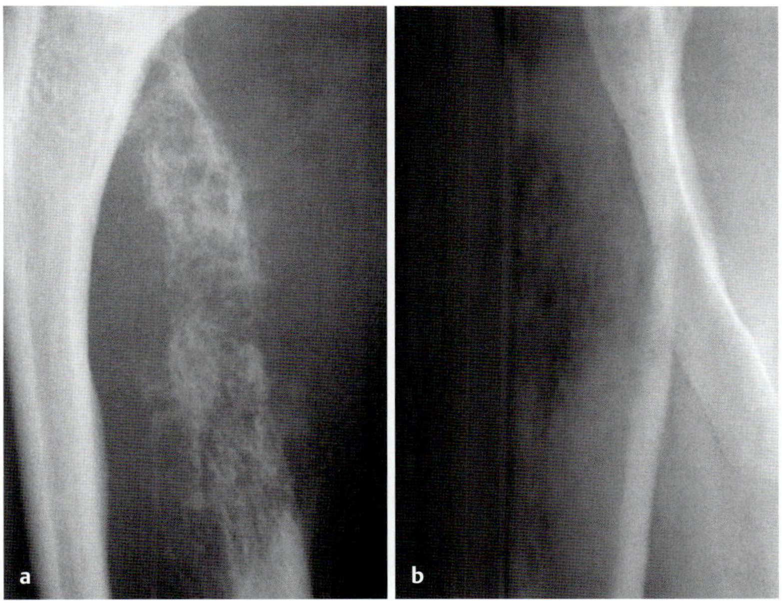

Fig. 4.3 Multiple radiolucencies. **(a)** Multiple irregular radiolucencies (moth-eaten pattern). **(b)** Multiple homogeneous radiolucencies ("permeative" pattern).

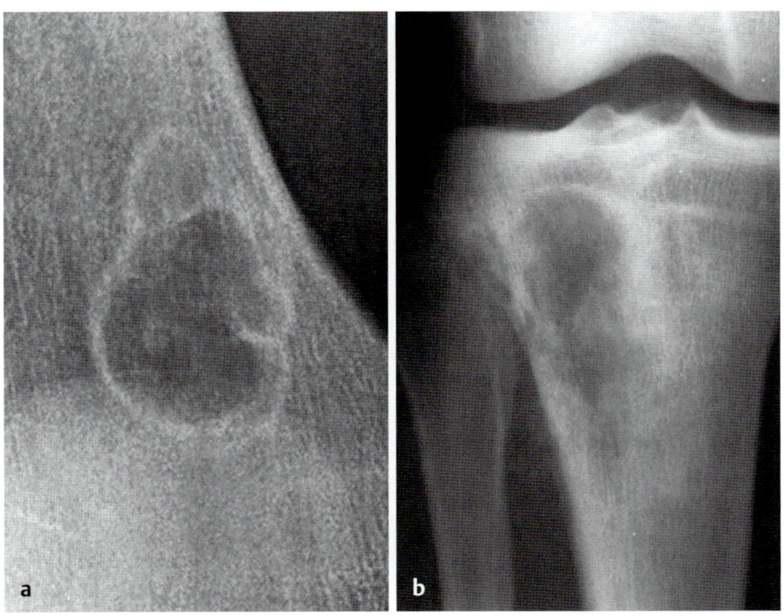

Fig. 4.4 Border of a bone lesion. **(a)** Well-defined border. **(b)** Ill-defined border.

4

Cortical Changes

The cortex of a tubular bone is widest in the diaphysis and gradually narrows toward the metaphysis and epiphysis. There is no cortex at the cartilage-covered joint surfaces but only an extremely thin layer of subchondral bone.

- **Endosteal cortical thinning**: the thinning from "within" may be linear or half-moon shaped. Lobular thinning is often found in the diaphysis (known as scalloping; ▸ Fig. 4.5 a).
- **Cortical bone destruction** (continuity disrupted or not disrupted): the comparison with a wall is suitable for explaining the alterations. "Continuity disrupted" means that there is a greater or lesser "hole" in the cortex (▸ Fig. 4.5b). "Not disrupted" means that the wall is still "standing" but it is already starting to crumble. This latter form of bone destruction often results in the impression of being "moth-eaten" (known as permeative osteolysis, ▸ Fig. 4.5 c).
- **Neocortex:** The original cortex has been replaced by an outer bony shell. The bone appears "ballooned" (▸ Fig. 4.5 d).

Periosteal Reaction

Stimulation of new bone production by the periosteum is primarily an adaptive process designed to preserve stability of the bone. This becomes particularly clear when periosteal reaction is induced by underlying osteolysis. However, hyperemia, disturbances of circulation of the surrounding soft tissues, or iatrogenic factors (e.g., prostaglandin administration in neonatales) can also stimulate a periosteal reaction.

Periosteal reaction is an extremely important indicator of the biological activity of a lesion. Aggressiveness and duration of the initiating process can be estimated by analyzing the periosteal reaction.

Periosteal reaction is possible in the presence of an intact as well as a disrupted cortex. On the other hand, the periosteal reaction itself can be interrupted. This latter process is an important sign of an aggressive growth pattern.

> **Note**
>
> Ten days is the minimum time before a periosteal reaction becomes radiographically visible: it must first mineralize. The older the patient the longer this takes. Periosteal reaction is absent in the following situations:
>
> - The lesion grows so slowly that it fails to stimulate the periosteum.
> - The lesion grows so rapidly that it is unable to develop a periosteal reaction.
> - The lesion is very small.

> **Note**
>
> Absence of periosteal reaction must not be misinterpreted as a sign of slow growth of a focal bone lesion.

Solid periosteal reaction. In this case, multiple layers of bone form a strong layer of new bone on a radiologically intact cortex or replace the original cortex (known as neocortex). Solid periosteal reactions may also take on an undulating, nodular, or trabeculated appearance. These are typically a sign of low biological activity (▸ Fig. 4.6a).

A single lamellar periosteal reaction. A single lamella consists of a discrete sheet of bone and can vary in thickness—the thicker it is, the slower the growth and accordingly the less aggressive the underlying lesion. The transition to solid periosteal reaction is smooth not discrete; a width of 2 mm and more indicates a solid periosteal reaction. The cortical bone may also be destroyed (▸ Fig. 4.6b). The term "lamella," however, does not mean that it is always a sharp line. A **Codman angle** refers to the interrupted pattern involving a single lamella or several lamellae (▸ Fig. 4.6b). It typically arises at the periphery of the lesion and the cortex is usually destroyed. A Codman angle must be clearly distinguished from a spur or projection of an uninterrupted solid periosteal reaction buttressing the periphery of a benign lesion.

A lamellated periosteal reaction ("onion skin"). This comprises multiple concentric lamellae of bone. It should be recognized that individual parallel lamellae may differ in thickness and—depending on the quality of the radiograph—may be difficult to separate (▸ Fig. 4.6c). For this reason, differentiation from a solid periosteal reaction is not always easy, but it can be of diagnostic importance. The identification of a lamellated periosteal reaction means that the growth rate of the lesion is ranked between that of a solid periosteal reaction and that of a single lamellar periosteal reaction. Benign entities (e.g., eosinophilic granuloma) should not be fundamentally ruled out.

Spicules. These are linear, parallel new bone formations, perpendicular to the cortex. The cortex is often morphologically intact (yet histologically already infiltrated [▸ Fig. 4.6d]).

Complex periosteal reactions. This term includes variants of spiculated periosteal reaction with or without a peripheral lamellar component. These may be termed the sunburst or hair-on-end phenomenon. The longitudinal bone densities of varying thickness and length are divergent, i.e., irregular in appearance. Reactive bony alterations can be difficult to distinguish from tumorous bone formation. Randomly organized or extensive periosteal reactions are classified as complex reactions (▸ Fig. 4.6e).

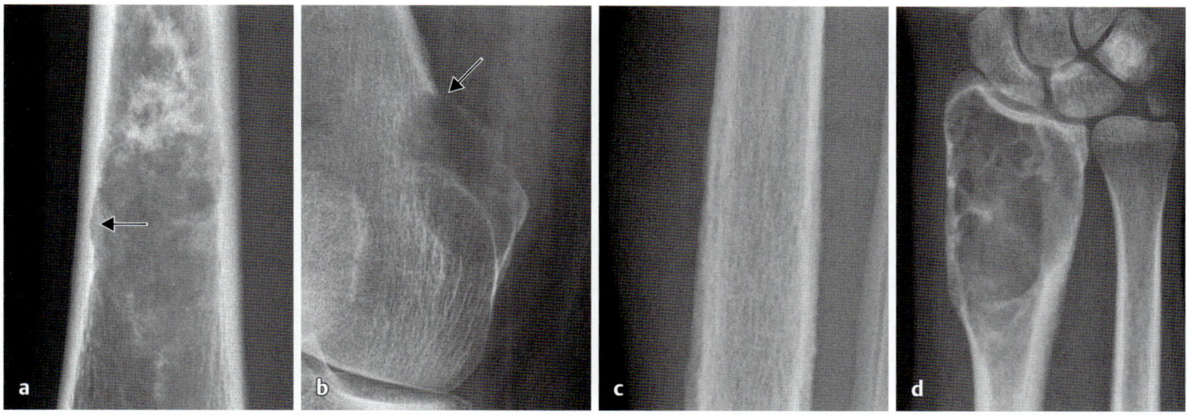

Fig. 4.5 Cortical changes. **(a)** Endosteal thinning, scalloping (arrow). **(b)** Partially interrupted, fine neocortex (arrow). **(c)** Uninterrupted, permeative cortical destruction. **(d)** Neocortex, "ballooning" of the bone.

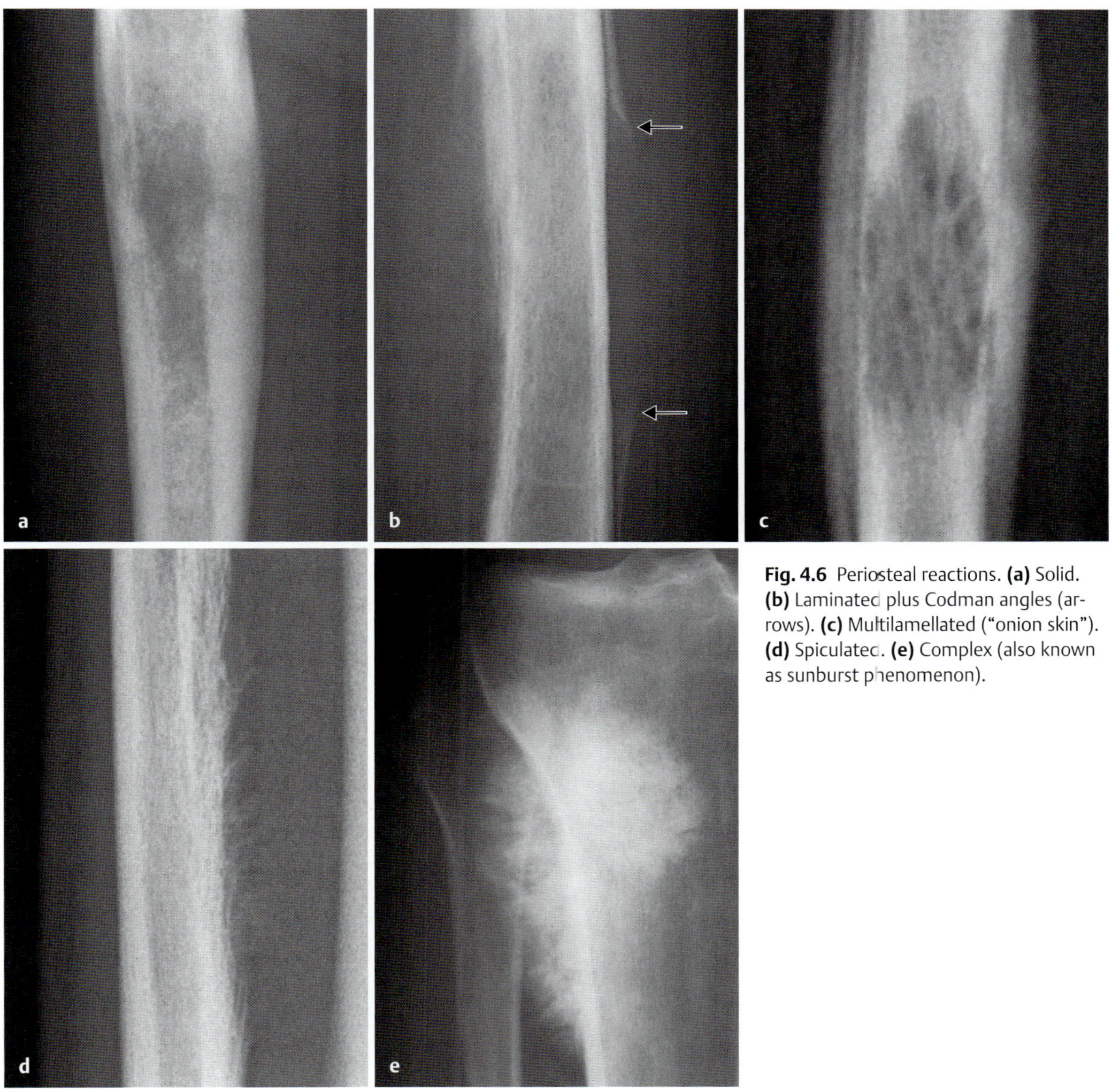

Fig. 4.6 Periosteal reactions. **(a)** Solid. **(b)** Laminated plus Codman angles (arrows). **(c)** Multilamellated ("onion skin"). **(d)** Spiculated. **(e)** Complex (also known as sunburst phenomenon).

Matrix Production

Assessment of the matrix on the radiograph can be difficult. It is often impossible to decide whether there is any matrix production at all or whether the calcified areas within a lesion represent the remains of the original bone or periosteal new bone seen en face. A CT can help here. A bony tumor matrix develops in one of two ways:

1. Bony tumor matrix is formed by the autonomous production of tumor osteoid by neoplastic cells—a classic process only seen with osteosarcoma, osteoid osteoma, and osteoblastoma.
2. Tumor-induced osteoblasts produce bone matrix that is typical of certain types of bone metastases. Only after mineralization of the tumor osteoid does it become radiographically visible. Because the tumor-stimulated bone production is extremely rapid (e.g., sclerotic metastasis from prostate cancer), the new bone lacks structure and appears amorphous and is less dense than, for example, osteomas.

A **bony matrix** may only be diagnosed radiographically if extensive areas of consolidation are present (▶ Fig. 4.7a). These may appear dense and ivorylike or even less dense and cloudy or latticed.

The radiological appearance of bone that has developed from **metaplastic new bone formation** (bone formation by pluripotential cells) differs from that of "normal" bone. The term **ground glass phenomenon** is used to describe its opaque appearance on the radiograph (▶ Fig. 4.7b). Unlike all forms of bony matrix, **chondroid matrix** displays primarily a focal, stippled, flocculent calcification pattern, resembling dots and "rings and arcs" (▶ Fig. 4.7c).

Dystrophic calcification, formed by the precipitation of calcium phosphates and carbonates in necrotic or degenerated tissue, has a heterogeneous pattern that can mimic chondroid matrix and metaplastic new bone formation (▶ Fig. 4.7d).

4.1.4 Assessment of the Aggressiveness of a Bone Lesion: Growth Rate

Assessment of the aggressiveness of a bone lesion, its rate of growth, and its expansion within the bone is a critical contribution of imaging. This is based on a precise description of the bone lesion (see Chapter 4.1.3). Determining growth rate will often form the basis for differentiating between benign and malignant lesions, providing additional support for differential diagnostic criteria. This applies primarily to bone tumors and tumorlike lesions, but also to inflammatory conditions. Determination of the growth rate from the radiograph also aids the histological assessment of the bony process.

This is based on the **classification system** proposed by **Lodwick** that describes the bone destruction pattern visible on radiographs (▶ Fig. 4.8).

This classification system has two disadvantages, however: on the one hand, it is restricted to osteolytic lesions; on the other, grading into five groups is somewhat laborious for everyday clinical practice.

The following **simplified classification** may be of assistance for those less experienced in arranging the radiographic patterns into different categories and preparing the way for further diagnostic steps:

- **Stage I:** Osteolytic lesion with a circumscribed, sharply defined margin; nonaggressive, slow-growing, or even stationary growth ("latent"; ▶ Fig. 4.9a).
- **Stage II:** Osteolytic lesion still demarcated in every direction but with an ill-defined margin; intermediate growth or intermediate rate of expansion ("active"; ▶ Fig. 4.9b).
- **Stage III:** Moth-eaten or permeative pattern of bone destruction; aggressive growth, rapidly expanding lesion ("aggressive"; ▶ Fig. 4.9c).

An aggressive growth pattern, Stage III, is a typical feature of malignancy but can also be seen in acute osteomyelitis. Similarly, it is also possible for a metastasis to be surrounded by a sclerotic margin and thereby be classified as Stage I.

One insight gained from advances in diagnostic and molecular imaging techniques is the fact that reality, as seen on radiographs, is relative. One must always bear in mind that it is primarily a question of developing an overview of the pathophysiological processes that are taking place. As the American pathologist, James Ewing, postulated, it is necessary to grasp the "concept" of the disease.

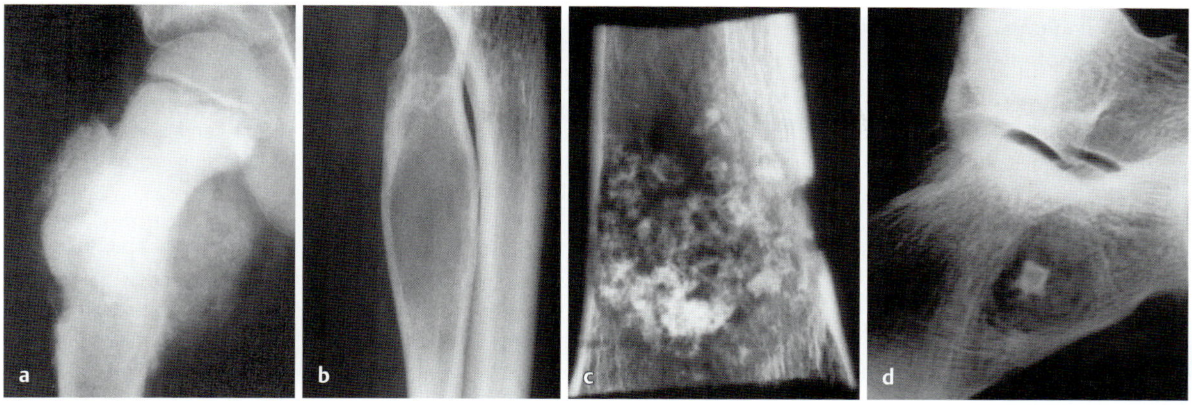

Fig. 4.7 Matrix production. **(a)** Bony matrix. **(b)** Ground glass phenomenon of metaplastic bone matrix. **(c)** Chondroid matrix with typical calcifications. **(d)** Dystrophic calcification.

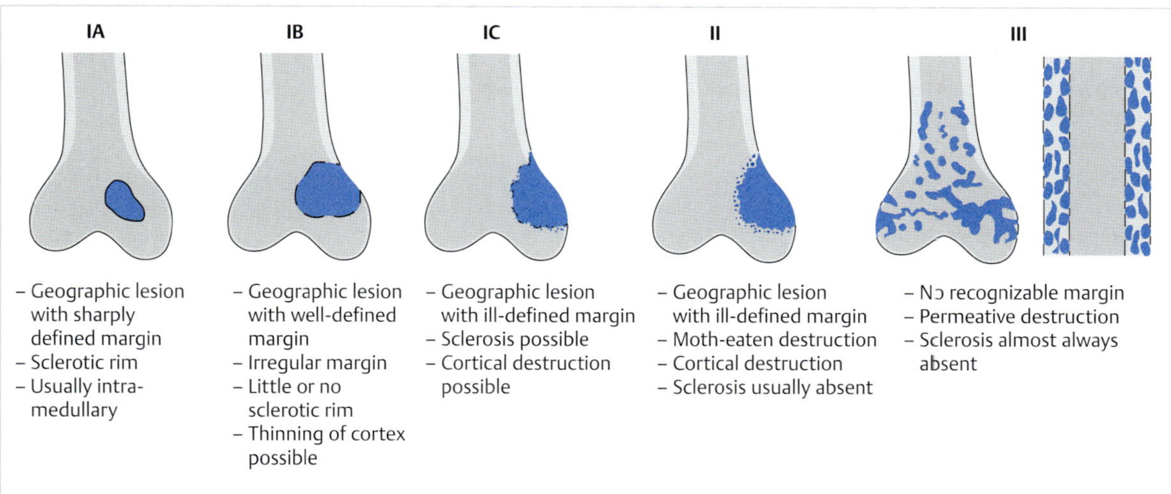

Fig. 4.8 Lodwick classification of the growth rate of tumors and tumorlike lesions.

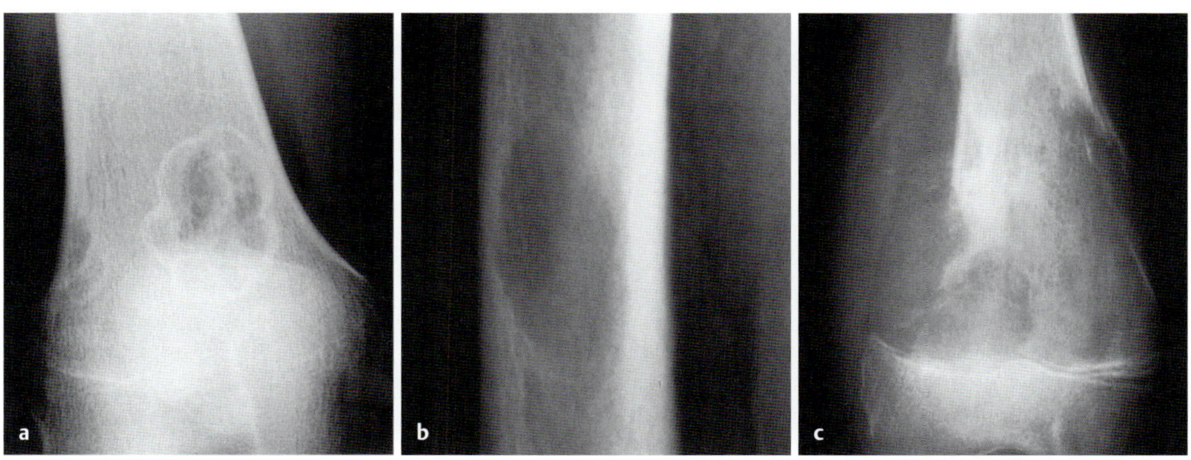

Fig. 4.9 Radiological morphology of osteolytic lesions: simple 3-stage assessment of growth rate. **(a)** Latent. **(b)** Active. **(c)** Aggressive.

Signs of a nonaggressive growth pattern on the radiograph or CT

- Solitary density.
- Well-defined border and marginal sclerosis.
- Only endosteal alteration of the cortical bone.
- Neocortex.
- Solid periosteal reaction.

Signs of an aggressive growth pattern on the radiograph or CT

- Moth-eaten pattern or permeative pattern.
- Ill-defined border.
- Cortical destruction.
- Spicules, lamellated, or complex periosteal reaction.
- Soft tissue infiltration.

4.1.5 Staging of Bone Tumors

Contemporary staging systems for primary bone tumors, in particular the malignant forms, are based on the UICC (Union for International Cancer Control) TNM Staging System in conjunction with histological grading (▶ Tables W4.1–W4.3). Apart from detecting metastases on bone scintigraphy and chest CT, it is particularly important for the radiologist to determine the extent of the primary tumor with MRI. The TNM classification of primary **bone tumors** defines T1 as a tumor of 8 cm or less in the greatest dimension, with T2 defined as a tumor of more than 8 cm in the greatest dimension. T3 is defined as a discontinuous tumor in the primary bone site ("skip metastasis"). The **classification according to Enneking** has established itself in the clinical surgical disciplines, taking into account above all the anatomical site, metastases, and histological grading (see specialized literature).

4.1.6 Imaging Modalities for Tissue Diagnosis, Assessment of Biological Activity and Staging of Bone Tumors

▶ **Radiography.** Radiography remains the primary imaging modality for diagnosing suspicious lesions. Given appropriate image quality, matrix calcification and ossification are usually easy to assess. The image is capable of displaying sometimes subtle changes such as bony destruction and periosteal reactions. An incidental finding on imaging, thought to be benign, will also require a radiograph as a baseline study for comparison with follow-up reviews (an enchondroma does not necessarily need to be followed up by MRI!).

▶ **NUC MED.** **Technetium Tc 99 m diphosphonate bone scintigraphy** is used for detecting multifocal involvement, for demonstrating metastases in malignant bone tumors, and for follow-up reviews of (chemo)therapy. Only in exceptional cases, such as Paget's disease and osteoid osteoma, does the bone scan display a diagnostic pattern of radionuclide uptake.

Fluorine-18 fluorodeoxyglucose PET (^{18}F-FDG-PET; also used as hybrid imaging together with CT and MRI) is gradually gaining favor over bone scintigraphy as a sensitive modality for the evaluation of primary bone tumors. T-, N-, and M-stages can be assessed in a single study However, CT is still indispensable for detecting lung metastases (e.g., secondary to osteosarcoma). One benefit of PET is in the detection of local tumor recurrence, particularly if metal implants adversely affect assessment by other modalities (such as CT und MRI). Individual reports are available in the literature showing that PET may be utilized for monitoring tumor response to chemotherapy. Initial hopes that the differentiation between malignant and benign bone tumors could be improved with the aid of PET imaging have been disappointed.

▶ **CT.** After the initial uncritical enthusiasm for MRI, CT has to an extent regained importance for staging purposes, in particular for those malignant tumors arising in complex anatomical areas such as the spine, pelvis, and shoulder. It also remains a good modality for assessing unclear radiographic and scintigraphic findings in terms of detection of lesions and differential diagnosis. Its greatest value lies in a subtle assessment of calcifications and ossifications. It demonstrates the presence and nature of any tumor matrix better than radiographs and certainly better than MRI. More recent CT-based developments, such as CAD (computer-assisted diagnostics), provide valuable additional information for detecting pulmonary nodules, 3D reconstructions of tumors, and computer-aided surgery.

▶ **US.** This modality is ideally suited at the bedside as a supplement to clinical examination of suspected soft tissue masses. It can improve the diagnostic yield of image-guided percutaneous biopsy and, utilizing the color-coded duplex function, it is suitable for simple differential diagnoses, such as "tumor versus hematoma."

▸ **MRI.** MRI is currently regarded as the gold standard for staging malignant tumors. This applies to the entire skeleton, but particularly the extremities. MRI also aids differential diagnosis by assessment of the different signal and contrast enhancement patterns as well as morphological features such as fluid–fluid levels.

Technique. As with all other clinical issues, differential diagnostic criteria are based on the signal pattern of T1W and water-sensitive sequences. The latter comprises "intermediate" (long TR and TE of 35–45 ms) T2W (TE > 70 ms) sequences, typically combined with fat saturation. Intravenous contrast administration together with T1W sequence (fat-suppressed) can be helpful in the work-up of bone tumors.

MRI confirmation of *peritumoral edema* within the bone or adjacent soft tissues is a nonspecific sign:

- Peritumoral edema can be seen with both malignant and benign tumors. Florid edema is typical of benign tumors such as osteoid osteoma and chondroblastoma.
- Edema is also found in with infection and trauma, and, to a lesser extent, around acute medullary infarction.
- It should be stressed that the peritumoral edema around malignant tumors may contain microscopic nests of tumor cells and so this zone should be included in any measurements of tumor extent when determining resection margins.

Monitoring. MRI is useful for assessing tumor response to chemotherapy. Simple measurement of size reduction is helpful in Ewing's sarcoma but not in osteosarcoma. Signal reduction of the lesion on water-sensitive sequences is an indicator for increasing ossification and/or increased proportion of fibrous tissue. If there is no increase in signal intensity within the lesion after IV contrast administration, then tumor necrosis may be inferred. Dynamic contrast medium examinations (observation of the increased signal intensity of a volume or a layer over predefined time intervals) have been successfully employed for distinguishing viable tumor tissue from the surrounding reactive tissue. More recent modalities, such as DWI and MR spectroscopy, may be useful additions, but are still the object of research and clinical studies (see specialized literature).

Note

MRI must always be assessed together with the radiograph and, if available, CT if a bone tumor is suspected! Matrix calcifications and matrix ossifications are difficult to differentiate by MRI. Instead, lipogenic, chondrogenic, and cystic structures are often indicative. Changes of signal intensity from pathologic fractures and biopsies as well as technical imaging artifacts should always be considered.

4

4.2 Primary Bone Tumors

4.2.1 Osteogenic Tumors

The common feature of all osteogenic tumors is their production of bone matrix. Radiologically, the picture is commonly characterized by bone destruction and osteolysis.

Osteoid Osteoma

An osteoid osteoma is a benign, bone-forming tumor. It is characterized by its small size (less than 1.5 cm) and slow growth. Perifocal sclerosis and edema are reactive and not part of the tumor itself.

► **Pathology.** The tumor comprises a small focus (the nidus) of highly vascularized fibrous tissue within an area of new bone formation surrounded by osteoblasts (► Fig. 4.10).

► **Clinical presentation.** Patients report slowly increasing severe pain (especially at night). Acetylsalicylic acid and other nonsteroidal anti-inflammatory drugs are effective for symptomatic relief. Systemic signs of inflammation, unlike acute osteomyelitis, are not present.

Age: First to third decades of life; males are more frequently affected than females. **Location:** Femur (30% of cases) and tibia (25%) are the most commonly affected. The location of the lesion is metadiaphyseal, eccentric, and commonly intracortical (80–90% of cases). **Treatment:** Therapy of choice is percutaneous radiofrequency or laser ablation.

> **Note**
> Clinically, juxta-articular, intracapsular osteoid osteomas present symptoms mimicking arthritis with joint effusion and reactive synovitis. In the spine, osteoid osteomas can present with a painful scoliosis, unlike adolescent idiopathic scoliosis which is typically painless.

► **Radiography.** The tumor produces focal osteolysis (nidus), surrounded by a varying degree of sclerosis. Once the osteoid formed by the tumor has mineralized, a punctate area of increased density develops within the nidus. This ossification and the surrounding sclerosis may obscure the focal lucency on the radiographs.

Site of the nidus

- **Intracortical** location of the nidus results in a strong, solid periosteal reaction (► Fig. 4.11) with an area of eccentric or fusiform sclerosis. Multiple or longitudinal nidi have been described but are rare.
- With a **medullary** location of the nidus (e.g., within the skeleton of the hand or foot), there is usually less marked sclerosis or even a local radiolucency (► Fig. 4.12). The nidus itself is commonly demarcated as a sclerotic lesion.
- An osteoid osteoma of the **spine** is most commonly located posteriorly in the neural arch or in the pars interarticularis (► Fig. 4.13).
- With **an intra-articular** location of the nidus, there is usually a relatively discrete, subarticular, round to ovoid radiolucency with only a minor sclerotic response. This is due to the absence of overlying periosteum at these sites.

► **NUC MED.** The double-density sign with higher activity in the center and lower activity toward the periphery is typical.

► **CT.** CT is the modality of choice when trying to identify this tumor (► Fig. 4.14; also ► Fig. 4.11) by its ability to detect the nidus, even with a nidus size of less than 3 mm. It is also the technique of choice when treating these cases with image-guided radiofrequency ablation.

► **MRI.** The nidus is hypointense on T1W, but of varying signal intensity on T2W sequences (regardless of the extent of the osteosclerosis). Strong central contrast enhancement is evident.

> **Caution**
> An osteoid osteoma can *appear* very "aggressive" on MRI due to the strong perifocal edema in bone and soft tissues. Unlike with malignant bone marrow infiltration, fatty marrow is still preserved in the immediate vicinity of the osteoid osteoma.

► **DD. Brodie abscess.** This displays a variable enhancement pattern.

Stress fracture. A spinal stress fracture is a differential diagnosis. Commonly only a CT allows a definite differentiation between nidus and fracture line.

Glomus tumor. A possible differential diagnosis is glomus tumor of the nail tuft.

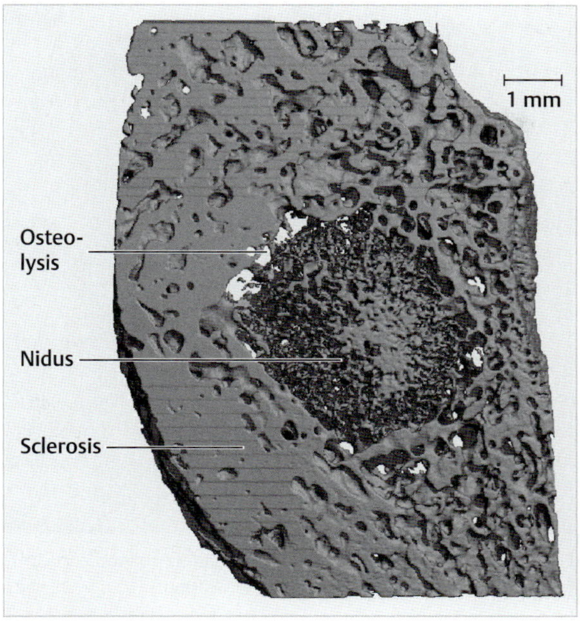

Fig. 4.10 Osteoid osteoma. Micro-CT with a resolution of ~ 20 µm clearly shows the radially arranged, mineralized structure of the nidus, surrounded by rarefaction of structure (osteolysis) and the typical sclerosis.

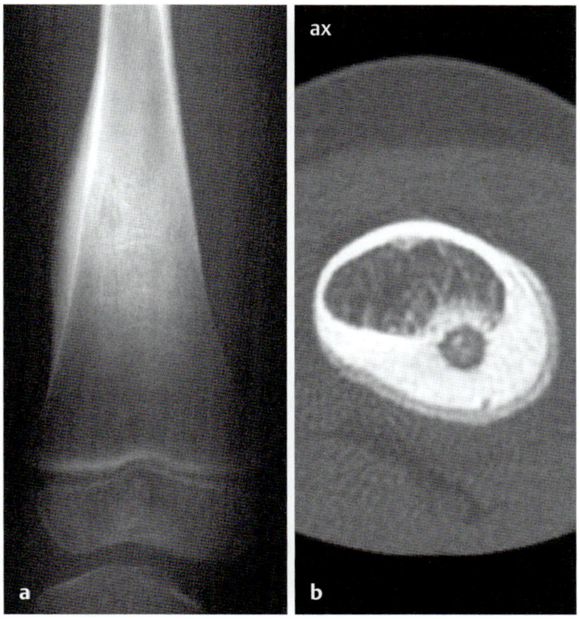

Fig. 4.11 Osteoid osteoma of the distal femur. **(a)** Solid periosteal reaction; the nidus is recognizable as a focal lucency. **(b)** Characteristic image: nidus with surrounding sclerosis.

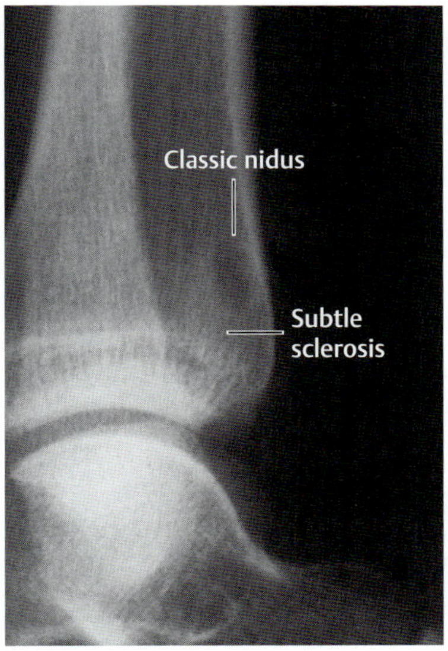

Fig. 4.12

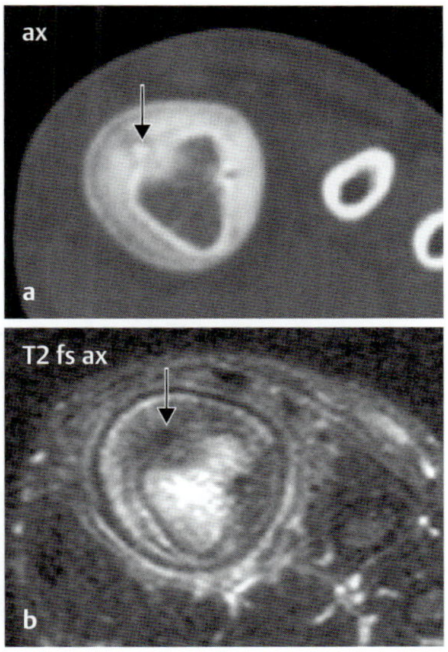

Fig. 4.14

Fig. 4.12 Osteoid osteoma of the distal tibia.

Fig. 4.14 Osteoid osteoma. **(a)** A calcified nidus (arrow) is evident on CT. **(b)** The nidus (arrow) is barely visible on MRI.

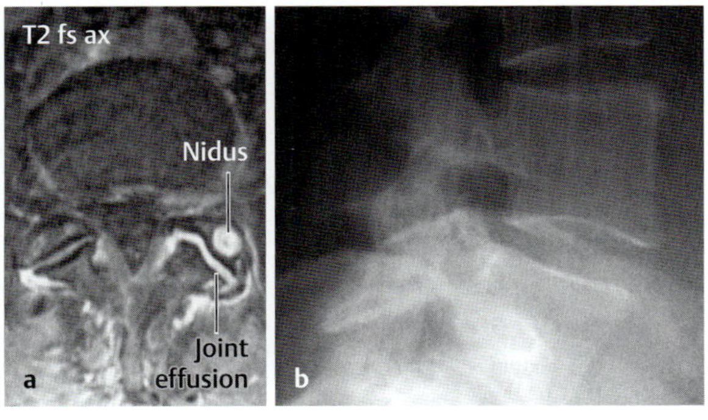

Fig. 4.13 Osteoid osteoma of the spine. **(a)** The nidus is hyperintense on the T2W image; typical periarticular location. **(b)** On the radiograph only a nonspecific density is recognizable at the facet joint.

4

Osteoblastoma

An osteoblastoma is a rare, benign, bone-forming tumor, histologically similar to osteoid osteoma (known as the big brother of osteoid osteoma, accordingly larger than 1.5 cm).

Location: More than 40% of cases are found in the spine, particularly thoracic and mostly posteriorly located. All other bones may potentially be affected.

Age: 1st to 5th decades of life.

▸ **Radiography.** Osteoblastomas lead to osteolysis (▸ Fig. 4.15), but do not always have a sclerotic margin. Expansion of the bone occurs with preservation of a fine external bone lamella. Intralesional ossifications are recognizable in just over one-half of cases (▸ Figs. 4.16 and ▸ 4.17).

▸ **CT/MRI.** Unlike osteoid osteoma, there is no discrete nidus. Signal intensity on T2W images depends strongly on the degree of matrix structure and is usually hypointense on T1W sequences. Perifocal bone marrow edema of varying degrees is evident in the surrounding bone and soft tissue.

▸ **DD.** **Aneurysmal bone cysts.** *Problem:* Osteoblastomas may be associated with cystic components and secondary aneurysmal bone cyst formation that can make differentiation difficult.

Osteoblastic, slowly growing osteosarcomas. CT is essential for demonstrating integrity of the cortex or the external bony shell and assessing the proximity of the lesion to important structures such as the spinal cord and nerve roots in the spine.

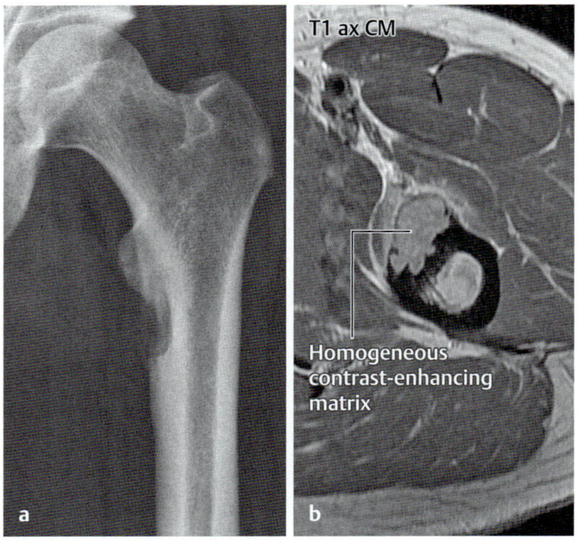

Fig. 4.15 Periosteal osteoblastoma. **(a)** Saucer-shaped cortical lysis. **(b)** The MRI shows the periosteal location.

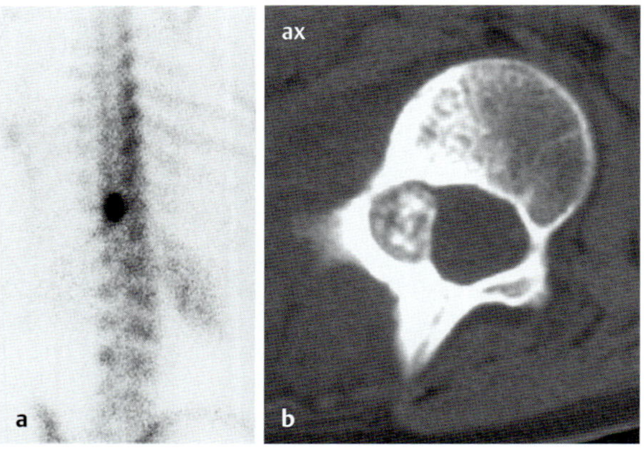

Fig. 4.16 Osteoblastoma. **(a)** Focal increased activity on the bone scan (late phase). **(b)** Sharply defined osteolytic lesion with matrix ossification.

Fig. 4.17 Osteoblastoma. **(a)** Focal lytic lesion in the talar neck with marginal sclerosis. **(b)** Perifocal bone marrow edema and reactive joint effusion on MRI. **(c)** Focal lysis with clear marginal sclerosis and central matrix ossifications, similar to a nidus on CT.

▼

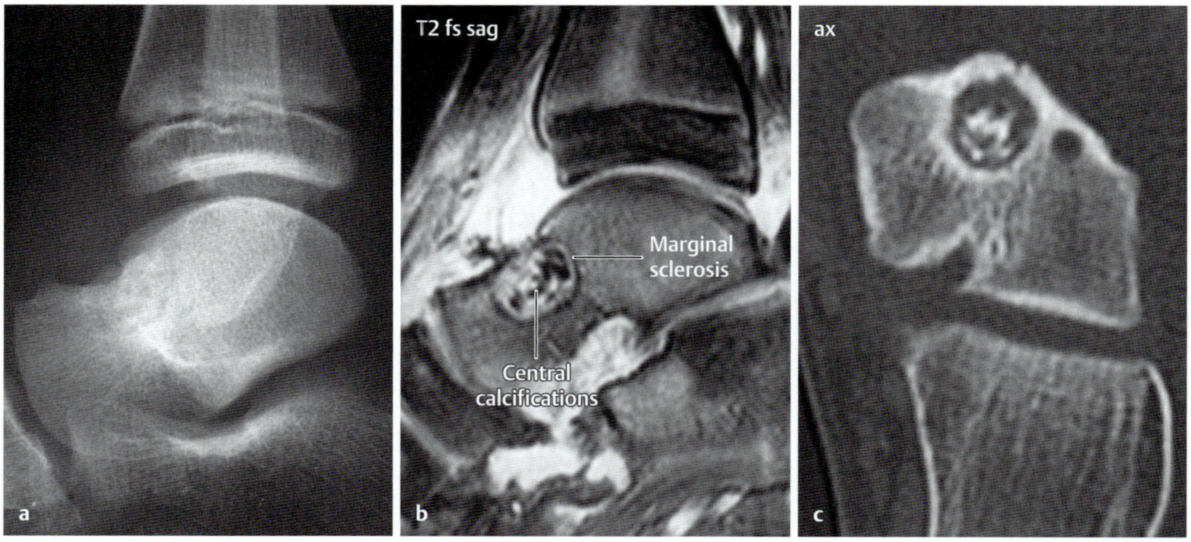

Osteosarcoma

Osteosarcoma is the most common primary malignant bone tumor, accounting for 40% of cases. The tumor has an intramedullary growth pattern and produces osteoid, albeit sometimes in only small amounts. There are numerous histological subtypes that vary from low grade to high grade.

► **Pathology.** Osteosarcomas are anaplastic, pleomorphic tumors with a complex variety of tumor cells (spindle cells, clear cells, epithelioid cells, round cells, etc.). The identification of malignant osteoid is the unifying feature. The tumor cells may also produce cartilage and fibrous matrix. This leads to further histological subtyping, such as osteoblastic, chondroblastic, or fibroblastic osteosarcoma and other variants.

Central Osteosarcoma

► **Clinical presentation.** Patients present clinically with pain increasing over weeks and months associated with local swelling. An unrelated minor injury is not uncommonly the reason for initial diagnostic investigations.

Age: About 60% of patients are under the age of 25 years. **Location:** This tumor can affect any bone. More than 80% of osteosarcomas develop in the metaphyses of the long tubular bones (femur, tibia). A diaphyseal location is always regarded as unusual. **Prognosis and treatment:** The most important prognostic factor is the degree of response to preoperative chemotherapy. Wide excision or amputation follows pre-operative (neoadjuvant) chemotherapy. The surgical procedure depends on local tumor staging (MRI!) and the detection of metastases (bone scan or whole-body MRI and chest CT).

► **Radiography.** The radiological morphology is variable, depending on the subtype and degree of osseous matrix formation. There is often a **mixed lytic/sclerotic pattern:**

- This involves a mixture of bone destruction of varying degrees (permeative to moth-eaten) and osteosclerosis (► Figs. 4.18–4.21).
- The tumor margin is ill-defined (Lodwick Grade II–III).
- Periosteal bone formation is almost always seen, with evidence of spicules being an important criterion for malignancy (see ► Fig. 4.18). Codman angles (elevation of the sclerotic periosteum with undermining cortical destruction) are found (see ► Fig. 4.21). Lamellated (onion skin), commonly interrupted, periosteal new bone formations are regularly to be seen (see ► Fig. 4.25).

Osteosclerotic osteosarcoma (ca. 10% of cases). Osteosclerotic osteosarcoma is characterized by ivory or "cloudlike" dense, sclerotic tumor matrix (► Fig. 4.22). Occasionally this variant remains confined within the borders of the affected bone for a relatively long time.

► **NUC MED.** Bone scintigraphy is important for detecting bone metastases. PET-CT can be used to assess prognosis after chemotherapy.

► **CT.** CT can differentiate better than radiography between periosteal reaction and the osteogenic tumor matrix. It should be noted when staging that metastases can display calcifications that—in this clinical context—are *not* signs of benign disease (chest CT; ► Fig. 4.23).

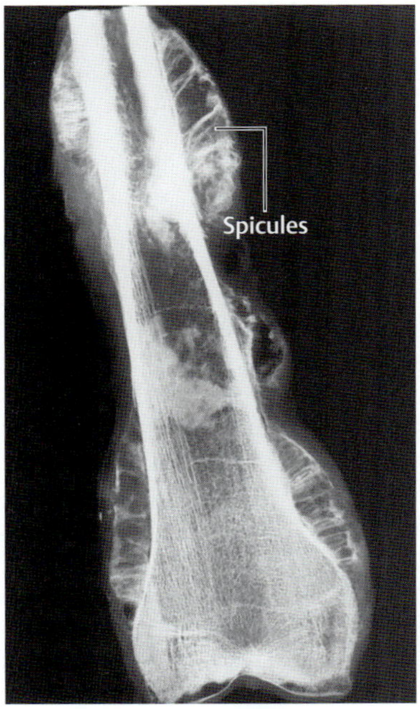

Fig. 4.18 Specimen radiograph of a central osteosarcoma following chemotherapy.

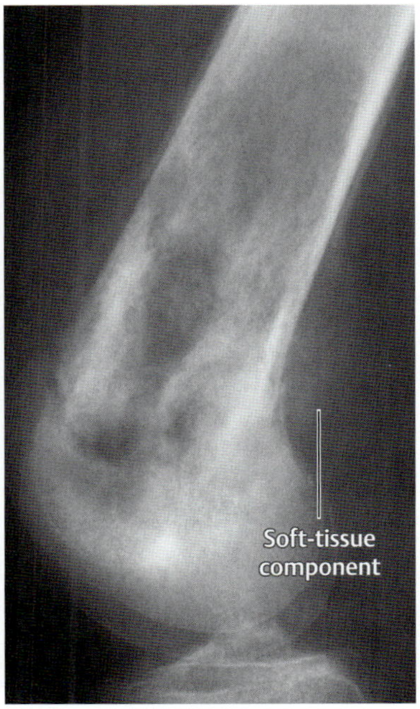

Fig. 4.19 Central osteosarcoma, mixed osteolytic/osteosclerotic.

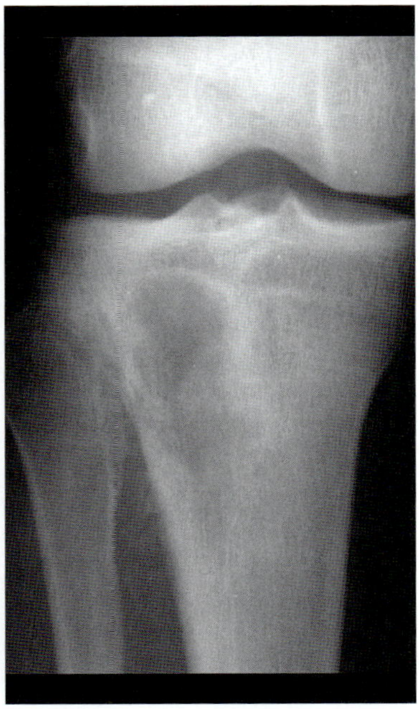

Fig. 4.20 Central osteosarcoma, mixed osteolytic/osteosclerotic.

▶ **MRI.** The signal alterations depend on the degree of matrix mineralization. The tumor enhances strongly after administration of gadolinium. MRI is the modality of choice for staging lesions in tubular bones (intramedullary extension, skip metastases, soft tissue infiltration, joint involvement; ▶ Figs. 4.24 and ▶ 4.25). The surgeon will be particularly interested in any possible association with neurovascular bundles.

▶ **DD. Ewing's sarcoma** (see Chapter 4.2.4). Ewing's sarcoma usually has a diaphyseal to metaphyseal location and does not demonstrate bone matrix or chondrogenic matrix.

CRMO (Chronic recurrent multifocal osteomyelitis). A chronic reactive form of osteomyelitis, in children and adolescents (see Chapter 10.7.1).

Chondrosarcoma. MRI characteristics of cartilage are to be found here (see Chapter 4.2.2).

High-grade pleomorphic sarcoma. See Chapter 4.2.3 for high-grade pleomorphic sarcoma.

> **Note**
> A primary malignant bone tumor in a patient over 30 years old is practically never a central osteosarcoma.

4

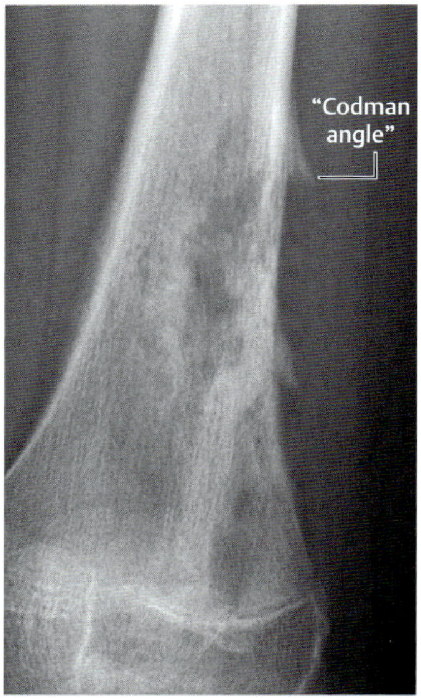

Fig. 4.21 Central osteosarcoma.

Other Osteosarcomas

Telangiectatic osteosarcoma (1–10% of osteosarcomas). This is a highly malignant tumor filled with hemorrhagic spaces (beware similarity with an aneurysmal bone cyst!). A moth-eaten pattern of osteolysis without osteogenic matrix is a predominant feature on the radiograph (▶ Fig. 4.26).

Small cell osteosarcoma. This osteosarcoma has an unfavorable prognosis. The predominant radiological features are bone destruction and sclerosis.

Low-grade central osteosarcoma (1–2% of osteosarcomas). This is a more slowly growing and prognostically more favorable variant occurring in the 2nd and 3rd decades of life. The lesion can simulate many other tumorlike lesions particularly fibrous dysplasia (▶ Figs. 4.27 and ▶ 4.28).

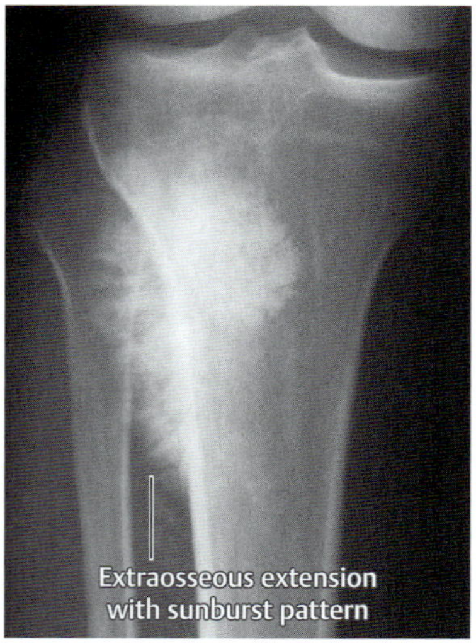

Fig. 4.22 Osteosclerotic central osteosarcoma.

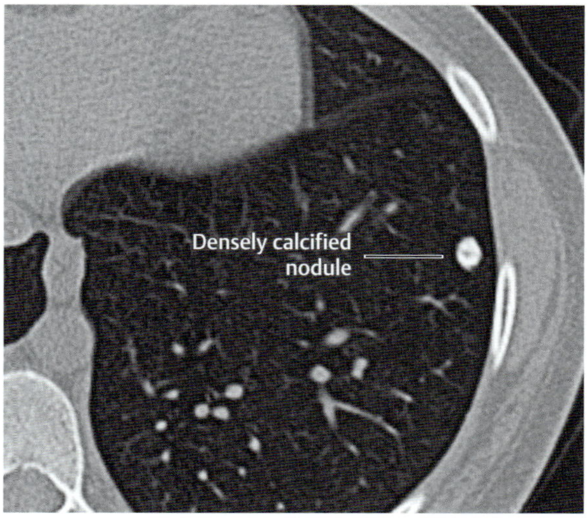

Fig. 4.23 Pulmonary metastasis from an osteosarcoma.

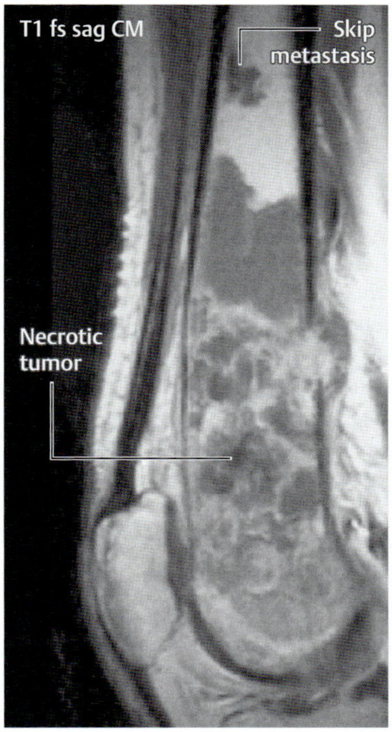

Fig. 4.24 Central osteosarcoma.

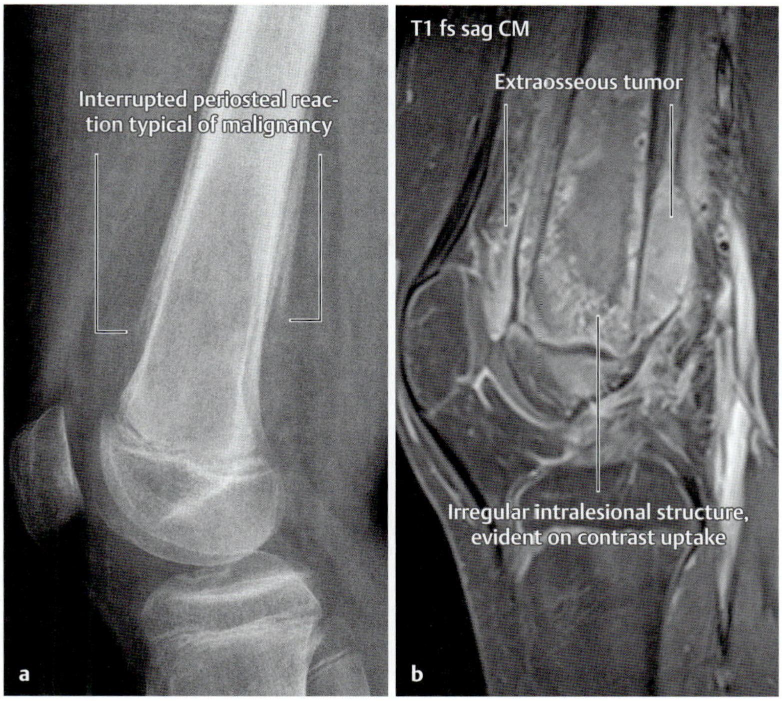

Fig. 4.25 Central, predominantly osteolytic osteosarcoma. **(a)** Large osteolytic lesion with soft tissue swelling. **(b)** Circular extraosseous component of the tumor.

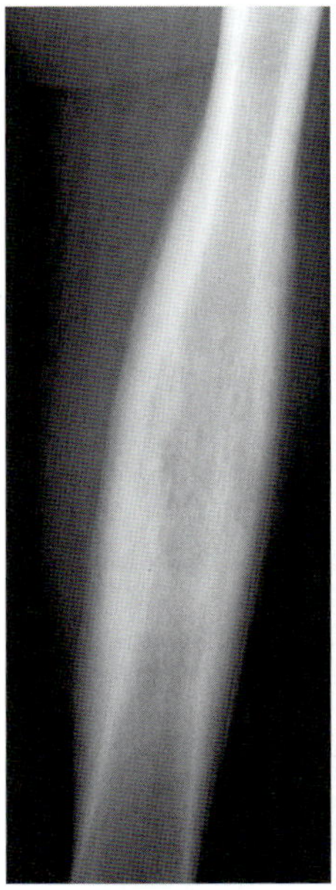

Fig. 4.26 Telangiectatic osteosarcoma with moth-eaten pattern of destruction.

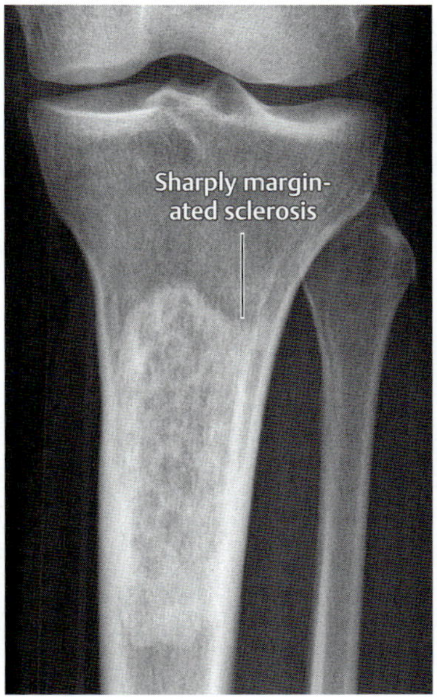

Fig. 4.27 Low-grade central osteosarcoma.

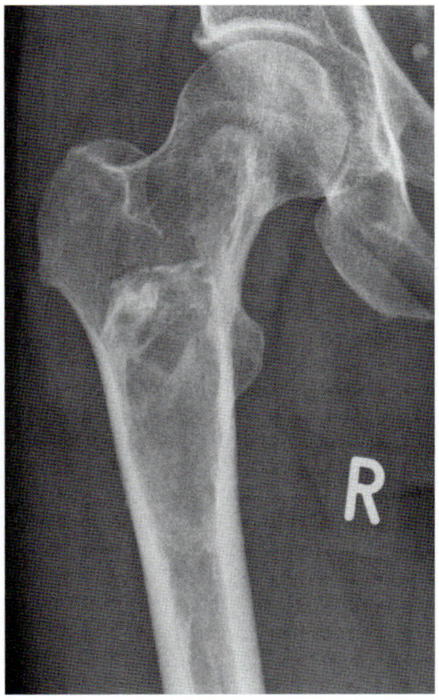

Fig. 4.28 Low-grade central osteosarcoma. The differential diagnosis from fibrous dysplasia is difficult.

Parosteal osteosarcoma. Parosteal osteosarcoma is the commonest form of surface osteosarcoma. It is a low-grade malignancy that develops slowly on the surface of the bone and only invades the medullary cavity secondarily. **Age:** 3rd and 4th decades of life. **Location:** Over 50% arise on the posterior distal femoral metaphysis. The main radiological feature is the eccentrically located density with solid internal structure (▶ Figs. 4.29–4.31). Cleft formations between cortical surface and tumor formation are identifiable by CT. **DD:** Cortical/periosteal desmoid (cortical irregularity), osteochondroma, heterotopic ossification.

Periosteal osteosarcoma. This is an osteoblastic or chondroblastic type that also arises from the surface of the bone, similarly to parosteal osteosarcoma. It has broad-based contact with the bone surface and may show marginal scalloping mimicking a periosteal chondroma or a spiculated periosteal reaction similar to central osteosarcoma (▶ Fig. 4.32). **Location:** Commonly diaphyseal. Secondary invasion of the medullary cavity is identifiable by MRI.

Secondary Osteosarcomas

Between 5 and 7% of osteosarcomas develop from a preexisting bony disorder:

Paget's disease. About 1% of patients with Paget's disease may undergo malignant transformation (95% of cases occur in the polyostotic form of Paget's). **Age:** 6th to 7th decades of life. Any change in the clinical symptoms of a patient with Paget's disease or a pathologic fracture raises the specter of a secondary osteosarcoma. Increasing levels of bone-specific alkaline phosphatase evident in the laboratory results may be an indicator. Increasing lysis and cortical destruction on the radiograph are important diagnostic signs (▶ Fig. 4.33). MRI confirms a soft tissue component. The prognosis is universally poor.

Radiation-induced osteosarcoma. The risk of developing an osteosarcoma after radiation therapy is reported to be 0.03 to 0.8% of cases with doses over 30 Gy required. The latent period before manifestation of the tumor is typically about 10 years and not less than 3 years (▶ Fig. W4.1).

Associations between osteosarcomas and medullary infarction or fibrous dysplasia, while recognized, are extremely rare.

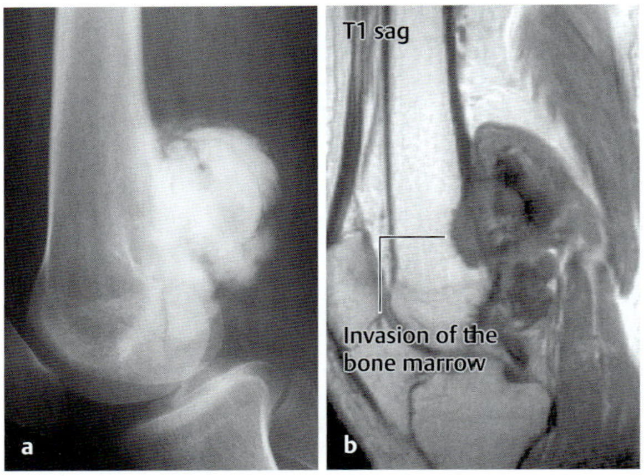

Fig. 4.29 Parosteal osteosarcoma. Compare ▶ Fig. 4.34. **(a)** Densely sclerotic parosteal mass. **(b)** Evidence of tumor infiltration of the medullary cavity.

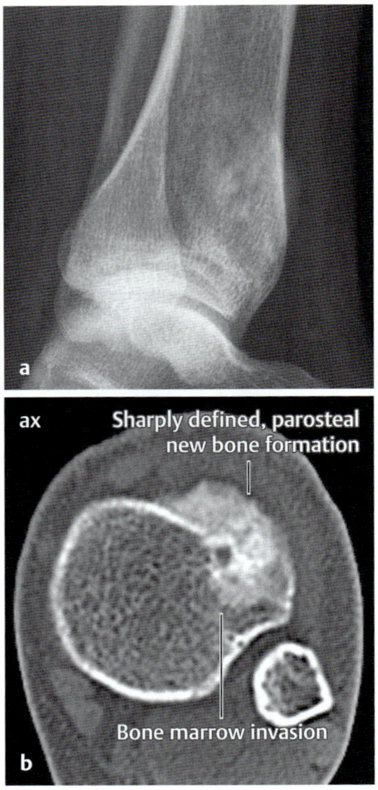

Fig. 4.30 Parosteal osteosarcoma. **(a)** Focal sclerotic zone in the distal tibia. **(b)** CT confirms the secondary invasion of the medullary cavity.

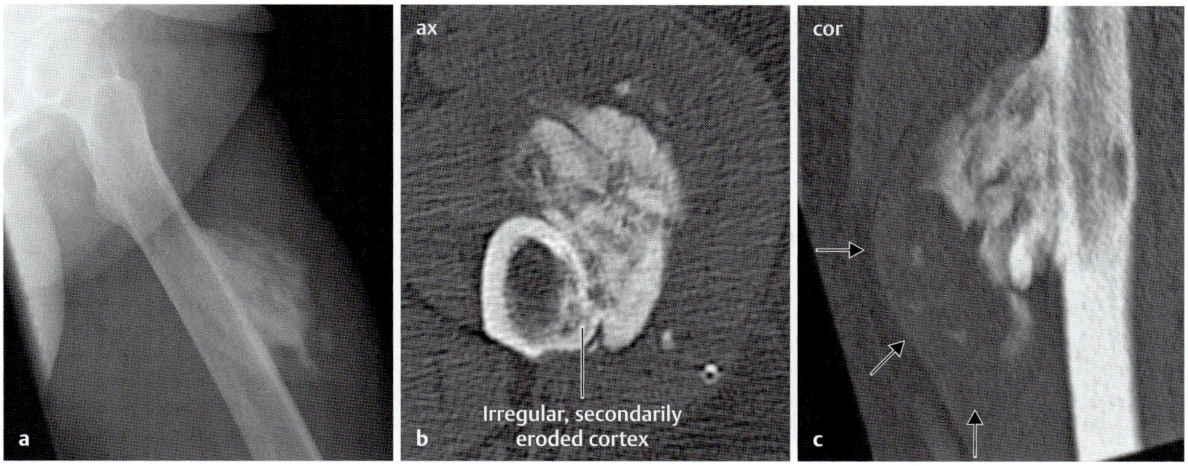

Fig. 4.31 Parosteal osteosarcoma. **(a)** Extraosseous density. **(b)** Broad-based, partly homogeneous, lobulated tumor. **(c)** Chondroid components (arrows) in the distal pole are hardly visible on CT.

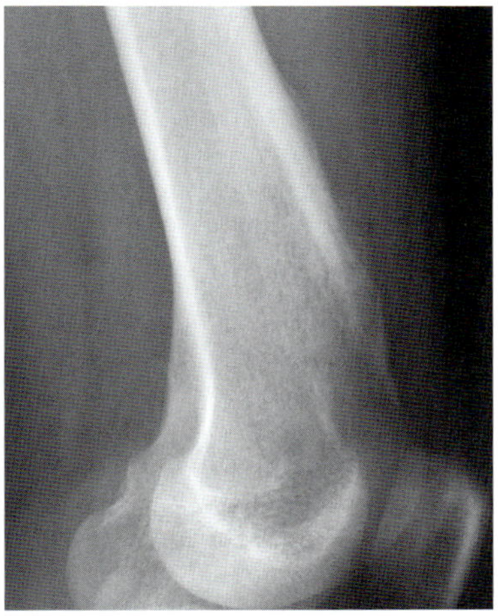

Fig. 4.32 Periosteal osteosarcoma. Broad-based, ill-defined invasion with evident periosteal reaction at the proximal margin of the lesion.

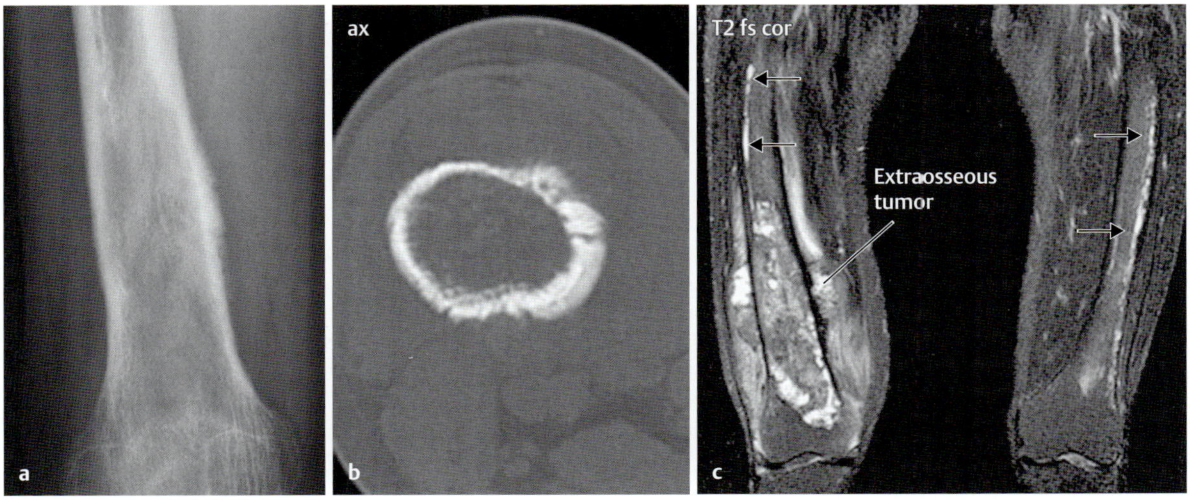

Fig. 4.33 Secondary osteosarcoma associated with Paget's disease. **(a)** Widening of the medullary cavity with ill-defined cortical margin. **(b)** Bone destruction and spiculation. **(c)** Contrast-enhancing tumor. The bilateral signal-intense, subcortical areas (arrows) and the bowing of both femurs are due to the underlying condition (Paget's disease).

4

4.2.2 Chondrogenic Tumors

Common to all cartilage tumors is their production of chondroid matrix, which sometimes may be only sparse and nestlike. Benign tumors are frequently asymptomatic and, as an incidental finding, represent the largest group among bone tumors.

Osteochondroma

Osteochondroma (synonym: cartilaginous exostosis) is the most common bone tumor. They are cartilage-covered bony outgrowths arising from the surface of the bone and containing bone marrow that has trabecular continuity with the central medullary cavity. Cytogenetic studies indicate that both sporadic as well as inherited osteochondromas are genuine benign tumors and not simply developmental abnormalities. Their growth ceases with completion of skeletal growth.

► **Pathology.** An osteochondroma displays a growth plate-like differentiation at the junction with a narrow cartilage cap. Calcifications are regularly found. Fatty marrow is found at the base.

> **Note**
> If the cartilage cap on imaging is thicker than 2 cm, malignant transformation to a secondary chondrosarcoma should be considered. It can occur in < 1% of solitary osteochondromas and < 5% of cases of the multiple form (hereditary multiple exostoses/diaphyseal aclasis); see ► Fig. 4.36). Increasing size or pain in an adult is suspicious for malignant transformation. Malignant transformation does **not** occur in children!

► **Clinical presentation.** It is frequently an incidental finding. Rarely do pain or problems secondary to mechanical compression occur.

Age: Predominantly the 1st to 3rd decade of life. **Location:** The metaphyseal region of the long tubular bones oriented away from the adjacent joint (~ 70% of cases; ► Fig. 4.34). The axial skeleton is also affected. **Treatment:** Leave alone or simple excision at the base of the osteochondroma.

► **Radiography.** The exostosis either arises as a relatively narrow-based bony projection from the underlying cortex (pedunculated) (see ► Fig. 4.34) or is connected to the bone by a broad base (sessile) in such a manner that the native cortex is hardly recognizable (widening of the bone; ► Figs. 4.35, ► 4.36c, and ► W4.2). Large osteochondromas can cause modeling deformity of the underlying bone and pressure erosion of adjacent bones. Calcifications are commonly found on the surface. The border with the surrounding soft tissue is sharp, but commonly of irregular configuration. The noncalcified cartilage cap is not visible on the radiograph.

► **US.** If the osteochondroma is superficial, then the cartilage cap is well visualized (hypoechoic). Ultrasound is particularly applicable in this respect in children.

► **CT.** The origin of the lesion is readily visualized, with depiction of the pathognomonic remodeling of the cortical bone, especially in the axial skeleton. The noncalcified cartilage cap is identifiable as a hypodense layer compared with surrounding muscle (see ► Fig. 4.35).

► **MRI.** As on CT, the direct continuity between the host bone marrow and the fatty marrow of a mature osteochondroma is diagnostic. MRI is the best modality for measuring precisely the thickness of the cartilage cap (see ► Fig. 4.34).

► **DD. Parosteal osteosarcoma.** Whereas osteochondromas have continuity with the normal medullary cavity, parosteal osteosarcomas show an intact cortex or direct tumor invasion with dense osteogenic matrix.

Chondrosarcoma. See “Chondrosarcoma,” page 280.

Nora lesion. This is a bizarre parosteal osteochondromatous proliferation (BPOP) affecting the tubular bones of the hand and foot (see Chapter 4.3.8). Again, there is no continuity between the lesion and the medullary cavity.

Periosteal chondroma. See ► Fig. 4.42.

Chondroma

Chondromas are the second most common benign bone tumor entities (incidence 2.5%). **Enchondromas** are usually solitary tumors of the medullary cavity. The less common **periosteal** (juxtacortical) **chondromas** develop on the surface of the bone, beneath the periosteum. **Enchondromatosis** is a disturbance of normal endochondral ossification.

> **Note**
> - Enchondromatosis = **Ollier's disease** (increased risk of malignant transformation; ► Fig. W4.3).
> - Enchondromatosis and multiple soft tissue hemangiomas = **Maffucci's syndrome.**

► **Pathology.** Chondromas are hypocellular tumors with only septal and peripheral vascularization and abundant hyaline cartilaginous matrix production. They usually grow in a clustered, lobulated fashion, with a bunch-of-grapes appearance displacing the original cancellous bone.

► **Clinical presentation.** In tubular bones, chondromas are typically painless; in the fingers they may present as swellings.

Age: 2nd to 5th decades of life. It is not uncommon for pathologic fractures to be the presenting complaint. **Location:** About 60% of all enchondromas are located in the small

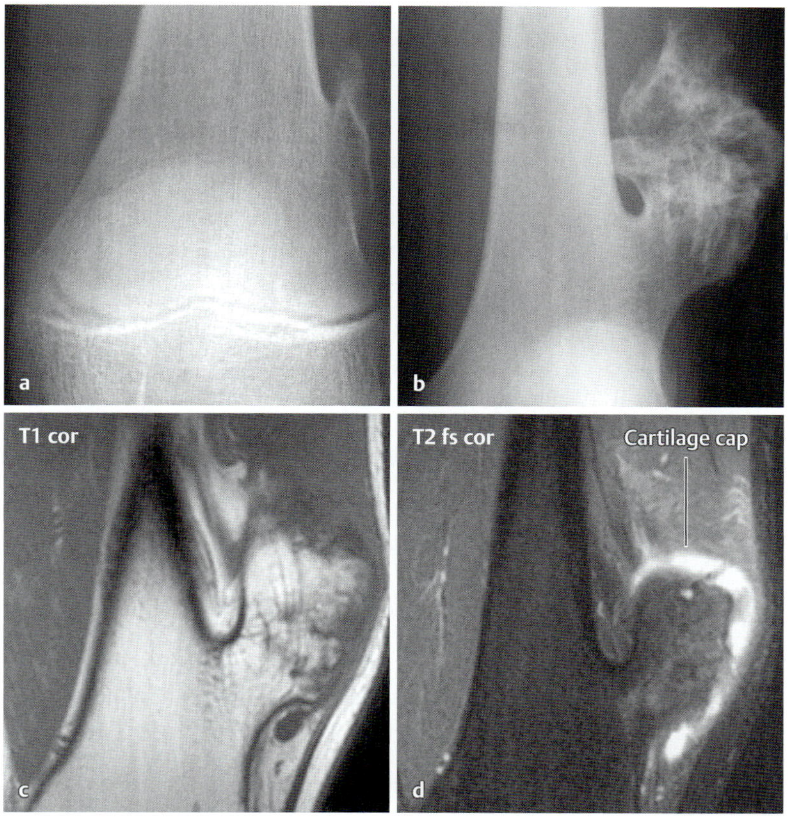

Fig. 4.34 Osteochondroma. **(a)** Pedicle-like primary finding. **(b)** Growth 6 years later. **(c)** Preserved continuity with the bone marrow is evident on MRI. **(d)** Hyperintensity of the cartilage on the fluid-sensitive sequence.

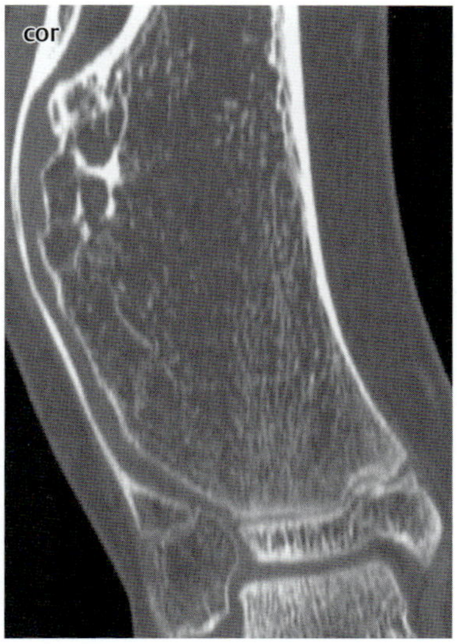

Fig. 4.35 Broad-based osteochondroma of the tibia with erosion/bowing of the fibula.

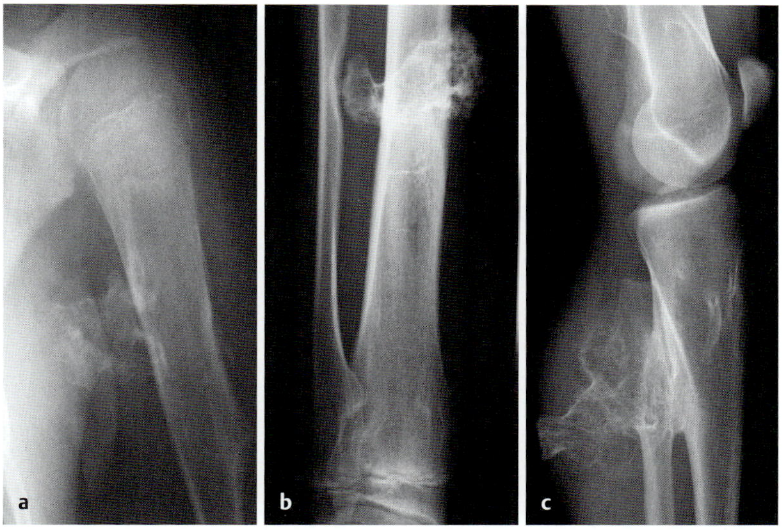

Fig. 4.36 Hereditary multiple exostoses. Multiple bony spur formations. **(a)** Pediclelike exostosis of the humerus. **(b)** Compression and deformation of adjacent bones of the lower leg. **(c)** Broad-based exostosis of the fibula.

tubular bones of the hands and feet. Long tubular bones and the ribs are also affected. Chondromas are rare in flat bones, as well as the spine. **Treatment:** There is currently no unified approach. A watchful waiting approach may be adopted for asymptomatic chondromas of the tubular bones up to a length of ~ 10 cm with yearly follow-up radiographs. Alternatively, careful curettage is performed. The general rule for small tubular bones is that chondroid tumors are practically always benign. Only slowly progressive pain and enlargement of the tumor as demonstrated by imaging should give cause for a generous biopsy.

In very rare cases, solitary enchondromas can undergo malignant transformation to a chondrosarcoma.

> **Note**
> Progressive enlargement and pain during adulthood are suspicious for chondrosarcoma. A more proximal or more central location of a cartilaginous tumor in the body implies a greater likelihood that it is malignant. Lesion length over 5 cm and unequivocal endosteal **scalloping** (= resorption of the inner cortex; see ▶ Fig. 4.41) are possible signs of malignancy.

▶ **Radiography.** The classic finding is a focus of osteolysis in which popcornlike, punctate, ringlike or arclike calcifications are interspersed (▶ Figs. 4.37–4.41). The transition to normal bone is sharp and commonly displays a fine sclerotic margin. In long tubular bones the tumor almost always has a central location. If scalloping and neocortex are present, then the lesion should be assessed for disruption of the cortical bone using CT or MRI. In the small bones of the hand, osteolysis is expansile and the cortex very frequently attenuated and sometimes no longer visible. In the hand, however, this is no proof of malignancy, because the bones are small and the tumor rapidly extends to the cortex.

▶ **CT.** Typical popcornlike calcifications are more readily recognizable (▶ Fig. 4.42). Unequivocal cortical destruction is indicative of malignant transformation into a chondrosarcoma.

▶ **MRI.** There is a hypointense signal pattern on T1W sequences; the signal on T2W sequences depends on the degree of calcification. A noncalcified enchondroma can appear so hyperintense that it is difficult to differentiate it from a cyst on T2W images. Intravenous administration of contrast agent is then helpful. There is a typical lobulated appearance with septation (▶ Figs. 4.37, ▶ 4.39, and ▶ Fig. W4.3). A chondrosarcoma should be considered where there is cortical destruction or extraosseous tumor components.

▶ **NUC MED.** Absent to mild increased activity is evident on the bone scan. Markedly increased uptake would suggest growing tumor and would be suspicious for malignancy. Increased uptake is regularly seen on PET, sometimes quite clearly depending on the proliferation rate. Differentiation from a low-grade chondrosarcoma is not possible. A threshold to higher-grade chondrosarcoma has been reported.

▶ **DD. Bone infarction.** Calcifications and infarctions are arranged more peripherally at the interface with healthy bone. On MRI, fat and/or cystic degeneration is found in a central location within the infarction area.

Chondrosarcoma G1 (well differentiated). This is a very difficult differentiation histologically and on imaging (see commentary of ▶ Fig. 4.41).

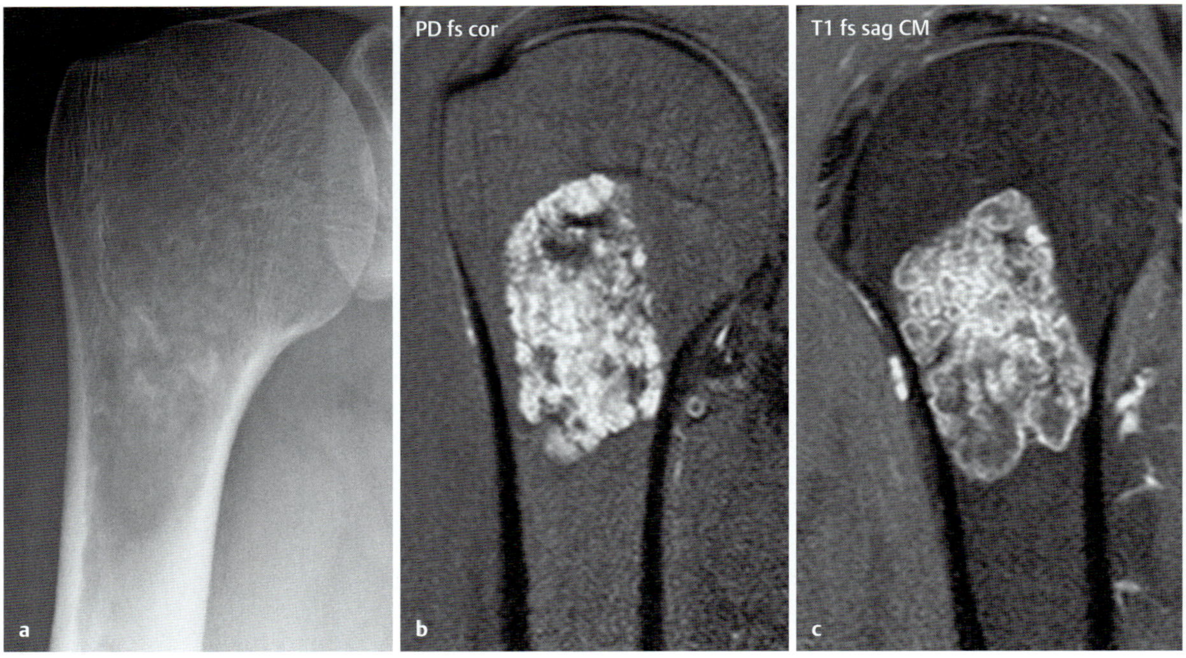

Fig. 4.37 Enchondroma. **(a)** Radiolucency with granular calcifications in the proximal humeral shaft evident on the radiograph. **(b)** Very hyperintense cartilage signal on the PDW image with grapelike configuration. **(c)** Septal contrast enhancement.

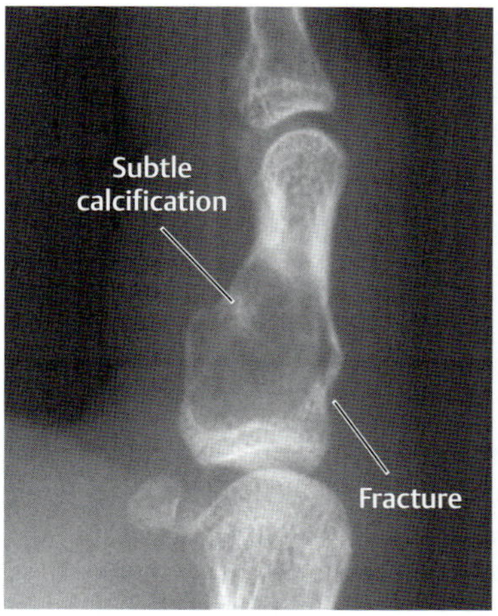

Fig. 4.38 Sharply defined osteolytic lesion with thinning of the cortex and (pathologic) fracture. Nevertheless, there are no concerns about diagnosing a "benign enchondroma" of the hand.

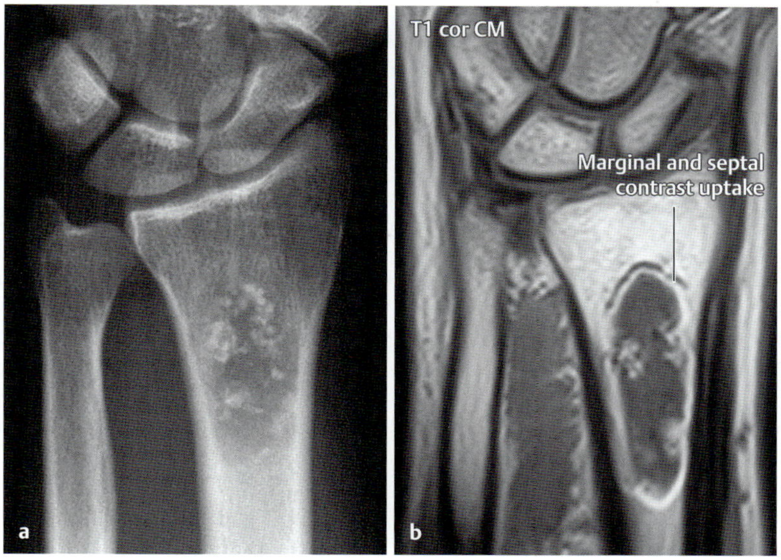

Fig. 4.39 Enchondroma of the distal forearm. **(a)** Osteolysis with popcornlike calcification. **(b)** Sharp margination; the cortex is preserved.

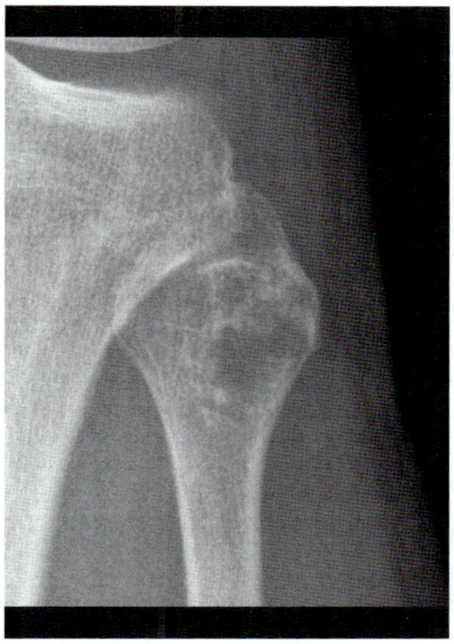

Fig. 4.40

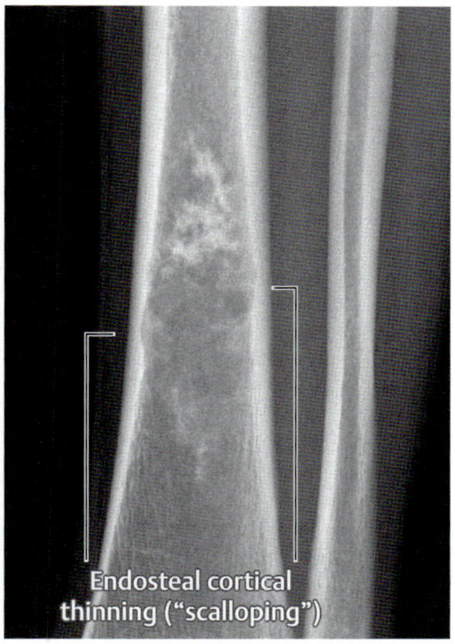

Fig. 4.41

Fig. 4.40 Enchondroma of the fibular head.

Fig. 4.41 Enchondroma of the distal tibia. The crucial clinical question—"Is this a slowly growing, but benign, tumor or has a growth spurt occurred?"—cannot be answered with this image alone. Is pain of increasing severity a feature? If so, generous biopsy and analysis at a bone tumor referral center are called for. A progressive increase in size as documented on imaging should also prompt a biopsy.

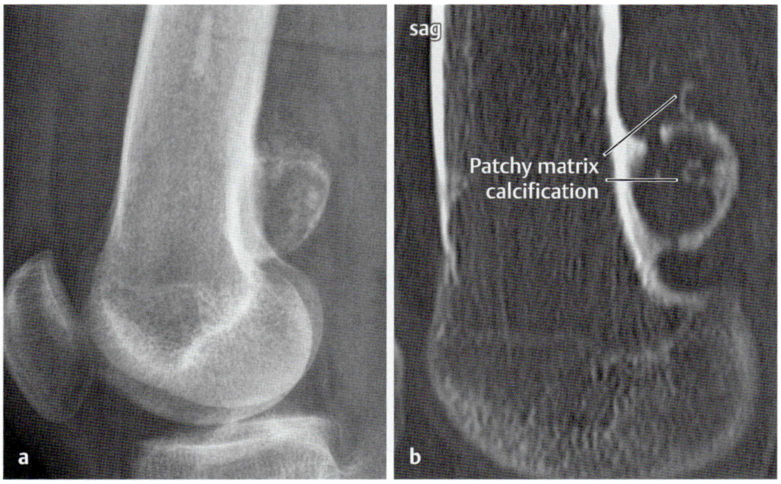

Fig. 4.42 Periosteal chondroma. **(a)** Egg-shaped periosteal tumor with a partly saucer-shaped border. **(b)** Typical saucer shape of the cortex.

Chondroblastoma

► **Pathology.** A chondroblastoma is a rare, benign, cartilage-producing tumor.

► **Clinical presentation.** **Age:** 1st to 3rd decades of life; males are twice as frequently affected as females. **Location:** Typically it arises in the epiphysis of long tubular bones, occasionally extending into the metaphysis. Chondroblastoma may arise in an apophysis and rarely at other sites such as the talus, calcaneus, patella (where it is the most common tumor!) and spine. **Treatment:** Curettage or, if small, radiofrequency ablation.

► **Radiography.** There is evidence of rounded radiolucency with sclerotic margin and intralesional calcifications in 30% of cases (► Figs. 4.43 and ► 4.44).

► **MRI.** The typical hyperintense cartilage signal on T2W sequences is absent because this is immature cartilage. A concomitant joint effusion is present in 30% of cases (see ► Fig. 4.43) with florid perilesional edema.

> **Note**
> The typical location in the epiphyses of tubular bones is the diagnostic key for a chondroblastoma, especially if intralesional calcifications are absent. The latter should be preferentially looked for using CT. MRI may well diagnose a tumor, but it is very nonspecific.

► **DD.** **Giant cell tumor.** A giant cell tumor does not show clear marginal sclerosis and occurs post skeletal fusion.

Low-grade osteosarcoma. Here, the matrix calcifications are decisive. If they are absent, then the differential diagnosis from a slowly growing osteosarcoma may be difficult.

Other differential diagnoses. Subchondral ganglion, chondromyxoid fibroma, clear cell chondrosarcoma, aneurysmal bone cyst (as a secondary finding commonly associated with a chondroblastoma), and epiphyseal abscess.

Chondromyxoid Fibroma

► **Pathology.** This is a very rare (less than 1% of cases) benign tumor that is characterized by abundant myxoid or chondroid intercellular substance.

► **Clinical presentation.** **Age:** 2nd to 3rd decade of life. **Location:** Frequently found in a metaphyseal, rarely diaphyseal, site around the knee joint (50% of cases). A chondromyxoid fibroma is practically only found in tubular bones.

► **Radiography.** Sharply delineated, solitary radiolucency, which demonstrates an elongated oval form along the longitudinal axis of the bone (► Figs. 4.45 and ► 4.46), are important diagnostic signs. The border of the tumor is not always sharp. Intratumoral calcifications are rare.

► **CT/MRI.** CT and MRI do not make any relevant contribution toward establishing a diagnosis other than determining the extent of the tumor.

► **DD.** Possible differential diagnoses are chondrosarcoma, chondroblastoma, and chondroblastic osteosarcoma. Histological confirmation before planning definitive therapy is essential.

Fig. 4.43 Chondroblastoma. **(a)** Sharply delineated, epimetaphyseal rounded lucency in the femoral head. **(b)** Note the intralesional calcifications on the radiograph. **(c)** MRI: The subchondral plate and the cartilage have been destroyed.

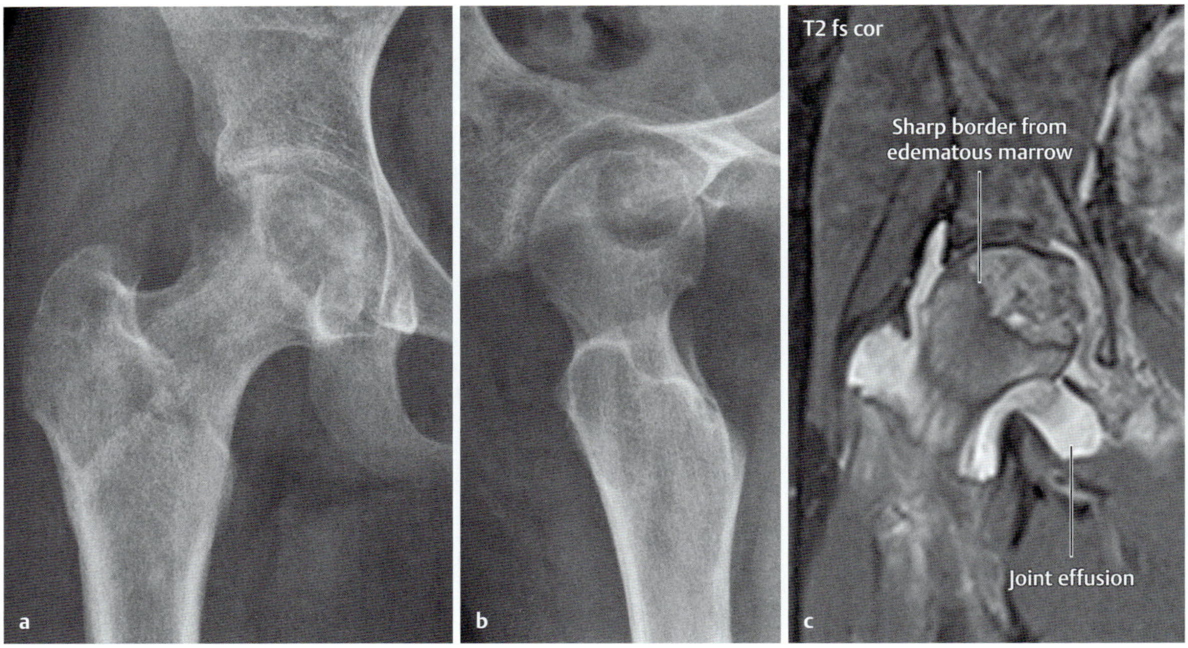

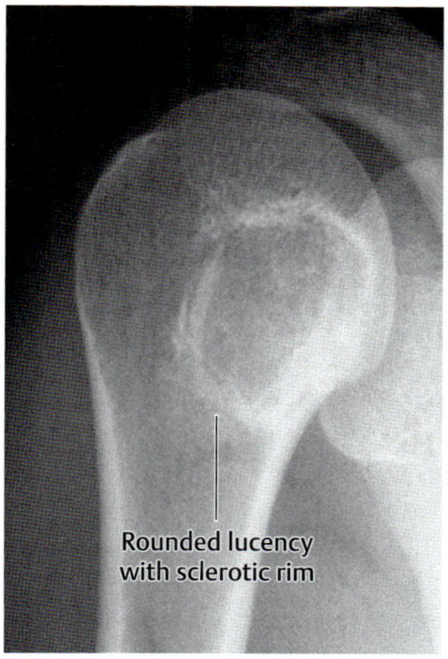

Fig. 4.44

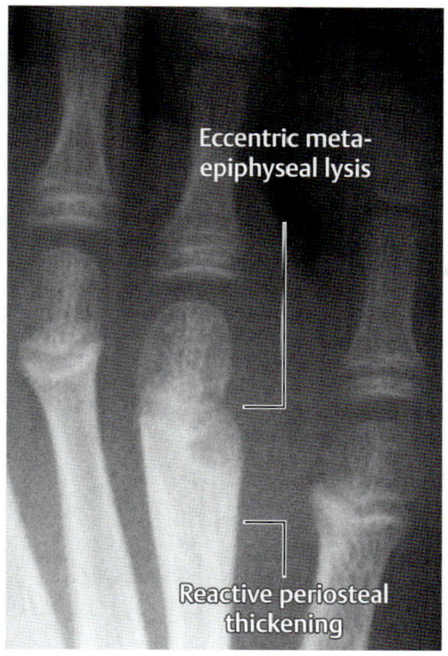

Fig. 4.45

Fig. 4.44 Chondroblastoma.

Fig. 4.45 Chondromyxoid fibroma. Large soft tissue component displacing the adjacent metatarsal.

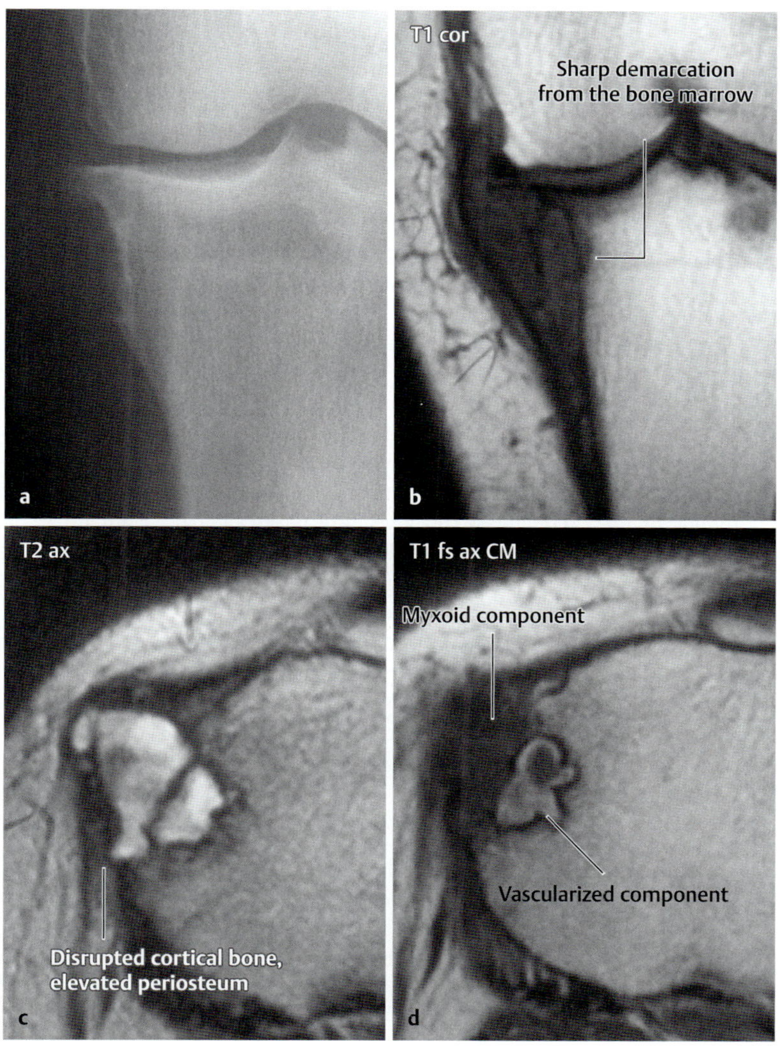

Fig. 4.46 Chondromyxoid fibroma. **(a)** Eccentric elongated oval areas of osteolysis in the metaphyseal region of the medial tibial plateau. **(b)** The tumor has two "parts" and extends in a cranial direction along the medial meniscus. **(c)** A signal-intense tumor matrix on the T2W image. **(d)** Contrast-enhancing vascularized tumor tissue on the internal aspect. The myxoid part does not enhance with contrast.

4

Chondrosarcoma

Chondrosarcomas are the second most common form of primary malignant bone tumors. They comprise a heterogeneous group of malignant cartilaginous tumors which differ both histomorphologically and clinically:

Primary central chondrosarcoma. This is the most common type of chondrosarcoma (▸ Figs. 4.47–4.49). The development of pulmonary metastases is dependent on the grade of the tumor.

Secondary chondrosarcoma. This develops as a result of malignant transformation of a primary benign chondroma to a central chondrosarcoma, or of a primary osteochondroma to a peripheral chondrosarcoma (▸ Fig. 4.50, ▸ Figs. W4.4 and W4.5).

Periosteal chondrosarcoma. This develops on the surface bone (▸ Fig. 4.51).

Dedifferentiated chondrosarcoma. This is a rare type of chondrosarcoma with a poor prognosis. It is characterized by two components: a well-differentiated cartilaginous tumor (enchondroma or low-grade chondrosarcoma, usually with typical matrix mineralizations) and a high-grade, noncartilaginous sarcoma, for example, osteosarcoma. The various radiologically differentiable parts of the tumor should be taken into consideration when determining the site for biopsy. **Age:** Over the age of 50 years.

Mesenchymal chondrosarcoma. This is a rare variant with undifferentiated small round cells and islands of well-differentiated cartilage (▸ Figs. 4.52 and ▸ 4.53). About 30% are extraskeletal. **Age:** From the second decade of life. **DD:** (Extraskeletal) Ewing's sarcoma.

Clear cell chondrosarcoma. This is a rare, low-grade variant with typically a subarticular location in long tubular bones of 20- to 40-year-olds. **DD:** Chondroblastoma; this occurs in 20- to 30-year-olds.

▸ **Pathology.** Myxoid and cystic changes are seen with **primary chondrosarcoma**, in addition to a dominant cartilaginous matrix production. Histological grading from 1 to 3—based on nuclear size, nuclear staining, and cellularity—has proven its worth with regard to prognostic value. The distinction between enchondroma and low-grade chondrosarcoma (G1) must be assessed using an adequate amount of biopsy material by judging the growth pattern with respect to the cortex and cancellous bone. This is difficult even for an experienced pathologist!

▸ **Clinical presentation.** Local swelling and pain that may last for weeks or months before the patient seeks medical attention.

Age: Over 50% of cases are over 50 years of age. All adult age groups, however, can be involved. **Location:** Pelvic bones, proximal femur, proximal humerus and ribs are primary locations. Chondrosarcomas are found in a metaphyseal (less commonly diaphyseal) location.

▸ **Radiography. Primary central chondrosarcoma:**

- A circumscribed radiolucency presents, sometimes with a permeative pattern. The cortical bone is destroyed (▸ Fig. 4.47) or remodeled.
- Only rarely is a sclerotic margin present.
- Periosteal reaction and widening of the bone occur (▸ Fig. 4.49).
- The tumors demonstrate calcifications in about 50% of cases. The calcifications of moderate and high-grade malignant tumors are usually more irregular and patchier than those of enchondromas or low-grade chondrosarcomas.

> **Note**
> Enchondromas and low-grade malignant chondrosarcomas are difficult to differentiate using radiographs alone.

▸ **CT.** CT can demonstrate bony expansion, destruction, and cortical breach (very important!) better than a radiograph (▸ Fig. W4.6; see also ▸ Figs. 4.47 and ▸ 4.53).

▸ **MRI.** MRI is of limited use in differentiating between low-grade chondrosarcoma and enchondroma. Demonstration of cortical breach and possible bone marrow edema can be helpful in individual cases. Large tumors may display central necrosis. The extent of the tumor can be exactly determined, especially if a soft tissue tumor is also present (▸ Figs. 4.47 and ▸ 4.53). There is often very little contrast enhancement of the hypovascularized chondrogenic tumor matrix.

▸ **NUC MED.** The uptake on bone scan is quite intense and depends on reactive cortical remodeling (▸ Fig. 4.49). PET is always positive; the increased uptake correlates with the grade of malignancy and thresholds for Grades II and III have been reported. The important differentiation between benign chondroma and low-grade chondrosarcoma is not so far possible.

▸ **DD.** Low-grade chondrosarcoma (G1) versus enchondroma and chondroblastic osteosarcoma.

> **Note**
> If the compact bone is focally destroyed (scalloping) and a soft tissue tumor is present, then a chondrosarcoma is highly likely, not an enchondroma. Other differentiating criteria are clinical presentation and progression in size as documented by serial imaging.

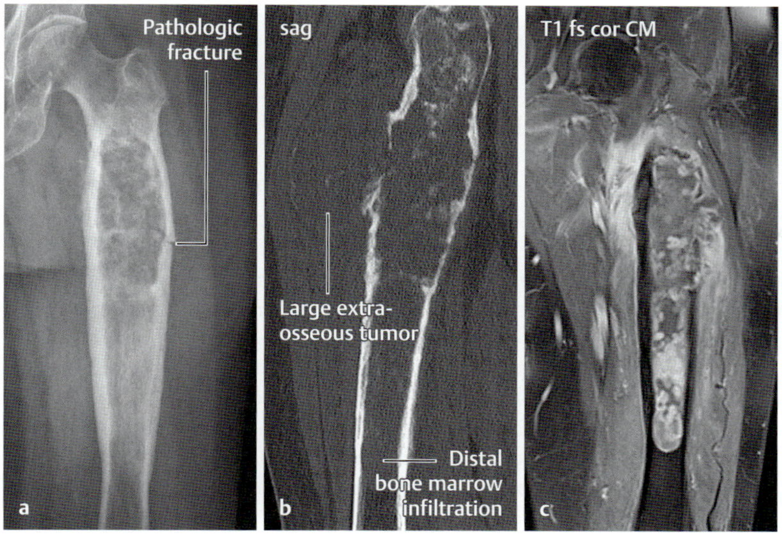

Fig. 4.47 Central chondrosarcoma. **(a)** Bony expansion of the proximal femur with thickening and remodeling of the cortex. **(b)** Endosteal scalloping and cortical destruction. **(c)** Inhomogeneous enhancement of the vascularized parts of the tumor.

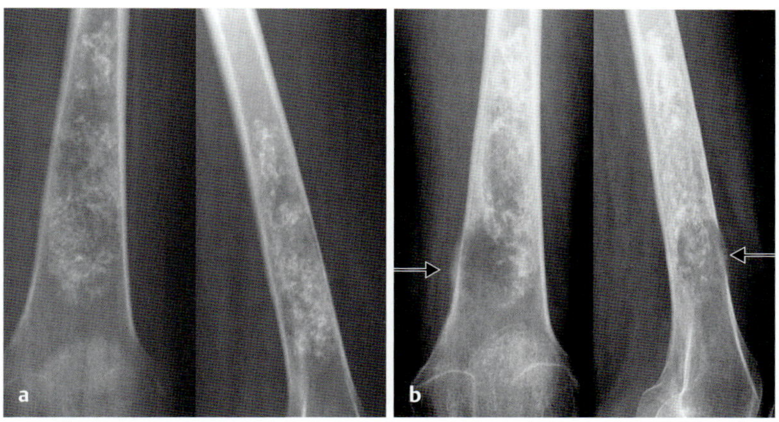

Fig. 4.50 Secondary chondrosarcoma. **(a)** An enchondroma in the distal femur that has remained unchanged for years. **(b)** Finally, development of a chondrosarcoma at the distal pole with a new area of osteolysis and periosteal reaction as signs of cortical invasion (arrows).

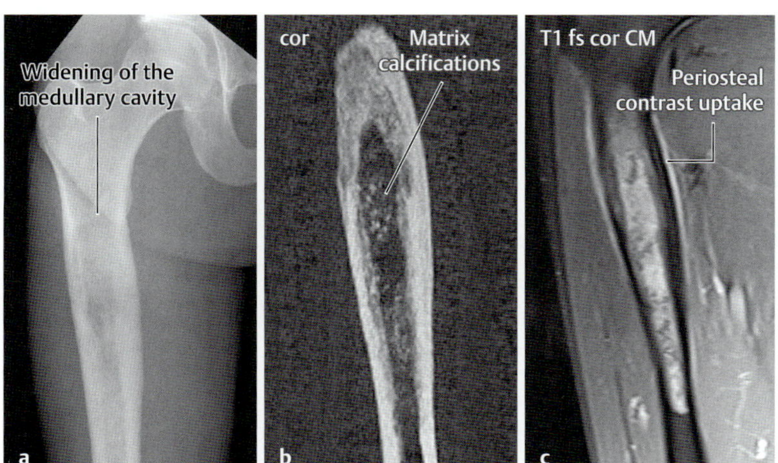

Fig. 4.53 Mesenchymal chondrosarcoma. **(a)** Metadiaphyseal tumor with thickened expanded cortex. **(b)** Cortical remodeling, including destruction of endosteal cortical bone. **(c)** Inhomogeneous but extensive contrast enhancement.

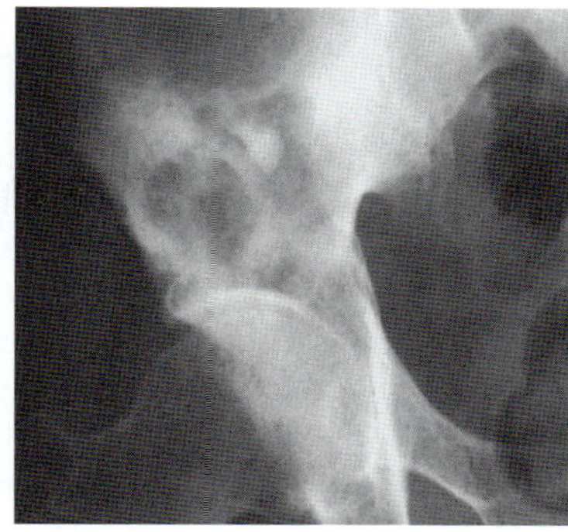

Fig. 4.48 Chondrosarcoma of the pelvis. Supra-acetabular radiolucencies together with areas of reactive sclerosis.

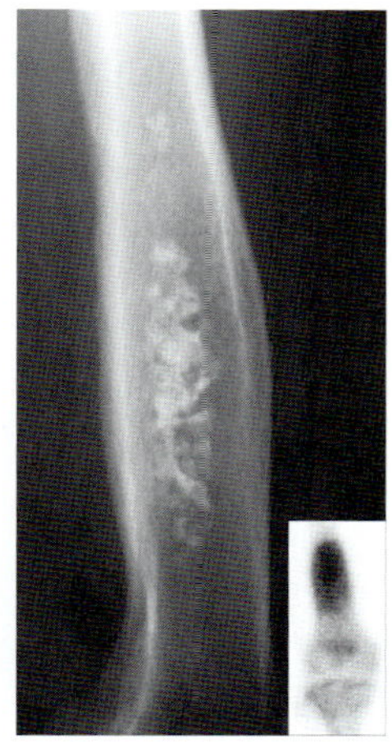

Fig. 4.49 Grade 1 chondrosarcoma. The presence of localized pain, cortical remodeling, and increased uptake on a bone scan are suggestive of malignancy.

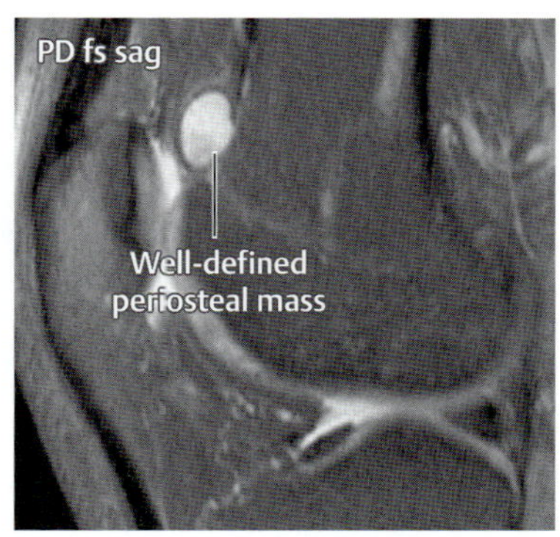

Fig. 4.51 Periosteal chondrosarcoma (G1). Histo ogical evidence of infiltrative growth adjacent to the cortical bone.

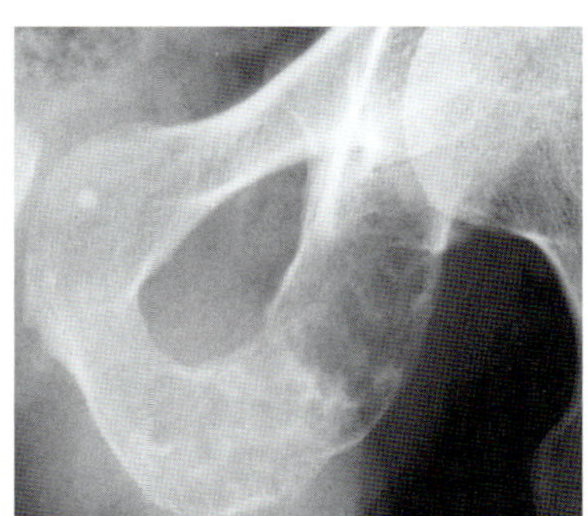

Fig. 4.52 Mesenchymal chondrosarcoma in a 35-year-old man with a 1-year history of pain.

4.2.3 Connective Tissue and Fibrohistiocytic Tumors

Desmoplastic fibroma. This is the intraosseous equivalent of the aggressive fibromatosis (desmoid) of soft tissues. It is considered benign according to the WHO (World Health Organization) classification system. It occurs in young adults and commonly affects the long tubular bones, especially the metadiaphyseal region, as well as the mandible and the pelvis. It has an expansile growth pattern. The radiograph displays a well-marginated area of osteolysis, usually with a neocortex (▶ Fig. 4.54). Low signal intensity on T1W sequences and T2W sequences is exhibited on MRI due to the high collagen content. Recurrences are rare when it is treated by curettage.

Benign fibrous histiocytoma. This is a very rare, benign bone tumor with a slow growth rate as seen on the radiograph. Bone expansion may be evident together with a sclerotic margin (Lodwick Grade Ic). Histologically, the tumor resembles a fibrous cortical defect (nonossifying fibroma) and can occur at all ages. Different skeletal parts are affected (among others, the sacrum and the diaphysis or epiphysis of tubular bones) than with an ossifying fibroma (▶ Figs. 4.55 and ▶ 4.56).

Undifferentiated high-grade pleomorphic sarcoma. Bone pathologists have changed the nomenclature of this category of sarcomas over the years. Originally the name fibrosarcoma was used, to be superseded later by malignant fibrous histiocytoma. In the latest WHO classification the term undifferentiated high-grade pleomorphic sarcoma (UPS) is preferred. The important thing for the radiologist to recognize is that the imaging features are similar. The histological appearance is that of a pleomorphic sarcoma without osseous matrix formation. It is often found around the knee. An important feature is that it can develop secondarily to bone infarction or Paget's disease. The radiograph is nonspecific; the predominant areas of osteolysis confirm the aggressive growth rate of the tumor (Lodwick Grade II; ▶ Fig. 4.57, ▶ Figs. W4.7 and W4.8). A rare variant is the intraosseous leiomyosarcoma, which is spindle cell sarcoma demonstrating immunohistochemically a smooth muscle cell differentiation. The site of predilection is again around the knee (more than 60% of cases); men are more commonly affected than women. If a leiomyogenic tumor manifests itself at a different location, then one should suspect a metastasis of a primary tumor located elsewhere. The tumor displays the radiological criteria of a high-grade osteosarcoma (Lodwick Grade II–III; ▶ Fig. 4.58), similar to malignant fibrous histiocytoma (differential diagnosis: metastasis).

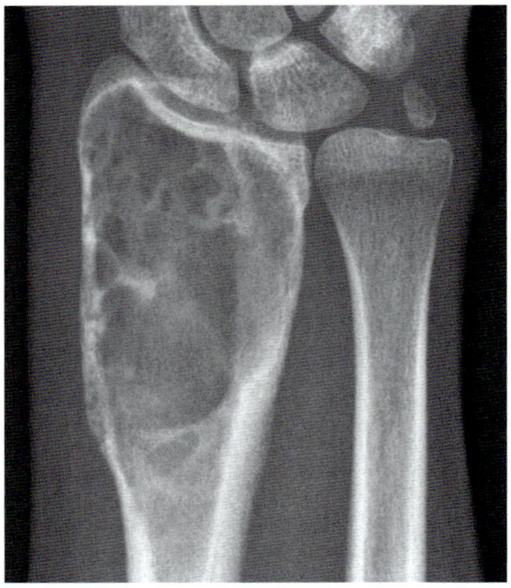

Fig. 4.54 Desmoplastic fibroma.

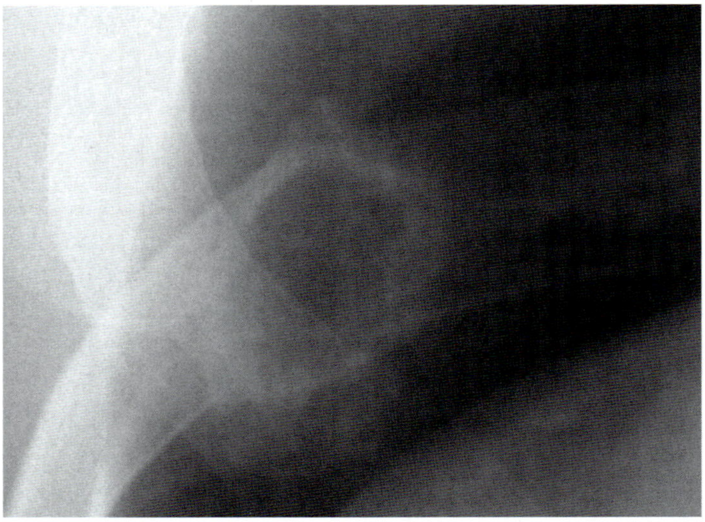

Fig. 4.55 Benign fibrous histiocytoma.

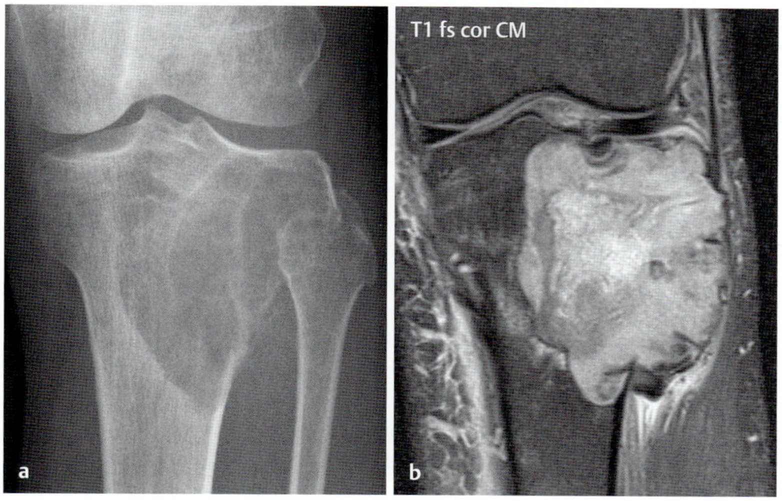

Fig. 4.56 Benign fibrous histiocytoma. **(a)** Sharply defined, epimetaphyseal lytic lesion with development of a neocortex. **(b)** The tumor clearly enhances homogeneously with contrast. Minimal perifocal bone marrow edema.

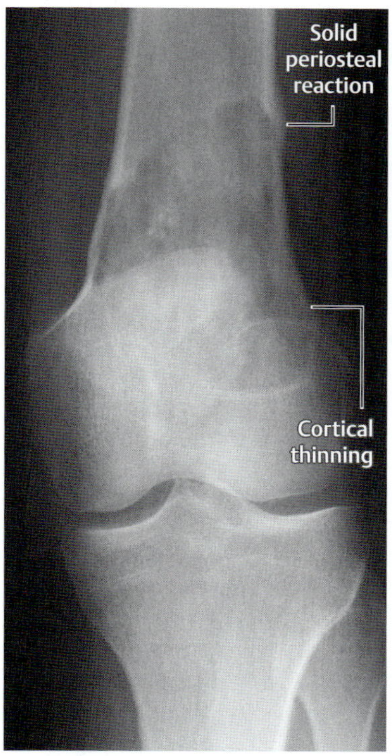

Fig. 4.57 Malignant fibrous histiocytoma.

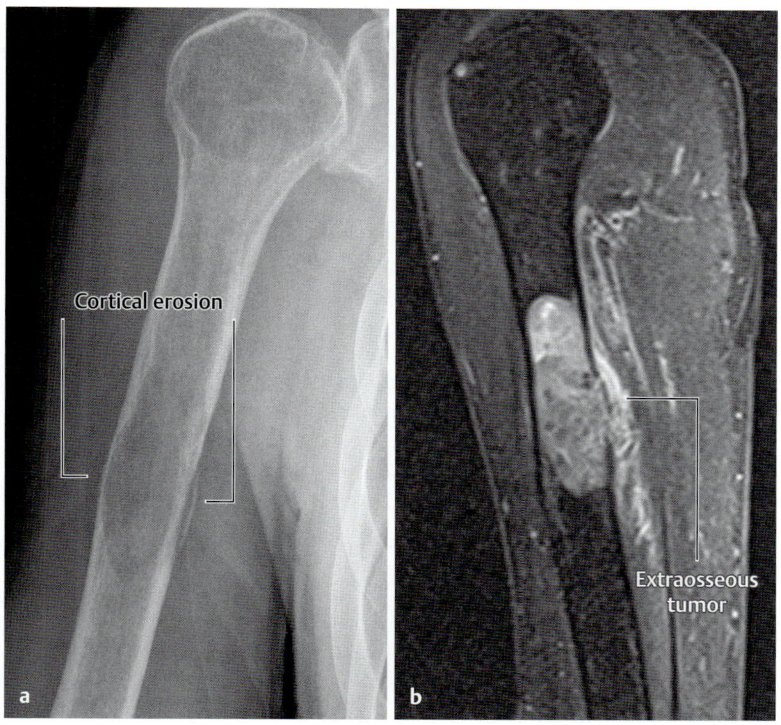

Fig. 4.58 Leiomyosarcoma of bone. **(a)** Nonspecific, diaphyseal lytic lesion. **(b)** Although the tumor is clearly demarcated from the medullary cavity, it already has an extraosseous tumor component.

4.2.4 Ewing's Sarcoma and Primitive Neuroectodermal Tumor

This is a high-grade sarcoma composed of round cells of neuroectodermal origin. Primitive neuroectodermal tumor and Ewing's sarcoma are the same tumor entity.

▸ **Pathology.** It is characterized by a uniform structure of densely packed, small monomorphic cells with round nuclei. The tumor does not produce matrix.

▸ **Clinical presentation.** Unlike patients with other bone tumors, Ewing's sarcoma patients can present systemic symptoms (fever, anemia, leukocytosis, elevated inflammatory parameters). Soft tissue swelling, localized pain and erythema are often seen mimicking infection.

Age: The majority of Ewing's sarcomas present between the ages of 9 and 18 years and this is the second most common sarcoma of bone in children and young adults after osteosarcoma. **Location:** As a rule, Ewing's sarcoma can develop in any bone, but sites of predilection are pelvic bone, femur, fibula, ribs, and humerus. In the long bones, diaphyseal location is classic although metadiaphyseal is frequent. **Treatment:** Preoperative chemotherapy to reduce the tumor size followed by the widest possible resection. This is followed by postoperative chemotherapy and, possibly, radiation therapy, especially after limb-preserving resection.

▸ **Radiography.** The radiological spectrum of Ewing's sarcoma can be very variable (a "chameleon" among bone tumors). Lytic bone destructions dominate in one-half of cases. Mixed forms of osteolysis are present in one-third of cases with more or less marked reactive osteosclerosis. New bone formation by the tumor itself is not found.

Changes in tubular bones

- Predominantly permeative destruction is present, ranging from a solitary radiolucency with a moth-eaten margin to multifocal fine areas of osteolysis.
- Permeative destruction lends the cortical bone a fibrous appearance (Lodwick Grade II–III; ▸ Fig. 4.59).
- The zone of transition between normal and pathologic bone is wide.
- Periosteal reactions are commonly found (▸ Fig. 4.60; see also ▸ Fig. 4.59). Interrupted, single or multilamellated forms (onion skin–like) predominate. Complex periosteal reactions are also possible.

Changes in flat bones

- The osteolytic lesions are usually irregular with ill-defined margins, or the lesions are purely moth-eaten destructions with intervening patchy reactive sclerotic zones spreading in an ill-defined manner into the surrounding tissue (▸ Fig. 4.61).
- "Sclerotic" Ewing's sarcomas are not uncommon in flat bones (~ 10% of cases; ▸ Fig. 4.62).

▸ **NUC MED.** Bone scan and PET serve in particular to exclude skeletal metastases. PET is eminently suitable for evaluating response to therapy and for detecting local recurrences.

▸ **CT.** CT is a suitable modality for demonstrating a permeative growth pattern (▸ Fig. 4.63), especially in the axial skeleton.

▸ **MRI.** The tumor displays a classic signal pattern (hypointense on T1W and hyperintense on T2W sequences) and strong contrast enhancement. The characteristic feature of tubular bones is the large soft tissue component of the tumor, which is almost always evident at the time of diagnosis (see ▸ Figs. 4.59 and ▸ 4.61). Whole-body MRI may be used as a substitute for both the bone scan and PET in the exclusion of skeletal metastasis.

> **Note**
> MRI with contrast administration is not capable of differentiating between necrosis with neovascularization and residual areas of viable Ewing's sarcoma post chemotherapy.

▸ **DD.** Acute hematogenous **osteomyelitis, eosinophilic granuloma** of tubular bones (= Langerhans cell histiocytosis), small cell **osteosarcoma, non-Hodgkin lymphoma,** mesenchymal **chondrosarcoma.**

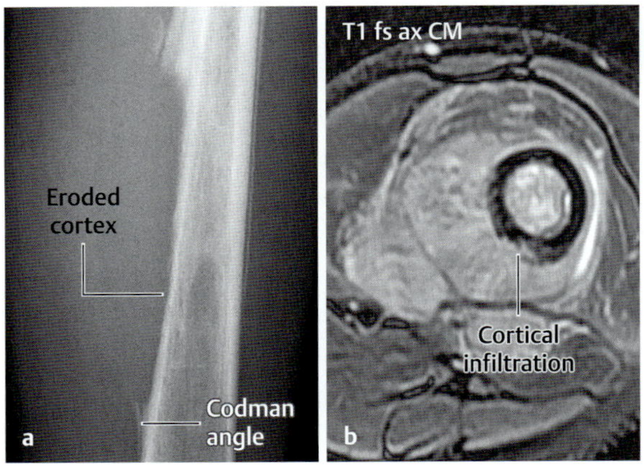

Fig. 4.59 Ewing's sarcoma of the femur. **(a)** Definite periosteal reaction and cortical bone destruction. **(b)** MRI displays the cortical infiltration and the extraosseous extent of the tumor.

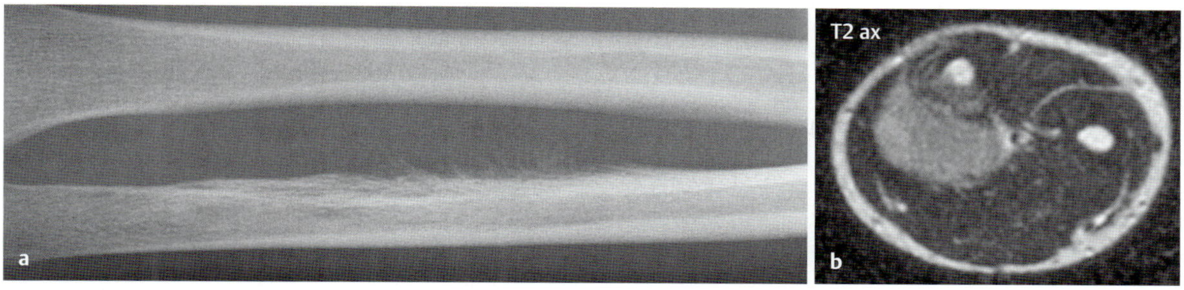

Fig. 4.60 Ewing's sarcoma. **(a)** Ill-defined ulnar cortex with spicules and sunburst phenomenon on the radial side. **(b)** Large extraosseous tumor component already evident.

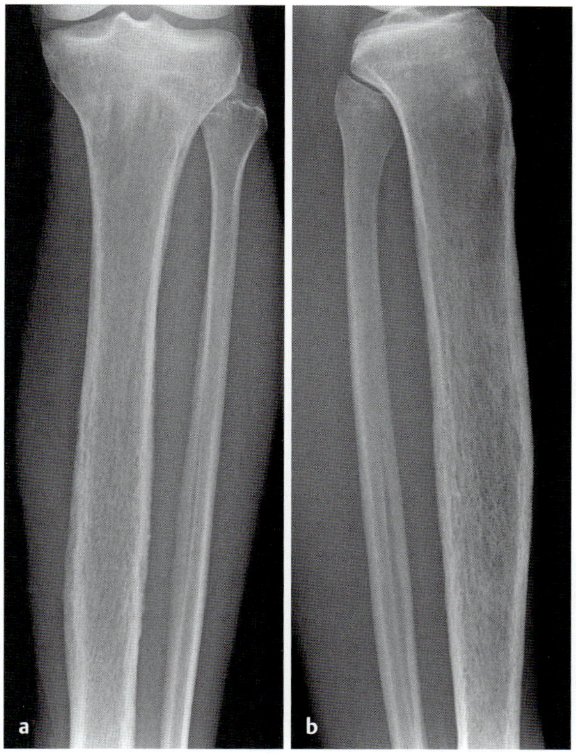

Fig. 4.61 Ewing's sarcoma. **(a)** Permeative growth pattern in the slightly expanded tibial shaft with ill-defined cortical destruction. **(b)** The tumor boundaries are not definable with certainty on the radiograph.

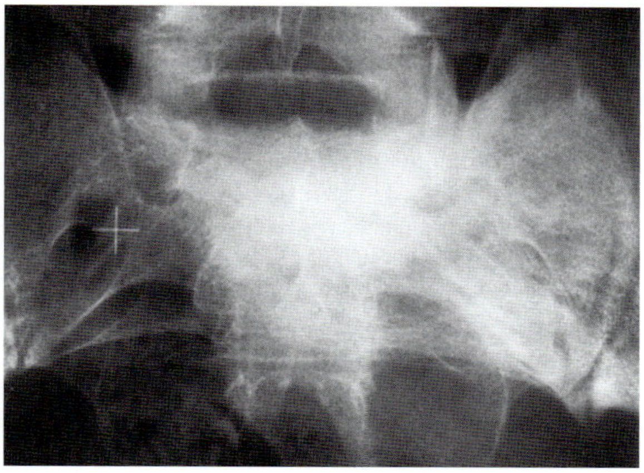

Fig. 4.62 Sclerotic form of Ewing's sarcoma. Not unusual in the pelvis.

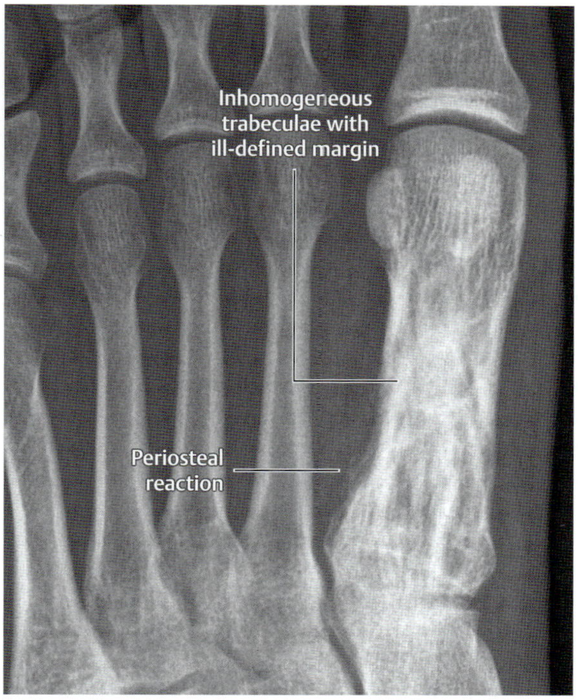

Fig. 4.63 Predominantly sclerotic lesion of a Ewing's sarcoma of the first metatarsal.

4

4.2.5 Giant Cell Tumor

► **Pathology.** This is a benign, locally aggressive tumor of bone. The lesion consists of a neoplastic, mononuclear component with round cells and giant cells that are relatively evenly distributed throughout the tumor. However, giant cells are also found in a large number of other skeletal lesions (e.g., in aneurysmal bone cyst), which may lead to histological misdiagnosis. The lesion does not produce matrix.

► **Clinical presentation.** The cardinal finding is local pain that increases over a period of months. Although it is categorized as a benign tumor, metastases to lung occur in < 5% of cases but do not alter the favorable prognosis.

Age: All age groups may be affected but age of predilection for a giant cell tumor is the 3rd decade of life when approximately 40% of all giant cell tumors present. **Location:** About one-half of all giant cell tumors are located around the knee. Other typical locations are the distal radius and the proximal humerus. The tumor is primarily eccentrically located in the subarticular zone of long bones extending into the metaphysis. **Treatment:** Curettage with the insertion of bone cement; wide excision in advanced stages.

► **Radiography.**

- The typical characteristic of a giant cell tumor on the radiograph is an eccentrically located osteolytic lesion in the subarticular bone without matrix ossifications (► Figs. 4.64, ► 4.65; ► W4.9 and W4.66).
- In about one-half of cases the intralesional structure appears in the form of fine or coarser septations (► Fig. 4.67).
- The border of the lesion is usually sharply defined (Lodwick Grade Ia–c) but without marginal sclerosis. The boundaries of rapidly growing tumors can be ill-defined and irregular.
- The cortical and subchondral margin is preserved for an extended time, but eventually it becomes eroded and is breached. Then either the cortex is completely destroyed or neocortex develops with preservation of the periosteum.
- Laminated or complex periosteal reactions are only rarely encountered.

► **CT.** This is a tumor that lacks matrix production. Isolated reactive calcifications (septations) should not be mistaken for matrix production (► Fig. 4.68). Evidence of re-ossification is possible during antiresorptive treatment (► Fig. 4.69).

► **MRI.** Classic signs of a tumor (low signal intensity on T1W and high signal intensity on T2W sequences) and strong contrast enhancement make differential diagnosis of the giant cell tumor from sarcoma difficult on MRI. Hemorrhage and necrosis produce inhomogeneous signal intensity and contrast enhancement. Fluid–fluid levels due to secondary aneurysmal bone cyst formation may be seen.

► **NUC MED.** There is a strong accumulation in all three phases of the bone scan.

► **DD.** Chondroblastoma, telangiectatic osteosarcoma, plasmacytoma, metastases, aneurysmal bone cyst, chordoma, **brown tumor** of hyperparathyroidism, large subchondral **ganglion.**

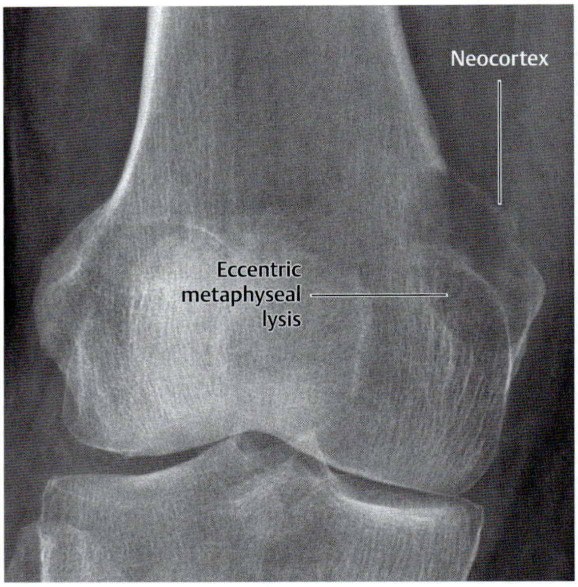

Fig. 4.64 Giant cell tumor with an early presentation.

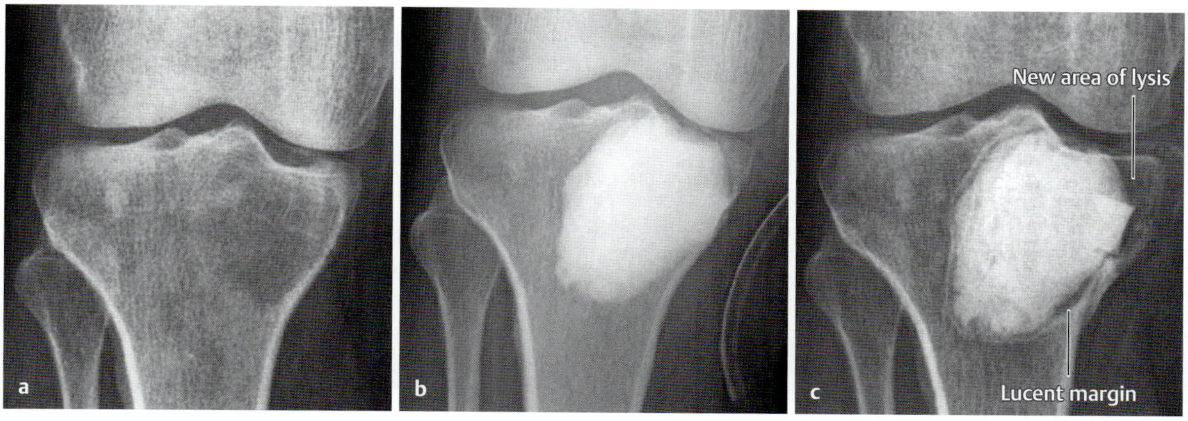

Fig. 4.65 Giant cell tumor. For additional images see ▶ Fig. W4.9. **(a)** Typical eccentrically located epimetaphyseal lytic lesion. **(b)** Appearance after curettage and filling with bone cement. **(c)** The follow-up review displays signs of recurrent tumor.

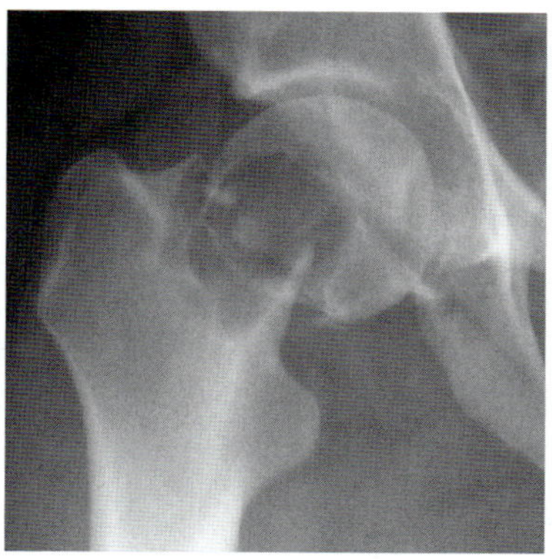

Fig. 4.66 Pathologic fracture secondary to a giant cell tumor of the femoral neck.

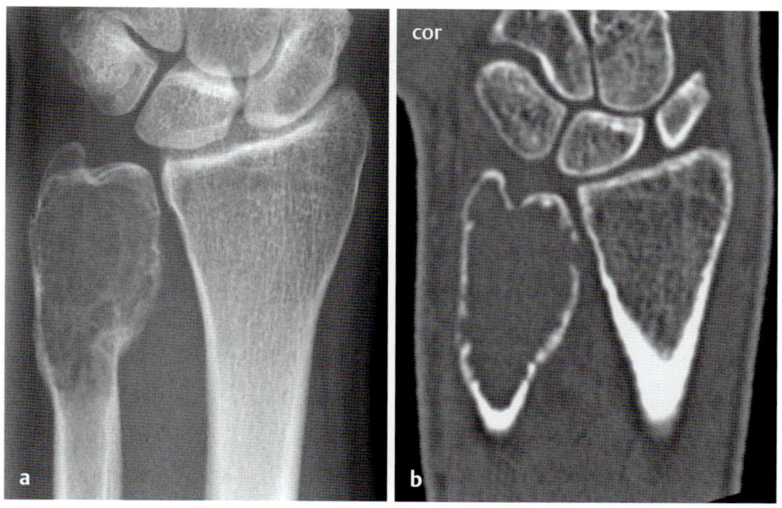

Fig. 4.67 Giant cell tumor. **(a)** Lysis within the ulnar head with irregular, but relatively sharp, proximal margin of the radiolucency. **(b)** Widening of the medullary cavity with development of a completely continuous neocortex.

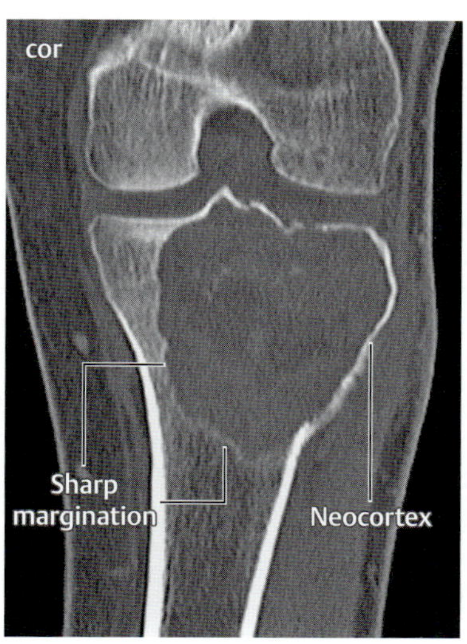

Fig. 4.68

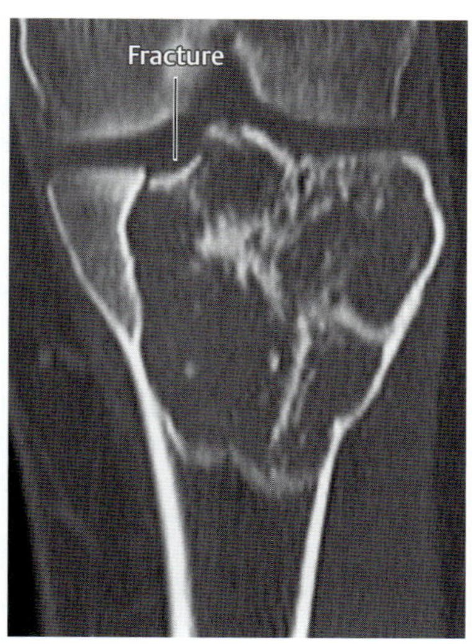

Fig. 4.69

Fig. 4.68 Giant cell tumor. Classically located, sharply circumscribed lytic lesion in the tibial plateau without matrix production.

Fig. 4.69 Sclerosis of a giant cell tumor in response to treatment with denosumab. Same patient as in ▶ Fig. 4.68. A fracture has occurred.

4.2.6 Vascular Tumors

► **Pathology.** Vascular tumors display endothelial hyperplasia with an increased endothelial proliferation rate. Immunohistochemical methods are extremely helpful in allowing differentiation between tumors and malformations.

Actual vascular tumors of the bone are very rare. They include epithelioid hemangiomas (benign), epithelioid hemangioendothelioma (low grade; ► Fig. 4.70), malignant angiosarcomas, and glomus tumors. Glomus tumors originating in the bone are extremely rare (as opposed to those in soft tissues). Reference is drawn here to special textbooks on bone pathology and bone radiology.

> **Note**
>
> A “hemangioma” of the vertebra is not a tumor but a vascular malformation! See also Chapter 4.3.7.
>
> Vascular tumors of bone may be multifocal within a limb (monomelic), thereby mimicking metastatic disease.

4.2.7 Lipogenic Tumors

Lipoma

Lipoma of bone, unlike its soft tissue counterpart, is a rare, benign tumor emanating from the adipocytes of the bone. Lipomas may calcify centrally or undergo cystic degeneration. Typical sites include the anterior calcaneus and less commonly the proximal femur.

► **Clinical presentation.** These are usually asymptomatic incidental findings.

► **Radiography.** Lysis with a discrete well-defined sclerotic margin is predominantly seen. In most cases the lesions are septated. Sometimes central calcifications are found (► Fig. 4.71) and/or bony expansion.

► **CT.** Density measurements confirm the fat content of the tumor.

► **MRI.** The signal intensity is hyperintense on T1W images confirming the diagnosis (► Fig. 4.72).

► **DD. Solitary bone cyst, hemangioma, and hemangioendothelioma.** Without central calcification, differentiation is not possible from the radiograph. Differentiation is achieved using MRI or CT (intralesional detection of fat within the lipoma).

Subchondral ganglion. Differentiation using MRI or CT (myxoid content with contact to the joint).

Intraosseous liposarcoma. These are extremely rare tumors, mostly at the distal femur (► Fig. W4.10). There are no specific radiographic or MRI features.

> **Caution**
>
> A sparse trabecular pattern on radiographs particularly in older patients, e.g., at the femoral neck and calcaneus, can mimic lysis but does not represent genuine space-occupying masses.

4.2.8 Miscellaneous Tumors

Chordoma

► **Pathology.** This is a low-to-intermediate grade malignant tumor of notochordal origin that only occurs along the clivus and spine and grows relatively slowly. The tumor resembles the immature structure of the notochord and has a lobular pattern.

► **Clinical presentation.** Neurologic symptoms usually develop when the tumor is located in the spine, comparable to those of a disk prolapse. Sacrococcygeal chordomas are usually palpable anterior to the sacral bone and, when of an appropriate size, can result in disturbances of voiding and defecation. Delineation from the surrounding structures remains possible for a relatively long time.

Age: The tumor can develop at all ages, with the age of predilection being around the 5th and 6th decades of life. **Location:** Sites of predilection are the spheno-occipital and sacrococcygeal regions. Chordomas are typically located in the midline. **Treatment:** Wide excision. Local recurrence is common because the surgical aim of wide excision is not always achieved due to desire to maintain bladder and bowel function.

► **Radiography.** Chordomas appear on radiographs as an area of osteolysis, possibly surrounded by an undulating sclerotic margin, and as a soft tissue mass. Matrix is not produced, but residual parts of bone (► Fig. 4.73) and calcifications (30–50%) are identifiable.

► **CT.** CT is a suitable modality for determining the extent of the tumor and the degree of bone destruction. Tumors of the sacrum usually already have a large anterior tumor component.

► **MRI.** The anatomical relationship to the contiguous soft tissues, especially the neurogenic structures, is best shown by MRI (► Fig. 4.74, ► Fig. W4.11, ► Fig. 4.75, and ► Fig. W4.12).

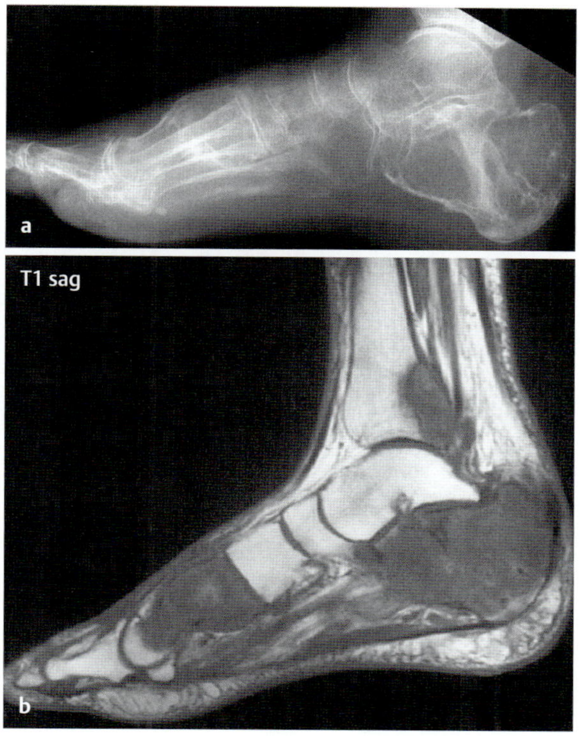

Fig. 4.70 Multiple hemangioendotheliomas. **(a)** Low expansile, in part honeycomb osteolytic lesions without sclerotic margin. **(b)** Hypointense matrix with delicate septations on the T1W image.

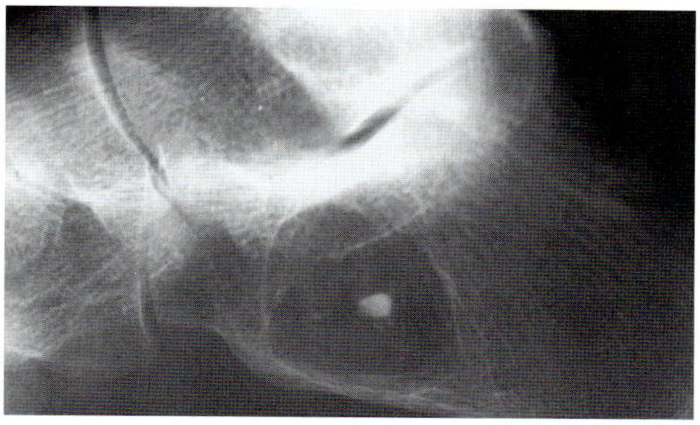

Fig. 4.71 Lipoma with typical central calcification.

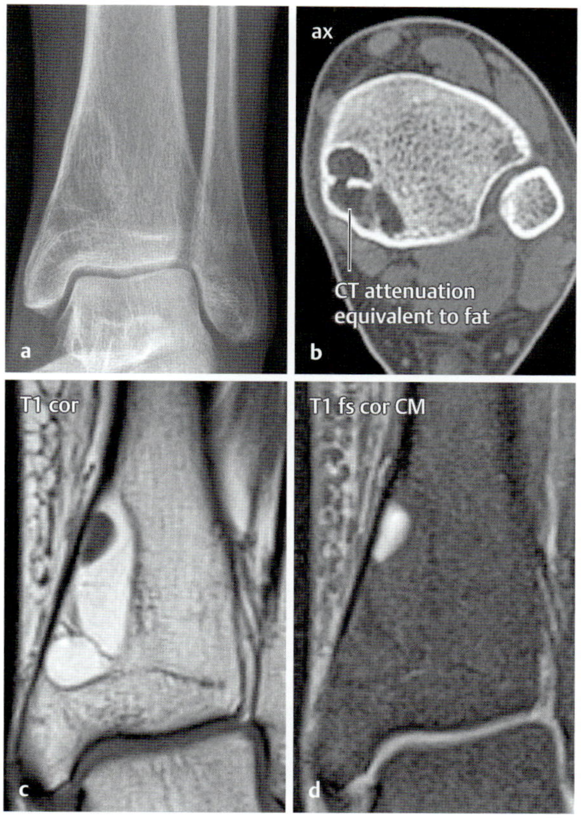

Fig. 4.72 Lipoma of the distal tibia. **(a)** Lucency with a sclerotic margin. **(b)** Negative fat density measurements on CT; isolated calcified septations. **(c)** Homogeneous hyperintense lesion with cranial focal hypointensity on the plain T1W image. **(d)** Isointense to bone marrow on the T1W FS (fat-suppressed) image after contrast administration. The small, contrast-enhancing area is consistent with a focal intralesional fibrosis.

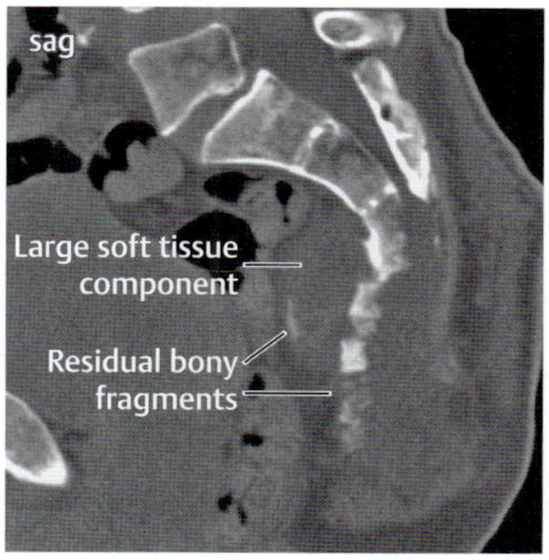

Fig. 4.73 Sacral chordoma. Typical midline location.

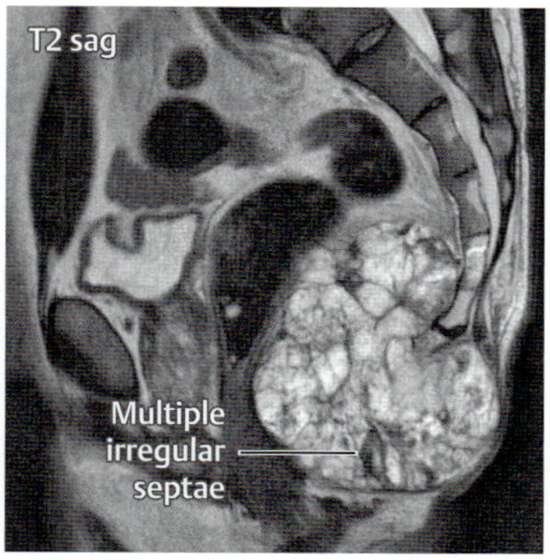

Fig. 4.74 Coccygeal chordoma. The T2W image illustrates the high fluid content of the chordoma. For another image see ▸ Fig. W4.11.

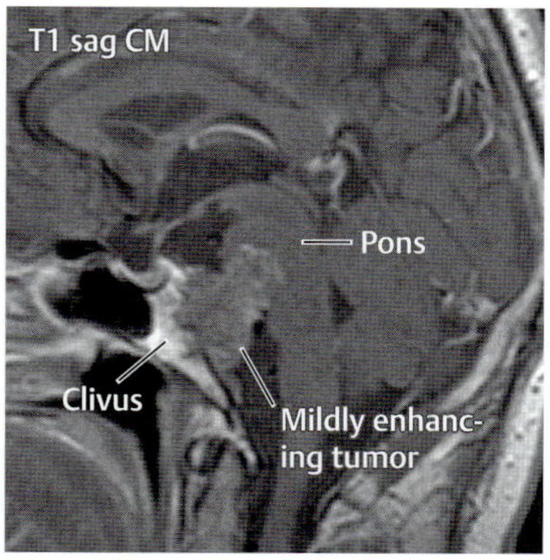

Fig. 4.75 Clival chordoma with penetration into the pons. For another image see ▸ Fig. W4.12.

▸ DD.

Sacrum. Giant cell tumors, chondrosarcomas, plasmacytomas, and carcinoma metastases are more common than chordomas.

Clivus/cervical spine. Carcinoma metastases and myxoid chondrosarcomas are essentially the main differential diagnoses of chordomas with partial chondroid differentiation. Craniopharyngeomas do not demonstrate calcifications.

Giant notochordal rest (giant notochordal hamartoma). Benign hamartomas; they contain trabecular bone, partly sclerotic. The bone boundaries are respected (▸ Fig. 4.76). The most common differential diagnosis is an osteoblastic metastasis.

Adamantinoma of the Long Tubular Bones

▸ **Pathology.** This is a slow-growing low-grade malignancy typically arising in the tibia. Metastasis to the lung is uncommon.

> **Caution**
> The name "adamantinoma" is derived from the histological similarity to adamantinoma (ameloblastoma) of the mandible. It is a distinct entity, however.

▸ **Clinical presentation.** The cardinal clinical finding of adamantinoma is local pain.

Age: Age peak is the 2nd to 3rd decades of life. **Location:** More than 90% of all adamantinomas are located eccentrically in the anterior tibial diaphysis. The fibula is also involved in about one-third of cases. Locations in other tubular bones are uncommon. Metastases occur in ~ 20% of cases. **Treatment:** Wide excision. Incomplete excisions result in high recurrence rates.

▸ **Radiography/CT.** Multifocal, confluent radiolucencies (soap-bubble appearance) with marginal sclerosis in the anterior cortex and medullary cavity of the tibia and fibula (Lodwick Grade Ib–c; ▸ Figs. 4.77 and ▸ 4.78). The development of a neocortex is due to a solid periosteal reaction. The metaphysis is also involved in 30% of cases.

▸ **MRI.** MRI serves to assess the exact extent of bone and soft tissue involvement.

▸ DD.

Fibrous dysplasia. Osteolysis or ground-glass appearance. Fibrous dysplasia tends to be more centrally located.

Osteofibrous dysplasia. This has a histological and radiological similarity to adamantinoma but occurs in children (see Chapter 4.3.8).

Carcinoma metastases. These particularly develop tumor fibrosis after treatment.

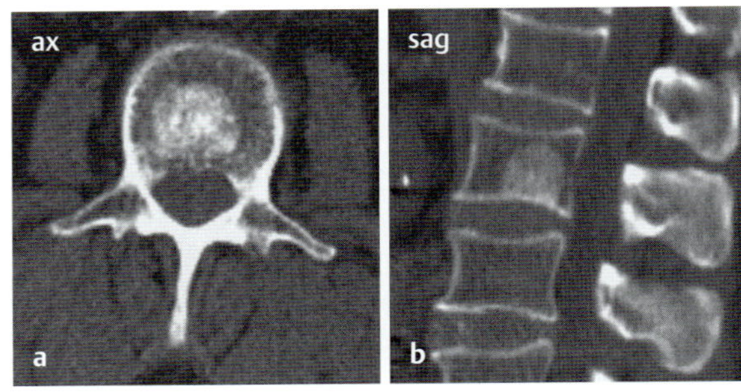

Fig. 4.76 Notochordal rest. **(a)** Sharply defined, central sclerosis in L2. **(b)** Bony boundaries are respected.

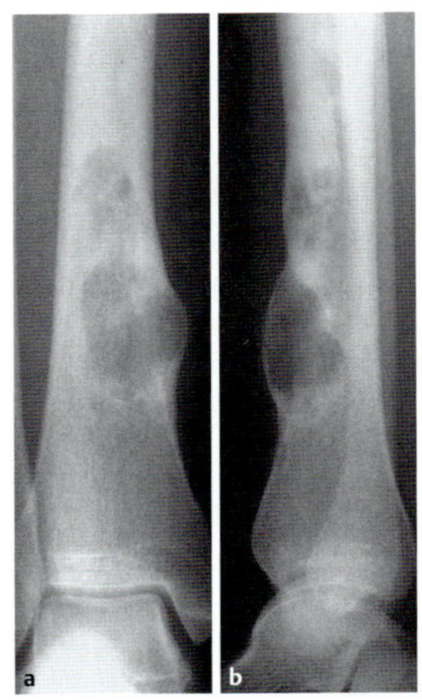

Fig. 4.77 Adamantinoma of the tibia. **(a)** Multifocal lucencies. **(b)** Reactive sclerosis around the lucencies.

Fig. 4.78 Juvenile adamantinoma. **(a)** Sharply delineated, intracortical osteolysis with marginal sclerosis in a typically diaphyseal location. **(b)** Soap bubble–like expansion of the cortical bone.

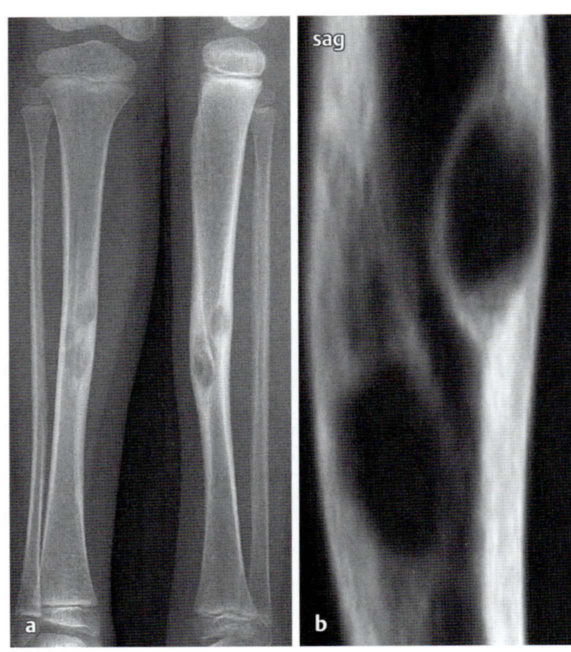

4.3 Tumorlike Lesions

4.3.1 Osteoma, Bone Islands, and Osteopoikilosis

Osteomas and bone islands are benign, bone-forming lesions that occur as monostotic or polyostotic forms.

► **Pathology.** Osteomas and bone islands consist of well-differentiated, mature compact bone with a predominantly lamellated structure and very slow, if any, growth. Osteomas are regarded as hamartomas (embryonal tumorlike malformation).

There are three types of osteomas:

- **Classic osteoma:** This develops almost exclusively in bones of the skull derived from condensed mesenchymal tissue (calvaria, frontal sinus, jaw bone). The lesion is seen from the 2nd decade of life and is clinically asymptomatic. It represents a distinct radiological entity, comprising an extremely dense and sharply delineated lesion of round, tear-drop, or ovoid configuration (► Fig. 4.79). Classic osteomas display no, or only mild, increased activity on the bone scan.
- **Parosteal osteoma:** These demonstrate dense (ivorylike) lesions attached to the tubular bones (femur!), but also to the skull (► Figs. 4.80 and ▶ W4.13). The differential diagnosis, albeit clinically irrelevant, from melorheostosis can be difficult. Calcified osteochondromas look similar to parosteal osteomas but at their base have continuity with the medullary cavity. Moreover, they are inhomogeneous and surrounded by a cartilage rim (MRI).
- **Medullary osteoma** (synonym: enostosis, bone island): These are sclerotic lesions of varying density, rarely up to 3 cm in size, that frequently adapt their form to the anatomy of the bone (► Fig. 4.81, ▶ Figs. W4.14 and ► W4.15). In tubular bones and the spine they are classically round or ovoid in shape. The initial radiological impression is that of a sharply delineated lesion, but on closer examination there are fine pediculate extensions (brush-border) that are characteristic for this dense lesion (▶ see ► Fig. W4.15). Bone islands are seen from the second decade of life onward. Any bone may be affected. Over the years, a slight increase in size is not uncommon (see ► Fig. 4.81). The lesions take up only small amounts of radionuclide on bone scans, with the intensity of activity increasing with size.

> **Note**
> The combination of classic osteomas, intestinal polyposis, and soft tissue fibromas is known as "Gardner syndrome."

► **DD.**

Osteoblastic metastases. Case history, laboratory results, and clinical presentation, together with the scintigraphic result, are the decisive differentiating features for osteoblastic metastases, especially those from prostatic carcinoma. The radiological distinction of a sharp versus ill-defined margin is not a definitive criterion. Elevated serum alkaline phosphatase, pain, and strong radionuclide uptake favors osteoblastic metastases.

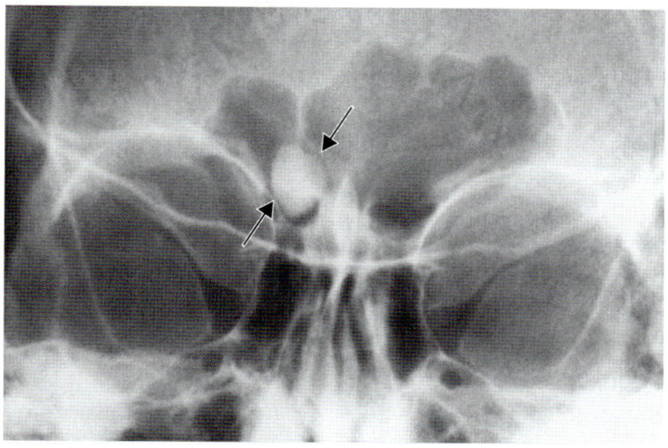

Fig. 4.79 Classic osteoma (arrows) of the frontal sinus.

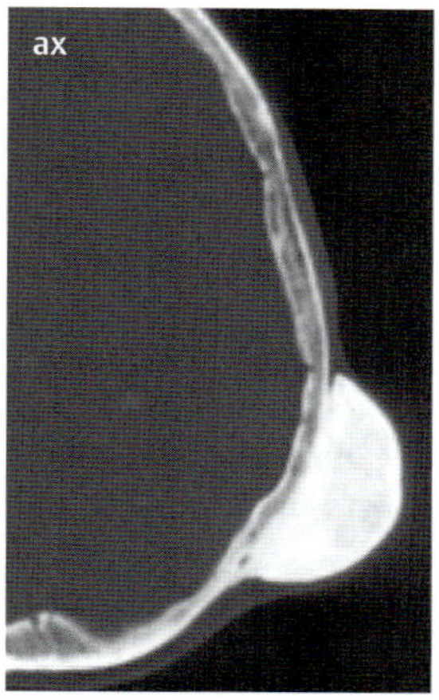

Fig. 4.80 Parosteal osteoma of the skull.

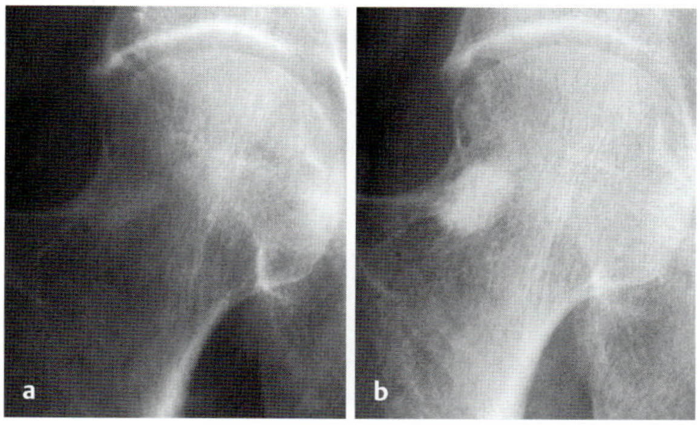

Fig. 4.81 Medullary osteoma. Development over 4 years. **(a)** Primary diagnosis (incidental finding). **(b)** Four years later.

Osteopoikilosis (synonym: "spotted bone disease"). This is an inherited autosomal-dominant bone dysplasia associated with multiple lentil- to pea-sized densities within the bone (► Fig. 4.82) that are found in the epiphysis of all bones, with a predilection for tubular bones. This dysplasia is usually an incidental finding of no clinical relevance.

4.3.2 Fibrous Cortical Defect and Nonossifying Fibroma

This is an eccentrically located, predominantly metaphyseal lesion, of long tubular bones in children. It usually heals spontaneously during bone development. If the lesion is small it is referred to as a "fibrous" cortical defect. Larger lesions are called "nonossifying fibromas."

► **Pathology.** The defect is filled with fibrous connective tissue, interspersed with multinucleate giant cells and macrophages.

► **Clinical presentation.** There are no symptoms; it is usually an incidental finding. Pathologic fractures are uncommon but may be the presenting complaint in larger lesions.

Age: Nonossifying fibroma is found in the 1st and 2nd decades of life. **Location:** The lesion has a metaphyseal location in long tubular bones. It migrates in a diaphyseal direction during growth. The site of predilection (90% of cases) is the lower limb around the knee and the lesions are often multiple. **Treatment:** None.

► **Radiography.** During the fibrous cortical defect stage, the eccentric lesion presents as an ovoid, sharply delineated, solitary radiolucency, with its longitudinal axis orientated parallel to the cortex. It is separated from healthy bone by a thin sclerotic margin (► Fig. 4.83). The lesion is commonly lobulated (► Fig. 4.84) and may expand the cortical boundary of the bone (► Fig. 4.85). Neocortex bridging the defect may be absent in places (► Fig. W4.16). The lesion can heal to become almost completely sclerotic (► Fig. 4.86).

► **CT.** CT does not provide much additional information to the radiograph (► Fig. 4.87).

► **MRI.** MRI does not contribute any essential additional information (► Fig. 4.88). It does occasionally display fat as well as residual cystic areas within the lesion in addition to connective tissue. The lesion enhances partly homogeneously and partly inhomogeneously with contrast.

► **DD.** The classic picture is unequivocal.
Benign fibrous histiocytoma (► **Fig. 4.89**). In elderly patients with pain at the site of the lesion and a positive bone scan, a benign fibrous histiocytoma with its similar histological finding should be considered.

Aneurysmal bone cyst. In certain cases an aneurysmal bone cyst should be considered in the differential diagnosis of the "large" nonossifying fibroma (differentiation by fluid–fluid levels detected on MRI).

Periosteal chondroma. On MRI, a chondroid tumor displays a very bright signal and only marginal contrast enhancement along the septations on T2W sequences.

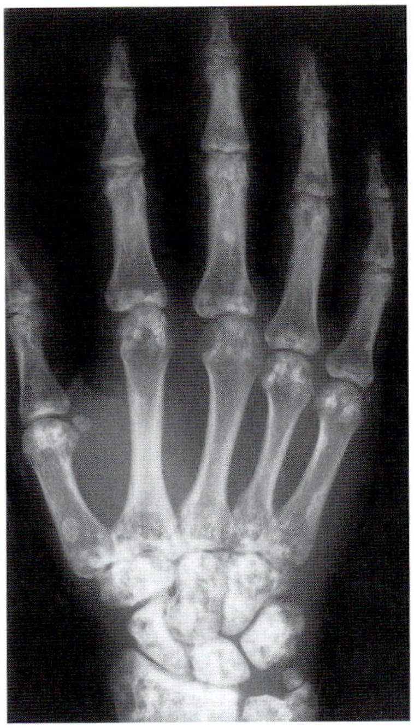

Fig. 4.82 Osteopoikilosis. Note the densities clustered in the epiphysis.

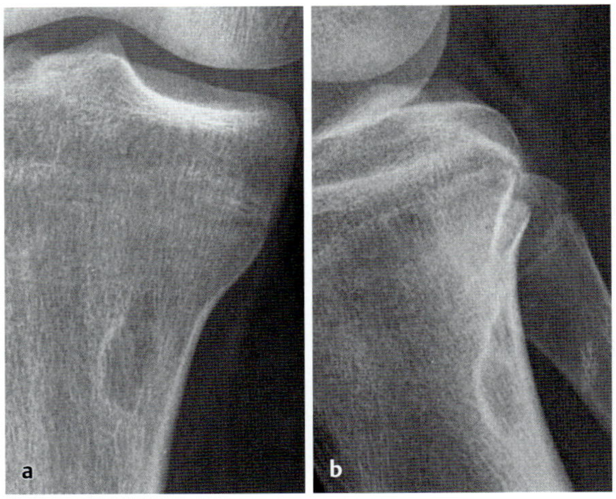

Fig. 4.83 Fibrous cortical defect. **(a)** Eccentrically located, longitudinal lucency. **(b)** Sharply demarcated border, marginal sclerosis.

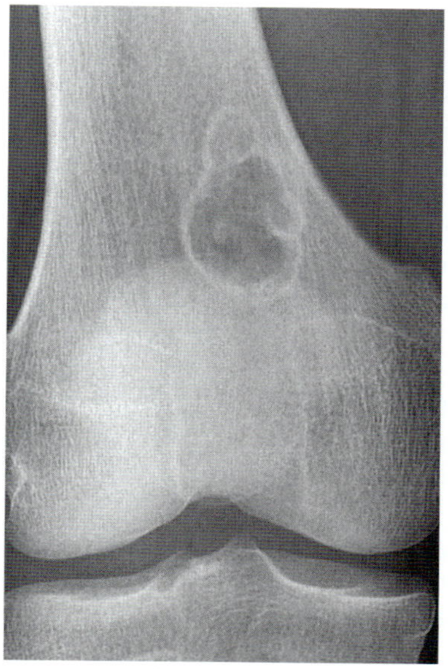

Fig. 4.84 Fibrous cortical defect. Lobulated form.

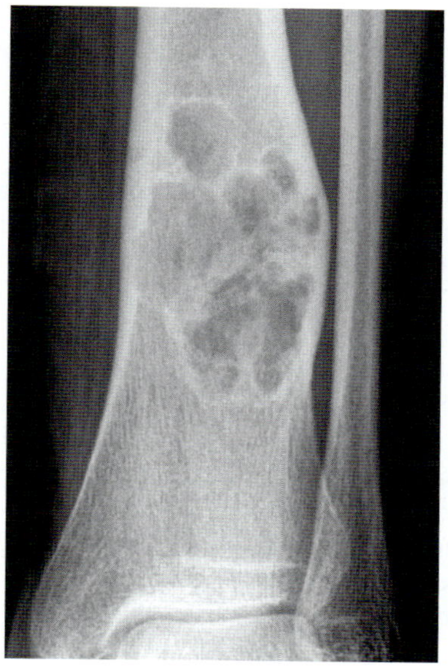

Fig. 4.85 Nonossifying fibroma.

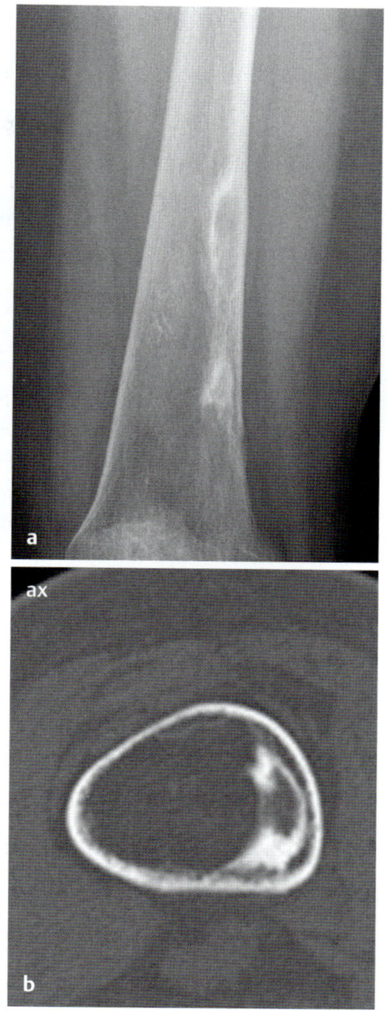

Fig. 4.86 Fibrous cortical defect after remodeling. **(a)** Eccentrically located sclerosis in the distal femur. **(b)** Presentation on CT, unobscured by overlying structures.

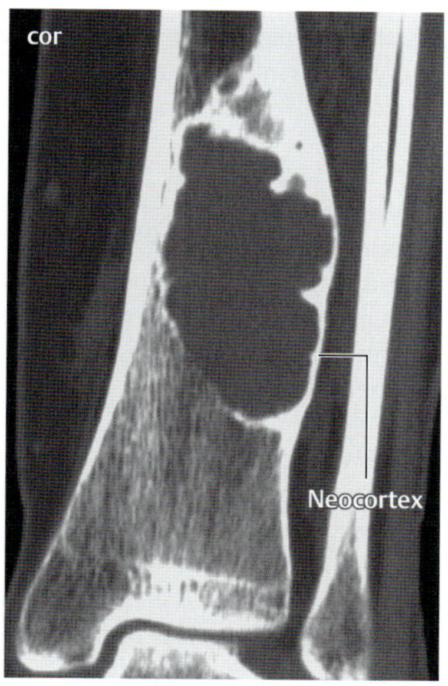

Fig. 4.87 Nonossifying fibroma.

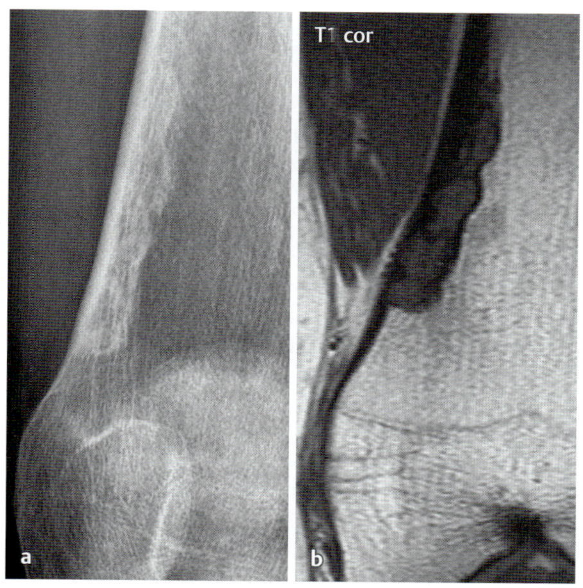

Fig. 4.88 Fibrous cortical defect in the distal femur. **(a)** Typical eccentric location. **(b)** Intermediate-to-hypointense signal on the T1W image.

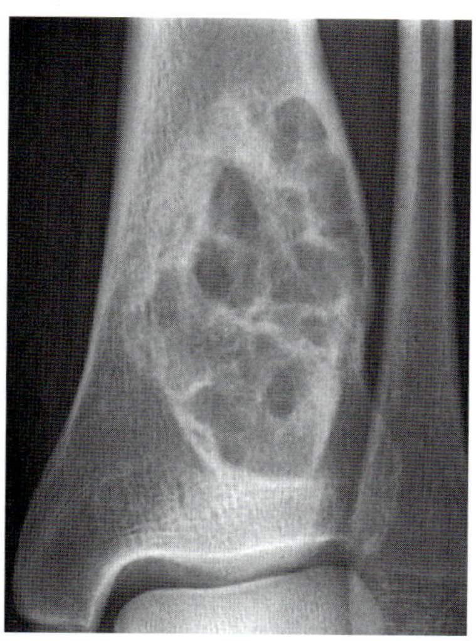

Fig. 4.89 Benign fibrous histiocytoma as a differential diagnosis of nonossifying fibroma. Note the great similarity to ▶Fig. 4.87. If it is an incidental finding, then a watch-and-wait policy is appropriate with follow-up reviews (initially after 6 months, then yearly). If there is localized pain then a biopsy is indicated.

4

4.3.3 Simple (Juvenile) Bone Cyst

The bone cyst is a benign, fluid-filled, and not uncommonly septated lesion.

▸ **Pathology.** It is primarily a single (unicameral) cavity containing clear or sanguineous fluid, lined with a membrane of varying thickness consisting of loose, vascularized connective tissue.

▸ **Clinical presentation.** Simple bone cysts usually only become symptomatic after spontaneous fractures.

Age: Between 70 and 80% of the lesions are discovered before the age of 20 years. **Location:** Sites of predilection are the proximal humerus (50% of cases) and proximal femur (25%). Simple bone cysts are primarily located in the metadiaphysis of tubular bones. With older patients, on the other hand, bones with intramembranous, direct ossification are usually affected. **Treatment:** Steroid injections and curettage plus cancellous bone graft, especially with multilocular cysts. A high recurrence rate is common to all methods.

▸ **Radiography.** On the radiograph the simple bone cyst appears as a centrally located, sharply defined, solitary radiolucency (▸ Fig. 4.90). A thin sclerotic margin is commonly seen. With larger cysts, solid periosteal reactions occur with concentric expansion of the bone due to erosion of the original cortex (neocortex; ▸ Fig. 4.91). Fractures may occur during the healing process of the cyst, making the lesion appear multilocular.

> **Note**
> The "fallen fragment sign" represents a fragment of the cortex that has fallen into the dependent portion of the fluid-filled cyst after a pathologic fracture (▸ Fig. 4.92).

▸ **CT.** Density measurements allow a CT diagnosis (attenuation equivalent to water). It is then easy to determine whether the cyst is unilocular or multilocular (see ▸ Fig. 4.91b).

▸ **MRI.** Proof of fluid in the cyst provides confirmation of the diagnosis (high signal intensity on water-sensitive sequences). The rim of the cyst as well as the membranous lining along the septations enhance with contrast (▸ Fig. 4.93). A single fluid–fluid level due to the layering out of blood products may be seen in the presence of a pathologic fracture (▸ Fig. 4.94).

▸ **DD.**

Aneurysmal bone cyst. This is located more eccentrically and extends into the soft tissues. Fluid–fluid levels tend to be multiple.

Fibrous dysplasia. This can look identical to bone cysts on the radiograph if reparative processes complicate the appearance of the bone cyst on the radiograph. Here too, the identification of fibrous soft tissue on MRI is the reliable distinguishing sign.

Lipoma. In the calcaneus, the differential diagnosis between cyst and lipoma is only possible radiologically if the lipoma demonstrates central calcification.

Enchondroma. Only MRI will allow a distinction in some cases. However, differentiation is not always possible even on T2W images (because cartilage may also display a very bright signal). Contrast administration is obligatory.

4.3.4 Aneurysmal Bone Cyst

The aneurysmal bone cyst is a benign cystic bone lesion. It develops de novo (primary aneurysmal bone cyst) or secondarily in association with other benign or malignant bone tumors.

▸ **Pathology.** The aneurysmal bone cyst consists of multiple blood-filled cavities separated by fibrous septae. An aneurysmal bone cyst can also display solid components that are usually due to other bone lesions, indicating a secondary aneurysmal bone cyst is present. The etiology and pathogenesis of aneurysmal bone cyst are unknown.

▸ **Clinical presentation.** Swellings and bone pain are nonspecific clinical findings. The lesion can grow very rapidly and mimic a malignant tumor.

Age: Aneurysmal bone cysts usually (more than 80% of cases) occur during the 1st and 2nd decades of life. **Location:** Any bone may be affected. Sites of predilection are the posterior spinal elements, femur, tibia, and pelvis. The cysts are located in the region of the meta- and diaphysis of long tubular bones. **Treatment:** Curettage (recurrence rate ~ 20–40%), denosumab (clinical trials).

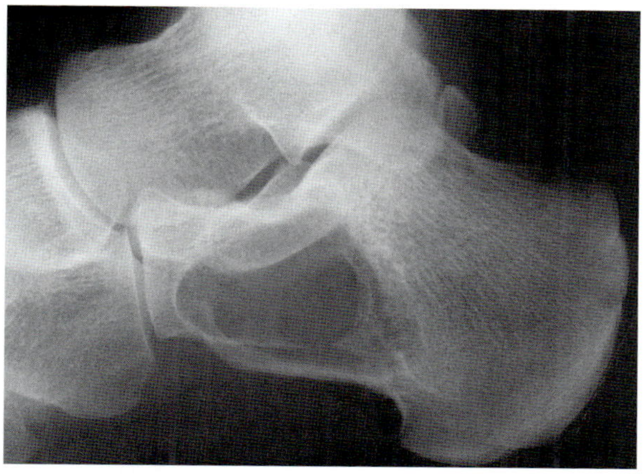

Fig. 4.90 Simple bone cyst of the calcaneus.

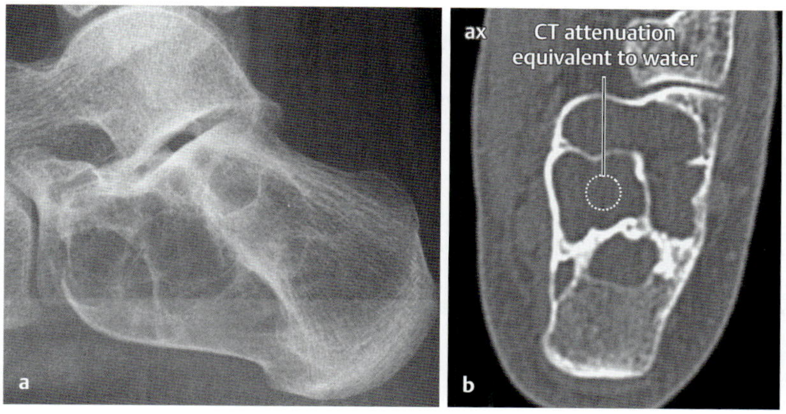

Fig. 4.91 Simple bone cyst of the calcaneus. **(a)** The radiograph already demonstrates signs of septation. **(b)** CT confirms multiple bony septations.

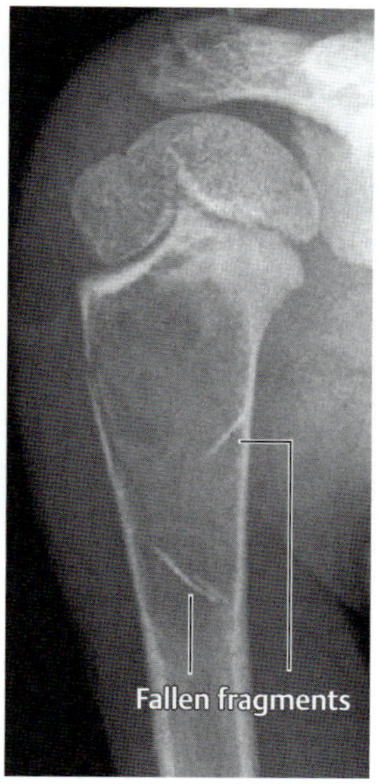

Fig. 4.92 Juvenile bone cyst. Pathologic fracture.

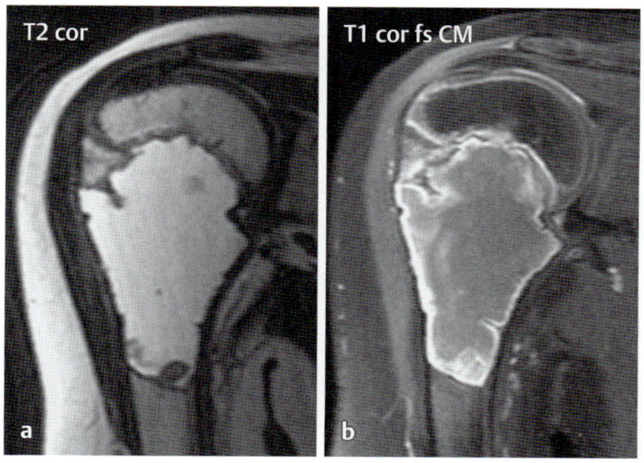

Fig. 4.93 Simple bone cyst **(a)** Strongly hyperintense on fluid-sensitive sequences. **(b)** Marginal and septated contrast enhancement.

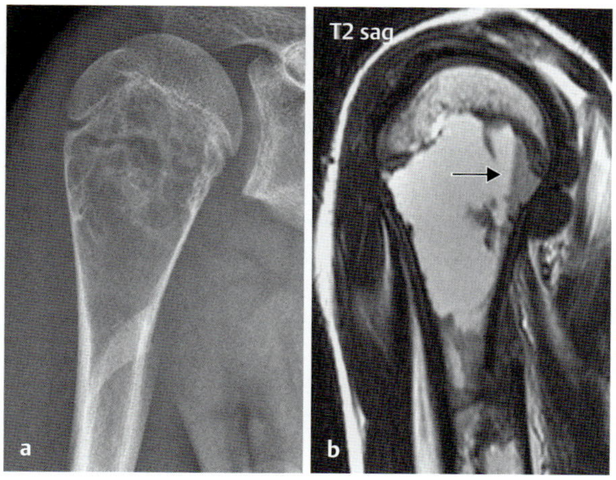

Fig. 4.94 Simple bone cyst. **(a)** Pathologic fracture. **(b)** Sedimentation can be visualized on MRI (arrow; investigation with the patient recumbent).

► **Radiography.** An aneurysmal bone cyst usually presents as a large, intramedullary or eccentrically located, sharply defined, solitary lucency (► Figs. 4.95–4.98). The area of osteolysis is partly surrounded by a sclerotic margin and is septated in many cases (see ► Fig. 4.95). Cysts without or with only sparse septations are possible (see ► Fig. 4.96). Expansion into the soft tissues is common. The component that is breaching the bone boundaries may display a bony shell (neocortex) (see ► Figs. 4.97 and ► 4.98) or it is not distinguishable radiologically from the soft tissues (► Fig. 4.99).

► **CT.** The neocortex usually remains evident as a fine sclerotic margin, even if the radiograph no longer displays this finding. It may, however, be absent altogether (see ► Fig. 4.99). Otherwise, CT does not provide any essential additional information in comparison with MRI.

► **MRI.** MRI is best capable of displaying cystic contents as fluid–fluid levels (see ► Fig. 4.95b). The borders of the cyst enhance strongly with contrast (see ► Fig. 4.95c). Sometimes extensive *solid*, soft tissue–dense areas of varying size are detectable in the aneurysmal bone cyst, which can also enhance with contrast (► Fig. 4.100).

> **Note**
> Careful histological examination of the curettage material taken from the aneurysmal bone cyst is particularly important as this is the only way of detecting tumors such as osteosarcomas or osteoblastomas.

► **DD.**

Giant cell tumor. CT and MRI are often capable of distinguishing between the two lesions. The giant cell tumor is usually “solid,” with the exception of central necrosis, and all or large parts of the tumor enhance with contrast, unlike cysts with their septations. Problems can arise with aneurysmal bone cysts with a high proportion of solid components. Giant cell tumors usually develop between the 3rd and 6th decades (more than 80% of cases). The appearance of giant cell tumors before skeletal fusion is rare.

Simple bone cyst. Differentiation is sometimes not possible radiologically, especially with multiple septated, “simple” cysts after spontaneous fracture. Simple bone cysts can exhibit fluid–fluid levels, albeit usually single; however, they do not have “solid” enhancing components.

Nonossifying fibroma. This has a well-defined sclerotic margin and appears more grapelike or as an area of osteolysis extending in a longitudinal direction. Delineation from the soft tissues by a bony shell is always evident with a nonossifying fibroma. MRT and CT allow confident differentiation between fibrous tissue and cystic contents.

Telangiectatic osteosarcoma This uncommon lytic variant of high-grade osteosarcoma may mimic on radiographs and MRI the more rapidly growing form of aneurysmal bone cyst. Again, correlation of imaging and histology is critical.

4.3.5 Langerhans Cell Histiocytosis

Langerhans cell histiocytosis represents a whole spectrum of disorders that affect not only the skeleton. **Eosinophilic granuloma** is the most common and clinically mildest variant. Other forms are **Hand–Schüller–Christian** disease and **Abt–Letterer–Siwe** disease. The latter are extremely rare systemic disorders (see specialized literature). Reference will be made here only to eosinophilic granuloma.

► **Pathology.** All of these lesions consist of fibrohistiocytic granulation tissue with a differing amount of Langerhans cells (specialized histiocytes) and eosinophilic granulocytes. Multinucleate giant cells, lymphocytes, and plasma cells are also detectable.

► **Clinical presentation.** Eosinophilic granuloma can be an incidental radiological finding, especially in the skull. Otherwise, swelling and local pain form the presenting complaint.

Age: Age of predilection is the 1st and 2nd decades of life. However, the finding can be made from infancy and, in exceptional cases, even up to the 5th decade of life. **Location:** Skull, femur, pelvic skeleton, ribs, and spine are primarily affected. All other locations of the skeleton are also possible. The disorder usually presents as a solitary lesion (monostotic), but multiple lesions (polyostotic) are found in ~20% of cases. **Treatment:** Spontaneous remission is commonly seen in the skull. Intralesional steroid injections have been attempted, with questionable success. Usually surgical curettage is performed in those bones where fracture is a risk and in cases of rapid progression.

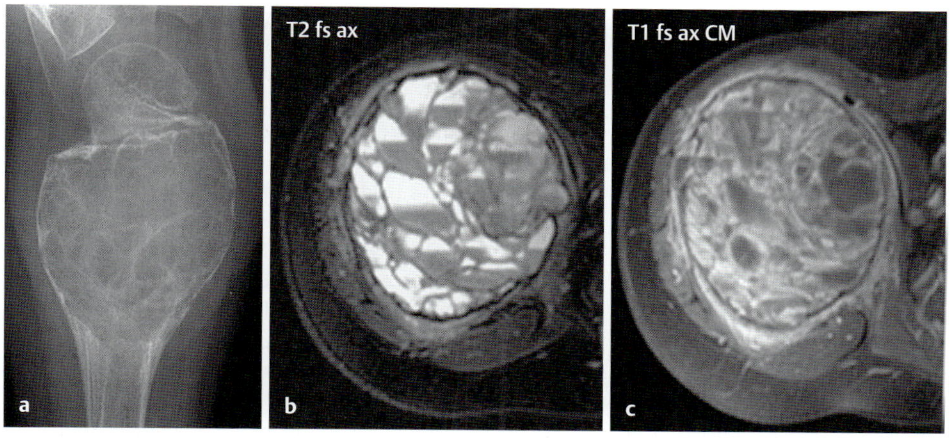

Fig. 4.95 Aneurysmal bone cyst of the proximal humerus. **(a)** Soap-bubble expansion of the bone. **(b)** Multiple fluid–fluid levels (sedimentation) in the multiseptated, cystic space-occupying lesion. **(c)** Strong contrast enhancement of the cyst wall.

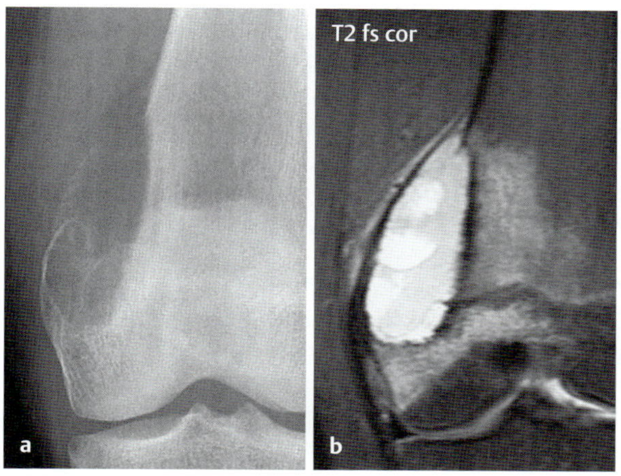

Fig. 4.96 Aneurysmal bone cyst. **(a)** Sharply defined, eccentrically located lucency. **(b)** Inhomogeneous signal intensity of the cystic contents.

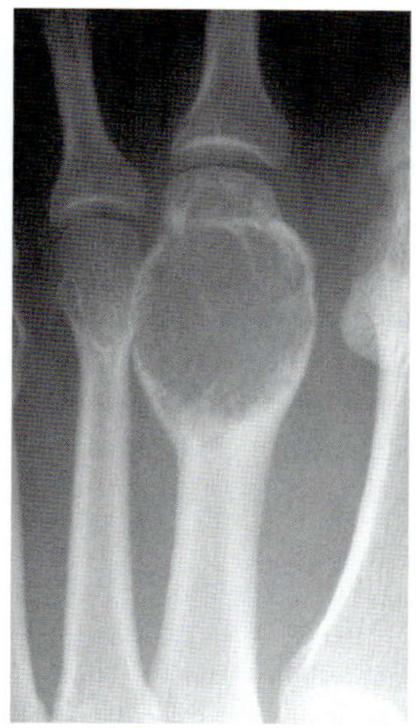

Fig. 4.97 Aneurysmal bone cyst in the second metatarsal bone.

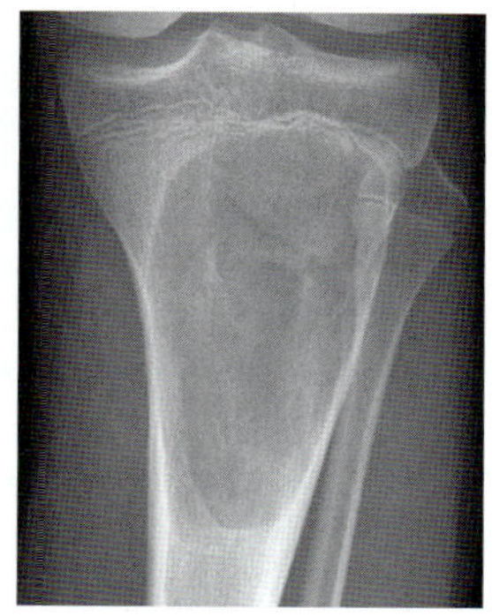

Fig. 4.98 Aneurysmal bone cyst of the proximal tibia.

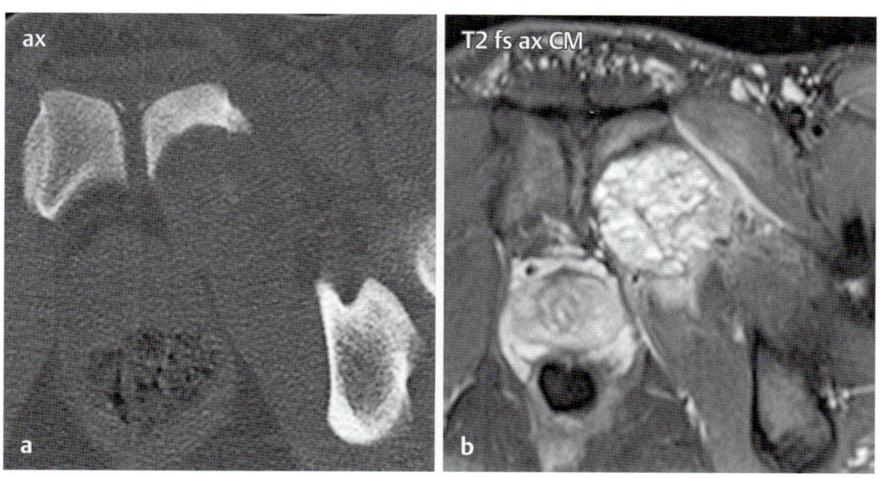

Fig. 4.99 Aneurysmal bone cyst. **(a)** Lysis within the left pubic bone without neocortex. **(b)** The T2W MRI image reveals the small cysts within the lesion.

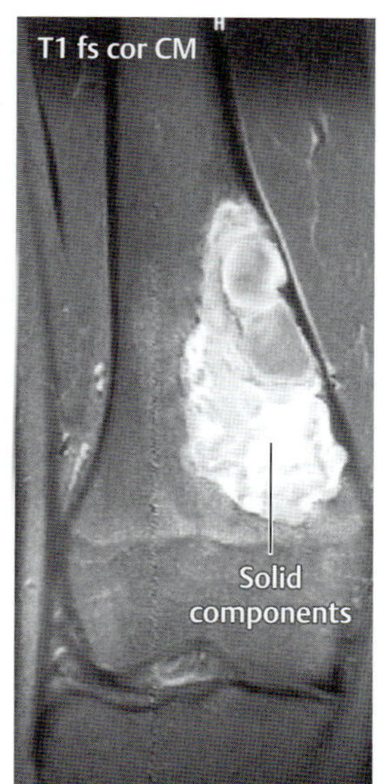

Fig. 4.100 Aneurysmal bone cyst with distinct solid components.

▶ **Radiography.** Morphological diversity is typical for eosinophilic granulomas, with the growth pattern ranging from latent, via active, to aggressive. The radiological morphology depends largely on the stage at which the eosinophilic granuloma is diagnosed. In the **skull**, they are generally round to ovoid osteolytic lesions with a diameter of up to 3 cm. The lesions appear clearly marginated, as if "punched out" (▶ Fig. 4.101). Residual bone within the lesions resembles sequestrum formation (known as "button sequestrum"). Although the border is sharply defined, a sclerotic margin is absent in the early stage. Geographic patterns are found in some cases.

Osteolytic lesions are also commonly seen in the **spine** and **pelvis** (sometimes traversed by trabeculae; ▶ Fig. 4.102). The vertebrae can collapse to form a vertebra plana ("pancake vertebra") (▶ Fig. W4.17).

Relatively sharply delineated foci are found in **tubular bones**, as well as moth-eaten osteolytic lesions (▶ Fig. 4.103). Cortical thickening with a lamellated periosteal reaction is typical. A sclerotic margin appears if the lesion heals spontaneously. Complete resolution of the abnormality may occur.

▶ **NUC MED.** This is an important modality for assessing whether a monostotic or a polyostotic form of the disorder is present. The uptake varies in relation to the activity of the lesion.

▶ **CT.** The type of foci, with their "punched out" appearance (± button sequestrum), is sometimes better visualized on CT than with radiography (▶ Fig. W4.18).

▶ **MRI.** MRI demonstrates the classic signal pattern of all tumors: low signal intensity on T1W, high signal intensity on T2W sequences (▶ Fig. W4.19). The lesion enhances with contrast (▶ Fig. 4.104) and perilesional edema is a frequent finding.

▶ **DD.**

Tubular bone

- **Osteomyelitis** can mimic an eosinophilic granuloma, although the latter commonly displays a relatively sharp delineation from the healthy bone.
- **Ewing's sarcoma:** Differentiation is sometimes not possible on imaging alone, leaving only the option of a biopsy.
- Slowly growing eosinophilic granulomas may possibly be mistaken for **fibrous dysplasia** or **cysts**.

Skull

- **Tuberculosis** can sometimes produce similar appearances in the presence of multiple lesions.
- An **epidermoid cyst** should be considered with solitary foci.

4.3.6 Fibrous Dysplasia

Fibrous dysplasia is a mono-, oligo-, or polyostotic developmental disorder in which normal bone marrow is replaced by fibro-osseous tissue.

▶ **Pathology.** This is a benign, tumorlike process based on a local disturbance in the differentiation of bone-forming mesenchymal tissue. The process is slowly progressive, but usually comes to a halt with puberty. Etiology and pathogenesis have yet to be finally clarified. Somatic mutation with an enzyme defect is proven, but the disorder is not inherited. Malignant transformation is reported but rare (< 0.5% of cases). The oligo- or polyostotic form of fibrous dysplasia is commonly associated with other developmental abnormalities. The most important of these associations is **Albright's syndrome** (polyostotic fibrous dysplasia, café au lait spots on trunk and extremities, precocious puberty).

▶ **Clinical presentation.** The monostotic form is frequently an incidental imaging finding. With the monostotic form, but above all with the polyostotic form, localized pain, spontaneous fractures, or deformity of the bone are seen.

Age: The disease is usually diagnosed before the age of 20 years, but diagnosis in adulthood is also possible. **Location:** Any bone may be affected; sites of predilection are femur, skull, and ribs. Vertebrae, shoulder girdle, and hand are almost exclusively involved in the polyostotic form. In long tubular bones the foci are commonly located in the diaphysis, but also extend into other parts of the bone. **Treatment:** Rarely necessary; possibly surgical in presence of fracture or increasing deformity.

▶ **Radiography.** The radiographic morphology of fibrous dysplasia is very variable and depends on the age of the patient, location in the skeleton, the degree of ossification, and the mineral content of the fibrotic tissue.

Fibrous dysplasia usually appears as a sharply defined, lytic destruction of the cancellous bone with loss of its normal trabecular pattern (▶ Figs. 4.105 and ▶ 4.106).

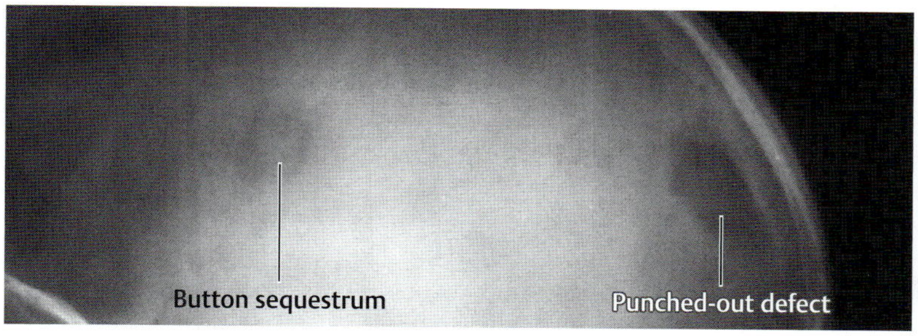

Fig. 4.101 Eosinophilic granuloma. Two lesions in the skull.

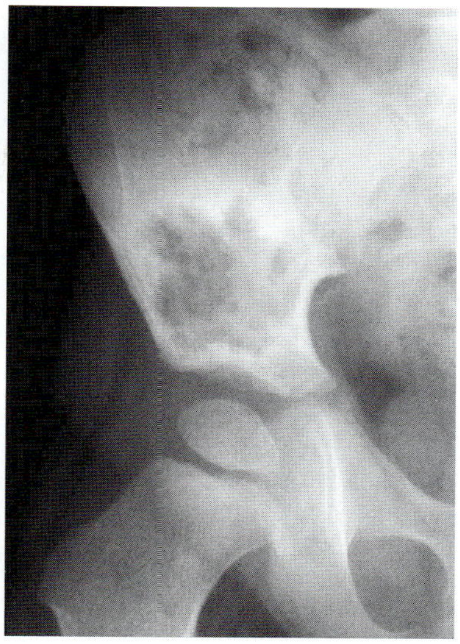

Fig. 4.102 Eosinophilic granuloma in an 8-year-old child. Sclerotic demarcation of the lesion in comparison with ▶ Fig. 4.103.

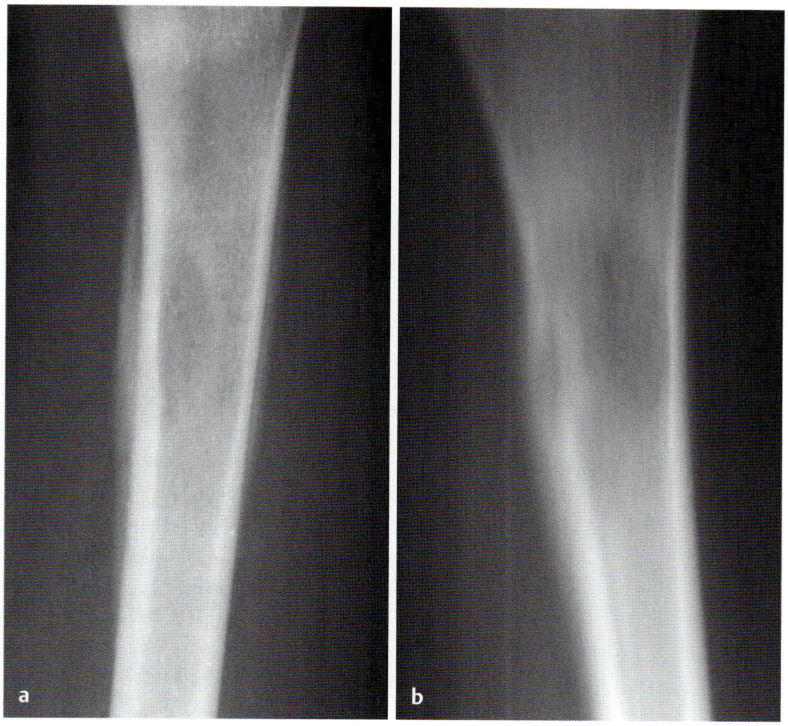

Fig. 4.103 Eosinophilic granuloma of the tibia of a 7-year-old boy. Difficult differential diagnosis from malignant tumor, especially Ewing's sarcoma. **(a)** Periosteal reaction. **(b)** Permeative destruction.

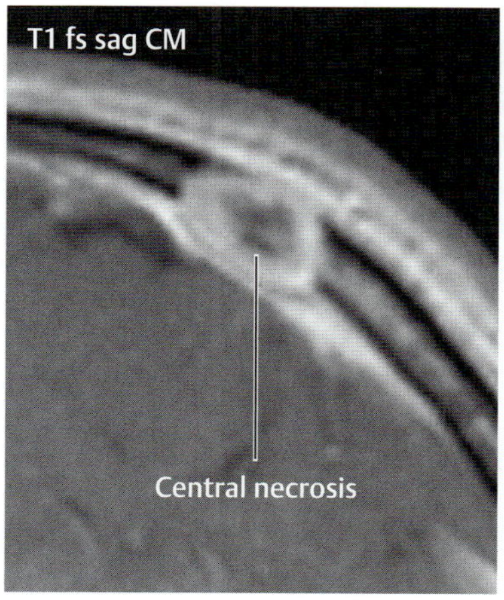

Fig. 4.104 Eosinophilic granuloma of the skull.

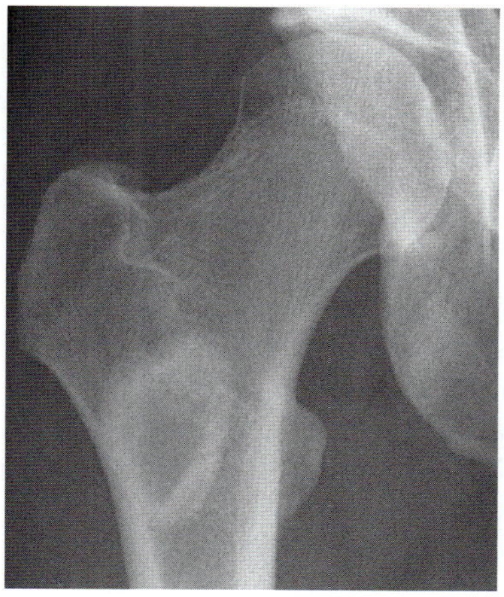

Fig. 4.105 Fibrous dysplasia.

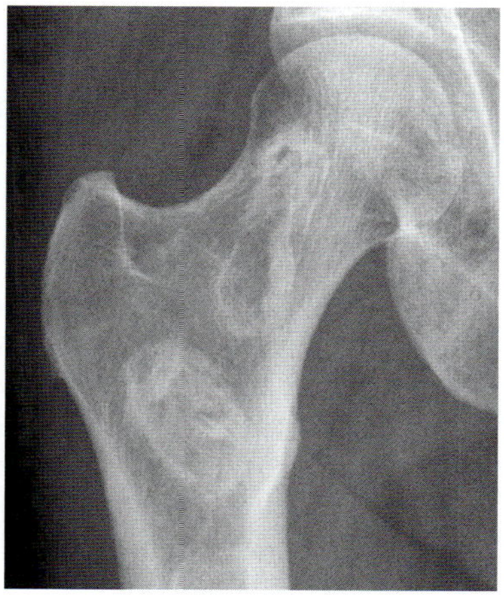

Fig. 4.106 Fibrous dysplasia.

Its concentric expansile growth pattern results in the formation of saucer-shaped periosteal new bone that is rarely breached. A sclerotic internal margin and cortical thickening are typical (▶ Fig. 4.107).

A **soap bubble–like pattern** is typical, but only found occasionally (▶ Fig. 4.108).

The **ground glass phenomenon** (▶ Fig. 4.109) is a classic feature of fibrous dysplasia, but depends on the nature of the matrix and degree of mineralization. The lesion can therefore also appear cystic or display irregular extensive or diffuse areas of sclerosis (▶ Fig. 4.110).

Bowing of long bones (see ▶ Fig. 4.110) and repeated fractures with callus formation are common findings. Necrosis and hemorrhage can give rise to genuine cysts. Older foci form rough, reparative sclerotic trabeculae as a sign that the bone is trying to regain its stability.

In the **ribs**, fibrous dysplasia appears as a sausagelike or soap-bubble expansion. In **tubular bones**, the main impression is that of multiloculation. In **flat bones** fibrous dysplasia has a mono- or polycystic appearance with an intralesional honeycomb structure. Three types have been described in the **skull**:

- **Pagetoid type** (▶ Figs. 4.111 and ▶ 4.112):
- Bubbling or blistering expansion of the diploic space.
- Ground glass appearance.
- Patchy cloudy sclerosis.
- **Sclerotic type:**
    - Sclerosis is dominant.
    - Almost no cystic components.
- **Cystic form:** multiple round or lobulated defects.

▶ NUC MED. Bone scintigraphy shows marked increased activity with fibrous dysplasia and can distinguish between the monostotic and polyostotic forms.

▶ CT. The ground glass phenomenon is best identified on CT, confirming the diagnosis of fibrous dysplasia and supplementing the radiographic results (see ▶ Figs. 4.111 and ▶ 4.112).

▶ MRI. The signal pattern of fibrous dysplasia conforms to the uniform pattern of all tumors (low signal intensity on T1W, intermediate to high signal intensity on T2W sequences). The fibrous tissue enhances with contrast. Both contrast-enhanced and T2W images can be relatively inhomogeneous because of blood, fat, and calcifications producing heterogeneous signal intensities.

▶ DD.

Tubular bone

Solitary or **aneurysmal bone cysts** should be differentiated from the monostotic forms of fibrous dysplasia if the latter does not involve large areas of bone. MRI usually enables differentiation.

Ribs

In younger patients **eosinophilic granuloma** and in older patients **chondrosarcoma.** CT can be helpful showing the characteristic ground glass phenomenon of fibrous dysplasia.

Skull

Paget's disease is a possible differential diagnosis only in the elderly patient. Meningioma should be considered with the predominantly sclerotic type (CT or MRI).

4.3.7 Vascular Malformations of the Bone (so-called Hemangioma)

See also Chapter 4.5.4.

▶ Pathology. Vascular malformation is the most common benign space-occupying lesion of the spine, with an occurrence of 10 to 12% of individuals, although it does occur in other bones such as the skull vault. The term "vertebral hemangioma," according to the ISSVA classification (International Society for the Study of Vascular Anomalies), has now been replaced by **intraosseous venous malformations.** Histological examination reveals mature endothelial cells without proliferation, together with multiple small channels (capillary hemangiomas) or larger venous vascular channels (known as cavernous hemangiomas), practically without any blood flow or arteriovenous shunts, interspersed with a varying number of fat cells. Growth has been reported in rare cases.

Variants. The variants include lymphatic malformations located in various bones that display either static cystic lytic lesions or progressive and extensive areas of osteolysis, and even complete resorption of the bone (Gorham–Stout syndrome, also known as vanishing bone disease).

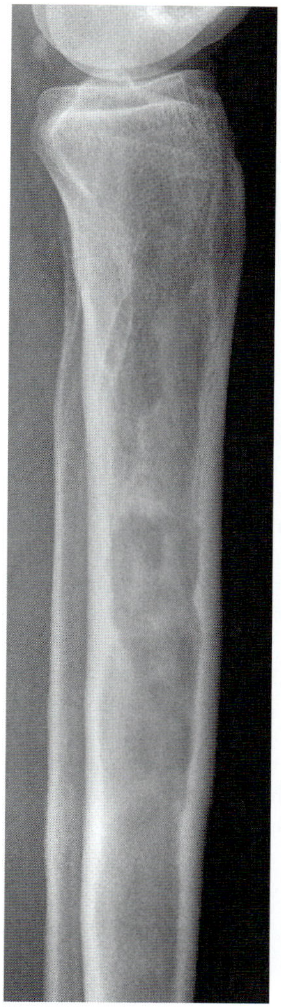

Fig. 4.107 Fibrous dysplasia.

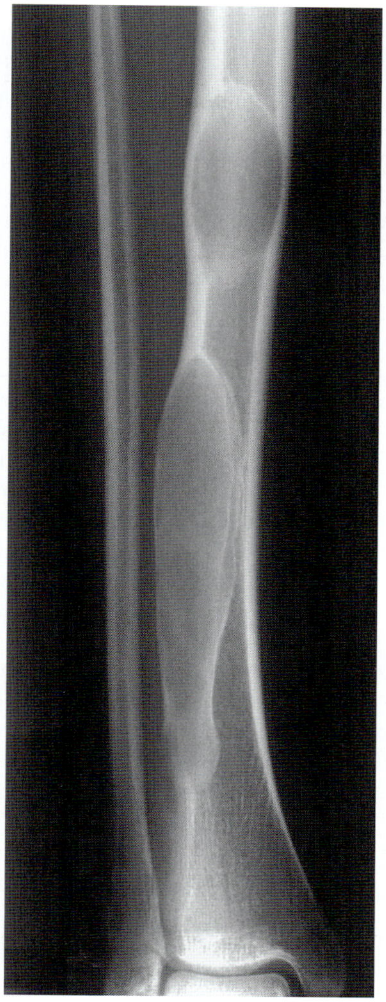

Fig. 4.109 Fibrous dysplasia. Classic ground glass pattern.

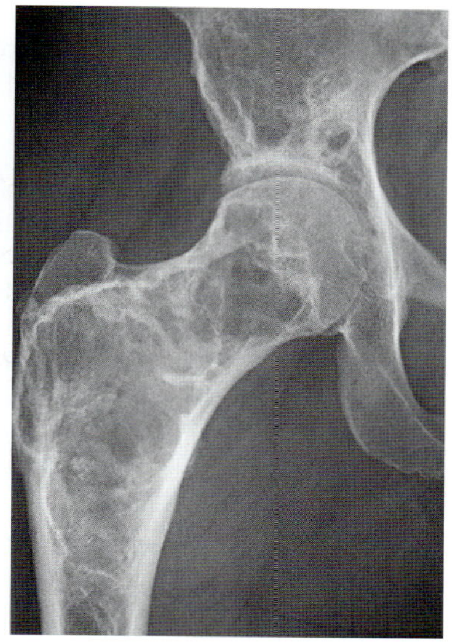

Fig. 4.108 Fibrous dysplasia.

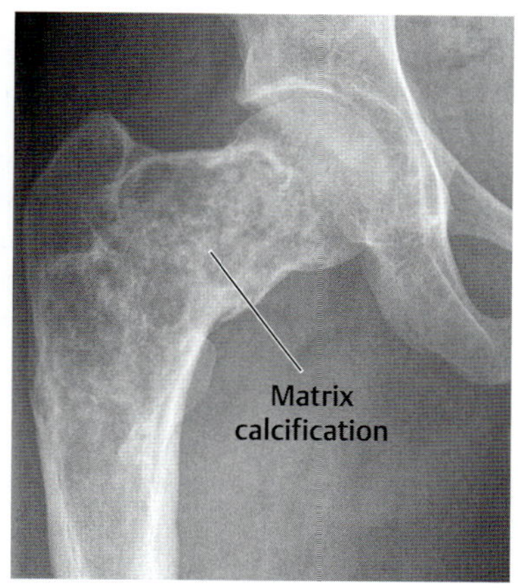

Fig. 4.110 Fibrous dysplasia. Coxa varus angulation of the proximal femur (final stage: shepherd crook deformity).

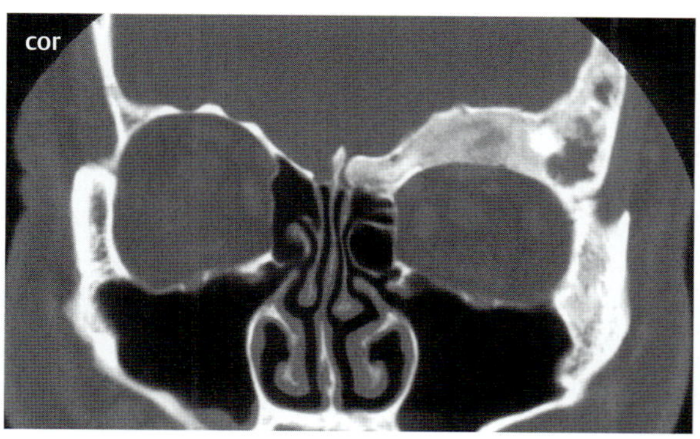

Fig. 4.111 Fibrous dysplasia. Pagetoid type with ground glass phenomenon.

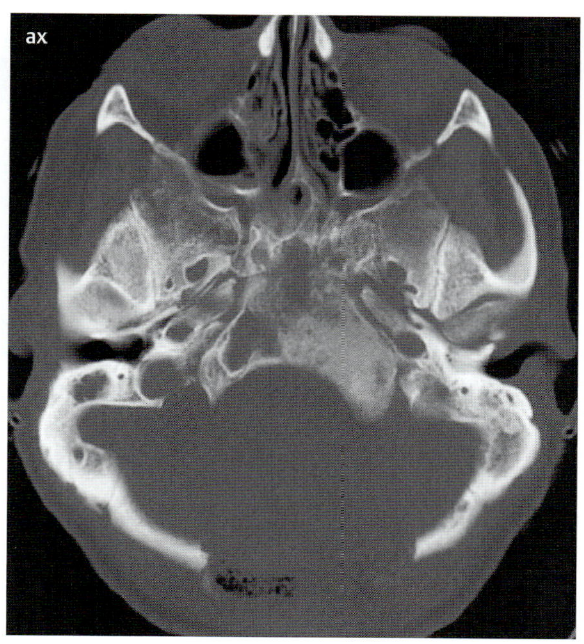

Fig. 4.112 Fibrous dysplasia. Pagetoid type involving the skull base. ▶

4

▶ Clinical presentation. A vertebral vascular malformation is symptomatic in only 1% of cases; patients complain of localized or radicular pain and rarely even of cord compression.

Age: All decades of life; the malformation is usually discovered in the 2nd to 5th decades of life. **Location:** In the thoracic spine more commonly than the lumbar; only 7% of cases occur in the cervical spine. Multifocal involvement in ~25% of cases. The second most common location is the cranial vault (▶ Figs. 4.113 and ▶ W4.20). **Treatment:** Usually no treatment is required. Vertebroplasty or surgery is undertaken for cord compression, preceded possibly by embolization (usually with little effect). Radiotherapy is rarely employed (pain therapy).

▶ Radiography.

- Resorption predominantly of the horizontal trabeculae in the vertebral body, with the vertical trabeculae often appearing more emphasized (corduroy or jailhouse pattern); this produces a "meshed" appearance on the radiograph (▶ Fig. 4.114).
- A honeycomblike appearance is also common (▶ Fig. 4.115).
- Marginal or also intralesional coarse osteosclerotic areas.
- In flat or tubular bones sharply defined osteolytic lesions, depending on the vascular type, possible thin sclerotic rim; no progression; often honeycomb pattern (▶ Fig. W4.21); periosteal reaction possible particularly in the ribs.

▶ CT. A vascular malformation is a common incidental finding on a spinal CT as a circumscribed, honeycomb patchy bone structure (▶ Figs. 4.116 and ▶ W4.22; see also ▶ Fig. 4.113). Any trabeculae still present are often spongelike and sclerotic. A paravertebral soft tissue component may be present in large lesions (▶ Fig. W4.23).

▶ MRI. A vascular malformation is a common incidental finding on spinal MRI, appearing hyperintense on T1W (fatty tissue) but more so on T2W sequences (blood). The fat component varies in intensity; sometimes it appears isointense to muscle on T1W sequences. A solid stroma component is hardy discernible; an image displaying small cysts is often seen (▶ Figs. 4.117, ▶ 4.118, and ▶ W4.24; and see ▶ Fig. W4.20). The intraosseous lesion displays moderate contrast enhancement, while any extramedullary component demonstrates marked contrast enhancement.

▶ DD.

Spine

- **Metastases, plasmacytoma:** Here thickened, coarse trabeculae are only rarely seen. A confident distinction is usually possible using MRI or CT.
- **Paget's disease:** Here there is a tendency to see bony expansion of the entire vertebra, with thickening and coarsening of the vertebral margins (picture frame). In Paget's disease the bone scan is strongly positive, whereas most so-called hemangiomas show normal skeletal activity.

Flat bones and tubular bones. Fibrous dysplasia, aneurysmal bone cyst, eosinophilic granuloma, enchondroma, plasmacytoma, metastases. These should be considered when classic trabecular patterns are absent. These entities are best differentiated using MRI. A fat component is contained in so-called hemangiomas; a soft tissue component is usually absent.

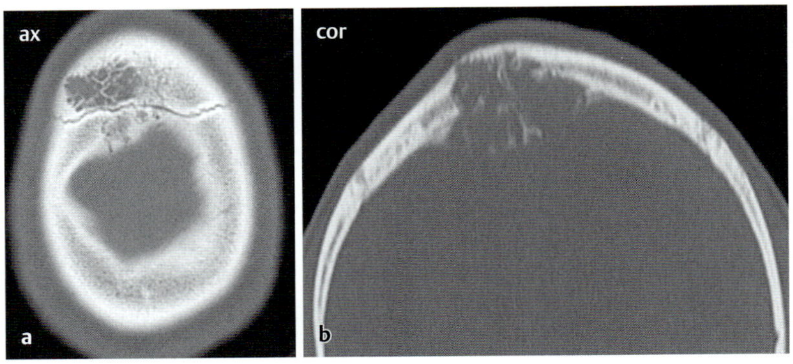

Fig. 4.113 Intraosseous venous malformation of the cranial vault. ▶ For additional MRI images see ▶ Fig. W4.20. **(a)** Honeycomb osteolysis. **(b)** The coronal plane demonstrates the expansile nature of the lesion.

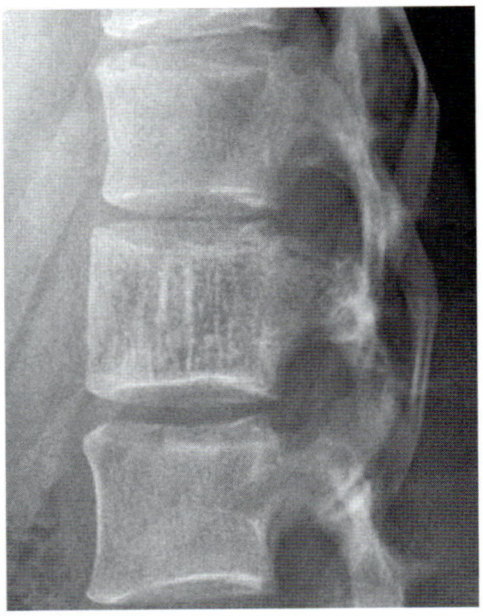

Fig. 4.114 Intraosseous venous malformation (hemangioma). Coarse trabecular pattern.

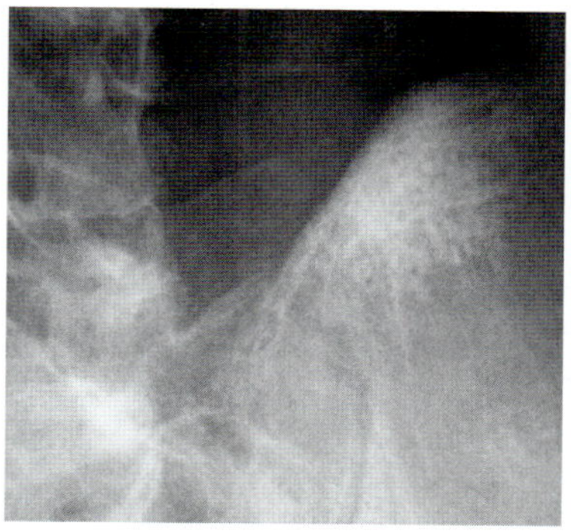

Fig. 4.115 Intraosseous venous malformation in the iliac bone.

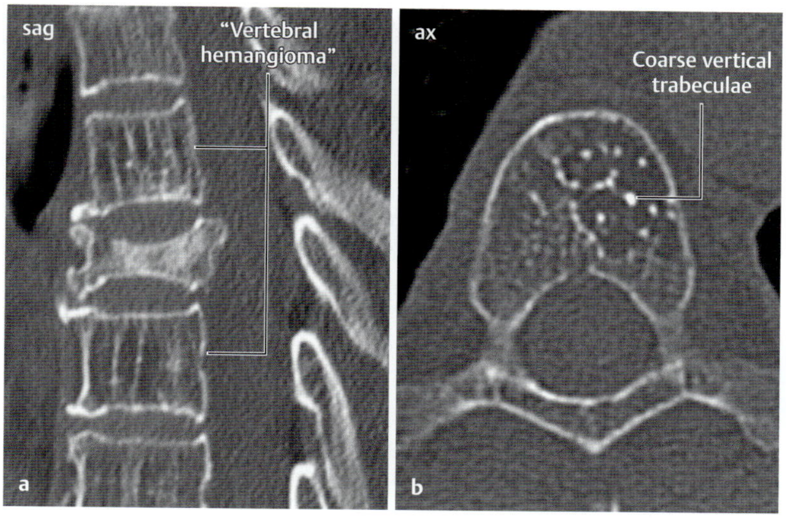

Fig. 4.116 "Vertebral hemangioma." **(a)** Osteoporosis-related collapse is assumed responsible for the compression fracture of the one thoracic vertebra. Vertebral hemangiomas rarely fracture. **(b)** Characteristic appearance of an intact so-called vertebral hemangioma on the axial CT.

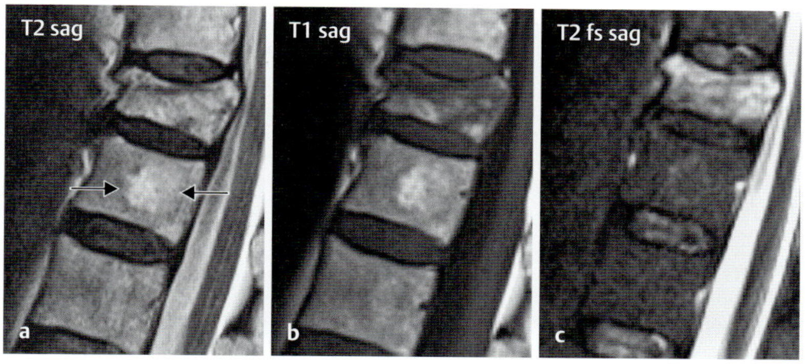

Fig. 4.117 Typical so-called vertebral hemangioma as an incidental finding of a compression fracture of the adjacent vertebra. **(a)** The lesion (arrows) is hyperintense on the T2W image. **(b)** The lesion also appears hyperintense on the T1W image (fat-containing). **(c)** Slight marginal hyperintensity on the T2W image after fat saturation.

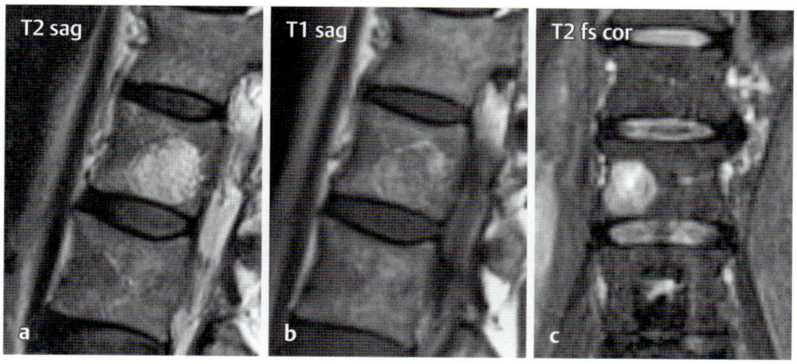

Fig. 4.118 "Vertebral hemangioma" with an atypical signal pattern on MRI. **(a)** Intermediate signal on the T2W image. **(b)** Nonclassic fat pattern on the T1W image. **(c)** Blood accumulating in the cavities of the lesion is the reason for the hyperintensity.

4

4.3.8 Less Common Tumorlike Lesions

Osteofibrous dysplasia. This is a rare, congenital fibrous tibial defect (very rarely in the fibula). The histological features overlap with those of adamantinoma, as well as ossifying fibroma of the facial bones. Almost all lesions are in the diaphysis where they are usually eccentrically/anteriorly located. The radiograph typically displays a lobulated area of osteolysis (▶ Fig. 4.119a). Sometimes a ground glass phenomenon is recognizable. Reactive peripheral and central sclerotic areas are almost always detectable.

4

> **Note**
> Some foci of osteofibrotic dysplasia remain small; others heal spontaneously, while others continue to grow. The majority of lesions heal spontaneously (▶ Fig. 4.120). A biopsy (to exclude adamantinoma) should only be taken if there is increasing pain and/or imaging displays unequivocal disease progression. Surgery should be avoided (even with a pathologic fracture), because recurrent tumor is inevitable, especially before the age of 5 years (▶ Fig. 4.119b).

Cortical (periosteal) desmoid. Unlike the desmoid tumor of the soft tissues (which is assigned to intermediate to low-grade soft tissue tumors), this is a cortical desmoid located around a reactive lesion involving the cortex (chronic overuse?) at the fibro-osseous insertion of muscles and may mimic a sarcoma to the unwary observer. The lesion occurs in children and adolescents during the growth phase (3–17 years of age). The classic site of a cortical desmoid is the posteromedial aspect of the distal femoral metaphysis (▶ Figs. 4.121, ▶ 4.122, and ▶ 4.123), but the distal humeral, radial, and ulnar metaphyses as well as the proximal tibial metaphysis (▶ Fig. W4.25) are also possible locations. There is probably an association with fibrous cortical defect (see Chapter 4.3.2). Radiographic and CT images of cortical desmoid are characterized by more or less flat cortical erosion. This is about 3 to 4 mm in depth and usually 1 to 2 cm long. The erosion is sharply defined and sometimes the periosteum also forms a thin bone covering on the lateral aspect of the process. Furthermore, the defect may present an irregular contour. The defect is also well defined on ultrasound (see ▶ Fig. 4.123). An important distinguishing feature of distal femoral cortical desmoids is that many are bilateral.

Epidermoid. This is an epithelial cyst beneath the periosteum producing a tumorlike bone lesion. Whereas epidermoids of the skull are asymptomatic, they cause pain at other locations. The lesions occur predominantly in the terminal phalanges of fingers, less commonly in the skull (▶ Fig. 4.124). Epidermoids produce a circumscribed expansion of the bone with thinning of the cortex. The inside of the lesion is usually structureless. Active epidermoids, associated with more severe pain, often have an ill-defined rim, whereas inactive lesions display a sclerotic margin.

Giant-cell reparative granuloma. This is a reactive, tumorlike accumulation of giant cells similar to giant cell tumor of bone. It arises primarily in the short tubular bones of the hands and feet (▶ Fig. 4.125). Local pain is the reason for radiological investigation. Radiological signs are most variable and comprise an osteolytic lesion with a sharp or ill-defined margin. Cortical destruction may also be evident so that an aggressively growing tumor must be assumed. Simple "bony expansions" with a neocortex are also possible.

Bizarre parosteal osteochondromatous proliferation (Nora lesion). Named after the pathologist who described it, Nora lesion is a rare, juxtacortical, proliferative lesion of unknown origin that can resemble a surface osteosarcoma or osteochondroma. The hands are most prominently affected, less often the feet, and very rarely other bones. Radiology demonstrates dense calcification directly attached to the outer cortex of bone. The involvement of the medullary cavity is merely reactive, as evident on MRI (▶ Fig. 4.126).

Posttraumatic bone cyst. A rare complication of healing fractures of tubular bones in children is the development of a bone cyst. The commonest site is the distal radius and the lesions resemble a simple bone cyst but tend to be cortically based. They tend to heal over time (see Chapter 1.7.1).

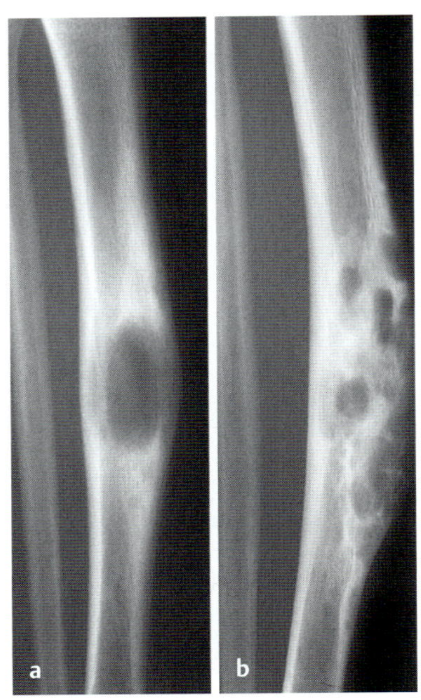

Fig. 4.119 Osteofibrous dysplasia. **(a)** Primary finding. **(b)** Recurrence after surgery.

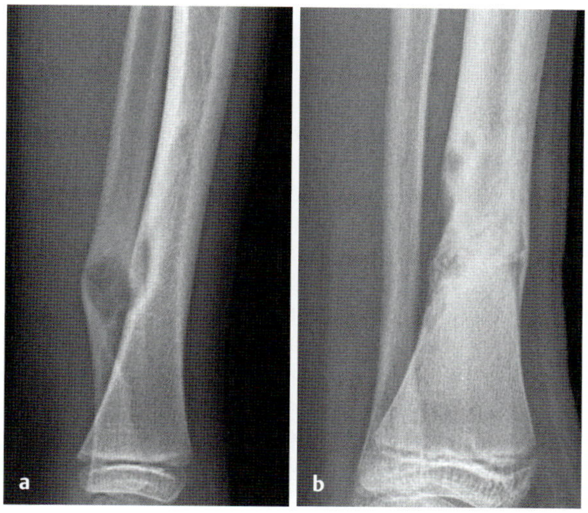

Fig. 4.120 Osteofibrous dysplasia of Campanacci. Monitoring of disease progression. **(a)** Initial diagnosis at the age of 6 years. **(b)** Follow-up review after 12 years.

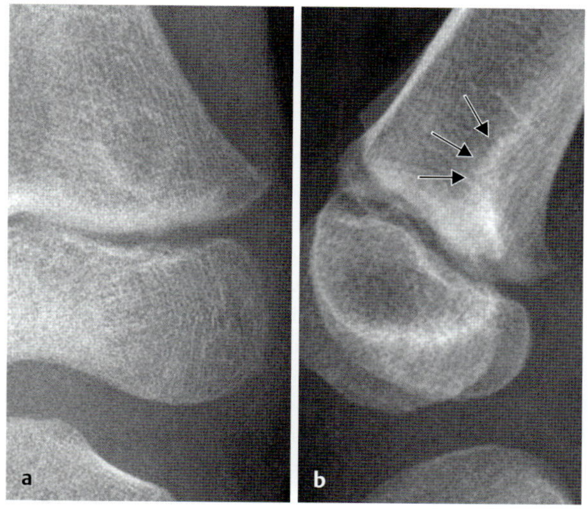

Fig. 4.121 Cortical desmoid. **(a)** Typical site at the distal femoral metaphysis. **(b)** Flat cortical erosion (arrows).

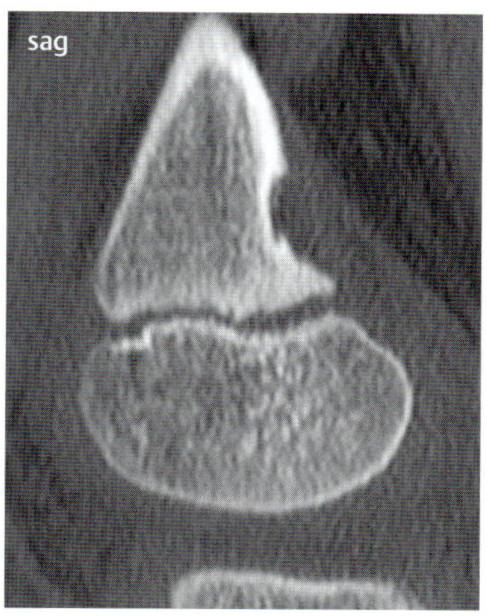

Fig. 4.122 Cortical desmoid.

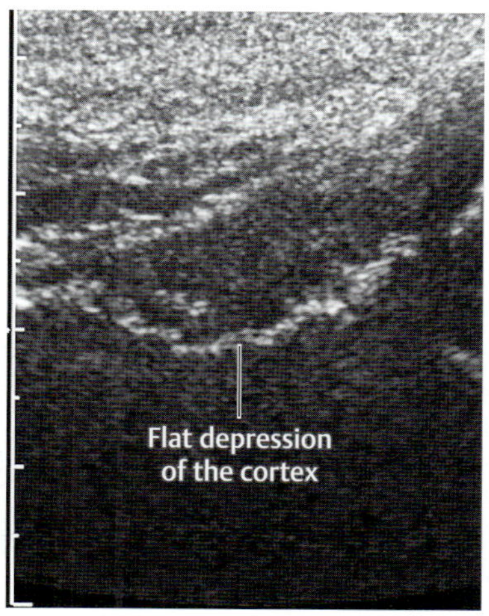

Fig. 4.123 Cortical desmoid. Ultrasound: posterior longitudinal section through the distal femoral metaphysis.

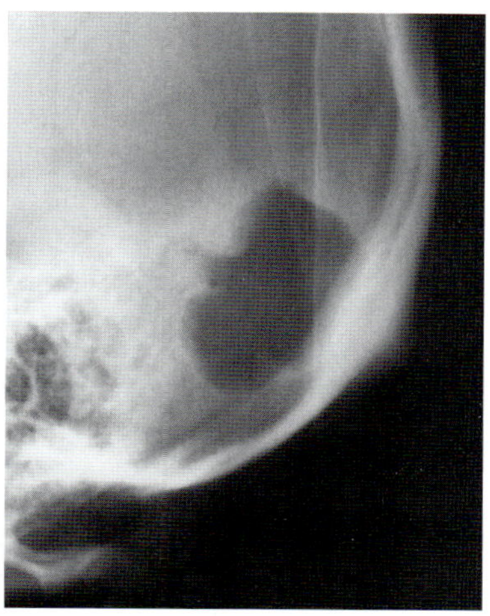

Fig. 4.124 Epidermoid of the skull.

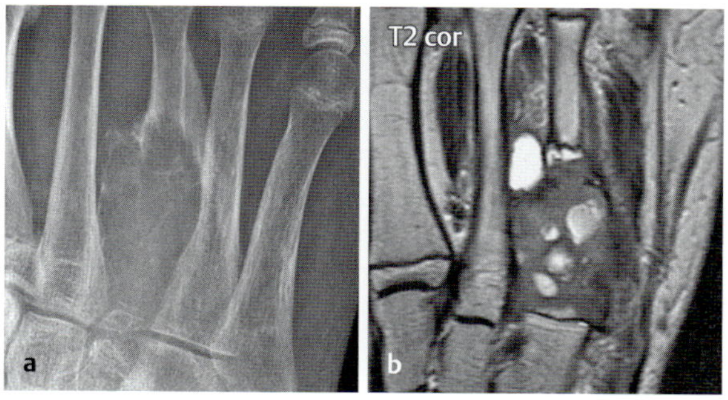

Fig. 4.125 Giant cell reparative granuloma. **(a)** Complete osteolysis without any significant neocortex. **(b)** Tumor with cystic components.

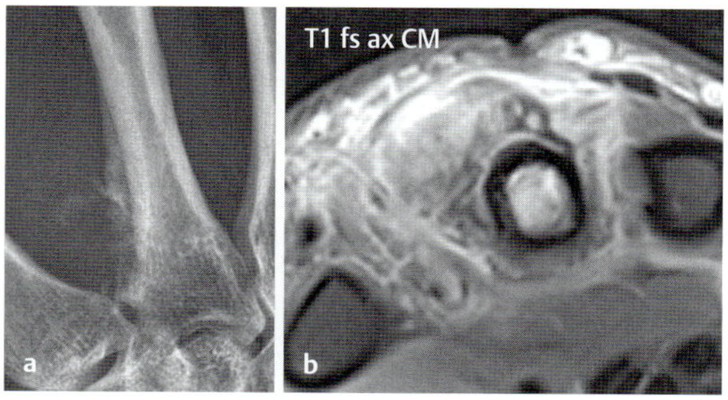

Fig. 4.126 Bizarre parosteal osteochondromatous proliferation (Nora lesion). **(a)** Nora lesion is the eponym for a disease for which the other term is self-descriptive. **(b)** The MRI is reminiscent of a malignant soft tissue tumor with its strong contrast enhancement and ill-defined border. A biopsy is mandatory to exclude osteosarcoma.

4.4 Metastases

Metastases are the most common tumors involving bone. They are the commonest differential diagnosis for bone destruction or sclerosis in patients over the age of 40 years.

► **Pathology.** The seeding and growth of tumor cells during metastatic bone disease is due to an imbalance of osteoclast and osteoblast activity. The seed and soil theory proposed by Paget is still valid, stating that tumor cells (the seed) have a special affinity for the suitable milieu within the bone (the soil). Tumor-specific factors of the primary tumor and the local response within the bone marrow determine the type of dysregulation of bone destruction and remodeling and, subsequently, the radiological image reflected in osteolytic, osteoblastic, or mixed osteolytic/osteoblastic metastases. Based on the current level of knowledge, the hematologic spread of tumor cells is clearly the predominant route. In principle, however, direct infiltration and lymphatic spread are also possible.

Primary tumors commonly involving the skeleton

- Breast cancer.
- Prostate cancer.
- Bronchogenic carcinoma.
- Renal cell carcinoma.
- Carcinoma of the gastrointestinal tract.
- Thyroid carcinomas.

► **Clinical presentation.** The cardinal symptom is dull, intermittent nonmechanical pain. Generalized symptoms, such as weight loss, weakness, and fatigue, are the result of systemic tumor spread. Inflammatory parameters may be elevated. Massive bone destruction secondary to metastases may lead to hypercalcemia and pathologic fracture.

Age: Skeletal metastases are not generally seen until after the age of 40 years. Exceptions include metastases of:

- Neuroblastoma in the child.
- Breast cancer in young women.
- Seminoma in young men.

Location: Metastases may develop in any bone, with a propensity for the spine, the axial skeleton and the skull where hematopoietic marrow persists in the adult. Here the rule applies: The more peripheral a bone is, the less likely it is to be affected by metastatic invasion. For this reason, metastases in the hands and feet are rarities. If present, they are then usually metastases from a bronchial carcinoma.

> **Note** !
>
> Only 10% of skeletal metastases present as a solitary lesion at the time of presentation—classically from renal cell carcinoma.

► **Radiography.** The radiographic findings are most variable:

- **Osteolytic type:** Solitary or multiple radiolucencies with an ill-defined, though occasionally sharp, border are common (► Fig. 4.127). The pattern of bone destruction ranges from the moth-eaten type to infiltrative-permeative findings (► Fig. 4.128). Sclerotic borders are only rarely encountered. The periosteal reaction is distinctly variable. The conventional radiograph commonly reveals metastatic involvement of the soft tissue secondary to cortical bone destruction. It is not uncommon for the diagnosis to be established from a pathologic fracture (► Fig. 4.128). Lytic destruction is primarily found in metastatic spread from bronchial, renal, and thyroid carcinomas, as well as from colorectal and breast carcinomas.
- **Osteoblastic type: Solitary or multiple foci of increased density** of various sizes: The increased density ranges from circumscribed small patchy areas to involvement of the entire bone (► Fig. 4.129). The sclerotic borders are usually ill-defined. This type of metastasis is seen in carcinoma of the prostate, breast, and, less frequently (~ 20% of cases), also in gastrointestinal tumors (e.g., colonic carcinoma, carcinoid).
- **Mixed osteolytic–osteoblastic type:** This is due to a combination of osteolytic and osteosclerotic foci which then become confluent (► Fig. 4.130). Breast and prostate carcinomas, gastrointestinal tumors, and bronchial carcinomas can be the cause of this type of metastatic spread.

Variants

- **Expansile cystic metastases:** The cortical bone is largely destroyed. The tumor components are surrounded by fine, periosteal new bone formation that can give the lesion a soap-bubble appearance. This type is rare and is typically seen in renal and thyroid metastases.
- **Cortical/periosteal metastases:** These are areas of osteolysis involving the cortical bone, with a permeative or moth-eaten appearance (see ► Fig. 4.136) commonest with bronchial metastasis.

► **NUC MED. Bone scintigraphy** using technetium Tc 99 m diphosphonate is the initial diagnostic procedure to screen the whole skeleton for bone metastases. Abnormal findings are supplemented by radiographs, at least as part of the initial diagnostic work-up, to reduce the chance of false-positive findings (degenerative disease, posttraumatic bone lesions) or to detect complications (imminent pathologic fracture). One problem remains: a large number of metastasis-related findings that are positive on the bone scan are not visible on the radiograph. If these discrepancies in findings are clinically relevant, then other imaging (MRI, PET-CT) must be utilized. In particular, the bone scan can remain false-negative with small osteolytic metastases. An important variant is the so-called superscan where there is intense symmetric activity throughout the skeleton due to diffuse or disseminated metastatic spread (commonly found with prostate cancer). A clue to this diagnosis is the reduced

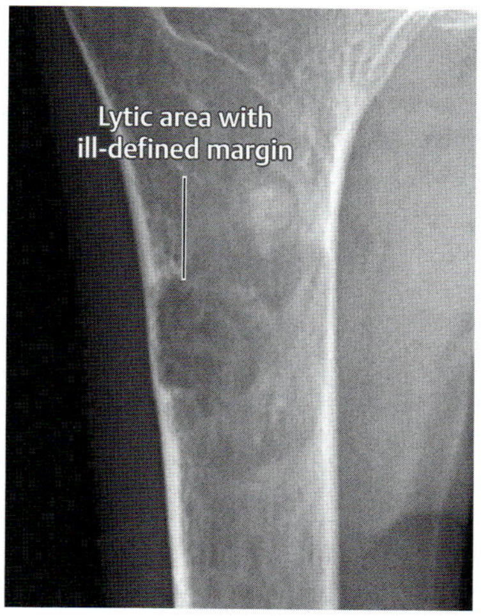

Fig. 4.127 Bone metastasis secondary to breast cancer.

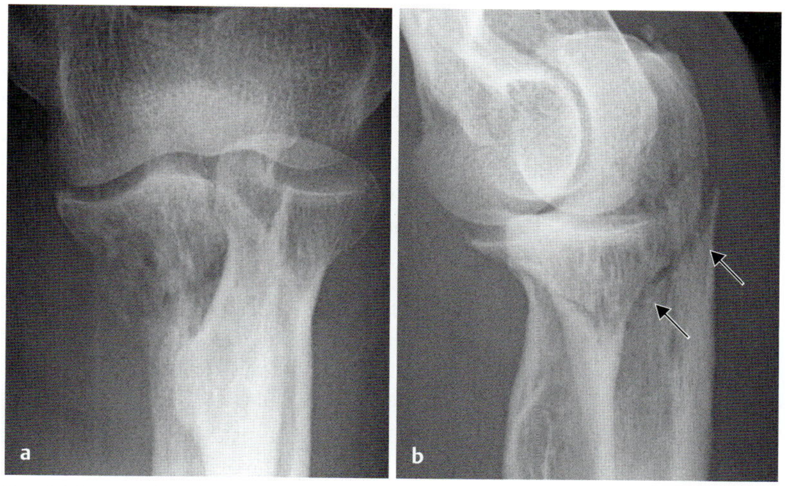

Fig. 4.128 Osteolytic bone metastasis in the proximal ulna from a malignant melanoma. **(a)** Moth-eaten pattern of osteolysis. **(b)** Attention was drawn to the osteolysis by a pathologic fracture (arrows).

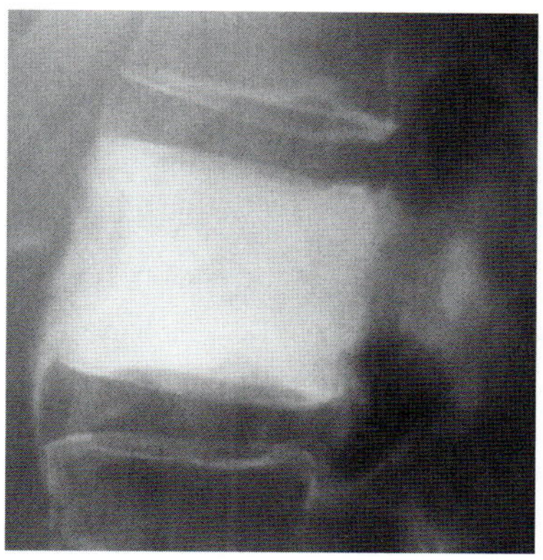

Fig. 4.129 Osteoblastic vertebral metastasis secondary to breast cancer.

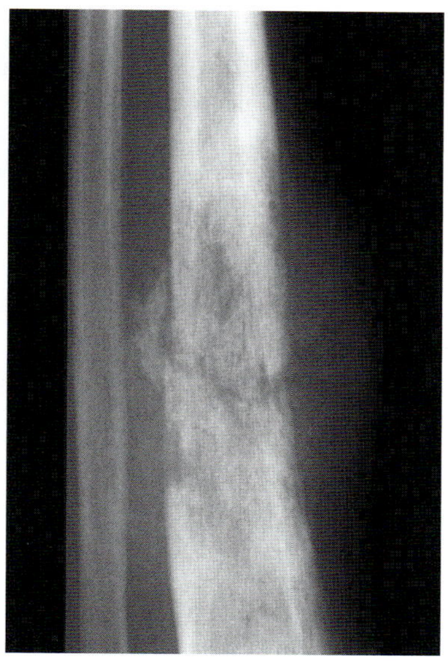

Fig. 4.130 Mixed osteolytic/osteoblastic bone metastases from a colonic carcinoma.

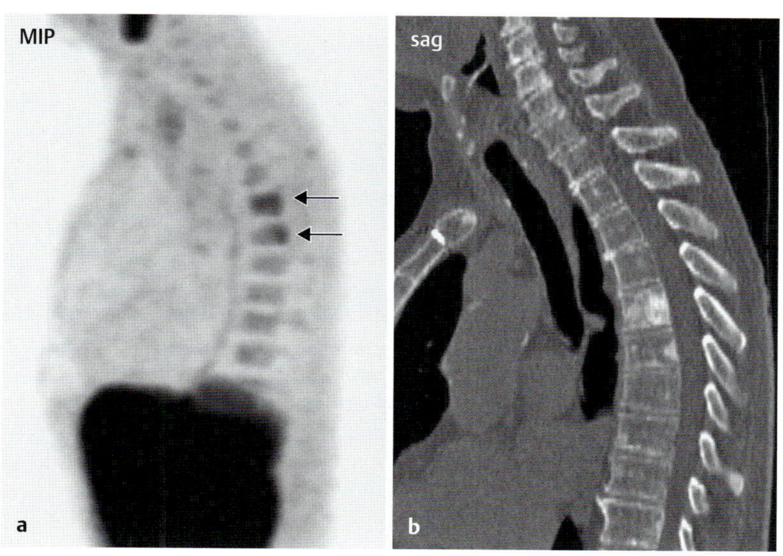

Fig. 4.131 Vertebral prostate cancer metastases. (Images courtesy of J. Scink, Augsburg, Germany.) **(a)** Hypermetabolic foci on ^{18}F-choline-PET (arrows). **(b)** Corresponding osteoblastic lesion on CT.

renal and bladder activity as the radionuclide is preferentially taken up by the metastases.

The importance of the **PET modality** in combination with CT for bone metastasis screening is increasing. Apart from ^{18}F-FDG and ^{18}F-choline (▶ Fig. 4.131) as tumor-specific tracers, sodium fluoride F18 is gaining increasing interest as a bone-specific tracer. PET-CT has higher sensitivity and specificity than bone scintigraphy. This applies above all to osteolytic bone metastases. However, the importance of PET-CT has not yet been conclusively determined in comparison with bone scintigraphy as definitive studies are still lacking. At the moment its general use for bone metastasis screening is not recommended. PET and MRI are regarded as similar with regard to sensitivity and specificity.

4

▶ **US.** In experienced hands, ultrasound is being successfully used in superficial bones (e.g., ribs, hands, feet) because cortical discontinuity is easily recognized with this modality (▶ Fig. 4.132).

▶ **CT.** CT is far superior to radiography for detecting bone destruction. It is used in the spine (vertebral arch, articular process), in facial bones, and in the pelvis. As a general rule: the diagnostic workup of unclear findings suspicious for metastasis in regions with complex skeletal anatomy is a good indication for CT (▶ Fig. 4.133).

▶ **MRI.** MRI is a very sensitive modality for detecting skeletal metastases. Signal intensity change due to metastases follows the classic pattern of most bone tumors (low intensity on T1W, high intensity on fluid-sensitive sequences). The signal depends greatly on the degree of reactive mineralization of the metastasis, so intermediate or hypointense lesions also appear on T2W sequences. Virtually all metastases enhance with contrast (▶ Figs. 4.134 and ▶ 4.135).

4.4.1 Monitoring

The response of osteolytic metastases to radiotherapy and/or chemotherapy is recognizable by progressive sclerosis toward the center (▶ Figs. 4.136, ▶ 4.137, and ▶ W4.26). Decrease in size of the osteolytic process is also a positive follow-up parameter, although it is seen less commonly in the absence of a change in bone density. PET-CT combines morphological and metabolic information and allows earlier assessment of the response to systemic treatment than the purely morphological modalities of radiography and CT or bone scintigraphy.

▶ **DD.** Establishing the diagnosis of metastatic bone disease is not a problem when multiple lesions appear on the bone scan in the presence of a known primary malignancy and their radiological finding is compatible with metastasis. Certain differential diagnoses should be considered with *solitary* lesions, depending on the type of metastasis:

Osteolytic lesions. It is not possible to differentiate malignant lymphoma of bone and plasmacytoma from metastases. Primary bony tumors may appear similar, but are a rarity compared with metastases.

Osteoblastic metastases. Osteoma and bone islands are difficult to define as solitary findings on conventional radiography. Strong uptake is found on the bone scan with metastatic foci, unlike with bone islands and classic osteoma.

Mixed osteolytic–osteoblastic metastases. Malignant lymphoma is the main consideration with this type of constellation.

Pathologic fracture due to metastasis. Refer to Chapter 2.2.7 for differentiation between metastatic fractures and osteoporotic fractures of the spine.

Instability. A common clinical question regards stability of the bone once a metastasis has been diagnosed. Instability may be assumed in the following cases:

- *In tubular bones:* if more than 50% of the cortical bone around the metastasis is destroyed.
- *In the spine:*
  - If the posterior margin of the vertebra is interrupted.
  - If a (tumor-related) reduction of vertebral height is present.
  - If MRI demonstrates that the entire vertebra is affected by the tumor, even though the cortical bone has not been breached.

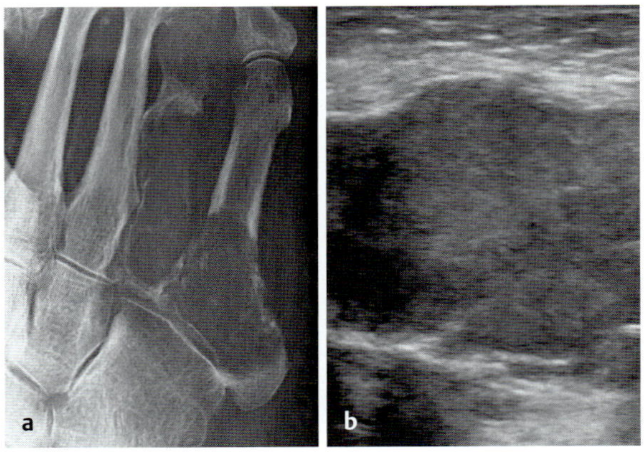

Fig. 4.132 Bone metastasis of a clear-cell renal carcinoma. **(a)** Soap bubble–like, mildly expansile osteolytic lesion. **(b)** Well demonstrated on ultrasound.

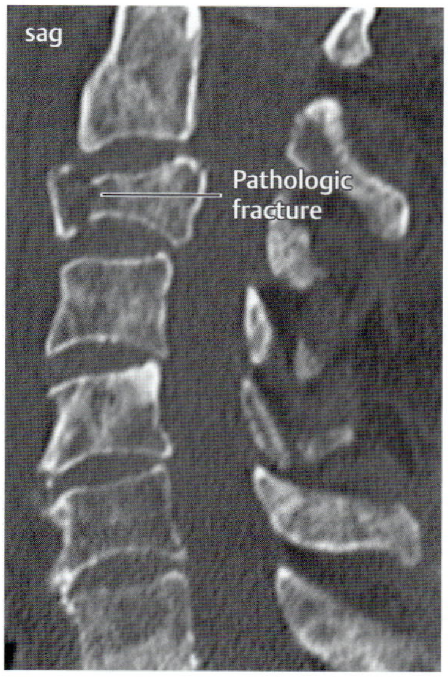

Fig. 4.133 Mixed osteolytic/osteoblastic metastatic spread of prostate cancer.

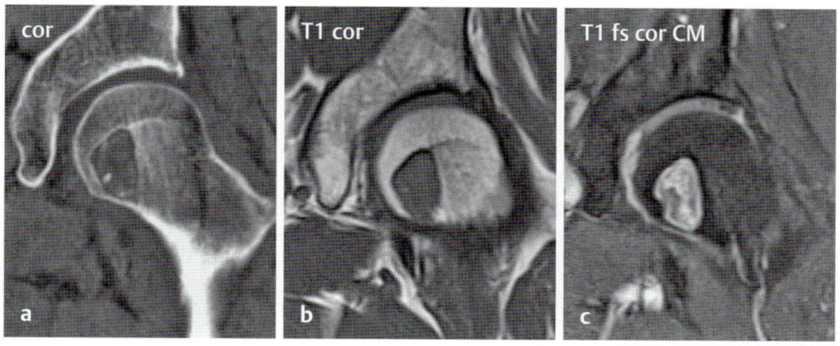

Fig. 4.134 Bone metastasis of a malignant melanoma. **(a)** Fine sclerosis in the center of the sharply marginated osteolytic lesion. **(b)** Relatively bright signal on the T1W image due to the melanin-containing lesion. **(c)** Identification of central necrosis after contrast administration.

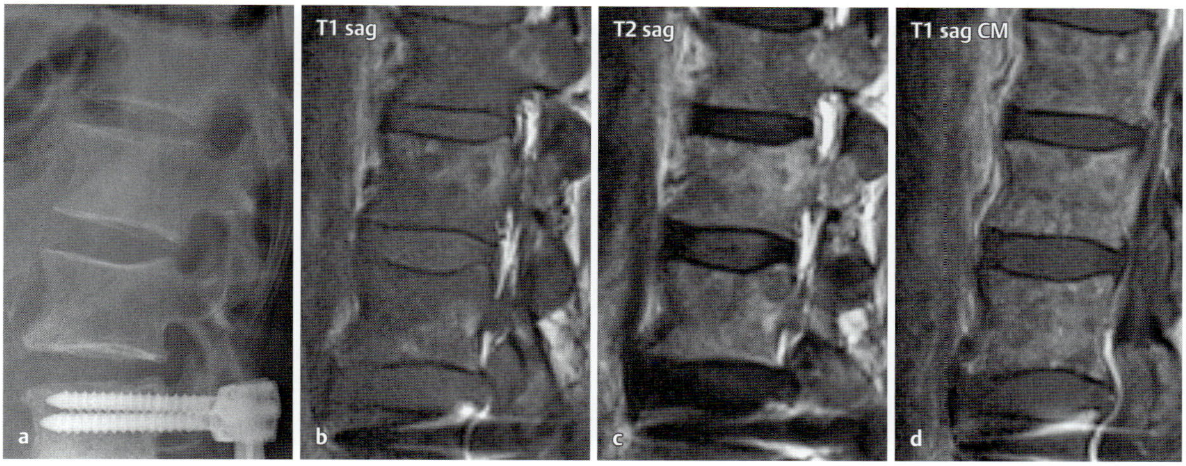

Fig. 4.135 Bone metastasis of prostate cancer. **(a)** On the radiograph there are, at most, discrete inhomogeneities. **(b)** Partial displacement of the fatty marrow by a hypointense tumor. **(c)** Increased signal intensity on the T2W image. **(d)** Increased signal intensity also on the T1W image after contrast administration (no fat saturation because of the implants).

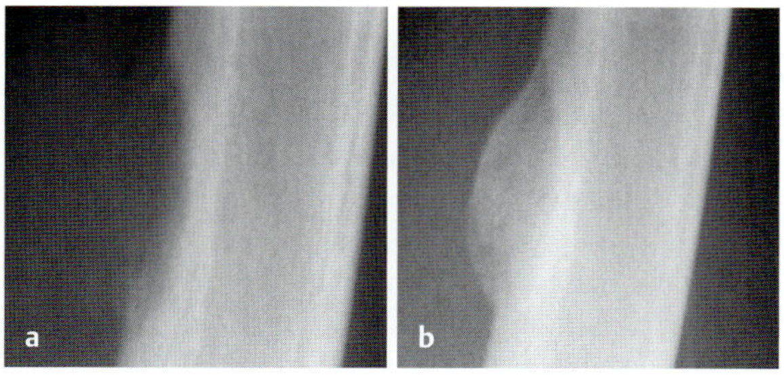

Fig. 4.136 Cortical bone metastasis from rectal carcinoma. **(a)** Moth-eaten pattern of cortical osteolysis. **(b)** Sclerosis following chemotherapy.

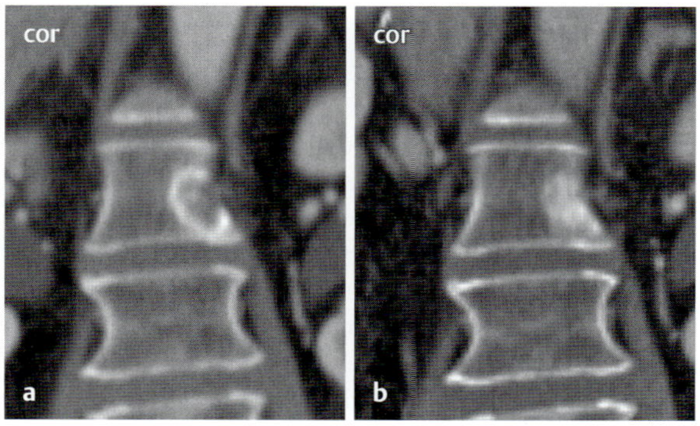

Fig. 4.137 Bone metastasis of an adenocarcinoma. See also the PET-CT image in ▶ Fig. W4.26. **(a)** Initial finding showing an osteolytic lesion with a sclerotic margin. **(b)** Sclerosis following chemotherapy.

4

4.5 Soft tissue Tumors

4.5.1 Introduction

Soft tissue tumors comprise ~ 50 histological subtypes and more than 100 different WHO diagnoses. In principle, they can originate in any soft tissue, peripheral (75% of cases), proximal (10%), or retroperitoneal. Benign tumors are 100 times more common than malignant tumors. That is why inadequate excisions of small tumors that are subsequently discovered to be malignant, without prior biopsy and even imaging, are unfortunately commonly performed outside specialist centers. Soft tissue sarcomas metastasize hematogenously, predominantly to the lungs.

▸ **Pathology.** The tumors are classified histologically according to cell type, tissue of origin, and matrix formation. However, classification according to tissue of origin has proven itself to be scientifically untenable. The WHO includes prognostic considerations and suggests dividing soft tissue tumors into three categories (▸ Fletcher et al. 2013):

- **Benign:** Lipomas, fibrohistiocytic and fibrous tumors, vascular tumors, nerve sheath tumors.
- **Intermediate** (locally aggressive, commonly locally recurrent or rarely metastatic): Desmoids (aggressive fibromatosis), special types of fibrohistiocytic tumors.
- **Malignant:** Soft tissue sarcomas.

New nomenclature. The tumor classification formerly known as "malignant fibrous histiocytoma" has been subdivided to include, for example, myxofibrosarcoma and the large group of undifferentiated sarcomas: known as NOS (not otherwise specified).

Soft tissue sarcomas hardly ever develop from a benign "precursor." An exception is the malignant peripheral nerve sheath tumor, which develops from transformation of a neurofibroma of Recklinghausen's disease (▸ Figs. 4.138 and ▸ 4.139). Transformation to a higher grade of malignancy is also possible, for example, after recurrence of liposarcoma and myxofibrosarcoma.

The **TNM Classification of Malignant Tumors** is also recognized for soft tissue tumors (see specialized literature).

Soft tissue tumors are today the domain of ultrasound and, above all, MRI. CT is used for staging and the detection or exclusion of calcifications and ossifications. Most soft tissue tumors can be identified on imaging but cannot be classified diagnostically with any degree of confidence. This applies in particular for relatively common tumors, such as neurinomas, neurofibromas, giant cell tumors of tendon sheaths, malignant fibrous histiocytomas, rhabdomyosarcomas, and many others. An image-guided biopsy is required for the majority of cases. Imaging allows for the detection or exclusion of a tumor and subsequent staging, biopsy planning, and treatment.

What supports malignancy in soft tissue tumors?

- **Size:** Maximum diameter over 5 cm.
- **Peritumoral edema** (differentiation between a solid tumor and edema of the surrounding tissue is best accomplished after contrast administration): What is known as the tumor pseudocapsule is in fact the active tumor front; in 66% of patients, tumor cells are detectable in the peritumoral edema (▸ Fig. 4.140). However, peritumoral edema is relatively subtle in sarcomas. It is more extensive in muscle tears, myositis ossificans, and infection than in sarcomas.
- **Sub- or transfascial** location: Infiltration or penetration of a fascia (especially between subcutaneous fatty tissue and muscle). Exceptions are intramuscular lipomas and benign vascular tumors. Although 99% of benign soft tissue tumors are superficial in location, this is not an exclusion criterion for malignancy (example: myxofibrosarcoma).
- **Extension** to include several muscle groups or anatomical sites.

> **Note**
> The report of sectional imaging findings on soft tissue tumors should always contain information on tumor size, location, affected compartments, and relationship to surrounding structures.

▸ **Radiography.** The radiograph can provide information on tumor calcifications and involvement of the bone adjacent to a soft tissue tumor:

- Erosion, abrasion.
- Periosteal bone reaction and/or invasion (▸ Fig. 4.141).

The radiograph can only provide initial indirect clues and information about extraosseous processes:

- Radiolucencies (lipoma; ▸ Fig. 4.142).
- Densities, phleboliths (arteriovenous malformations, lipomas, lymph nodes, chondromas, sarcomas, and tumor metastases; ▸ Fig. 4.143).
- Ossifications, calcifications (synovial sarcoma, leiomyoma; ▸ Fig. W4.27).

▸ **Angiography.** Angiography is used (now rarely) preoperatively to display vascular structure and as a prelude for embolization.

▸ **US.** Ultrasound is used as the primary modality for superficial tumors. Lipomas are usually hyperechoic; occasionally the surrounding capsule is recognizable by ultrasound. All other soft tissue tumors usually appear as inhomogeneous, hypoechoic space-occupying masses. Cystic parts of the tumor, necroses, or fresh hemorrhages may show as anechoic regions. Ultrasound is of no help with differential diagnosis.

▸ **CT.** CT has only a limited role unless MRI is contraindicated. Its use for lipogenic tumors may help in differentiating healthy fatty tissue with the aid of density measurements.

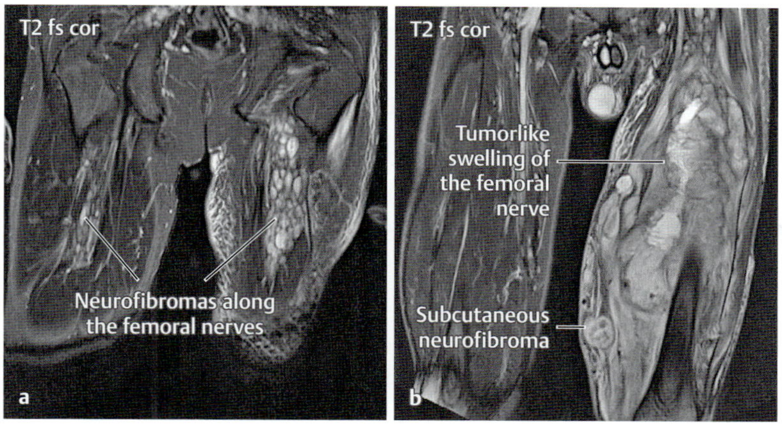

Fig. 4.138 Malignant peripheral nerve sheath tumor in neurofibromatosis (von Recklinghausen). **(a)** Symmetrical, nodular neurofibromas of the thigh. **(b)** Large soft tissue space-occupying mass on the left, along the distended femoral nerve. In addition, subcutaneous neurofibromas that originate in cutaneous nerves and are clinically palpable.

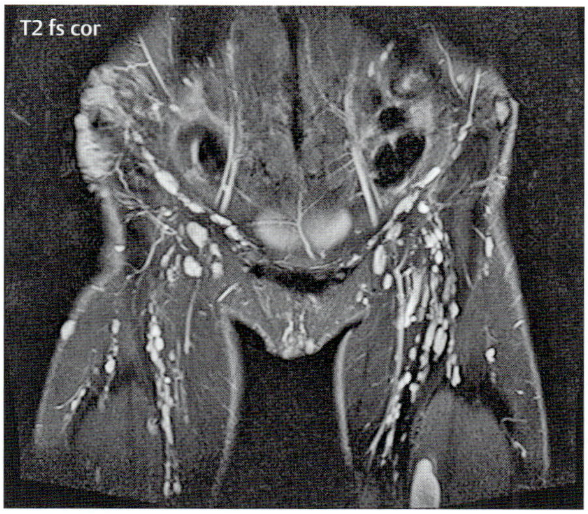

Fig. 4.139 Neurofibromatosis arranged in a chainlike manner. Hyperintense on the T2W image. **Caution:** These are not lymph nodes!

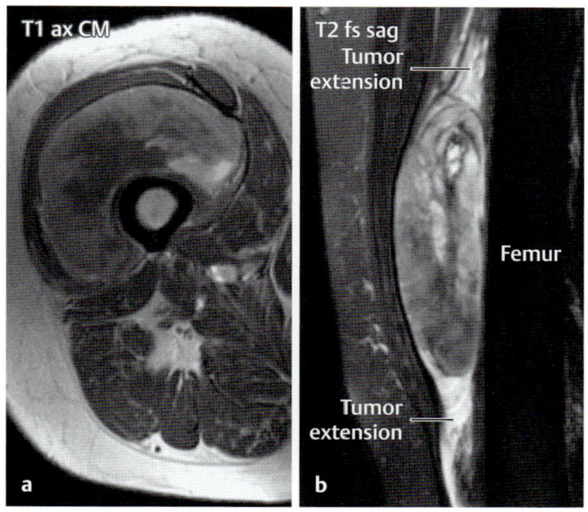

Fig. 4.140 Leiomyosarcoma of the thigh. **(a)** Predominantly peripheral contrast enhancement. **(b)** The hypointense signal on the T2W sequence is an expression of the high tissue density. The craniocaudal, edemalike signal raises the suspicion of tumor spread.

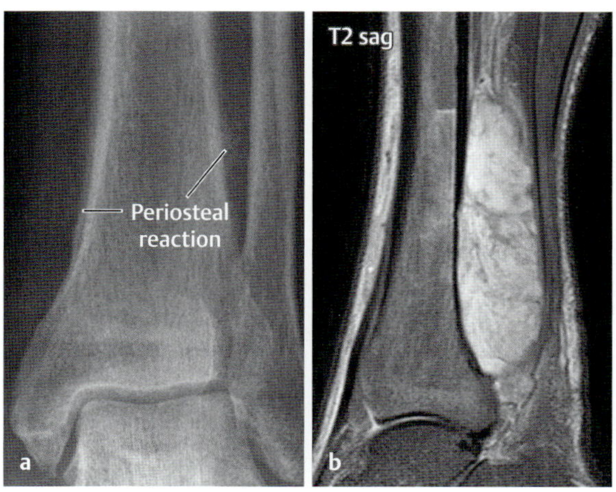

Fig. 4.141 Periosteal, high-grade pleomorphic soft tissue sarcoma (NOS). **(a)** A periosteal reaction of unknown origin is evident on the radiograph. **(b)** MRI confirms the inhomogeneous soft tissue mass.

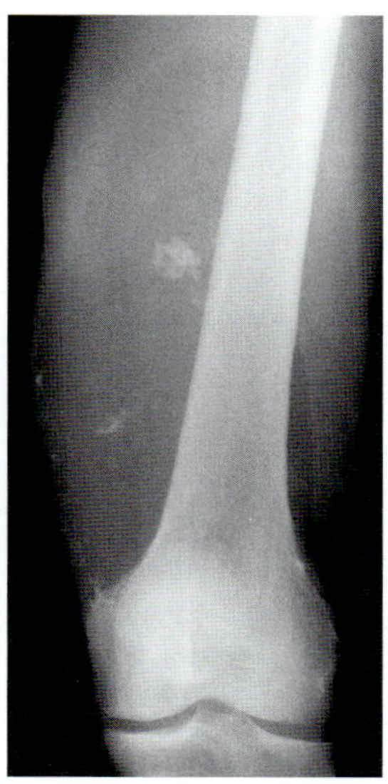

Fig. 4.142 Lipoma. Radiolucent mass with calcification.

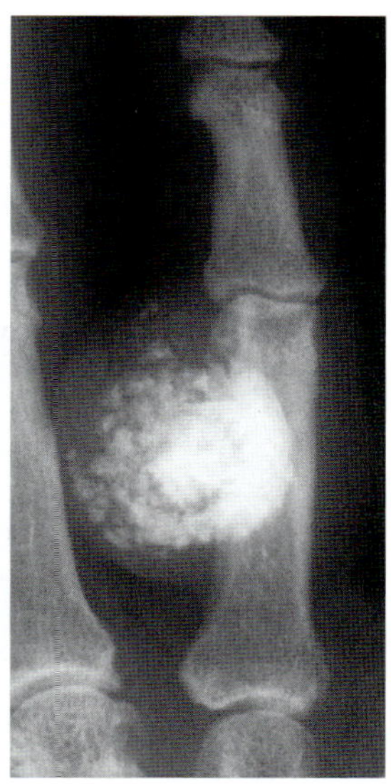

Fig. 4.143 Tendon sheath chondroma.

▶ NUC MED. Current studies on PET-CT and also, of late, on PET-MRI do not yet provide any conclusive assessment. The use of PET-MRI, e.g., for the diagnostic work-up of recurrences, is promising (▶ Figs. 4.144 and ▶ W4.28).

Note

Postoperative reparative processes can demonstrate nonspecific increased metabolism for up to 3 months after surgery.

▶ MRI. The majority of soft tissue tumors are of low intensity on T1W and of high intensity on intermediate weighting or T2W sequences. They vary in their enhancement with contrast; *contrast enhancement is not a specific criterion for malignancy*. The use of contrast has proven to be helpful for differentiating local recurrence from postoperative seroma. More recent techniques, such as diffusion-weighted imaging (DWI) and perfusion-weighted imaging (PWI) have already found their way into clinical diagnostics, but need further validation, as does MR spectroscopy.

Caution

- Pulsation artifacts from vessels can give rise to unclear findings and this should be taken into consideration, or selection of a different read-out direction should be considered (▶ Fig. 4.145).
- Unlike with bone tumors, an irregular tumor border and an inhomogeneous tumor signal are not definite indications for malignancy on MRI.
- Homogeneous hyperintense internal structure of a cartilaginous tumor on T2W sequences is easily mistaken for fluid (▶ Fig. 4.146). **Caution:** Not every tumor in the popliteal fossa is a Baker's cyst (▶ Fig. 4.147)!
- Irregular margins of a lesion and perilesional edema on MRI are nonspecific signs. They are also encountered in soft tissue injuries, myositis ossificans (early form), and soft tissue inflammations.
- Postoperative contrast enhancement of the former tumor site is nonspecific within the first 3 months of surgery and is commonly of reparative nature (granulation tissue and neovascularization). Postoperative seromas are a regular finding.

4.5.2 Clinically Important Soft Tissue Tumors, also Partially Amenable to Classification Using Imaging Procedures

Lipoma. Lipomas account for ~ one in three benign tumors. Most are of superficial location and appear as a sharply defined mass on MRI. They display a homogeneous, high signal on T1W and T2W sequences. Fine, hypointense capsules may be recognized in some cases (▶ Fig. 4.148). Intramuscular lipomas and fatty tissue are also found (▶ Figs. 4.149–4.151).

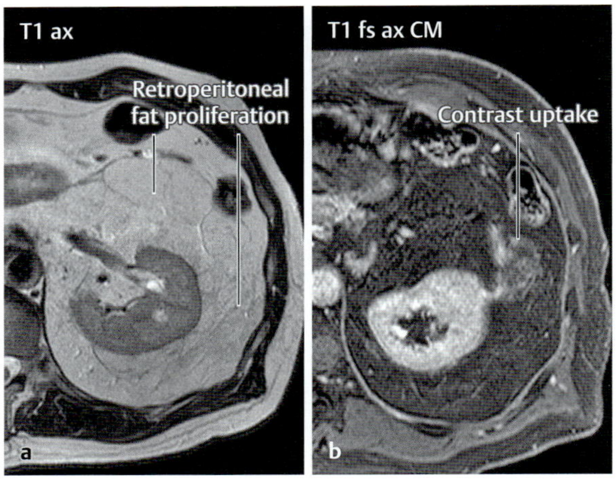

Fig. 4.144 Retroperitoneal liposarcoma. ▶ See supplementary PET-CT in ▶ Fig. W4.28. **(a)** It is not possible to differentiate the tumor from the surrounding retroperitoneal or mesenteric fat on plain MRI (T1W). **(b)** Contrast enhancement of poorly differentiated, pararenal parts of the liposarcoma.

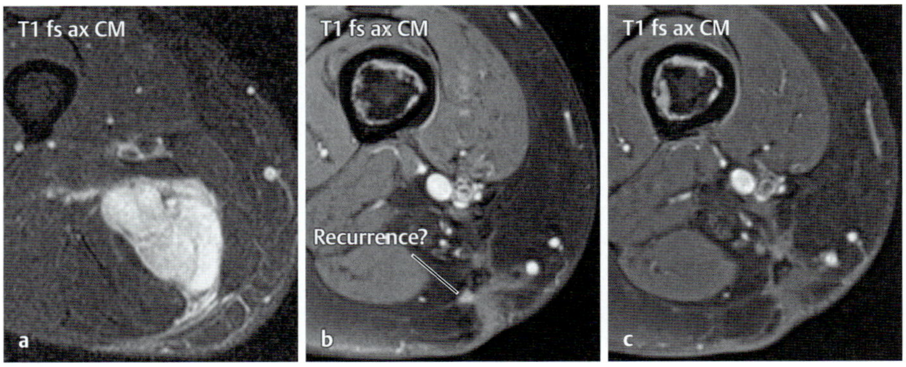

Fig. 4.145 Pitfall in the follow-up of a soft tissue sarcoma of the thigh on MRI. Pulsation artifacts. **(a)** Initial preoperative finding. **(b)** Follow-up after 3 years. Focal hyperintensity in the scar tissue is suspicious for recurrence (read-out direction posteroanterior). **(c)** Repeated acquisition with altered read-out direction (left–right) reveals the finding to be a pulsation artifact of the femoral artery.

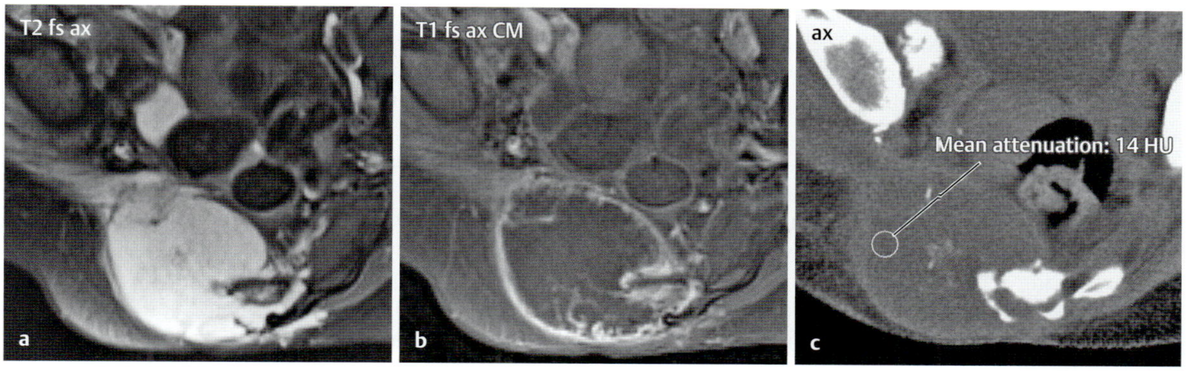

Fig. 4.146 Soft tissue recurrence following excision of a chondroblastic osteosarcoma of the sacrum. **(a)** Parasacral space-occupying mass on the right with a high signal in the center on the T2W image. **(b)** Almost exclusively peripheral enhancement. **(c)** The CT reveals fine septal calcifications inside the lesion and density values of around +14 HU; this excludes a purely cystic space-occupying lesion and confirms the predominantly chondroblastic recurrent tumor.

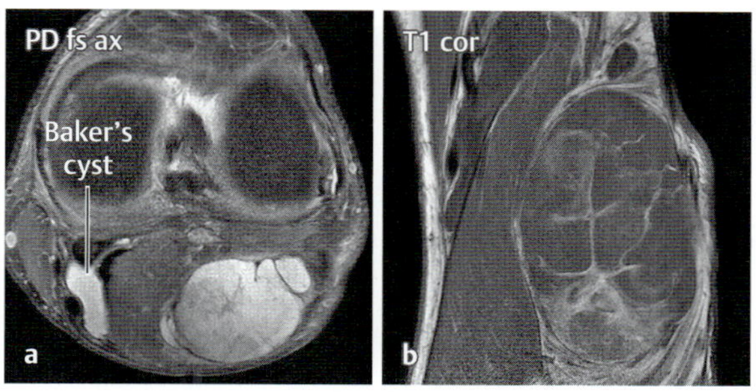

Fig. 4.147 Myxoid liposarcoma and Baker's cyst. **(a)** In addition to the typical Baker's cyst, there is another "cystic" space-occupying lesion evident. **(b)** This demonstrates multiple hyperintense septations (fat-containing) on the T1W image; the intralesional fluid signal is fairly isointense to the muscle. This is the myxoid component of the liposarcoma.

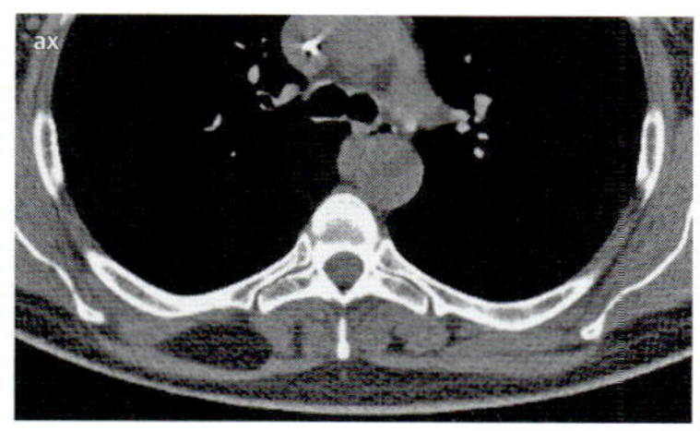

Fig. 4.149 Lipoma deep to the right trapezius.

Fig. 4.148 Lipoma. **(a)** CT displays a homogeneous, hypodense space-occupying mass. **(b)** The space-occupying mass appears predominantly homogeneously hyperintense and isointense to fat on the T1W image. **(c)** No focal enhancement. However, a biopsy should be considered in view of the subfascial location and size over 5 cm.

▼

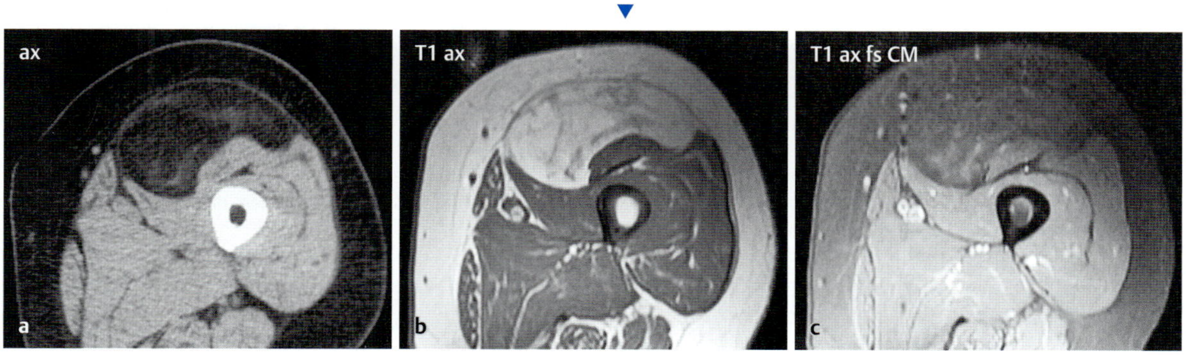

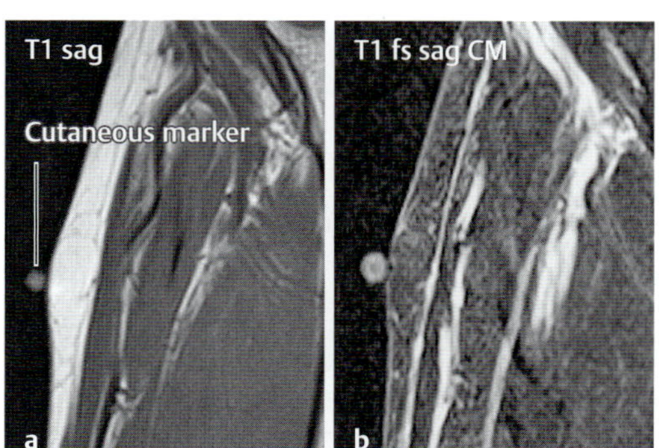

Fig. 4.150 Subcutaneous lipoma of the lower arm. **(a)** The clinically palpable lesion is barely distinguishable from the adjacent subcutaneous fat. **(b)** No contrast enhancement.

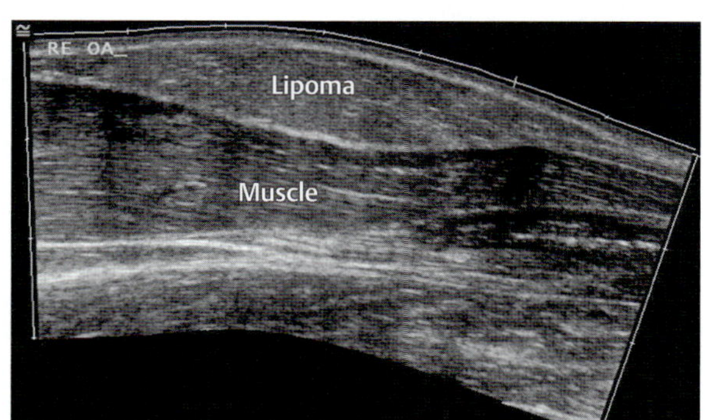

Fig. 4.151 Subcutaneous lipoma on ultrasound. Homogeneous pattern, clearly marginated and hyperechogenic.

Hibernoma. Hibernomas are benign brown fat tumors, commonly found in the shoulder region of young adults. Other sites are possible (► Figs. 4.152 and ► 4.153). The tumors are more hypointense than subcutaneous fat on T1W and T2W sequences.

Liposarcoma. Small, fatty elements can be detected within the tumor in this entity. In general, the higher grade the tumor the less the fatty component. Myxoid components (common!) are very hyperintense on T2W sequences (► Fig. 4.154). Increased and thick septations as well as deep location are signs of malignancy. Retroperitoneal tumors are usually malignant.

4

> **Caution**
> Liposarcomas of the inguinal canal (► Fig. 4.155) can be mistaken for commonly found hernias of fat tissue on the axial image and vice versa. Many liposarcomas do not present a characteristic pattern as only solid parts are recognizable.

Myxomas. These are benign tumors with little vascularization but rich in myxoid ground substance. The space-occupying masses are hypointense on T1W and hyperintense on T2W sequences and commonly display a margin of fat. Hypercellular myxomas can enhance in various ways with contrast. A myxoid-rich soft tissue sarcoma must be included in the differential diagnosis.

Synovial sarcoma. This is a relatively common sarcoma (10% of all sarcomas), usually appearing during the first three decades of life. The tumor primarily arises in the peripheral extremities, in close proximity to but rarely in a joint. A synovial origin has been refuted. The tumor boundaries are usually sharp, without signs of peritumoral edema (► Fig. W4.29). Calcification, dispersed throughout the tumor, is seen in 30% of cases.

Leiomyosarcoma. Apart from synovial sarcoma, this is the third most common soft tissue tumor entity, with the majority being retroperitoneal or associated with vessels. Women in middle to advanced age are more commonly affected. A well-recognized but rare variant can arise from a vein, typically the femoral.

Glomus tumor. A glomus tumor is a benign and usually very painful soft tissue tumor. Glomus tumors are vascular tumors that in their structure resemble glomus bodies (thermoregulation). They occur primarily in the terminal phalanges with a subungual location, usually measuring only a few millimeters in size. The lesion is very signal intense on T2W sequences and enhances strongly with contrast (► Fig. 4.156). The tumor is readily detectable with ultrasound (hypoechoic lesion).

Tumors of the peripheral nerves (schwannomas and neurofibromas). Morphology and signal behavior on MRI (as well as ultrasound) are basically nonspecific. Necrosis and cysts are typically found in association with ancient schwannomas (► Fig. 4.157), and the so-called target sign (strongly enhancing rim, surrounding a less strongly enhancing center on T1W and hypointense center with hyperintense periphery on T2W images) is seen in neurofibromas (► Fig. 4.158)—albeit not universally.

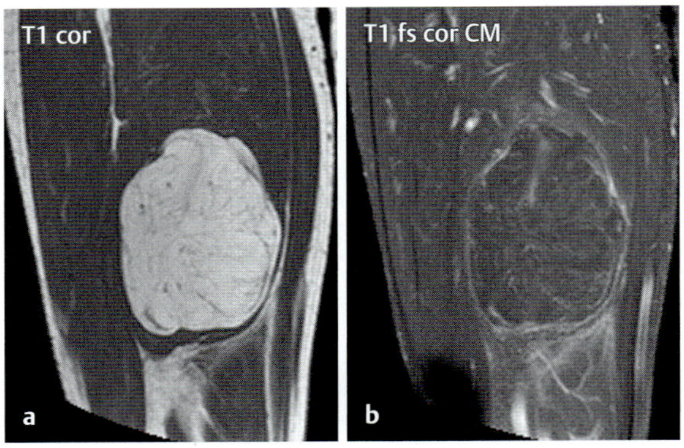

Fig. 4.152 Hibernoma. **(a)** Clearly marginated lipomatous mass within the muscle of the thigh. **(b)** The intralesional structure with septations and vessels also allows the differential diagnosis of a liposarcoma; a biopsy should be taken for clarification.

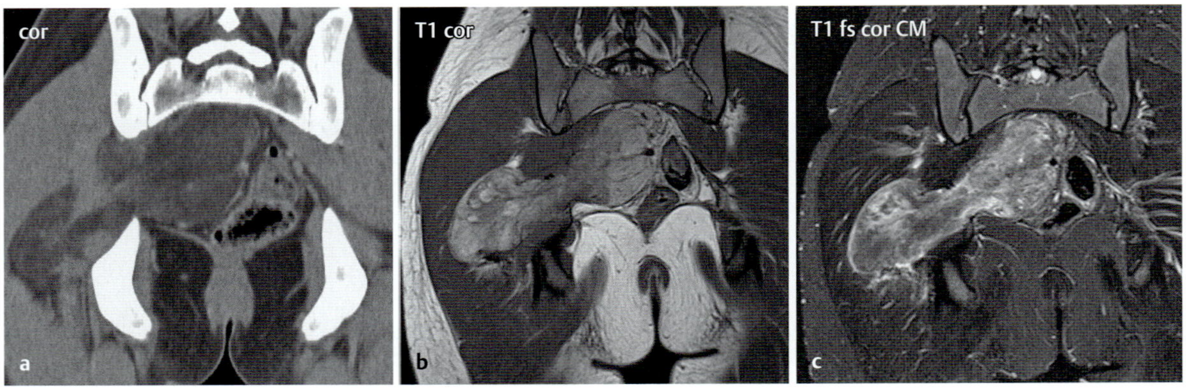

Fig. 4.153 Hibernoma. **(a)** Fatty intrapelvic mass on CT. **(b)** On the plain T1W and T2W images, the mass is less signal intense than the subcutaneous fat. **(c)** The intralesional pattern displays fine septations and vessels; and enhances relatively homogeneously with contrast.

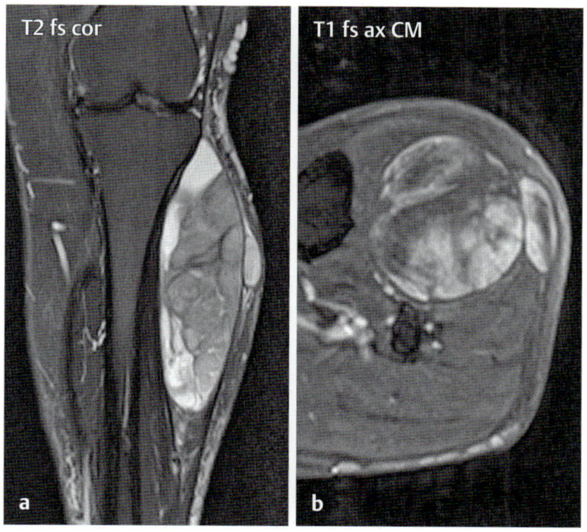

Fig. 4.154 Myxoid liposarcoma. **(a)** The T2W image shows hypointense solid components in addition to hyperintense myxoid tissue in the cranial parts of the tumor. **(b)** Heterogeneous contrast enhancement.

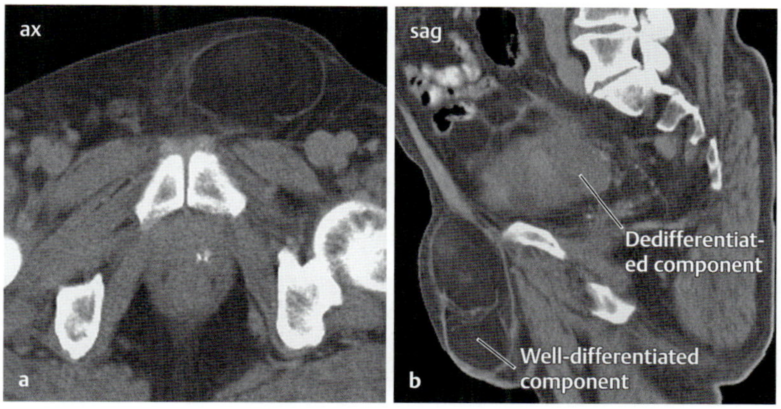

Fig. 4.155 Liposarcoma of the inguinal canal. **(a)** A highly differentiated, hypodense lipogenous part is located in the inguinal canal; the differential diagnosis from an inguinal hernia is difficult. **(b)** Another solid space-occupying mass has an intraperitoneal location and is consistent with a dedifferentiated component.

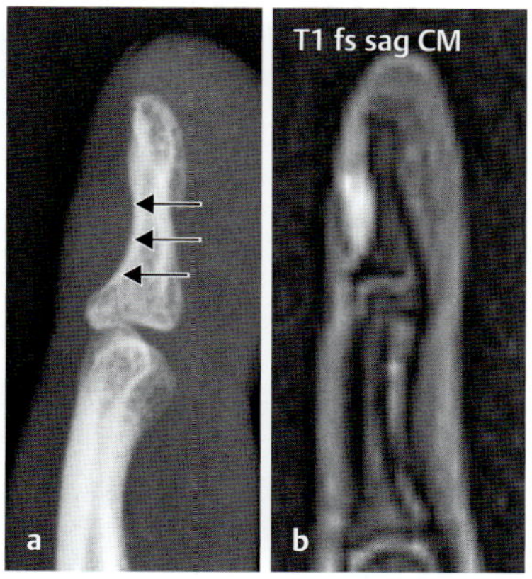

Fig. 4.156 Glomus tumor. **(a)** Dorsal soft tissue mass over the terminal phalanx of the finger that has eroded the cortex (arrows). **(b)** The hyperintensity of the lesion is an indication of the vascular origin of the tumor.

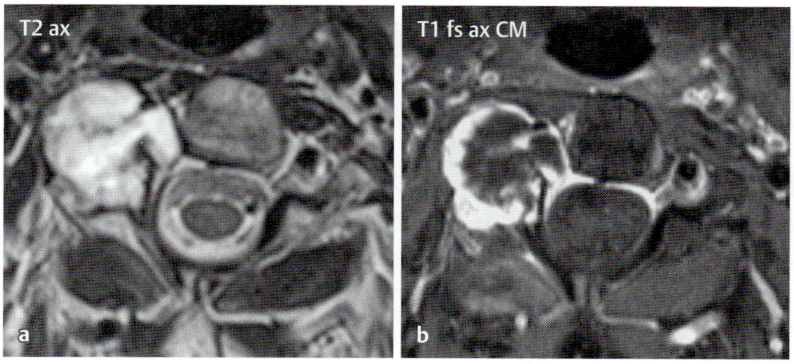

Fig. 4.157 Schwannoma. **(a)** Tumor of the right neural foramen at C2–C3. **(b)** A central necrotic part of the tumor becomes evident after administration of contrast.

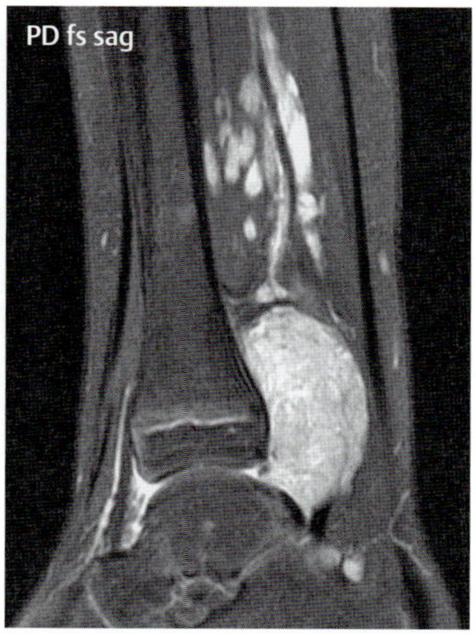

Fig. 4.158 Neurofibromas. Multiple lesions appearing hyperintense on the PDW image along the course of the tibial nerve.

Fibromatoses. These are a group of fibrous tumors that differ in the time point and site of their occurrence. A local infiltrative growth pattern is characteristic for this tumor group. A capsule is only rarely recognizable on ultrasound and above all on MRI. They do not respect fasciae as barriers. MRI displays these tumors as very hypointense on T1W sequences and almost always hypointense on T2W sequences. Fibromatoses enhance with contrast. The **subgroup "aggressive fibromatosis (desmoid)"** is found in the abdominal wall and extremities; they affect all age groups (▶ Figs. 4.159 and ▶ 4.160). The tumor tissue is very dense and hard with a clearly reduced signal on T2W images due to the small number of freely mobile water molecules.

Elastofibroma dorsi. This benign fibroelastic space-occupying mass classically develops deep to the scapula and is frequently bilateral. The patients are usually asymptomatic. Their incidence on CT scans is ~ 2%. MRI shows intermediate signal intensity with typical linear fatty strands, evident on T1W and T2W sequences. Contrast enhancement varies considerably (▶ Fig. 4.161).

4.5.3 Follow-up Reviews and Diagnostics for Recurrences of Soft Tissue Tumors

MRI is the modality of choice for the detection of local recurrence. MRI interpretation can be difficult due to postsurgical and radiotherapy changes. Contrast medium administration may be required to distinguish local recurrence from other masses such as hematoma and seroma (▶ Fig. 4.162). Most soft tissue sarcomas will metastasize first to the lungs. Follow-up usually relies on chest radiography with chest CT reserved for those cases with abnormal radiographic findings.

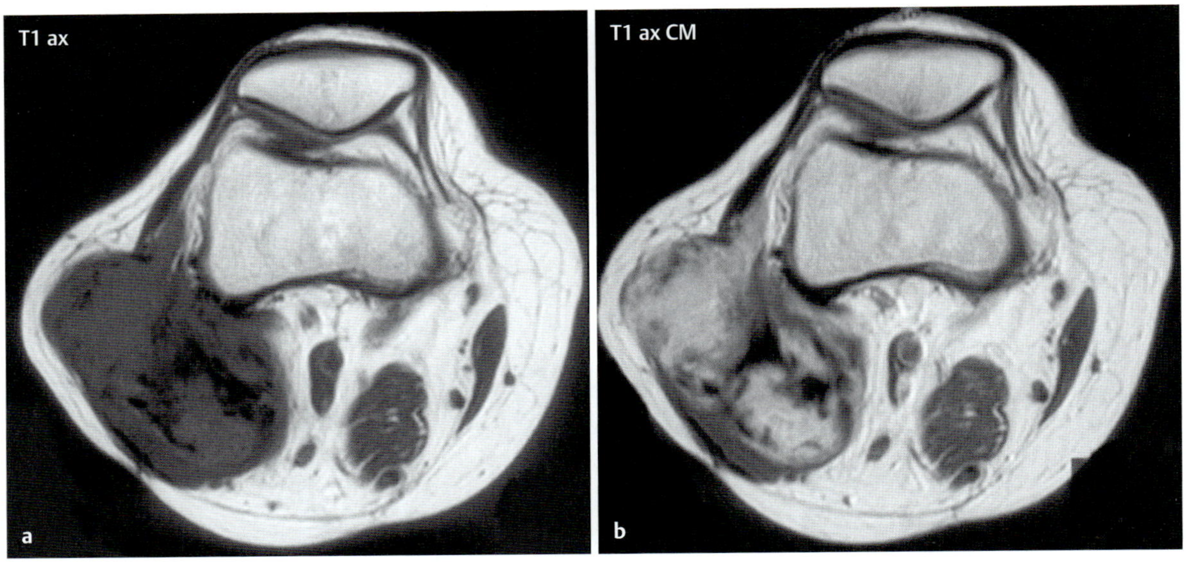

Fig. 4.159 Aggressive fibromatosis. **(a)** These have intratumoral components with very low signal intensity (collagen). **(b)** Clear enhancement after IV contrast administration, interspersed with areas of low signal.

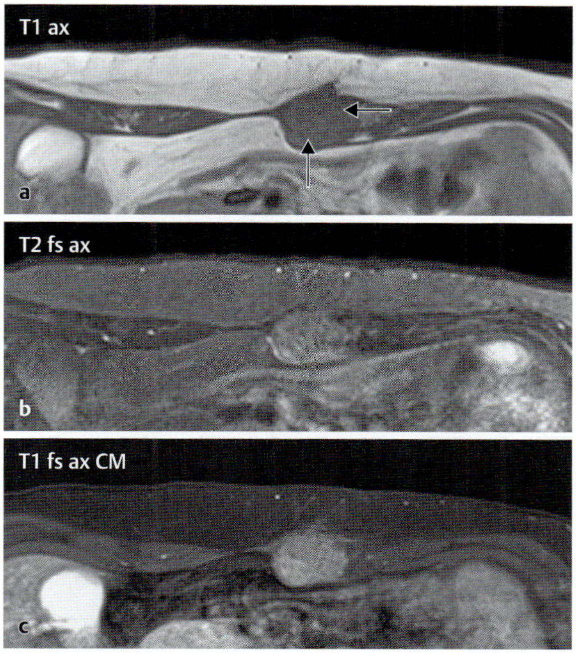

Fig. 4.160 Desmoid tumor of the abdominal wall. **(a)** Hypointense on the T1W image (arrows). **(b)** Also hypointense on the T2W image. **(c)** Clear contrast enhancement.

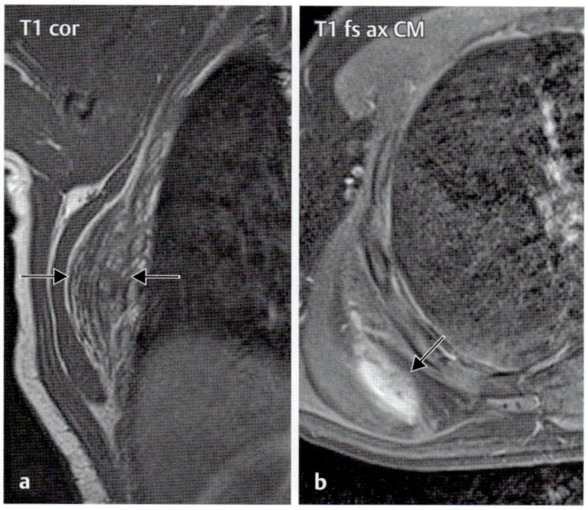

Fig. 4.161 Elastofibroma dorsi (arrows). **(a)** Soft tissue mass with linear fatty strands in a typical location on the T1W image. **(b)** Contrast enhancement.

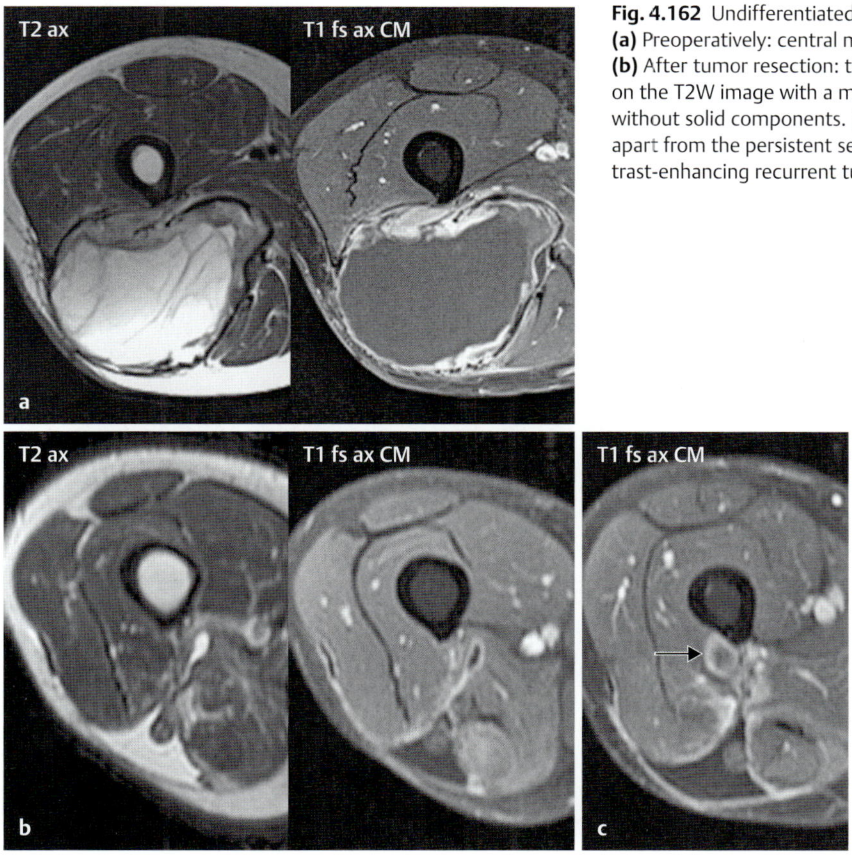

Fig. 4.162 Undifferentiated sarcoma of the posterior thigh. **(a)** Preoperatively: central myxoid, peripheral solid tumor. **(b)** After tumor resection: the hyperintense seroma is evident on the T2W image with a mild marginal contrast enhancement without solid components. **(c)** Follow-up review after 3 months: apart from the persistent seroma, there is also new, solid, contrast-enhancing recurrent tumor posterior to the femur (arrow).

4.5.4 Vascular Malformations

▸ **Pathology.** The current valid worldwide classification of peripheral congenital vascular malformations of the ISSVA differentiates between vascular tumors (usually infantile hemangiomas) and vascular malformations. Vascular malformations are defects of vascular morphogenesis. Based on the underlying type of vessels, they are divided into predominantly venous, capillary, lymphatic (both being low-flow), and arterial or arteriovenous (both high-flow), or combined vascular malformations.

> **Caution**
> Lesions generally referred to as "hemangiomas" are usually vascular malformations! See ▸ Table 4.2 for differentiation.

Venous Malformations

▸ **Radiography.** The identification of phleboliths is almost pathognomonic (▸ Fig. 4.163a). The draining venous system (communication with the trunk veins?) and the lesion itself (often grapelike polycystic in appearance) are examined using phlebography (▸ Fig. 4.163b) and varicography (▸ Fig. 4.164).

▸ **MRI.** MRI is the gold standard for the diagnosis of extension. Strongly hyperintense honeycomb lesions are identified on T2W sequences that are isointense to the muscles on the plain T1W image and enhance strongly with contrast (▸ Figs. 4.165 and ▸ W4.30).

Lymphatic Malformations

▸ **MRI.** Circumscribed lymphatic malformations are macrocystic (cyst diameter greater than 5 mm) or microcystic and are hyperintense on T2W sequences. The cysts show minimal enhancement with contrast, predominantly in the periphery (▸ Fig. 4.166).

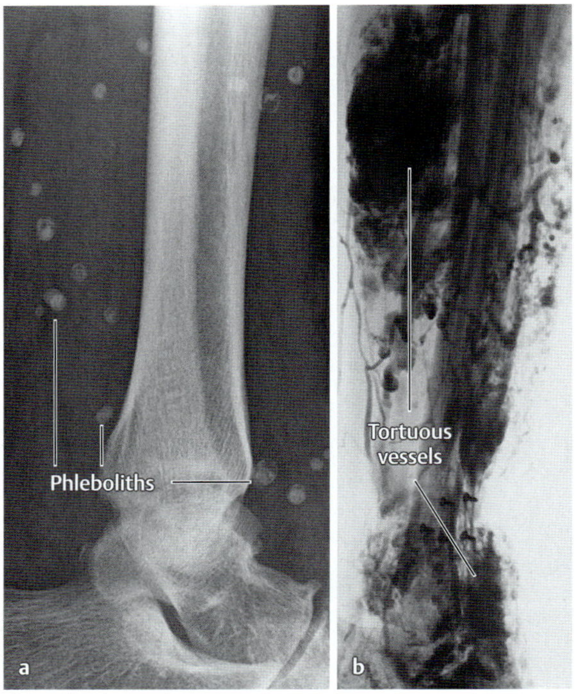

Fig. 4.163 Venous vascular malformation of the lower leg. **(a)** Lateral radiograph. **(b)** Phlebography.

Arteriovenous Malformation

▸ **MRI.** A typical finding is the detection of strongly serpiginous hypointense flow voids as a result of the rapid flow-through in the afferent feeder arteries in an arteriovenous malformation. The contrast-enhanced MR angiography provides a good overall view of the extent of the arteriovenous malformation (▸ Fig. 4.167).

▸ **DSA.** DSA (digital subtraction angiography) is the gold standard; it best reflects the true flow conditions with its accurate temporal and spatial resolution. A distinction is made between the afferent feeder arteries, known as the nidus (a reticular network of arteriovenous shunts) and dilated draining veins (▸ Fig. 4.168).

▸ **DD.** Others **soft tissue tumors** (e.g., sarcomas, schwannomas, juxta-articular myxomas).

Table 4.2 Clinical features distinguishing hemangiomas from vascular malformations

Clinical presentation/ Treatment	Hemangioma	Vascular malformation
Patient age and sex distribution	Infant and young child ♀ >> ♂	Life-long (often asymptomatic during childhood) ♀ ≈ ♂
Natural course	Rapid growth (1st year of life), spontaneous resolution	Growth proportional to the patient
Treatment	Spontaneous resolution (watchful waiting), pharmacological (beta-blockers), laser/cryotherapy	Interventional radiology (sclerotherapy, embolization), laser therapy, open surgery

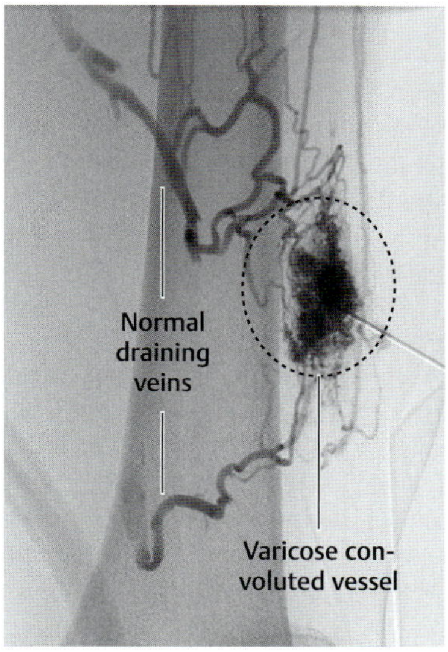

Fig. 4.164 Varicography of a venous vascular malformation of the foot.

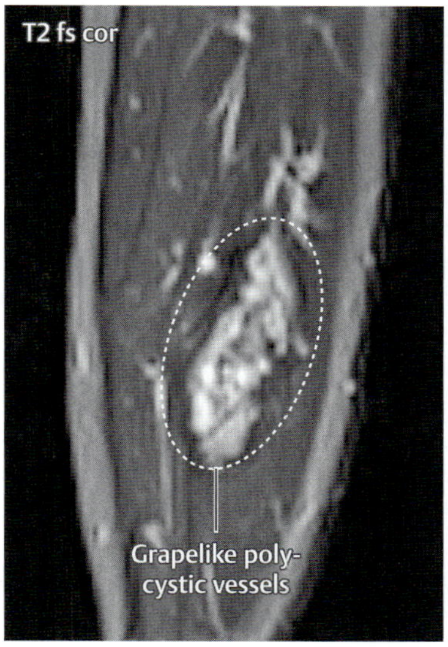

Fig. 4.165 Venous vascular malformation of the lower leg.

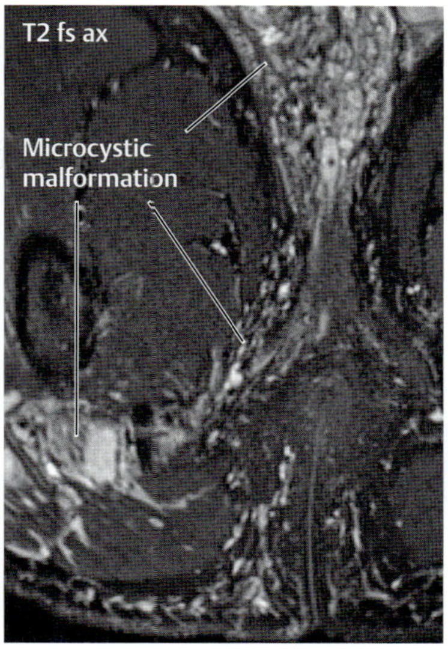

Fig. 4.166 Microcystic lymphatic malformation in the pelvis.

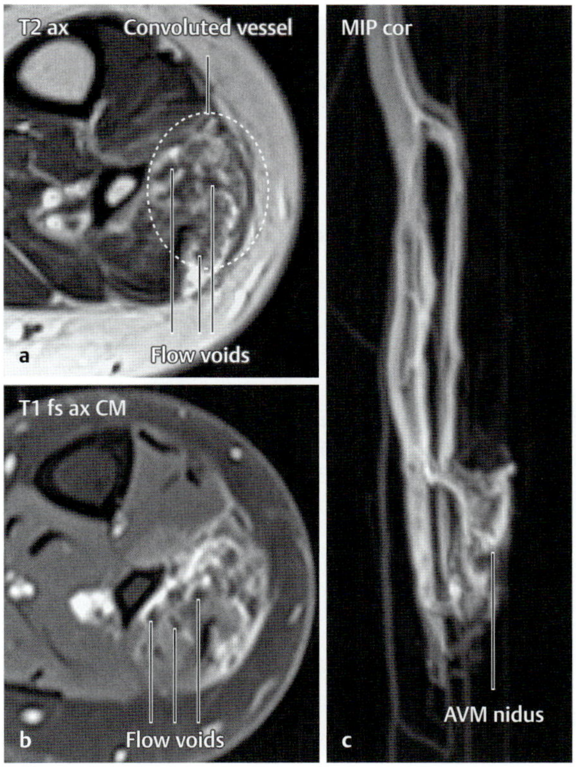

Fig. 4.167 Arteriovenous malformation of the lower leg. **(a)** Identification of hypointense flow voids as a sign of rapid blood flow. **(b)** These are recognizable after contrast administration. **(c)** The anatomy of the arteriovenous malformation is clearly evident on the MIP of the MR angiography. AVM, arteriovenous malformation.

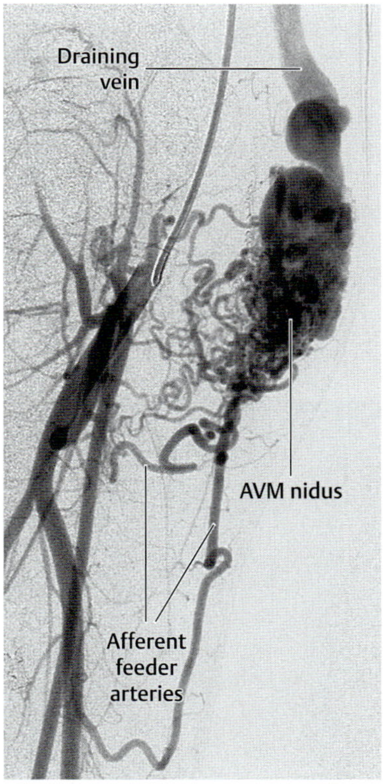

Fig. 4.168 Digital subtraction angiography (DSA) of an arteriovenous malformation of the elbow. AVM, arteriovenous malformation.

4.6 Intra-articular Tumors and Tumorlike Lesions

4.6.1 Loose Joint Bodies

▶ **Pathology.** Loose joint bodies have various etiologies and methods of development. A distinction is made between the following variants:

- Trauma-induced avulsions of bone and/or cartilaginous fragments.
- Degenerations of the meniscus or labrum secondary to trauma or repetitive overload.
- Disintegration of the cartilage in osteoarthritis.
- Chondromas arising from synovial osteochondromatosis (cf. Chapter 4.6.2).
- Loose joint bodies secondary to osteochondritis dissecans and osteonecrosis.
- Rice bodies (fibrin deposits from the synovial membrane) in rheumatoid arthritis (cf. Chapter 10.5).

Loose joint bodies congregate according to the anatomy of the articular cavities and are also found in synovial outpouchings (e.g., Baker's cyst) or in bursae with a joint connection (see ▶ Fig. 4.173).

▶ **Radiography.** Only those loose bodies of bone or cartilaginous/fibrous tissue with calcification or ossification are radiologically visible (▶ Figs. 4.169 and ▶ 4.170).

▶ **US.** Calcification-free chondromas or hyaline cartilage tend to be hypoechoic and are difficult to differentiate from an effusion that is also hypoechoic. The same applies to fibrin deposits (rice bodies). Even small calcifications alter echogenicity, rendering the findings more hyperechoic. Ossifications will produce acoustic shadows. Occasionally it is possible to distinguish the hyperechoic bone from the more hypoechoic cartilage cap in osteocartilaginous avulsions secondary to trauma.

▶ **CT.** In comparison with conventional radiography, CT improves the detectability as well as anatomical location (intra- versus para-articular) of loose joint bodies, provided they are calcified or ossified (▶ Figs. 4.170 and ▶ 4.171). CT arthrography increases sensitivity for detection of loose bodies: hyaline cartilage and fibrous loose bodies are also recognizable (▶ Fig. 4.169).

▶ **MRI.** Nonmineralized cartilage fragments or chondromas are indeed bright on T2W sequences, but are still darker than joint fluid. Windowing of the images is critical to show the distinction. They are hardly distinguishable from water on T1W images. Fibrin deposits (rice bodies) are smaller and more uniform in size; their signal is low on T2W sequences. Loose joint bodies with calcified components are hypointense on T1W and T2W sequences (▶ Figs. 4.172–4.174). If chondromas have become completely ossified, they behave like bone fragments that still have a fatty marrow component: The fat signal predominates in the center (T1W sequence), surrounded by margins with absent signal intensity.

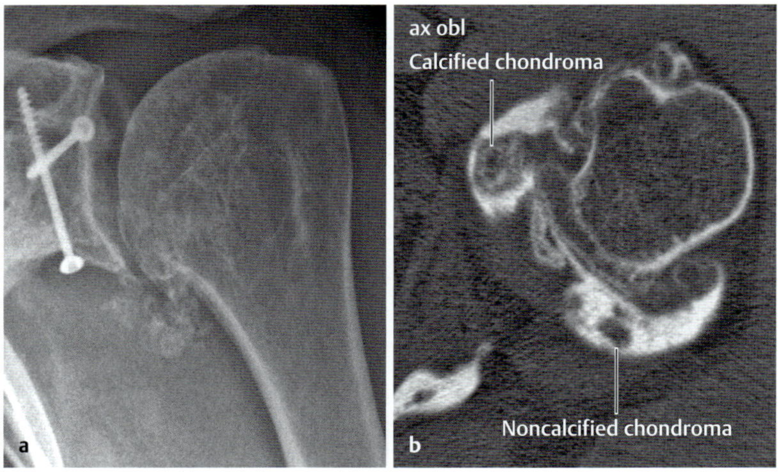

Fig. 4.169 Osteochondromatosis of the shoulder with posttraumatic osteoarthritis. **(a)** Multiple calcified chondromas located in the axillary recess. **(b)** CT arthrography demonstrates the intra-articular location with additional noncalcified loose joint bodies.

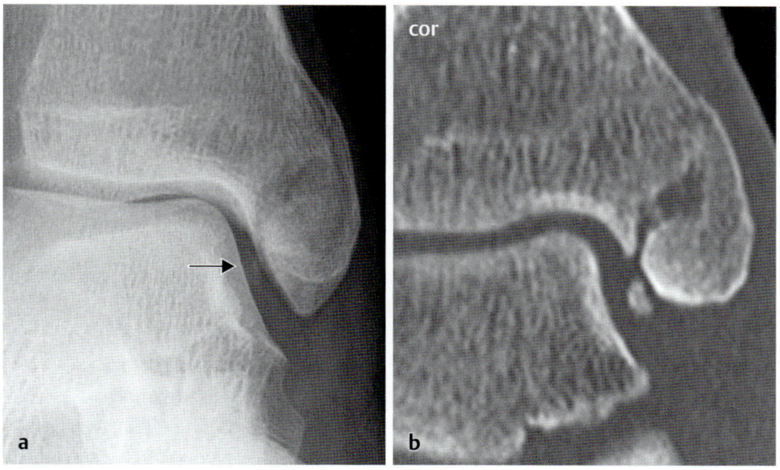

Fig. 4.170 Loose body in the ankle joint secondary to trauma. (a) Detection of a fragment of bone (arrow) in the posterior tibiotalar joint space. (b) CT confirms the intra-articular location.

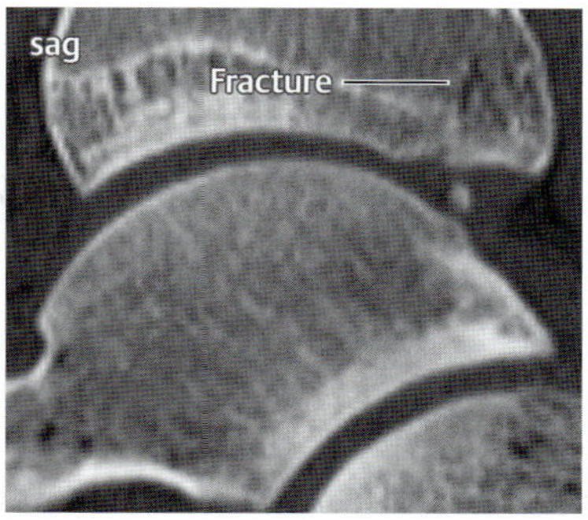

Fig. 4.171 Posttraumatic loose body in the ankle joint.

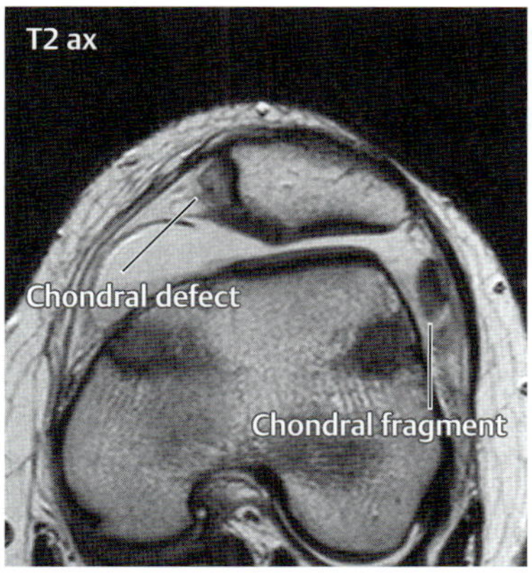

Fig. 4.172 Loose chondral fragment in the knee joint secondary to dislocation of the patella.

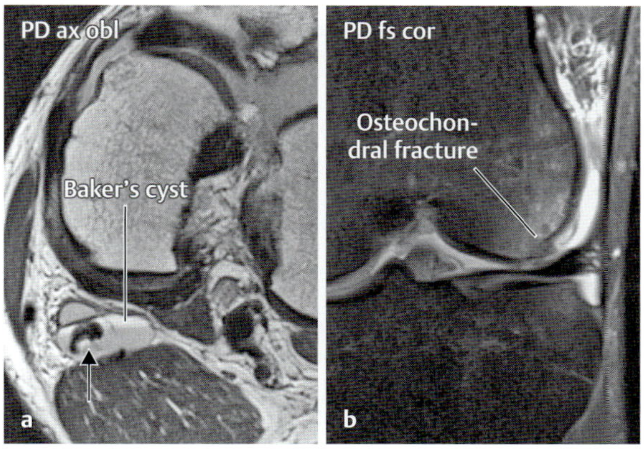

Fig. 4.173 Unusual location for a loose joint body. (a) Osteochondral fragment (arrow) in a Baker's cyst. Fluid level indicative of a fresh hemorrhage. (b) The source of the fragment was an osteochondral fracture of the lateral femoral condyle secondary to patellar dislocation.

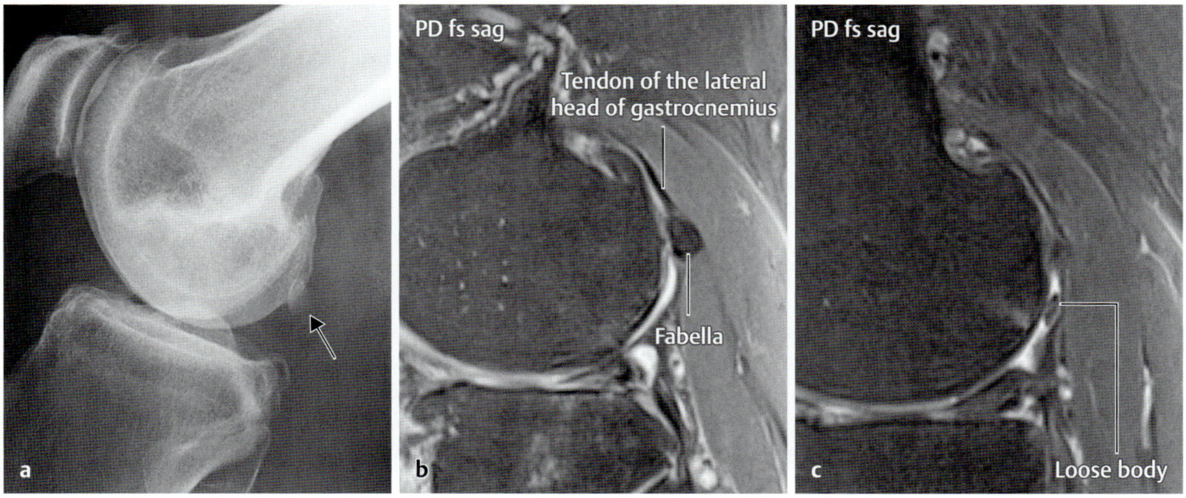

Fig. 4.174 Pitfall: pain after knee injury, preexisting osteoarthritis of the knee. (a) Loose joint body (arrow)? (b) No. This is a sesamoid (fabella). (c) However, MRI demonstrates an adjacent, noncalcified, loose body not visible on the radiograph.

4.6.2 Synovial Chondromatosis

Synovial chondromatosis (synonym: osteochondromatosis) is a benign nodular cartilaginous proliferation. It takes origin from the synovial lining of joints, bursae, and tendon sheaths.

▶ **Pathology.** Synovial metaplasia of unknown origin leads to the formation of tumorlike cartilaginous proliferation. These chondromas appear in varying numbers and receive nourishment from the synovial membrane as long as they remain in contact with it, sometimes via a pedicle. Ultimately, they separate from the synovial membrane and form loose joint bodies. Chondromas can also become completely ossified. The **primary (idiopathic) form** is distinguished from the considerably more common **secondary form** of the disorder that can develop in association with **osteoarthritis**.

▶ **Clinical presentation.** The disorder is associated with nonspecific articular pain, limitation of motion, and effusion.

Age: Any age group, especially during the 3rd to 5th decades of life (primary form). **Location:** Usually monoarticular involvement, especially in the knee, hip, elbow, and shoulder joints. Other locations are possible. **Treatment:** Surgical excision and synovectomy.

▶ **Radiography.** If calcifications or ossifications are absent, synovial chondromatosis is only recognizable in exceptional cases as a soft tissue mass. Calcification can be tiny and/or also display a ring- or comma-shaped to popcornlike configuration. Ossifications finally result in the formation of cortical bone and cancellous bone. If many chondromas are present, then the diagnosis is straightforward from the radiograph. Pressure erosion of adjacent bone is evident in ~ 10% of cases (▶ Fig. 4.175).

▶ **US.** An effusion is always detectable in sonographically easily accessible joints. Round foreign bodies of quite varying echogenicity "float" within the effusion (depending on the degree of calcification).

▶ **CT.** Calcifications and erosions not clearly visible on the radiograph are often recognizable on CT. Clearly marginated pressure erosions can be well differentiated from tumor-related bone destruction.

▶ **MRI.** MRI displays well both purely cartilaginous and already ossified chondromas (▶ Figs. 4.175 and ▶ 4.177); variable signal intensities are to be expected, depending on the degree of calcification and ossification. The spectrum on PDW and T2W sequences ranges from hyperintense to absent signal intensity and their mixed forms. If ossification is present, then the fatty bone marrow may be visualized on T1W images.

Problems may arise with multiple, completely noncalcified chondromas that "float" around in an effusion. Chondromas and water both display a strong signal on T2W sequences. Differentiation is possible by varying the window setting. IV application of gadolinium may also help in establishing a diagnosis as this will result in a characteristic peripheral enhancement around the chondroma (which itself does not enhance with contrast; ▶ Fig. 4.177b).

MRI displays pressure erosions of the intracapsular parts of the bone much more clearly than the radiograph.

▶ **DD.**

Primary and secondary forms of chondromatosis. Differentiation of the primary from the secondary form of chondromatosis is usually readily possible since the secondary form occurs often (but not always) bilaterally in older patients (above 50 years of age) and almost exclusively in association with osteoarthritis.

Rice bodies. Rice bodies (fibrin–collagen particles in rheumatoid arthritis) can resemble chondromatosis on MRI but they are uniformly small, hypointense on T2W sequences, and do *not* calcify. Thus, taking radiograph and MR image into consideration, together with knowledge of the case history, it should be possible to establish a specific diagnosis of rice bodies.

4.6.3 Ganglion and Synovial Cyst

Ganglia are cystic formations comprising a mucinous, gelatinous mass, enclosed in a connective tissue capsule. Ganglia tend to develop in close proximity to joints, although they can also take origin from tendon sheaths, bursae, and ligamentous structures. Their size can range from a few millimeters to several centimeters.

The term **synovial cyst** should be reserved for those lesions which represent a protrusion of the joint capsule, demonstrate a broad connection with the joint cavity, and lack the viscous, gelatinous contents of a ganglion. Typical locations of synovial cysts are, for example, facet joints.

Since a proper epithelial lining of the lumen is absent in ganglia and synovial cysts, they are, strictly speaking, pseudocysts.

Location. Basically, ganglia can occur in any joint of the body but they are most commonly found in the wrist. The knee joint plays a special role, where ganglia and synovial cysts can also take origin from the cruciate ligaments or the menisci, in addition to the joint capsule (e.g., the proximal tibiofibular joint). A **Baker's cyst** is not a ganglion but is regarded as a (synovial) cyst.

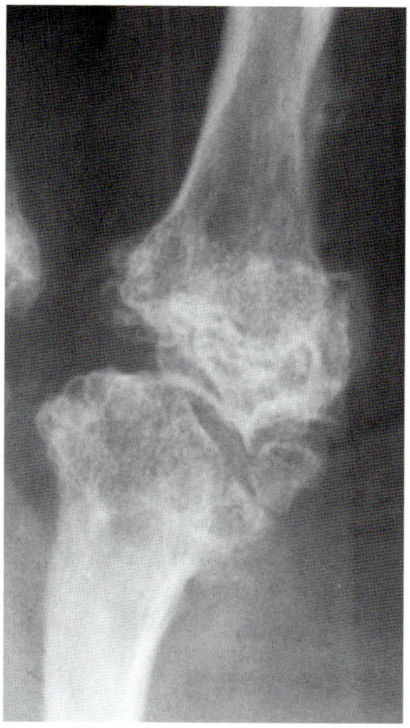

Fig. 4.175 Primary synovial chondromatosis of the second metacarpophalangeal joint.

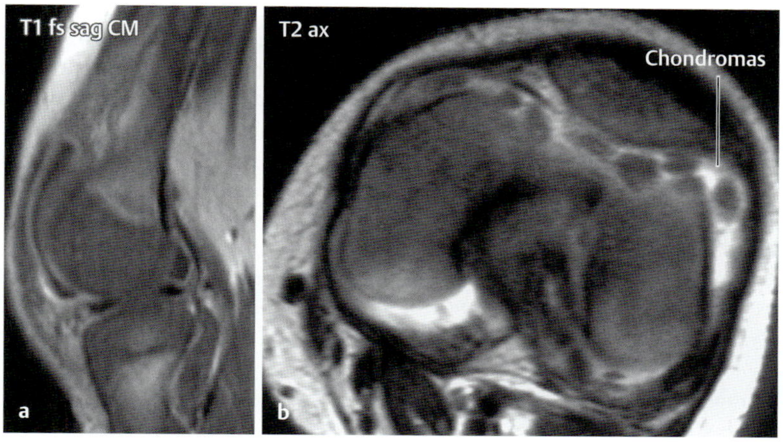

Fig. 4.176 Synovial chondromatosis in a 2-year-old boy. **(a)** Only synovitis is identifiable on the contrast sequence. **(b)** Multiple intra-articular chondromas.

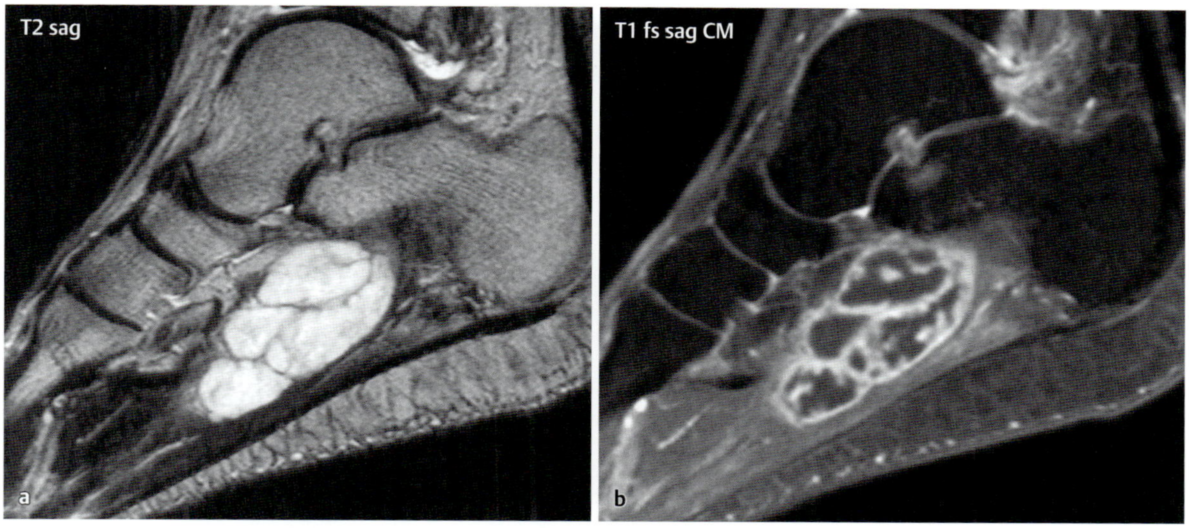

Fig. 4.177 Synovial chondromatosis of the tendon sheath of flexor hallucis longus presenting with tarsal tunnel syndrome. **(a)** Chondromas are barely calcified, hence a bright signal here on the T2W image. No definite delineation from the effusion. **(b)** Only the septations between the chondromas enhance with contrast.

▶ **Pathology.** There are a number of theories about the development of ganglia: When locally increased intra-articular pressure causes the hyaluronic acid–rich synovial joint fluid to escape into the adjacent connective tissue, cavities develop and, with increasing mucoid thickening, a ganglion is formed. This may extend further to penetrate the adjacent structures. A ganglion is usually connected via a pedicle (often tortuous) with its origin at the joint capsule or at another connective tissue structure. Another theory of the development of ganglia assumes herniation of an intact synovial membrane through a weak point in the adjacent connective tissue.

Intraosseous ganglia may develop in one of two possible ways:

- A parosteal soft tissue ganglion breaches the cortex and then extends further into the trabecular bone. If the cortical bone is only eroded, without being completely breached, then a **periosteal ganglion** develops.
- Joint fluid invades the medullary cavity after disruption of the cartilage and the subchondral bone plate. The communication is commonly visualized on MRI or arthrographically. If it obliterates secondarily, then a completely intraosseous ganglion develops, which some authors refer to as "idiopathic."

▶ **Radiography.** **Soft tissue ganglia** are usually not detectable on radiographs. **Intraosseous ganglia** appear as a round or ovoid, sharply delineated lucency usually with a clear sclerotic margin (▶ Fig. 4.178). Intralesional calcifications are absent as a rule, although the lesions can be divided and may appear septated or lobulated.

▶ **US.** Ganglia appear on ultrasound as cystic, usually hypoechoic or anechoic structures. They may be septated or lobulated (complex ganglia). Ultrasound can provide an exact positional relationship of the lesion to adjacent tendons, ligaments, and other anatomical landmarks. The origin of the ganglion pedicle is often to be visualized as a tapering cone or as a narrow, comma-shaped extension (▶ Fig. 4.179). Tendon (sheath) ganglia, on the other hand, often display a broad-based connection with their origin (see ▶ Fig. 4.186).

▶ **CT.** Ganglia appear on CT as sharply demarcated hypodense lesions (10–20 HU [Hounsfield units]). Depending on the viscosity and composition of the contents, density values on plain images can rise to over 60 HU, especially after hemorrhage. Furthermore, CT is capable of identifying the connection of intraosseous ganglia with the joint better than is radiography (▶ Fig. 4.180).

▶ **MRI.** Typically, ganglia have a low signal intensity on T1W sequences, being isointense or slightly hypointense in comparison with muscle, whereas they have a high signal intensity on T2W images (▶ Figs. 4.181–4.186). The wall of the cyst is hypointense on the T2W sequence. After IV contrast administration, ganglia display peripheral enhancement while their contents do not enhance (see ▶ Fig. 4.182).

▶ **DD.**

Osteoarthritic subchondral cysts (geodes). Differentiation can be difficult. Unlike subchondral cysts, ganglia usually do not appear at both articulating parts of the joint and are primarily eccentrically located, outside the main load-bearing area. Typical signs of osteoarthritis, such as joint-space narrowing and osteophyte formations, may also be absent with intraosseous ganglia. However, it should be noted that distinction between the two conditions is of little clinical importance.

Juvenile and aneurysmal bone cysts. These may be distinguished by their position and the size. Aneurysmal bone cysts are noted for their typical fluid–fluid levels on sectional imaging.

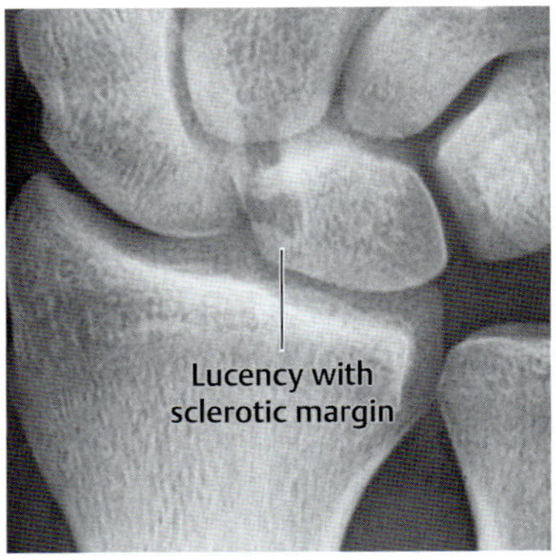

Fig. 4.178 Intraosseous ganglion of the lunate.

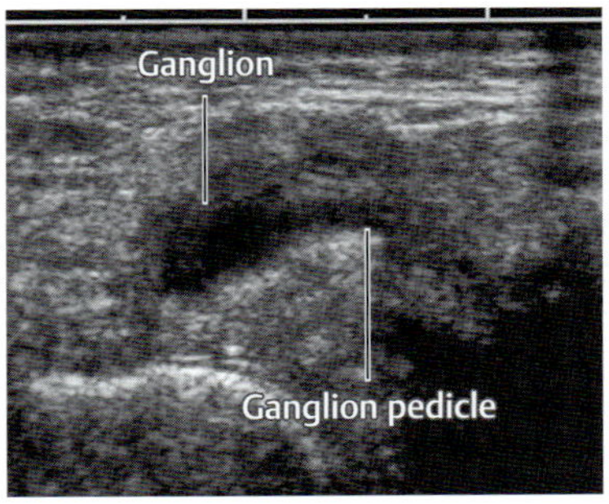

Fig. 4.179 Dorsal wrist ganglion on ultrasound.

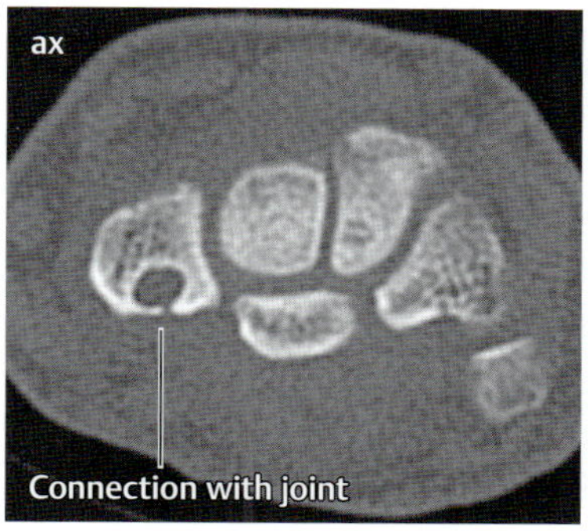

Fig. 4.180 Intraosseous ganglion of the scaphoid.

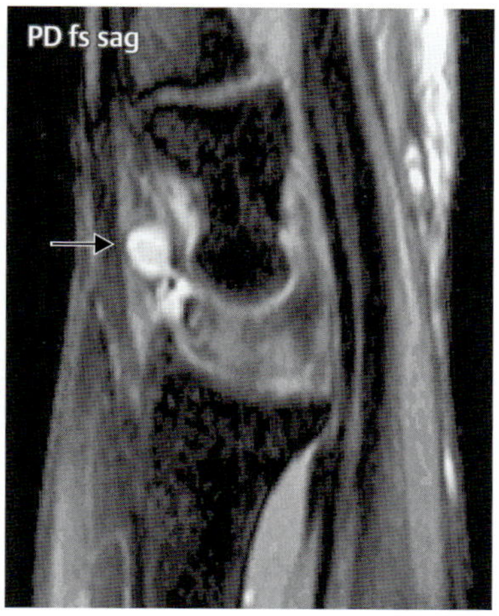

Fig. 4.181 Dorsal wrist ganglion (arrow).

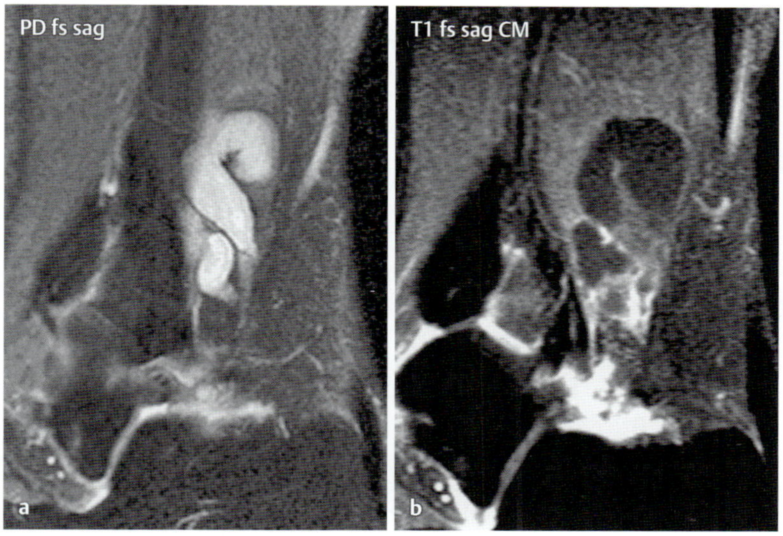

Fig. 4.182 Ankle ganglion. **(a)** Large, tortuous, cystlike mass. **(b)** The contents do not enhance with contrast.

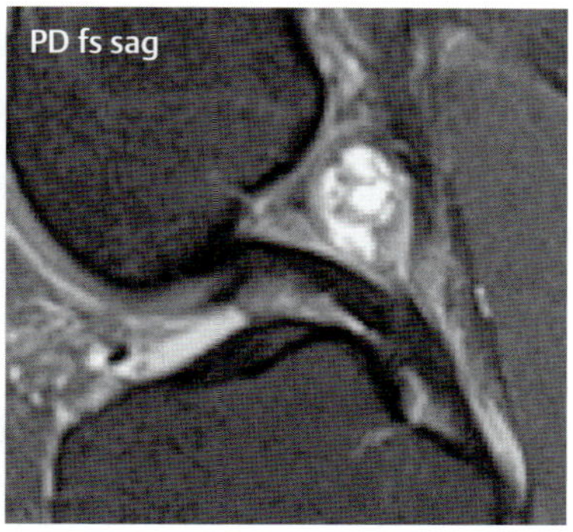

Fig. 4.183 Lobulated ganglion of the posterior cruciate ligament.

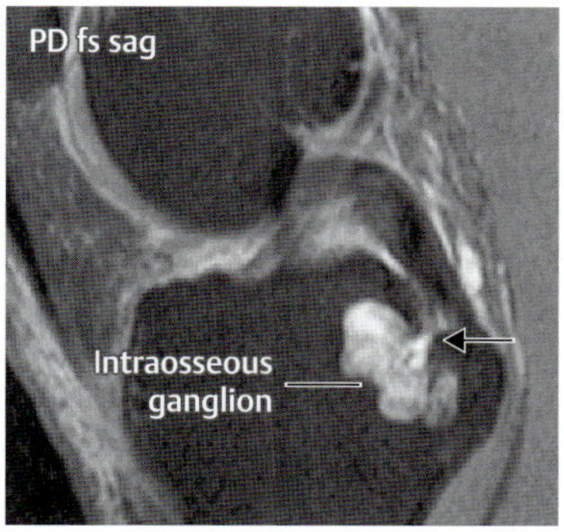

Fig. 4.184 Intraosseous ganglion at the attachment of the posterior cruciate ligament. Note the connection (arrow) with the joint at the insertion of the ligament.

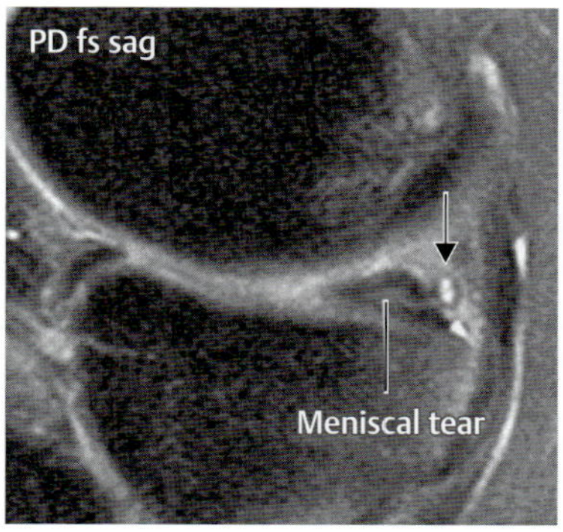

Fig. 4.185 Small meniscal ganglion/cyst (arrow). The ganglion originates from a horizontal tear of the posterior horn.

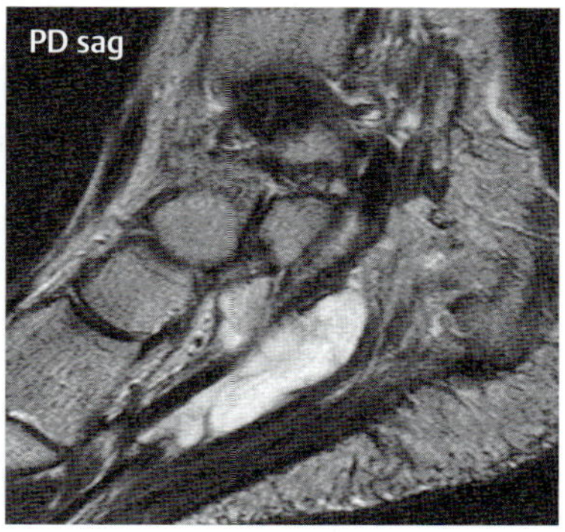

Fig. 4.186 Ganglion of the tendon sheath of flexor hallucis longus. No chondromatosis. Compare ▶ Fig. 4.177.

4.6.4 Lipoma Arborescens

A lipoma arborescens is a rare, intra-articular, villous, synovial proliferation. Subsynovial tissue is replaced by fat cells. This is probably not a genuine tumor but a nonspecific, synovial reaction of unknown etiology. A lipoma arborescens arises mainly in the knee, usually in the 5th to 7th decades of life.

▸ **US.** The lesion is readily identified on ultrasound.

▸ **MRI.** MRI can establish a specific diagnosis: the frondlike/branching fat content of the lesion may be identified on T1W images (▸ Figs. 4.187 and ▸ 4.188). When location is also taken into consideration there should not be any difficulty in diagnosis.

4.6.5 Pigmented Villonodular Synovitis/Giant Cell Tumor of the Tendon Sheath

Pigmented villonodular synovitis (PVNS) is a benign proliferative disease of the synovial membrane. It develops **diffusely** or **focally** in structures with synovial lining. When located in the tendon sheath, it is traditionally referred to as a "giant cell tumor of the tendon sheath."

▸ **Pathology.** A large number of cell types (among others, hyperplastic synoviocytes and the giant cells from which the disorder derives its name) are located in a fibrous stroma. Intra- and extracellular hemosiderin deposits are fundamental, representing the histological correlate for the brownish "pigmentation." Depending on the point in time of the diagnosis, bony erosions may result from the PVNS, especially if the joint is involved. The frequency and size of the erosions depends on whether a large-volume joint (knee) or a joint with a tight capsule (hip, wrist) is affected.

▸ **Clinical presentation.** The degree of pain and swelling depends on the type (focal versus diffuse) and location.

Age: Every age group is affected, especially the third to fourth decade of life. **Location:** The whole hand, followed by the foot, is predominant when tendon sheaths are involved. The type of joint primarily affected by PVNS is the knee; although other joints may be involved. PVNS manifests itself almost exclusively in monoarticular sites. In the knee it may be focal (e.g., in Hoffa's fat pad or the intercondylar notch) or diffuse involving the whole joint. **Treatment:** Excision and synovectomy of the joints. Recurrence rates are high (up to 40%).

▸ **Radiography.** When the joint is involved, the following findings may be expected with varying frequency and severity:

- A soft tissue–dense space-occupying mass is evident (relatively well recognizable from the hemosiderin deposits); there are no calcifications present.
- The intracapsular parts of the skeleton display isolated or multiple erosions of varying sizes (▸ Fig. 4.189a). They are sharply defined and usually surrounded by a sclerotic margin. They are sometimes arranged in mirror-image fashion on either side of the joint (▸ Fig. 4.190). The noncartilaginous parts of the intra-articular parts of the skeleton are primarily affected.
- Joint space is usually preserved.

Giant cell tumor of the tendon sheath results in secondary pressure erosions in ~10 to 20% of cases involving hands and feet. This produces radiolucencies with fine sclerotic margins.

▸ **US.** Ultrasound is primarily used in peripheral lesions (tendon sheaths of the hand and foot). A perfused space-occupying mass is evident (▸ Fig. W4.31).

▸ **CT.** PVNS demonstrates high attenuation on CT. The secondary bony alterations are better visualized and appear unobscured by overlying structures (▸ Fig. 4.189b). It usually becomes evident that the bone is affected secondarily and the space-occupying mass takes origin from the joint.

▸ **MRI.** MRI is the primary diagnostic modality. All forms of PVNS have a partly homogeneous, partly inhomogeneous signal pattern in common, depending on the amount of hemosiderin deposits and collagen content. A classic finding is present when the tissue appears hypointense on T1W and T2W sequences and enhances inhomogeneously with contrast (▸ Fig. 4.191).

▸ **DD.**

Synovial osteochondromatosis. This can be well differentiated by MRI because PVNS commonly enhances inhomogeneously with contrast and there is *no* calcification on radiographs in PVNS.

Hemosiderotic synovitis. Any cause of repeated intra-articular hemorrhage will cause synovial proliferation with hemosiderin deposition, e.g., hemophiliac arthropathy.

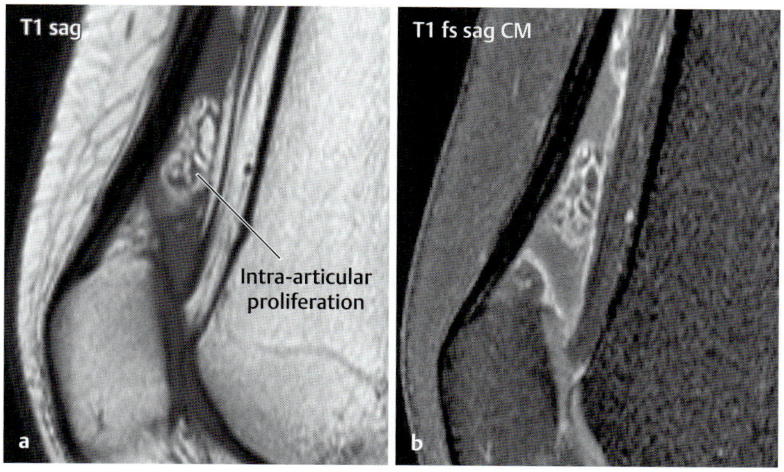

Fig. 4.187 Lipoma arborescens. (a) The signal appears isointense to fat on the T1W image. (b) Synovial contrast enhancement of the fat proliferation.

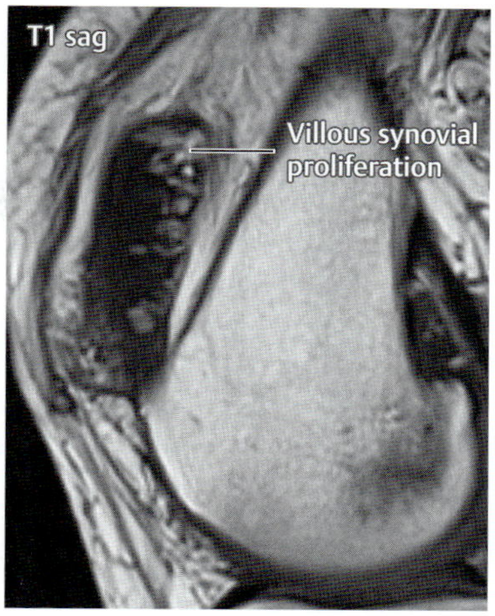

Fig. 4.188 Lipoma arborescens. Villous intra-articular proliferation with signal isointense to fat.

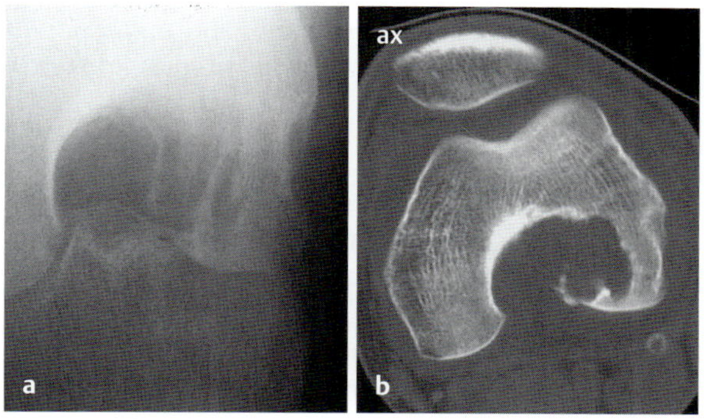

Fig. 4.189 PVNS with destruction of the femoral condyle. (a) Frick's tunnel view. (b) Focal osteolytic lesion with minimal marginal sclerosis.

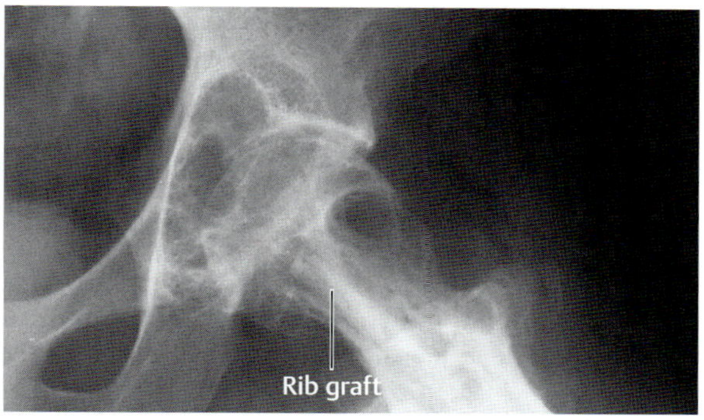

Fig. 4.190 Recurrent PVNS. Appearance after insertion of a rib graft into the femoral neck. Both sides of the joint are affected.

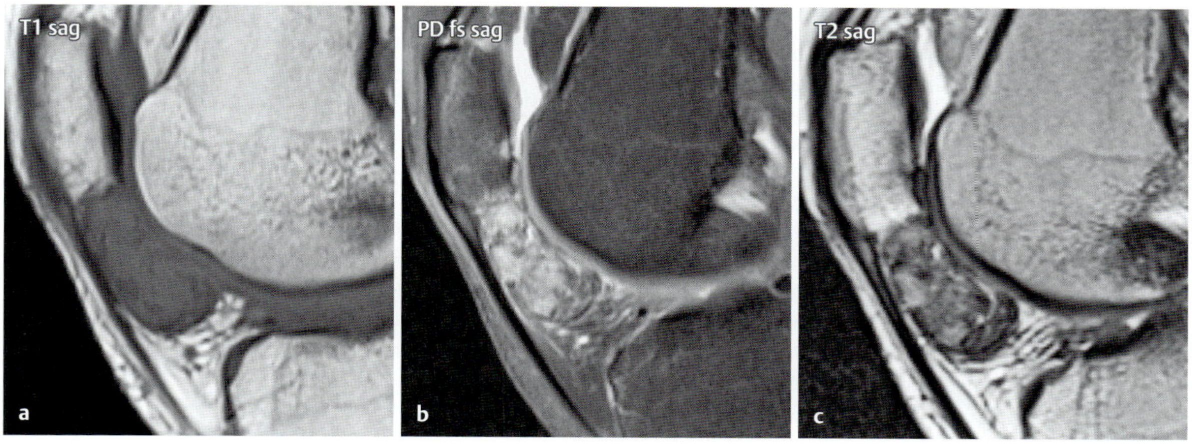

Fig. 4.191 Focal PVNS of the knee joint. (a) Soft tissue mass arising in Hoffa's fat pad. (b) Erosion of the tip of the patella. (c) Typical hypointense signal of the lesion on the T2W image due to hemosiderin deposits.

5 Bone Marrow

5.1 Normal Bone Marrow

Bone marrow is divided into two types (with a smooth transition between the two):

- **Yellow marrow** (fatty marrow) has a high fat content and a poorly developed capillary bed.
- **Red marrow** (hematopoietic marrow) is composed of a mixture of hematopoietic cells and fat with a highly developed network of sinusoids.

5.1.1 Distribution and Age-dependent Physiological Conversion of Red to Yellow Marrow

Red marrow predominates at birth and is increasingly replaced by fatty marrow with aging This normal process follows a typical distribution pattern:

1. In the peripheral skeleton it proceeds in a distal-to-proximal manner (i.e., the forearm before the upper arm, for example).
2. Within the peripheral bone, this conversion occurs initially in the epiphyses and apophyses, followed by the diaphysis and finally the metaphysis; in turn, the distal metaphysis converts first (even in adults, proximal bones maintain residual hematopoietic marrow; ▸ Fig. 5.1).
3. In adults, hematopoietic marrow is still predominantly located in the axial skeleton where gradual fatty conversion of the marrow is a life-long process (▸ Figs. W5.1 and ▸ W5.2).
4. A diagnostically important feature is an (almost) symmetrical distribution at any age.

▸ **CT.** The distribution of red and yellow marrow may be vaguely discerned from the lower attenuation value of fat (fatty marrow, approximately100 HU; hematopoietic marrow, approximately 50 HU; ▸ Fig. 5.2). Any objective measurement based on the trabeculation pattern is very limited and most likely only possible for long tubular bones.

▸ **MRI.** MRI is best suitable for demonstrating bone marrow composition owing to its high soft-tissue contrast. A high contrast between fat and fluid content may be achieved by using the following sequences:

- Fat appears hyperintense on T1W sequences, while fluid is hypointense.
- Fluid-sensitive fat-saturated sequences (T2W and PDW sequences with fat saturation, inversion recovery with bright fluid and dark fat) produce high contrast between fat and fluid.
- Contrast between fluid and fat is poor on T2W sequences without fat saturation. Fibrosis and sclerosis are hypointense.
- Contrast agent uptake is higher in hematopoietic marrow. It should be noted that the administration of contrast is not reliable for differentiating between diffuse infiltrations and normal red marrow.

> **Note**
> A patchy pattern may be evident as a normal variant, with focal nodular hyperplasia (the epiphyses remain uninvolved; ▸ Fig. 5.3) or dense pockets of fat in the bone marrow of elderly patients, especially in the spine (▸ Figs. 5.4 and ▸ 5.5). Patchy bone marrow signal alterations in the skeleton of the foot are normal in children between the ages of 4 and 12 years (▸ Fig. 5.6).

▸ **NUC MED.** Metabolic activity (e.g., FDG uptake in PET imaging) is somewhat higher in hematopoietic marrow than in fatty marrow.

5.1.2 Reconversion of Yellow to Red Marrow/Bone Marrow Hyperplasia

This process takes place in a direction opposite to that of conversion. Marrow within the proximal portion of a bone is recruited first for hematopoiesis, i.e., the proximal metaphyses in the long tubular bones (▸ Fig. 5.7). Typically, reconversion does not take place in the epiphyses and apophyses.

> **Caution**
> Physiological bone marrow conversion may be delayed in children!

Causes of reconversion

- If the existing **hematopoietic marrow** is **insufficient** (e.g., in the presence of fibrosis, cell infiltration), fatty marrow regions are at once recruited for new blood formation.
- Reconversion is also seen in the "healthy": an **increased demand for hematopoietic marrow** can exist, for example, in marathon runners and in those taking hematopoietic factors, as well as in smokers and obese patients.
- **Compensatory hypertrophy** of hematopoietic marrow is seen e.g., in cases of anemia, infection, heart failure, and lung disease.

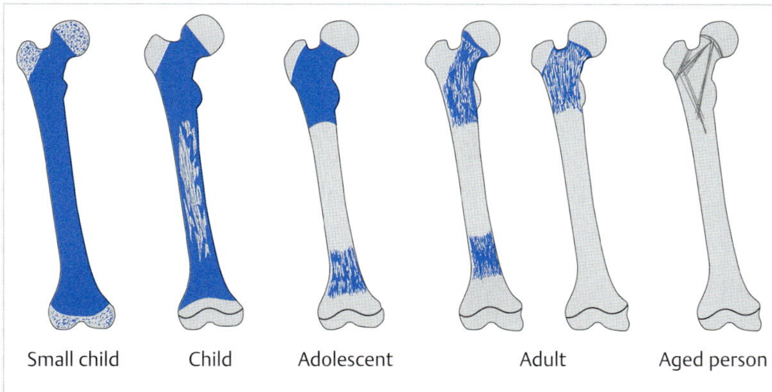

Fig. 5.1 Normal age-dependent distribution of red and yellow marrow in the femur.

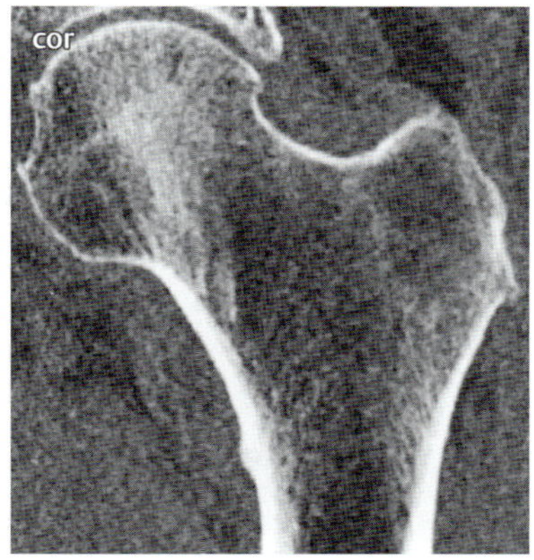

Fig. 5.2 Bone marrow on CT; 1-mm CT slice. The comparison between muscle and bone marrow gives a semiquantitative assessment of the presence of fatty marrow. Fine trabeculae will falsify the measurement of a region of interest.

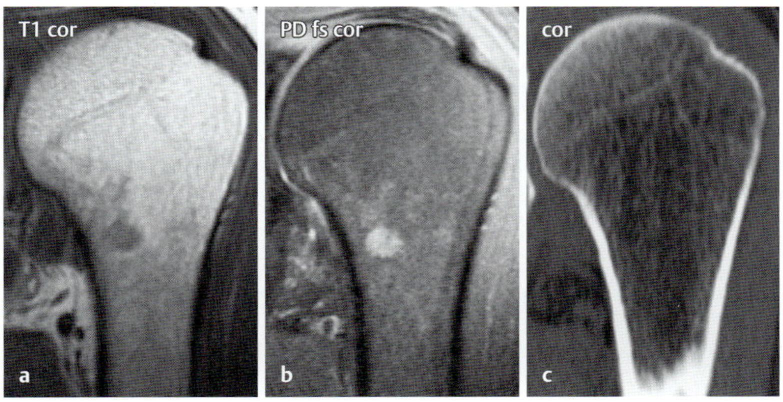

Fig. 5.3 Nodular hyperplasia of the bone marrow. Normal variant. **(a)** Nodular red marrow in the surgical neck of the humerus (T1W image). **(b)** Corresponding PDW image. **(c)** CT demonstrates a rounded lucency and reduced trabeculae at the site of the MRI finding; no marginal sclerosis.

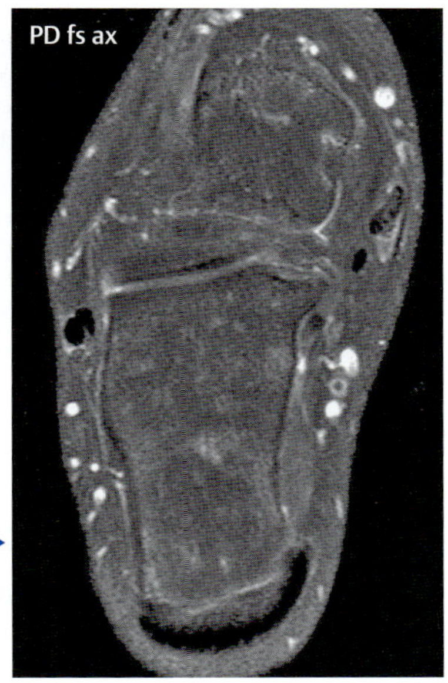

Fig. 5.6 Patchily increased bone marrow signal within the foot of a 12-year-old child. Normal variant.

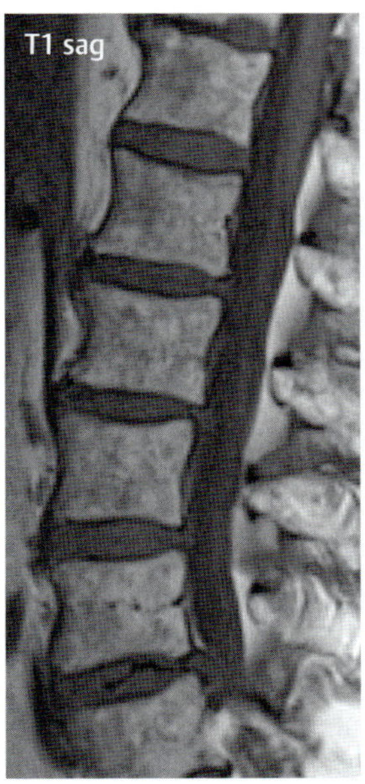

Fig. 5.4 Female breast cancer patient after chemotherapy. A definite differentiation between red marrow reconversion and tumor infiltration is not possible.

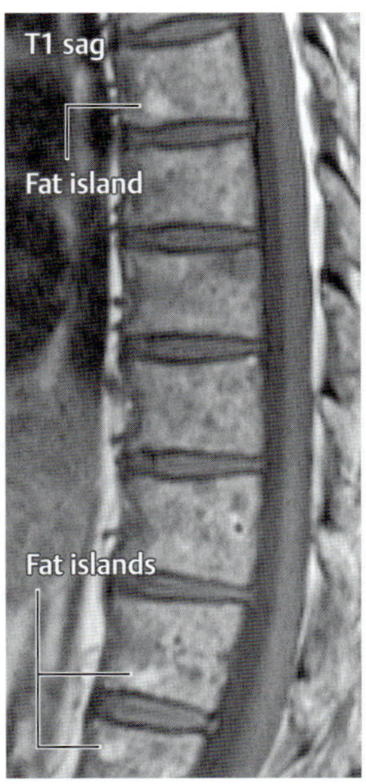

Fig. 5.5 Diffuse, in part nodular, infiltration of the bone marrow by plasmacytoma. Residual hyperintense islands of fat are also seen.

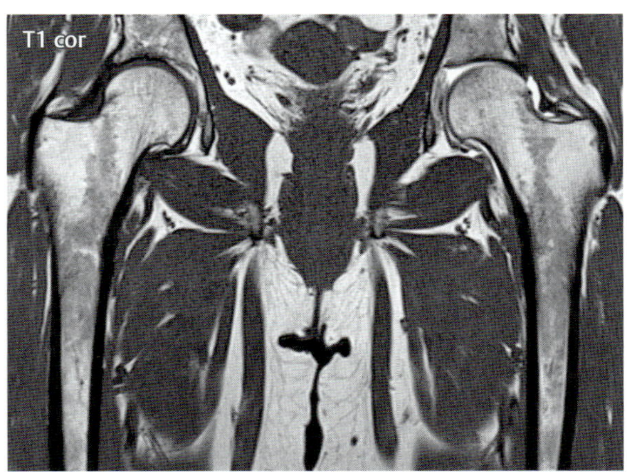

Fig. 5.7 Symmetrical residual hematopoietic marrow in the proximal femurs in this 40-year-old obese female smoker.

> **Note**
> In order to better evaluate diffuse alterations of the bone marrow, T1W contrast may be compared with normal skeletal muscle or, in the spine, with the signal of the intervertebral disks. Bone marrow that is darker than skeletal muscle or disk is an indication of diffuse marrow infiltration, which is usually pathologic. This is also referred to in the spine as the "bright disk sign" (▸ Figs. 5.8 and ▸ W5.3).

5.2 Anemias and Hemoglobinopathies

5

5.2.1 Anemias

▸ **Pathology.** Anemias develop from abnormal blood loss (acute or chronic hemorrhage), reduced production (e.g., aplastic anemia; deficiency of iron, vitamin B_{12}, or folic acid; erythropoietin deficiency), ineffective hematopoiesis (hemoglobinopathies), and increased degradation (e.g., hemolytic anemia).

Aplastic Anemia

▸ **Pathology.** This is a rare disorder. Aplastic anemia is associated with inadequate blood-cell formation within the bone marrow and blood. There can be a number of causes for this, such as radiotherapy, chemotherapy, paroxysmal nocturnal hemoglobinuria, Fanconi anemia, hepatitis, pregnancy, and thymoma. However, aplastic anemia may also be idiopathic.

▸ **MRI.** There are signs of cellular depletion as evidenced by extensive fatty marrow. Hematopoietic marrow is once again identified after successful therapy, appearing as diffuse or patchy islands of cellular marrow. Hemosiderosis (Chapter 5.3.1) may develop after multiple blood transfusions.

5.2.2 Hemoglobinopathies (Thalassemia, Sickle Cell Anemia)

▸ **Pathology.** All hemoglobinopathies have a similar effect on the skeletal system and result in alterations of bone and bone marrow that are the result of bone marrow hyperplasia due to insufficient hemoglobin production.

▸ **Radiography.** Expansion of the medullary cavity, coarsened trabeculation, and cortical thinning are typical radiographic signs. The so-called hair-on-end phenomenon is seen on skull radiographs (▸ Fig. 5.9). "Fish vertebrae" occur in the spine secondary to decreased bone density.

▸ **MRI.** MRI will demonstrate reconversion of bone marrow or—in children and adolescents—delayed fatty marrow conversion. Extramedullary blood production may develop, producing typical symmetrical, lobulated, paravertebral and presacral space-occupying lesions that have intermediate signal intensity on T1W images and enhance moderately with contrast (▸ Fig. W5.4).

Acute and chronic complications involving bone are mainly the result of vascular occlusion, infection, or a combination of the two.

Vascular occlusion. In the growing skeleton, this results in a disturbance of bone growth due to premature closure of the growth plates (H-shaped vertebra; ▸ Fig. 5.10). Infarctions occur in all regions of the tubular bones (▸ Fig. 5.11) and less commonly in flat bones. Infarction may also occur in muscles and other soft tissues.

Osteomyelitis. Osteomyelitis is commonly caused by *Staphylococcus aureus* or *Salmonella typhi*. It is usually not possible to discriminate between septic infarction (osteomyelitis) and aseptic infarction.

5.3 Metabolic Bone Marrow Alterations

5.3.1 Hemosiderosis and Hemochromatosis

▸ **Pathology.** Hemochromatosis is a hereditary disorder leading to iron deposition in organs as well as in the bone marrow as a result of excessive iron absorption. "Hemosiderosis" is the more general term for increased iron deposition in tissues, most commonly after multiple blood transfusions, but may also occur secondarily to hemolytic anemia and other disorders.

▸ **MRI.** Iron deposition renders the bone marrow hypointense on T1W and T2W sequences. T2* GRE sequences demonstrate particularly low signal intensity. An almost complete loss of signal may be seen in marked cases (known as "black marrow"; ▸ Fig. 5.12).

5.3.2 Lipidoses and Lysosomal Storage Diseases

These disorders are due to a genetic defect resulting in the accumulation of partially degraded, insoluble metabolites within the lysosomes.

▸ **Pathology.** One example is **Gaucher's disease** (glucocerebrosidosis), in which glucocerebrosides accumulate in the reticuloendothelial cells of liver, spleen, and bone marrow.

▸ **Radiography.** Typical features include reduced tubulation of long tubular bones (Erlenmeyer flask deformity), osteoporosis (with subsequent fractures), and osteonecrosis (H-shaped vertebrae; see ▸ Fig. 5.10). Less commonly seen are sharply marginated or moth-eaten osteolytic lesions and very rarely osteosclerosis.

▸ **MRI.** The areas of cellular deposition are hypointense, both on T1W and T2W sequences. Initially the signal alteration tends to be patchy. Typically the region around the basivertebral veins still demonstrates normal bone marrow signal in less severe cases. The signal becomes diffusely hypointense in advanced stages. Subsequently, bone marrow recruitment with reconversion takes place. These alterations regress in patients who respond to enzyme replacement therapy.

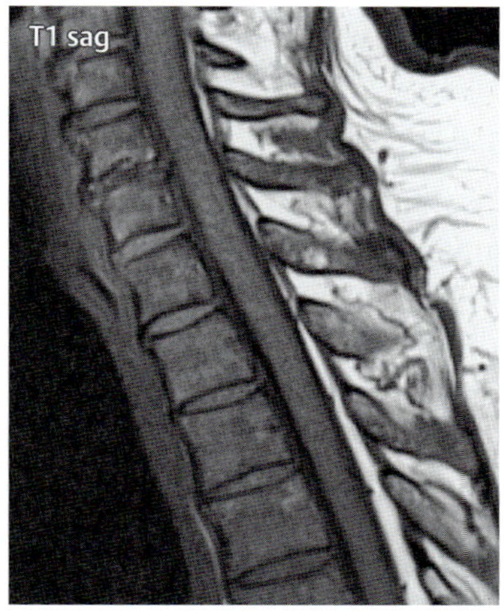

Fig. 5.8 Bright disk sign due to diffuse hematopoietic marrow in a 74-year-old patient with anemia. Note the hypointensity of the bone marrow compared with the disks (and with the subcutaneous fat).

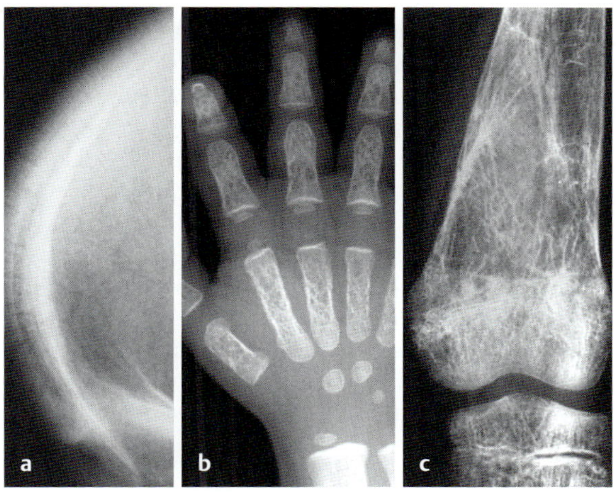

Fig. 5.9

Fig. 5.9 Thalassemia. **(a)** Typical hair-on-end appearance of the skull. **(b)** Coarsened trabeculation and expanded medullary cavities in a child's hand. **(c)** Erlenmeyer flask deformity (metaphyseal flaring in long bones).

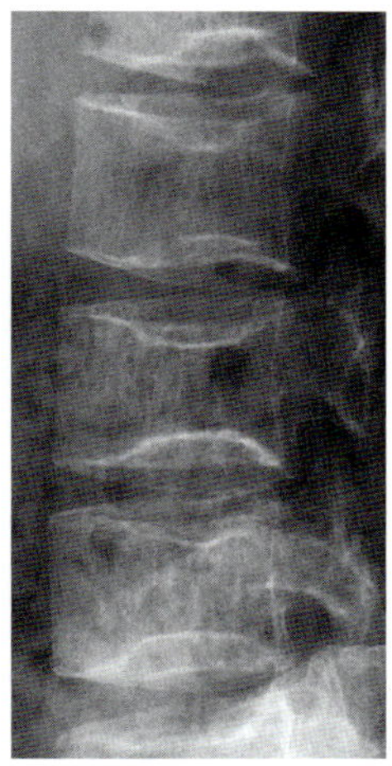

Fig. 5.10

Fig. 5.10 H-shaped vertebra (also known as Lincoln log vertebra) in sickle cell anemia.

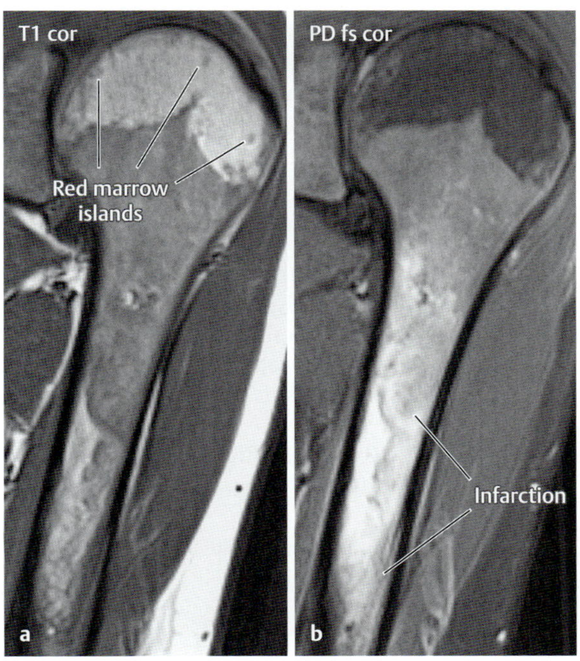

Fig. 5.11 A 25-year-old patient with known sickle cell anemia. Sickle-cell crisis 3 weeks previously; since then pain in the upper arm. **(a)** Hyperplastic red marrow extending as far as the epiphysis. **(b)** Extensive infarctions, presumably developed over time, in the proximal diaphysis.

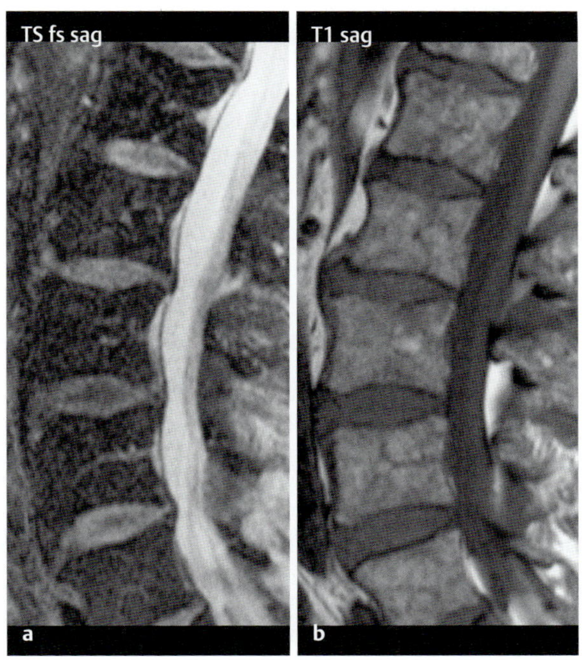

Fig. 5.12 Hemosiderosis. **(a)** Significantly decreased signal intensity of the bone marrow on the T2W fs image. **(b)** Smaller, nonspecific, areas of low signal intensity on the T1W image.

Complications. The disease can result in infarction, epiphyseal osteonecrosis, osteomyelitis and fracture.

5.3.3 Serous Atrophy

Gelatinous material (mucopolysaccharides) instead of fat is found in the bone marrow in patients with severely reduced body fat content, e.g., in cases of tumor cachexia, anorexia nervosa, or chronic infections such as HIV. The signal pattern is similar to that of fluid on T1W and T2W images; there is no enhancement with contrast. The subcutaneous tissues of these patients consist of vascular connective tissue and therefore exhibit a loss of subcutaneous fat signal, and contrast enhancement.

5.3.4 Fat Accumulation Secondary to Osteoporosis

Reduction of bone mineral density is associated with a subsequent increase in marrow fat content (hyperintense on T1W and T2W, hypointense on fat-saturated sequences; ▸ Fig. 5.13). At the same time perfusion on dynamic sequences is reduced.

5.4 Chronic Myeloproliferative Diseases

5.4.1 Myelodysplastic Syndrome (Also Known as Preleukemia)

This is a heterogeneous group of diseases that result in ineffective production, or dysplasia, of myeloid cells. These may be idiopathic or may result from secondary causes (e.g., radiotherapy, chemotherapy, toxic substances). About one-third of patients later develop acute myeloid leukemia.

▸ **MRI.** Signs of marrow reconversion are found on T1W images; fat-suppressed T2W sequences may appear normal in the spine or may have altered signal intensity.

5.4.2 Polycythemia Vera

This is a pre-neoplastic condition originating from granulocytic and megakaryocytic cell lines. Characteristic features include hepatosplenomegaly, thrombosis, and hemorrhage.

▸ **Radiography/MRI.** Radiographs may reveal diffuse osteoporosis and osteosclerosis (often associated with secondary myelofibrosis). Bone infarctions and gouty arthritis may also develop. Diffuse cellular infiltration and myelofibrosis or myelosclerosis demonstrate nonspecific homogeneous, hypointense signal intensity on T1W images.

5.4.3 Myelofibrosis/ Osteomyelofibrosis

Osteomyelofibrosis is a rare chronic disorder of middle and advanced age, characterized by an abnormal maturation process of erythrocytes and granulocytes with fibrosis and later sclerosis of the medullary cavity. It either appears secondarily to other bone marrow diseases or is idiopathic, commonly as a precursor of leukemia.

▸ **Radiography/MRI.** Focal or diffuse sclerosis is evident, especially within the axial skeleton and proximal portions of the humeri and femurs. Signs of bone absorption are only rarely present; instead diffuse, nonspecific cellular infiltration or fibrosis is found, with diffuse low signal intensity within the bone marrow on T1W and variable signal intensity on T2W sequences. A more typical finding on MRI is osteomyelofibrosis in which the fibrotic tissue appears hypointense on all MRI sequences, yet the architecture of the bone marrow is preserved. The result of osteomyelofibrosis is that blood-forming marrow is recruited in the periphery (reconversion) and extramedullary hematopoiesis may also be seen (▸ Fig. 5.14).

▸ **DD.** The differential diagnosis of increased bone density on radiographs includes other bone marrow disorders such as lymphoma, leukemia, osteoblastic metastases, and sarcoidosis, or metabolic disorders such as fluorosis, renal osteodystrophy and osteopetrosis, (pseudo-) hypoparathyroidism, myelofibrosis in polycythemia, and mastocytosis.

5.4.4 Essential Thrombocythemia

Together with polycythemia vera and osteomyelofibrosis, essential thrombocythemia is one of the group of Philadelphia-negative, chronic myeloproliferative disorders. Platelet counts are elevated, with an associated increased risk of myocardial infarction and stroke. Myelofibrosis is commonly found.

5.4.5 Systemic Mastocytosis

This disorder is associated with abnormal mast cell proliferation in bone marrow, skin, lymph nodes, gastrointestinal tract, liver, and spleen. Clinical findings include urticaria, skin erythema, tachycardia, anaphylactic reactions, chronic weight loss, weakness and gastric ulcer.

▸ **Radiography/CT.** Osteolysis, diffuse loss of bone mineral density and sclerosis are seen (▸ Figs. 5.15 and ▸ Fig. 5.16).

▸ **MRI.** Signs of patchy or diffuse cellular infiltration are apparent on T1W images (▸ Fig. 5.17).

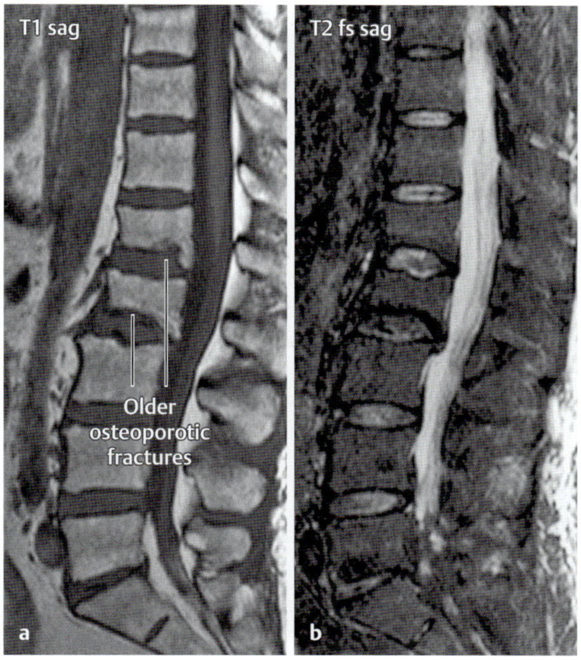

◀ **Fig. 5.13** Osteoporosis in a 47-year-old woman. The bone marrow of the spine demonstrates increased fat accumulation for the patient's age. **(a)** Increased bone marrow signal (fatty marrow) on the T1W image. **(b)** Significantly decreased signal intensity on the corresponding fat saturated image.

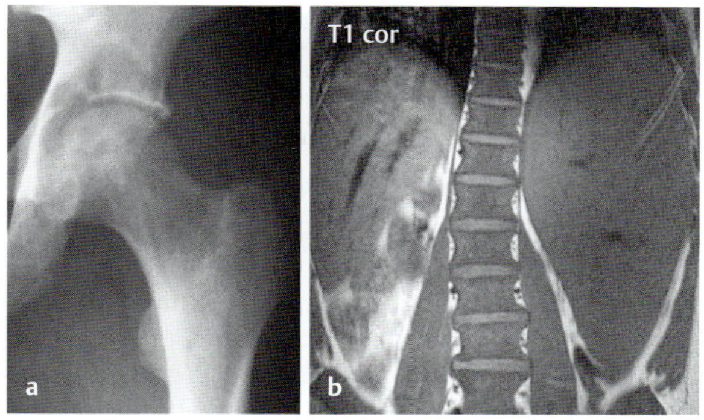

Fig. 5.14 Osteomyelofibrosis. **(a)** Sclerosis of the axial skeleton, here in the hip joint. **(b)** MRI confirms diffuse bone marrow infiltration and splenomegaly.

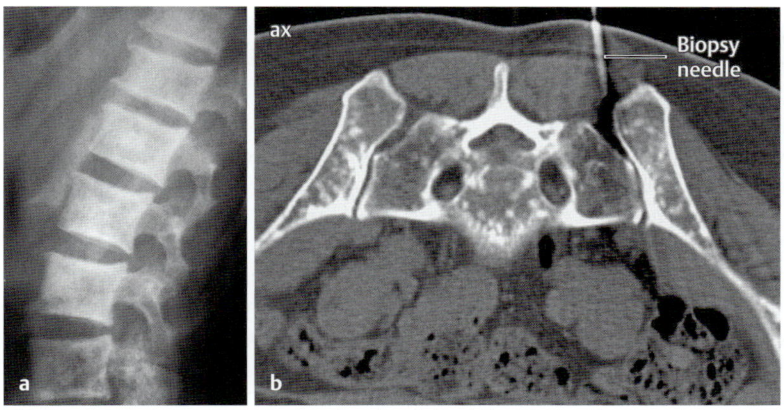

Fig. 5.16 Systemic mastocytosis. (Images courtesy of B. Jobke, Heidelberg, Germany.) **(a)** Significantly increased sclerosis of the vertebrae. **(b)** Patchy sclerosis of the bone marrow.

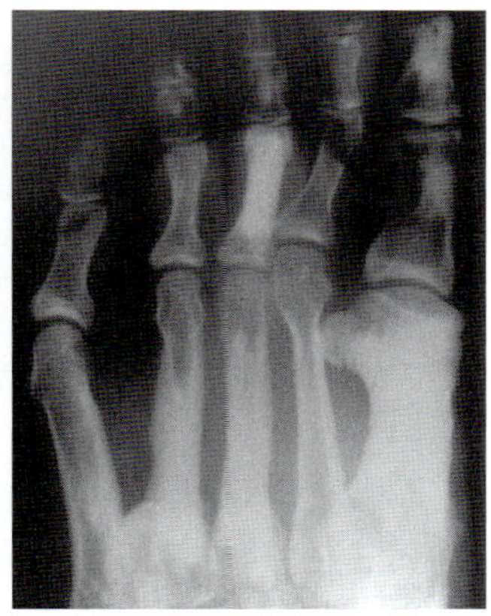

Fig. 5.15 Mastocytosis. Peripheral focal osteosclerosis. The image is not specific, but manifestation and location are certainly typical.

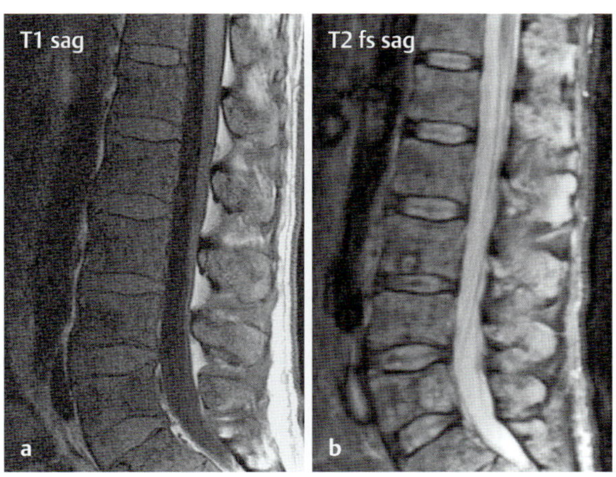

Fig. 5.17 Systemic mastocytosis. (Images courtesy of B. Uffmann, Vienna, Austria.) **(a)** Hypointensity of the bone marrow on the T1W image in the presence of diffuse infiltration. **(b)** Patchy hyperintensity of the bone marrow on the fat-saturated T2W image.

5.5 Malignant Disorders of the Bone Marrow

5.5.1 Multiple Myeloma/ Solitary Plasmacytoma

▸**Pathology.** Myeloma arises from an asymptomatic premalignant proliferation of monoclonal plasma cells. Multistep genetic and microenvironmental changes lead to the transformation of these cells into a malignant neoplasm. Myeloma is thought to evolve most commonly from a monoclonal gammopathy of undetermined clinical significance (usually known as MGUS) that progresses to smoldering myeloma and, finally, to symptomatic multiple myeloma. Myelomatous plasma cell proliferation leads to displacement of the hematopoietic stem cells within the bone marrow. Multiple myeloma accounts for approximately 1% of neoplastic diseases and 13% of hematologic cancers and usually develops in older age.

5

A solitary plasmacytoma is less common (~ 5% of cases) and is distinguished from multiple myeloma. Solitary plasmacytoma is characterized by a mass of neoplastic monoclonal plasma cells in either bone or soft tissue without evidence of systemic disease attributed to myeloma (increased calcium, renal insufficiency, anemia, or multiple bone lesions). The most common location of a solitary plasmacytoma in bone is in the axial skeleton. The incidence increases exponentially with advancing age. Solitary plasmacytoma of bone carries a significant risk of progressing to multiple myeloma.

The osseous pattern of involvement of multiple myeloma is quite variable. Usually there is diffuse involvement of varying degree that is not always evident on imaging, but it may exhibit multifocal micro- and/or macronodular lesions or a mixed picture. Depending on location, the lesions may destroy the cortex and invade adjacent soft tissues. The axial skeleton and proximal tubular bones (regions with hematopoietic marrow) are primarily affected. Extraosseous manifestation is rare.

Typically, a bone marrow biopsy is taken from the iliac crest, and if this proves to be negative then a biopsy of a focal lesion is performed (best done under CT guidance).

▸**Clinical presentation.** Apart from nonspecific general symptoms (B symptoms), bone pain, and pathologic fractures occur as a result of increased bone absorption. Displacement of normal blood-forming cells in the bone marrow results in anemia, a tendency to bleed, and infections.

Complications

- Fractures.
- Bone infarctions and osteonecrosis.
- Amyloidosis (in 5–10% of cases of multiple myeloma) (Chapter 8.6).

▸**Radiography.** Purely osteolytic foci (absent intralesional matrix calcifications) without marginal sclerosis are evident and create the impression of being circumscribed, as if "punched out" (▸Figs. 5.18 and ▸5.19). An infiltrative, moth-eaten pattern is also possible. Cortical bone is commonly destroyed. Abnormal soft tissue opacity adjacent to an involved bone is suspicious for soft tissue invasion. A periosteal reaction creating the impression of a so-called neocortex is possible. Diffuse involvement may express itself in the form of "osteopenia," together with corresponding subjective symptoms. A sclerotic margin may form around the lesion during and after chemotherapy (▸Fig. 5.20).

> **Note**
>
> The still commonly used classification of multiple myeloma according to **Durie and Salmon** includes radiographic evidence of osteolytic lesions as one criterion. Standard radiography, however, is not commonly used for detecting osteolytic lesions, and has been replaced by what is known as plasmacytoma CT (see following text). Standard radiography should only be used for clarifying localized pain (circumscribed lytic lesion, fracture?). It is also not suitable for monitoring therapy.

▸**CT.** Plain low-dose spiral CT from the vertex to the thigh (plasmacytoma CT) has established itself as a fast and, in comparison with radiography, more sensitive examination for diagnosing and staging myeloma of the axial skeleton. Radiation exposure is no greater than it is for screening with conventional radiographs (axial skeleton, head, bilateral proximal humerus, and proximal femur). With the option of generating multiplanar reconstructions, osteolytic lesions of the spine at risk of fracture can be detected and assessed significantly earlier (▶ Figs. W5.5–W5.7).

▸**Important findings.** The findings in ▸Table 5.1 have proven useful for judging whether the osteolytic lesions detected are typical for multiple myeloma.

▸**MRI.** The MRI appearance of the lesions is nonspecific (hypointense on T1W, hyperintense on fluid-sensitive sequences, contrast enhancement; ▸Fig. 5.21; ▶ Figs. W5.8 and ▶ W5.9; see also ▶ Fig. W5.7). The bright disk sign (Chapter 5.1) in the spine is helpful in cases of diffuse involvement.

> **Caution**
>
> The marrow changes can be so subtle in some cases of multiple myeloma that in the early stages, the MRI may appear "normal." A typical, albeit rare, feature is the "salt and pepper" (variegated) pattern caused by minute cell clusters and islands of fat (see ▸Fig. 5.5). Follow-up studies

Table 5.1 Myeloma CT findings based on the Durie-Salmon radiographic staging system

Evaluation	Finding
Normal	No cortical bone destruction, no intratrabecular radiolucencies > 1 cm
Unclear finding ("nonspecific")	No cortical bone destruction, circumscribed intratrabecular radiolucencies > 1 cm
Pathologic finding ("typical" for plasmacytoma)	Evidence of cortical destruction associated with intratrabecular radiolucencies
Fracture risk	• In tubular bones: cortical bone destruction of > 50% of the circumference • In vertebrae: cortical bone destruction of > 50% of the lateral, anterior or posterior wall

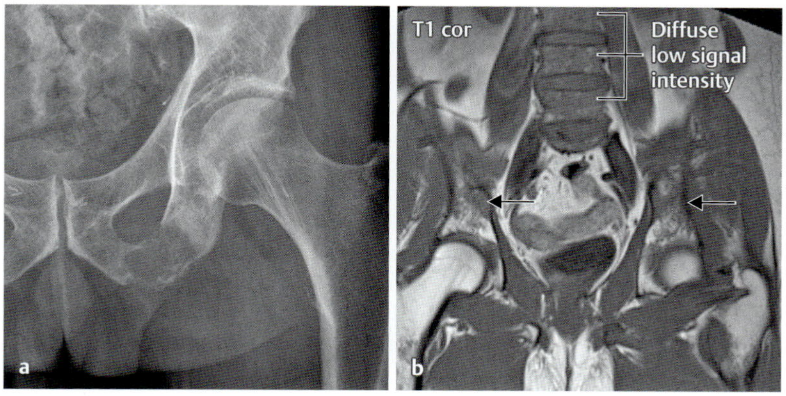

Fig. 5.18 Multiple myeloma. **(a)** Sharply defined osteolytic lesions of the ischial tuberosity and the lesser trochanter. **(b)** As well as these lesions, whole-body MRI clearly demonstrates a multifocal involvement of the pelvis (arrows) and a diffuse infiltration of the spine.

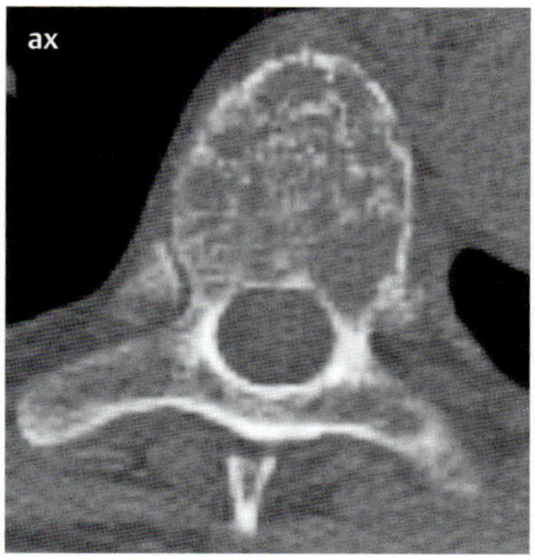

Fig. 5.19

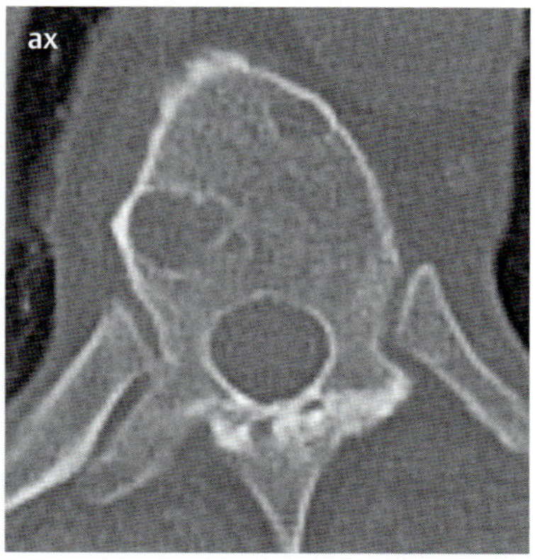

Fig. 5.20

Fig. 5.19 Plasmacytoma. Patchy osteolytic lesions without marginal sclerosis.

Fig. 5.20 Plasmacytoma. Osteolytic lesions with thin sclerotic margins after treatment.

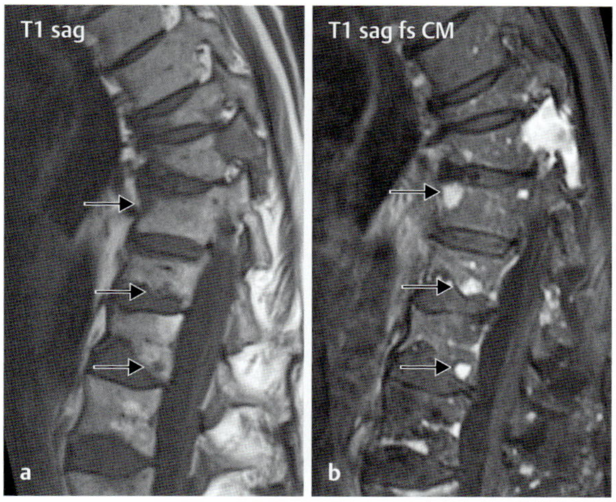

Fig. 5.21 Plasmacytoma. **(a)** Multiple chronic vertebral fractures, smaller nodular lesions (arrows). **(b)** Additional involvement of the pedicle and posterior elements of T10.

after successful treatment show regression of the lesions and replacement with fatty marrow over the longer term.

Note

MRI is currently the most sensitive imaging modality for identifying marrow involvement with multiple myeloma and is particularly useful in detecting diffuse involvement. Whole-body MRI is also capable of detecting peripheral lesions, which is important because this may alter the stage of the disease (see, for example, ▶ Fig. W5.9). Dynamic contrast-enhanced and diffusion-weighted MRI are new and promising quantitative methods for classifying the disorder and monitoring therapy, but these are not yet used in routine clinical practice.

▸ **NUC MED.** FDG-PET CT has the advantage of demonstrating osteolytic lesions by CT, while at the same time providing a scintigraphic quantification of the activity of the lesion. The latter is also used for monitoring therapy. FDG-PET CT is very well suited for detecting extramedullary lesions. However, diffuse alterations are less well detected than by MRI.

In many centers an extended staging system (Durie-Salmon PLUS) is used instead of the classic Durie-Salmon staging system (▶ Table W5.1). This system relies on MRI and PET-CT as the decisive imaging modalities. In these cases routine screening CT is superfluous.

Note

A technetium bone scan is not indicated for multiple myeloma since there is little if any osteoblastic activity with these lesions.

▸ **DD.**

- *Diffuse pattern on MRI and PET:* **Reconversion** (Chapter 5.1.2), **leukemia**, and **bone marrow stimulation** cannot be distinguished from each other by MRI and PET.
- *Multifocal lesions on MRI:* Atypical **hemangiomas** (coarse longitudinal trabeculae on CT help with differentiation.) **Metastases.**
- *Osteolytic lesions on the radiograph and CT:* **Metastases**, especially from thyroid and renal cell carcinoma. The latter are usually well vascularized and have a peripheral and cortical location.

Further differential diagnoses. Lymphoma, leukemia, primary bone tumors, hyperparathyroidism.

Related Disorders

MGUS (monoclonal gammopathy of unknown significance). This is a common condition in older patients, characterized by monoclonal gammopathy in the blood and a very low tumor load. There is only a very low risk of developing full-blown multiple myeloma over time.

POEMS (polyneuropathy, organomegaly, endocrinopathy, M-proteins, skin changes). This is a rare paraneoplastic syndrome associated with monoclonal gammopathy. The radiographs may show numerous, variably sized sclerotic bone lesions.

Caution

Not all components of POEMS syndrome may be present, but there should be a minimum of three to make the diagnosis.

PEST (papilledema, extravascular volume overload, sclerotic bone lesions, and thrombocytosis/erythrocytosis). Imaging demonstrates sclerotic lesions (known as sclerotic myeloma).

Waldenstrom macroglobulinemia. This disorder involves the production of immunoglobulin M paraprotein by lymphoplasmacytic cells. Skeletal manifestations are nonspecific and resemble those of plasmacytoma, but are less marked.

5.5.2 Lymphoma

Lymphomas are a heterogeneous group of disorders characterized by the proliferation and accumulation of abnormal lymphocytes, particularly in lymphatic organs (lymph nodes, spleen) and occasionally in other organs. By definition, Stage IV includes any involvement of bone marrow.

▸ **Pathology.** Lymphomas are divided into two main categories: Hodgkin's and non-Hodgkin's lymphomas. The prevalence of bone involvement is quite varied. It is low in Hodgkin's lymphoma at the time of diagnosis, but is more common with recurrences. It is variable with non-Hodgkin's lymphoma, depending on the histological subtype. Bone involvement is diffuse and multifocal, or it results from direct invasion by adjacent nodal masses. Solitary bone lesions are less common. Pure bony involvement of lymphoma is rare (non-Hodgkin's lymphoma) but can develop in any part of the skeleton.

Lymphomas may develop anywhere in the musculoskeletal system, including the subperiosteal space, epidural space, and muscles.

▸ **Clinical presentation.** Lymphadenopathy and possible hepatosplenomegaly are the main features. General symptoms, such as fever, night sweats, and weight loss (B symptoms) are indicative of a poorer prognosis.

▸ **Radiography.** Osteolytic and/or osteoblastic lesions are encountered. Osteolytic lesions often display a highly aggressive pattern of bone destruction, moth-eaten or permeative, to such an extent that the cortex might even appear preserved on standard radiographs, even though an adjacent soft-tissue shadow is already present. Complex or malignant types of periosteal reaction are common.

► **CT.** CT reveals that bone destruction and osteosclerosis often coexist, even in lesions that appear predominantly lytic on the radiograph (► Figs. 5.22–5.24).

► **NUC MED.** The bone scan may identify focal bone involvement, although this would presuppose an osteoblastic reaction of the bone lesion. FDG-PET is very well suited for staging, monitoring of therapeutic response, and follow-up of lymphomas. FDG-PET CT well demonstrates any therapeutic response to therapy of Hodgkin's disease and diffuse large B-cell lymphoma.

► **MRI.** MRI is the modality of choice for assessing any symptomatic regions in order to establish the diagnosis and for assessing cases in which there is clinical suspicion of spinal cord or nerve root compression.

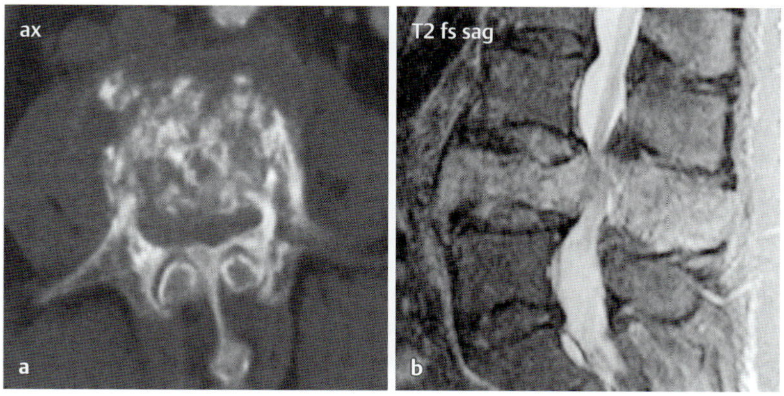

Fig. 5.22 Lymphoma infiltration of the entire L4 vertebra exhibits a pathologic fracture. **(a)** Lytic and sclerotic alterations. **(b)** Bulging of the posterior margin past the posterior spinal line resulting in severe spinal stenosis, typical for tumor-related vertebral collapse.

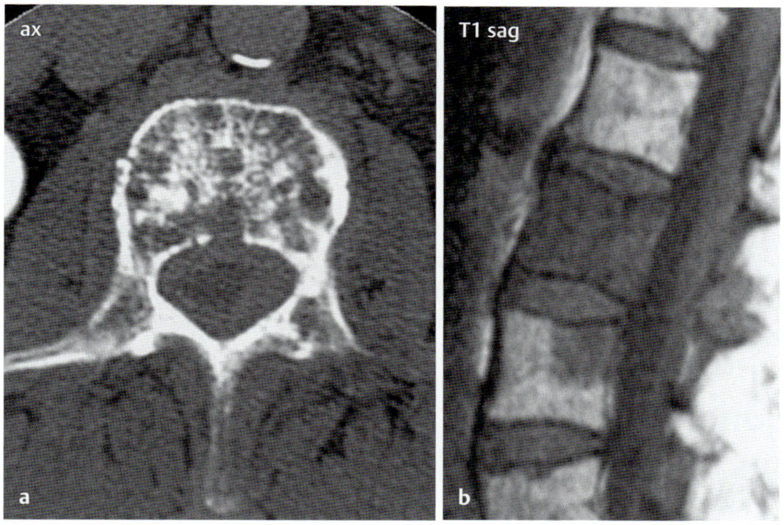

Fig. 5.23 Non-Hodgkin's lymphoma. **(a)** Axial CT slice through L2 displays a mixed osteolytic/osteosclerotic lesion. **(b)** Hypointense tumor on a T1W image infiltrating the normally fatty marrow.

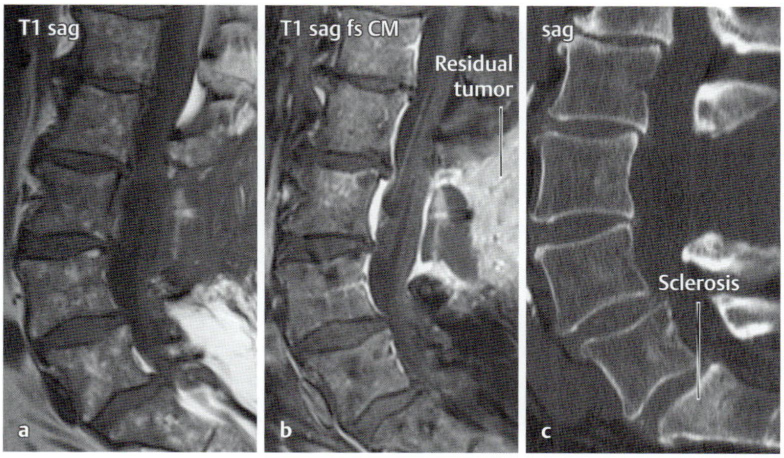

Fig. 5.24 Non-Hodgkin's lymphoma. **(a)** Diffuse patchy hypointensity of the bone marrow. (note also evidence of prior laminectomy of L3) **(b)** Irregular contrast enhancement of the bone marrow. Large amount of residual tumor posteriorly. **(c)** CT demonstrates only localized sclerosis in S1.

The appearance of bone involvement is nonspecific and includes diffuse bone marrow infiltration, a diffuse variegated picture or focal bone marrow displacement (▶ Fig. W5.10; ▶ Figs. 5.22–5.24). The alterations may resemble those of plasmacytoma.

Caution

Typically, MRI will often demonstrate a large soft-tissue component despite seemingly preserved cortical bone (known as the wrap-around sign, i.e., the soft-tissue component appears to surround the intact cortical bone), when in actual fact there is permeative bone infiltration (▶ Fig. 5.25).

5

5.5.3 Leukemia

Leukemia arises as a result of an uncontrolled proliferation of malignant hematopoietic cell clones. The result is the spread of these lymphoid or myeloid cells in the bone marrow, ultimately leading to the infiltration of extramedullary organs and the invasion of the peripheral blood. Imaging is not employed for the primary diagnosis of leukemia. The use of radiography, CT, and MRI is limited to the diagnostic work-up of localized pain or possible complications of therapy. Illness- and therapy-related complications include gout (Chapter 10.9), septic arthritis (Chapter 3.3), avascular necrosis (Chapter 6), bone infarction (Chapter 6) and osteomyelitis (Chapter 3.1).

A **chloroma** (granulocytic sarcoma) is a variant of leukemia with a localized accumulation of blasts in the bone (lytic lesions), periosteum, lymph nodes, or soft tissues. MRI displays a mass demonstrating nonspecific signal intensity (▶ Fig. 5.26).

5.6 Therapy-related Bone Marrow Alterations

Blood transfusions. Multiple blood transfusions may cause bone marrow hemosiderosis (Chapter 5.3.1).

Glucocorticoids. Imaging plays an important role in demonstrating complications related to steroid use. Bone infarction and osteonecrosis are commonly seen during steroid therapy, especially with long-term administration of steroids after bone marrow transplantation (Chapter 6). Osteomyelitis also occurs more frequently in these patients.

Chemotherapy. The reaction of the various bone marrow disorders to chemotherapy is complex, depending on the underlying condition and the substances used (▶ see References for Chapter 5).

Bone marrow–stimulating factors. These substances increase the number of hematopoietic cells in the marrow (thus shortening the duration of aplasia after chemotherapy, for example); that is, they lead to marrow reconversion. Here too, the pattern may be patchy, with focal islands of red marrow or a nodular appearance.

Caution

The type of cells involved cannot be reliably differentiated on the MRI sequences currently available. It is therefore not possible to distinguish between stimulated or regenerative bone marrow from malignant cell infiltration.

Radiotherapy. In the acute phase (1–3 days) bone marrow reacts with the development of edema (known as radiation osteitis: hypointense on T1W images and hyperintense on fluid-sensitive sequences with somewhat increased contrast enhancement). Eventually (the time span is variable, depending on the dose, possibly beginning after only 10–14 days), the number of hematopoietic cells in the marrow is reduced after successful radiotherapy and fat degeneration occurs (▶ Figs. 5.27 and ▶ W5.11). The latter is irreversible at over 40 Gy. Typically the radiation margins are clearly demarcated within the marrow

Caution

The probability of an insufficiency fracture occurring as a complication of radiotherapy is increased (▶ Fig. W5.12); this should not be mistaken for tumor recurrence. Avascular necrosis may also result from radiation.

Bone marrow transplantation. Focal lesions may persist after preparatory high-dose induction chemotherapy; it is still not certain whether this has any effect on survival. An edematous pattern appears within the first week of bone marrow transplantation (autologous or allogenic stem-cell transplantation). Regeneration of blood-forming marrow takes place over the next 3 months, especially in the periphery of the vertebrae, resulting in a typical bandlike ("picture-frame") pattern. The central vertebral marrow is not recruited until later. In the long term, conversion back to fatty marrow takes place.

See Chapter 8.5 for possible toxic complications from various substances during therapy.

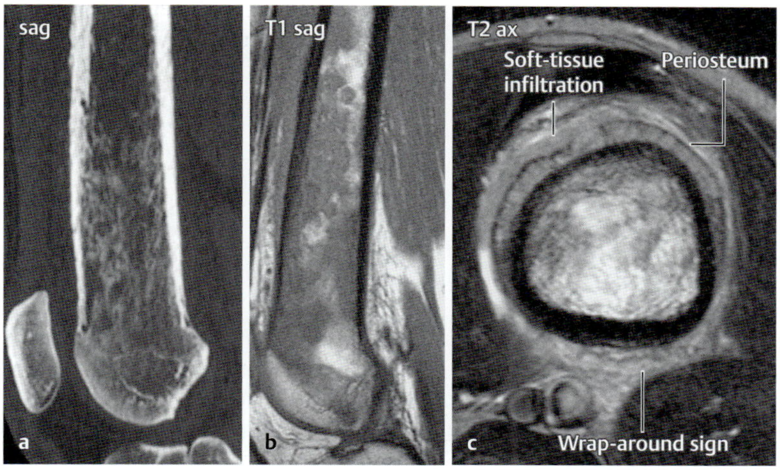

Fig. 5.25 Non-Hodgkin's lymphoma. **(a)** Extensive, ill-defined permeative bone destruction. The cortex is also infiltrated. **(b)** Bone marrow infiltration is evident on the T1W image. **(c)** On the T2W sequence, tumor has infiltrated into the subperiosteal region and adjacent soft tissues. The extent of cortical destruction is not fully recognizable on MRI (wrap around sign).

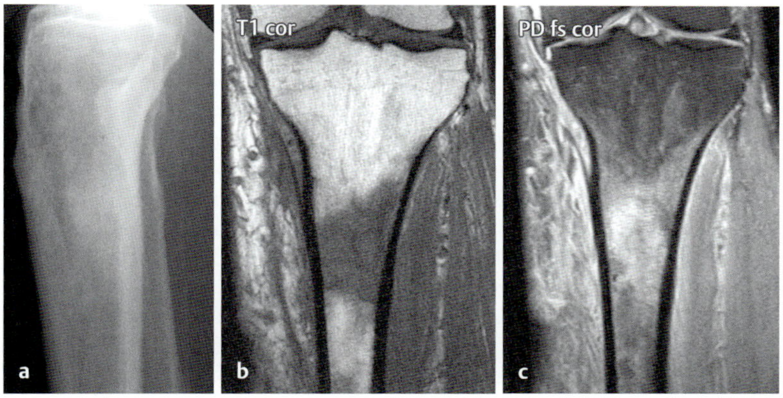

Fig. 5.26 Chloroma in chronic lymphocytic leukemia. **(a)** Sclerosis of the proximal tibia. **(b)** Focal infiltration of the bone marrow. **(c)** Nonspecific contrast enhancement.

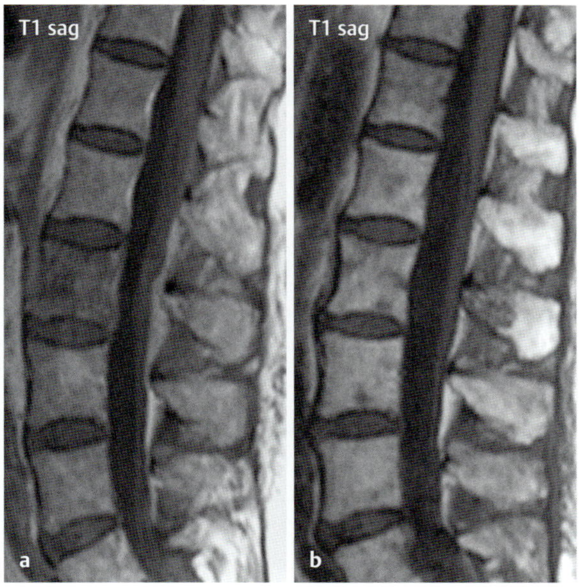

Fig. 5.27 Non-Hodgkin's lymphoma with manifestation in the lumbar spine. **(a)** MRI prior to radiotherapy. **(b)** Follow-up after radiotherapy. The bone marrow within the radiation field has undergone fatty degeneration.

6 Osteonecroses of the Skeletal System

6.1 Anatomy, Etiology, and Pathogenesis

▸ **Anatomy.** Bone varies significantly in its composition, depending on age and location. It has an organic matrix, comprised of primarily collagen (osteoid), into which inorganic mineral components (especially calcium hydroxyapatite) are incorporated. The mineralized matrix is subject to constant resorption and formation by specific cells (osteoblasts and osteoclasts). This matrix harbors both red (hematopoietic) and yellow (fatty) marrow. These are the components that, together with the mineralized bony matrix, constitute the *organ* "bone." Survival of the bone is not possible, however, without arterial inflow and venous drainage.

6

For purposes of clarification. *Osteonecrosis* takes place at a *cellular* level and only histopathology can identify the cellular alterations. Fat cells and hematopoietic marrow are always involved where ischemia is present. Cellular death in bone is a nonspecific, commonly subclinical, process that occurs more often when bone cells are subjected to abnormal stress. Therefore, histopathology will reveal small areas of necrosis along with severe osteoarthritis, stress or insufficiency fracture, an acute fracture, tumor, or infection. This chapter addresses clinically relevant forms of osteonecrosis which can be readily demonstrated by imaging studies. Imaging reflects macroscopic anatomy and reveals the effects of cell death on the bone (or parts of it). Common terms such as "osteonecrosis," "bone infarction," "avascular necrosis," and "aseptic necrosis" are poorly defined and are applied inconsistently. These terms do not provide information about *prognosis* or *etiology*.

> **Note**
>
> In everyday language, the term **"osteonecrosis"** generally refers to bone necrosis located in the epiphysis or apophysis or involving the entire bone (▶ Fig. W6.1). If the osteonecrosis is located in the metaphysis or diaphysis, then this is referred to as **"bone infarct."** A task for the future is to devise a classification system for bone necrosis that provides prognostic information independent of the skeletal location.

▸ **Etiology.** In many cases **the etiology** and pathogenesis are obvious, such as interruption of blood supply secondary to a dislocation. If an etiology cannot be clearly defined, then it is better to refer to **risk factors** that may result in bone necrosis. ▸ Table 6.1 presents important risk factors. Additionally, some genetic factors that may predispose to bone necrosis have been identified.

Osteonecrosis without a clear etiology is referred to as **"primary," "idiopathic,"** or **"spontaneous"** osteonecrosis.

▸ **Pathology.** A number of theories have been advanced to describe the processes involved in the pathogenesis of osteonecrosis. It is generally accepted that all of them ultimately end in a reduced or interrupted supply of oxygenated blood to the bone. Ischemia prevents the normal repair processes of microfractures; results in the death of osteocytes, fat cells, and cells of hematopoiesis; and culminates in the loss of normal bone architecture.

Revascularization of an area of bone necrosis starts from the periphery. Osteoclasts are activated to absorb dead trabeculae. Fibrovascular tissue is formed to enclose the dead bone. This tissue is partially converted to bone. If the zone of necrosis involves the metaphysis or diaphysis, it will have no biomechanical impact. The same holds true for small epiphyseal lesions. If a larger necrotic zone and/or a lesion located within a weight-bearing area of a joint is placed under significant stress, then disruption of bone architecture will lead to functional failure with subsequent subchondral fracture and collapse of the joint surface.

Table 6.1 Risk factors for necrosis of the skeletal system

Pathogenesis	Risk factors
External factors	• Trauma • Surgery • Decompression sickness (caisson disease)
Iatrogenic	• Corticosteroids • Bisphosphonates • Radiotherapy
Nutritional	• Alcohol
Hematologic/ oncologic	• Previous renal transplant (even without steroids) • Hemoglobinopathies (sickle cell anemia, thalassemia) • Leukemia
Metabolic	• Gaucher's disease • Pancreatitis with fat embolism
Rheumatological	• Systemic lupus erythematosus • Necrotizing arteritis
Infections	• Osteomyelitis

> **Note**
> Beware of simplification. A "multiple-hit hypothesis" is now favored for the common cortisone-induced osteonecrosis. Cortisone results in an imbalance between osteoblasts and osteoclasts related to fatty degeneration and damage to the cell membrane. Steroids damage endothelial cells of blood vessels within bone. Thrombophilia and hypofibrinolysis are augmented by steroids; the latter are also responsible for alterations in fat metabolism resulting in increased adipogenesis, fat cell hypertrophy, and fat emboli.

6.2 Bone Infarction

► **Pathology.** A bone infarction involving fatty marrow presents as a circumscribed lesion, while an infarct involving red marrow tends to be a poorly marginated lesion within the hematopoietic marrow. Ultimately, the necrotic area slowly becomes surrounded by a reparative margin. Bone infarcts may become smaller over time (this is common; see ► Fig. 6.5), or may even be completely absorbed.

> **Note**
> From a prognostic viewpoint, a bone infarction located in the metaphysis or diaphysis may be regarded as a "benign" form of osteonecrosis. Because of their location, with little cancellous bone and strong cortex, infarcts here are irrelevant for the structural integrity of the bone and are often clinically occult. Similar areas of necrosis in the epiphysis of tubular bones, in flat bones such as the ilium, and in irregularly formed bones such as the sacrum resemble metaphyseal infarctions but are referred to as osteonecrosis merely because of their location.

► **Clinical presentation.** As a general rule, infarcts are often incidental findings. In the majority of cases these lesions are asymptomatic; however, they may be associated with chronic or acute pain, with the latter often occurring with acute infarctions related to a hemoglobinopathy (especially sickle cell anemia).

► **Radiography/CT.** The early stage of bone infarction/osteonecrosis is radiographically undetectable, with subsequent poorly marginated rarefaction of the trabeculae (► Fig. 6.1). Reparative tissue develops at the edge of the infarct and slowly mineralizes to become evident as a peripheral sclerotic margin surrounding an area of central lucency (► Fig. 6.2). Extensive, intralesional calcifications are recognizable in the later stages. In very rare cases, metaphyseal and diaphyseal infarcts result in periosteal reaction and a widening of the bone.

► **NUC MED.** In the initial phase a "cold spot" (i.e., decreased uptake) will be present in the area of necrosis, and eventually a "cold in hot spot" (► Fig. 6.3a) will be seen owing to the increased peripheral uptake related to the vascularized reparative tissue along its margin.

► **MRI.** An **infarction within yellow, fatty marrow**, will demonstrate fat-equivalent signal in its center on T1W sequences. The area is typically bordered by a low-signal intensity margin, although the appearance may vary depending on the age of the infarct (► Figs. 6.3c, ► 6.4b, and ► 6.5). A hyperintense line (granulation tissue; ► Figs. 6.3b and ► 6.4a) is often present around the zones of necrosis on fat-suppressed water-sensitive sequences (see ► Fig. 6.3c). On T2W sequences without fat suppression (not routinely used) a "double-line sign" may be seen. Areas of cystic degeneration (fluid signal intensity on T2W images) and amorphous calcifications (hypointense on all sequences) may be present within the necrosis.

An **infarction** in areas with predominantly hematopoietic marrow or with pathologic bone marrow infiltration displays an area of low signal intensity on T1W images (provided it is visible at all against the already dark marrow) and increased signal intensity on fat-saturated PDW or T2W sequences (► Fig. 6.6). The enhancement pattern of an infarct after contrast administration reflects its pathophysiology: If the diagnosis is made early, there is little or no contrast enhancement within the center of the infarction. Later, strong marginal enhancement of the entire border zone will be seen. With advancing age of the infarction, the nonenhancing region becomes progressively smaller.

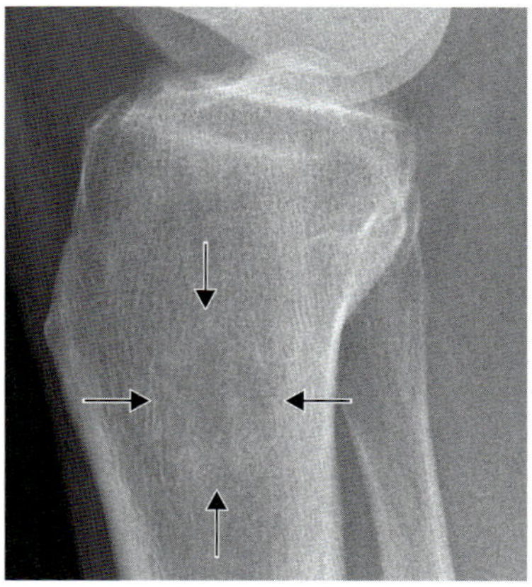

Fig. 6.1 Bone infarction in the tibial plateau. Fine sclerotic margin (arrows).

► **DD.** A confident diagnosis of a **bone infarct within yellow marrow** is established by the detection of fat within the lesion on MRI. Other lesions containing fat include:

- Bone lesions with the potential for spontaneous remission (fibrous cortical defect, a brown tumor in renal osteodystrophy).
- Intraosseous lipomas.

The differential diagnosis of an **infarction within red marrow** is particularly difficult. Osteomyelitis, stress fractures, and necrotic tumors must be differentiated with the aid of the clinical history and presentation, laboratory findings, and follow-up imaging studies.

Enchondroma. If intralesional fat is not identified within an infarct due to a large amount of reparative fibrous tissue (rare), then it is not always distinguishable on T1W sequences from a chondroid tumor. Differentiation is also difficult on T2W images due to the juxtaposition of bright (cysts, cartilage) and dark signal intensity (calcifications). The typical lobular pattern of an enchondroma is often helpful in diagnosis (► Fig. 6.7). After contrast administration, an enchondroma demonstrates a number of "septations," reflecting its lobular structure. Enhancement in bone infarction is more marginal or—when within the lesion—patchy.

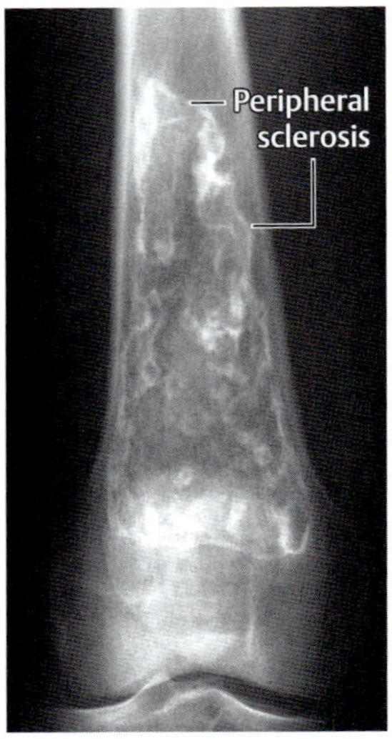

Fig. 6.2 Bone infarction of the distal femur.

6

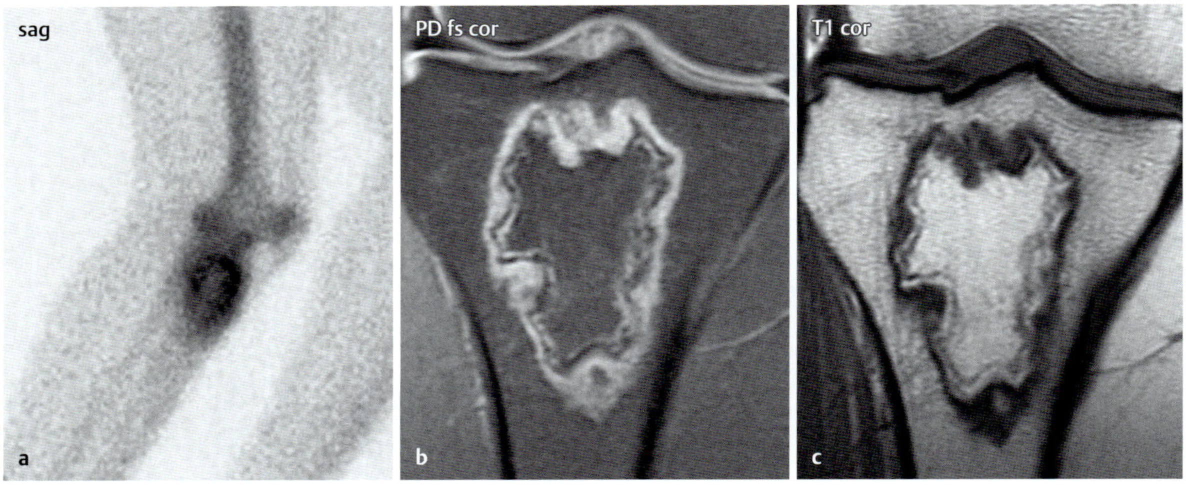

Fig. 6.3 Bone infarction of the tibial plateau. **(a)** Classic "cold in hot spot" appearance on the bone scan. **(b)** Serpentine, high-signal intensity margin surrounds the central necrosis on this fluid-sensitive, fat-saturated image. **(c)** The central necrosis is even brighter than the surrounding bone marrow due to cell death of the fat cells.

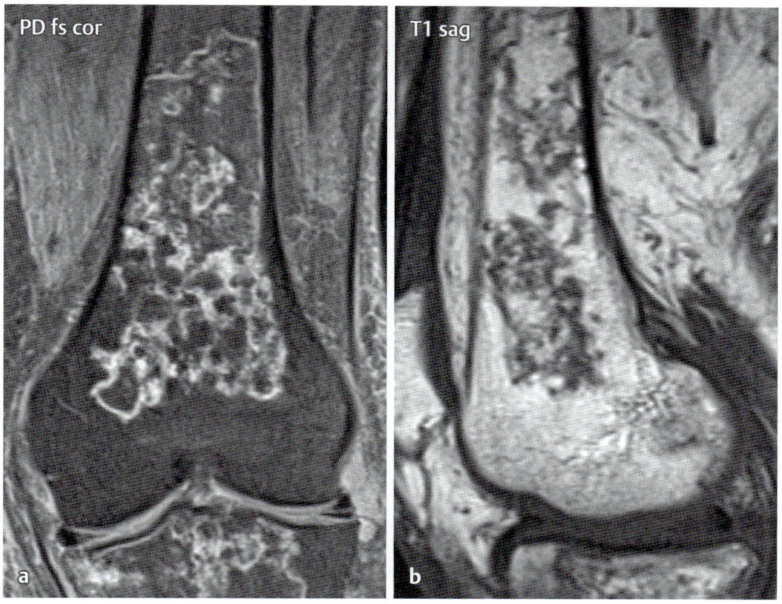

Fig. 6.4 Typical bone infarctions in femur and tibia. **(a)** Multilobular signal-intense lines, similar to an enchondroma, predominate on the fat-saturated PDW image. **(b)** Markedly irregular margins surround the extensive central necrosis.

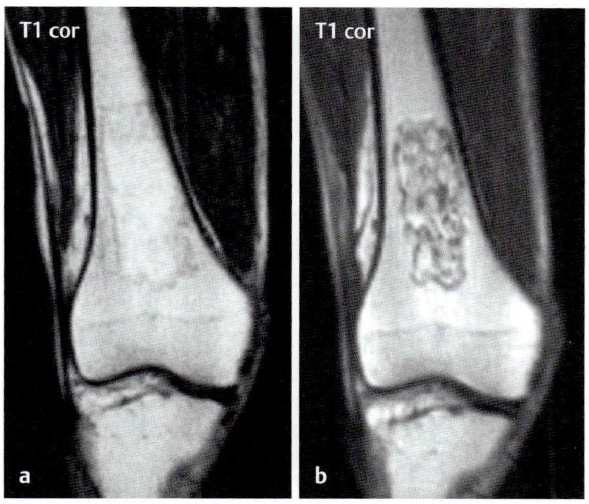

Fig. 6.5 Radiological course of a bone infarction in the distal femur. **(a)** Initial appearance. **(b)** After one year, reduction in size and increasing marginal sclerosis is evident.

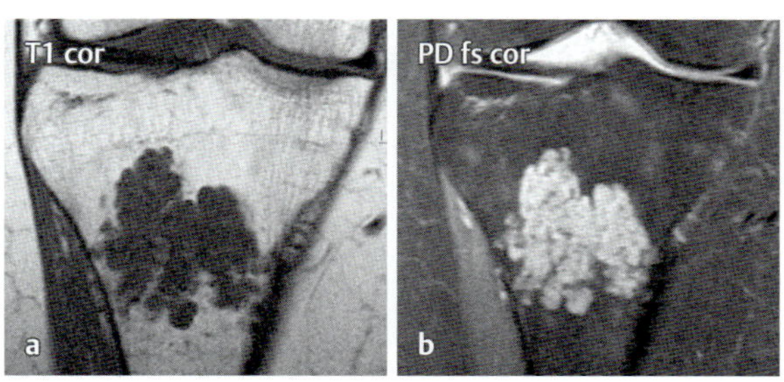

Fig. 6.7 Enchondroma versus bone infarction. **(a)** The center of the lesion appears hypointense on the T1W image (cartilaginous matrix). **(b)** Typical lobular high signal intensity architecture of an enchondroma.

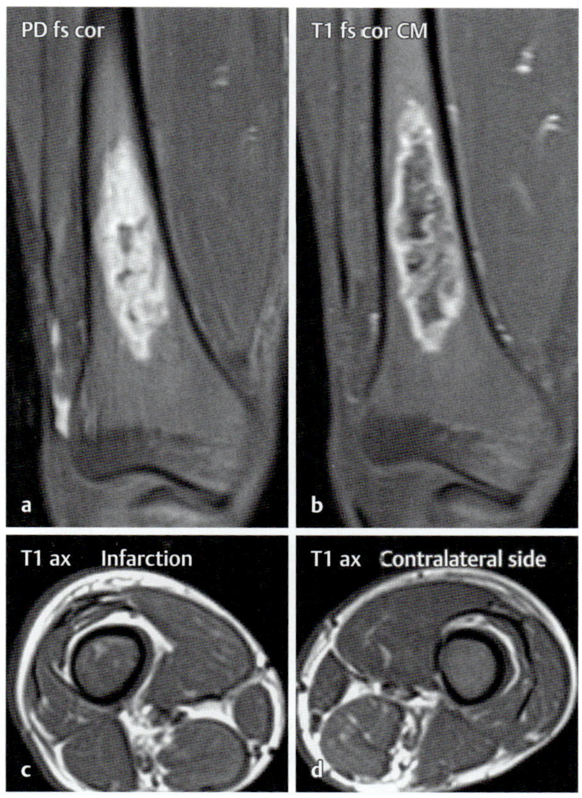

Fig. 6.6 Bone infarction of red marrow in sickle cell anemia. **(a)** Extensive increased signal intensity in the metaphysis. **(b)** The necrosis becomes visible after contrast administration due to the lack of enhancement of the central components. **(c)** It is not possible to differentiate the red infarction on the unenhanced T1W image due to the diffuse bone marrow infiltration in sickle cell anemia. **(d)** "Normal" contralateral side without infarction.

6.3 Osteonecrosis

▶ **Pathology.** The term "osteonecrosis" is used when an area of necrosis occurs within an epiphysis. Alterations involving an entire bone are also covered by the term "osteonecrosis" (e.g., necrosis of the lunate). From a pathophysiological aspect, there is no difference from a bone infarction. If the necrosis takes up large areas of the epiphysis or is situated in the weight-bearing part of the bone, the subchondral bone plate may collapse in that area. The entire subchondral bone then collapses into the necrotic zone, together with the overlying cartilage.

Location. Common sites of osteonecrosis related to the risk factors and pathogenesis described in Chapter 6.1 include the femoral head, humeral head (▶ Figs. 6.8, ▶ W6.2 and ▶ W6.3), scaphoid, lunate, femoral condyles (▶ Figs. 6.9, ▶ W6.4 and ▶ W6.5), and talus. Other less commonly involved sites include the proximal tibia, patella, navicular bone of the foot, and vertebrae.

6

> **Note**
>
> Osteonecrosis of the **talus** related to the risk factors in Table 6.1 is not uncommon. Trauma (especially talar neck fractures, cf. Chapter 2.15.4), and corticosteroids are the most common causes. Chronic osteochondral lesions of the talar dome (cf. Chapter 2.15.3) are not true osteonecroses, but are posttraumatic injuries sometimes associated with small, necrotic fragments. Osteochondritis dissecans of the talar dome is considered an osteochondrosis and not osteonecrosis (cf. Chapter 7.2.5).

6.3.1 Osteonecrosis of the Femoral Head

Osteonecrosis of the femoral head is the most common form of epiphyseal osteonecrosis; however, the same features may be seen in other locations, such as the femoral condyles and humeral head, and will therefore not be repeated for those sites.

▶ **Clinical presentation.** The clinical spectrum ranges from a total lack of symptoms to severe pain and an inability to walk. The vast majority of symptomatic patients have a poor prognosis, with subsequent loss of function of the hip joint. There is also a risk of progression in asymptomatic cases discovered by MRI; however, these lesions may remain constant over a long period of time or may sometimes heal spontaneously (▶ Fig. W6.5).

▶ **Pathology.** Osteonecrosis of the femoral head is found more commonly in men than in women, usually between the ages of 35 and 55 years. It is commonly bilateral. See Chapter. 6.1 regarding the etiology and pathophysiology of osteonecrosis of the femoral head. Progression results in collapse of the femoral head and subsequent secondary osteoarthritis of the hip joint.

Prognosis. Prognosis depends on the underlying risk factors (e.g., steroid therapy) and the degree of mechanical stress. As a rule, osteonecrosis with *joint surface collapse* does not regenerate over time nor is it influenced in its progression by surgical measures. With an intact joint surface, the risk of a poor outcome is related to the *size of the necrotic area*, so that MRI findings are helpful for predicting prognosis. The literature does provide some rules for determining the size of the affected area of the femoral head (expressed as a percentage), picturing the femoral head as an idealized hemisphere:

- If only 15 to 25% of the joint surface of the femoral head is involved, then a stable lesion without tendency to collapse may be expected.
- If over 25% of the joint surface is involved, then the development of a collapse is probable; surgery should be considered.
- If the area of necrosis is situated in the medial third of the stress distribution zone (on the coronal image), then prognosis is favorable. The "best" lesion, therefore, is small and located medially in the femoral head.

Classification systems. The presence of a fracture involving the joint surface is an important feature in all current classification systems because this typically portends collapse of the femoral head. Fractures of the joint surface correspond in almost all classification systems to Stage III. **Ficat's classification** (▶ Table 6.2) is based on radiographic findings and functional evaluation of bone (by intraosseous phlebography and measurement of bone marrow pressure). The **ARCO** classification system (Association Internationale de Recherche sur la Circulation Osseuse) introduced MRI into the classification and took the size and site of the necrotic zone into account (▶ Table. 6.3). The Steinberg classification is also a modification of the Ficat system, with stages ranging from 0 to VI. As with the ARCO system, the extent of involvement is also taken into consideration.

Treatment. Currently, surgical treatment of the early stages primarily involves core decompression of the femoral head, with or without the insertion of a bone graft. If the femoral head has collapsed, then total hip replacement is basically the only therapeutic option. If the collapsed area is small, then a displacement osteotomy may be attempted.

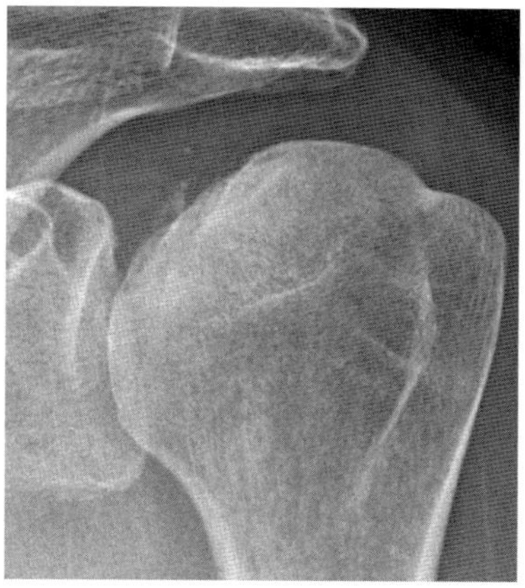

Fig. 6.8

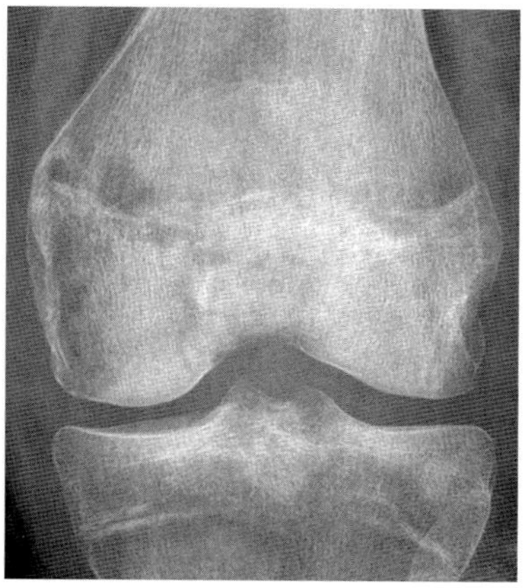

Fig. 6.9

Fig. 6.8 Osteonecrosis of the humeral head with collapse of a portion of the articular surface.

Fig. 6.9 Signs of osteonecrosis of the medial femoral condyle. Trabecular rarefication, produces apparent "sclerosis" centrally and along its margin. This is defined as "osteonecrosis" due to the site of involvement.

Table 6.2 Radiographic classification of osteonecrosis of the femoral head according to Ficat

Stage	Radiology
0	• Normal radiograph
I	• Normal, equivocal findings or only mild alterations (extensive reduced density, loss of trabecular detail, bone structure no longer recognizable)
II	• Diffuse or focal alterations (reduction of density, abnormal trabecular structure, diffuse or bandlike sclerosis, round radiolucencies; see ▸ Fig. 6.10) • Normal contour and form of the femoral head (see ▸ Fig. 6.11) • No joint-space narrowing
III	• Steplike collapse of the contour of the femoral head without any, or only slight, flattening (see ▸ Fig. 6.13b) • Bandlike and sector-shaped sclerosis of the femoral head • Formation of areas of lytic resorption and/or formation of a curvilinear subchondral zone of radiolucency parallel to the articular surface of femoral head (crescent sign; see ▸ Figs. 6.12 and ▸ 6.14) • Normal or slightly widened joint space
IV	• Collapse of the femoral head with complete loss of the bone structure • Large, subchondral lucencies and diffuse sclerosis • Narrowing of the joint space with development of arthritis deformans

Table 6.3 ARCO staging system of necrosis of the femoral head

Stage	Clinical presentation, pathology and imaging procedures
0	• Normal findings on radiography, MRI and scintigraphy • Histological signs of necrosis
I	• Normal radiography/CT • MRI or scintigraphic abnormalities • Subclassification based on MRI according to affected part of the femoral head (lateral, medial, or anterior) and amount of involvement of the femoral head circumference (< 15%, 15–30%, > 30%)
II	• Structural radiographic changes in the bone without alterations in the contour of the femoral head • Normal joint space • MRI findings specific for necrosis of the femoral head • Subclassification according to affected part of the femoral head (lateral, medial, or anterior) and amount of involvement of the femoral head circumference (< 15%, 15–30%, > 30%)
III	• Structural radiographic changes in the bone with subchondral fracturing, appearing as a curvilinear zone of radiolucency in the subchondral bone (crescent sign) • Flattening of the contour of the femoral head • Normal width of the joint space • Subclassification according to the part of the head involved (lateral, medial, or anterior), amount of involvement of the femoral head circumference (< 15%, 15–30%, > 30%), and extent of femoral head flattening (< 2 mm, 2–4 mm, > 4 mm)
IV	• Development of arthritis deformans • Flattening of the femoral head • Joint-space narrowing

► **Radiography.** The radiographic findings of osteonecrosis of the femoral head are presented in ►Table 6.2 (►Figs. 6.10–6.15). A curvilinear focus of subchondral lucency (crescent sign; see ►Figs. 6.12 and ►6.14) or contour changes of the femoral head are late-stage findings. Development of (secondary) osteoarthritis typically progresses more or less parallel with the collapse of the femoral head. Classification of the radiographic changes listed in ►Table 6.2 does not address the prognostically important factors of the size and location of the necrosis since these cannot be determined with radiography.

► **CT.** CT findings correlate with those seen on radiographs. Osteolytic and sclerotic changes as well as the change of contour of the femoral head may be recognized earlier and more confidently than with radiographs using multiplanar reconstructions (►Fig. 6.16). CT is better than MRI at demonstrating abnormalities in contour of the subchondral bone plate and, in particular, subchondral fractures running parallel to the articular surface (crescent sign).

A simple formula for calculating the amount of joint surface affected is:

Affected joint surface (%)

$$= \left(\frac{\text{angle of the affected surface in the sagittal plane}}{180}\right) \times \left(\frac{\text{angle of the affected surface in the coronal plane}}{180}\right) \times 100$$

► **NUC MED.** A 3-phase bone scan with technetium Tc 99 m diphosphonate will demonstrate reduced uptake at the site of necrosis (cold spot) in the early stages and, over time, increased uptake along the reactive border (cold in hot spot; cf. ►Fig. 6.3a), which are considered to be specific signs of osteonecrosis of the femoral head. A more common, nonspecific, finding is diffuse uptake as a sign of a repair process. With this type of pattern, however, differentiation from transient bone marrow edema syndrome or other types of pathology is difficult.

► **MRI.** MRI is the modality of choice for suspected osteonecrosis of the femoral head.

> **Note**
> Understanding pathophysiology of osteonecrosis of the femoral head is critical for understanding its appearance on MR imaging.

In its early stages, osteonecrosis of the femoral head resembles an infarct within the metaphysis (yellow infarction; ►Fig. 6.17), but again, by definition, when it occurs in the epiphysis (subchondral bone) it is termed osteonecrosis rather than infarct (Chapter 6.1). An area of fat-equivalent signal surrounded by a dark line is present in this early stage on T1W images. On fluid-sensitive sequences without fat saturation a "double line sign" (hypointense/hyperintense) is seen along the periphery (►Fig. 6.18). The latter enhances strongly with contrast, and this bandlike margination is the decisive criterion for diagnosing osteonecrosis of the femoral head.

In its later stages, collapse of the subchondral plate overlying the necrotic focus into the necrotic zone, together with the overlying cartilage.

This appearance changes from ARCO Stage III onward. The lesion is still well defined but now displays mixed intralesional signal intensity, although some fat-equivalent signal is identifiable on T1W images. The zone of demarcation ("reactive interface") between the infarct and the normal surrounding fatty marrow is bandlike, similar to the early stages, albeit more commonly ill-defined. Sometimes the entire area of necrosis is also completely hypointense on T1W sequences. A fracture of the joint surface may appear as follows:

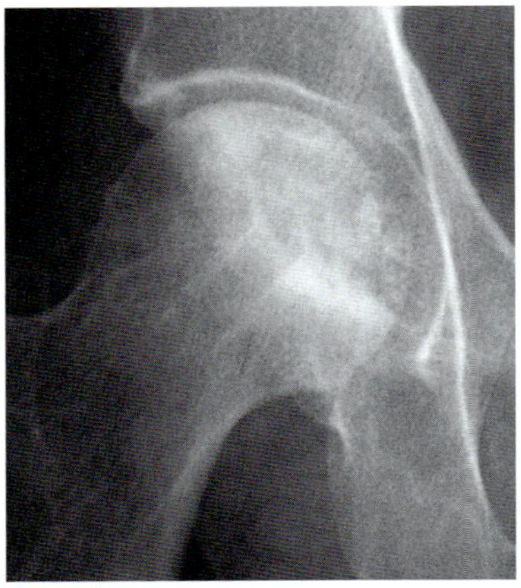

Fig. 6.10 Osteonecrosis of the femoral head. Ficat Stage II.

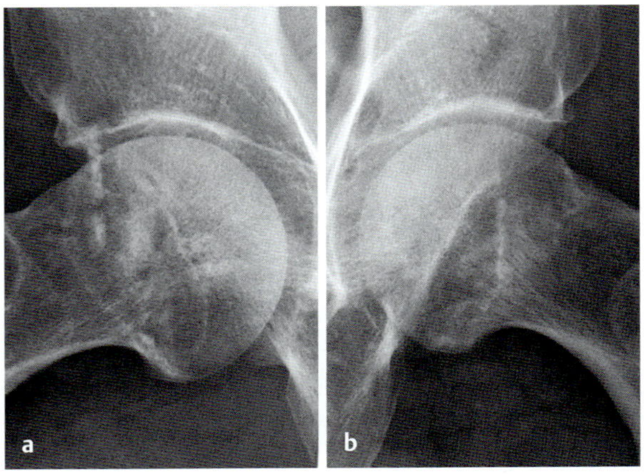

Fig. 6.11 Bilateral osteonecrosis of the femoral heads. Lauenstein views. **(a)** Irregular sclerosis of the femoral head. **(b)** No evidence of subchondral infraction. Normal joint space.

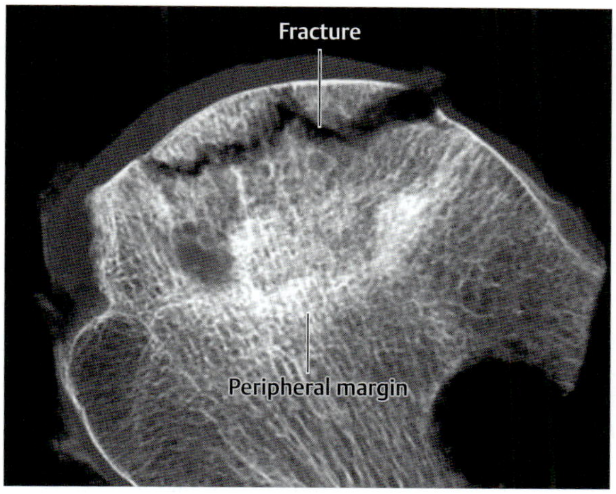

Fig. 6.12 Osteonecrosis of the femoral head. Specimen radiography. The subchondral fracture produces the characteristic crescent sign.

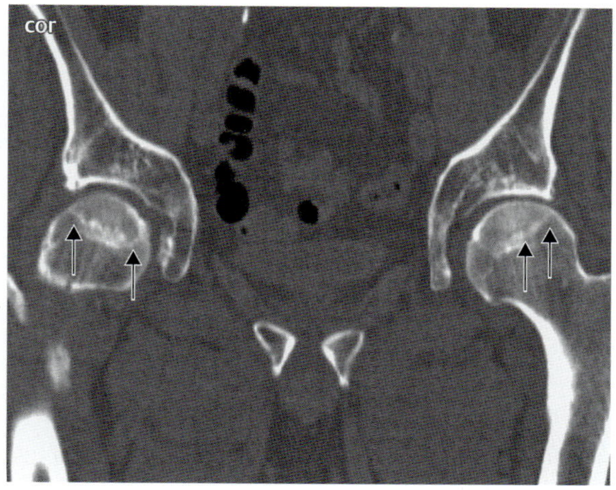

Fig. 6.16 Bilateral Ficat Stage II osteonecrosis of the femoral head. Discrete sclerotic margins (arrows).

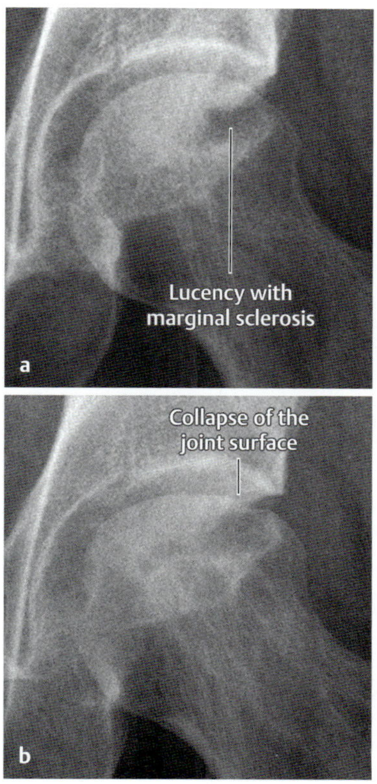

Fig. 6.13 Osteonecrosis of the femoral head. **(a)** Ficat Stage II. **(b)** Despite decompression, there is eventually progression to Stage III.

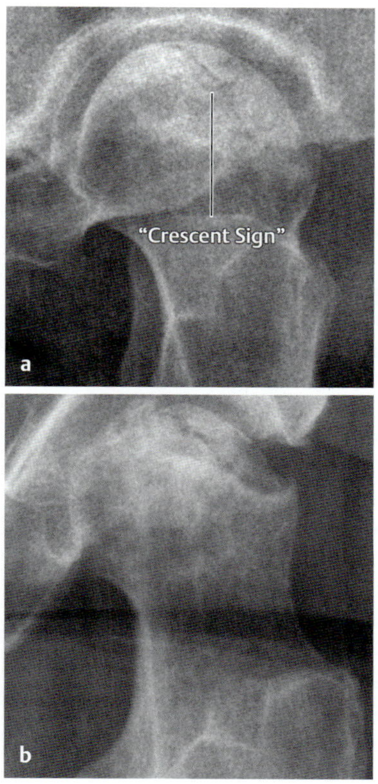

Fig. 6.14 Osteonecrosis of the femoral head. **(a)** Ficat Stage III. **(b)** Progressive deformation of the femoral head is eventually seen.

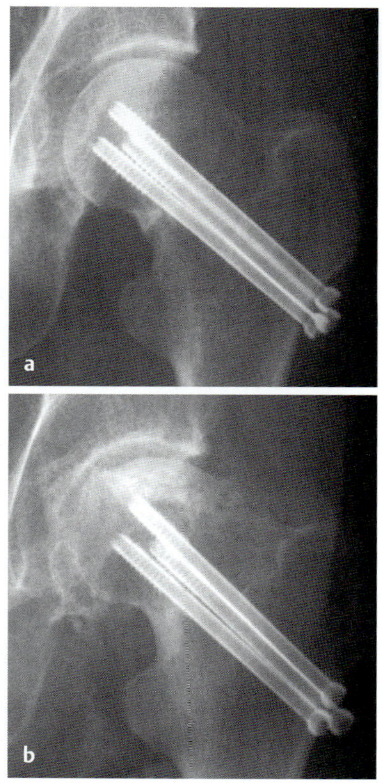

Fig. 6.15 Posttraumatic osteonecrosis of the femoral head. **(a)** Screw fixation of a subcapital femoral neck fracture. **(b)** Subsequent development of osteonecrosis and collapse of the femoral head.

- As a slight step-off on the articular surface (especially on T2W sequences without fat saturation or on GRE sequences; ▶ Fig. 6.19).
- As a subchondral band of high signal intensity on T2W images (crescent sign; ▶ Figs. 6.20 and ▶ 6.21)
- In the presence of increased syncvial contrast enhancement (▶ Fig. 6.22).

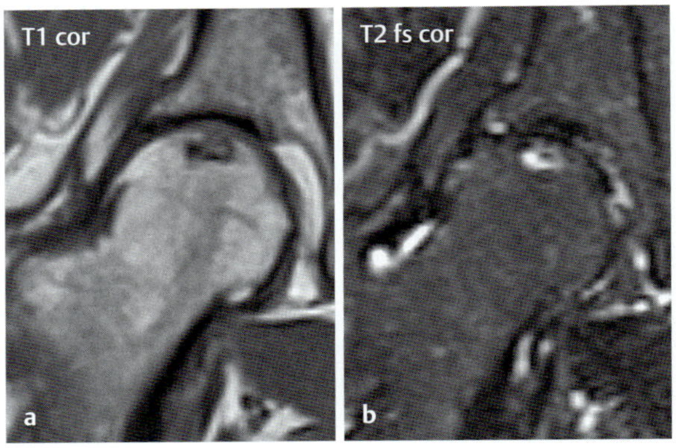

Fig. 6.17 Small area of osteonecrosis of the femoral head as an incidental finding on an MRI performed for myositis. **(a)** Small oval-shaped abnormality demonstrating MRI findings of an infarct. **(b)** The finding is referred to as osteonecrosis because of its epiphyseal location.

> **Note**
>
> If the osteonecrosis is advanced (beyond ARCO III) or if large areas of the femoral head are involved, even in an early stage, additional edemalike signal may be evident in some patients outside of the zone of osteonecrosis. Its origin is not yet fully clarified. It was assumed for a long time that this represented additional areas of necrosis, but with a different MRI appearance. Histological evidence, however, contradicts this, and these changes are more commonly seen in patients with a relatively "fresh" fracture of the articular surface (as opposed to patients without a fracture or with more chronic collapse). These edemalike areas may resolve or change location and are therefore classified as reactive and transient.

▶ DD.

Transient bone marrow edema (cf. Chapter 1.5.4). Even with osteonecrosis a prominent edemalike pattern may be present adjacent to the necrotic area with extension into the femoral neck, making differentiation between transient bone marrow edema and osteonecrosis sometimes difficult. However, in transient bone marrow edema the edema pattern is mostly homogeneous. Strong, relatively homogeneous contrast enhancement is seen after IV contrast administration in transient bone marrow edema as well.

Stress reaction or insufficiency fracture. A stress reaction corresponds to many small trabecular fractures, without a fracture line being visible on radiographs, CT, or MRI. Accordingly, diffuse bone marrow edema on fluid-sensitive sequences characterizes a stress reaction (similar to what is seen with transient bone marrow edema). Linear signal abnormality corresponding to a fracture line is seen with an insufficiency fracture, running parallel with the articular surface in the majority of cases (as opposed to concave) (cf. Chapter 1.5.1). The femoral head enhances relatively homogeneously and strongly with contrast in cases of stress reaction and insufficiency fracture (▶ Fig. W6.6).

It should not be forgotten that steroids predispose both to osteonecrosis and to decreased bone density which may result in insufficiency fractures. As a result both osteonecrosis and insufficiency fractures may be found in patients with a history of steroid use.

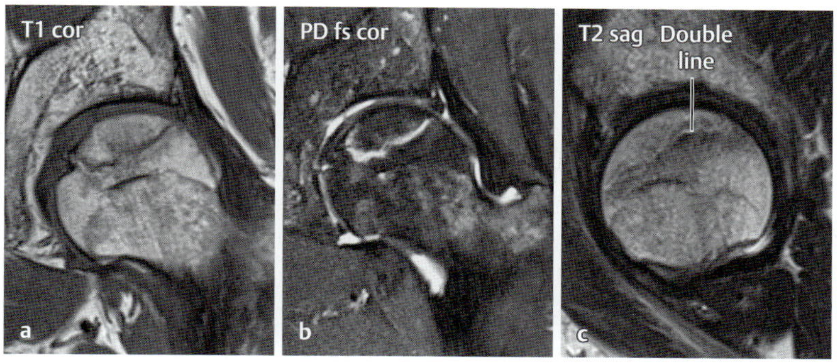

Fig. 6.18 Osteonecrosis of the femoral head Stage II according to the ARCO classification system. Same patient as in ▶ Fig. 6.16. **(a)** Fat-equivalent signal, surrounded by a low signal intensity margin on the T1W image. This margin looks like a mirror image of the joint surface. **(b)** The margin demonstrates increased signal intensity on fat-saturated and water-sensitive sequences. **(c)** There is a double-line sign with increased signal intensity along the inner margin of the necrosis on this T2W image without fat saturation.

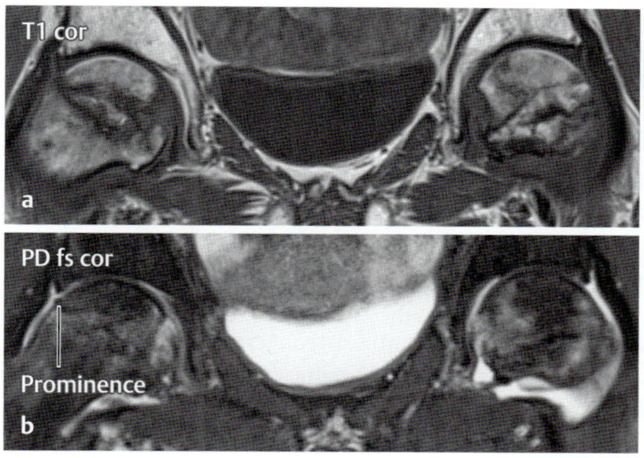

Fig. 6.19 Bilateral osteonecrosis of the femoral heads. The same patient as in ▶ Fig. 6.12. **(a)** The T1W image demonstrates very large bilateral necrotic areas. **(b)** Focal contour irregularity along the lateral aspect of the right femoral head indicates an ARCO Stage III on this side.

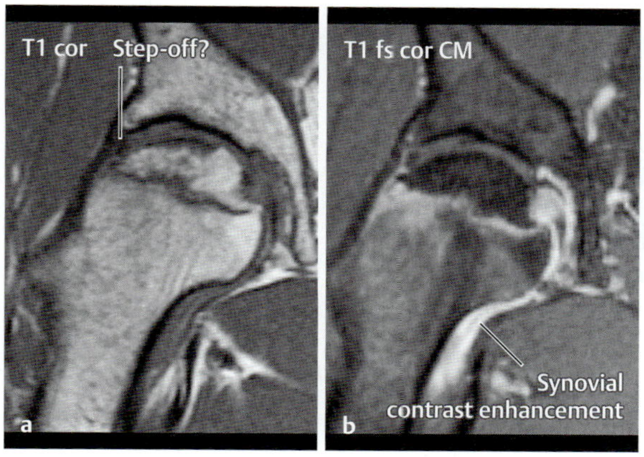

Fig. 6.22 Osteonecrosis of the femoral head, ARCO Stage III. **(a)** Equivocal step-off of the lateral joint surface on the T1W image. **(b)** The presence of synovitis is highly suspicious for some articular collapse.

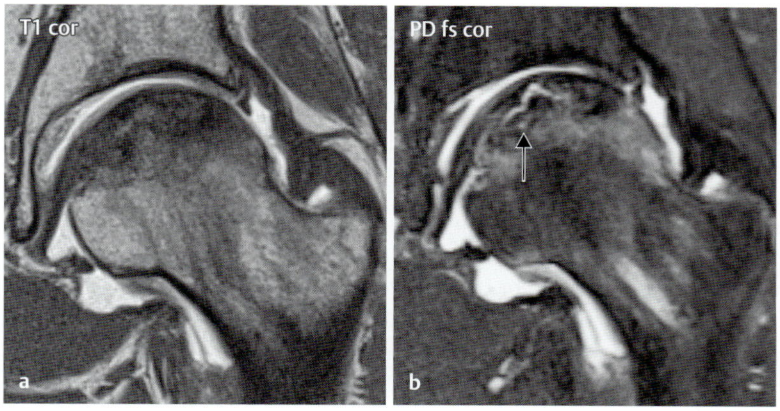

Fig. 6.20 Appearance after core decompression for osteonecrosis of the femoral head. **(a)** Extensive subchondral hypointensity. **(b)** Fluid accumulating in a subchondral fracture manifests itself as a crescent sign (arrow) on MRI. There is already minimal flattening of the femoral head medially compatible with ARCO Stage III.

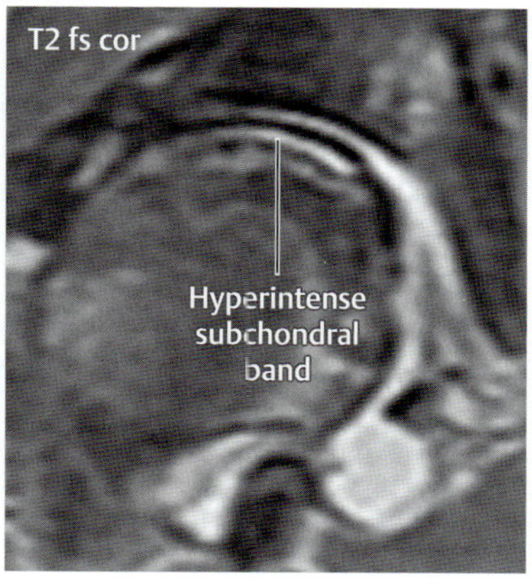

Fig. 6.21 Crescent sign on MRI as an indication of a fracture involving the joint surface.

6.3.2 Osteonecrosis of the Lunate

▶ **Pathology.** The precise pathogenesis of this disorder is unclear (synonyms are Kienbock's disease and lunatomalacia). Chronic repetitive trauma has been implicated as the cause of Kienbock's disease, but this view is currently being strongly contested. There is general consensus only about the final pathophysiological pathway—ischemia of the bone. Why the ischemia/infarction develops and why, over time, the activity of osteoclasts predominates over that of osteoblasts remain unknown. Males between the ages of 20 and 40 years are primarily affected. Unequivocal **posttraumatic osteonecrosis** of the lunate may be distinguished from Kienbock's disease by the duration of symptoms and findings on posttraumatic imaging (perilunate dislocation fractures).

The **staging system for Kienbock's disease according to Lichtmann and Ross** is based on radiographic findings. Supplementary information provided by contrast-enhanced MRI and CT is very helpful in making a more exact assessment:

- **Stage I:** Normal radiographs with diffuse bone marrow edema on MRI.
- **Stage II:** Diffuse sclerosis and cystic foci with normal bone morphology.
- **Stage III:** Transition to Stage III is characterized by infarction of the lunate, usually starting at the proximal joint surface (Stage IIIA). With progressive collapse, loss of carpal height and carpal instability become recognizable (Stage IIIB). The scaphoid goes into palmar flexion while the triquetrum deviates in a dorsal direction.
- **Stage IV:** Complete collapse of the lunate and secondary osteoarthritis.

▶ **Radiography/CT.** A conventional radiograph is usually sufficient to classify Stages II to IV (▶ Fig. 6.23). Cinefluoroscopy may be helpful in distinguishing between Stages III a and III b in cases with equivocal findings, since dynamic carpal instability is sometimes only recognized with movement. Subtle bony changes are better detected by high-resolution CT which is important for distinguishing between Stages II and III a (evidence of incipient collapse of the articular surface; ▶ Fig. 6.24) and between Stages III b and IV (evidence of osteophyte formation and joint space irregularities).

▶ **MRI.** MRI is used in Kienbock's disease to answer two questions:

- *Is **Kienbock's disease** present?* Clinical suspicion with an unremarkable radiograph is an indication for MRI to clarify this question. MRI demonstrates edemalike signal (low signal intensity on T1W, increased signal intensity on fluid-sensitive sequences).
- *How viable is the lunate?* Lunatomalacia is not the result of a sudden, complete interruption of perfusion. Initially, reparative fibrovascular tissue causes the edemalike signal changes and results in significant contrast enhancement (▶ Fig. 6.25). Perfusion only decreases over time, resulting in more heterogeneous signal intensity after IV contrast administration. Ultimately, complete infarction typically results in low signal intensity on all sequences.

> **Caution**
> The degree of lunate viability is not synonymous with the stage of lunate necrosis, which is based on bone morphology. Thus, for example, a completely nonviable bone may be present in Stage II, whereas partially vascularized regions may still be recognizable in Stage III.

▶ **DD.** Ulnar **impaction syndrome** should be distinguished from Kienbock's disease. That condition is dealt with in Chapter 2.9.5.

6.3.3 Osteonecrosis of the Scaphoid

Preiser's disease (idiopathic osteonecrosis of the scaphoid) is much less common than Kienbock's disease. It is also much less common than—and should not be mistaken for—osteonecrosis related to a fracture of the scaphoid (▶ Fig. 6.26; see also Chapter 2.9.2).

6.3.4 Osteonecrosis of the Vertebrae

It should be noted that osteonecrosis may occur in the spine as a result of a systemic disorder or medication or after radiation therapy. In 1895, the surgeon Hermann Kummell reported on adult patients who had suffered vertebral collapse without a history of significant trauma. Later histological studies revealed that areas of osteonecrosis were present in these vertebrae, but it should always be kept in mind that traumatic fractures are also associated with osteonecrotic areas. The intravertebral vacuum phenomenon and the fluid sign visible on MRI (cf. Chapter 10.1.3) are found in osteoporotic fractures as well as in Kummell's disease, illustrating the overlap between these two disorders.

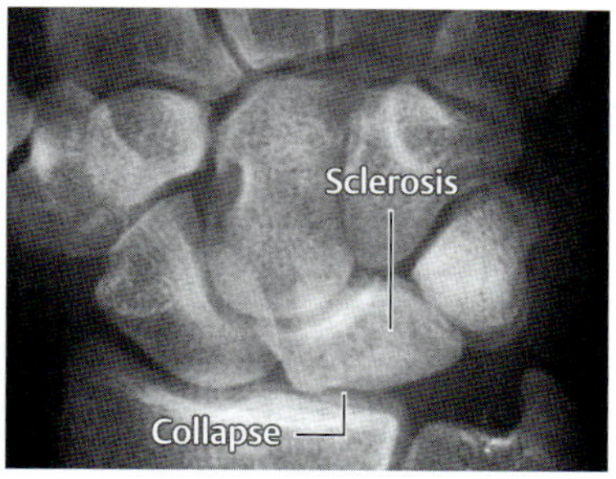

Fig. 6.23 Necrosis of the lunate. Stage III a.

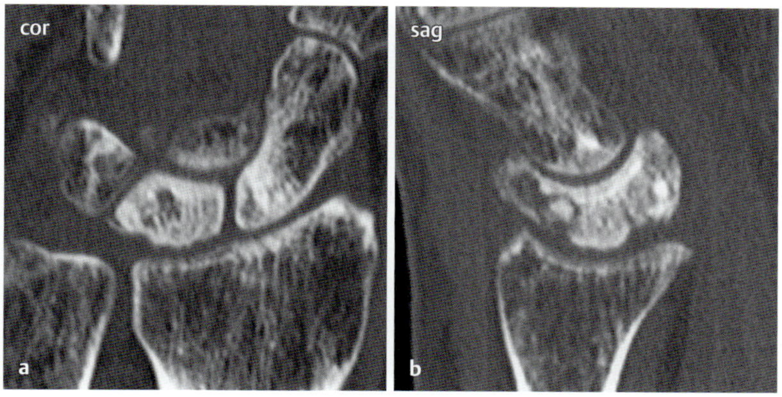

Fig. 6.24 Necrosis of the lunate. Stage III a. **(a)** Sclerosis of the lunate. **(b)** Collapse of the proximal joint surface.

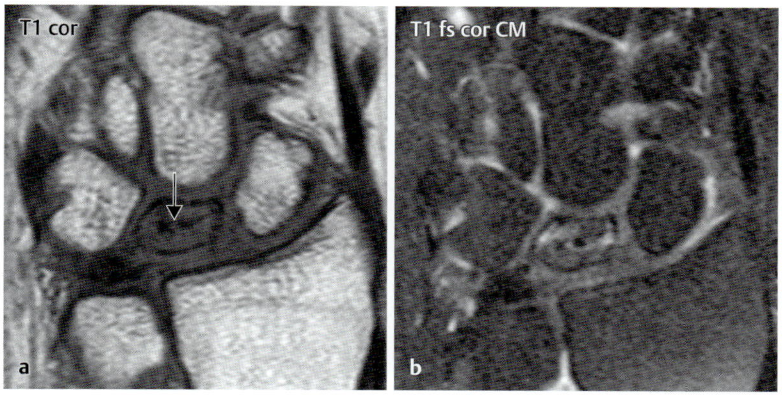

Fig. 6.25 Kienbock's disease. **(a)** Diffuse hypointensity on this T1W image; the dark line (arrow) likely represents a small trabecular condensation or fracture. **(b)** Areas of mixed enhancement suggest there is some residual vascularity in the lunate.

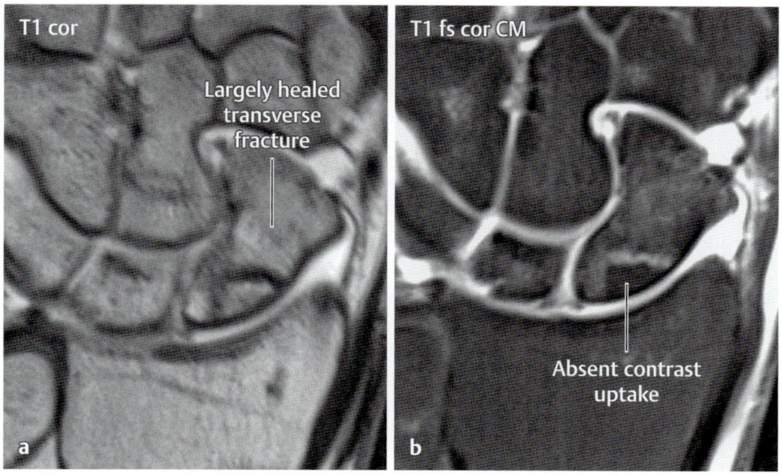

Fig. 6.26 Posttraumatic avascular necrosis of the proximal pole of the scaphoid. MR arthrography and IV contrast application. **(a)** A hypointense border surrounds the infarcted area. **(b)** The border enhances with contrast, the necrotic area does not.

6.4 Sequelae of Radiotherapy

A distinction is made between **expected postradiation changes**, such as fatty degeneration of the bone marrow and muscular atrophy, and radiation-related **complications**, such as osteonecrosis, insufficiency fractures, soft tissue necrosis, radiation-induced tumors, and growth arrest.

▸ **Pathology.** In an adult, ionizing radiation affects the nuclei of osteoblasts, resulting in reduced matrix production, followed by bone atrophy. Depending on the dose, cell death may occur, triggering reparative mechanisms; but if these are unsuccessful, **osteoradionecrosis** is the result. Although osteoradionecrosis is rare, it usually develops several years after very high radiation doses. **Insufficiency fractures** are considerably more common due to reduced osteoblastic activity. In soft tissues, muscle atrophy and, in some cases, myonecrosis may develop. The majority of **radiation-induced tumors** are malignant; occasionally, however, benign tumors may also develop (typically osteochondromas).

6

▸ **Clinical presentation.** The most important causes of pain are insufficiency fractures and osteoradionecrosis in the radiation field. Typical fracture locations are marrow-rich bones, such as the pubic rami, iliac wing, sacrum, and spine.

▸ **Special features in children.** Radiotherapy prior to skeletal maturity can lead to growth arrest, resulting in shortening of limbs, pelvic hypoplasia or scoliosis. Epiphysiolysis of the femoral head and delayed osteoradionecrosis are also seen.

▸ **Radiography/CT.** Osteoradionecrosis and associated reparative mechanisms result in mixed lytic and sclerotic changes along with coarsened trabeculae (▸ Figs. 6.27–6.31). Slowly progressive osteolysis develops in severe forms. Pathologic fractures and nonunions may also occur (see ▸ Figs. 6.28 and ▸ 6.29).

Caution

Fractures may remain radiographically occult due to the absence of callus formation.

▸ **NUC MED.** A bone scan may reveal radiographically occult insufficiency fractures and osteonecrosis.

▸ **MRI.** Areas of osteoradionecrosis are either fatlike or hypointense on T1W images. The signal intensity on T2W images depends on the degree of fluid and fibrosis within the affected bone (see Chapter 6.3.1). If the radiotherapy occurred more than 2 years previously, no increased contrast enhancement should be seen after IV administration of gadolinium.

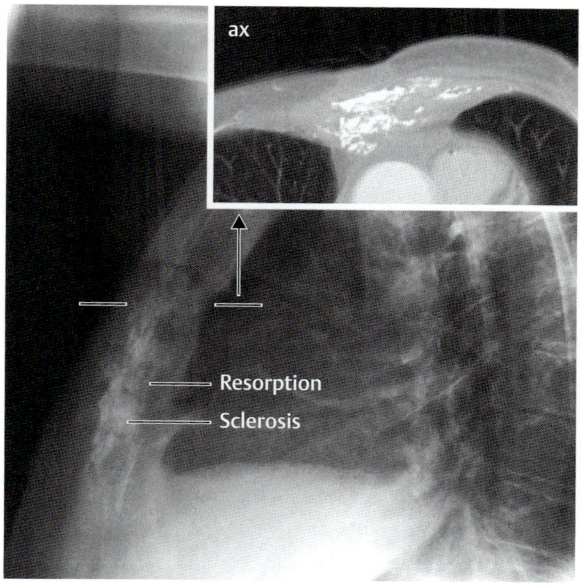

Fig. 6.27 Postradiotherapy osteonecrosis of the sternum.

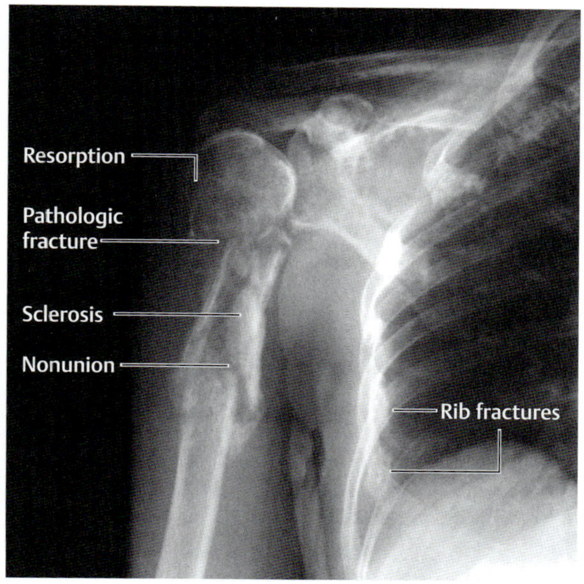

Fig. 6.28 Osteonecrosis of the humerus with pathologic fracture after high-dose radiotherapy of the axilla for breast cancer.

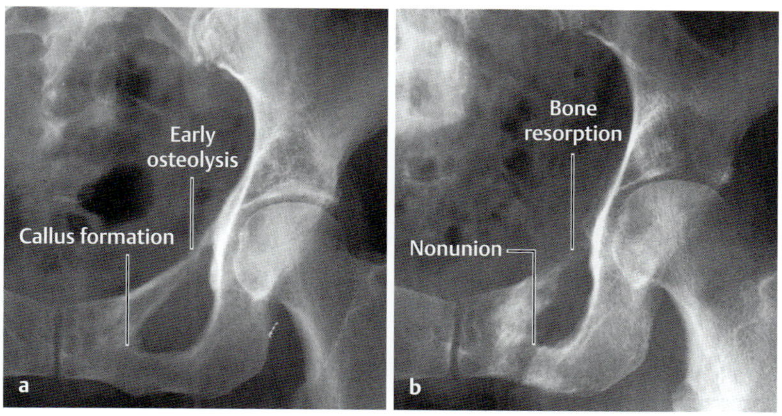

Fig. 6.29 Osteoradionecrosis over time following irradiation of a gynecological tumor. **(a)** At the onset of pain. **(b)** One year later.

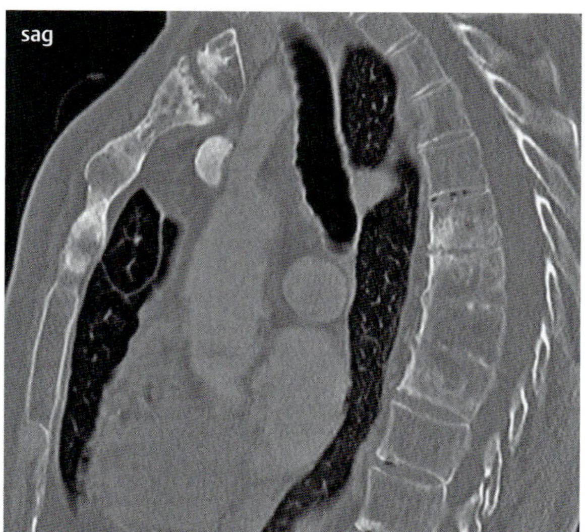

Fig. 6.30 Osteoradionecrosis within the radiation field in a case of lung cancer. Heterogeneous mixed lytic and sclerotic areas in the sternum and thoracic spine.

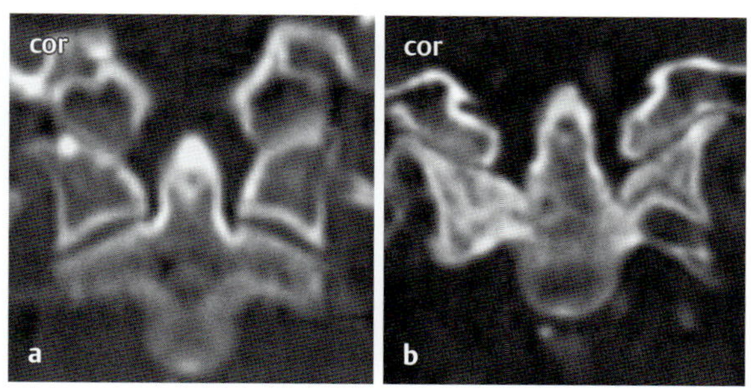

Fig. 6.31 Course of osteoradionecrosis of C1. **(a)** Initial finding after radiotherapy of a head and neck tumor. **(b)** One year later: collapse and destruction of C1 with protrusion of the dens into the foramen magnum.

6.5 Pseudo-osteonecroses

This term refers to disorders that are, strictly speaking, not true osteonecrosis but are still included under this name. SONK (spontaneous osteonecrosis of the knee) is a classic example. This is a destructive arthropathy affecting a femoral condyle and is considered to be a complication of a nonhealing subchondral insufficiency fracture (Chapter 1.5). In these cases, histology will indeed detect osteonecrotic cells from the unhealed fracture, but a circumscribed area of necrosis of a significant size is not present. Furthermore, as MRI clearly demonstrates, compromise of perfusion is only recognizable for very small subchondral areas (▸ Fig. 6.32). An insufficiency fracture located directly beneath the joint surface can create such a disruption of the load-bearing capacity of the bone that the joint surface eventually *collapses* if not adequately protected. Confusion with osteonecrosis is possible at this stage since the affected bones are similar in both entities (e.g., femoral head, femoral condyle; cf. ▶ Fig. W6.6).

True "**Freiberg's disease**" is a disease of childhood (Chapter 7.2.2). However, insufficiency fractures of a metatarsal head in an adult (usually in the presence of osteoporosis) may look similar on radiographs and MRI (▶ Fig. W6.7).

The theory persists that "**transient osteoporosis**," i.e., **transient bone marrow edema**, has something in common with osteonecrosis. The reason is related to the histopathological identification of necrotic bone cells associated with this disease (cf. Chapter 1.5.4). For the sake of completeness, it should be mentioned that there have been individual reports of true osteonecrosis developing in the femoral head following transient bone marrow edema after inadequate (non–weight bearing) therapy. Increased intraosseous pressure arising from long-standing edema is feasible as a possible mechanism in these cases.

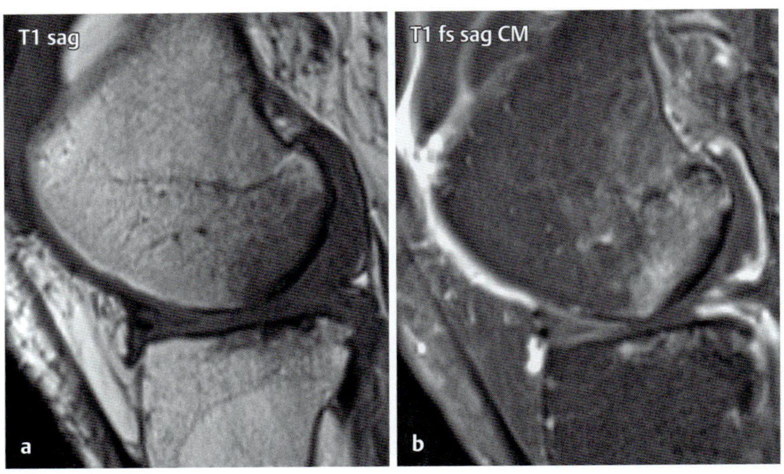

Fig. 6.32 Pseudo-osteonecrosis of the lateral femoral condyle. "Ahlback's disease." **(a)** Absence of an underlying hypointense border. **(b)** Mild articular collapse with only a thin, nonenhancing subchondral zone.

Chapter 7

Osteochondroses

7 Osteochondroses

7.1 Anatomy, Etiology, and Pathogenesis

▶ **Anatomy.** See Chapter 7.1 for anatomy (Fig. W7.1).

"Osteochondrosis" is a very general term which, strictly speaking, means nothing other than "disorder of cartilage and bone" (Greek *-osis* = process or condition). The decisive feature is involvement of bone *and* cartilage in the epiphysis, apophysis, and growth plate of the growing skeleton. It is considered probable that a failure of blood supply sets off a disturbance of enchondral ossification. Osteochondrosis has nothing to do with acute injury to the growth cartilage.

7.1.1 What Do the Different Forms of Osteochondrosis Have in Common?

They develop primarily in **children** and **adolescents** during the **growth phase. Risk factors** play an important role in osteochondrosis:

- **Inheritance:** This is supported by the presence of osteochondroses in members of one family or in twins.
- **"Metabolic" and "hormonal" changes:** Although difficult to define, these alterations must also play a role. Thus, osteochondrosis develops in particular in growth-delayed children (especially boys) or in children with congenital skeletal dysplasias. Osteochondrosis is also seen particularly during strong growth spurts.
- **Anatomy:** This appears to play a role. Certain bones and joints may be affected because of some incongruence of the joint surfaces leading to abnormal forces at those sites. Children with a congenitally abnormal discoid meniscus are more commonly affected with osteochondritis dissecans than other children. Similarly, osteochondrosis of the elbow develops much more commonly in the capitulum than in the trochlea.

Osteochondrosis is a **disease** and not a normal variant of ossification, but it is striking that the sites of predilection for variants coincide with locations of osteochondrosis.

Osteochondrosis appears in many epiphyses and apophyses as well as in the region of the growth plate. There are currently approximately 75 known entities and most are named after those who first reported them. For good reasons, osteochondritis dissecans is assigned to the articular osteochondroses in this book. ▶Table 7.1 intentionally specifies only the most important disorders; for other disorders see References for Chapter 7.1.

Table 7.1 Classification of the osteochondroses based on Siffert

Description		Location
Articular (epiphyseal) osteochondroses	Legg–Calvé–Perthes' disease	Femoral head
	Freiberg's disease (Köhler's disease Type II)	Metatarsal heads II–IV
	Köhler's disease Type I	Navicular bone
	Panner's disease	Humeral capitellum
	Osteochondritis dissecans	Any joint, especially knee, talus, and elbow
Nonarticular (apophyseal) osteochondroses	Osgood–Schlatter disease	Tibial tuberosity
	Sinding–Larsen–Johansson disease	Inferior patellar pole
	Sever's disease	Calcaneal apophysis
Osteochondroses of the growth plate	Scheuermann's disease	Hyaline cartilage end plate, and subchondral superior end plate of the spine
	Blount's disease	Medial part of the proximal tibial epiphysis

7.1.2 To Which Disorders is the Term "Osteochondrosis" Not Applicable?

Of course, the cartilage and subchondral bone may also be affected in adults, but there is usually a history of some form of injury. For this reason, the following common cases are *not* assigned to the osteochondroses:

- Posttraumatic osteoarthritis.
- Posttraumatic osteonecrosis (e.g., of the talar dome).

These are usually secondary to a fracture involving the articular surfaces (e.g., intra-articular radial fracture or osteochondral fracture).

7.2 Articular Osteochondroses

7.2.1 Perthes' Disease

Perthes' disease (synonym: Legg–Calvé–Perthes' disease) is an osteochondrosis of the femoral head. Its etiology remains unclear; its pathogenesis is slowly becoming understood. Perthes' disease has a self-limiting clinical course that proceeds in stages and carries a risk of incomplete recovery.

▸ **Pathology.** It is not known why the vessels supplying the femoral head fail. It also remains unclear whether one or several ischemic attacks are required to initiate the disease. The concept of "osteonecrosis" does not go far enough; in this condition, the epiphyseal cartilage, the ossification center of the epiphysis, the growth plate, and even the metaphysis are all affected. The necrotic ossification center is extremely vulnerable to mechanical loading and there is an imbalance between bone degradation and regeneration. The disorder is self-limiting; spontaneous revascularization occurs.

There are four **characteristic stages:**

- **Early stage:** Cell death in the bony epiphysis, resulting in the development of microfractures. The deep layer of the epiphyseal cartilage becomes necrotic and enchondral ossification ceases.
- **Condensation stage:** Condensation and narrowing of the ossified epiphysis. The cartilage undergoes early revascularization and becomes hypertrophic.
- **Fragmentation stage:** Fibrotic bony remodeling and trabecular absorption result in an unstable structure with fragmentation and further reduction in size of the bony epiphysis. Epiphyseal contour deformity and exuberant growth of the epiphyseal cartilage lead to decentralization of the femoral head and thus to lateral subluxation. Concomitant involvement of the metaphysis leads to widening and shortening of the femoral neck.
- **Regeneration phase:** Revascularization of the femoral head occurs with new bone formation, usually associated with incomplete recovery, though rarely with complete restoration.

▸ **Clinical presentation.** The disorder presents between the ages of 3 and 12 years, with a peak between the ages of 5 and 6 years. The cardinal symptom is a limp. The signs and symptoms in the early stage are indistinguishable from transient synovitis. The prognosis of Perthes' disease depends on early detection.

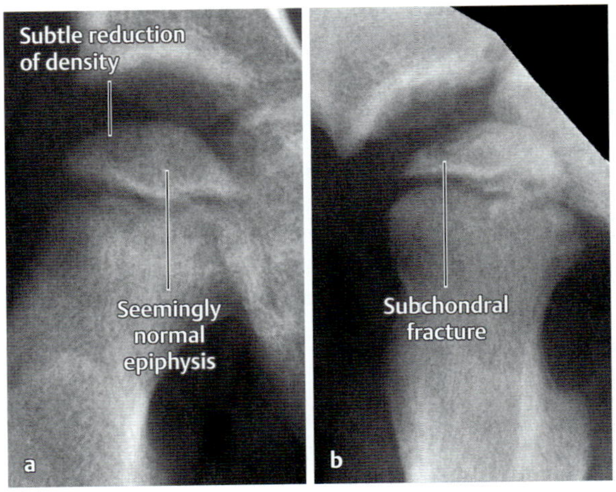

Fig. 7.1 Perthes disease. Initial stage. **(a)** Very subtle alterations on the AP image. **(b)** Typical subchondral fracture on the frog lateral view.

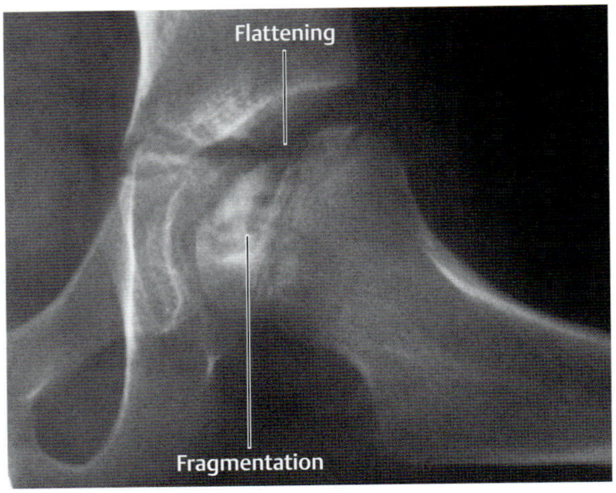

Fig. 7.3 Perthes' disease. Fragmentation stage. As well as the fragmentation, flattening of the epiphysis is typical for this stage.

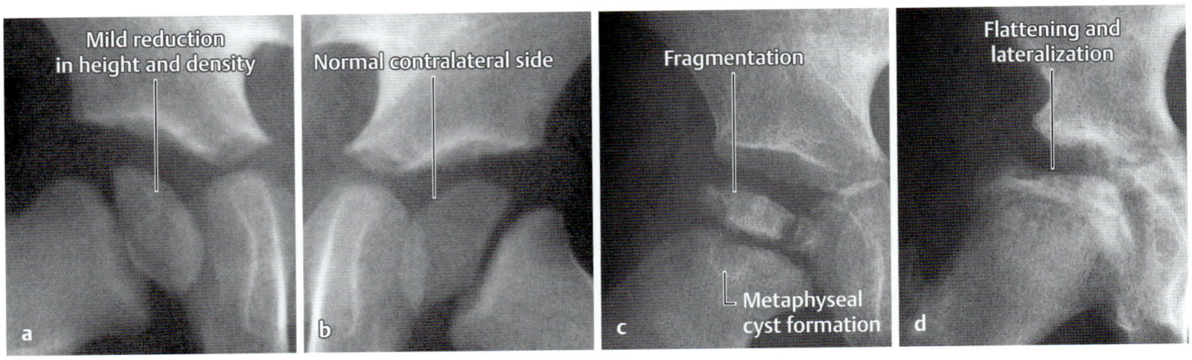

Fig. 7.2 Radiological course of Perthes' disease. **(a)** Condensation stage. **(b)** Healthy contralateral side for comparison. **(c)** Fragmentation stage. **(d)** Final stage with remodeling, flattening, and lateralization of the femoral head.

▸ **Radiography/CT.** Radiographic diagnostic examinations are inadequate during the early stage. However, over the course of the disease, AP and frog-leg lateral views are helpful for establishing the diagnosis and determining prognosis. Classification of the radiographic abnormalities is based on the disease course outlined above. The use of 3D-reconstruction CT is primarily reserved for operative planning.

- **Initial stage:** Minimal radiographic signs:
  - Joint-space widening.
  - Periarticular soft-tissue swelling.
  - Subtle irregularity of structure and contour of the epiphysis (▸ Fig. 7.1).
- **Condensation stage:** Increased density and decreased size of the bony epiphysis (▸ Figs. 7.2a and ▸ 7.2b).
- **Fragmentation stage:** Decreased size and fragmentation of the epiphysis (▸ Figs. 7.2c–7.5 and ▸ W7.2).
- **Regeneration stage** (▸ Figs. 7.6, ▸ 7.7, and ▸ W7.3):
  - Fusion of the ossification centers with a tendency for remodeling of the bone.
  - Irregular widening of the physeal plate; later premature physeal closure as a result of epiphyseal–metaphyseal bridging.
  - Metaphyseal involvement with radiolucent bands, densities, and cystic lesions.
- **Final stage** (▸ Figs. 7.2d and ▸ 7.8):
  - Complete restoration *or*
  - Widening, flattening, and subluxation of the femoral head (mushroom deformity, "coxa plana") with secondary acetabular hypoplasia (predisposition for degenerative osteoarthritis, see ▸ Fig. 7.8).
  - Widening of the metaphysis and shortening of the femoral neck.

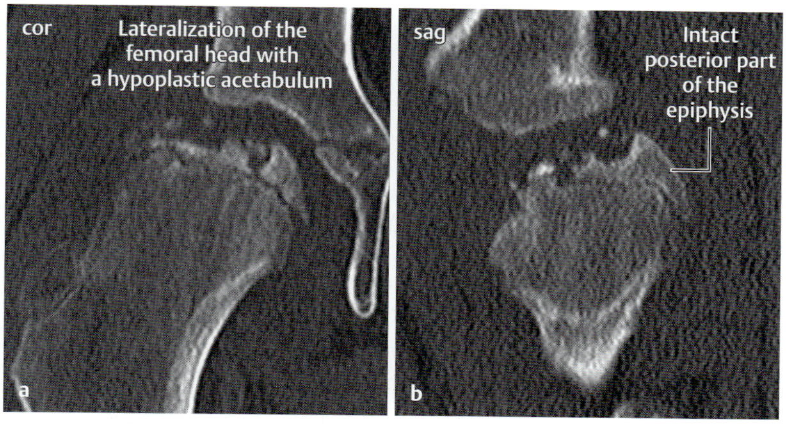

Fig. 7.4 Perthes' disease. Fragmentation stage. **(a)** Fragmentation and flattening of the epiphysis. **(b)** The fragmentation does not involve the entire epiphysis.

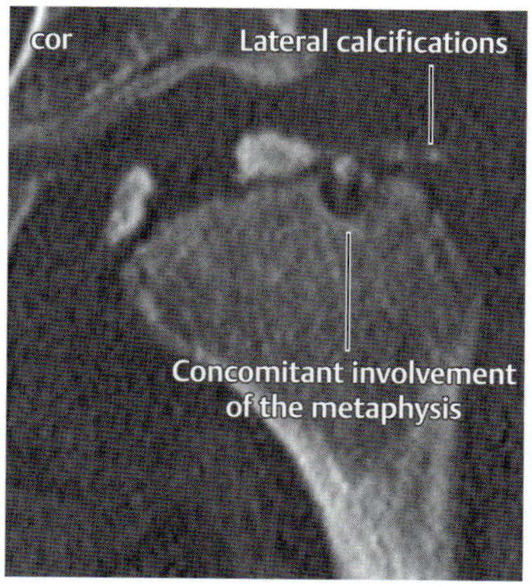

Fig. 7.5 Perthes' disease. Fragmentation stage (▶ see also ▸ Fig. W7.2).

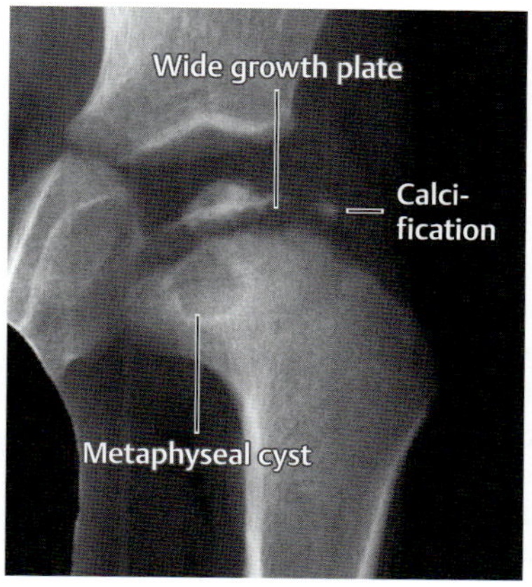

Fig. 7.6 Perthes' disease. Regeneration stage. Lateral calcification of the epiphyseal plate and the metaphyseal cysts are regarded as head-at-risk signs and suggest a poor prognosis.

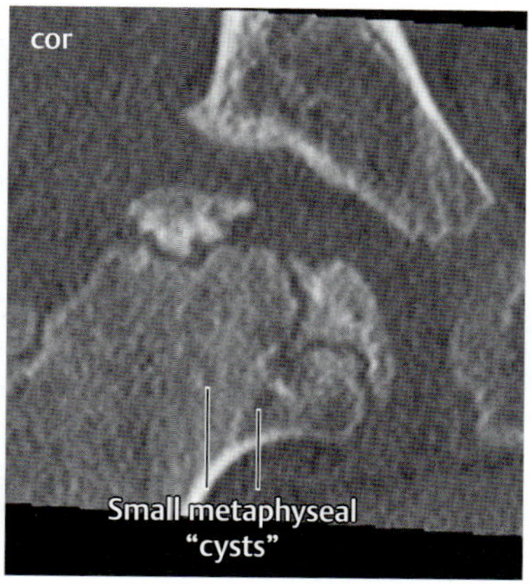

Fig. 7.7 Perthes' disease. Regeneration stage (▶ see also ▸ Fig. W7.3).

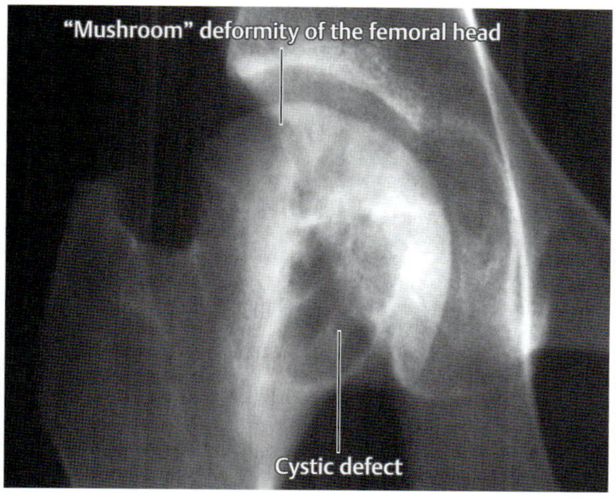

Fig. 7.8 Perthes' disease. Final stage. As well as the mushroom deformity of the femoral head (pre-osteoarthritis), this example also demonstrates a large defect in the femoral head.

7

The **Catterall Classification** (▶ Fig. 7.9) provides prognostic information for possible surgical intervention. Stages III and IV represent severe forms in which more than one-half of the femoral head is involved. In addition, these prognostically unfavorable radiological signs (**head-at-risk signs**) should also be reported:

- Decentralization of the femoral head in a lateral direction (▶ Fig. 7.4a).
- Lateral calcification of the physeal plate (▶ Figs. 7.5 and ▶ 7.6).
- Metaphyseal involvement (▶ Figs. 7.5 and ▶ 7.6).
- Horizontalization of the physeal plate.

The final stage may be further classified according to Stulberg and co-workers (▶ see References for Chapter 7.2.1).

▶ **US.** Ultrasound provides confirmation of a joint effusion.

▶ **MRI.** In the initial stage, MRI allows an early diagnosis with evidence of bone marrow edema in the ossification center of the epiphysis while the radiograph is still unremarkable (▶ Fig. 7.10a, b). Coronal fat-suppressed, fluid-sensitive, and coronal and sagittal T1W sequences are useful for diagnosis. In the presence of bone marrow edema, an additional fat-suppressed, contrast-enhanced T1W sequence, or even better a dynamic contrast MRI, is helpful for determining the stage (early stage, revascularization stage) and for early detection of compromised perfusion (▶ Fig. 7.11).

Serial MRI examinations reveal development of the necrotic area and hypertrophy of the epiphyseal cartilage and, thus, the decentralization of the epiphysis within the acetabulum. The final stage shows fat-equivalent signal (▶ Fig. 7.10c) or—depending on the severity of the course—increased sclerosis with loss of signal.

Functional MRI (neutral position, abduction and internal rotation) is helpful for preoperative planning in the incomplete recovery phase in order to document the degree of incongruence and risk of impingement between acetabulum and deformed femoral head.

▶ **NUC MED.** Bone scan is sensitive during the early stages by detecting absent or reduced tracer uptake in the anterolateral portion of the femoral head. However, it has been largely replaced by MRI.

▶ **DD.**

Transient synovitis and synovitis of other etiologies. MRI is helpful to further investigate equivocal radiographic findings and/or laboratory findings and the detection of a joint effusion on ultrasound.

Other origins of osteonecrosis of the femoral head. Simultaneous development of bilateral osteonecrosis of the femoral heads suggests a systemic disease (sickle cell anemia, hypothyroidism, Gaucher's disease).

Meyer dysplasia. This is associated with delayed, irregular ossification of the femoral head that results in multiple ossification centers. If the clinical and radiological findings are unclear, differentiation can be achieved using MRI.

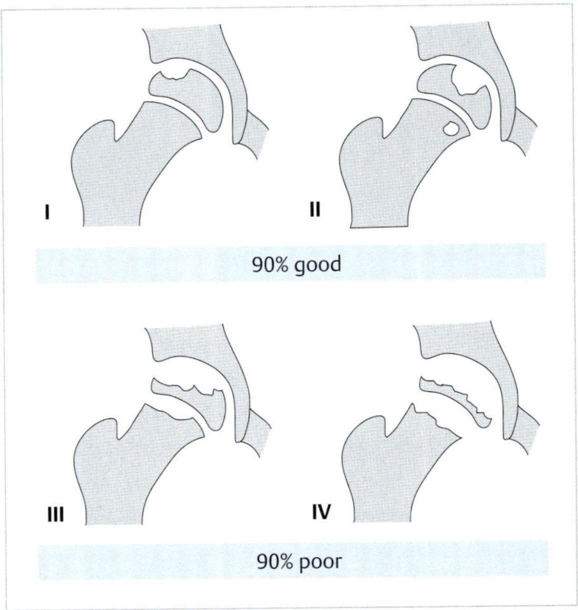

Fig. 7.9 Classification of Perthes' disease according to Catterall.

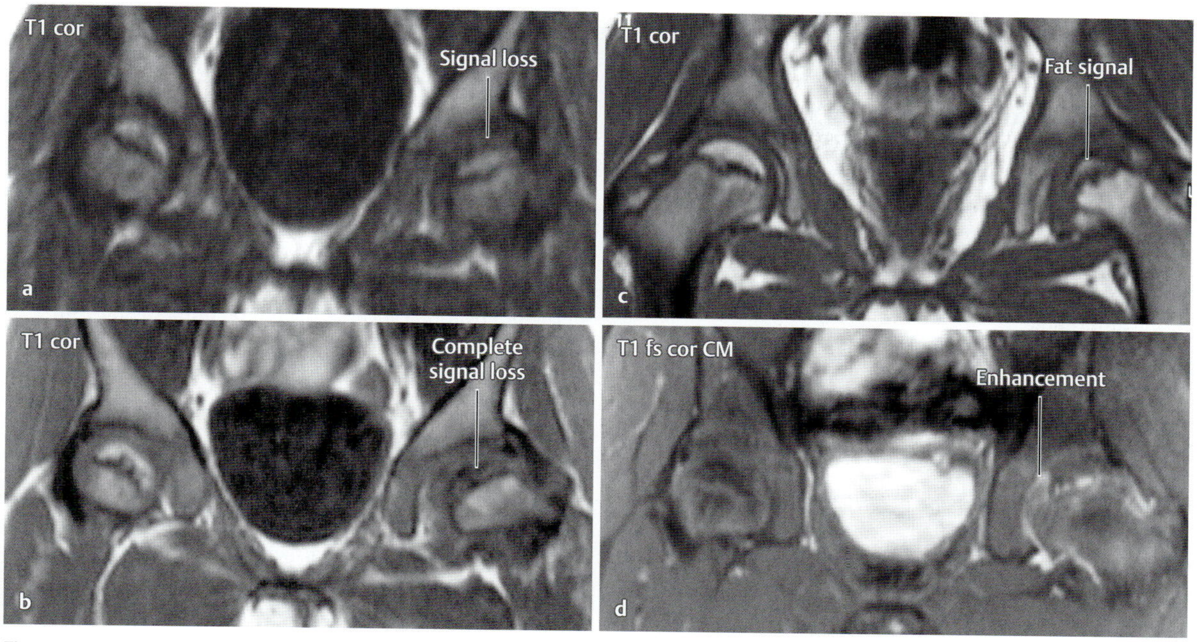

Fig. 7.10 Monitoring of disease progression in a case of left-sided Perthes' disease. **(a)** Early stage. **(b)** Eventually, there is complete loss of signal. **(c)** Finally, fatty marrow evident in the center and reactive deposition of fatty marrow in the metaphysis. **(d)** Contrast enhancement in the medial part of the epiphysis as a sign of repair.

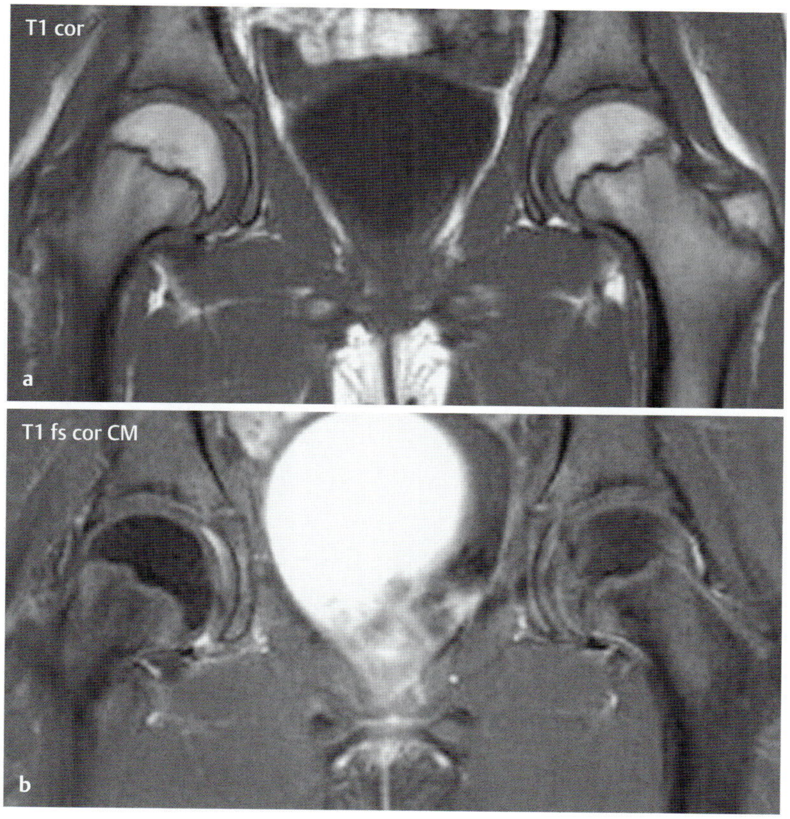

Fig. 7.11 Early diagnosis of Perthes' disease in the initial stage. (Courtesy of M. Anderson, Charlottesville, Virginia, USA.) **(a)** No definite detection of edema on the T1W image. **(b)** However, there is evidence of compromise of perfusion of the right femoral head based on absent contrast uptake.

7.2.2 Freiberg's Disease (Osteochondrosis of the Metatarsal Heads)

The term "Köhler's disease Type II" is also used for this condition. The cause of osteochondrosis of the metatarsal heads (primarily the second metatarsal) is unclear. The diagnosis is usually made in adolescence (girls are more commonly affected than boys), but is also seen as an incidental finding during adulthood.

▶ **Radiography.** Depending on when the diagnosis is made, the following radiographic signs are seen:

- Flattening and widening of the head (▶ Fig. 7.12).
- Fragmentation.
- Possible premature closure of the growth plate.
- Reactive sclerosis.
- The joint space is usually maintained.
- Widening of the opposite base of the proximal phalanx is seen in marked cases.

7

▶ DD. **Overuse-related insufficiency fractures** with subsequent collapse of the joint surface may result in a similar appearance of a metatarsal head (▶ Fig. 7.13).

7.2.3 Köhler's Disease Type I

Osteochondrosis of the navicular bone can occur from age 2 years onward, being most common during the 4th and 5th years of age. The prognosis of Köhler's disease Type I is very good. The navicular bone assumes a normal appearance after spontaneous healing (~6–18 months after diagnosis). Only rarely does pain persist after skeletal maturity.

▶ **Radiography/CT.** Conventional radiography demonstrates mixed areas of sclerosis and lucency in the ossification center. In other cases the ossification center is collapsed and sclerotic (▶ Fig. 7.14), sometimes only sclerotic, and sometimes fragmented.

▶ **MRI.** MRI is frequently employed even before radiographic examination for a painful foot of unknown origin, so the radiologist may also be confronted with the findings of Köhler's disease type I on MRI, typically those of sclerosis and bony remodeling (▶ Fig. 7.15).

▶ DD. **Muller–Weiss syndrome.** The age of the patient prevents confusion with the rare Muller–Weiss syndrome (osteonecrosis of the tarsal navicular in the adult; ▶ Fig. 7.16).

7.2.4 Panner's Disease and Hegemann's Disease

Panner's disease is an osteochondrosis of the humeral capitulum in children up to the age of about 10 years; boys are more commonly affected. The majority of these osteochondroses heal spontaneously. Cases in which collapse of the capitulum results in secondary osteoarthritis are very rare. Radiographic findings include diffuse sclerotic changes of the ossification center of the lateral humeral joint surface —similar to Köhler's disease although in some cases mixed lytic and sclerotic changes are seen along with irregularity of the joint surface. During spontaneous healing, a lytic lesion without contour irregularity is seen in adolescents just prior to complete fusion of the ossification center (▶ Figs. 7.17 and ▶ W7.4). Patients with Panner's disease present without a history of significant injury or chronic overuse. It may, however, also be associated with chronic overuse in throwing sports.

The more **focal osteochondritis dissecans** is also found in the capitulum and the trochlea and must be distinguished from Panner's disease, although it does tend to affect an older age group: adolescents up to the age of 15 to 16 years (Chapter 7.2.5).

If the trochlea is involved instead of the capitulum (Panner's disease), this is known as **Hegemann's disease** (▶ Fig. 7.18), which is rare.

> **Caution**
>
> The term "Little Leaguer's Elbow," used by many authors globally for all types of overuse injuries of the elbow joint, but should be reserved for chronic traction apophysitis (either as epiphysiolysis and/or as osteochondrosis) of the medial epicondyle (cf. Chapter 2.7.1).

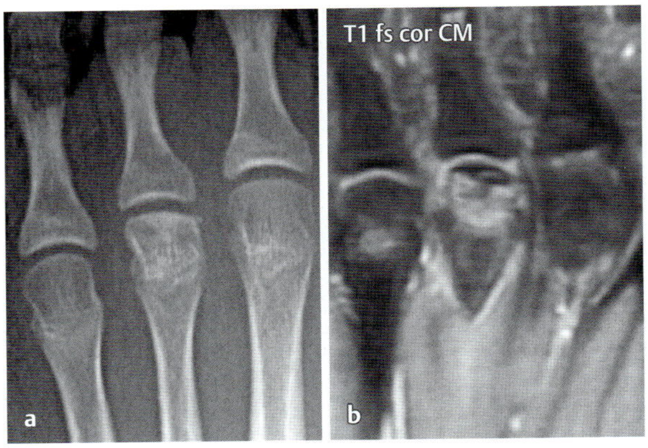

Fig. 7.12 Freiberg's disease (Köhler's disease Type II). (Courtesy of R. Whitehouse, Manchester, UK.) **(a)** Subtle flattening and density of the third metatarsal head. **(b)** Narrow, nonenhancing subchondral zone.

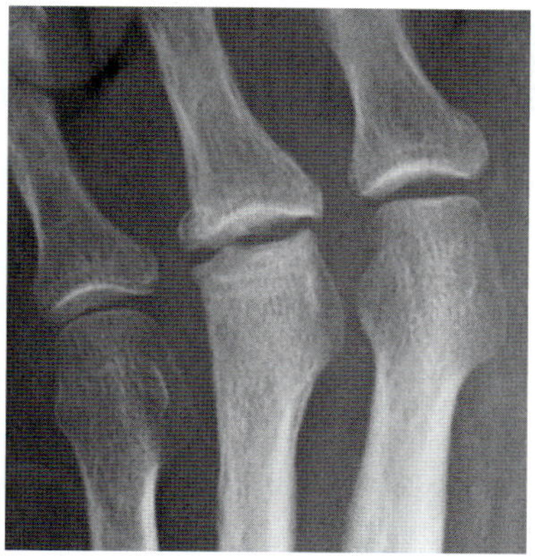

Fig. 7.13 Differential diagnosis of Freiberg's disease. Incomplete recovery after an insufficiency fracture of the third metatarsal head 5 years previously. The cause was most probably steroid therapy. Subtle findings with flattening also of the second metatarsal.

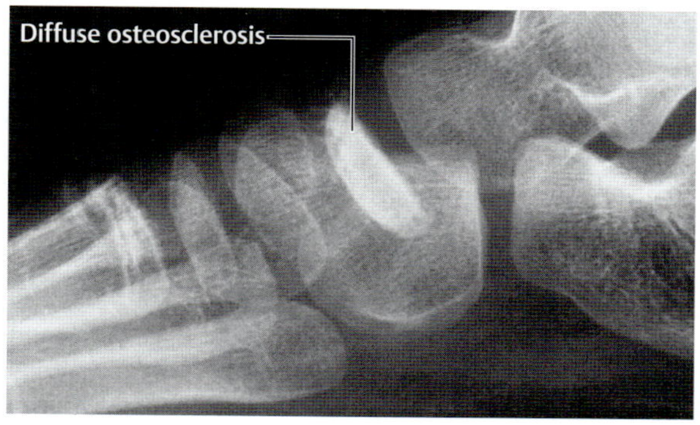

Fig. 7.14 Köhler's disease Type I. Markedly increased density of navicular bone.

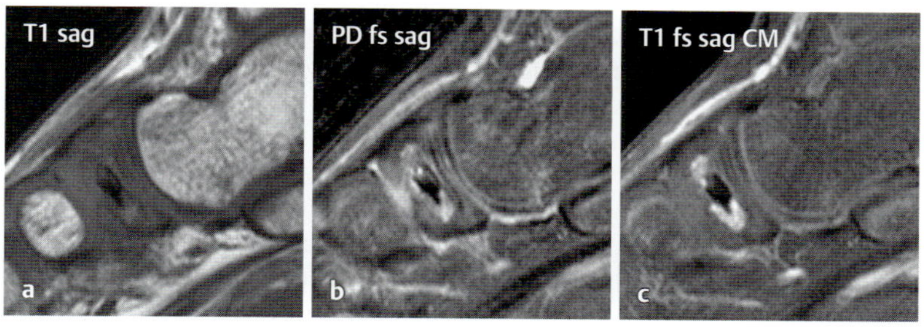

Fig. 7.15 Köhler's disease Type I. **(a)** The navicular bone is condensed and sclerotic centrally. **(b)** The edema is a sign of a reparative process. **(c)** Another sign is contrast enhancement.

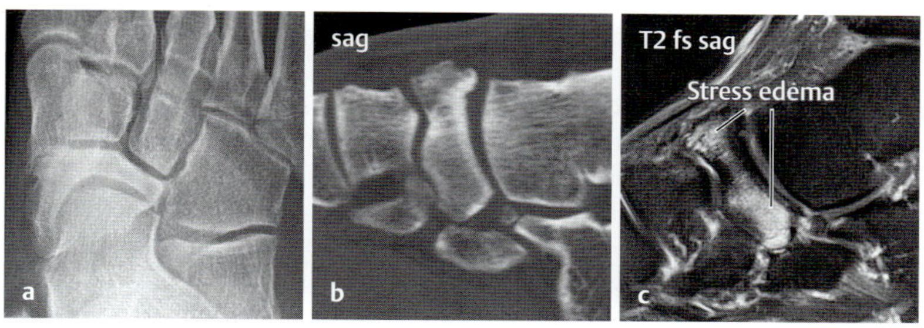

Fig. 7.16 Incidental finding in a 30-year-old man after injury to the tarsus. **(a)** Dense navicular bone with an irregular contour. **(b)** The chronic appearing deformity of the adjacent bone suggests juvenile Köhler's disease Type I rather than Muller–Weiss syndrome. **(c)** The largely preserved articular cartilage is also more suggestive of a juvenile Köhler's disease Type I than of Muller–Weiss syndrome.

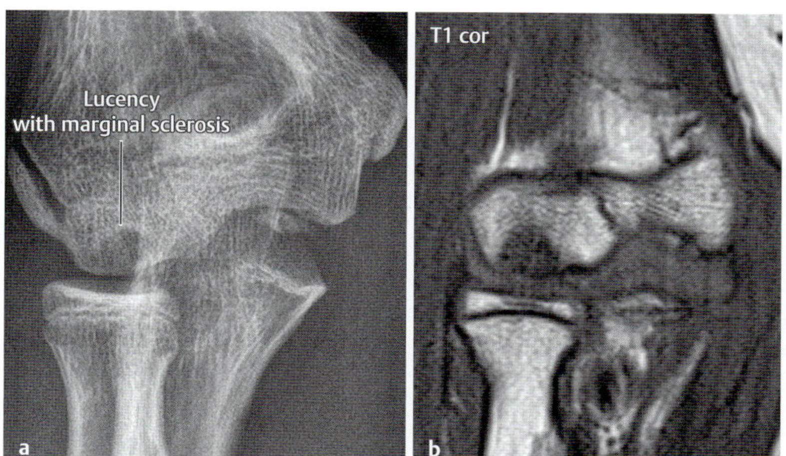

Fig. 7.17 Panner's disease. ▶ For additional images see ▶ Fig. W7.4. **(a)** Subchondral radiolucency of the humeral capitulum with a sclerotic margin. **(b)** A half-moon–shaped area of subchondral low signal intensity evident on the T1W image correlates with the radiograph.

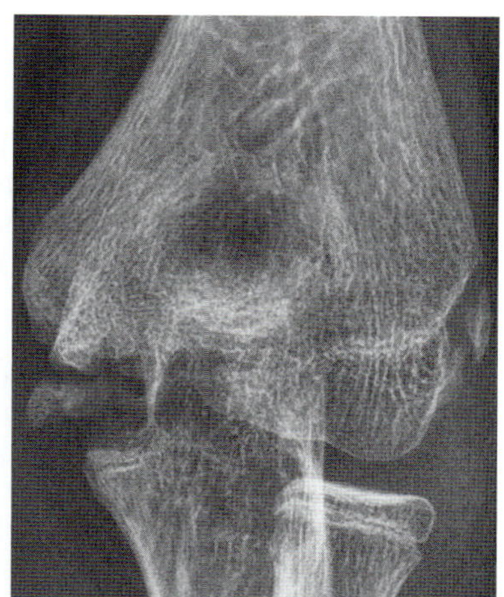

Fig. 7.18 Hegemann's disease. Irregularity of the ossification center of the humeral trochlea. (Courtesy of R. Whitehouse, Manchester, UK.)

7.2.5 Osteochondritis Dissecans

Osteochondritis dissecans is a disturbance of enchondral ossification of the growing skeleton. Most cases of osteochondritis dissecans heal with conservative treatment. In the majority of cases a real osteochondral fragment does not develop.

▸ **Pathology.** Modern doctrine, largely based on animal experiments, assumes that the disease originates from **chondronecrosis** of the epiphyseal cartilage as its starting point. The cause is most likely a disturbance of vascular supply in the zone of transition between the already ossified epiphysis and the epiphyseal cartilage ("ossification front"). This results in a disturbance of enchondral ossification, which—as the epiphyseal growth cartilage becomes thinner with advancing age—*may* involve the articular surface with its hyaline cartilage. The primary features, which are particularly well visible histopathologically, are chondronecroses and repair processes around the necroses within the epiphyseal growth plate. If these chondronecroses are larger in size and located near the joint surface, then discoloration of the joint surface may occur, later developing chondral tears. Eventually, fissures appear at the border between osteochondral lesion and normal cartilage/bone. The final stage is an osteochondral fragment that can spontaneously detach itself from the underlying bone.

The current theory of its etiology implicates physical (over-) loading, possibly acting synergically with a genetic predisposition.

▸ **Clinical presentation.** Primarily children and adolescents between the ages of 8 and 16 years are affected, although the disease is also diagnosed in young adults—but by then it is usually at an advanced stage. A basic rule is: The older a patient is when osteochondritis dissecans is discovered, the more advanced are the abnormalities. Clinical symptoms consist of pain on loading and recurrent effusions. In the final stage, a loose body ("joint mouse") can lead to intermittent pain and locking of the joint. In its early stages (i.e., without an actual osteochondral fragment), osteochondritis dissecans is sometimes asymptomatic and for this reason is not uncommonly discovered as an incidental radiographic finding (especially at the talus).

Location. Weight-bearing parts of all major, and some minor, joints are affected. The classic locations are the inner aspect of the medial femoral condyle and the medial and lateral facet of the talus and the capitulum humeri.

Treatment. Treatment depends largely on clinical presentation and the appearance of the joint surface (arthroscopy). A finding that is only visible on MRI and not arthroscopy (Stage I in all classification systems) should be treated conservatively, with avoidance of any excessive loading. The majority of classifications include four grades, but the higher grades are not uniformly classified nor is there any wide consensus regarding treatment.

▸ **Radiography.** The following radiographic signs are recognizable:

- Subchondral radiolucency without a sharp border (early sign; ▸ Fig. 7.19a).
- Subchondral fragment with normal or increased bone density, surrounded by a radiolucent border (▸ Fig. 7.19b).
- Bandlike sclerosis along the radiolucent zone (▸ Fig. 7.20).
- Poorly marginated subchondral sclerosis with irregular joint contour (late sign).
- Round, cystoid radiolucencies with sclerotic margins (late sign).
- Loose bodies and a subchondral defect (late sign).

▸ **CT.** CT documents the radiographic signs unobscured by overlying structures and is helpful for differentiating between chronic osteochondritis dissecans, in which case there may be evidence of a sclerotic margin, and an acute osteochondral fracture (cf. Chapter 1.4.3).

▸ **MRI.**

Stage I. A hypointense zone immediately beneath the joint surface is seen on T1W images (▸ Figs. 7.21a and ▸ 7.22a), usually appearing crescentic or oval-shaped in configuration, depending on whether the sagittal or coronal plane is being viewed. The subchondral plate between bone and cartilage is interrupted in this region. On fat-saturated, fluid-sensitive sequences, there is a signal-intense halo around a zone of heterogeneous signal intensity (▸ Fig. 7.22b). This halo does not have the same intensity as intra-articular fluid. The important feature for the diagnosis of Stage I is that the *joint surface* is *completely intact* (▸ Fig. 7.21b). This can be verified exactly by using fluid-sensitive sequences in two projections. It should also be confirmed that the lesion does not "bulge" into the intra-articular space.

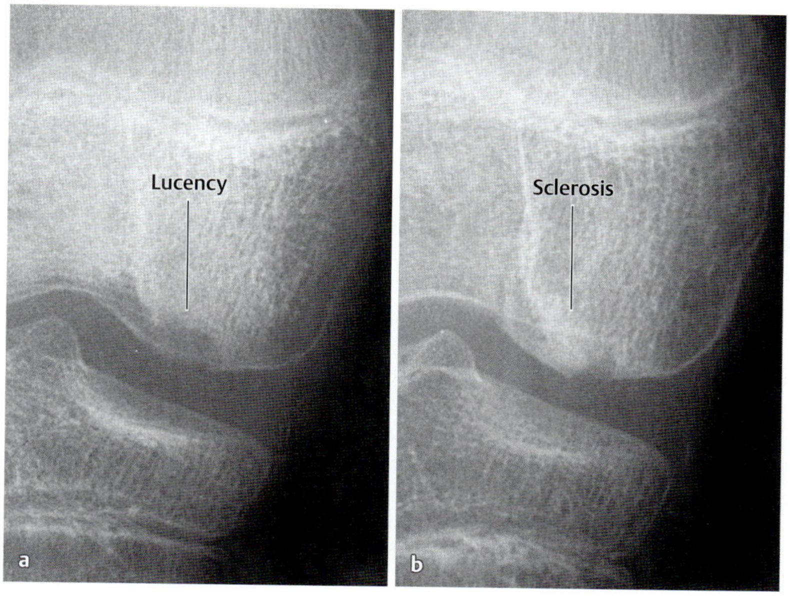

Fig. 7.19 Osteochondrosis dissecans of the medial femoral condyle. **(a)** Early stage. **(b)** Four months later.

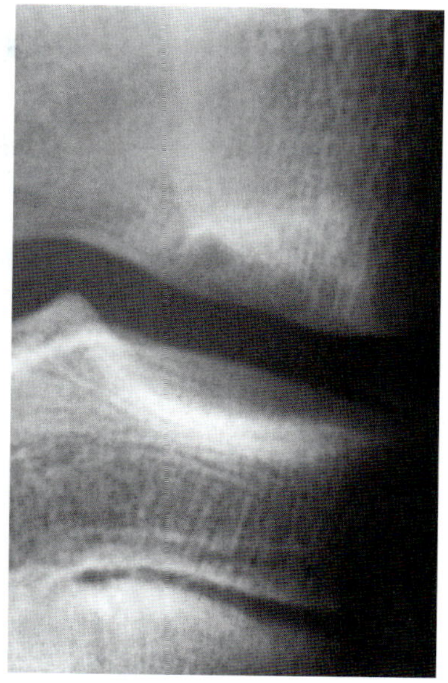

Fig. 7.20 Ostecchondrosis dissecans of the medial femoral condyle. Arthroscopy confirmed intact cartilage.

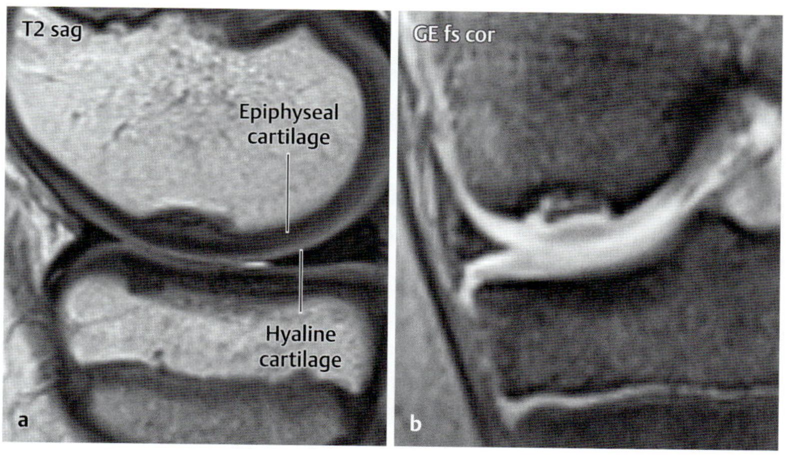

Fig. 7.21 Osteochondritis dissecans. Stage I. **(a)** Hypointense, oval-shaped finding with sha-p demarcation from the bone. **(b)** The GRE sequence demonstrates mildly heterogeneous signal characteristics of normal cartilage. The "osteochondral fragment–like" character of the lesion is evident, but no real osteochondral fragment is present; the overlying cartilage is ir tact.

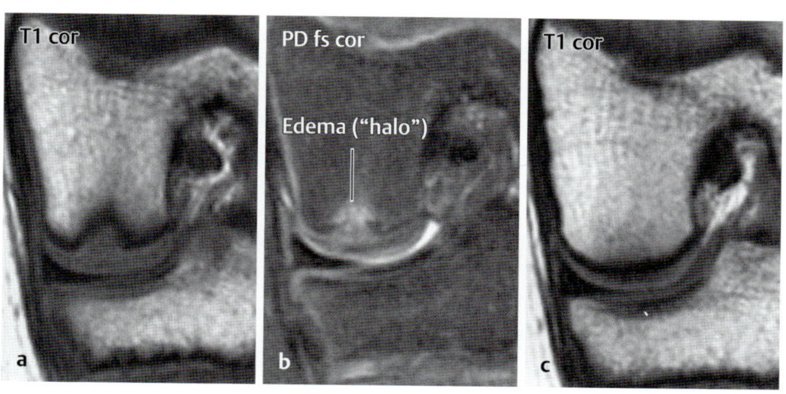

Fig. 7.22 Osteochondritis dissecans. Course of Stage I. **(a)** Initial appearance of the early stage. **(b)** A signal-intense halo on this fluid-sens tive, fat-saturated sequence. **(c)** Complete restoration subsequently occurred over the course of 18 months.

Stages II–IV. Depending on the stage, the cartilage appears *irregular* (**Stage II**; ▶ Fig. 7.23), demonstrates *tears* (**Stage III**) and in some cases *osteochondral defects* (**Stage IV**). The zone of transition between hypointense zone and normal bone is always hyperintense on fluid-sensitive sequences (see ▶ Fig. 7.23b); it also enhances with contrast. If there is a fissure in the cartilage, then joint fluid may intrude into this zone of transition between fragment and underlying bone (▶ Fig. 7.24).

Since patients with osteochondritis dissecans also have an effusion, its arthrographic effect will adequately demonstrate the cartilage on MRI. The (albeit superior) direct intra-articular administration of a contrast agent may be dispensed with, particularly in the knee, although, if there is any diagnostic uncertainty with an ankle, hip, or elbow joint, then it is advisable to resort to MR arthrography or, alternatively, to CT arthrography.

A large number of **MRI classification systems** have been proposed that are related to arthroscopic classifications systems. Distinction between the following findings is important for treatment and prognosis:

7

- **Osteochondrosis dissecans with completely intact joint surface** without chondral fissure or bulging (Stage I, stable osteochondritis dissecans).
- **Osteochondritis dissecans with pathologic articular surface:** the spectrum of findings includes chondral bulging into the joint space (▶ Fig. 7.25), cartilage irregularity and tearing, a nondisplaced osteochondral fragment ("trap door"; see ▶ Fig. 7.24), and an empty defect bed.

If it is not possible to evaluate the articular cartilage with certainty (e.g., the thin cartilage of the talus), the following features are **signs suggesting fragment instability**:

- Larger (more than 3–4 mm), circumscribed cysts in the zone of transition between osteochondral fragment and healthy bone.
- Fluid-equivalent signal (effusion) in the zone of transition beneath the fragment.
- Absent contrast agent uptake in the zone of transition.

▶ **DD.** Differentiating juvenile osteochondritis dissecans from **disorders and variants of ossification** can be very difficult (cf. Chapter 1.1.2). It can be argued that variants of ossification are disturbances of enchondral ossification (= osteochondroses) that heal spontaneously over the course of skeletal development and therefore do not become apparent. Osteochondritis dissecans is the unhealed, or not yet healed, form of osteochondrosis.

A basic rule for the **knee** is: The younger the patient (at least if younger than 8 years) and the farther posterior the lesion is located in the femoral condyle, the more likely that it is a self-healing variant of the ossification (Chapter 1.1.2).

With the **talus**, differentiation from a fresh osteochondral fracture is based on clinical features (cf. Chapter 2.15.3):

- An osteochondral fracture is almost always associated with bone marrow edema (on MRI), whereas it is seen with osteochondritis dissecans only in higher stages.
- Osteochondritis dissecans is usually located in the medial talar dome; acute fractures, in contrast, are more often found laterally. Acute osteochondral fractures have a longitudinal configuration, whereas osteochondritis dissecans of the talus is typically a more round, crater-shaped lesion (▶ Fig. 7.26).

Differentiation of an old posttraumatic osteochondral lesion of the talus from osteochondritis dissecans can be difficult. A basic rule is that posttraumatic changes are almost always found in patients over 25 to 30 years of age regardless of whether the patient can recall an injury. Osteochondritis dissecans usually manifests clinically during adolescence or, at the latest, in early adulthood. Differentiation may also be achieved with radiography and MRI. A round-to-oval shaped, sharply circumscribed lesion on the radiograph, possibly surrounded by a fine radiolucent margin, suggests osteochondritis dissecans. Poor margination and heterogeneous signal on MRI are more suggestive of an old osteochondral injury (cf. Chapter 2.15.3).

7.3 Nonarticular (Apophyseal) Osteochondroses

7.3.1 What do Apophyseal Osteochondroses Have in Common?

Nonarticular osteochondroses are disturbances of ossification of apophyses. These do not occur until normal enchondral ossification of the affected apophysis has started (at the tibial tuberosity, for example, between the 7th and 9th years of age). Unlike epiphyses, apophyses are subject to strong traction forces from muscles, which likely disrupts the vascular supply of the apophysis. All apophyseal osteochondroses present with swelling and tenderness around the apophysis and associated tendon insertions. Prompted by these clinical factors, an apophyseal osteochondrosis is often referred to as a "traction apophysitis," although this does not correctly describe the pathogenesis. Apophyseal osteochondroses are chronic, self-limiting processes that come to a halt spontaneously at the completion of growth, unless the chronic overuse continues uninterrupted. An acute, traumatic tear of the apophyseal growth plate corresponds to a Salter–Harris Type I fracture (cf. Chapter 1.3.1) and is not considered to be a true osteochondrosis.

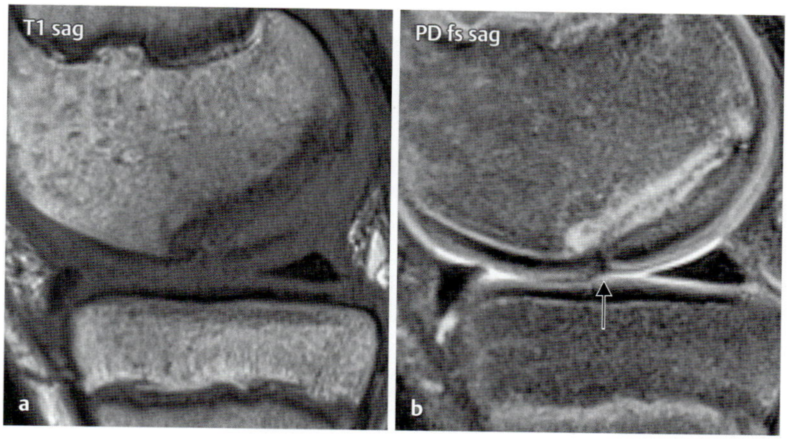

Fig. 7.23 Osteochondritis dissecans. Stage II. **(a)** The T1W image demonstrates the extent of the lesion. **(b)** The irregularity (arrow) of the articular cartilage becomes evident because of the arthrographic effect of the joint effusion.

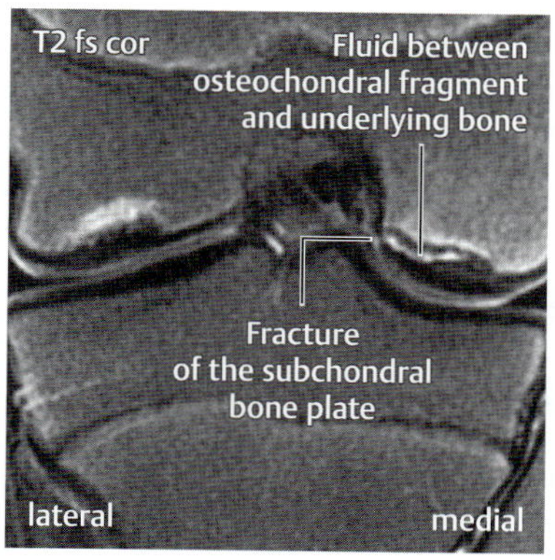

Fig. 7.24

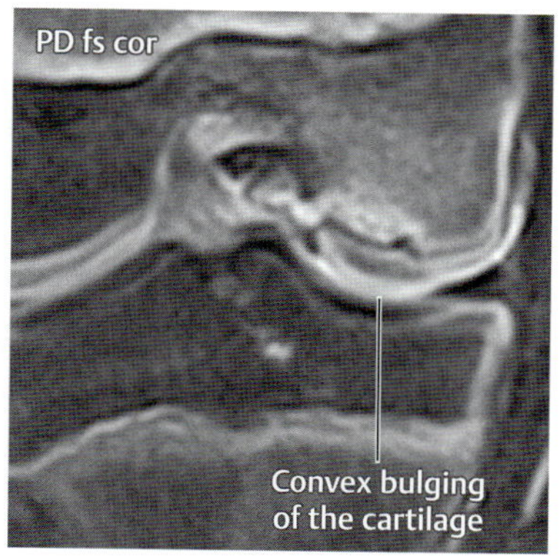

Fig. 7.25

Fig. 7.24 Osteochondritis dissecans of both femoral condyles. Medial Stage III, lateral Stage I.

Fig. 7.25 Osteochondritis dissecans. Stage II. The abnormal cartilage is "suspended" into the intra-articular space.

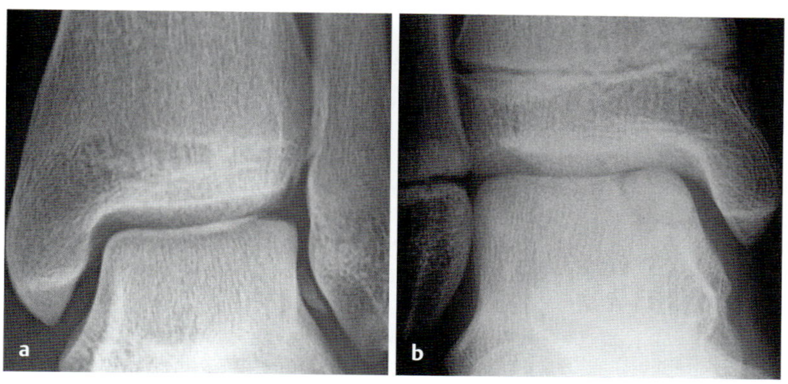

Fig. 7.26 Differential diagnosis "fresh osteochondral fracture versus osteochondritis dissecans" of the talus. **(a)** The osteochondral fracture is usually located laterally; there is a longitudinal fragment between talus and fibula. **(b)** Round, well-fitted lesion of the medial talar shoulder in a case of osteochondritis dissecans. Note the smooth surface of the osteochondral fragment.

7.3.2 Osgood–Schlatter Disease

This involves the apophysis at the anterior-superior margin of the tibia where the patellar ligament inserts. Boys between 11 and 15 years of age and girls between 8 and 13 are affected. It occurs bilaterally in 30% of cases. Many of the affected children and adolescents play sports. Parts of the apophysis can become detached as a result of the disturbance of ossification and develop into ossicles.

▸ **Radiography.** On radiographs the apophysis appears poorly marginated, fragmented, or sclerotic, depending on the stage of the condition (▸ Fig. 7.27).

▸ **MRI.** Fluid-sensitive MRI sequences reveal increased signal intensity in the apophysis and surrounding soft tissues, including the insertion of the patellar tendon (▸ Fig. 7.28).

▸ **DD.** **Enthesopathy at the patellar tendon** insertion on the proximal tibia in an adult (after closure of the apophyseal growth plate) is by definition not Osgood–Schlatter disease.

7.3.3 Sinding–Larsen–Johansson Disease

The description of this osteochondrosis as "Osgood–Schlatter disease of the inferior patellar pole" almost says it all. Physically active adolescents are affected prior to complete ossification of the patella. Radiographically, calcifications are recognizable at the attachment of the patellar tendon up to the end of the growth zone. The osteochondrosis can lead to deformation of the inferior pole of the patella (▸ Figs. 7.29 and ▸ 7.30), or result in an infrapatellar ossicle.

▸ **DD.** **Insertional tendinopathy of the patellar tendon** occurring after skeletal maturity (**jumper's knee**) should be not be confused with Sinding–Larsen–Johansson disease.

7.3.4 Sever's Disease

This osteochondrosis is also known as "calcaneal apophysitis" and affects children and adolescents between the ages of 7 and 15 years. Patients usually experience chronic, low grade pain. Diagnosis is primarily based on clinical findings and this disease heals spontaneously.

▸ **Radiography.** Increased fragmentation of the apophysis is evident in comparison with healthy children and adolescents and also in comparison with the patient's unaffected side.

▸ **MRI.** In certain cases where the clinical presentation is insufficient to make a diagnosis MRI may be obtained. On fluid-sensitive sequences an irregular increase in signal intensity of the calcaneal apophysis should suggest the need for a targeted physical examination (▸ Fig. 7.31).

▸ **DD.** Density of the calcaneal apophysis is nonspecific and is not a sign of Sever's disease.

7.3.5 "Little Leaguer's Elbow"

This disorder is generally known as "traction apophysitis" and involves the medial epicondylar apophysis of young baseball players (cf. also Chapter 2.7.1). Valgus stress during the late phase of an overhead throw results in medial traction forces and disturbance of the development of the apophysis. The ulnar collateral ligament inserts distal to the growth plate of the apophysis and may or may not be injured as well.

▸ **Radiography.** Radiography demonstrates separation and fragmentation of the medial epicondyle. These findings correlate with pain and swelling of the medial epicondyle in only about half of the cases, i.e., the osteochondrosis may not result in symptoms.

7.4 Physeal Osteochondroses

7.4.1 Scheuermann's Disease

Scheuermann's disease affects adolescents (synonyms: adolescent kyphosis, juvenile kyphosis) and is a disturbance of growth of the vertebral end plates of the thoracic and/or lumbar spine, associated with narrowing of the disks, wedging, and kyphosis.

▸ **Pathology.** Genetic and mechanical factors (competitive sports) are recognized etiological factors. Schmorl's theory of a herniation of disk material into the vertebral body during an adolescent growth spurt is widely agreed upon, but does not explain "why." The loss of height due to the herniation in the anterior part of the vertebra combined with continued growth of the posterior part of the vertebra results in a kyphotic deformity.

▸ **Clinical presentation.** Incidence rates vary between 1 and 8% of all adolescents, most commonly between 12 and 15 years of age. Male adolescents are 4 to 5 times more frequently affected than are female adolescents. Only one-third of those affected complain of back pain. Whereas thoracic involvement leads to kyphosis but may not cause any symptoms, thoracolumbar involvement tends to produce pain early. The latter form of the disease is referred to as "atypical Scheuermann's disease" and is commonly found in competitive adolescent athletes. The physiologic lumbar lordosis is lost, eventually transitioning to a lumbar kyphosis.

Prognosis. Prognosis is usually favorable; severe clinical forms are rare. The kyphosis ceases to progress after completion of growth.

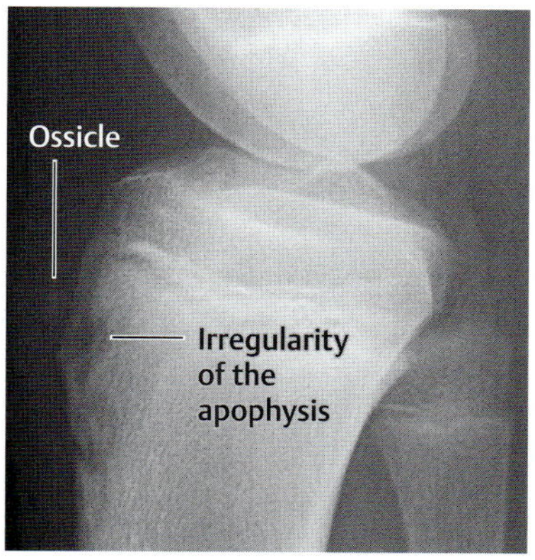

Fig. 7.27 Osgood–Schlatter disease.

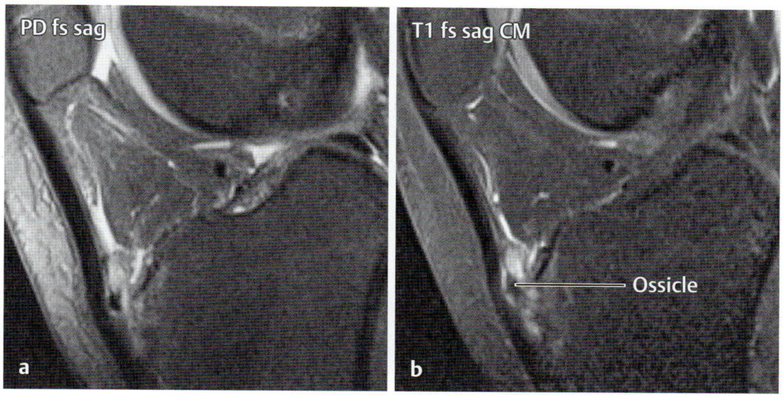

Fig. 7.28 Osgood–Schlatter disease. **(a)** The patellar tendon is thickened and demonstrates increased intensity due to edema. **(b)** Increased contrast enhancement in the apophysis as a sign of the remodeling process.

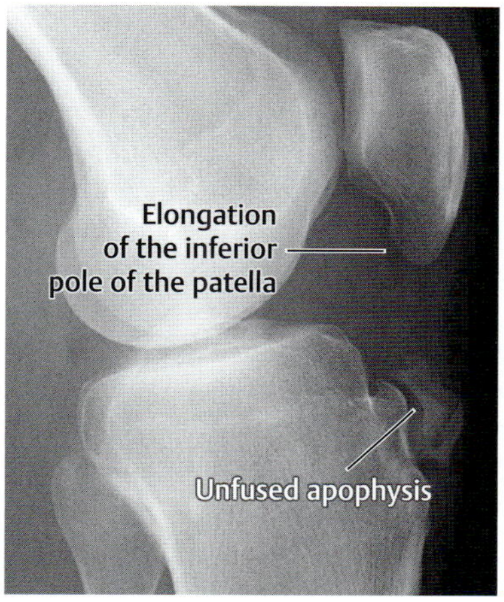

Fig. 7.29 History of Sinding–Larsen–Johansson disease and Osgood–Schlatter disease.

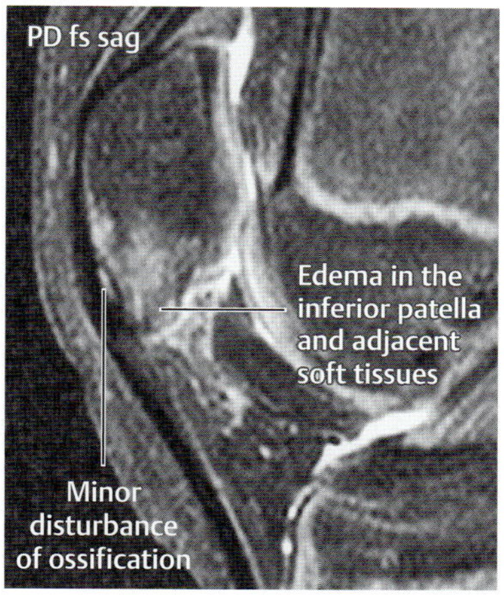

Fig. 7.30 Sinding–Larsen–Johansson disease.

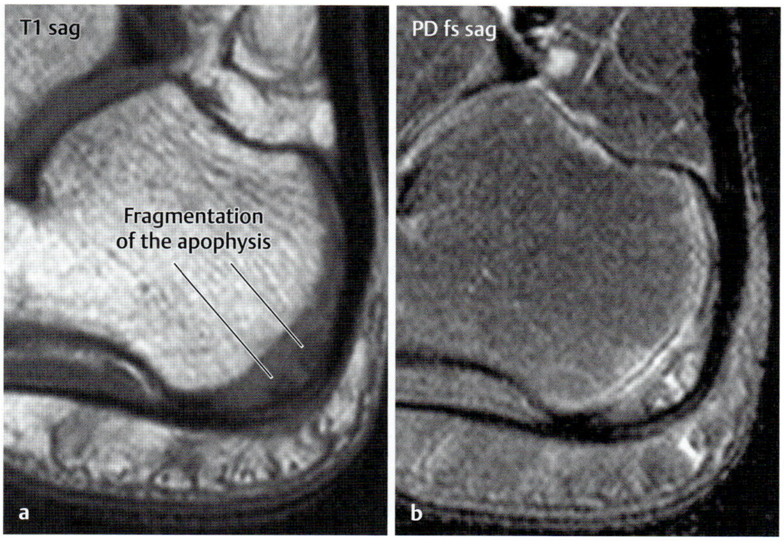

Fig. 7.31 Sever's disease. **(a)** Increased fragmentation of the calcaneal apophysis. **(b)** Edema secondary to bony remodeling.

▶ **Radiography/CT.** Conventional radiographs of the entire thoracic and lumbar spine in two projections while standing are needed and allow assessment of the degree of kyphosis. The following typical radiographic abnormalities are found:

- Kyphosis of the thoracic spine of more than 40° (as measured in the standing position according to Cobb; ▶ Fig. 7.32).
- Anterior flattening of two or more contiguous vertebrae by more than 5° (▶ Fig. 7.33).
- Intervertebral disk space narrowing.
- Circumscribed disk herniation in the central superior and inferior end plates (Schmorl's node) or as limbus vertebrae (▶ Fig. 7.34; see also Chapter 10.1.3).
- Edgren–Vaino sign reflecting the compensatory bony overgrowth of the adjacent inferior end plate (Chapter 10.1.3).
- Irregular appearance of the end plates (see ▶ Fig. 7.33).

Caution

Disk space narrowing and end plate irregularity alone are not enough to make the diagnosis of Scheuermann's disease. Kyphosis, vertebral flattening, and Schmorl's nodes must also be seen.

The kyphotic angle of the lumbar spine is irrelevant; the diagnosis can already be established from the presence of wedge-shaped vertebrae or Schmorl's nodes.

Note

Schmorl's nodes are located in the middle of the end plate or anteriorly as limbus vertebrae (retromarginal diskal prolapse; see ▶ Fig. 7.34) in the majority of cases. Posteriorly, more segmental arched indentations of the superior end plate usually represent remnants of the notochord and are normal variants (▶ Fig. 7.35; Chapter 10.1.3). However, posterior limbus vertebrae also occur.

▶ **MRI.** MRI directly demonstrates herniation of disk material into the end plate and is important for differentiating this from other inflammatory, traumatic, and occasionally neoplastic disorders. With an acute Schmorl's node, bone marrow edema is present around the herniated disk material (Chapter 10.1.3).

▶ **DD.**

Juvenile round back. In this condition the radiological alterations of the vertebrae described above are absent.

Spondylodiskitis. This occurs in childhood between the ages of 2 and 8 when the disk still has its own blood supply. However, in childhood and adolescence spondylodiskitis can also start in the end plate as in adults. MRI is able to detect edema originating from the disk and invading both adjacent vertebrae.

Posttraumatic compression fractures. These do not demonstrate any disk-space narrowing or Schmorl's nodes.

Osteoporosis-related loss of vertebral height. Analysis of the superior end plate will allow this to be differentiated from Scheuermann's disease. Masharawi and co-workers (▶ see References for Chapter 7.4.1) have developed a simple method for analyzing the angulation of the center of the end plate for this purpose (▶ Fig. 7.36).

7.4.2 Blount's Disease

Blount's disease is an epiphyseal or metaphyseal growth disturbance involving the medial aspect of the proximal tibia. It may be unilateral or bilateral and results in the progressive development of genu varum. Blount's disease is found more commonly in overweight children. A distinction is made between infantile and juvenile forms of this condition (▶ Table 7.2).

▶ **Radiography.** An AP radiograph of both legs will demonstrate the degree of varus deformity of one or both knees. The abnormalities involve the posteromedial epimetaphysis of the tibia. The contour of the physis is irregular, inferiorly sloped, and widened medially (▶ Fig. 7.37). The medial epiphysis is narrow and in part fragmented. During later stages, a bone bridge is seen at the medial aspect of the physis, while the lateral growth plate has not yet ossified. The severity of the radiographic alterations is classified according to the Langenskiold classification system (▶ see References for Chapter 7.4.2).

▶ **MRI.** MRI can precisely demonstrate the anatomy of the growth disturbance. The development of the medial tibial epiphysis is reduced with compensatory enlargement of the physeal cartilage. The physis is inferiorly sloped and widened; there is a protrusion of the epiphyseal cartilage in the metaphyseal defect zone. There is usually thickening of the medial meniscus, and stress-related bone marrow edema may be present (▶ Fig. 7.38).

▶ **DD.**

Physiologic genu varum. This is a self-limiting phenomenon of infancy that normalizes during early childhood.

Rickets. Metaphyseal alterations as a result of vitamin D-resistant rickets are not confined to the knee joint only.

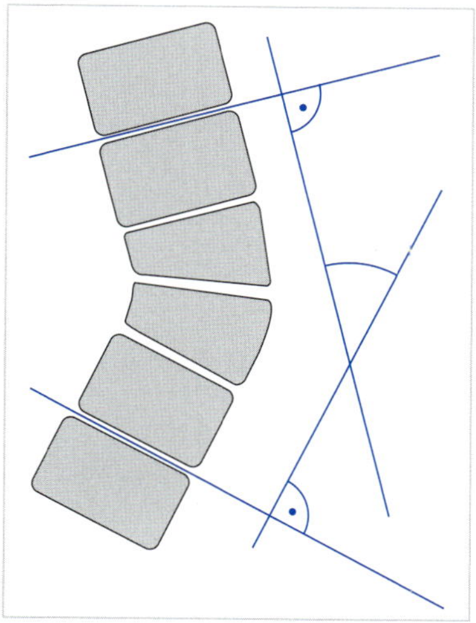

Fig. 7.32 Cobb technique for measuring kyphosis using the lateral spinal radiograph or sagittal MR/CT images.

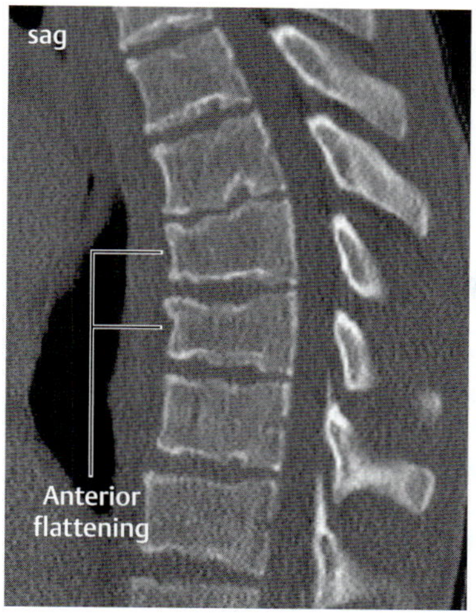

Fig. 7.33 Appearance of Scheuermann's disease. Note the irregularity of the end plates.

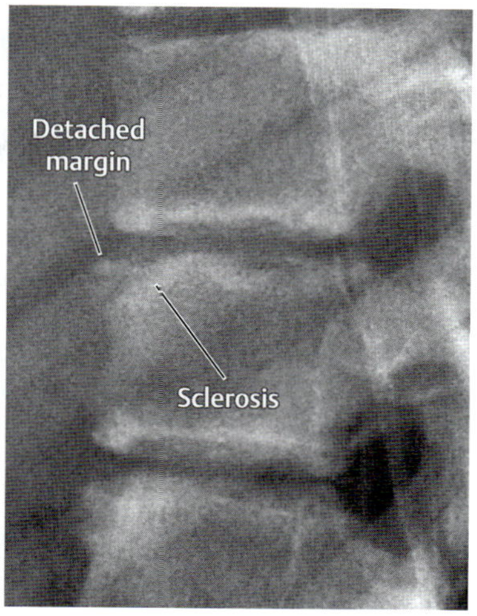

Fig. 7.34 Limbus vertebra in a case of Scheuermann's disease.

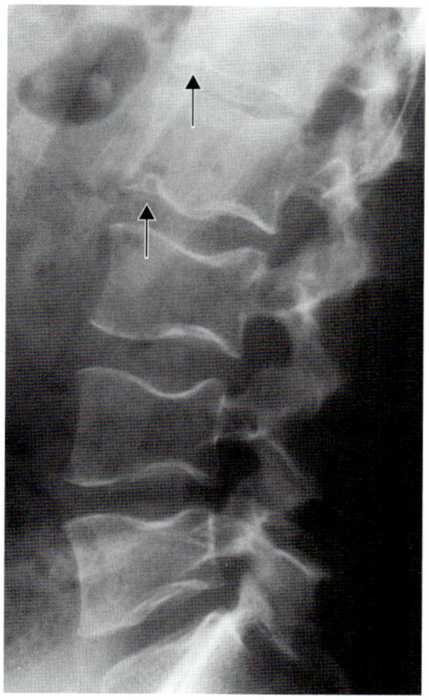

Fig. 7.35 Notochord involution disorder with a concave depression in the dorsal vertebral end plates. Additional Schmorl's nodules (arrows).

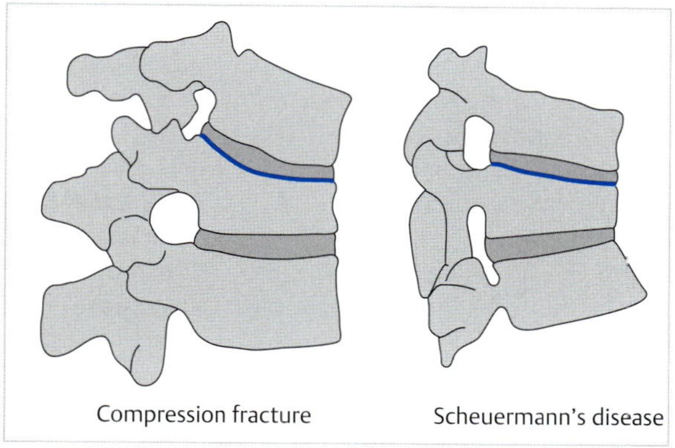

Fig. 7.36 Osteoporosis-related loss of vertebral height. The superior end plate of a compression fracture usually displays a typical "buckling," which is absent in Scheuermann's disease.

Table 7.2 Clinical forms of Blount's disease

Characteristic	Infantile form	Juvenile form
Start	1st–3rd year of age	> 4 years of age
Frequency	Rare	Very rare
Location	Usually bilateral	Usually unilateral
Prognosis	Progressive deformity	Mild deformity

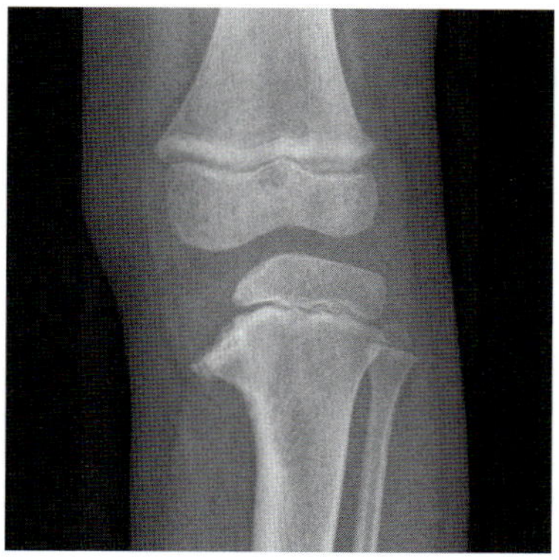

Fig. 7.37

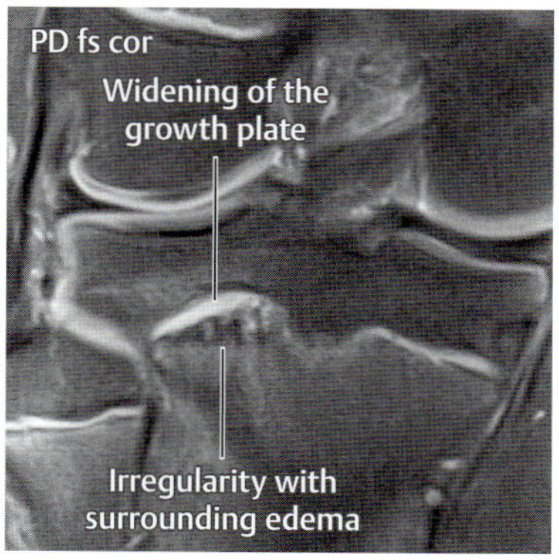

Fig. 7.38

Fig. 7.37 Blount's disease.

Fig. 7.38 Dorsolateral physeal osteochondrosis of the proximal tibia instead of dorsomedial as with Blount's disease. Development of knock-knees (genu valgus) is to be expected in this case.

8 Metabolic, Hormonal, and Toxic Bone Disorders

8.1 Osteoporosis

Osteoporosis is a systemic skeletal disease characterized by low bone mass and microarchitectural deterioration of bone tissue, leading to enhanced bone fragility (WHO definition from 1994; ▶ see References for Chapter 8.1).

▶ **Pathology.** Osteoporosis is a **multifactorial disease** requiring a careful diagnostic work-up. Basically, osteoporosis is due to an imbalance between bone resorption and bone formation (remodeling). A distinction is made between types of osteoporosis with increased bone turnover (high turnover) and those with reduced bone turnover (low turnover).

Whereas the bone mass of an adult consists of about 80% compact/cortical bone and only 20% cancellous (trabecular) bone, the latter is considerably more active with regard to bone metabolism. Trabecular bone is particularly susceptible to processes involving bone resorption because of its 10-fold greater surface area compared with cortical bone.

Osteoporosis involves not only a loss of bone mass but also thinning and a conversion of the originally plate-shaped trabeculae into rod-shaped trabeculae and the appearance of perforating resorptive lacunae, resulting in a loss of 3D networking (▶ Figs. 8.1 and ▶ 8.2). The result is loss of biomechanical competence and increased fragility; this is the reason for pathologically increased bone fragility. Trabecular microfractures indicate a failure of the bone when subjected to load-bearing. The formation of microcallus is an attempt to produce healing (▶ Fig. 8.3), although this process is not capable of restoring the destroyed microarchitecture.

8.1.1 Classification and Clinical Presentation of Osteoporosis

There are several classification and grading systems for osteoporosis, some of which overlap. Osteoporosis may be classified using the following criteria:

- Location and extent (e.g., disuse osteoporosis, transitory osteoporosis, complex regional pain syndrome [CRPS]).
- Age at initial onset (e.g., idiopathic juvenile osteoporosis, postmenopausal osteoporosis, senile osteoporosis).
- Bone turnover rate (high and very high turnover, low turnover).
- Severity of the osteoporosis (normal, osteopenia, preclinical osteoporosis, and clinically manifest osteoporosis; severity Grades 0–3 according to Minne).
- Bone histology.
- Etiology.

An **etiological classification** based on more practical features:

- **Primary osteoporosis:** This includes postmenopausal and senile osteoporosis as well as primary osteoporosis of the male. It is the most common form and has many causes and risk factors, although some single pathogenetic factors are known. Although it involves the entire skeleton, it primarily affects the spine and proximal extremities.
- **Secondary osteoporosis:** This is considerably less common (about 5% of cases), but more often leads to osteoporotic fractures. It may be related to an underlying condition or medication (e.g., glucocorticoids) or may be of a genetic origin (e.g., Turner's syndrome, osteogenesis imperfecta). Typical disorders with an increased risk of osteoporosis include hypogonadism, hyperparathyroidism, Cushing's disease, hyperthyroidism, chronic malabsorption syndrome, chronic inflammatory diseases, malignancies (especially multiple myeloma), and storage diseases.

▶ **Clinical presentation.** Osteoporosis is a silent condition, with few exceptions. Only after the development of macrofractures, either spontaneously or after minor injury, does the disease become apparent. Typical osteoporotic fractures involve a vertebral body, the proximal femur, distal radius, proximal humerus, and sacrum. Vertebral and hip fractures, in particular, result in increased mortality of those, typically older, patients who are affected since they have an additive effect with preexisting comorbidities. Osteoporotic vertebral fractures may also cause considerable back pain that is resistant to therapy. Referred pain can occur in a pseudoradicular distribution, but neurologic deficits are not part of the typical clinical course.

Clinical screening using bone density testing to identify individuals at risk for osteoporosis are becoming increasingly important given the typical asymptomatic course of the disease. Risk factors include hereditary predisposition, steroid therapy, nutritional calcium and/or vitamin D deficiency, reduced mobility, reduced exposure to sunlight, nicotine abuse, and cachexia, as well hormonal factors such as late menarche, early menopause, amenorrhea, and hypogonadism in men.

8.1.2 Bone Density Testing

Because bone density correlates most strongly with fracture risk, noninvasive bone density testing is of great importance in the diagnostic work-up for osteoporosis. The WHO has constructed a stratification tool based on the standard deviation (SD) of the patient's bone density from the average maximum bone density in the third decade of life (peak bone mass) of a sex- and race-matched normal population ("T-score"; ▶ Fig. 8.4). About 95% of all patients who suffer a fracture have a T-score below −2.5 SD. This value was defined as the statistical reference value for "osteoporosis."

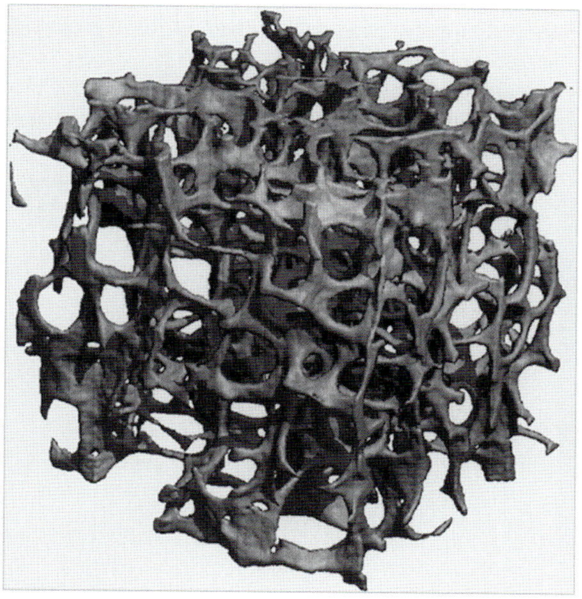

Fig. 8.1 Normal trabecular bone with predominantly platelike, well-connected trabecular networks. 3D CT of a bone-block specimen (4 mm × 4 mm × 4 mm) with ultra-high resolution.

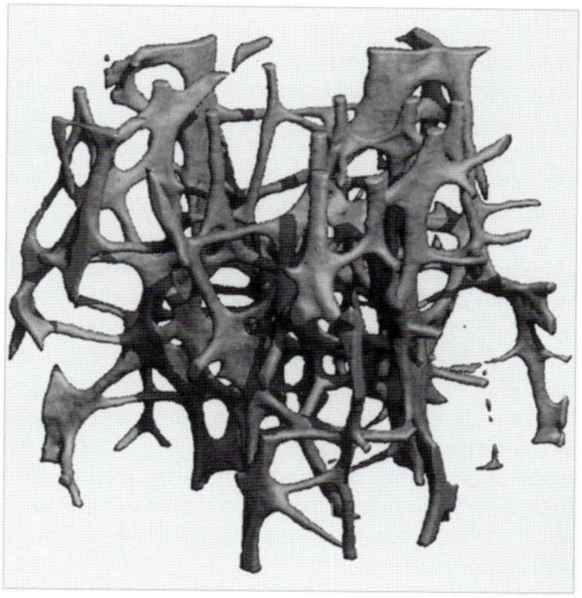

Fig. 8.2 Senile osteoporosis with thin, rodlike trabeculae, reduced number of trabeculae, and decreased cross-linking. 3D CT of a bone-block specimen (4 mm × 4 mm × 4 mm) with ultra-high resolution.

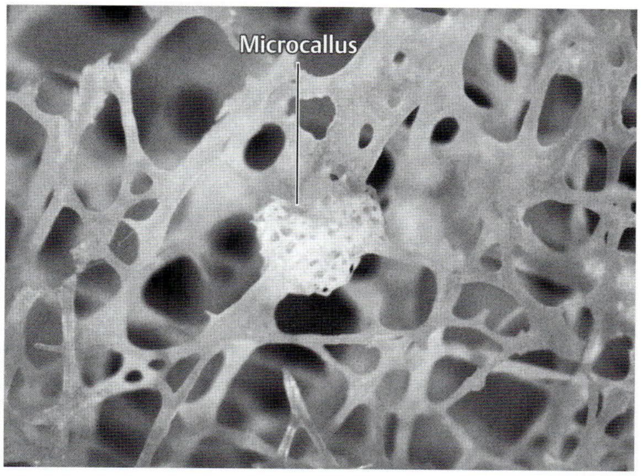

Fig. 8.3 Reparative microcallus after trabecular microfracture. Enlarged view of a specimen. (Image courtesy of Dr. B. Jobke, Heidelberg, Germany.)

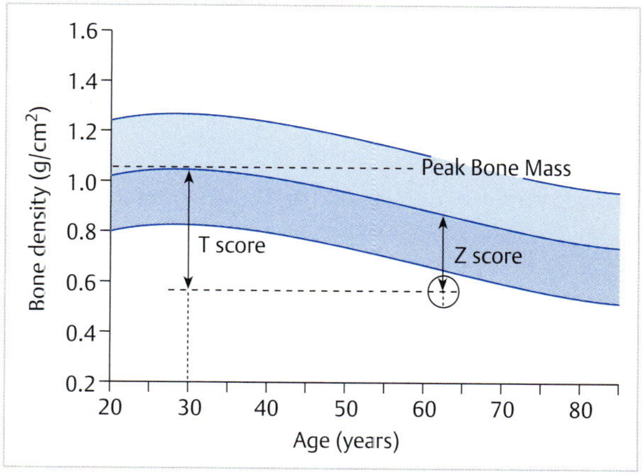

Fig. 8.4 Bone mineral density curve for a normal female population (by DXA [dual energy X-ray absorptiometry] of the lumbar spine). Bone density is plotted against age. A patient's actual bone density value is compared with a reference curve with standard deviations. The measured values are stated as the deviation from the peak bone mass (T-score) and as the deviation from the age-matched mean value (Z score).

According to the WHO definition:

- T-score less than −2.5 SD: **osteoporosis.**
- T-score between −1.0 and −2.5 SD: **osteopenia.**
- T-score more than or equal to −1.0 SD: **normal.**

> **Note**
> This T-score–based osteoporosis stratification by the WHO is only valid for DEXA (dual energy X-ray absorptiometry) measurements.

DEXA. Dual energy X-ray absorptiometry (DEXA) is currently regarded as the method of choice for bone density analysis. Measurements are usually made in the spine and proximal femur. The patient is scanned using low dose x-rays at two different energy levels, which then allows for correction for overlying soft tissues of variable thickness by subtracting the two absorption spectra. Bone mineral density (BMD) is calculated as mass per unit surface area (g/cm^2) (▶ Fig. 8.5a). The most important limitation of the method is that degenerative changes in the lumbar spine (osteophytes, discogenic sclerosis), aortic calcifications, and hyperostoses of the ligaments and joints are also measured and are very common, especially in patients over the age of 65 years. The presence of these types of changes must be assessed by performing an initial "scout" x-ray examination of the lumbar spine since including theses nonstructural types of calcium will result in falsely elevated BMD measurements (see ▶ Fig. 8.3).

QCT. Quantitative computed tomography (QCT) is conducted using standard clinical CT scanners with special software. Axial slices are obtained through the middle of three or four vertebrae (T12 to L4) and the bone mineral density is determined in the trabecular bone, excluding overlying structures (in g/cm^3; ▶ Fig. 8.5b). Included in the image, behind the patient, is an external reference phantom of known density. The actual value is calculated by comparing the absorption coefficients in bone with the absorption coefficients in the phantom.

QUS. Quantitative ultrasound (QUS) is a more recent method for assessing the risk of fracture. Sound waves are pulsed along the bone and the attenuation of the ultrasonic amplitude as it passes through bone is used to assess bone stiffness. Measurements are typically made in the calcaneus, less commonly the tibial shaft and the phalanges. Major studies have confirmed reliable correlation between these parameters and the risk of fracture, especially with regard to the femoral neck region. However, this method has not yet been adopted for routine use.

8.1.3 Radiographic Findings in Osteoporosis

▶ Radiography. The typical radiographic findings in osteoporosis are **increased lucency, trabecular rarefaction**, and **thinned but sharply defined cortex** (▶ Fig. 8.6). Conventional radiographs (thoracic and lumbar spine) are an essential part of the diagnostic work-up for osteoporosis. They allow recognition of structural changes:

- Marked **lucency** (evident when there has been about 30% loss of calcium; ▶ Fig. 8.7).
- Accentuation of the **cortical rim of the vertebrae** ("picture framing") and increased prominence of the vertical trabeculae.

> **Caution**
> These radiographic criteria for osteoporosis are unreliable since they are dependent upon the individual subjectivity of the imager. Furthermore, they also depend upon technical factors (image parameters, physical dimensions of the patient, etc.). Radiographs allow the diagnosis of vertebral body fractures, which should be diagnosed when there is a loss of height of at least 20% relative to the expected vertebral height. The presence of vertebral fractures implies clinically relevant osteoporosis and has an immediate effect on therapeutic decisions.

> **Note**
> It is imperative to report vertebral body fractures (also on lateral chest radiographs and on chest or abdominal CT) because the presence of one vertebral body fracture increases the risk of subsequent fractures 4-fold, and two vertebral body fractures increases the risk up to 12-fold.

Fracture types typical for **osteoporosis** of the spine:

- Wedge fracture (most commonly found in the thoracic spine).
- Biconcave compression fracture (codfish vertebra; most common in the lumbar spine).
- High-grade compression fracture (vertebra plana, pancake vertebra; common in secondary osteoporosis).

The degree of vertebral height loss may be classified according to Genant (▶ Figs. 8.8 and ▶ 8.9).

For the differential diagnosis of osteoporotic fractures versus traumatic or tumor-related fractures, see also Chapter 2.2.7.

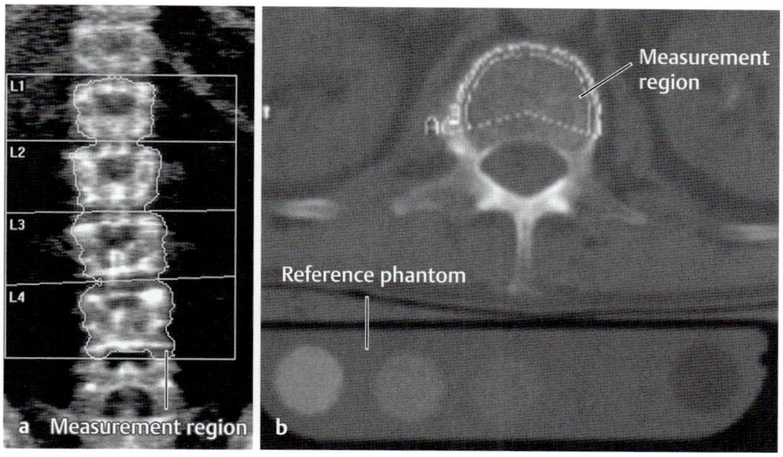

Fig. 8.5 Comparison between DXA (dual energy X-ray absorptiometry) and QCT (quantitative CT). **(a)** DXA is a planimetric procedure; bone density is expressed in g/cm^2. **(b)** QCT is a volumetric procedure; bone density is expressed in g/cm^3.

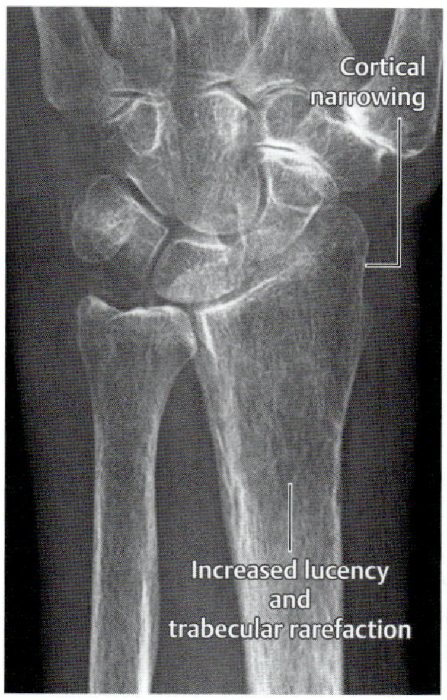

Fig. 8.6

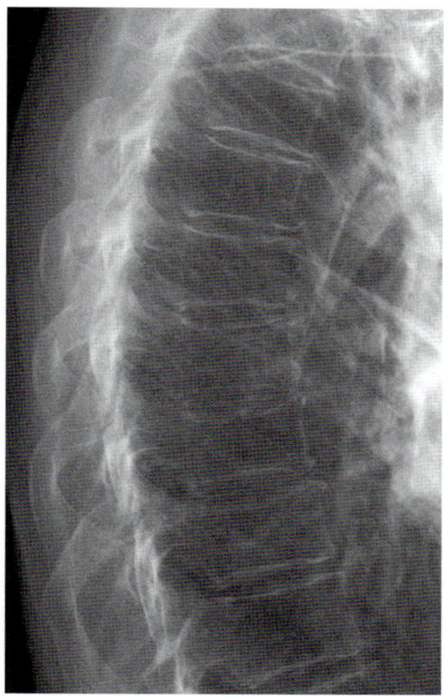

Fig. 8.7

Fig. 8.6 Generalized osteoporosis in a 92-year-old woman.

Fig. 8.7 Osteoporosis with typical "structureless" spine and increased radiolucency of the vertebrae.

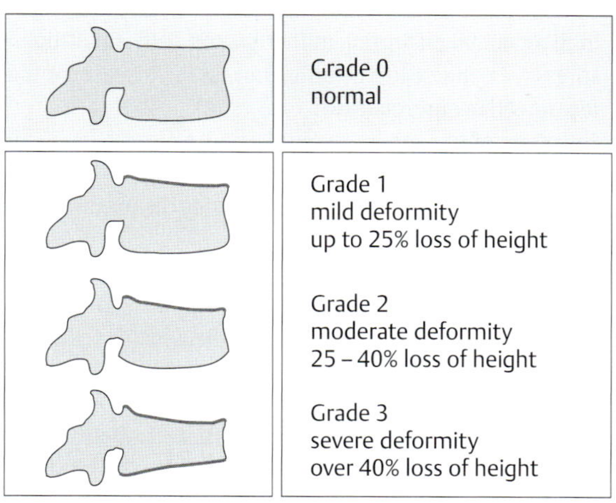

Fig. 8.8 Classification of osteoporosis-related vertebral body deformities according to the degree of anterior, medial, and/or posterior loss of height.

Fig. 8.9 The course of osteoporosis. **(a)** Initial finding. **(b)** One year later: multiple osteoporotic vertebral body fractures displaying typical morphology.

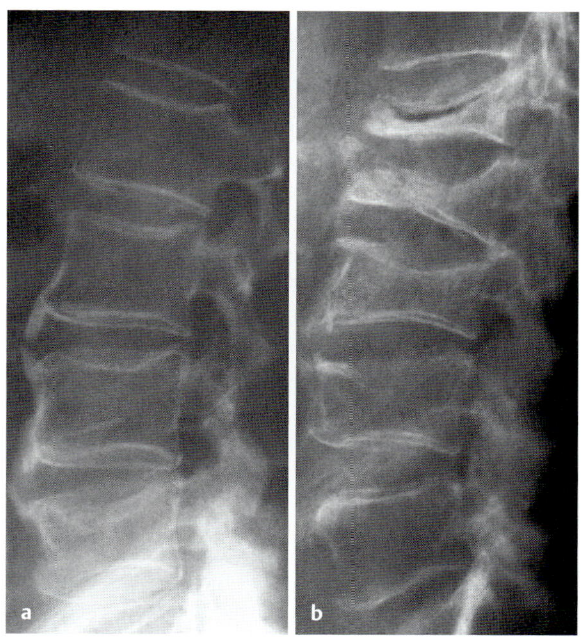

► **CT.** CT findings are the same as on radiographs, yet without being obscured by overlying structures (► Fig. 8.10). CT is important for assessing any cortical disruption and posterior wall involvement in vertebral fractures and for identifying osteolysis as a sign of a malignant (pathologic) fracture. The most specific sign of an osteoporotic vertebral fracture is an intravertebral vacuum phenomenon (due to the release of nitrogen; Chapter 2.2.7). Bandlike sclerosis and focal intravertebral calcifications are usually a sign of preexisting trabecular callus formation and suggest a subacute fracture, although they may also represent impacted trabeculae of a fresh fracture.

► **MRI.** MRI is the best modality for identifying acute vertebral body fractures and also helps to differentiate benign from malignant fractures. An acute osteoporotic vertebral fracture produces marrow edema that is easily detected on fat-suppressed fluid-sensitive sequences as a hyperintense bone marrow signal. It is *typically found in a bandlike distribution* near the affected vertebral end plate (► Fig. 8.11). It may occupy the entire vertebral body, *but never the whole pedicle* (an important differential diagnostic criterion). A corresponding bandlike area of decreased signal intensity is evident on T1W sequences, sometimes with a hypointense fracture line as well.

8

Differentiation from tumor. With an osteoporotic fracture, the vertebral body rarely appears hypointense in its entirety, but there are often *areas with a (bright) fat marrow signal.* The detection of focal, usually round, hypointense marrow lesions on T1W sequences, not in continuity with the fracture, is not typical for osteoporotic fractures and is more in keeping with vertebral metastases.

The administration of intravenous contrast provides very little additional differential diagnostic information: osteoporotic fractures occasionally display strong, linear or bandlike areas of contrast enhancement paralleling the end plates. Diffuse vertebral enhancement is nonspecific, whereas pedicle involvement on the other hand is suspicious for malignancy. In any case, pathologic extravertebral soft tissue components that make a malignant fracture probable should be carefully looked for. See ► Table 2.1 for an overview of the differentiation of "osteoporotic versus malignant fractures."

More recent special MR imaging techniques, such as DWI (diffusion weighted imaging), are supposed to make differentiation between benign and malignant vertebral body fractures easier. Refer to specialized literature for further details.

► **NUC MED.** Fractured vertebral bodies due to neoplastic infiltration are expected to display more uptake on FDG-PET than osteoporotic vertebral body fractures. The degree of overlap is large, however, so that the positive predictive value of malignant fractures is only about 71% while the negative predictive value is approximately 91%.

► **DD.** For the differential diagnosis of *systemic osteoporosis*, see Chapter 8.1.1.

Differential diagnosis of *focal osteoporosis* includes the following:

- **Disuse osteoporosis:** This affects skeletal regions less subject to load bearing such as when they are immobilized (Chapter 1.7.3).
- **Para-articular demineralization** secondary to an inflammatory arthritis, in which case the clinical presentation is very helpful.
- **CRPS:** An initiating injury is usually reported.
- **Transient regional osteoporosis:** see Chapter 1.5.4.

8.2 Rickets and Osteomalacia

Both of these are diseases in which vitamin D deficiency or metabolic disturbances result in insufficient mineralization of osteoid (► Fig. W8.1). In the growing skeleton the normal development of the growth plates is disrupted (rickets), while in the mature skeleton mineralization of cortical and cancellous bone is delayed (osteomalacia).

► **Pathology.** Calcium metabolism is regulated by parathyroid hormone, calcitonin, and vitamin D, each of which can also be used therapeutically (► Fig. W8.2).

Rickets or osteomalacia develops when there is insufficient vitamin D or calcium available:

- Due to inadequate absorption of calcium related to gastrointestinal malabsorption (after gastric and small-bowel surgery, in pancreatic insufficiency, celiac disease, or gluten-sensitive enteropathy).
- From loss of phosphate in renal tubular disease (congenital, hemodialysis, transplant).
- In preterm infants who have 3 to 6 times the requirements of full-term infants.
- In liver diseases.
- In cases of inadequate exposure of the skin to sunlight, e.g., from cultural/religious restrictions (such as skin covering) or domestic causes (e.g., in nursing home residents).

► **Clinical presentation.** The most striking findings in children are the disproportionately short stature (the growth of the extremities lags behind that of the trunk) and bony deformities.

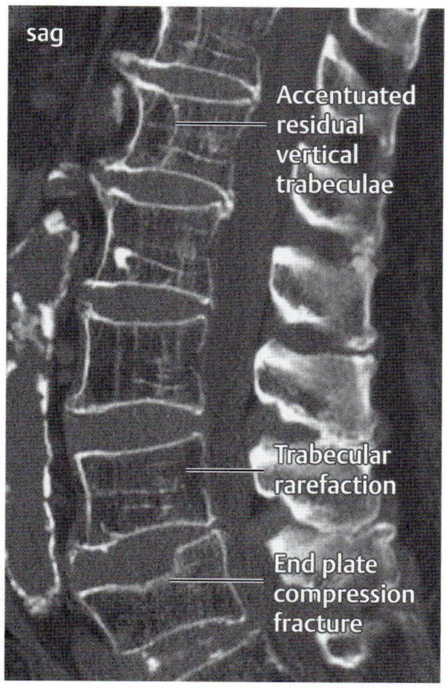

Fig. 8.10 Typical CT morphology of osteoporosis of the spine.

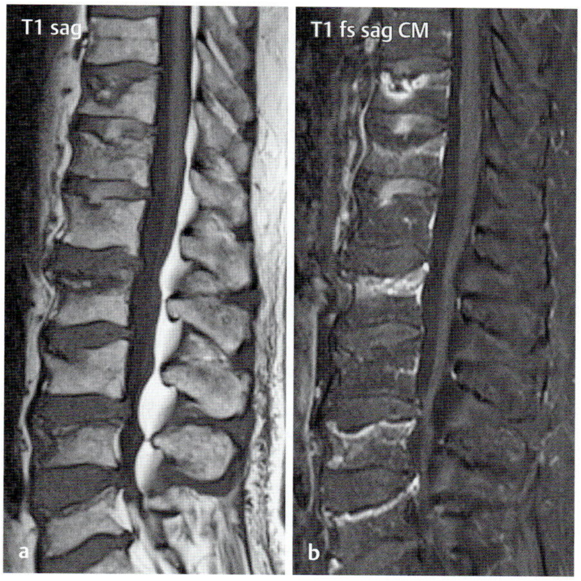

Fig. 8.11 Osteoporosis. **(a)** Multiple end plate compression fractures in the lumbar spine and at the thoracolumbar junction. **(b)** Typical bandlike contrast enhancement (edema) along the fractured end plates.

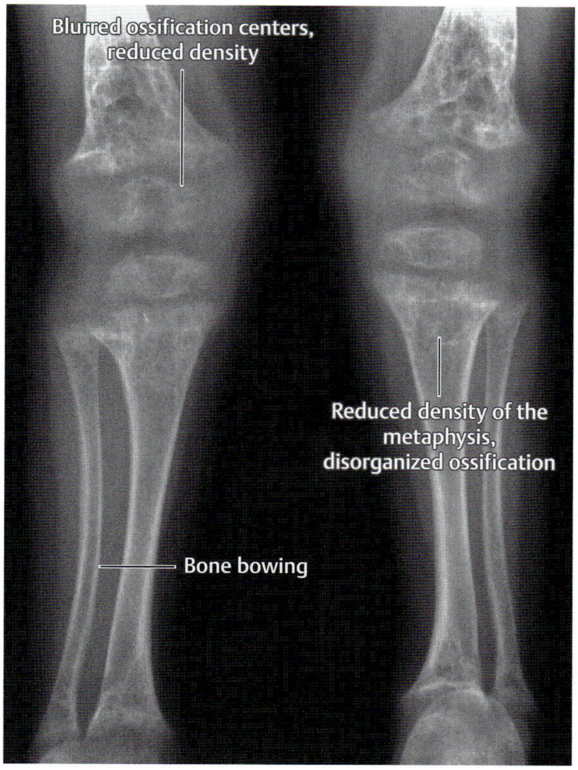

Fig. 8.12 Knee and lower leg of a 10-year-old boy with rickets. Cupping and widening of the epiphyseal plates.

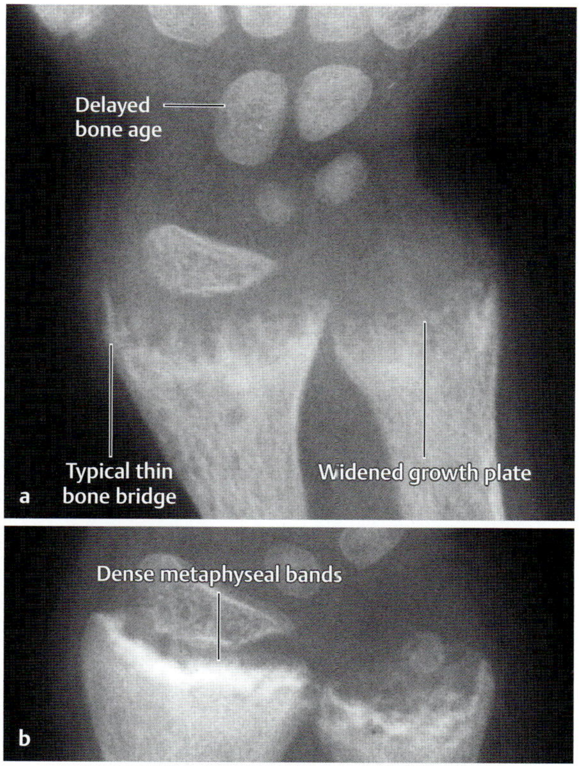

Fig. 8.13 Wrist of a 10-year-old boy with rickets. **(a)** Typical marginal bone bridges are evident because the periosteal reaction is significantly more pronounced than the endosteal reaction. **(b)** After 1 year of vitamin D therapy, metaphyseal bands of increased density have developed as a result of massive ossification of the bony matrix.

▸ **Radiography.** **Rickets.** The radiographic abnormalities are most pronounced in zones of increased bone turnover. The epiphyseal plates demonstrate cupping and widening, and appear fragmented and frayed (▸ Figs. 8.12 and ▸ 8.13) and possibly invaginated into the adjacent metaphyses due to the lack of load bearing. Bowing of bones is possible and bone development is delayed.

Osteomalacia. Nonspecific osteopenia, a fuzzy/blurred appearance of the trabeculae, and poor corticomedullary differentiation become evident as a result of a decreased number of mineralized trabeculae and surplus of unmineralized osteoid (▸ Fig. 8.14). Looser zones are a characteristic feature of osteomalacia (▸ Fig. W8.3; see also ▸ Fig. 8.14). They represent incomplete insufficiency fractures. They are often multiple and symmetric and perpendicular to the cortex, and typically involve only part of the bone circumference. They are commonly found in the parasymphyseal region, femur, proximal dorsal ulna, scapula, and ribs.

▸ **NUC MED.** On a radionuclide bone scan, multiple foci of abnormal uptake are seen with obvious osteomalacia. This reflects increased osteoblastic activity at the sites of insufficiency fractures, which commonly appear in a linear pattern in the ribs—unlike bone metastases (▸ Fig. 8.15).

▸ **DD.** **Tumor-induced osteomalacia** in conjunction with mesenchymal or other types of tumors.

8.3 Hyperparathyroidism and Hypoparathyroidism

8.3.1 Hyperparathyroidism

▸ **Pathology.** **Primary hyperparathyroidism** is caused by autonomous overactive parathyroid glands (solitary or multiple adenomas, hyperplasia, carcinoma) and is characterized by hypercalcemia. It is commonly found beyond the 6th decade of life; women are three times more frequently affected than men. There is an increasing number of asymptomatic and normocalcemic forms. In rare cases, primary hyperparathyroidism is associated with multiple endocrine neoplasia (MEN)-I or MEN-II syndrome.

Secondary hyperparathyroidism is caused by long-standing hypocalcemia, the causes of which include chronic renal failure, malabsorption, and disturbances of phosphate metabolism. Hyperplasia of the parathyroid glands is found in the majority of cases.

Tertiary hyperparathyroidism develops when a parathyroid gland becomes autonomous due to long-standing secondary hyperparathyroidism, essentially turning into a hyperplastic parathyroid gland.

The development of bone mass in hyperparathyroidism may vary, depending on skeletal location and the type of bone (cortex versus cancellous). Radiographic abnormalities are rarely encountered in the early stages and bone mass remains stable. Typical abnormalities and osteopenia appear in advanced disease and may be treated by parathyroidectomy.

> **Note**
> "Brown" tumors are tumorlike, osteoclastic resorption zones, named after their macroscopic appearance. They are the tip of the iceberg of the pathophysiologically dominant feature of bone resorption found in hyperparathyroidism.

▸ **Clinical presentation.** Patients demonstrate symptoms related to nausea, vomiting, and kidney stones. The clinical presentation of peptic ulcers of the stomach and small intestine or pancreatitis (calcifications on radiography or CT) has become rare. Paraneoplastic hypercalcemia must be ruled out in the differential diagnosis.

> **Note**
> The diagnosis of primary hyperparathyroidism is based on laboratory results (rising parathyroid hormone levels, constant or rising calcium levels, creatinine clearance); clinical symptoms associated with hypercalcemia are rare at the time the diagnosis is established. Radiologists and nuclear medicine physicians therefore primarily play a role in finding the parathyroid adenoma in cases of primary hyperparathyroidism. The radiologist should nevertheless be familiar with the classic radiographic abnormalities since some patients will demonstrate marked osteoarticular symptoms at the time of presentation.

▸ **Radiography.**

- Bone resorption is found in subperiosteal, endosteal, subchondral, and subligamentous and/or subtendinous locations. The classic location is the radial aspect of the middle phalanx of the **fingers** (see ▸ Fig. 8.18). Cortical tunneling is also found (▸ Fig. W8.4).
- Trabecular bone resorption produces a diffuse reduction of density.
- Lytic lesions without a sclerotic margin (▸ Fig. 8.16) correspond to a "brown tumor"; these lesions become sclerotic after treatment.
- Chondrocalcinosis is found most commonly within the menisci and the triangular fibrocartilage complex (▸ Fig. 8.17).
- Rarely a "salt-and-pepper" pattern is also encountered in the skull.

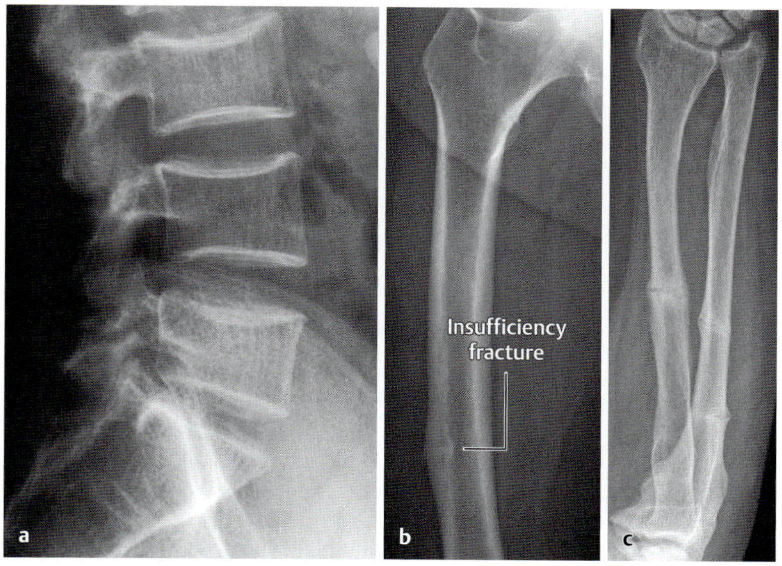

Fig. 8.14 Osteomalacia. **(a)** Blurred cancellous bone pattern. **(b)** Looser zone of the lateral femoral cortex with surrounding callus formation. The fine infarction usually remairs preserved as a line. **(c)** Multiple insufficiency fractures with Looser zones of the forearm of a patient with phosphate diabetes (hypophosphatasia).

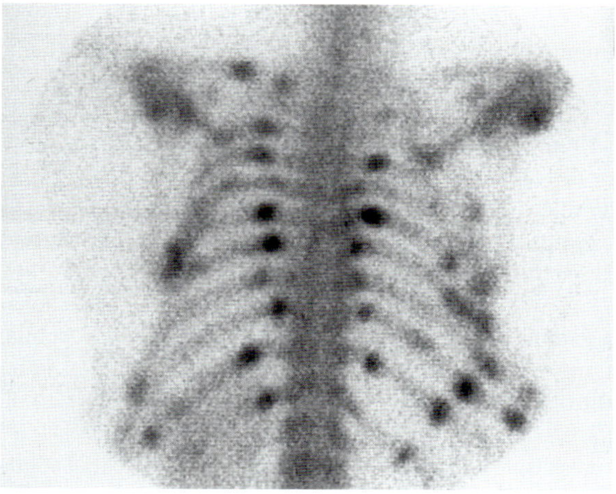

Fig. 8.15 Multifocal hot spots on the bone scan of the thorax as an indication of fractured ribs. Note the commonly found linear patterns of the fractures.

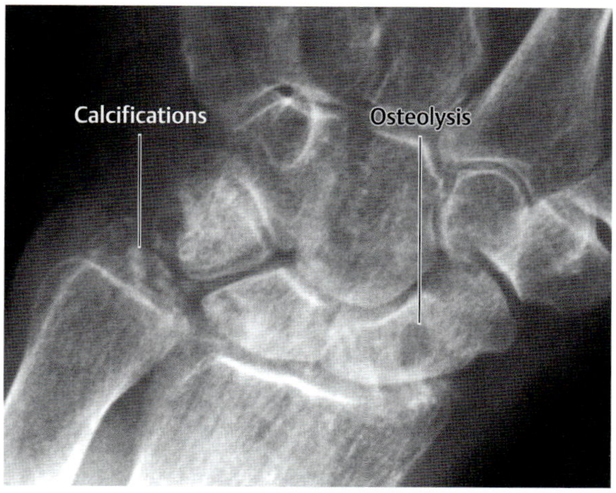

Fig. 8.17 Secondary hyperparathyroidism in a 72-year-old woman with renal osteodystrophy. The osteolytic lesion may either be due to a "brown tumor" or amyloid.

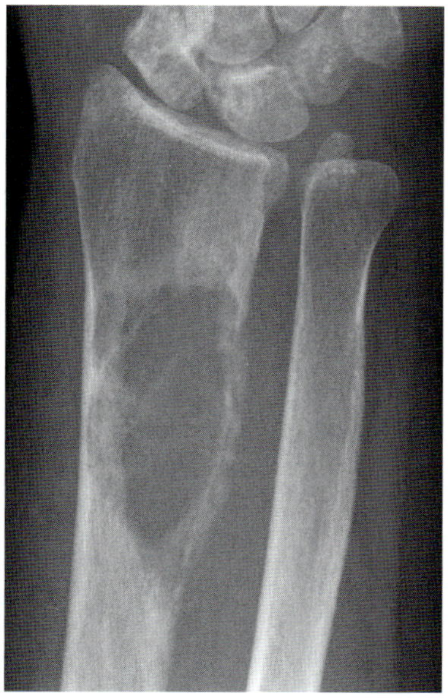

Fig. 8.16 Brown tumor in a case of primary hyperparathyroidism. The metadiaphyseal location makes improbable the differential diagnosis of a giant cell tumor; the demonstration of additional skeletal lesions and a typical constellation of laboratory findings confirmed the diagnosis of primary hyperparathyroidism.

8.3.2 Hypoparathyroidism

Hypoparathyroidism involves a reduction of serum parathyroid hormone levels, resulting in hypocalcemia and hyperphosphatemia. Parathyroid hormone deficiency can result from iatrogenic factors, aplasia or atrophy of the parathyroid glands, or secondarily to an autoimmune disorder.

Pseudohypoparathyroidism is a genetic end-organ resistance with a characteristic phenotype (Albright's osteodystrophy).

Imaging has no role in its early diagnosis. Late radiographic findings include osteosclerosis, enamel defects in the teeth, calcifications in the soft tissues and basal ganglia, dwarfism due to premature closure of the epiphyseal plates, and hypertrophy of the cranial vault. Decreased bone density is another late effect.

Pseudohypoparathyroidism also presents with shortening of the metacarpals and metatarsals as well as exostoses protruding perpendicular to the longitudinal axis of the bone, and bowing of the bones.

8.4 Renal Osteodystrophy

► **Pathology.** Renal osteodystrophy is the osteoarticular manifestation of chronic renal failure, characterized by the following findings:

- Renal failure causes a reduction in vitamin D production. This leads to hypocalcemia (osteomalacic component of renal osteodystrophy; ▶ Fig. W8.5) and secondary hyperparathyroidism.
- Renal osteodystrophy is also characterized by the deposition of hydroxyapatite in subcutaneous fat, periarticular tissues, and vessel walls.

► **Radiography.** The radiographic features associated with primary hyperparathyroidism are also found in renal osteodystrophy. Subperiosteal resorption in the hands (► Fig. 8.18) and subchondral loss of bone mass (particularly in the acromioclavicular joints) predominate (► Fig. 8.19). In contrast to primary hyperparathyroidism, "brown tumors" are very rarely found in renal osteodystrophy; osteosclerosis, periosteal new bone formation, and vascular calcifications, on the other hand, are more common. The pattern of osteosclerosis in the spine often demonstrates a layered (rugger-jersey spine) or diffuse appearance (► Figs. 8.20 and ▶ W8.6).

The osteomalacic components of renal osteodystrophy produce the following findings:

- Osteopenia.
- Looser zones.

Particular attention should be paid to deposits of calcium hydroxyapatite in the soft tissues (► Fig. 8.21; see also ► Fig. 8.17).

8.5 Drug-induced Changes to the Bone

8.5.1 Corticosteroids

► **Pathology.** The pathogenesis of the skeletal side effects is not fully understood. Osteoporosis is the main result of steroid therapy. Even with low doses, the risk of secondary osteoporosis is significantly increased. With higher doses, a rapid loss of bone mass within the first months is characteristic (▶ Fig. W8.7). The risk of developing osteonecrosis increases with high-dose therapy and long-term treatment (over 6 months).

Important musculoskeletal side effects of steroid treatment are listed in ► Table 8.1.

► **Clinical presentation.** Insufficiency fractures (secondary to osteopenia) may remain asymptomatic for a long time. Steroid-induced osteonecrosis often affects multiple sites in a symmetric distribution. Common sites include the femoral and humeral heads, distal femur, and talus.

► **Radiography.** Insufficiency fractures produce subtle, transverse sclerotic bands, primarily in the femoral neck, the tibia, or calcaneus. Exuberant callus formation is typical, particularly in the pelvis (► Fig. 8.22) and ribs. Vertebral fractures display a fracture pattern that is identical to that of idiopathic osteoporosis, including wedge-shaped vertebral fractures, collapse of the inferior and superior end plates and, later, sclerosis of the end plates (Chapter 8.1).

► **MRI.** MRI is the modality of choice for distinguishing between infection, fracture, and osteonecrosis.

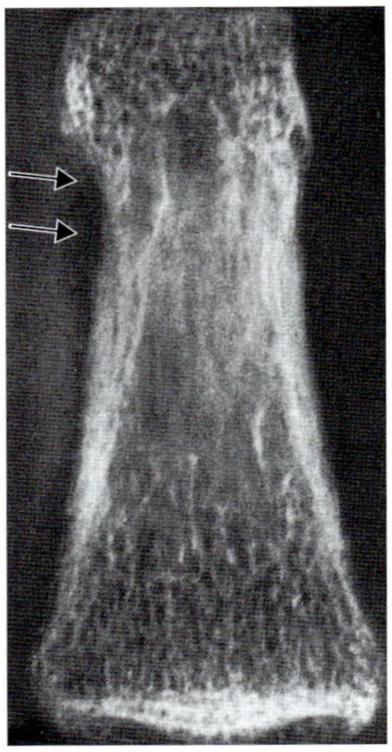

Fig. 8.18 Subperiosteal resorption (arrows) in a case of renal osteodystrophy. Enlarged view.

Table 8.1 The effects of steroids on the musculoskeletal system

Effect	Theory of development
Osteoporosis	Inhibition of osteoblasts, increased bone resorption secondary to activation of osteoclasts; secondary hyperparathyroidism due to hypercalciuria and reduced intestinal calcium absorption
Osteonecrosis	Microfractures due to osteocyte apoptosis; vascular compromise from fat emboli; vascular compression by fat cells
Neuropathic joints (pseudo-Charcot)	Damage to cartilage due to intra-articular infections; reduced pain sensation leads to overuse
Osteomyelitis, septic arthritis	Immunosuppression; sterile joint effusions also occur, albeit rarely; *Staphylococcus aureus* is the most common pathogen
Tendinopathy	Impaired tendon healing and tendon tension; direct injections can produce degeneration and necrosis
Atrophy of skin and soft tissue	Due to the application of topical agents and injections
Intra-/periarticular calcifications	Hydroxyapatite deposits may be due to systemic steroid administration or local injections

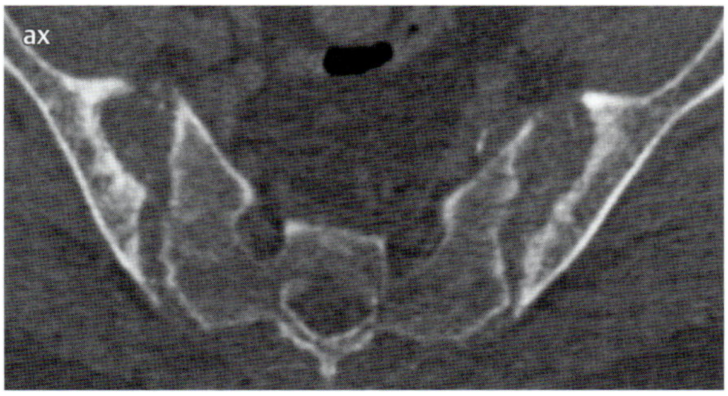

Fig. 8.19 Renal osteodystrophy. Uniform bilateral subchondral resorption at the sacroiliac joints.

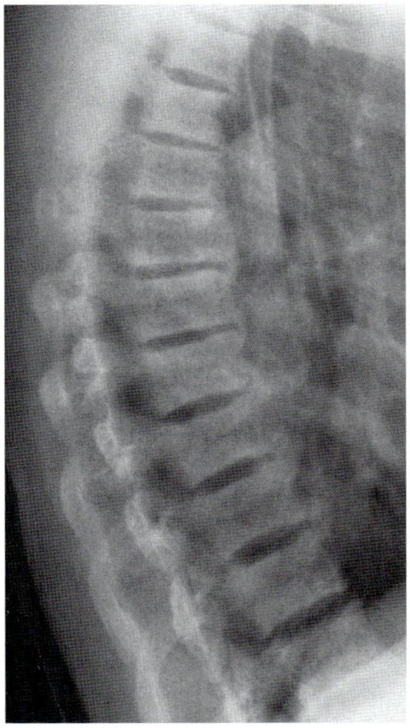

Fig. 8.20 Renal osteodystrophy. Osteosclerosis of the spine (rugger-jersey spine). ▶ For additional images see ▶ Fig. W8.6.

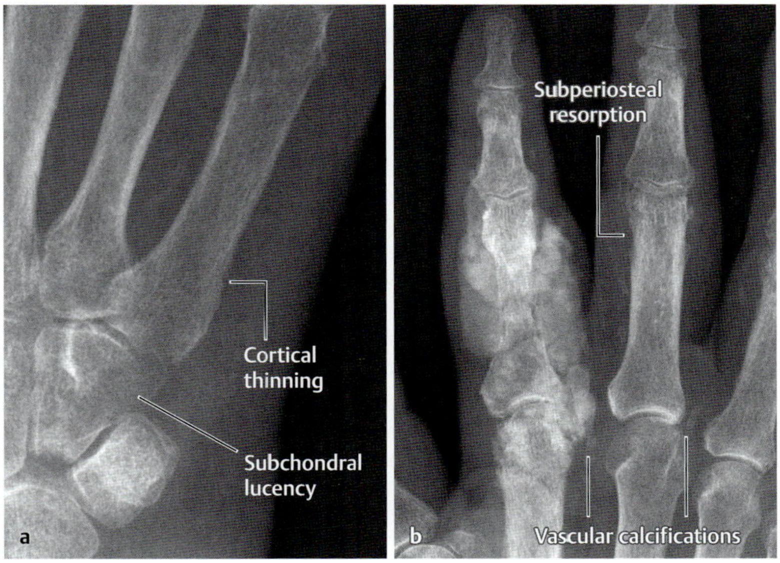

Fig. 8.21 Monitoring of disease progression in a case of secondary hyperparathyroidism. **(a)** Initial finding. **(b)** The eventual appearance of progressive cloudy soft tissue calcifications around the second ray. There is also generalized vascular calcification.

8.5.2 Other Drugs

Alterations to the musculoskeletal system caused by other medications and substances are to be found in ▶ Table 8.2.

8.6 Amyloidosis

Amyloidosis is the focal or generalized deposition of amyloid, a heterogeneous group of proteins, characterized by the formation of fibrils. The skeleton, joints, and peripheral soft tissues are rarely involved in comparison with other organs.

▶ Pathology. A distinction is made between various types of amyloidosis, each involving different specific proteins:

- **Primary form** (known as AL amyloidosis): This can develop without a known previous disease, although it is primarily associated with a monoclonal gammopathy, e.g., multiple myeloma.
- **Secondary form** (known as AA amyloidosis): The most common causes include chronic rheumatic disorders as well as tuberculosis.
- **Familial (or hereditary) type:** Localized tumorous forms, among others, are found in this group.
- **Dialysis-related amyloidosis** (AB amyloidosis): This type is particularly associated with osteoarticular manifestations. The proteins are deposited in periosteum, joint capsule, synovial membrane, articular cartilage, bone marrow, tendons, and periarticular soft tissue (▶ Fig. W8.9).

8

▶ Clinical presentation. Amyloid osteoarthropathy often follows an insidious course and is characterized by the development of pain, swelling, limitation of motion and the development of nodules involving both major and minor joints. There are no clinical signs of inflammation. At the wrist it can cause carpal tunnel syndrome.

▶ Radiography.

Wrist, hip, shoulder, elbow, knee

- Multiple subchondral radiolucencies or erosions are found, usually associated with a narrow sclerotic margin (▶ Figs. 8.23 and ▶ 8.24). The erosions can become large and result in, for example, an apple-core appearance of the femoral head (▶ Fig. W8.10).
- The joint space may appear normal, widened because of amyloid deposits, or narrowed from a destructive arthropathy.
- Periarticular soft tissue masses are also possible (see ▶ Fig. 8.24).
- There may be osteopenia.

Spine

- The cervical spine is usually involved.
- Disk space narrowing.
- End plate erosions or destruction.
- Absent or only minimal paravertebral soft tissue swelling.
- Minimal sclerosis or spondylophyte formation.

▶ US. Ultrasound reveals joint effusion, synovial and periarticular tissue proliferation, and thickening of the tendons.

▶ MRI. Amyloid lesions are typically of low to intermediate signal intensity on both T1W and, most characteristically, T2W sequences. Only very rarely do they demonstrate increased signal intensity on T2W and STIR sequences. They do not enhance with contrast.

▶ DD.

Rheumatoid (or other inflammatory) arthritis. It can be very difficult to distinguish rheumatoid arthritis from destructive amyloid osteoarthropathy, especially since both disorders may occur simultaneously. Preservation of the joint space, extensive soft tissue masses, sclerosis, and absence of juxta-articular osteopenia suggest amyloidosis.

PVNS. Pigmented villonodular synovitis is a disorder with monoarticular involvement that affects the major joints (in 80% of cases the knee) and is characterized by hemosiderin deposits that are evident on MRI.

8.7 Other Osteopathic Diseases

8.7.1 Hemophilic Arthropathy

Hemophilia A and B are congenital coagulation disorders that cause recurrent bleeding into joints. Coagulation does not occur because prothrombin and fibrinogen are not present in the articular cavity. Plasma is only slowly resorbed and the red cells are phagocytosed via the synovial membrane. This results in hemosiderin deposits and a chronic proliferative synovitis. It is associated with the development of lysosomal enzymes and cytokines (e.g., tumor necrosis factor alpha), which result in cartilage damage.

Intra-articular hyperdensity (due to fresh hemorrhage), enlargement of the intercondylar notch of the knee, and early osteoarthritis are evident on radiographs or CT images. "Ballooning" of the epiphyses is a typical sign in children. MRI confirms intra-articular hemorrhage, synovial deposition of hemosiderin (areas of absent signal on T2W sequences), proliferative synovitis, and cartilage damage.

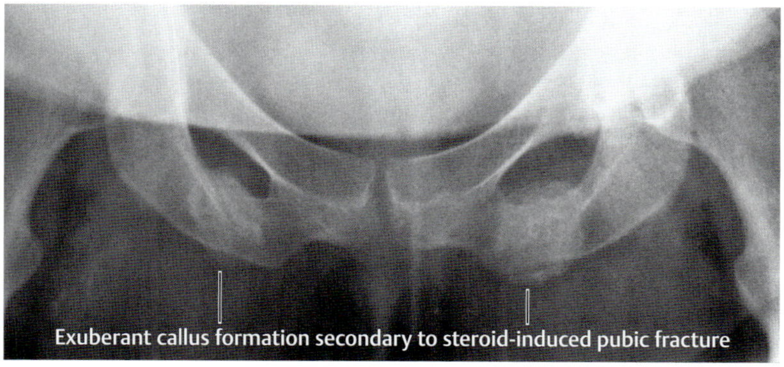

Fig. 8.22 Pelvis of a 34-year-old woman with steroid-induced Cushing's syndrome.

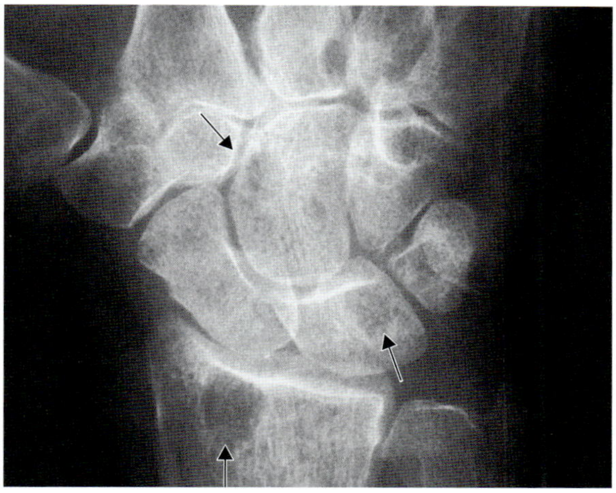

Fig. 8.23 Amyloidosis secondary to long-term hemodialysis. Multiple subchondral osteolytic lesions (arrows).

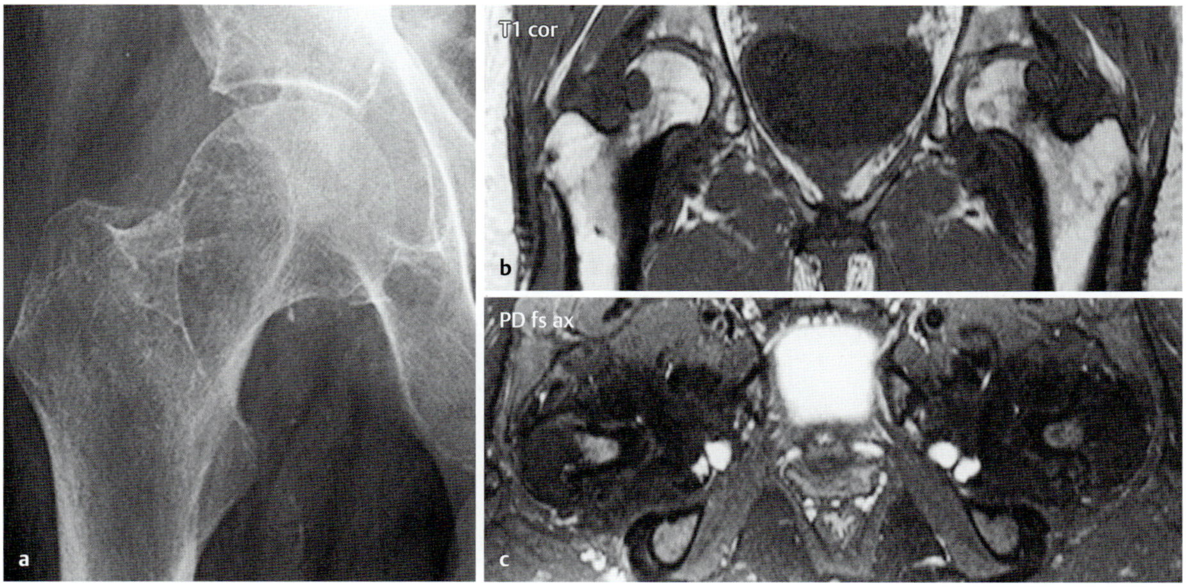

Fig. 8.24 Amyloid deposits in the hip joint. (Courtesy of H. Rosenthal, Hannover, Germany.) **(a)** Osteolytic lesions with sclerotic margins in the proximal femur, and periarticular soft tissue densities. **(b)** Bilateral, nearly symmetric intraosseous and periosseous space-occupying lesions. **(c)** The lesions are typically hypointense on fluid-sensitive sequences.

Table 8.2 Musculoskeletal complications of other drugs and incorporated substances

Substance	Effect
Dopamine	Gangrene, avascular necrosis
Calcium gluconate	Soft tissue calcifications
Heparin	Osteoporosis, stress/insufficiency fractures
Phenytoin	Rickets, osteomalacia, thickening of the skull, increased heel pad thickness
Vitamin A, retinoids	Increased bone resorption, soft tissue calcifications in adults, sclerosis of the metaphyseal ligaments, cortical thickening and interference with growth in children
Prostaglandins	Periostitis (in a newborn), delayed closure of cranial sutures
Chemotherapy (cisplatin, bleomycin, vinblastine, etoposide)	Osteonecrosis
Aluminum	Rickets, osteomalacia (▶ Fig. W8.8), periostitis, fractures
Quinolone	Tendinosis, tendon tear
Fluoride, voriconazole (fluorinated antifungal agent)	Osteosclerosis, hyperostosis, calcification of ligaments, periostitis
Bisphosphonates	Sclerotic horizontal, metaphyseal bands, epiphyseal/apophyseal sclerosis, "bone in bone" appearance of the vertebrae of children, osteonecrosis of the mandible (high dose), atypical fractures (particularly the femur)
Phenylbutazone, indomethacin	Osteonecrosis, arthropathy
Alcohol	Avascular osteonecrosis (crosses the placenta and can cause dysplasia of the hip and milder skeletal anomalies); ethanol toxicity causes osteoporosis

8.7.2 Acromegaly

An adenoma of the anterior pituitary gland produces excess growth hormone. Clinical symptoms usually present in the 3rd to 4th decades of life, typically pain in the extremities and lumbar spine.

Radiographic findings are manifold. Coarsening of the osseous structures with widening of the phalanges are evident in the hand and foot. Especially characteristic is the finding of prominent osteophytes with preserved, or even widened joint spaces (▶ Fig. 8.25). Eventually "ordinary" osteoarthritis develops.

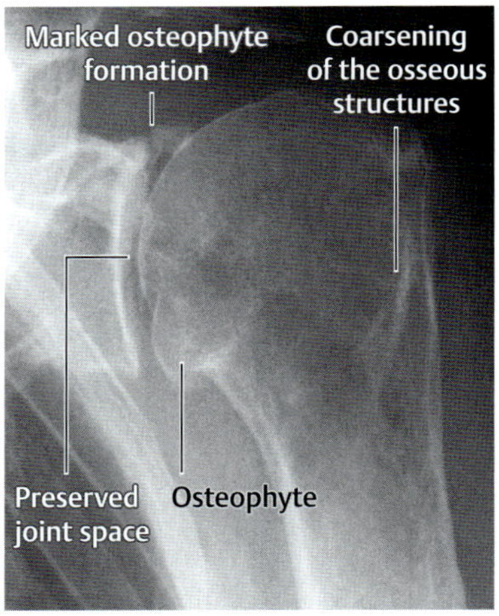

Fig. 8.25 Acromegaly. Marked structural alterations of the humerus and discrepancy between severe osteophyte formation and preserved width of the joint space.

Chapter 9

Congenital Disorders of Bone and Joint Development

9

9 Congenital Disorders of Bone and Joint Development

9.1 Bone Age Assessment in Growth Disorders

Skeletal maturity is closely associated with physical maturation, especially growth rate and sexual maturity. Disturbances of physical maturation may occur secondary to a genetic, hormonal, nutritional, or other cause. Clinical monitoring of growth is done with age-related **percentile graphs**. If longitudinal growth or somatic maturity demonstrates progressive deviation from the norm or if the patient's height falls below the 3rd percentile or above the 97th percentile, then skeletal age should be determined. Assessment of skeletal development provides prognostic information with regard to further development.

▸ **Radiography.**

- **Neonates/infants:** In newborns, the presence and form of ossification centers are analyzed using a radiograph of the lateral lower leg (including knee and ankle joints) according to the method of Sénécal and a special points system. The skeletal age is then expressed in percentiles. This can assess the severity of, for example, congenital hypothyroidism. A possible alternative is the determination of skeletal maturation of the newborn by ultrasound of the distal femur and proximal tibial epiphysis.
- **Two years of age and older:** A dorsopalmar radiograph of the left hand, including the distal portions of the radius and ulna, is needed for assessing skeletal age. Skeletal age is determined using the method of Greulich and Pyle or that of Tanner and Whitehouse.

The **Greulich and Pyle** method for bone age assessment evaluates the extent of ossification of the carpal bones and is the more practical method for daily clinical practice. The development of the ossification centers within the initially cartilaginous carpal bones is tracked and their maturation is assessed according to form and size. The growth plates of the first to fifth digits and radius and ulna as well as the maturation of the epiphyses are employed in a similar way. The skeletal age of the child can be determined by comparison with standard radiographs provided in the Greulich and Pyle atlas. The more elaborate method proposed by **Tanner and Whitehouse** is more suitable when skeletal development of the bones of the hand is asynchronous. This method assigns an individual score to each ossification center of the carpus and the epiphyses based on their current stage of development. A total maturity score is calculated by summing all these scores. This score is correlated with the bone age separately for males and females. The Tanner and Whitehouse method is the more complex and requires more time but it is more accurate and more reproducible than the Greulich and Pyle method.

Deviations of skeletal age from the norm by more than a year either way are rated as "retarded" or "accelerated." The corresponding tables by Bayley and Pinneau (in the appendix of the Greulich and Pyle atlas) list what percentage a child has reached of their final height. The child's expected final height (ultimate height) may be determined using this information. The standard deviation (SD) of the predicted values from the actual height reached was only ±2.5 cm in children up to the age of 14 years, and only ±1 cm in older children in the series reported by Bayley and Pinneau.

Additionally, digital applications using the method of Tanner and Whitehouse can calculate both bone age and future adult height with considerable time-saving by evaluating a digital radiograph and entering the child's chronological age and current height.

By the age of 18 years, bone age cannot be computed from hand and wrist radiographs, therefore the medial end of the clavicle is used for bone age calculation in individuals aged 18 to 22 years. Radiographs or CT are used for visualization of the clavicle. MRI-based methods are being developed but require more research.

9.2 Congenital Dysplasia of the Hip

Congenital dysplasia of the hip involves abnormal development of the acetabular roof and the acetabular rim. The result is an unstable joint with subluxation or even dislocation of the femoral head.

▸ **Pathology.** This is a multifactorial disorder that may be secondary to a mechanical cause such as breech presentation or oligohydramnios, an endogenous cause, or familial disposition. Congenital dysplasia of the hip results from a disturbance of growth and ossification of the acetabular roof, especially of its cranial margin so that it no longer supports the femoral head. This leads to instability of the hip joint, subluxation, and a shift of the hip's center of rotation (▸ Fig. 9.1). Complete dislocation can occur and result in the formation of a secondary pseudoacetabulum. With subluxation or dislocation, an elongated ligamentum teres and/or entrapped joint capsule and adipose tissue may impede adequate reduction of the joint.

▶ **Clinical presentation.** Girls are six times more commonly affected. Although the left hip is most commonly involved, bilateral involvement is seen in 25% of cases. The Ortolani and Barlow maneuvers are important functional tests to assess stability.

Treatment. Treatment depends on the age of the patient and stage of the disorder. The aims of treatment are to retain the femoral head within the acetabulum, resulting in remodeling of the acetabulum and prevention of subluxation. Reduction is required in the presence of subluxation or dislocation.

▶ **US.** Ultrasound provides a direct demonstration of the cartilaginous femoral head, the hyaline cartilage of the acetabular rim and fibrocartilaginous labrum, and the bony and cartilaginous acetabular roof. Coronal slices produce images comparable to a radiograph with better detail and the option of dynamic testing of mobility and stability of the femoral head.

Ultrasound or radiography?

- **Ultrasound:**
  - In newborns with risk factors (familial disposition, breech presentation, unusual clinical presentation).
  - Obligatory in the 4th to 6th weeks of life.
  - Still useful to the age of approximately 1 year.
- **Radiograph:** from the 9th month onward or when ultrasound assessment is limited.

Ultrasound **classification** of developmental dysplasia of the hip is generally performed using the **Graf** technique; it is divided into four basic types. After definition of the standard plane, the joint is assessed using the acetabular roof line (through the bony acetabular roof) and the acetabular inclination line (from the osseous acetabular rim through the acetabular labrum). These two reference lines each form an angle with a baseline parallel to the contour of the iliac wing. These angles are used to classify dysplasia of the hip (▶ Fig. 9.2a). The ultrasound assessment of hip maturity therefore takes into consideration both the bony architecture of the acetabulum and acetabular rim and the extent of coverage of the femoral head by the cartilaginous acetabular roof. With a displaced femoral head, the labrum is moved cranially (▶ Fig. 9.2b).

Ultrasound assessment requires an experienced examiner since even a minimally suboptimal imaging plane (tilt, shift) will produce an aberrant measurement result and the potential for misdiagnosis.

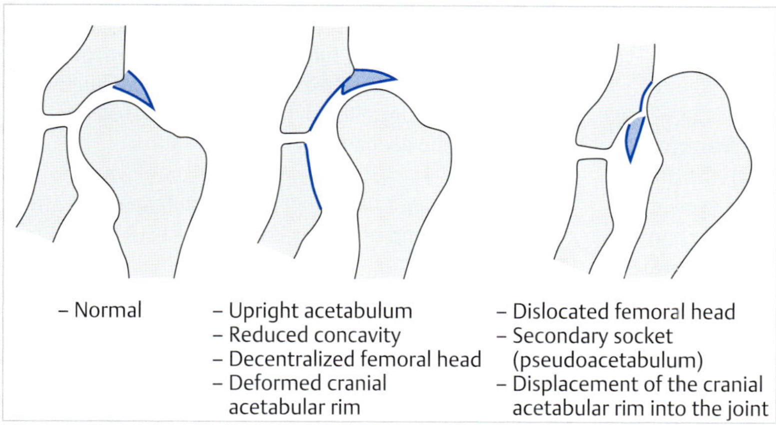

Fig. 9.1 Configuration of the acetabular cup and the labrum.

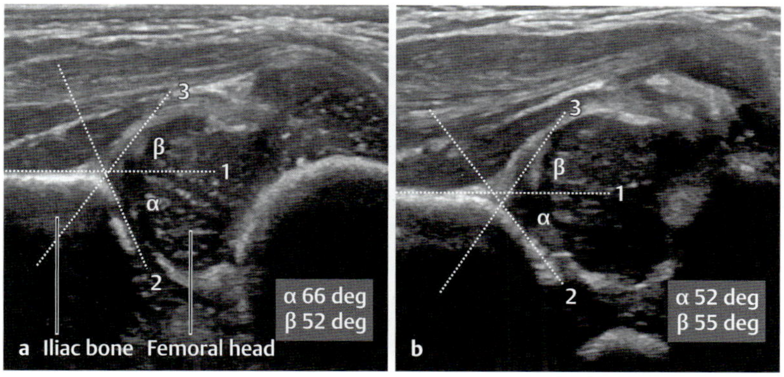

Fig. 9.2 Ultrasound of the infant hip. **(a)** Normal finding. **(b)** Dysplasia with reduced alpha angle (Graf Type II). 1, baseline; 2, acetabular roof line; 3, inclination line.

▸ **Radiography/CT.** Given the availability of ultrasound, radiographs are only indicated in exceptional cases in the first nine months of life, e.g., in clinical courses with an unclear differential diagnosis or on completion of treatment for developmental dysplasia of the hip.

Between 3 and 6 months, ossification of the hip progresses to the extent that dysplasia of the hip can be confidently identified. A diagnosis is reached by measuring the geometry of the acetabular cup and the centering of the ossification of the femoral head within the acetabulum (▸ Fig. 9.3). The acetabular roof angle decreases with increasing ossification of the acetabular cup. Depending on the severity of the hip dysplasia, the bony roof of the femoral head deteriorates, the acetabular inclination angle becomes steeper, and ultimately the femoral head becomes displaced and subluxated (▸ Figs. 9.4 and ▸ 9.5). With chronic dislocation a secondary, "pseudoacetabular cup" develops where the femoral head abuts the lateral margin of the acetabulum and/or ilium.

▸ **MRI.** Indications for MRI include failure of conservative treatment and preoperative planning. Causes of a failure to be able to reduce the hip such as displacement of the margin of the acetabular roof into the joint (inverted limbus), entrapped parts of the capsule or fatty tissue, are more readily identified with MRI than with ultrasound (▸ Fig. 9.6). Another indication is suspected osteonecrosis of the femoral head, which can develop after forced attempts at reduction.

9

9.3 Congenital Deformities of the Foot

The foot of the neonate and the infant has a characteristic pattern of development: until early childhood, the arch of the foot is flat because it is filled with a fat pad. A mild talipes calcaneus position of the hindfoot and a supination position of the forefoot are also temporary. Weight bearing during the standing phase results in an apparent pes planovalgus (flat valgus foot), which corrects itself by the age of 7 to 8 years.

Congenital foot deformities must be distinguished from these physiological and age-related changes within the child's foot. From an etiological standpoint, congenital deformities occur with higher familial frequency or may be associated with underlying neurogenic or myogenic conditions (e.g., meningomyelocele, cerebral palsy, arthrogryposis).

Early initiation of treatment is crucial for providing optimal therapy because the mobility of the infant foot is still great but ossification and fixation of the foot skeleton progresses rapidly in the first 2 years.

Club foot (pes equinovarus). This is a complex deformity of the foot which cannot be corrected passively and comprises four components:

- Pes equinus (horse foot) with a vertical calcaneus and shortened Achilles tendon.
- Pes varus (varus position of the heel).
- Metatarsus adductus (sickle foot) with inward turning of the midfoot.
- Pes cavus (hollow foot) with a high arch of the foot.

Club foot is the second most common congenital skeletal deformity after congenital dysplasia of the hip, affecting 0.1% of all newborns. It may be unilateral or bilateral and is commonly associated with other malformations, especially congenital dysplasia of the hip.

Metatarsus adductus (sickle foot). Metatarsus adductus is a foot deformity with adduction or varus position of the forefoot relative to the hindfoot.

Flat foot (vertical talus). This malformation involves an increased vertical position of the talus and dislocation of the navicular on the talus (not to be confused with a flexible flat foot deformity and physiologic pes planovalgus [flat valgus foot]).

Hollow foot (pes cavus). Pes cavus refers to a foot deformity with a deepened (high) longitudinal arch and increased vertical position of the metatarsals, especially the first ray.

Talipes calcaneus. This term refers to a malalignment with the dorsum of the foot fully dorsiflexed toward the lower leg. Congenital talipes calcaneus should be distinguished from the often encountered, harmless and transient talipes calcaneus of the neonate.

Pes equinus. A foot fixed in plantar flexion due to tightness of the Achilles tendon is referred to as pes equinus.

▸ **Radiography.** Radiography serves to assess the axes of the tarsal bones in the dorsoplantar and lateral projections (▸ Figs. 9.7 and ▸ 9.8).

▸ **CT/MRI.** The tarsal bones are largely preformed in cartilage at birth and in early infancy—at a time when important decisions should be made regarding therapy. The calcaneus, talus, and cuboid initially have small ossification centers. At this time MRI provides an exact demonstration of malalignment in three planes.

As ossification of the bones of the foot progresses, CT with 3D-reconstructed images provides a good spatial overview of the foot deformity.

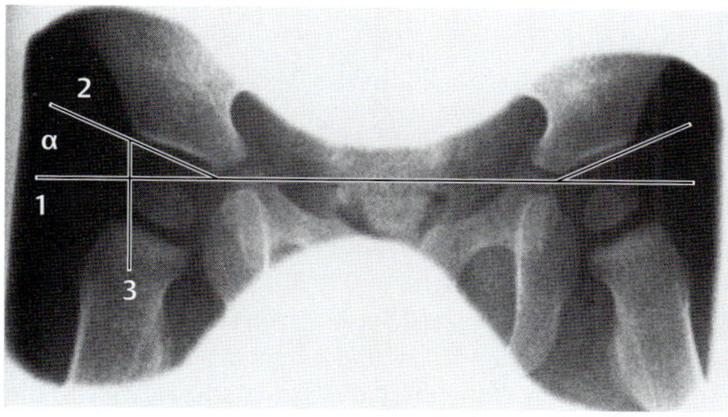

Fig. 9.3 Measurement of the acetabular roof angle. 1, Hilgenreiner line; 2, acetabular roof line; 3, Ombredanne's vertical line; α = acetabular angle.

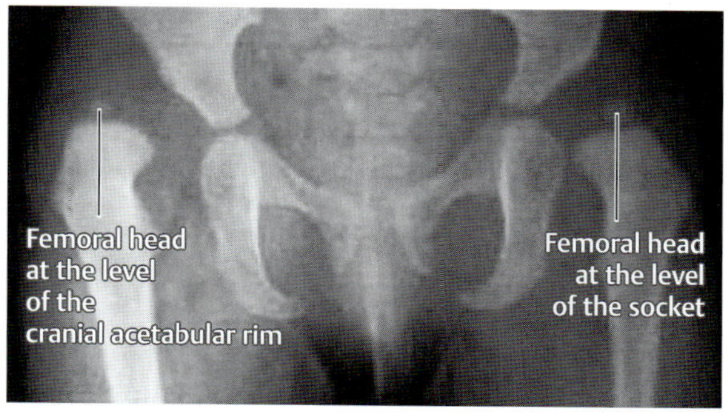

Fig. 9.4 Bilateral dislocation of the hips with vertical acetabulae and displaced femoral heads, lateral to Ombredanne's line.

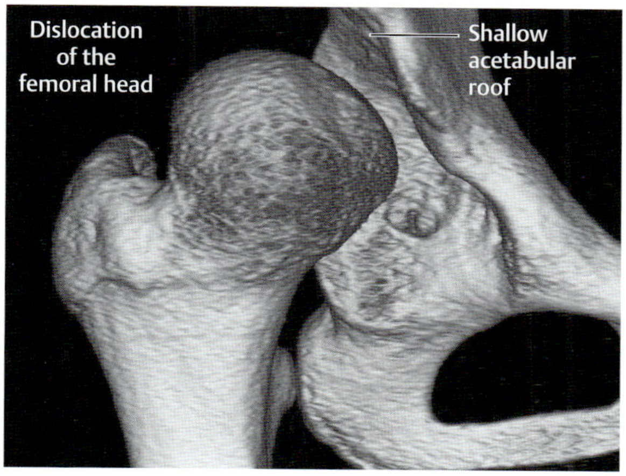

Fig. 9.5 Dysplasia of the hip. 3D reconstruction obtained from one CT data set.

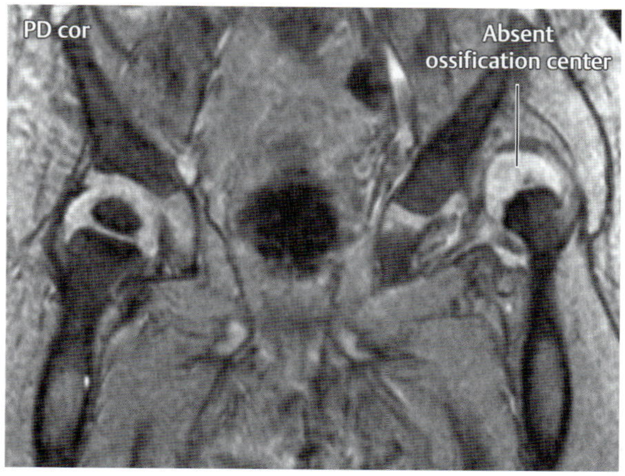

Fig. 9.6 Left hip dislocation with dysplasia. The development of the femoral head lags behind the normal right side.

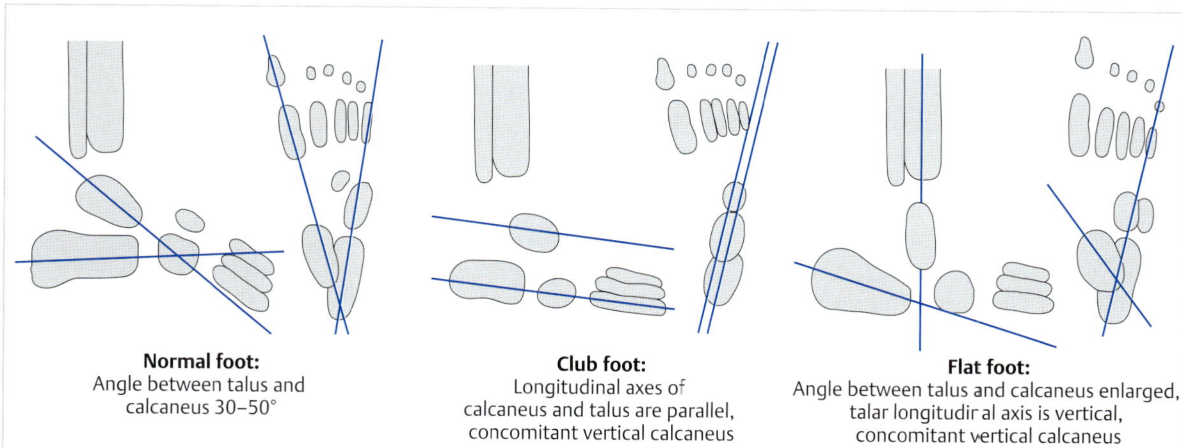

Fig. 9.7 Schematic diagram of radiographic criteria for the normal, club, and flat foot.

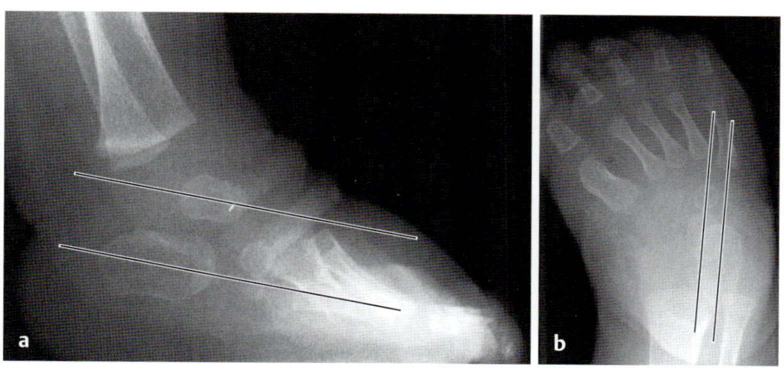

Fig. 9.8 Clubfoot. **(a)** The longitudinal axes of talus and calcaneus are orientated parallel to each other in the lateral projection. **(b)** The longitudinal axes of talus and calcaneus are also orientated parallel to each other in the dorsoplantar projection.

9.4 Patellofemoral Dysplasia

In the field of traumatology, lateral patellar dislocation is a common indication for imaging, with patellofemoral dysplasia representing a risk factor for patellofemoral instability.

▸ Pathology. **Patellar dysplasia** refers to hypoplasia of the medial facet, with significant asymmetry (hunter's cap), or widening ("pebble-shaped"). Wiberg's variations in shape (Types 1–3) are not considered to be dysplasias. The shape of the patella alone is not the decisive factor; rather it is cartilage congruence within the trochlear groove. With patellar **malalignment**, congruence is absent; with patellar **maltracking**, there is incorrect patellar engagement within the trochlear groove. Apart from extensive lateral compression syndrome (ELPS), this can also cause patellofemoral instability with the risk of lateral patellar dislocation. Main risk factors include patella alta; abnormal, typically lateral, patellar tilt (abnormal tilting of the patella in the horizontal plane); trochlear dysplasia; and abnormal lateralization of the tibial tuberosity.

▸ Radiography. Apart from plain films of the knee in two projections, an additional sunrise view of the patella in 30° flexion is obtained. Series of axial views in 30°, 60°, and 90° flexion are now obsolete.

Vertical malalignment (dystopia) may be determined from the lateral view using various indices, the most commonly used being the Insall–Salvati index (▸ Fig. 9.9). As a general rule:

- Insall–Salvati index smaller than 0.8: **patella alta.**
- Insall–Salvati index 0.8 to 1.2: **normal.**
- Insall–Salvati index greater than 1.2: **patella baja.**

An axial view may be obtained in cases of horizontal malalignment to determine the patellofemoral congruence angle and degree of patellar tilt, whereas the sulcus angle is used to assess for trochlear dysplasia (see specialized literature).

▸ CT/MRI. The above measuring techniques (Insall–Salvati index, etc.) may be similarly applied to sectional imaging. Since younger patients are usually involved, MRI is preferred. The imaging study should include the tibial tuberosity.

Apart from the sulcus angle, the depth of the trochlea may be used to assess for trochlear dysplasia (pathologic is 3 mm and less; measured 3 cm proximal to the femorotibial joint). An important parameter, not measurable on radiographs, is the TT–TG distance (tibial tuberosity–trochlear groove distance), which expresses the distance between the deepest point of the femoral trochlea and the most anterior part of the tibial tuberosity, vertical to the femoral condylar line (see specialized literature). Values greater than 20 mm are associated with patellar instability; values from 15 to 20 mm are within the gray zone.

> **Caution**
>
> Abnormal TT–TG values can also be caused by rotational malalignment.

In addition to identifying static parameters of patellar maltracking, a **dynamic MRI examination** may be obtained. However, this is only useful in 0 to 30° flexion. According to McNally's method (▸ see References for Chapter 9.4), extension under resistance occurs in the region of 20 to 0° of flexion. The position of the middle of the patella relative to the trochlea in comparison with the contralateral side is determined and the degree of lateralization is classified.

Furthermore, patellar tilt without lateralization is recognizable during dynamic examinations and is referred to as "ELPS" (▸ see References for Chapter 9.4). Edema within the superolateral aspect of Hoffa's fat pad may also be seen in these patients.

▸ Important findings. After a patellar dislocation (▸ Fig. 9.10) or in cases of chronic anterior knee pain, risk factors such as patella alta, abnormal patellar tilt, trochlear dysplasia, or abnormal lateralization of the tibial tuberosity should be determined, since these can be addressed therapeutically. However, according to more recent studies, the reliability and validity of measurement techniques should not be overrated. Dynamic examinations using MRI can often provide better information.

9.5 Scoliosis and Kyphosis

9.5.1 Kyphosis

Kyphosis is a dorsally convex curvature of the spine. Mild kyphosis of the thoracic spine is physiologic, kyphosis of the cervical or lumbar spine or increased thoracic kyphosis, however, are pathologic. The degree of kyphosis can be quantified using various measurement techniques (see ▸ Fig. 7.32). Apart from Scheuermann's disease, other causes of pathologic kyphosis include traumatic, osteoporotic, and postinflammatory vertebral wedging.

9.5.2 Scoliosis

Scoliosis is a fixed axial deviation of the spine in the frontal plane with additional rotation of individual vertebrae (rotatory scoliosis).

The idiopathic form is further subdivided into infantile, juvenile, and adolescent forms. This must be distinguished from other, secondary causes (e.g., spinal cord injury, rheumatic disorders, infections).

Scoliosis is assessed clinically and radiographically (Cobb angle and vertebral rotation using the Nash and Moe technique; see specialized orthopaedic literature).

9.6 Congenital Disorders of Skeletal Development

A large number of congenital disorders affect skeletal growth and development.

A distinction is made between **skeletal dysplasia** (synonym: osteochondral dysplasia), which represents a generalized disorder of cartilage and bone development resulting in dwarfism, and **dysostosis**, which results in the abnormal development of individual bones (singly or in combination). Dwarfism is rarely encountered in the latter.

▶ Pathology. The classification of skeletal dysplasias is based on the "Paris Nomenclature" of 1986, but this has been revised several times since then, most recently in 1997. The number of known skeletal dysplasias is large and has continued to expand over the last two decades, thanks in large part to the enormous progress achieved in the field of molecular biology. New disorders have been discovered, along with unexpected insights into connections between different skeletal dysplasias. For example, the same genetic mutation can result in skeletal dysplasias that have completely different clinical and radiomorphological phenotypes.

Whereas the earlier classification was based on radiomorphological criteria and the age of appearance, the new classification emphasizes the etiopathological aspects. This type of etiopathogenetic differentiation is of little help for making a diagnosis based on radiographic findings. Nevertheless, a detailed, specific diagnosis is necessary to be able to provide genetic counseling to parents along with important prognostic information. For this purpose, a conventional radiographic examination still serves as a basic diagnostic tool for confirming the presence of a skeletal dysplasia and for determining its most likely family or subgroup.

For the purpose of this book, individual presentations of the various skeletal dysplasias will not be provided and reference is made to the specialized literature that is available. The following section, however, will present a five-step diagnostic pathway to assist in arriving at a radiomorphological classification.

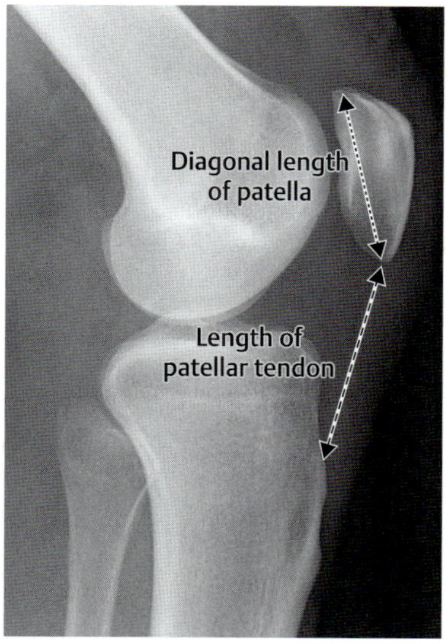

Fig. 9.9 Measurement of the Insall–Salvati index (ratio of the diagonal length of the patella to the length of the patellar tendon). Normal finding.

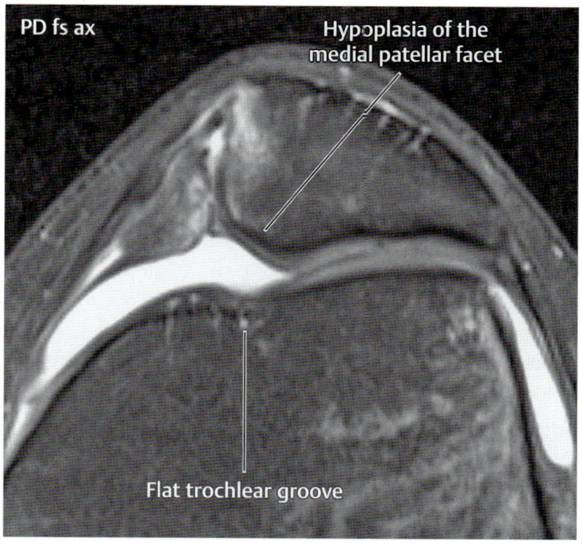

Fig. 9.10 Appearance after patellar dislocation. History of recurrent dislocations with patellar dysplasia, hunter's cap deformity, and dysplastic flat femoral trochlea.

9.6.1 Diagnostic Pathway for Classification of Skeletal Dysplasia

Step 1: Analysis of Pathognomonic Radiological Alterations

Appropriate radiographic examinations are necessary for systematically identifying skeletal alterations. The minimum projections obtained should include:

- PA hand.
- AP pelvis.
- AP and lateral lumbar spine and sacrum.
- Whole-body survey of the skeleton ("babygram") in the neonate and infant as well as in the case of a stillbirth.
- AP chest using rib technique.

Consider:

- Lateral view of the skull.

Long Tubular Bones

Length and Proportion. Bone length of the extremities is usually reduced, with the exception of Marfan's syndrome and homocystinuria. Disproportionate limb growth can result in *rhizomelic* (humerus or femur; ▶ Fig. 9.11), *mesomelic* (ulna, radius or tibia, fibula; ▶ Fig. 9.12), or *acromelic forms* (hand or foot; ▶ Fig. 9.13) of micromelia (short limbs). Isolated forms of acromelia are rare and are then regarded as peripheral dysostoses. Acromelia is usually associated with mesomelic dwarfism.

9

Growth zones of the epiphyses, metaphyses, and diaphyses. Skeletal growth of epiphysis and metaphysis must be regarded as one unit; disturbances of growth always involve both parts. Nevertheless, there are skeletal dysplasias in which the epiphyseal disturbance of growth is more prominent than in those in which the metaphyseal disturbance of growth is paramount.

Epiphyseal disturbance of growth. The ossification centers are small, irregular, and fragmented. Calcifications can develop within the epiphyseal cartilage (▶ Figs. 9.14 and ▶ 9.15).

Metaphyseal disturbance of growth. The metaphyseal zone appears elongated and widened, cup-shaped, and irregularly contoured (▶ Fig. 9.16; see also ▶ Fig. 9.14).

Diaphyseal disturbance of growth. It manifests in various ways:

- Slender tubular bones with thin cortex, usually as a result of a neuromuscular disease.
- Short, stubby, and wide extremity bones with thickened cortices and narrow medullary cavities (▶ Fig. 9.17).

Spine

The most common forms of skeletal dysplasia are associated with alterations of the spine. The following vertebral features should be evaluated:

- The shape of the vertebral bodies and neural arches.
- Flattened vertebral bodies as seen in platyspondyly (▶ Fig. 9.18).
- Beaklike anterior margins (▶ Fig. 9.19).
- Barrel vertebrae.
- Concavity of the posterior vertebral margins.
- Decreasing interpedicular distance and associated narrowing of the spinal canal (▶ Fig. 9.20).
- Vertebral clefts, hemi-, block, and butterfly vertebrae (see ▶ Fig. 9.18).
- Kyphoscoliosis (a common finding in the skeletal dysplasias).

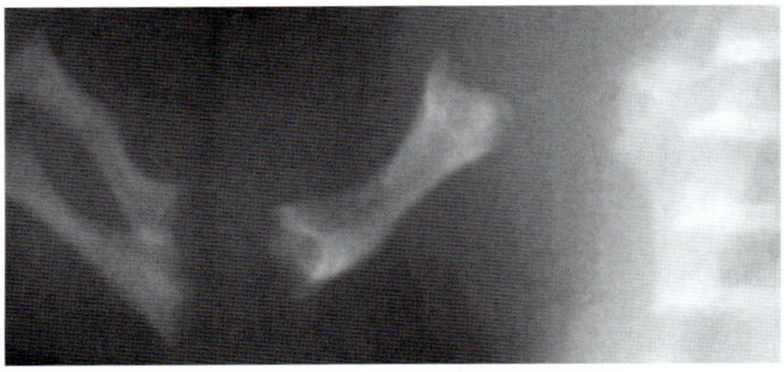

Fig. 9.11 Rhizomelic and mesomelic dwarfism with shortening and widening of the humerus and the forearm bones. Example: thanatophoric dysplasia.

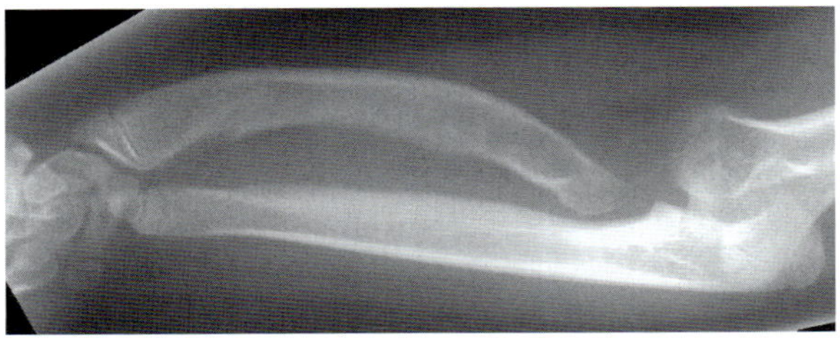

Fig. 9.12 Mesomelia with shortening of the forearm bones and bowing of the radius. Example: dyschondrosteosis.

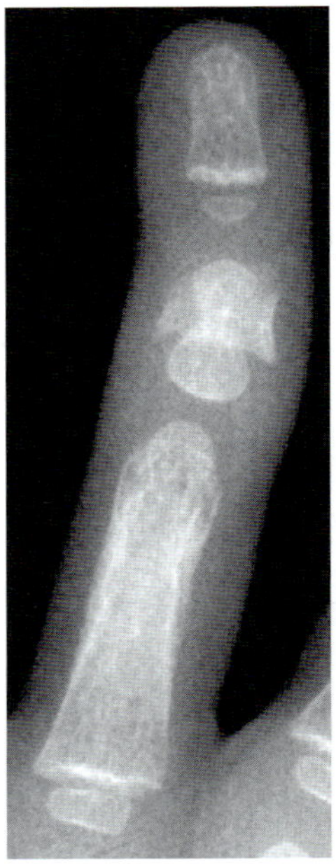

Fig. 9.13 Shortening of the middle phalanx due to marked cone-shaped epiphysis and cufflike ("winglike") diaphysis. Example: angel-shaped phalangoepiphyseal dysplasia (ASPED).

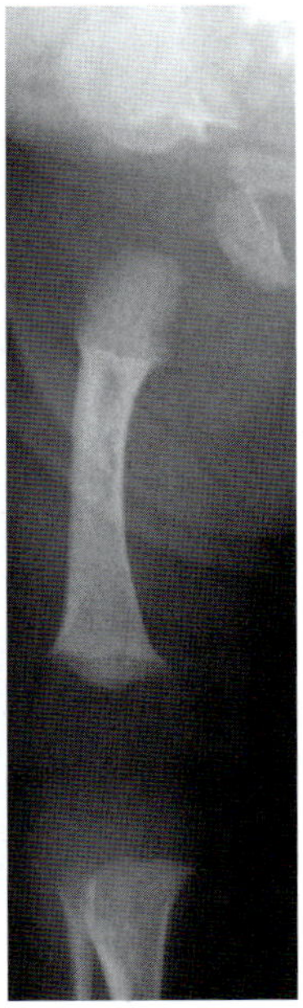

Fig. 9.17 Short and broad femur with a wide cortices and narrow medullary cavity. Example: achondroplasia.

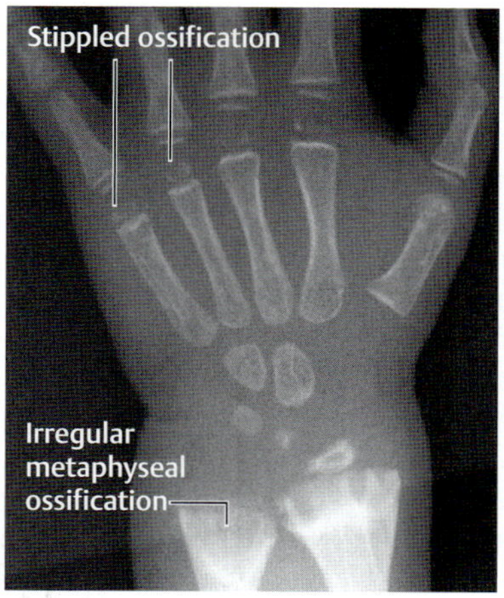

Fig. 9.14

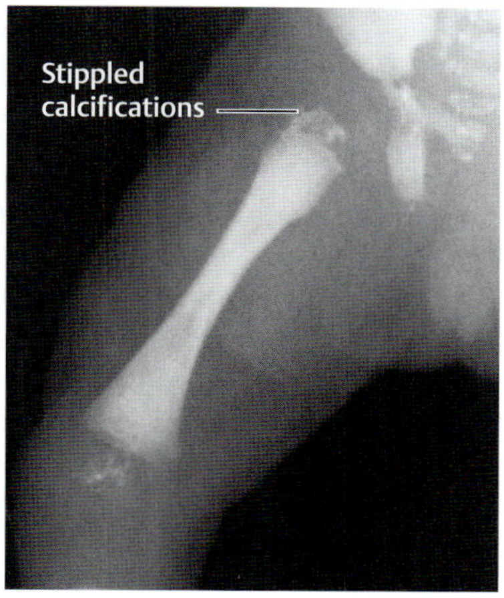

Fig. 9.15

Fig. 9.14 Stippled ossification of the metacarpal epiphyses, small, irregularly marginated and ossified radial epiphysis, severe disturbance of metaphyseal ossification. Example: the group of spondylo-epiphyseal and spondylometaphyseal dysplasias.

Fig. 9.15 Stippled calcification of the epiphyseal cartilage and the joint capsule of the proximal and distal femoral epiphyses. Example: epiphyseal chondrodysplasia punctata, Conradi–Hünermann type.

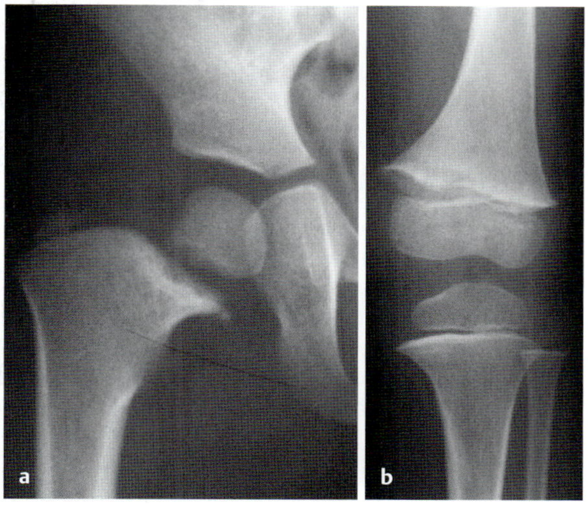

Fig. 9.16 Metaphyseal growth disturbance. Example: Schmid-type metaphyseal chondrodysplasia. **(a)** Shortened femoral neck in varus with widened, somewhat cup-shaped, irregularly contoured, fragmented metaphysis. **(b)** Mild widening and irregularity of the metaphyses of the knee joint.

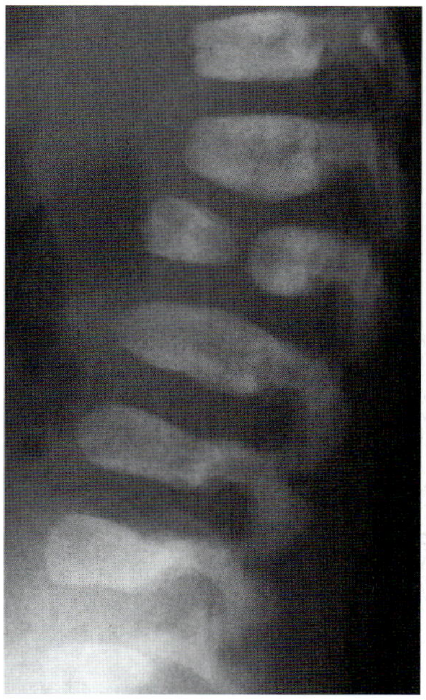

Fig. 9.18 Coronal cleft of L2 with platyspondyly and mildly ovoid vertebral morphology. Example: Kniest dysplasia.

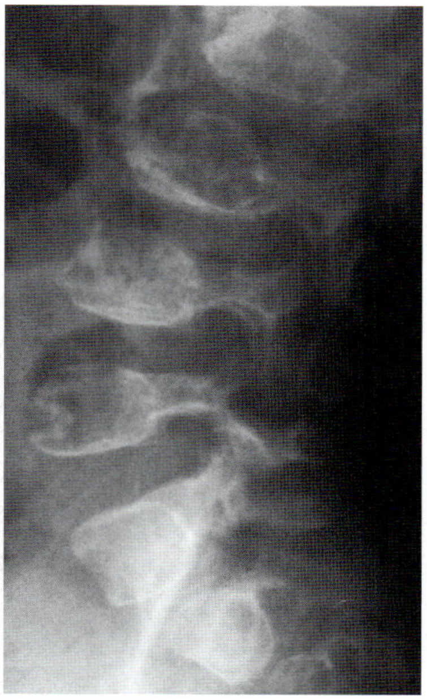

Fig. 9.19 Ovoid vertebrae with anterior beaking due to an anterosuperior ossification defect at L2 and L3. Reduced mineralization. Example: gangliosidosis Type I.

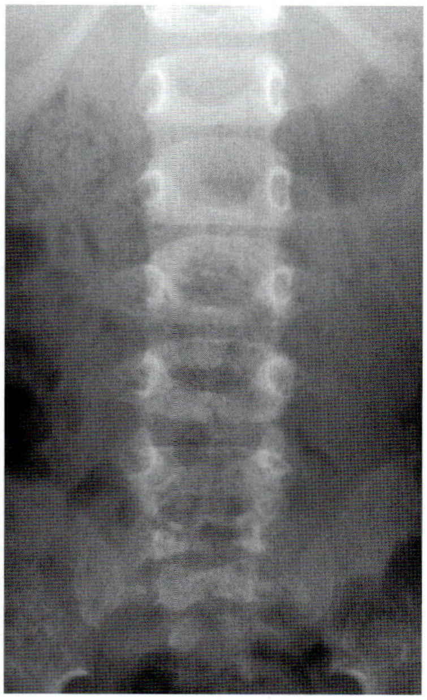

Fig. 9.20 Progressive decrease in interpedicular distance. Example: hypochondroplasia.

Pelvis

Some skeletal dysplasias demonstrate special features in the pelvis. Two **characteristic shapes** of the iliac bones are found: Type 1 with short and stubby, square iliac bones (▶ Fig. 9.21) and Type 2 with narrow, tapered acetabular roofs (▶ Fig. 9.22). In addition to these characteristic forms, measurements of the acetabular roof angle and the iliac angle are also of diagnostic value (▶ Fig. 9.23).

A wide pubic symphysis in the first year of life is found in many forms of skeletal dysplasia due to delayed ossification; this is particularly noticeable in cleidocranial dysostosis.

Hand

Number, length, and morphology of the individual bones of the hand must be analyzed:

- Changes in the number of fingers resulting in oligodactyly or polydactyly.
- Shortening of all phalanges, a row of phalanges, or individual phalanges is found in a large number of congenital diseases. Isolated shortening of the fourth and fifth metacarpals results in a positive metacarpal sign (▶ Fig. 9.24).
- Fusions are commonly seen. **Syndactyly** is fusion between two adjacent fingers (membranous or osseous); **symphalangy** refers to fusion between two phalanges of the same ray (▶ Fig. 9.25). Carpal synostosis of one row is regarded as a normal variant; carpal fusion crossing both carpal rows is an indication of a syndrome.
- Abnormal morphology of phalanges and carpal bones such as cone-shaped epiphyses, widening or narrowing of the phalanges or metacarpals, and irregularity of the carpal bones may be an important diagnostic clue (▶ Figs. 9.26 and ▶ 9.27).

Step 2: Age at the Time of the Manifestation of Radiographic Abnormalities

The patient's age at the time of manifestation of radiographic abnormalities is another diagnostic key. A large number of abnormalities will occur in infancy. Here a distinction is made between fatal early skeletal dysplasias, such as achondrogenesis and thanatophoric dysplasia, and the usually nonfatal dysplasias, such as achondroplasia (see ▶ Table 9.2). Another group of dysplasias becomes clinically manifest after the first year of life.

It is possible for skeletal alterations of a skeletal dysplasia that manifests in infancy to disappear over time. Therefore, chondrodysplasia punctata (Conradi–Hünermann type), with its characteristic epiphyseal and periarticular, punctate calcifications (see ▶ Fig. 9.15), can usually be diagnosed only in infancy. With time, the fine calcifications regress and any residual asymmetric disturbances of growth are nonspecific and often no longer help with arriving at the diagnosis.

Step 3: Analysis of Skeletal Distribution Pattern and Resulting Bone Abnormalities

A single anomaly usually excludes the presence of skeletal dysplasia. Two or more variations may allow for the diagnosis of a particular skeletal dysplasia. Analysis of the skeletal distribution and the resulting skeletal abnormalities allows for classifying a disorder as an epiphyseal, metaphyseal, epimetaphyseal, spondylometaphyseal, or spondyloepimetaphyseal dysplasia. Within these individual groups there are yet further options for differentiation based on regional involvement. For example, with the Schmid type of metaphyseal dysplasia, the proximal femoral metaphysis is more altered than the distal (see ▶ Fig. 9.16).

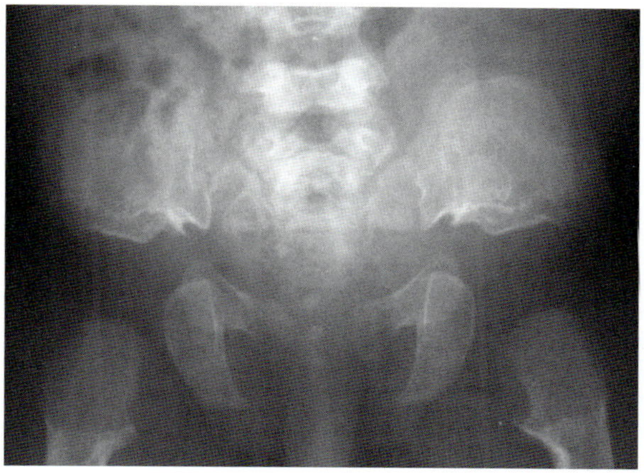

Fig. 9.21 Pelvis Type 1 with short and stubby squared iliac wings. Example: achondroplasia.

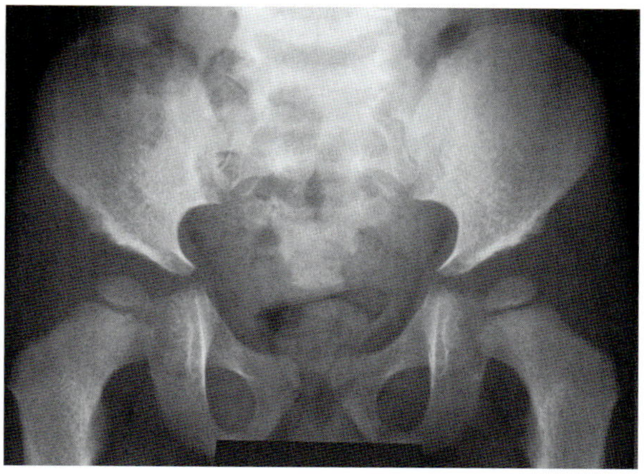

Fig. 9.22 Pelvis Type 2 with a narrow, tapered acetabular roofs (iliac wings resembling Mickey Mouse ears). Example: dysostosis multiplex group.

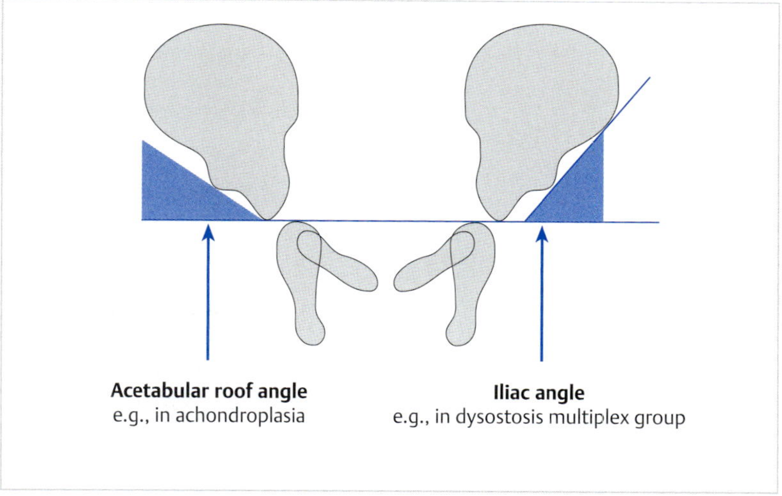

Fig. 9.23 Schematic diagram of the acetabular roof angle and the iliac angle.

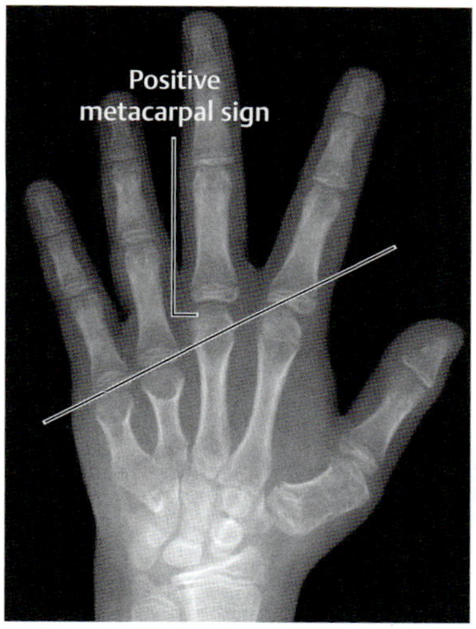

Fig. 9.24 Shortening of metacarpals IV and V. Example: Albright's hereditary osteodystrophy.

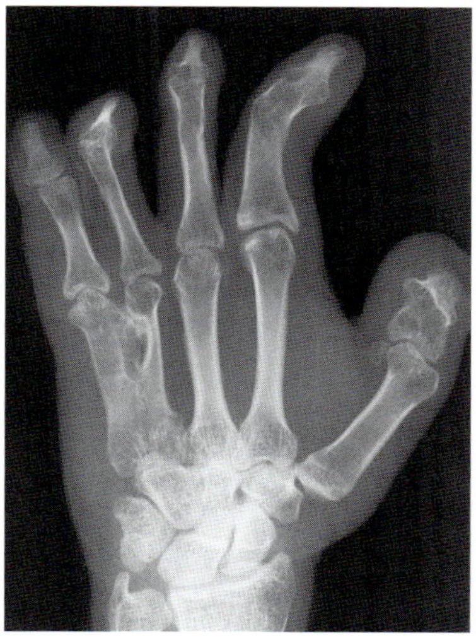

Fig. 9.25 Syndactyly involving the fourth and fifth metacarpals, fusion between second to fourth terminal and middle phalanges. Example: Apert's syndrome.

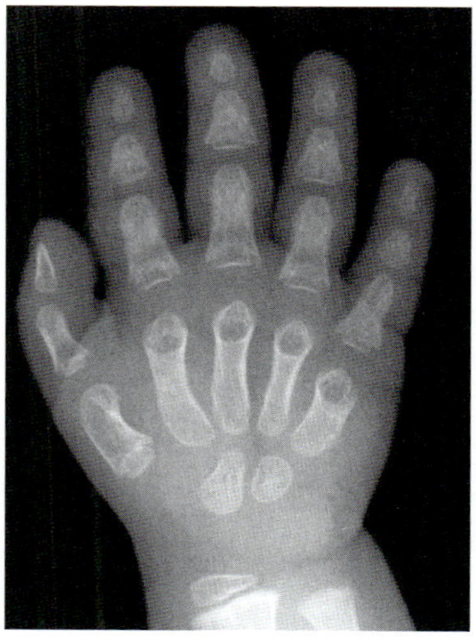

Fig. 9.26 Shortened, wide, and stubby metacarpals, proximal and middle phalanges; cone-shaped epiphyses of the second to fourth metacarpals and proximal phalanges. Example: achondroplasia.

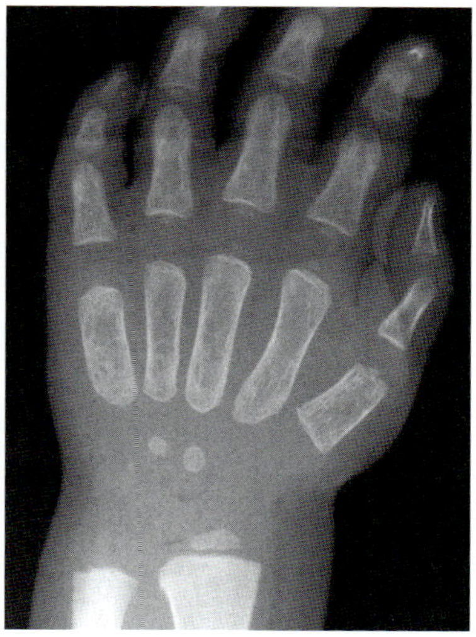

Fig. 9.27 Short and stubby metacarpals without diaphyseal wasp waisting; short and stubby proximal and middle phalanges, proximal ends of the metacarpals narrowed. Example: Type II mucopolysaccharidosis.

Step 4: Analysis of the Density and Fracture Potential of the Bone

Analysis of bone density when a skeletal dysplasia is suspected allows for differentiation between dysplasias with reduced bone density (osteopenia) and those with increased bone density (osteosclerosis). Alteration of bone density may result in abnormal bone function such as fractures more commonly occurring after minor injury. Osteogenesis imperfecta is an example of a dysplasia with reduced bone density (▸ Figs. 9.28 and ▸ 9.29), while increased bone density is seen with osteopetrosis (Albers–Schönberg disease; ▸ Fig. 9.30).

Step 5: Integration of Radiological and Clinical Findings

Rarely are the findings of skeletal dysplasias confined exclusively to the skeleton. There are often associated abnormalities of other organ systems, such as the skin, heart, abdominal organs, or central nervous system, that may result in other nonskeletal complications (▸ Table 9.1).

Integrating the radiological abnormalities with clinical findings is often a key to diagnosis. Relevant literature, tables, and directories are available for reference. Internet databanks with the possibility of entering key radiographic and clinical findings can also be useful diagnostic aids.

9.6.2 The Most Common Neonatal Skeletal Dysplasias

The majority of skeletal dysplasias are rarely encountered clinically. ▸ Table 9.2 provides an overview of the ten most common skeletal dysplasias with neonatal manifestation; they represent approximately 80% of all skeletal dysplasias.

Table 9.1 Early complications of skeletal dysplasias

Skeletal	Extraskeletal
• Atlanto-occipital instability • Spinal canal stenosis • Kyphoscolioses • Dislocations • Contractures • Fractures • Extremity malalignments • Foot deformities	• Ophthalmological complications (myopias, detached retinas among others) • Hearing loss • Neurologic disturbances (hydrocephalus, spinal cord compression) • Nephropathies • Maldigestion • Immune deficiencies • Pulmonary complications

9

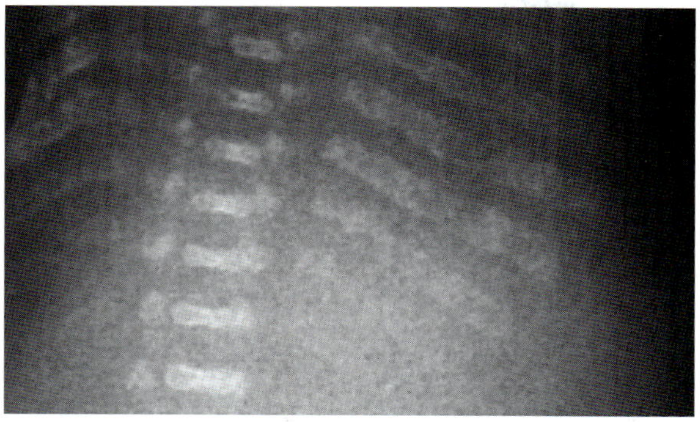

Fig. 9.28 Type II c osteogenesis imperfecta (fatal). Compression fractures of the vertebrae with diffuse rib fractures.

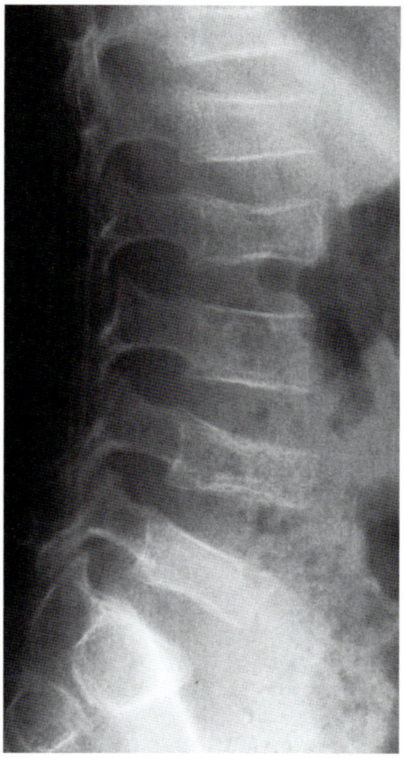

Fig. 9.29 Type III osteogenesis imperfecta (nonfatal). Flattening of the vertebral bodies in the presence of osteopenia.

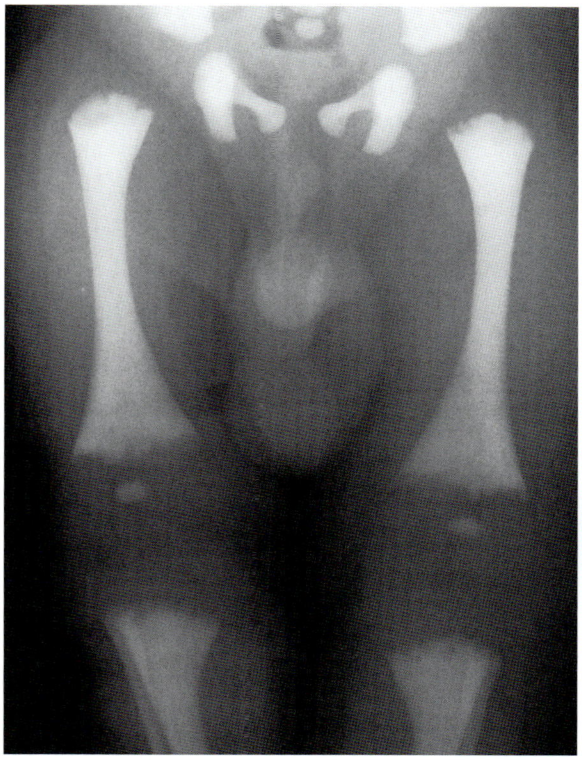

Fig. 9.30 Infantile osteopetrosis. Symmetrically increased bone density, irregularly ossified metaphyseal zones.

Table 9.2 The 10 most common neonatal manifestations of skeletal dysplasias

Skeletal dysplasia	Fatal	Fatality dependent upon subtype	Nonfatal	Frequency per 100 000 births
Osteogenesis imperfecta		+		3.64
Achondroplasia			+	2.77
Thanatophoric dysplasia	+			1.68
Chondrodysplasia punctata		+		0.78
Jeune's syndrome		+		0.51
Campomelic dysplasia		+		0.47
Diastrophic dysplasia			+	0.37
Spondylothoracic dysplasia			+	0.35
Achondrogenesis	+		+	0.31
Cleidocranial dysplasia			+	0.31

10 Rheumatic Disorders

10.1 Introduction

10.1.1 Common Pathogenic Features

Rheumatic disorders affect primarily the musculoskeletal system, although any organ may be involved.

A large number of disorders are subsumed under the term "rheumatism" but present quite different manifestations and pose different diagnostic and therapeutic challenges. The WHO defines the term "rheumatism" as diseases occurring in the locomotor system, almost always associated with pain and commonly also with restriction of movement.

The **four main WHO groups** comprise:

1. Inflammatory rheumatic disorders.
2. Degenerative articular and spinal disorders.
3. Soft tissue rheumatic disorders.
4. Metabolic disorders with rheumatic symptoms.

This broad classification of rheumatic diseases is based in part on the various disease causes and in part on organ systems.

We have arranged this chapter on rheumatological disorders according to this classification scheme and shall present the wide variety of associated clinical characteristics and imaging findings that occur with these disorders. This includes inflammatory and degenerative arthropathies, as well as those of the spine and crystal-induced alterations. Osteoporosis is often assigned to the topic of "rheumatism," but for didactic reasons is dealt with in Chapter 8.1 under the general heading "Metabolic, Hormonal, and Toxic Bone Disorders."

10

10.1.2 Radiographic Features of the Peripheral Joints and their Role in Differential Diagnosis

To minimize repetition in the following chapters, fundamental radiographic features will now be presented, together with a brief discussion of differential diagnostic considerations.

Soft Tissue Swelling

Soft tissue swelling is recognized by a change in contour and by displacement or loss of fat planes:

- The characteristic sign of **active arthritis** is the voluminous, fusiform soft tissue swelling (▶ Fig. 10.1), which becomes apparent a few days after onset of the arthritis and is therefore the only "early" radiographic sign, typically affecting the hands and, in some patients, also the forefeet.
- In **osteoarthritis** soft tissue swelling is less pronounced and is usually asymmetric, with a firm and nodular clinical appearance in the fingers and toes. During an acute inflammatory exacerbation (known as "erosive" osteoarthritis; cf. Chapter 10.2) the appearance is that of an "arthritic" soft tissue swelling.
- In periarticular **soft tissue inflammation** (bursitis, tenosynovitis, fasciitis, abscess, infection) soft tissue swelling is even more asymmetric.

> **Note**
>
> **Synovitis:** This is an inflammation of the synovial membrane of the joints and tendon sheaths. The finding is nonspecific and most commonly seen in cases of rheumatic diseases, osteoarthritis, and infection as well as after trauma.
>
> **Pannus:** In rheumatic disorders this term is used synonymously for synovitis, although it truly refers to chronic fibrovascular tissue. Modern literature no longer uses the term.
>
> **Effusion:** An effusion is a nonspecific phenomenon associated with synovitis.

Juxta-articular Loss of Bone Mineral Density

Juxta-articular, heterogeneous, patchy or even bandlike demineralization develops; the cancellous bone loses its "sharpness," the number of trabeculae is reduced. Those isolated trabeculae that remain therefore appear accentuated (▶ Fig. 10.2).

- In the context of **arthritis**, this is referred to as a "collateral phenomenon." It is the arthritis that triggers this process of bone resorption (via neurocirculatory reflexes, increased perfusion, and activated osteoclasts). Initially, this is *not* related to the direct bone destruction by joint inflammation, which does not become radiographically evident until some weeks after the onset of the arthritis. These collateral phenomena are only detectable during an acute inflammatory flare and are completely reversible.
- Morphologically, **disuse osteoporosis** is indistinguishable from demineralization related to long-standing arthritis (pain-related immobilization) or prior trauma.

- The osteoporosis of **CRPS** (complex regional pain syndrome; Sudeck's dystrophy), like soft tissue swelling, is a diffuse phenomenon and is not confined to the joints. It usually involves several bones of one limb.
- In self-limiting **transient osteoporosis** only one bone (most commonly the proximal femur) and one joint are involved.
- Juxta-articular loss of bone mineral density is not seen in **osteoarthritis**. Yet osteoarthritis and diffuse senile or disuse osteoporosis may of course be associated with one another.

Loss of the Subchondral Bone Plate

Loss of the subchondral bone plate (▶ Figs. 10.3 and ▶ 10.4) precedes erosion and is regarded as the first direct sign of arthritis. The cause may be either disuse demineralization (as part of a collateral phenomenon) or secondary to pus or synovitis.

- Absence of the subchondral bone plate is a specific sign of **arthritis**; this is particularly the case when the other parts of the joint contour remain preserved ("partial" loss).
- Loss of the subchondral bone plate is seen in **osteoarthritis** only where there is more significant destruction.

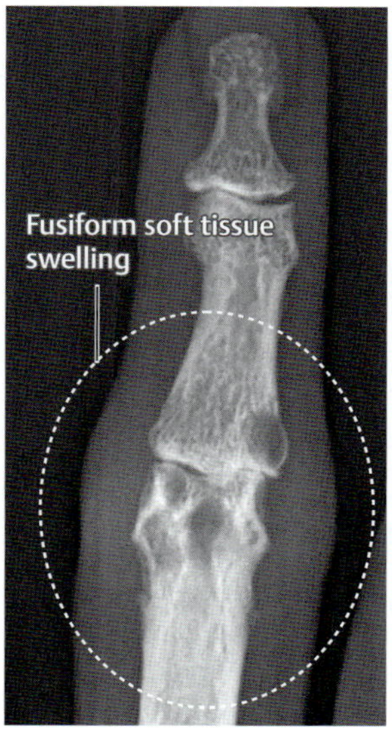

Fig. 10.1 Rheumatoid arthritis with involvement of the proximal interphalangeal joint.

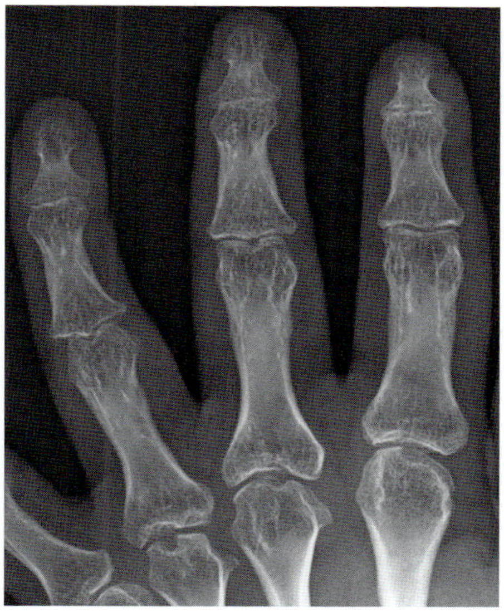

Fig. 10.2 Juvenile chronic polyarthritis. Juxta-articular, as well as less marked diffuse osteopenia; the patient is 30 years old.

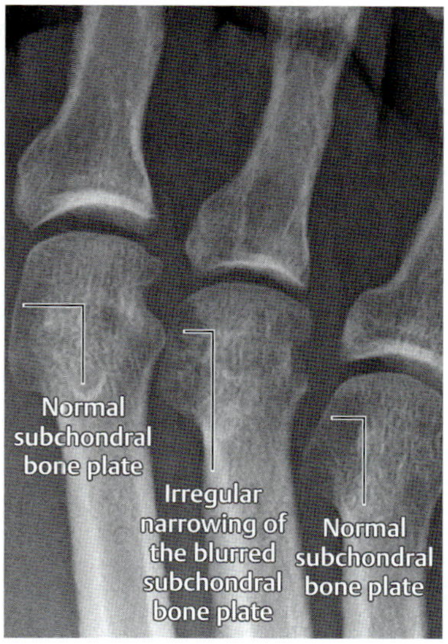

Fig. 10.3 Partial loss of the subchondral bone plate at the site of a developing erosion in a patient with rheumatoid arthritis.

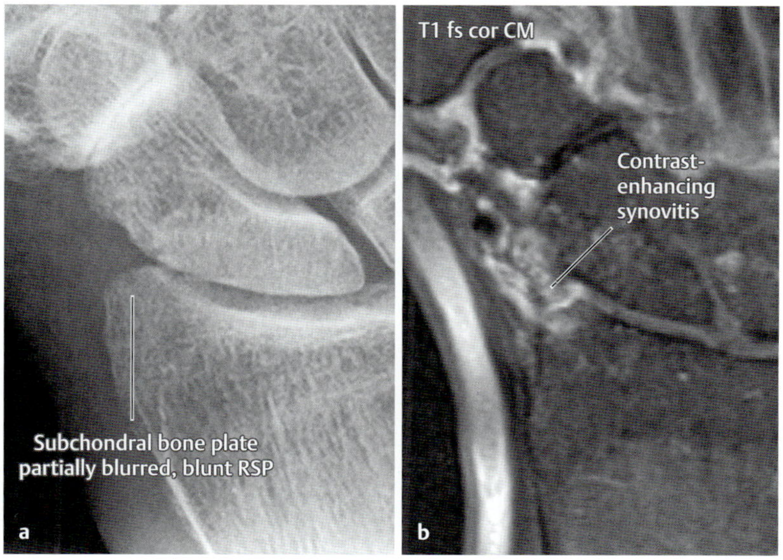

Fig. 10.4 Rheumatoid arthritis. **(a)** Partial loss of the cortical margin of the radial styloid process. **(b)** MRI reveals synovitis and associated erosion at the radial styloid process. MRI demonstrates that loss of the bone plate is often caused by an erosion that is not viewed tangentially on standard radiographs. RSP, radial styloid process.

- **Systemic demineralization** (e.g., in cases of hyperparathyroidism, rickets, osteomalacia) is associated with destruction of the entire subchondral bone plate.
- In **transient osteoporosis** (transient bone marrow edema), the bone plate is lost, as in arthritis. This finding is usually confined to one joint and the joint space is not narrowed.

Erosion

An erosion is a focal bone defect involving the articular portions of the bone. Seen in profile, it is a defect; looked at end on, it appears as a rounded lucency, simulating a cyst. Depending on the activity of the disease process, the erosion can display a blurred, distinct, or even sclerotic border (▸ Fig. 10.5). In **arthritis**, erosions begin at the "bare areas," i.e., the portions of the bone within the joint capsule that are not covered with articular cartilage. Outside of a joint, inflammatory tenosynovitis may produce superficial defects in adjacent bones. This can be a relatively specific indication of a synovial origin of the disease.

- In **osteoarthritis**, "pressure erosions" may be seen at the site of maximum loading; the abnormal loading associated with articular destruction can induce bone resorption and subsequently "cyst formation."
- Erosions and bone destruction associated with **gout** are very often located "para-articularly," some distance away from the joint. They can become quite large. Usually—but not always—gouty erosions are demarcated by a fine sclerotic margin.
- **Destruction caused by an adjacent tumor** presents as a solitary, broad-based bone defect or erosion, without any other joint alterations.

10

Subchondral Osteolytic Lesions (Geodes, "Signal Cysts")

These are *round* (partially confluent) defects in the subarticular regions at the end of a bone (▸ Fig. 10.6). In arthritic conditions, these are also referred to as "signal cysts."

- In **rheumatoid arthritis** they are rarely larger than 1 cm. Marginal sclerosis only appears after treatment or spontaneous healing. The finding must be seen in context with other radiographic features in order for a subchondral cyst to be regarded as a direct sign of arthritis.
- Subchondral cysts in association with **osteoarthritis** ("detritic cysts") are usually multiple, are found at the main load-bearing sites, may be larger than 1 cm, and usually display marginal sclerosis.
- Intraosseous **gouty tophi** are characterized by a variety of features: punched-out defects may be seen alone or together with longitudinal oval osteolytic areas and may appear septated or demonstrate a trabecular pattern.
- In pigmented villonodular synovitis (**PVNS**), the osteolytic areas develop at the margins of the joint. There is nearly always marginal sclerosis but joint space narrowing and juxta-articular osteoporosis are absent (Chapter 4.6.5).
- A connection with the joint space is proof of an **intraosseous ganglion**, although this may not always be observable (Chapter 4.6.3).

Joint Space Narrowing

Joint space narrowing (▸ Fig. 10.7) is an indication of cartilage destruction.

- In **arthritis** narrowing is usually harmonic and symmetrical and involves the entire joint space, or large portions of it.
- Asymmetrical joint space narrowing, in particular the main weight-bearing area, is characteristic of **osteoarthritis**.
- Joint space narrowing also occurs in **CPPD** (calcium pyrophosphate deposition disease). Associated cartilage calcification (chondrocalcinosis) may be seen and can assist in arriving at the correct diagnosis.

Subchondral Sclerosis

This is reactive osteosclerosis.

- Subchondral sclerosis is unusual in active **arthritis**; however, it is found after reparative intervals in chronic forms of arthritis and following drug therapy as well as in cases where secondary osteoarthritis has developed.
- Subchondral sclerosis is a characteristic sign of **osteoarthritis** (Chapter 10.2).

Periarticular Periosteal Reaction

This is found at an epimetaphyseal location, but can also extend to the diaphysis, especially in small tubular bones.

- Periosteal new bone formation is often associated with **spondylarthritis** (e.g., psoriatic arthritis).
- A **lamellated periosteal reaction** (▸ Fig. 10.8) occurs in active, *acute* inflammatory joint processes, but may persist after healing.
- *Chronic* inflammatory arthropathies tend to develop **solid,** sometimes undulating, **periosteal reaction** (▸ Figs. 10.9 and ▸ 10.10).

▸ **DD.** The differential diagnosis includes osteoarthritis, posttraumatic alterations, tumors, hematologic disorders, forms of vasculitis, and chronic venous insufficiency.

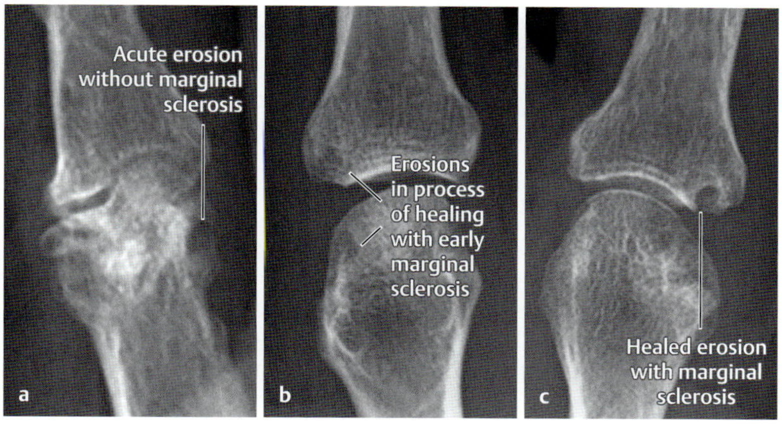

Fig. 10.5 Radiographic morphology of erosions over time. **(a)** Fresh erosion in a patient with gouty arthropathy with preexisting osteoarthritis. **(b)** Erosion in the process of healing in a patient with rheumatoid arthritis. **(c)** Healed erosion in a patient with psoriatic arthropathy.

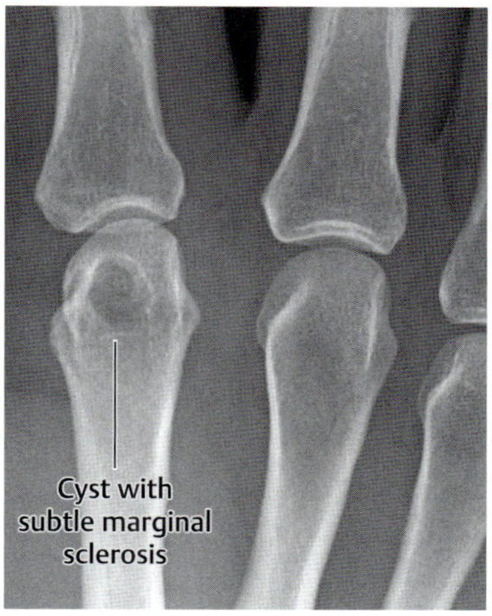

Fig. 10.6 Signal cyst in a patient with rheumatoid arthritis.

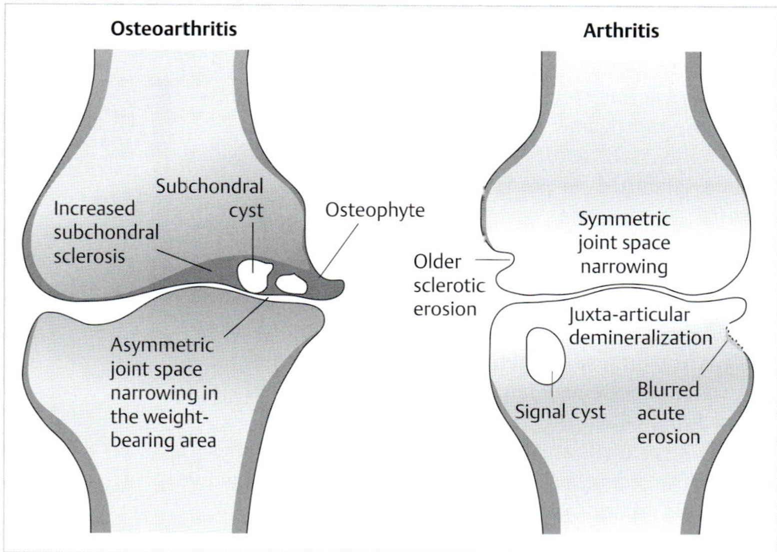

Fig. 10.7 Comparison of the characteristic radiographic features of degenerative and inflammatory arthropathies.

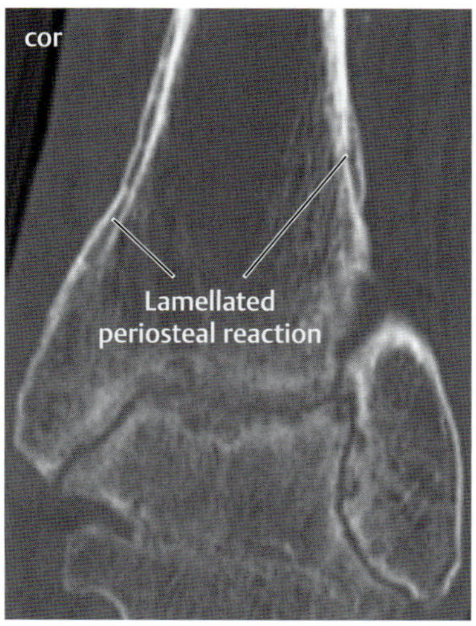

Fig. 10.8 Periosteal reaction in a patient with spondylarthritis. Although this is a lamella, its thickness is an indication of a chronic process.

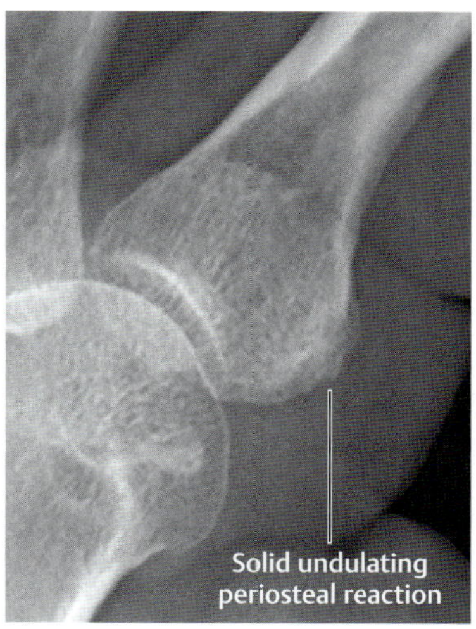

Fig. 10.9 Periosteal reaction in a patient with psoriatic arthropathy.

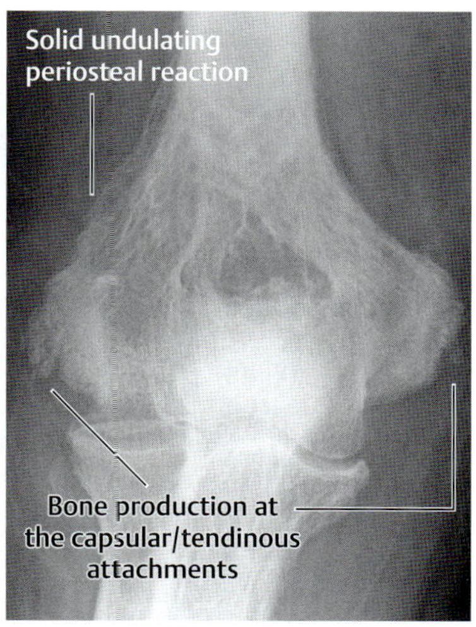

Fig. 10.10 Reactive bone production and periosteal reaction in a patient with psoriasis.

Reactive Bone Formation

Reactive bone formation may produce **osteophytes, bony protuberances**, and **ossification at tendon insertions**. The shape and distribution of these often provide clues for differential diagnosis. Some types of arthritis, such as psoriatic arthritis, tend to develop osseous proliferation in the region of the capsule and at tendon insertions. Blurred, "cotton wool–like" margins and rather faint radiopacity are characteristic.

- *Osteophytes* are typical for **osteoarthritis.** They originate typically at the margin between cartilage and bone (Chapter 10.2) and have a narrow cortex.
- *"Protuberances"* are small bony proliferations at the joint-capsule insertion or in a nearby extra-articular location of fingers and toes (▸ Figs. 10.11 and ▸ 10.12a). They are typical for **psoriatic arthritis** and in rare cases are also found in Reiter's syndrome.
- Irregularly formed *insertional ossification* of joint capsule, tendons, and ligaments during fibro-osteotic processes (see ▸ Figs. 10.10 and ▸ 10.12b) are commonly found in **spondylarthritis**, yet practically never in rheumatoid arthritis.

Mutilation (Severe Destruction and Disfiguration) and Ankylosis

Erosions may progress to mutilations or even end in ankylosis with fibrous or bony bridging.

- Some types of **arthritis** tend to develop *mutilations* very early (e.g., psoriatic arthritis; ▸ Fig. 10.13). Otherwise, mutilations and ankylosis are usually a sign of advanced stages of a disease (▸ Fig. 10.14).
- In **osteoarthritis** *ankylosis* is only seen after long-standing disease, and then predominantly in the sacroiliac joints. Ankylosis is also a feature of spondylarthritis and chronic juvenile arthritis.

10.1.3 Radiographic Features of the Spine and Sacroiliac Joints and Their Differential Diagnosis

Vertebral Osteophytes

Vertebral osteophytes are commonly found at the vertebral margins of a **degenerating** intervertebral disk (▸ Fig. 10.15).

- A distinction is made between a **submarginal osteophyte,** which arises, initially horizontally, at the insertion of the anterior longitudinal ligament a few millimeters from the intervertebral disk, to later curve in a superior or inferior direction, and a **marginal osteophyte**, which continues to grow horizontally into the superior or inferior end plate.
- Osteophytes of two adjacent vertebrae can fuse together to form a bony bridge within the motion segment.
- Exuberant osteophyte formation is found primarily in cases of **DISH** (diffuse idiopathic skeletal hyperostosis; Chapter 10.4) in the form of **spondylosis hyperostotica.**

Syndesmophytes

A syndesmophyte refers to ossification of the outer fibers of the anulus fibrosus, caused by a progressive **inflammatory process** associated with all forms of **spondylarthritis** (Chapter 10.6). Initially syndesmophytes are thin vertical outgrowths along the contour of the juvenile disk; at a later stage they take on a more concave course (▸ Fig. 10.16). Eventually they thicken and incorporate the anterior longitudinal ligament. The end result of this polysegmental process is the **"bamboo spine"** (▸ Fig. 10.17).

> **Caution**
> Sometimes syndesmophytes are asymmetric in their distribution; they are thicker and not exactly vertical but rather more curved or comma-shaped and are separated from the edge of the vertebral body. They are commonly called nonmarginal syndesmophytes (▸ Fig. 10.18). These forms are more often found with psoriasis or reactive arthritis.

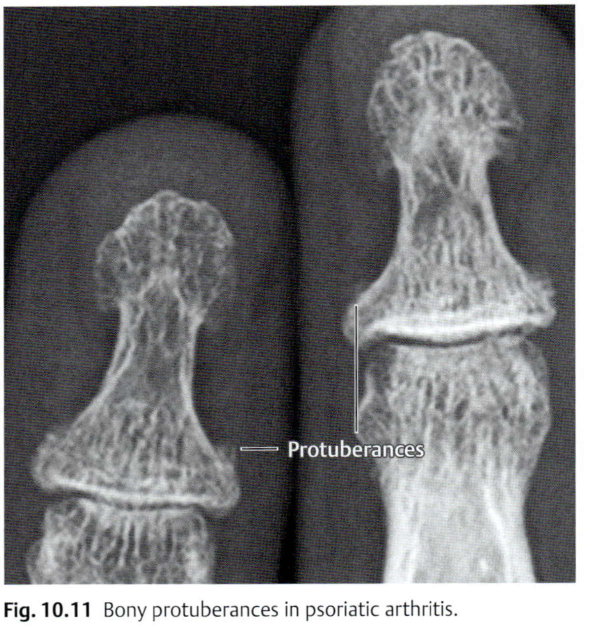

Fig. 10.11 Bony protuberances in psoriatic arthritis.

10

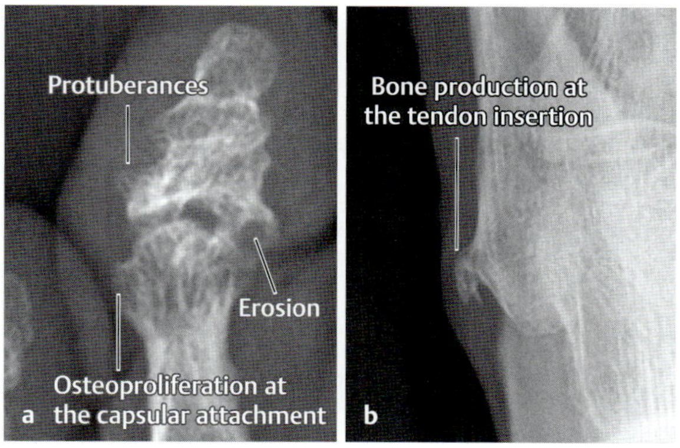

Fig. 10.12 Psoriatic arthropathy. **(a)** Bony changes at the distal interphalangeal joint of the fourth toe. **(b)** Bone production at the base of the fifth metatarsal at the peroneus brevis tendon insertion.

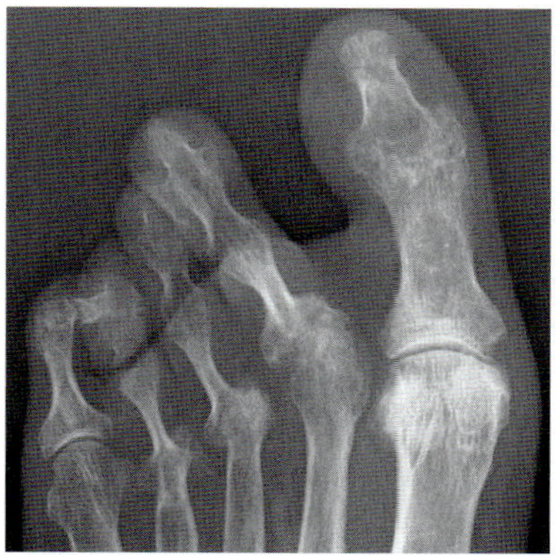

Fig. 10.13 Mutilation of the metatarsophalangeal joints of the second to fourth rays in psoriatic arthropathy. The proximal interphalangeal joints and the interphalangeal joint of the big toe are ankylosed.

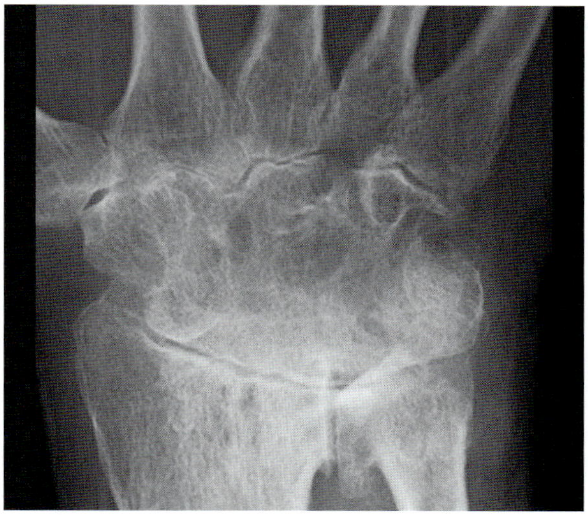

Fig. 10.14

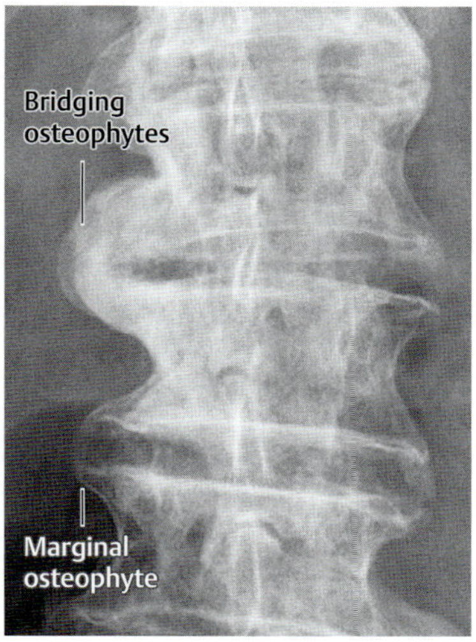

Fig. 10.15

Fig. 10.14 Ankylosis of the carpus producing an os carpale, a late result of rheumatoid arthritis.

Fig. 10.15 Osteophytes.

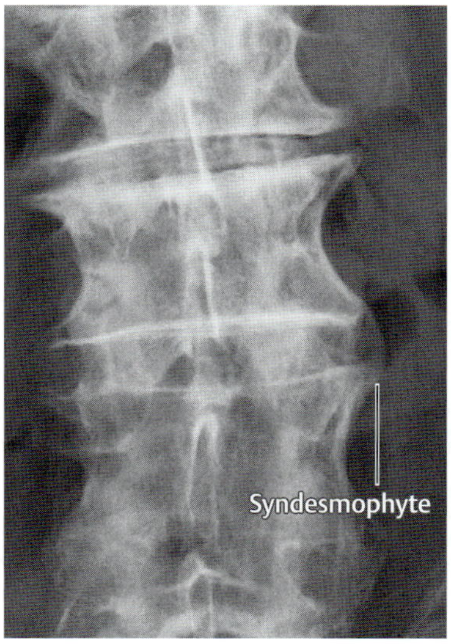

Fig. 10.16 Syndesmophyte in a patient with ankylosing spondylitis. Additional finding of smaller osteophytes.

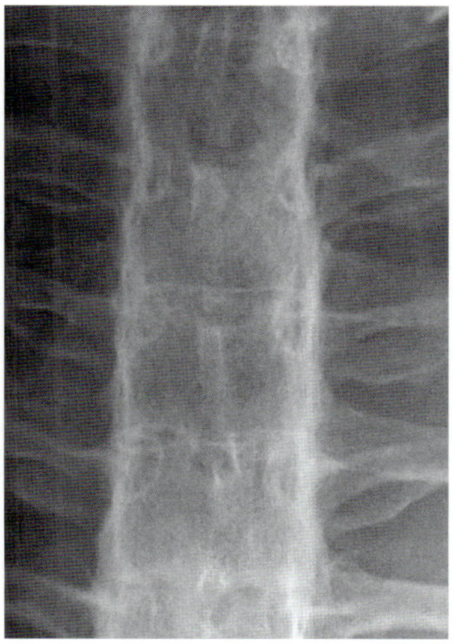

Fig. 10.17 Bamboo spine in ankylosing spondylitis.

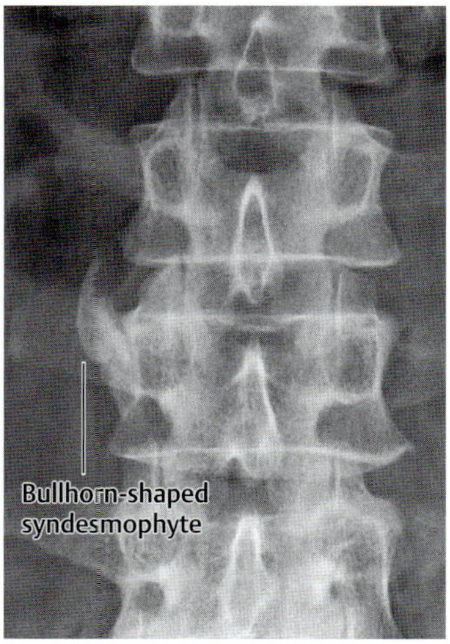

Fig. 10.18 Singular, and thus actually nonspecific, clearly asymmetric nonmarginal syndesmophyte. The patient had a known history of psoriatic spondylarthropathy.

Schmorl's Nodes

A "Schmorl's node" is a herniation of disk tissue through the vertebral end plate and into the cancellous bone of the vertebral body. Older Schmorl's nodes usually demonstrate prominent marginal sclerosis (▶ Figs. 10.19 and ▶ 10.20).

- In **Scheuermann's disease** (Chapter 7.4.1) these herniations are commonly found in the thoracic spine, characteristically in the anterior third of the vertebral body. If this intratrabecular herniation occurs in a still-growing spine, compensatory hyperostosis of the opposing end plate may develop (**Edgren–Vaino sign;** ▶ Figs. 10.21 and ▶ 10.22).
- Schmorl's nodes must be differentiated from **normal variants** of the vertebral end plates that are of no **clinical significance** and represent **notochord remnants**. These usually focal depressions are typically located in the posterior third, usually in two opposing end plates, and have a linear configuration over several segments of the thoracic spine or the thoracolumbar junction (see ▶ Fig. 10.21).
- Similarly, in the lower lumbar vertebrae, broad-based, paramedian depressions of the end plates are located more posteriorly, creating the **Cupid's bow sign** on the AP view, but are of no clinical significance (▶ Fig. 10.23).

Vacuum Phenomenon

Sometimes negative pressure forces nitrogen gas bubbles to escape from the degenerative disk (▶ Fig. 10.24).

- Such a vacuum phenomenon can also develop in **osteoporotic fractures**, especially when bone healing is delayed. This finding argues against a pathologic fracture due to underlying tumor.
- Accumulation of gas in the facet joints is a sign of **joint degeneration**—as in the sacroiliac joints.

Baastrup's Sign

This often painful condition results from contact between the spinous processes related to an excessive lordosis of the lumbar spine. It is further compounded by degenerative loss of disk height. Increased sclerosis and cysts as well as new bone formation may develop in the contact zone (▶ Fig. 10.25). Occasionally, interspinal synovial pseudoarticulations or bursae develop.

Romanus Lesion (Anterior Spondylitis)

This refers to focal inflammation of the anterior or posterior borders of the vertebral body and is predominantly found in the thoracic spine. It occurs in spondylarthritis, especially in **ankylosing spondylitis.** It may also be associated with small, focal areas of osseous destruction (▶ Fig. 10.26). Sclerosis appears later, producing the "shiny corner" sign (▶ Fig. 10.27) due to its typical triangular shape on radiographs and CT. It should be noted that the term "Romanus lesion" was coined at a time when only radiographs were available, for which reason a classic Romanus lesion is characterized by the presence of sclerosis. However, MRI has shown that anterior inflammation can also develop, as evidenced by focal edema-like signal intensity at these sites, even without any sign of destruction. With time, this inflammation heals and leads to fat conversion (▶ Fig. 10.28; see also ▶ Fig. 10.26). Evidence of more than five such fatty Romanus lesions is highly specific for ankylosing spondylitis.

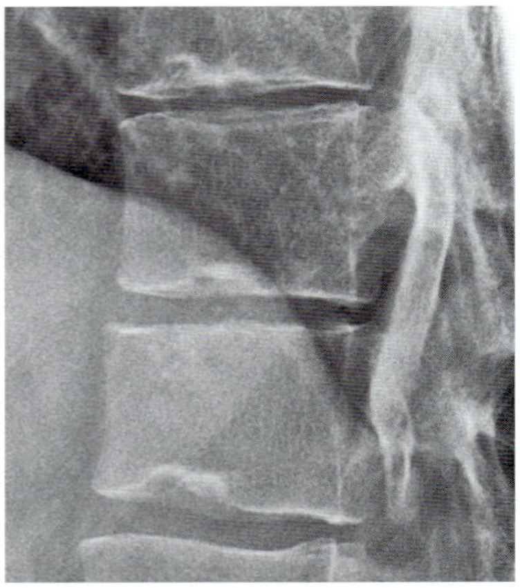

Fig. 10.19 Multisegmental Schmorl's nodes in the inferior end plates. The prominent marginal sclerosis is an indication of a chronic condition.

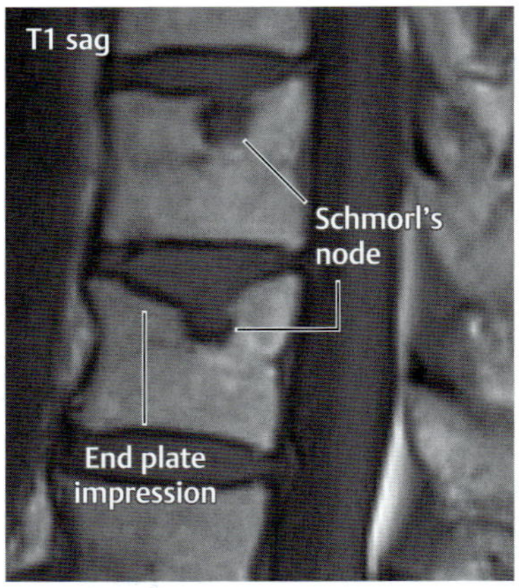

Fig. 10.20 Schmorl's nodes in two vertebrae. There is also chronic depression of the superior end plate of the lower vertebral body (sclerotic end plate, no vertebral body edema).

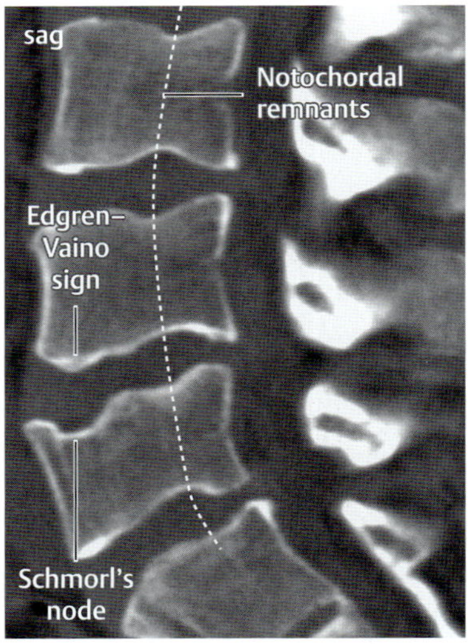

Fig. 10.21 Notochordal remnants. Additional Schmorl's node in the superior end plate of L4 with compensatory bony protrusion of the opposing inferior end plate (Edgren–Vaino sign).

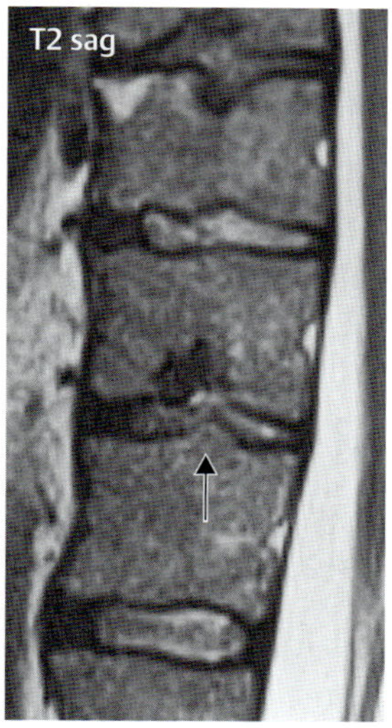

Fig. 10.22 Multiple Schmorl's nodes. The relatively anterior site of the lesions and the obvious Edgren–Vaino sign (arrow) argue against a notochordal remnant.

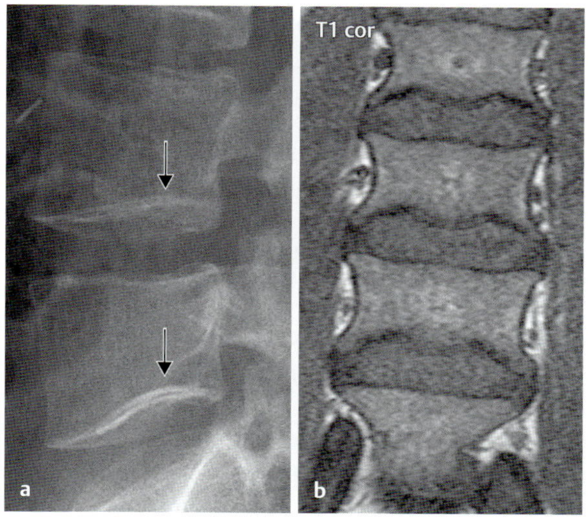

Fig. 10.23 Cupid's bow sign. ▶ **(a)** Broad-based depressions (arrows) of the posterior end plates. **(b)** Cupid's bow sign is evident on the coronal view.

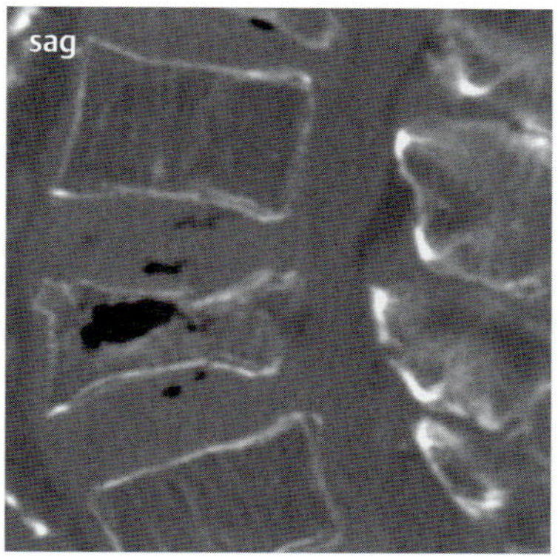

Fig. 10.24 Vacuum phenomenon. Gas within multiple intervertebral disks. Note also the compression fracture with intravertebral gas; this is supportive of an osteoporotic fracture.

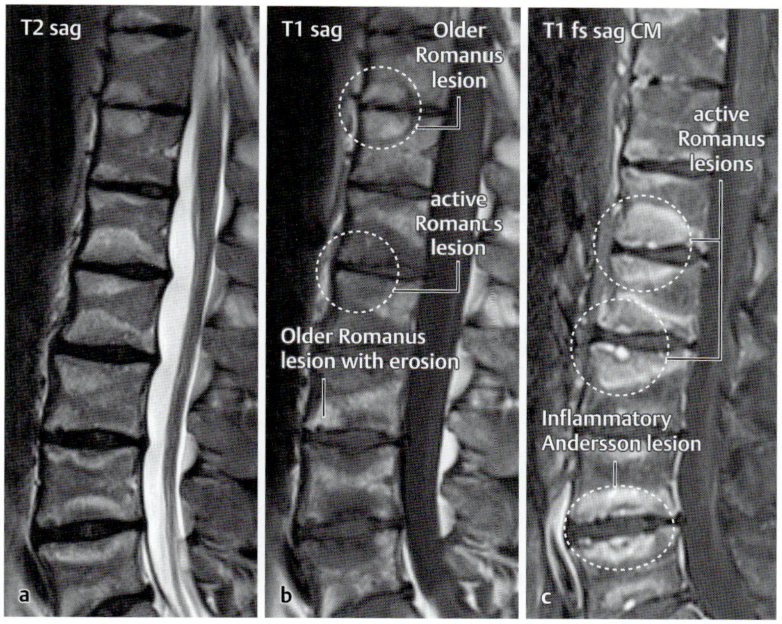

Fig. 10.26 Ankylosing spondylitis. **(a)** Multisegmental hyperintense changes along the end plates. **(b)** The T1W view allows for differentiation between fat and edemalike inflammatory bone marrow changes. **(c)** The acute inflammatory lesions enhance with contrast.

Fig. 10.25 Baastrup's disease (arrows). Note also the vacuum phenomenon in two intervertebral disk spaces. ▼

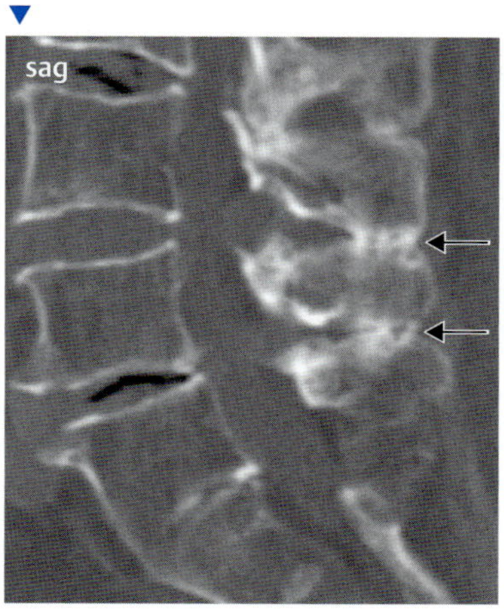

Fig. 10.25

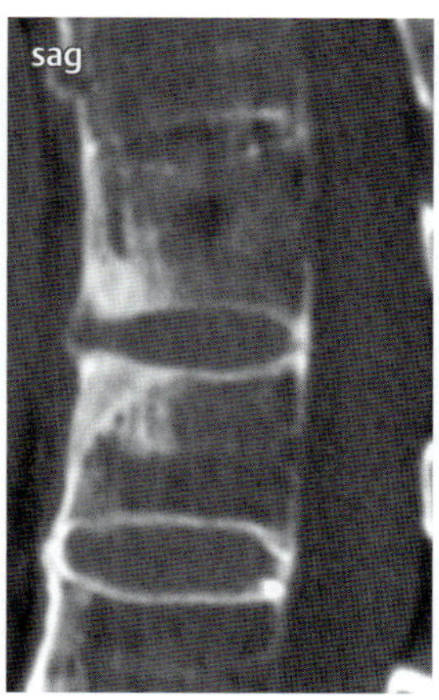

Fig. 10.27

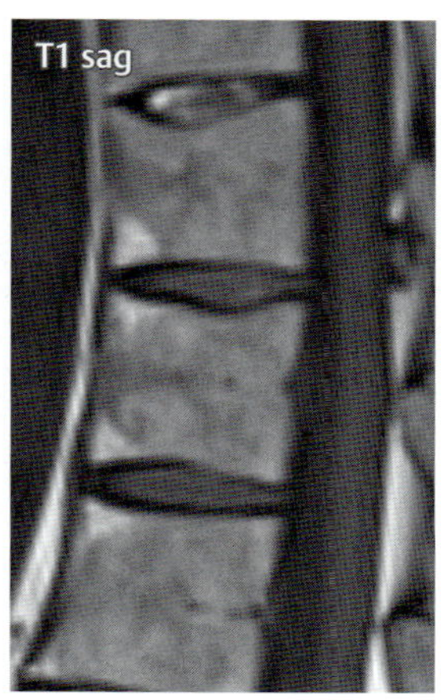

Fig. 10.28

Fig. 10.27 Romanus lesion. Typical postinflammatory triangular regions of sclerosis (shiny corner sign) with multilevel syndesmophytes.

Fig. 10.28 Multiple fatty Romanus lesions, related to multilevel anterior spondylitis.

Andersson Lesion (Inflammatory Type)

Inflammatory lesions can occur with spondylarthritis that destroy the osteochondral junction between vertebral body and intervertebral disk (see ▶ Fig. 10.26). A characteristic feature is circumscribed central or paracentral destruction, which is later usually surrounded by an extensive perilesional sclerotic zone.

- Degenerative types of **osteochondrosis** look similar. Bandlike subchondral sclerosis is more suggestive of osteochondrosis.
- An irregular pattern of bone destruction without sclerosis is found in acute **bacterial spondylodiskitis**.

Andersson Lesion (Noninflammatory, Pseudarthrosis Type)

This is a pseudarthrosis secondary to a transdiskal or transvertebral fatigue fracture with involvement of the posterior vertebral elements in a largely stiff spine (as found in the late stages of ankylosing spondylitis; ▶ Fig. 10.29).

Much more common, however, is an **acute fracture** of a spinal column that has developed in a rigid spine secondarily to ankylosing spondylitis, even in the absence of a significant injury. It is usually found at the cervicothoracic or thoracolumbar junction, is almost always unstable, and involves all three columns. This is not an Andersson lesion, however.

Vertebral Body Enlargement and Deformity

10

Vertebral body deformity and enlargement are typically seen in **Paget's disease** and **vertebral hemangioma** (▶ Fig. 10.30; also Chapter 4.3.7). It must be differentiated from the pure deformity of **vertebral body squaring** and **barrel-shaped vertebrae** (▶ Fig. W10.1), which develop secondary to inflammatory destruction of the vertebral margins and bone apposition found in advanced spondylarthritis. **Compression fractures** can increase the sagittal or transversal diameter of a vertebra, but usually result in a significant loss of height as well.

Block Vertebrae

The expression "block vertebrae" refers to osseous fusion of two or more adjacent vertebrae. Partial block vertebra formation occurs when the vertebrae are fused across a portion of the disk or, for example, only via the facet joints.

- Acquired **postinflammatory** or **degenerative block vertebrae** characteristically display bone apposition (bridging osteophytes) at the site of fusion (▶ Fig. 10.31).
- **Congenital block vertebrae** often demonstrate a tapered appearance at the level of the fusion and are not associated with bridging osteophytes (▶ Figs. 10.32 and ▶ 10.33).

Sacroiliitis

Sacroiliitis (bi- or unilateral; ▶ Figs. 10.34 and ▶ 10.35) is the key symptom of **spondylarthritis**. A bacterial origin should also be included in the differential diagnosis when there is evidence of unilateral sacroiliitis with significant marginal destruction (initially without sclerosis).

The radiographic appearance of sacroiliitis includes the following signs:

- Thinning of the subchondral cortex.
- Erosions (more severe on the iliac than on the sacral side).
- Irregular pseudo-widening of the joint space secondary to confluent erosions, preceded by joint-space narrowing.
- Irregular subchondral sclerosis.
- Osseous bridging and later bony ankylosis.
- Capsular and ligamentous ossification later in the course.

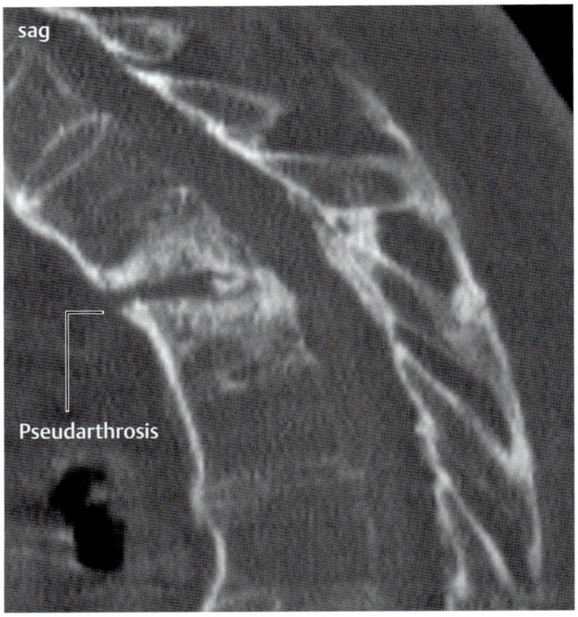

Fig. 10.29 Andersson lesion (pseudarthrosis type) in ankylosing spondylitis.

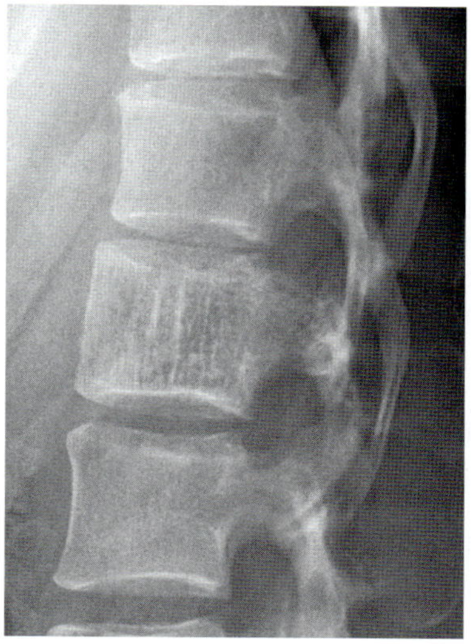

Fig. 10.30 Vertebral enlargement in a patient with "vertebral hemangioma." Note the loss of concavity of its anterior margin.

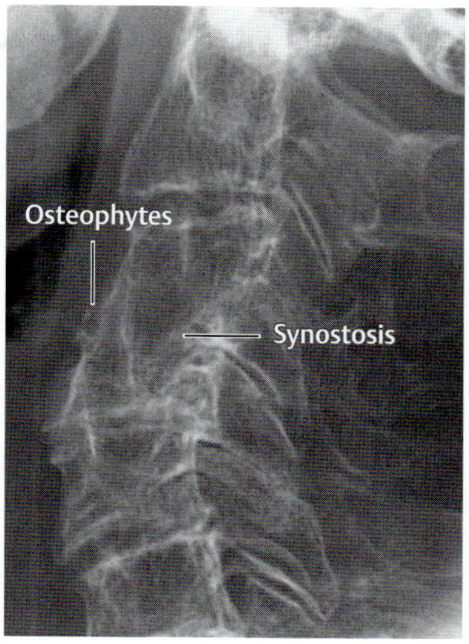

Fig. 10.31 Acquired, degenerative block-vertebra formation. This finding is indistinguishable from a postinflammatory ankylosis, but the patient was never known to have suffered from a local or systemic inflammatory disease.

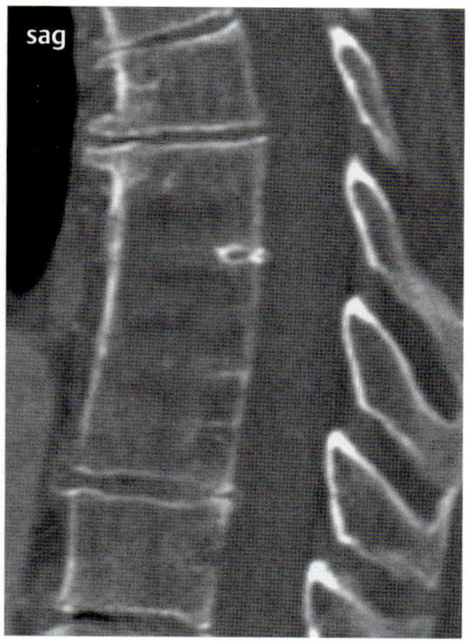

Fig. 10.32 Congenital block vertebrae covering three vertebrae and two disk spaces. Note the degeneration of the adjacent segments superior and inferior to the block vertebrae as a result of the increased movement and stresses in these segments.

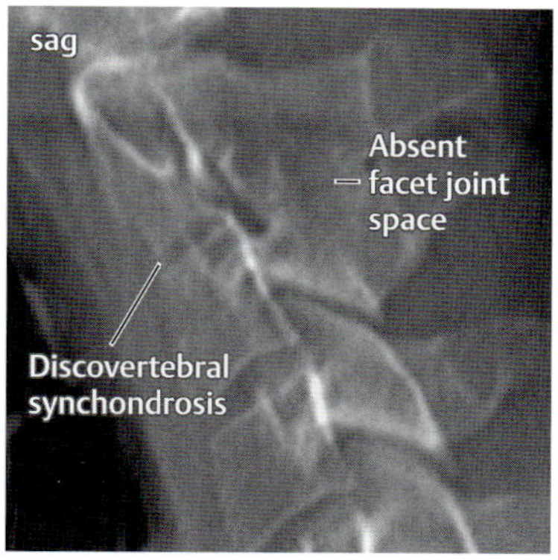

Fig. 10.33 Congenital, partial block vertebrae formation with fusion of the facet joints. Thick-slice MPR obtained from one CT dataset.

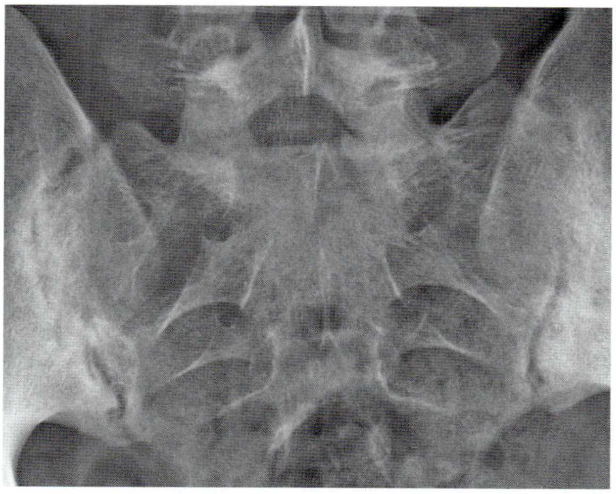

Fig. 10.34 Sacroiliitis. Multiple abnormalities of the sacroiliac joints including irregular subchondral sclerosis, destruction, and areas of bridging ossification, especially in the right lower third of the joint.

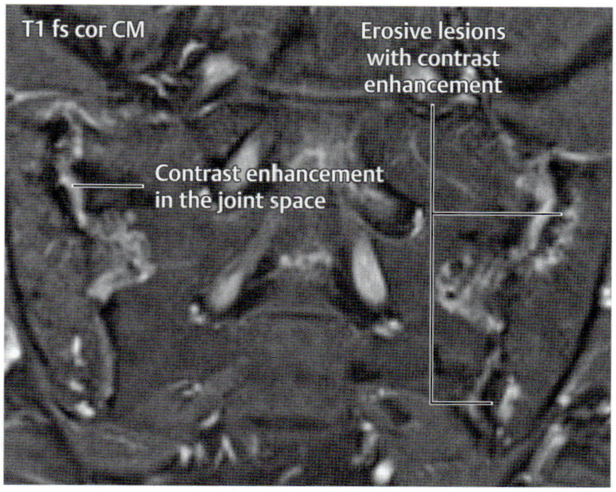

Fig. 10.35 Bilateral sacroiliitis on MRI. Increased intra- and periarticular contrast enhancement, as well as irregularity of the joint spaces.

10.2 Osteoarthritis of the Peripheral Joints

10.2.1 Basic Principles of Imaging Techniques

The term "osteoarthritis" refers to various "degenerative" joint diseases that are characterized by progressive articular dysfunction. A distinction is made between **primary (idiopathic)** and **secondary osteoarthritis.** Although osteoarthritis has so far been classified as a noninflammatory arthropathy, many authors are now asserting that **intermittent episodes of inflammation** strongly affect the disease course and clinical presentation. For this reason osteoarthritis, as a slowly progressive chronic arthropathy, will be included in the rheumatological section.

▸ Pathology. For purposes of clinical classification, idiopathic and secondary types of osteoarthritis should be distinguished. From a pathophysiological view, however, this concept must be called into question. Today it is assumed that a **trigger** causes early changes to the joint and subsequently initiates catabolic as well as reparative mechanisms. Such triggers include, for example, direct or indirect injury to the joint, joint inflammation, chronic overuse, and other systemic factors.

The concept of a primary cartilage disease has been abandoned, given that **multiple structures within a joint** are involved in the disease process. In particular, a close link between articular cartilage and subchondral bone has been recognized. The term "osteoarthritis" therefore appears appropriate. Nevertheless, osteoarthritis is phenotypically characterized by a progressive loss of cartilage.

Multiple risk factors have been defined over the years that would suggest progressive articular damage. Joint-related factors include joint malalignment (knee, hip), impingement, congenital or hereditary malformations (e.g., dysplasia of the hip), intrinsic degeneration, such as meniscal and labral damage, focal cartilage defects, ligamentous laxity, and subchondral bone marrow lesions (as detected by MRI). Systemic factors include obesity, genetic predisposition, nutrition (e.g., vitamin D deficiency), metabolic diseases (e.g., gout), age, and sex. A diagnosis of osteoarthritis is based on both radiographic and clinical features. The radiographic diagnosis of osteoarthritis is based on the presence of osteophytes (see also Kellgren–Lawrence classification); the clinical diagnosis rests on a combination of symptoms listed below under "Clinical presentation." There is currently no universally accepted MRI-based definition of osteoarthritis.

▸ Clinical presentation. Pain with weight bearing, limitation of motion, crepitation, and morning stiffness are primary symptoms. Osteoarthritis is characterized by intermittent episodes of increased pain ("flares") that are associated with acute "inflammatory" changes, such as joint effusion and synovitis. The appearance, or increase in size, of bone marrow lesions as seen in MRI correlates with the degree of pain. Other typical clinical symptoms of osteoarthritis include joint malalignment, deformity, instability, and muscular weakness.

A discrepancy between the degree of radiographic abnormalities within the joint and clinical symptoms has long been recognized.

Commonly used (but not exactly defined) clinical terms

- **"Activated" osteoarthritis,** known osteoarthritis with acute, renewed pain. Synovitis, joint effusion, and bone marrow edema usually develop. The cause of the synovitis and pain is usually related to acutely sloughed fragments of articular cartilage and bone, known as detritus.
- **Erosive osteoarthritis** is characterized by an acute episode of inflammation and radiographic evidence of progressive central erosions, especially in the hands.

▸ Radiography. **Technique.** Standing (weight-bearing) views of the joints of the lower limbs should be obtained. This is particularly important to assess for associated limb malalignment ("long-leg view").

Conventional radiography remains the diagnostic standard for osteoarthritis. It serves to establish the diagnosis, to narrow the differential diagnosis, and for follow-up studies to assess the progression of disease. A radiograph is not capable of demonstrating directly the articular cartilage, unless chondrocalcinosis (CPPD) with (secondary) calcification of the hyaline cartilage matrix is present. However, it does allow indirect conclusions to be drawn about cartilage integrity. It should be borne in mind that only more advanced cartilage loss is demonstrated radiographically when there is evidence of joint-space narrowing.

Radiographic signs of osteoarthritis

(▸ Figs. 10.36 and ▸ 10.37)

- Osteophytes.
- Joint space narrowing.
- Subchondral sclerosis.
- Subchondral cysts.
- Loose joint bodies.
- Soft tissue swelling and/or effusion.
- Chondrocalcinosis and meniscal calcifications.
- Joint deformity and attrition (increased concavity or flattening of the joint surfaces).

Atlases with illustrative examples can be of great assistance for reporting purposes (e.g., the atlas by Altman and coworkers from 1995 or the revised version from 2007 ▶ see References for Chapter 10.2 under "Grading Osteoarthritic Changes").

The **Kellgren–Lawrence classification** is used to grade the severity of osteoarthritis; it is assessed from a plain AP radiograph:

- **Grade 0:** No osteophytes, no joint space narrowing.
- **Grade 1:** Possible small, marginal osteophyte.
- **Grade 2:** Definite osteophyte formation.
- **Grade 3:** Joint-space narrowing.
- **Grade 4:** Complete loss of the joint space (bone-to-bone contact).

▶ **CT.** CT is also not capable of displaying cartilage directly but it can reveal radiographic abnormalities at an earlier time. CT can depict subchondral cysts and osteophytes unobscured by overlying structures (▶ Fig. 10.38) and assist in locating loose joint bodies. CT arthrography is an excellent modality for demonstrating surface alterations involving the articular cartilage surfaces. CT is of particular value for differentiating between changes of osteoarthritis and classical rheumatological disorders (Chapter 10.2.2). This applies in particular to the axial skeleton and to joints with complex anatomy, such as the wrist and tarsus (see also the corresponding text sections in Chapter 10.2.2).

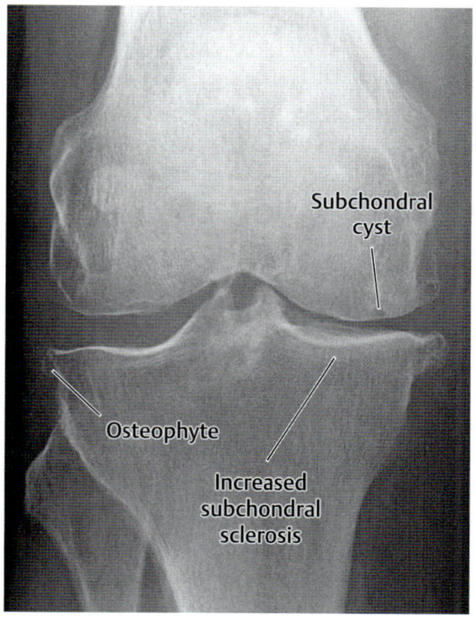

Fig. 10.36 Classic appearance of primarily medial ("varus") osteoarthritis of the knee.

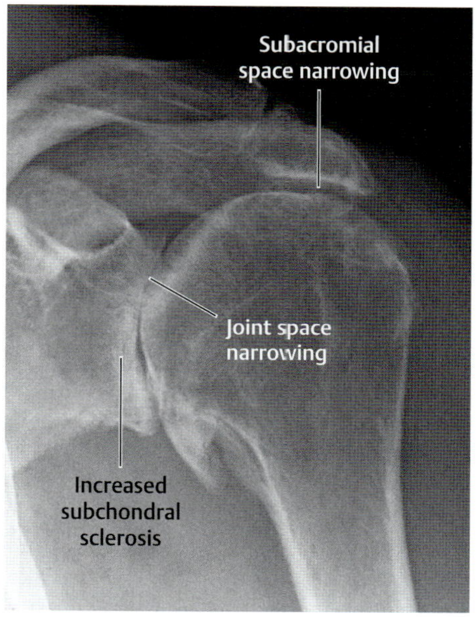

Fig. 10.37 Markedly advanced osteoarthritis of the shoulder.

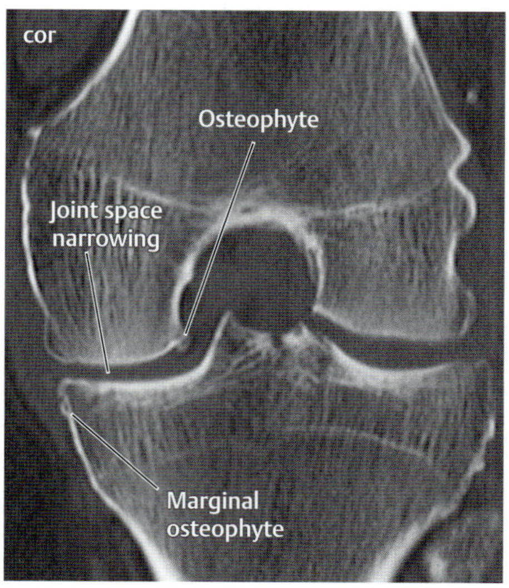

Fig. 10.38 Medial tibiofemoral osteoarthritis. Since the CT view is obtained with the patient supine, the actual degree of cartilage loss can only be partially assessed. Additiona ly, there is a fracture of the tibial plateau.

10

▶ MRI. **Technique.** With regard to sequence selection, PDW (echo time 15–25 ms) and intermediate FSE sequences (echo time 35–40 ms) are the clinical standard. These are usually acquired with fat suppression to obtain better contrast between subchondral bone and hyaline cartilage. Without fat suppression, it is not possible to sufficiently capture bone marrow alterations. The earliest alterations to cartilage are recognizable on PDW, intermediate, and T2W FSE sequences as increased intrachondral signal intensity (corresponding to edematous changes) (▶ Fig. W10.2).

High-resolution 3D-GRE sequences (e.g., FLASH, SPGR, DESS, MEDIC [Multi-Echo Data Image Combination], etc.) may be helpful supplements but have not yet become established in clinical routine. The disadvantages of these gradient sequences are the relatively long acquisition times, susceptibility artifacts, lack of sensitivity for displaying subchondral lesions, and poorer demonstration of focal cartilage defects (▶ Fig. W10.3). These sequences are primarily used for cartilage segmentation and for 3D-volumetric analysis during research projects.

Contrast-enhanced sequences are sometimes useful for assessing the degree of synovitis, which can be quite pronounced in clinically acute episodes of osteoarthritis (▶ Fig. W10.4). Subchondral bone marrow lesions may display strong contrast enhancement and cysts ("geodes") are readily apparent.

The role of MRI in clinical practice is less for arriving at a specific diagnosis than for excluding associated complications such as osteonecrosis or insufficiency fractures; it may be used in some cases for assessing the degree of joint abnormality during preoperative planning (cartilage transplantation).

Findings. Subchondral bone marrow signal. Common findings on MRI of osteoarthritis are subchondral areas of focal increased signal intensity, evident on water-sensitive fat-suppressed sequences (as well as on T1W fat-suppressed sequences after contrast agent application), which are associated with overlying cartilage lesions. The term "bone marrow lesion" has become established for these subchondral areas of high signal.

Cartilage. Many MRI classification systems of cartilage damage use a scale ranging from 0 to 4 in accordance with a classification system used for arthroscopy that is based on the suggestions proposed by Outerbridge (1961) (see References for Chapter 10.2 under "Reviews on Osteoarthritis and Imaging of the Cartilage"). However, these classifications have only limited application to daily clinical practice. Close communication with the referring clinician is imperative. Ideally, the report should describe any cartilage pathology and include at least the following points:

- Anatomical site (e.g., medial trochlea, medial patellar facet, central weight-bearing part of the medial tibia, etc.).
- Surface involvement in two dimensions (in millimeters or centimeters).
- Maximal depth (superficial or full thickness, extending to bone).

Any associated pathologic features relevant for prognosis should also be included (▶ Figs. 10.39 and ▶ 10.40):
- Osteophytes.
- Joint effusion.
- Synovitis (best recognized as an increase in synovial thickness and signal intensity after IV contrast administration).
- Bone marrow lesion (definition above).
- Meniscal pathology, including meniscal extrusion.
- Plicae.
- Patellar malalignment.
- Subchondral cysts.
- Ligament pathology.

▶ NUC. Technetium 99 m multiphase bone scan demonstrates areas of focally increased perfusion (blood pool phase; ▶ Fig. 10.41) and increased bone turnover (osseous late phase). Bone marrow lesions detected on MRI display increased uptake on bone scans and a significantly increased carbohydrate turnover on PET scanning.

▶ DD. The large group of **arthritic conditions**—especially **psoriatic arthritis, infectious arthritis**, and **crystal arthropathies**—should be considered in the differential diagnosis, which may be particularly difficult in the presence of *erosive osteoarthritis.*
- **Osteophytes** in osteoarthritis are "marginal" in location, in the direct vicinity of the joint space, whereas the new bone production such as is seen in **psoriatic arthritis** is found in the region of the capsule and tendon insertions.
- **Subchondral sclerosis** is a characteristic sign of osteoarthritis, and is an unusual finding in other types of **arthritis** and, if present, is then the result of a reparative process of a chronic disease course.
- Marginal erosions in the immediate vicinity of capsular insertions, as are seen in **rheumatoid arthritis**, are not found in osteoarthritis.
- **Joint-space narrowing** is usually located in the region of a loaded part of the joint and is therefore often **asymmetric.** In the inflammatory **arthritides**, on the other hand, the narrowing tends to be symmetrical and involves all parts of the joint space.

Chapter 10.1.2 provides a schematic comparison of the most important signs of osteoarthritis in comparison with an inflammatory arthritis.

Significant increased signal intensity or enhancement of the joint capsule and reinforcing ligaments on water-sensitive or postcontrast images can pose differential diagnostic problems. These changes may occur in osteoarthritis as a result of synovial irritation by cartilage and bone detritus and can sometimes mimic the appearance of an inflammatory arthritis. This applies particularly to minor joints (fingers, small vertebral joints) and joints with complex anatomy (wrist, tarsus). Correlation with radiographs or, if need be, CT allows for a confident diagnosis of osteoarthritis by demonstrating subchondral sclerosis, osteophytes, and, in some cases, a vacuum phenomenon.

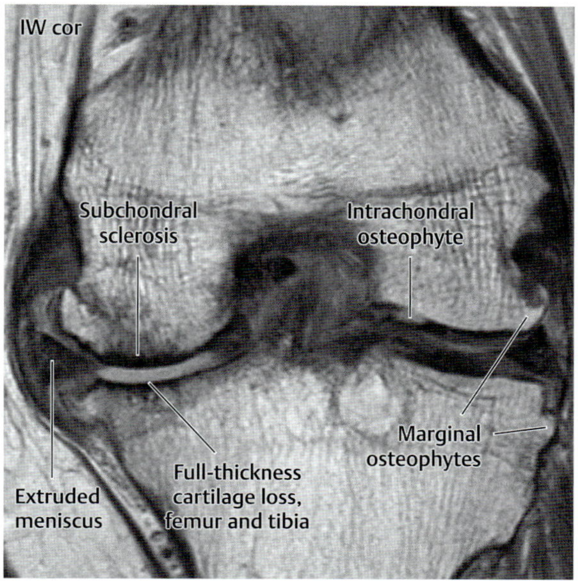

Fig. 10.39 Advanced tibiofemoral osteoarthritis.

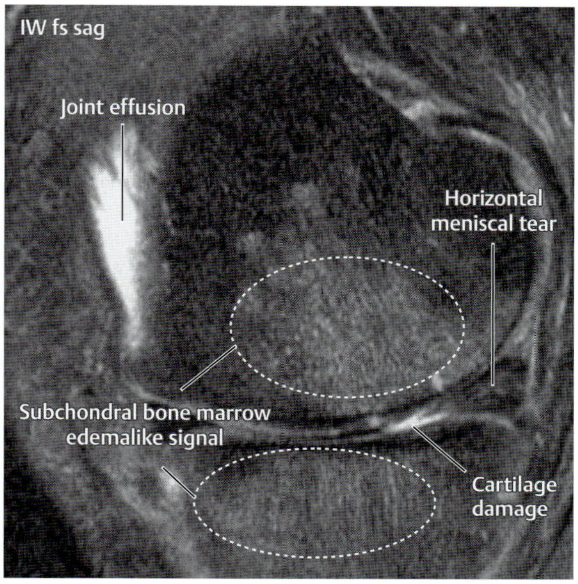

Fig. 10.40 Medial tibiofemoral osteoarthritis.

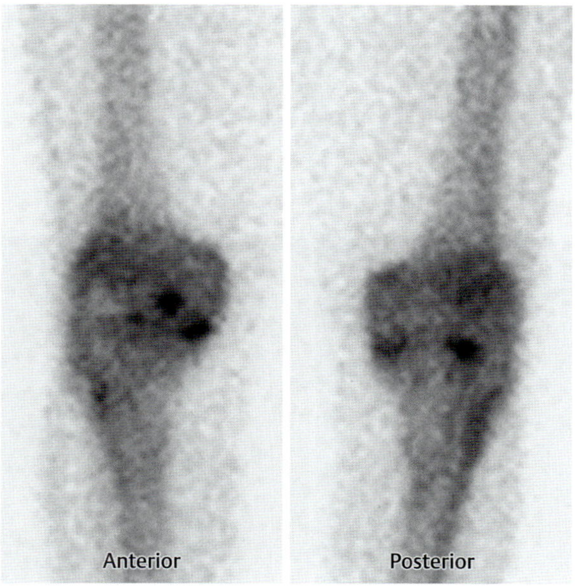

Fig. 10.41 Bone scan. Abnormal, increased tracer uptake in the medial right knee during the blood pool phase.

Imaging Procedures after Surgical Cartilage Replacement

Several surgical procedures have been developed to address cartilage repair, including **microfracture surgery, osteochondral transplantation**, and **matrix-associated chondrocyte transplantation.** Microfracturing of the subchondral bone using fine drilling promotes the formation of fibrous repair cartilage at that site. With osteochondral transplantation, a cylinder of bone and its overlying articular cartilage is harvested from a non–weight-bearing portion of the articular surface and then fitted into the area of cartilage defect. The aim of the procedure is the complete integration of the cylinder to achieve a smooth surface (also referred to as "mosaicplasty"). Chondrocyte transplantation is a two-stage procedure that involves the harvest of cartilage cells that are then cultured in vitro where they multiply. The artificially generated chondrocytes are then introduced into the cartilage defect in a second arthroscopic procedure.

All repair procedures are particularly successful for circumscribed defects and in younger patients (under 50 years of age). Imaging evidence of success is defined as the complete filling of the defect with complete marginal integration and without signs of cartilage hypertrophy (▸ Fig. 10.42). Although clinical improvement is often achieved, long-term results are still lacking as to whether osteoarthritis can be prevented or delayed by these procedures.

10.2.2 Individual Joints

Hip Joint

10

Osteoarthritis of the hip is common (▸ Figs. 10.43–10.45 and ▸ Fig. W10.5). Surgical treatment of early and precursor forms of osteoarthritis of the hip is increasingly being advocated, on the basis of the concept of femoroacetabular impingement (FAI) (Chapters 2.11.3 and 2.11.4). Another recognized risk factor for osteoarthritis of the hip is developmental hip dysplasia, which today usually receives early treatment as a result of ultrasound screening in the neonatal period.

The joint space narrowing is primarily of a superolateral location, and less commonly mediocaudal. Periosteal thickening at the femoral neck is referred to as **Wiberg's sign.** If the femoral head migrates into the acetabulum with increasing depth of the joint socket, this is referred to as **"protrusio acetabuli,"** whereas migration of the femoral head in a lateral direction is known as **"decentralizing osteoarthritis of the hip."**

▸ DD. The diagnosis of an **infectious arthritis** is suggested by the presence of a joint effusion, characteristic marked osteopenia, and the rapid progression of osteolytic areas. In bacterial arthritis, the pattern of bone destruction is clearly more irregular than in rheumatic arthritic conditions. The diagnosis can be confirmed with joint aspiration.

Knee Joint

A distinction is made between tibiofemoral and patellofemoral osteoarthritis, with the latter being promoted by anatomical variations of the patellofemoral joint (patellar and trochlear dysplasia, patella alta, lateralization of the patellar tendon insertion at the tibial tubercle).

Characteristic features of osteoarthritis of the knee include the following:

- The patellofemoral and the medial femorotibial joint compartments are most commonly affected (▸ Figs. 10.46–10.48, ▸ Figs. W10.6–W10.8).
- Meniscal injury and extrusion as well as joint malalignment are important risk factors.
- Loose joint bodies are common sequelae of osteoarthritis.

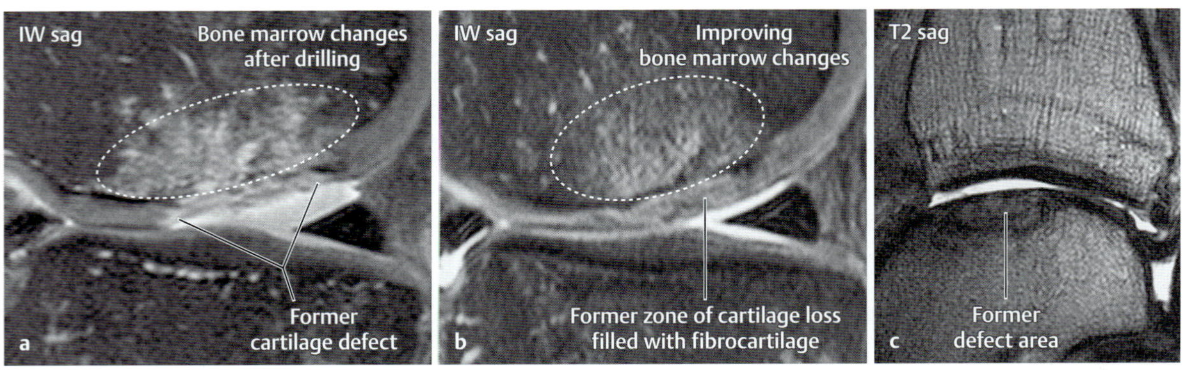

Fig. 10.42 Cartilage repair procedures. **(a)** and **(b)** are from follow-up studies after microfracture surgery, and **(c)** after autologous chondrocyte transplantation. (Courtesy of Dr. W. Fischer, Augsburg, Germany). **(a)** Six weeks after drilling of the femoral condyle, subchondral bone marrow alterations are clearly visible with regenerative tissue already starting to form. **(b)** After 12 weeks an almost complete filling of the defect with fibrocartilage regenerate tissue is evident. **(c)** Complete filling in of an extensive defect in the talar dome.

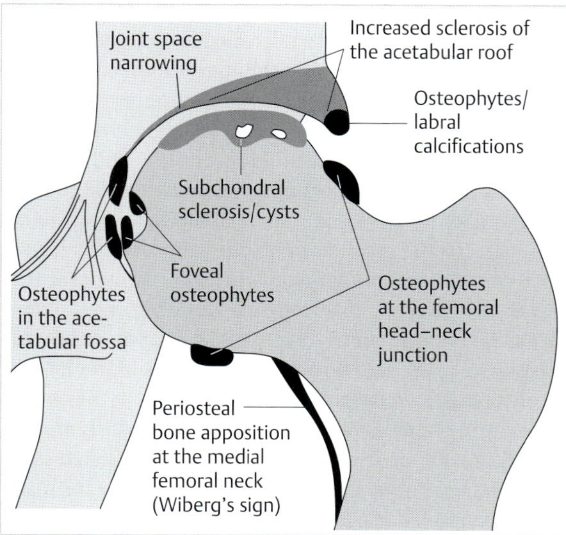

Fig. 10.43 Signs of osteoarthritis of the hip.

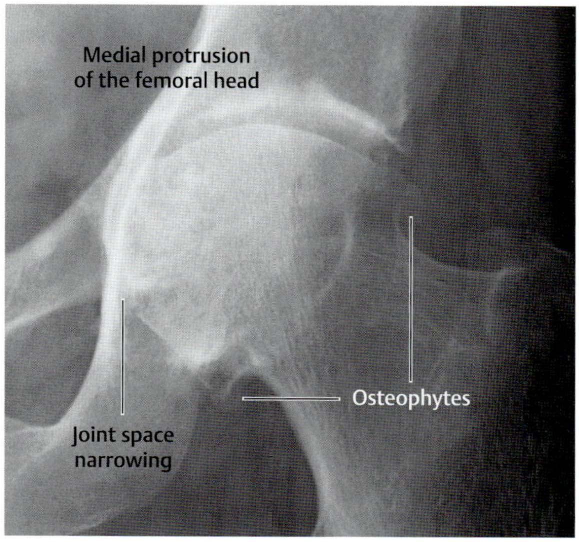

Fig. 10.44 Predominantly medial osteoarthritis of the hip with mild acetabular protrusion.

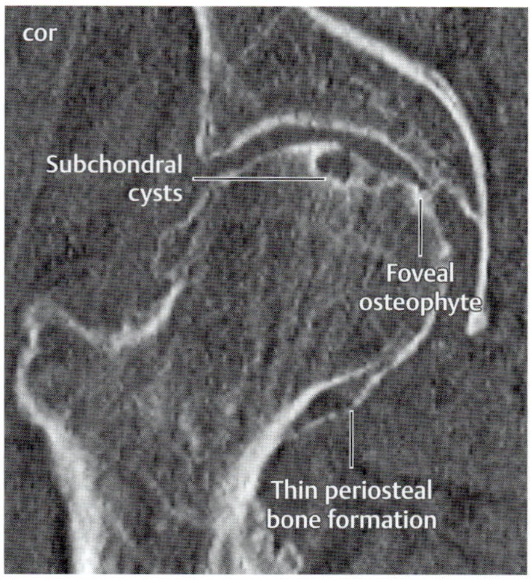

Fig. 10.45 Osteoarthritis of the hip.

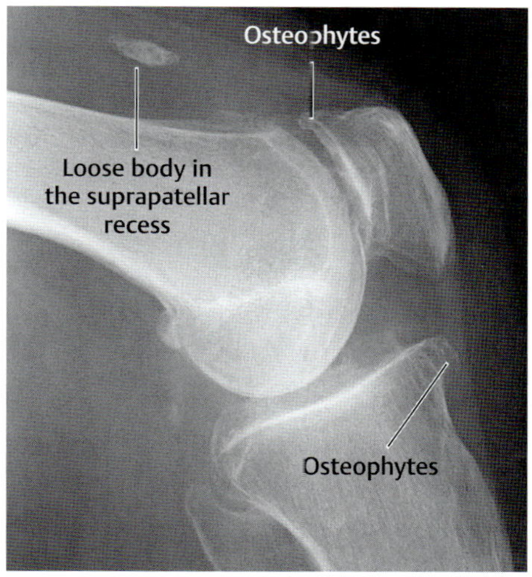

Fig. 10.46 Tibiofemoral and patellofemoral osteoarthritis.

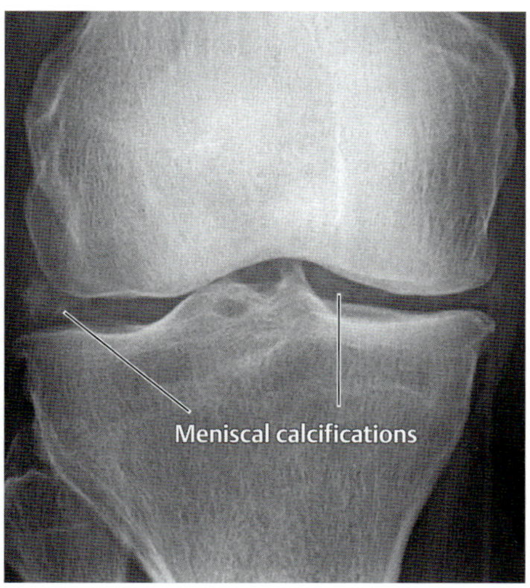

Fig. 10.47 Tibiofemoral osteoarthritis and meniscal calcification.

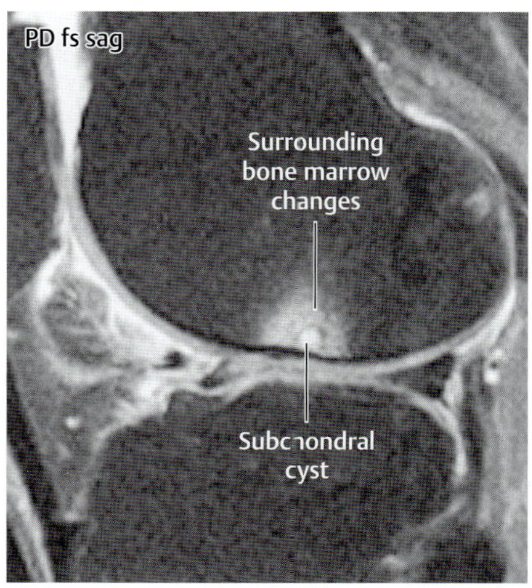

Fig. 10.48 Subchondral bone marrow alteration in osteoarthritis of the knee. These lesions are often a combination of diffuse "edemalike" changes and cystic components. A concomitant effusion is present.

Ankle Joint and Foot

Osteoarthritis of the ankle is comparatively rare. It is usually related to an earlier injury or other predisposing factors (osteonecrosis, osteochondrosis dissecans, malalignment, extensive sporting activities with recurrent microtrauma, etc.; ▸ Figs. 10.49 and ▸ W10.9). The talar head often displays a dorsal hooked or beaklike osteophyte in the region of the talonavicular joint or at the junction of the talar body and the talar neck (▸ Fig. 10.50). The body may be deformed and demonstrate numerous cysts and subchondral sclerosis. A posttraumatic etiology is often recognizable by additional well-corticated ossific fragments at the sites of ligament insertions.

The most common cause of degenerative arthritis in the region of the metatarsal phalangeal and interphalangeal joints is malalignment of the toes. **Hallux valgus** produces a rotation of the base of the proximal phalanx around its longitudinal axis with an associated lateral shift in the position of the hallux and the sesamoid bones (▸ Fig. 10.51). Subsequently, osteoarthritis develops between the metatarsal head and the sesamoids, which is not necessarily visible on the dorsoplantar view. Often extreme hyperostoses of the metatarsal heads and “cystoid” bone remodeling are noticeable in later stages. Additional associated soft tissue swelling (bursitis) is not uncommon.

Wrist and Fingers

The distal (**Heberden's osteoarthritis;** ▸ Figs. 10.52 and ▸ 10.53) and proximal interphalangeal joints (**Bouchard's osteoarthritis**) are the most common sites of involvement of osteoarthritis; women are significantly more often affected than men.

A genetic component appears to play a larger role in its development in the interphalangeal joints of the fingers than is the case in the lower limbs and the other joints of the upper limbs. The clinically noticeable **Heberden and Bouchard nodes** are caused by osteophytes covered by a thickened layer of soft tissue and by mucoid soft tissue nodules or cysts. A characteristic feature is also the “gullwing” appearance, mostly seen in erosive osteoarthritis (see ▸ Fig. 10.53). This includes osteoarthritis of the carpus, which is usually most prominent along its radial aspect and most commonly involves **STT osteoarthritis** between scaphoid, trapezium, and trapezoideum (▸ Fig. 10.54) and **basal thumb osteoarthritis** of the first carpometacarpal joint (▸ Fig. 10.55).

Erosive osteoarthritis is of particular significance in the hand. The distribution is irregular and moves from interphalangeal joint to interphalangeal joint in phases, often with a break of several months. The clinical picture resembles that of an inflammatory arthritis with swelling, erythema and severe pain. Women between the ages of 40 and 60 years are affected. Typical radiographic features include marked erosions and cysts in the interphalangeal joints (▸ Fig. 10.56). The erosions of erosive osteoarthritis have a more central location and combine with marginal osteophytes to produce a characteristic “gullwing” appearance. They may transform into (sometimes large) cysts or become sclerotic. Another rare type of osteoarthritis of the hand is the **osteoclastic subtype**. Subchondral areas of lucent remodeling of the medullary cavity are characteristic, extending over at least one-third of the length of the affected small tubular bones. Primary locations are the proximal and distal interphalangeal joints. These alterations cannot be regarded as detritic cysts, but are probably the result of an imbalance of local bone metabolism (▸ Figs. 10.57 and ▸ W10.10). This type of osteoarthritis often poses differential diagnostic difficulties. Chronic tophaceous gout, superimposed inflammatory arthritis (secondary rheumatoid arthritis with preexistent osteoarthritis), and osteoarthritis of the hand combined with an additional process such as fibrous dysplasia, intraosseous ganglion, or benign tumor should all be considered.

Risk factors for osteoarthritis of the wrist include positive ulnar variance (congenital or posttraumatically acquired) with subsequent overloading of the triangular fibrocartilage and the lunate (ulnolunate impaction syndrome) and ligamentous lesions (most commonly scapholunate and lunotriquetral). Scaphoid fractures and tears of the scapholunate ligament also often result in subsequent osteoarthritis, the end stages of which are referred to as SNAC and SLAC wrist, respectively (Chapter 2.9.3).

▸ DD. **Gouty arthropathy, psoriatic arthritis, superimposed arthritis** (secondary rheumatoid arthritis with preexistent osteoarthritis), and **infectious arthritis** should be excluded. Ankylosis can also develop in the fingers, which is not typical for osteoarthritis.

10

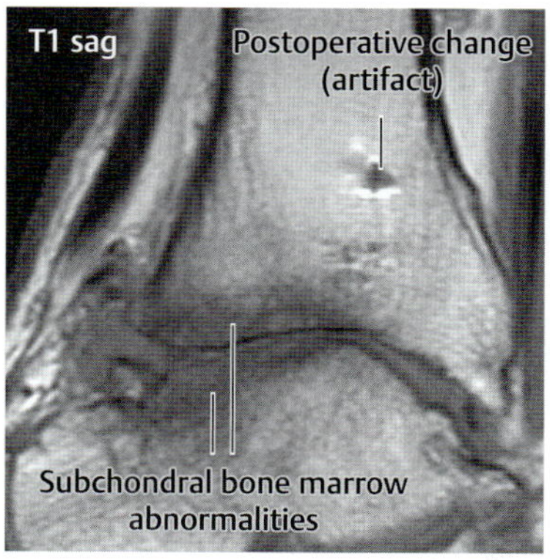

Fig. 10.49 Posttraumatic osteoarthritis of the ankle. Almost complete loss of the tibiotalar joint space and significant anterior as well as posterior osteophyte formation is evident (▶ see also ▶ Fig. W10.9).

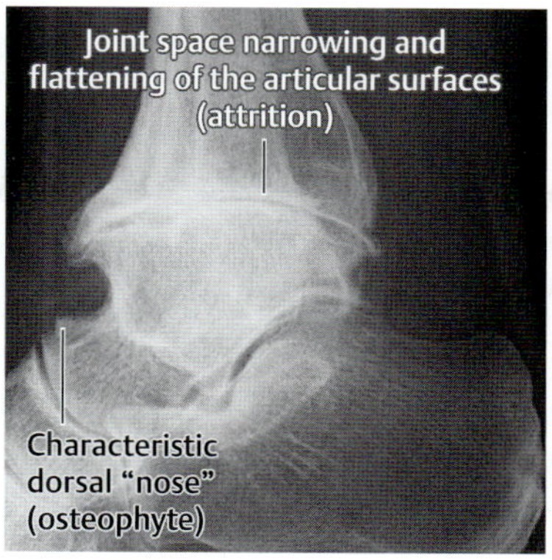

Fig. 10.50 Osteoarthritis of the ankle joint. Lateral radiograph.

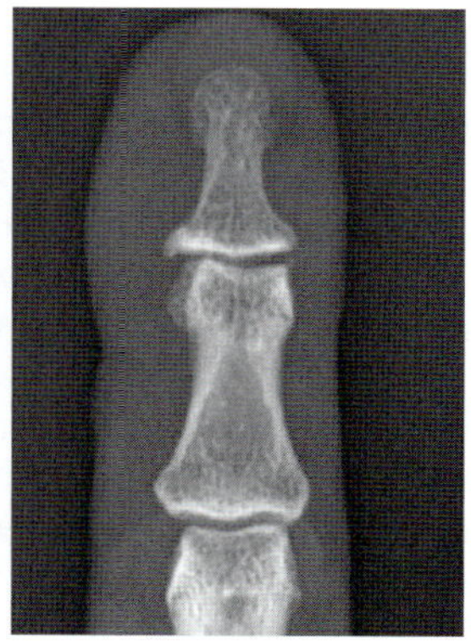

Fig. 10.52 Heberden's osteoarthritis of the fingers. Evidence of an osteophyte of the terminal phalanx and asymmetric joint space narrowing.

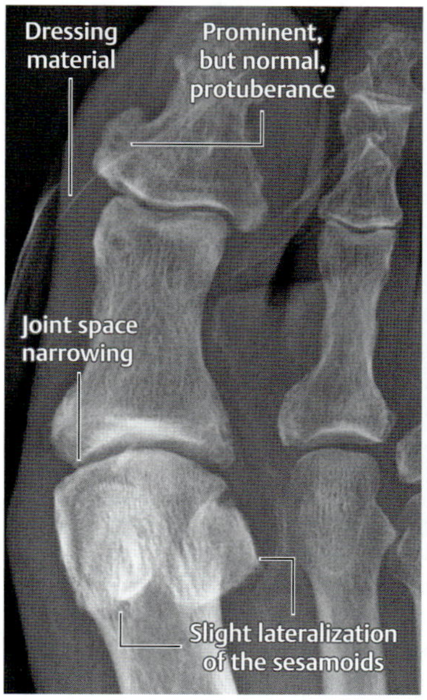

Fig. 10.51 Early osteoarthritis of the first metatarsophalangeal joint in the presence of mild hallux valgus.

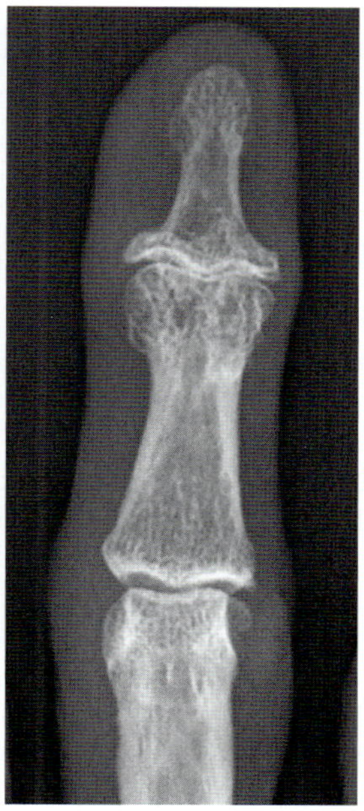

Fig. 10.53 Heberden's osteoarthritis of the little finger with deformity of the joint surface.

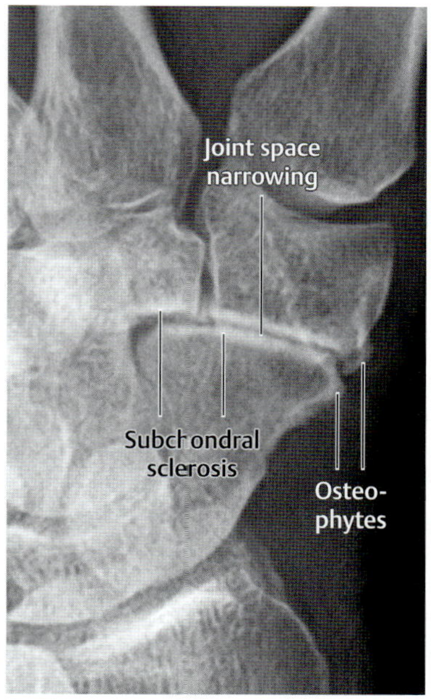

Fig. 10.54 STT osteoarthritis.

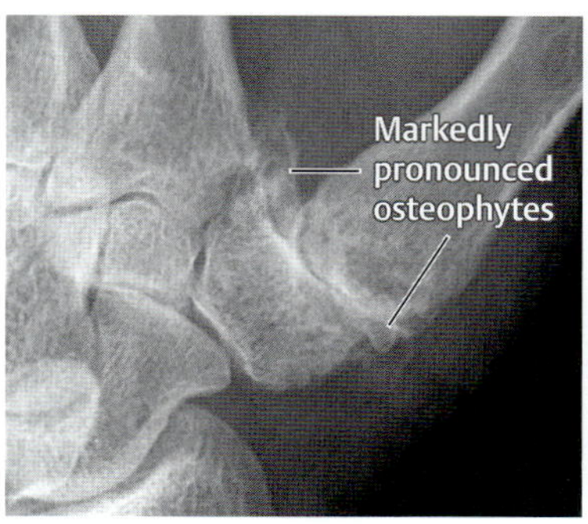

Fig. 10.55 Basal thumb osteoarthritis.

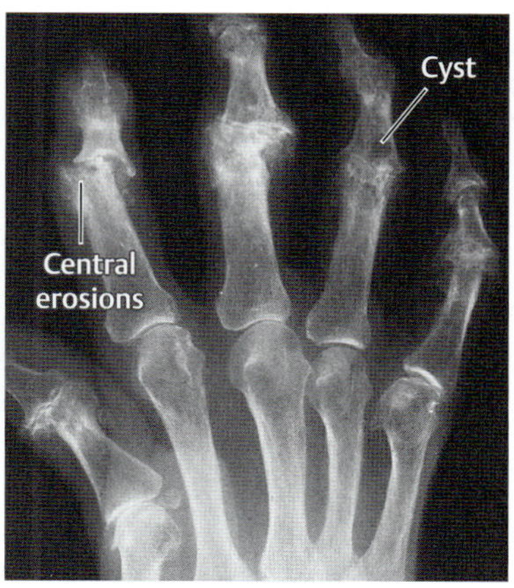

Fig. 10.56 Osteoarthritis of several finger joints with erosive components.

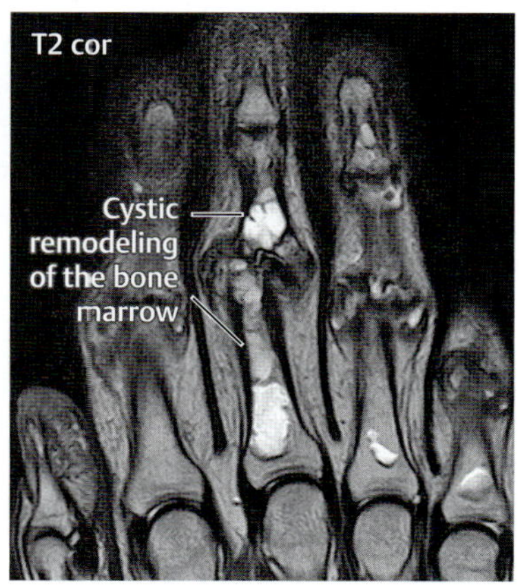

Fig. 10.57 Cystic ("osteoclastic") osteoarthritis of the hand. ▶ See also ▶ Fig. W10.10.

10

Shoulder and Elbow

Osteoarthritis of the acromioclavicular joint is common, albeit usually clinically asymptomatic (▶ Fig. 10.58). Hypertrophy of the capsule and osteophytes with caudad projection can result in narrowing of the subacromial space and in development of subacromial impingement syndrome.

Osteoarthritis of the glenohumeral joint is less common and is often associated with advanced chronic pathology of the rotator cuff. Osteophytes are commonly located at the inferior humeral head (▶ Fig. 10.59).

Rapid destructive arthritis of the shoulder (Milwaukee shoulder) is the result of an idiopathic destructive inflammatory process. This disabling disease develops secondarily after phagocytosis of hydroxyapatite crystals. It usually presents bilaterally and primarily affects older women.

Osteoarthritis of the elbow joint is rare. It usually develops as a result of mechanical occupational overuse (mining industry, pneumatic drills) or secondary to injury. Associated loose bodies are commonly found within the joint (▶ Fig. 10.60).

10.2.3 Treatment of Osteoarthritis

There is still no drug capable of healing osteoarthritis. For this reason, all therapeutic approaches are "symptomatic." Treatment of osteoarthritis follows a graduated approach, starting with counseling for the patient, physiotherapy, weight reduction, and increased muscle tone, backed up by nonsteroidal analgesics as required (see also OARSI [Osteoarthritis Research Society International] and EULAR [European League Against Rheumatism] guidelines in the References for Chapter 10.2 under "Clinical Diagnosis of Osteoarthritis"). Intra-articular injection of corticosteroids may be beneficial in advanced stages. The topical application of analgesics (e.g., capsaicin) may also be indicated. Intra-articular viscosupplementation is controversial. Nutritional supplementation with chondroitin and glucosamine has no positive effect on cartilage loss. Likewise, arthroscopic "lavage" does not demonstrate a significant advantage compared with placebo. Arthroscopic repair of an unstable meniscal tear or removal of a loose joint body may be beneficial, however. Surgical joint replacement has become an established procedure for treatment of osteoarthritis of the hip and knee joints in particular. There are no hard and fast criteria for surgical intervention, so it becomes an individual decision as to when a potential replacement should be considered.

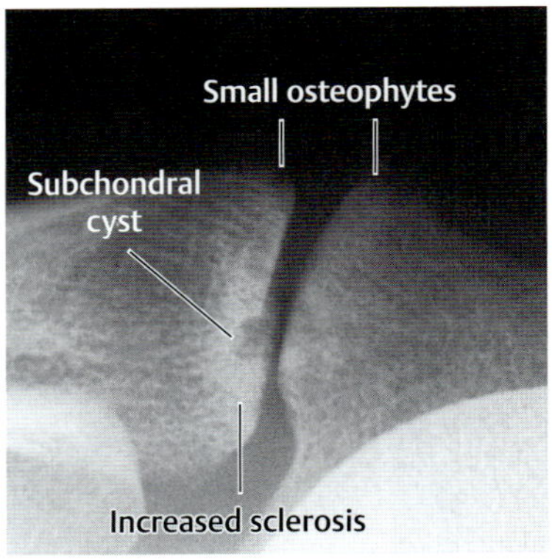

Fig. 10.58 Early stage of acromioclavicular osteoarthritis.

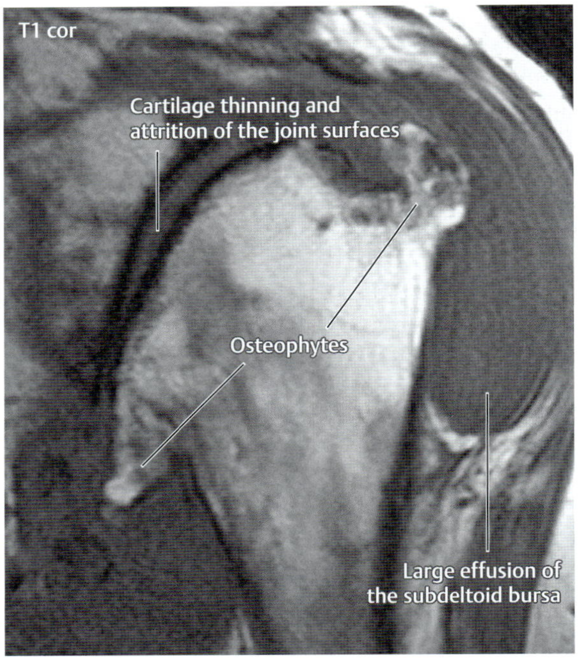

Fig. 10.59 Advanced osteoarthritis of the shoulder. Large osteophytes at the medial humeral head and in the region of the greater tubercle, diffuse thinning of the glenohumeral cartilage and massive subdeltoid bursitis.

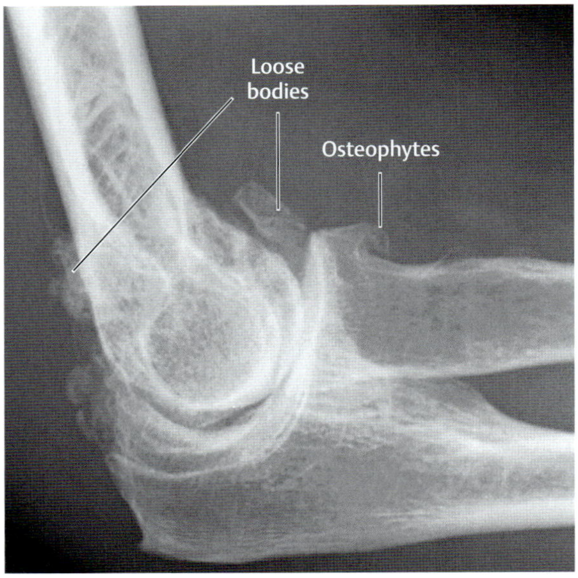

Fig. 10.60 Osteoarthritis of the elbow. In addition to joint space narrowing and osteophyte formation, multiple loose bodies are also evident.

10.3 Degeneration of the Spine

Degenerative disease of the spine is extremely common. Vertebral bodies and intervertebral disks, the facet joints, and the surrounding true synovial joints demonstrate the same degenerative alterations as other joints of the human body. The lower cervical and lumbar spines are subjected to the most weight bearing and motion and are therefore primarily affected. Isolated osteoarthritis of the facet joints (synonym: intervertebral joints) can occur, but is usually related to degenerative disk disease, which also has an effect on the integrity and mechanical properties of the surrounding musculoligamentous structures.

According to Kirkaldy-Willis, a "degenerative cascade" develops in the **"three-joint complex"** (comprised of the discovertebral complex and the two facet joints), which is associated with three successive stages of dysfunction, instability, and stabilization. This process of degeneration is the result of a complex interaction between an intervertebral disk and the facet joints at that level, whereby the initial event can begin at any of the three sites.

Four basic components are involved in spinal degeneration and they both influence and also augment each other:

- Degenerative disk disease.
- Osteophytes.
- Facet joint osteoarthritis and uncovertebral osteoarthritis.
- Ligamentous and soft tissue changes (ligamentous hypertrophy, ligamentous calcification and ossification; epidural lipomatosis).

10.3.1 Anatomy, Variants, and Information on Imaging and Technique

▸**Anatomy.** The spine is embryonically established as a system of multiple motion segments. Each motion segment has a **three-joint complex** comprising the intervertebral disk between two adjacent vertebral end plates anteriorly and the two facet joints in the posterior column.

The facet joints adopt a sagittal direction at the upper lumbar spine. These change in orientation both cranially and caudally so that in the upper thoracic spine they are oriented in a coronal plane and in the lower lumbar spine the joints are obliquely oriented. On an AP view, therefore, only the intervertebral joints of the upper lumbar spine are viewed in profile, and on a lateral view only those of the upper thoracic spine.

The arrangement of articular processes, neural arches, and spinal processes produces dorsal overlapping of the vertebral bodies, resembling the tiles of a roof and producing an "interlaminar window" and a route of access to the spinal canal that is not covered by bone.

The **motion segment** is surrounded and supported by ligaments and muscles. Facet joints (and the atlanto-axial joint) are true synovial joints. The intervertebral disk is a cartilaginous joint and consists of the nucleus pulposus, the anulus fibrosus, and the cartilaginous plates (▸ Fig. 10.61).

Structures sensitive to pain within the motion segment include (apart from the spinal nerve itself), the vertebral body periosteum, the peripheral portion of the anulus fibrosus, the posterior longitudinal ligament, the facet joint capsule, and the surrounding musculoligamentous structures.

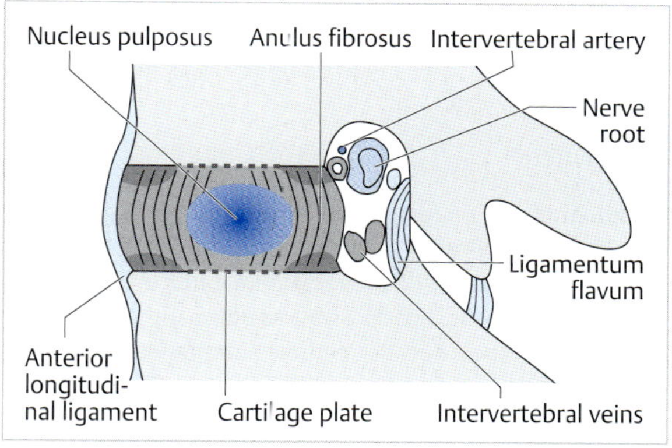

Fig. 10.61 Schematic architecture of the intervertebral disk and the intervertebral foramen.

Normal Variants

Congenital variations are common in the spine. The exact labeling of a transitional vertebra at the lumbosacral junction (lumbarized sacral or sacralized lumbar) may only be possible if all vertebrae are counted, starting from C1 downward. If this is not possible, then it is referred to as a "lumbosacral transitional vertebra."

- **Cranial variations:** cervical rib, sacralization of the fifth lumbar vertebra.
- **Caudal variations:** shortened first rib, lumbarization of the first sacral vertebra, rudimentary ribs at L1.

> **Note**
>
> Given that there are seven cervical vertebrae but eight cervical nerve roots, the following applies to the correct anatomical delineation of nerve roots in relation to their neural foramina:
>
> - **Cervical:** exit of the nerve root *above* the corresponding vertebra (e.g., C6 nerve root exits in the C5–C6 neuroforamen.
> - **Thoracic and lumbar:** exit of the nerve root below the corresponding vertebra (e.g., L4 nerve root exits in the L4–L5 neuroforamen, ▶ Fig. 10.62).
>
> If it is not possible to label a certain vertebral level unequivocally, this must be taken into consideration when annotating the film and explicitly stated in the report since confusion as to an exact level, e.g., for a planned surgical procedure, could have catastrophic consequences.

Technique

▶ Radiography. Images of the spine should, wherever possible, be obtained with the patient standing. Oblique views allow demonstration of the facet joints and the neural foramina. However, it is not possible to optimally demonstrate both of these anatomical structures simultaneously as they have different angles in the sagittal plane (▶ Fig. 10.63). See Chapter 10.3.8 for functional studies.

▶ CT. CT is better suited to displaying bony changes than is radiography because it is not hampered by overlapping structures. This is particularly important when assessing the facet joints, the neural foramina and the width of the spinal canal. A maximal slice thickness of 2 mm is recommended. The ability of modern CT devices to produce isotropic voxels allows for high-quality reconstructions at all levels. Axial and sagittal reconstructions, in a bone and soft tissue algorithm, are routinely obtained, with the axial reconstructions being acquired parallel to the intervertebral disks in cases of degenerative disease. Exact measurements of osseous features (e.g., spinal canal stenosis) should only be performed using bone windows since measurement errors are too great otherwise.

▶ Myelography/CT Myelography. Currently, myelography is usually combined with CT myelography. Its use is largely confined to the preoperative assessment of patients in whom it is uncertain whether the changes detected on CT or MRI adequately explain their symptoms. This technique is able to more accurately display the degree of root or spinal cord compression (▶ Fig. 10.64). With disk herniation, therefore, a good filling of the nerve root sheath argues against significant nerve root compression. Myelography without CT can provide important additional information since it allows for a dynamic examination in functional positions (flexion, extension).

▶ Discography. This involves "pressurizing" a disk by injecting radiographic contrast directly into the nucleus pulposus under fluoroscopic or CT guidance and assessing the patient's pain response to this provocative test. In cases of multilevel disease or in patients with discordant or equivocal findings on sectional imaging studies relative to the clinical examination, discography may identify the exact disk level responsible for the patient's symptoms. Discography is very rarely performed because it often does not add significant information to the clinical picture and there is some evidence that it may be harmful to the injected disks.

▸ **MRI.** MRI is the method of choice for detecting disk herniation. With the option of multiplanar reconstructions, CT achieves adequate accuracy in the lumbar spine but it is clearly inferior to MRI in the cervical spine. Calcification within the intervertebral disk or spinal ligaments and bony changes, on the other hand, are the much better assessed with CT. If CT or MRI of the spine is obtained, supplementary radiographs only rarely add any useful information.

MRI is primarily indicated for acute radicular symptoms with neurologic deficits; multiplanar reconstruction CT with or without intrathecal contrast (myelography) is an alternative imaging option when MRI is not available.

Newer MRI techniques are providing additional physiological and functional information, beyond the current anatomical imaging. This has not yet established itself, however, in daily clinical practice.

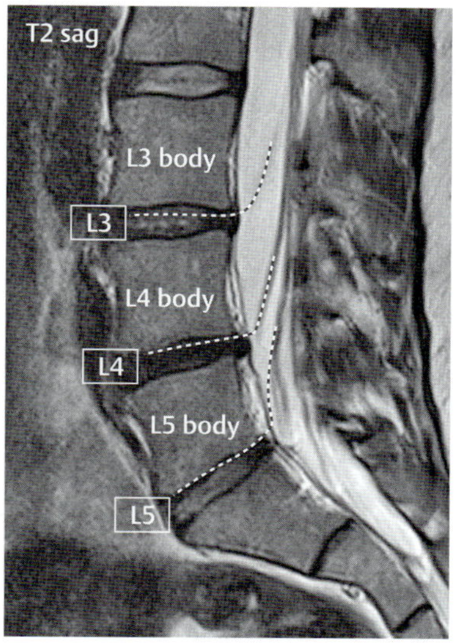

Fig. 10.62 Anatomical relationship of lumbar nerve roots to their respective neural foramina.

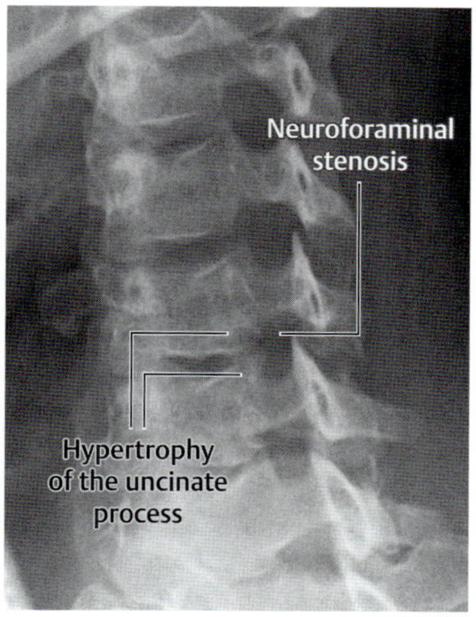

Fig. 10.63 Oblique view of the cervical spine to assess the neural foramina.

10.3.2 Clinical Presentation of the Degenerative Spine

Back pain is the main reason for time lost from work in Western industrialized nations. With low back pain, **psychosocial factors** should be considered in addition to true **somatic abnormalities** with regard to pathogenesis and disease prognosis. This also impacts the use of diagnostic investigations and treatment: problem-solving skills, anxiety-related avoidance behavior, passive pain behavior, pessimistic attitudes, social situation, care level, job satisfaction, and entitlements for pension and/or insurance claims all need to be considered.

Degeneration of spinal segments per se is not painful. Initiating factors for pain include irritation associated with dysfunction and segmental hypermobility. On the other hand, degenerative processes based on bony, ligamentous, or discogenic causes can lead to mechanical compromise of neural structures.

The **main causes of back pain** secondary to degenerative spinal disease are, apart from facet joint osteoarthritis, Modic 1 changes and irritation of the posterior longitudinal ligament, e.g., in association with disk herniation. These usually manifest clinically as load-dependent symptoms. Associated or isolated pain of musculoligamentous origin should not be ignored and needs to be included in differential diagnostic considerations.

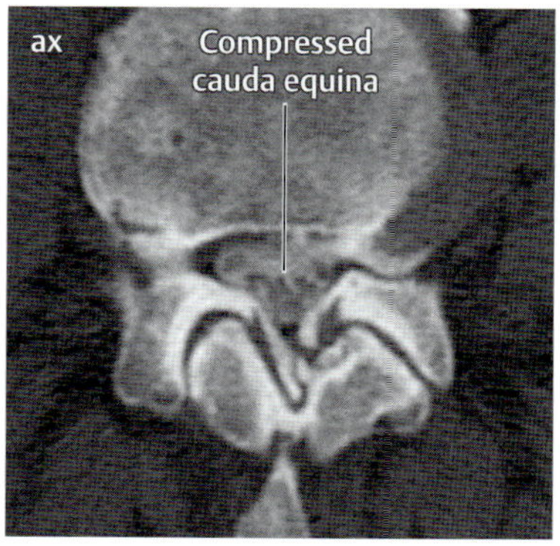

Fig. 10.64 CT myelography displaying facet joint osteoarthritis and associated bony spinal canal stenosis.

Disk herniations produce radicular symptoms secondary to **nerve root compression**, which may also be related to bony narrowing of the neuroforamina or the spinal canal from spondylarthritis or uncovertebral osteoarthritis. Radicular compression results in venous congestion, edema, and ultimately intra- and perineural fibrosis. The segments L3–S1 are by far the most commonly affected, followed by the cervical spine, especially C5–C7. Usually sensory disturbances predominate in the form of radicular pain, dysesthesia, and possibly hypoesthesia. Paralysis is classified clinically according to degrees of strength, ranging from 0/5 (no movement) to 5/5 (normal strength) (▶ Table W10.1).

Radicular distribution allows a precise clinical determination of level (▶ Table 10.1 and ▶ Fig. 10.65).

A distinction is made between the following types of low back pain with regard to the time course of back pain:

- Acute low back pain: less than 6 weeks.
- Subacute low back pain: more than 6 weeks up to 12 weeks.
- Chronic or chronic recurrent low back pain: longer than 12 weeks.

Furthermore, a distinction should be made between the following types of low back pain:

- **Nonspecific low back pain:** No clear indications of a specific cause are evident.
- **Specific low back pain:** A cause is identified (e.g., infection, tumor, osteoporotic fracture, disk herniation, spondylarthrosis, spinal canal stenosis, etc.).

"Red flags" are symptoms or previous illnesses that serve as warning signs for a specific underlying cause, possibly requiring urgent treatment. A radiculopathy, for example, would also be considered a "red flag."

Caution

Acute **conus medullaris and cauda equina syndromes** (pain, flaccid paralysis, saddle anesthesia, absent reflexes, sphincter dysfunction, urinary and fecal incontinence, absent pyramidal signs) are a spinal emergency necessitating *immediate* diagnostic evaluation with imaging. The cause is often a massively prolapsed disk, less commonly a hematoma, a decompensated spinal canal stenosis, or, even less frequently, tumor or infection.

Possible causes of the discrepancy between clinical presentation and radiographic findings are manifold:

- Many **morphological alterations,** such as osteochondrosis, facet joint osteoarthritis, disk herniations, and sometimes even higher-grade stenosis of the spinal canal and/or the neural foramina, are asymptomatic and therefore **clinically irrelevant.**

Table 10.1 Overview of the most commonly affected nerve roots and their function. The most important key regions are in bold type

Nerve root	Motor function	Key muscles	Key sensory structure	Key reflex
C5	Arm elevation	Deltoid muscle	Anterolateral shoulder, proximal lateral upper arm	
C6	Elbow flexion	Biceps brachii muscle	Lateral upper arm, forearm to **first digit** + radial aspect second digit	BTR
C7	Elbow extension	Triceps brachii muscle	Posterior upper arm, forearm to **third digit** + ulnar aspect of second digit and radial aspect fourth digit	TTR
C8	Finger spreading	Interosseous muscles	Dorsomedial upper arm, forearm to **fifth digit** + ulnar aspect of fourth digit	
L2	Hip flexion	Adductor and iliopsoas muscles	Antero**medial** proximal **thigh** beneath inguinal ligament	
L3	Knee extension	Quadriceps femoris muscles	**Antero**medial **thigh**	PTR
L4	Knee extension, elevation of medial foot	Quadriceps femoris, tibialis anterior muscles	Anterolateral distal thigh, anteromedial lower leg (**anterior margin of tibia**)	
L5	Foot and toe extension	Extensor hallucis longus muscle	(Postero-)lateral thigh, (antero-)lateral lower leg, **instep, great toe**	
S1	Plantar flexion of foot and toes	Triceps surae muscle	Dorsal/dorsolateral thigh, dorsal/dorsolateral lower leg, **lateral margin of foot, sole of foot**	ATR

BTR, biceps tendon reflex; TTR, triceps tendon reflex; PTR, patellar tendon reflex; ATR, Achilles tendon reflex.

- **Nerve root irritation** is not only caused by mechanical compression. The causes of radicular pain have not yet been finally clarified; however, local biochemical alterations certainly play a significant role (changes of prostaglandin levels, increased levels of tumor necrosis factor, interleukin, and cyclooxygenase-2, etc.) with cascadelike inflammatory processes.
- Pain radiating, for example, from the facet, sacroiliac, or hip joints can create the impression of nerve root irritation (**pseudoradicular pain**).
- Anomalous nerve-root exit levels, transitional anomalies, and **normal variants** of innervation create the wrong clinical impression of a "false" level of the lesion.

Note

In order to avoid treating insignificant additional findings, the radiologist should refrain from giving a clinical opinion regarding the imaging findings without an adequate knowledge of the clinical presentation. A statement as to whether the imaging findings correlate with clinical symptoms presupposes sufficient knowledge regarding the clinical presentation.

10.3.3 Degenerative Disk Disease

▸**Pathology.** Disk degeneration results from the combined effects of mechanical and metabolic causes, which are mutually dependent and reinforce each other. Genetic factors also play a role.

The metabolism of the disk is maintained by diffusion, either from the bone marrow of the adjacent vertebral bodies via the subchondral bone lamella and the cartilaginous end plate or from the surrounding blood vessels via the anulus fibrosus. Age-related or degenerative alterations of the vertebral bodies and the cartilaginous end plates can interfere with the nutritive supply of the disks and exacerbate the degenerative changes. If this process emanates from the vertebral bodies, then it usually begins in the periphery where the cartilaginous plates are absent. Reparative tissue extends into the disk and may lead to revascularization of the disk (the disk is partially vascularized only up to the fourth year of life).

In the natural course of aging, the nucleus pulposus loses its capacity to take up water and its inner pressure is reduced. Degenerative damage and deformity of the cartilaginous end plates and leakage of disk material through the end plates (Schmorl's nodes) result in a loss of intradiscal pressure and increased mechanical loading of the anulus fibrosus and facet joints. Additionally, the reduced perfusion of the end plates also results in impaired metabolism of the intervertebral disk. There is also a positive correlation between impaired arterial circulation due to arteriosclerosis and disk degeneration.

The degenerative process of the disk appears initially as horizontal bands in the nucleus pulposus; water content and integrity of the proteoglycans decrease and disk height is reduced. In later stages disk calcification (▸Fig. 10.66) and gaping anular fissures parallel to the superior and inferior end plates may become evident. These cavities then fill with gas (nitrogen; "vacuum phenomenon"). In rare cases degradation of the disk can lead to fusion of two adjacent vertebral bodies.

During the process of degeneration and increased mechanical loading, splitting and fragmentation of the otherwise spirally arranged fibers of the anulus fibrosus occurs. The fibers can only resist the high pressure of the nucleus pulposus (~8 bar [800 kilopascals]) to a certain extent; the result is an **anular tear** (▸Figs. 10.67 and ▸10.68). Recurrent overloading can result in abrupt or slowly developing displacement (**herniation**) of disk material beyond the margins of

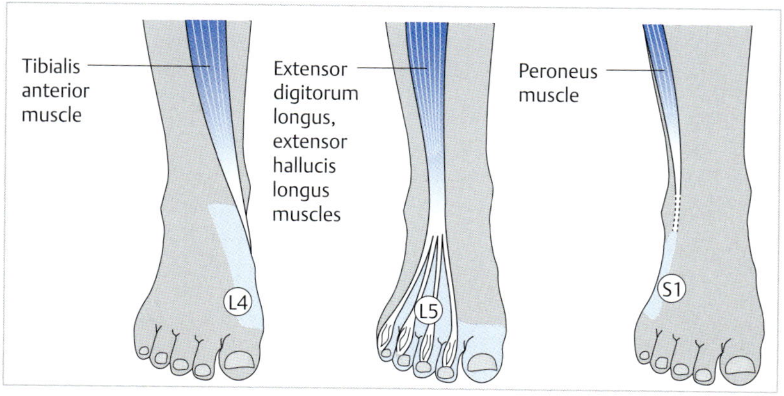

Fig. 10.65 Peripheral dermatomes and key muscles of the most important lumbosacral nerve roots. However, keep in mind that the muscles also receive contributions from other nerves (e.g., the extensor digitorum longus is innervated mainly by L5, but also from L4 and S1).

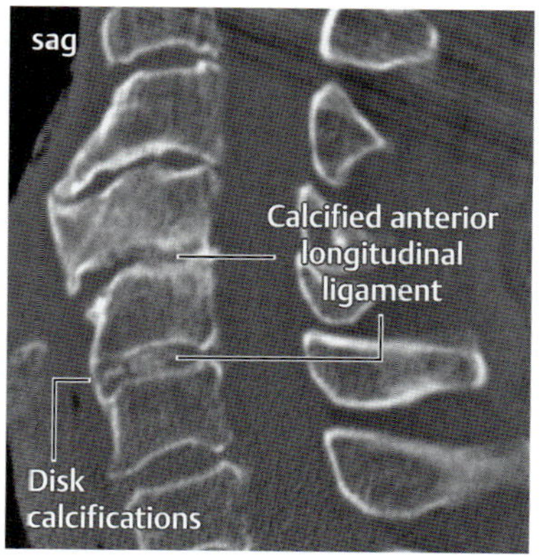

Fig. 10.66 Disk and ligamentous calcifications. Bridging anterior osteophytes in the presence of osteochondrosis.

the disk space (see ▸ Fig. 10.67). This can occur in any direction, but herniations in dorsal and dorsolateral directions are of particular clinical importance since these are the sites where there is a risk of compression of neural structures.

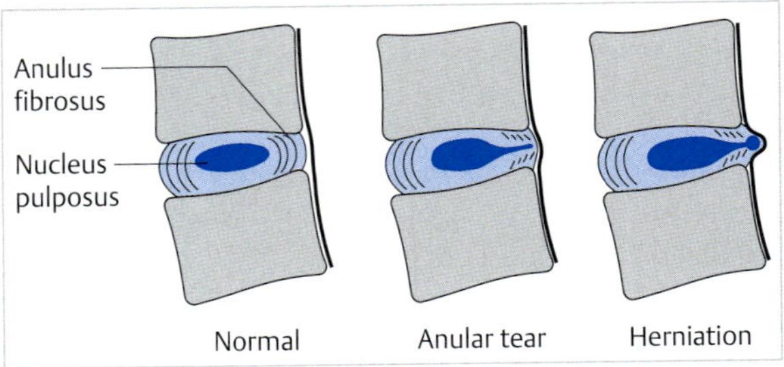

Fig. 10.67 Pathogenesis of disk hernias. Herniation of the nucleus pulposus follows a tear of the anulus fibrosus.

Disk Herniations

A simplified nomenclature of disk herniations was clearly defined for the first time in 2001 (see References for Chapter 10.3). However, common parlance is often inconsistent and adheres to old habits. The terms used refer exclusively to the **imaging results** and not to their effect on neural structures:

- **Herniation:** A herniation is the displacement of disk material beyond the normal margins of the intervertebral disk space, maximally 180° of the disk circumference. There is a further division into focal hernias (less than 90°) and broad-based hernias (90–180°).
- **Bulging:** A bulging disk is a broad-based protrusion extending more than 180° of the disk circumference.
- **Protrusion:** This refers to a herniation in which the greatest distance, in any plane, between the ends of the disk material is less than the distance between the edges of the base of the herniation in the same plane (corresponding to the confines of the disk space) (▸ Figs. 10.69–10.71 and W10.11).
- **Extrusion:** A herniation in which the greatest distance between the ends of the disk material *in at least one plane* is greater than at the base of the bulge is referred to as an "extrusion." This finding is more or less consistent with what is commonly known as "prolapse" (▸ Figs. 10.70–10.72).
- **Sequestration:** There is a loss of continuity between the herniated disk material and the disk of origin (▸ Figs. 10.69 and ▸ 10.73).

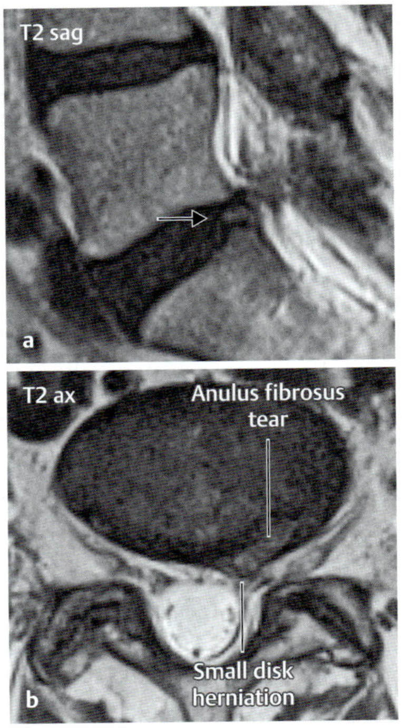

Fig. 10.68 Anular tear. **(a)** The tear (arrow) is hyperintense on the T2W image. **(b)** Small herniation of the nucleus pulposus through the tear.

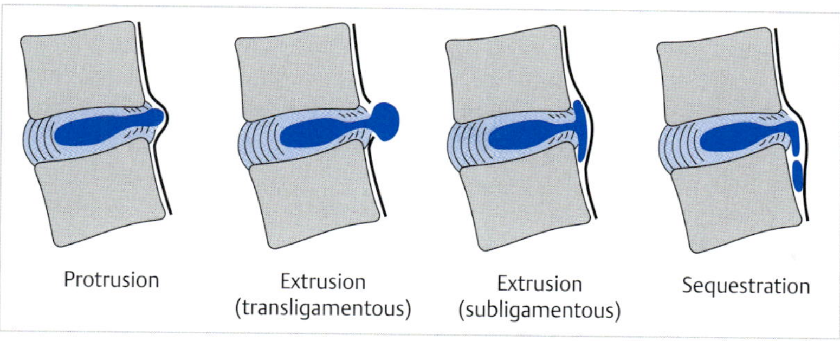

Fig. 10.69 Illustration of the different terms used to describe disk pathology.

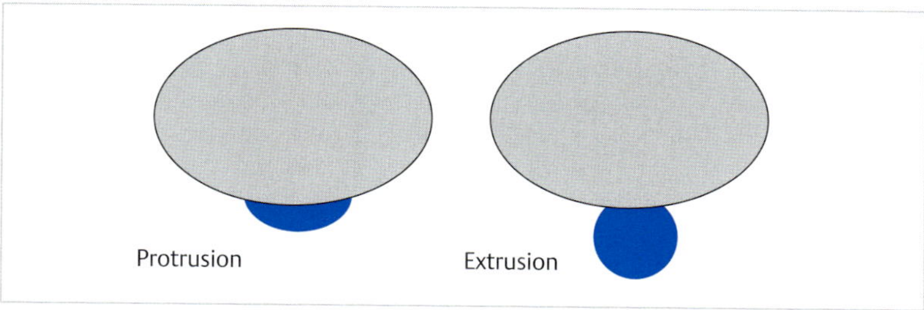

Fig. 10.70 Protrusion versus extrusion. In a protrusion, the base of the disk hernia is broader than the length of the protruding material. The opposite is the case with an extrusion.

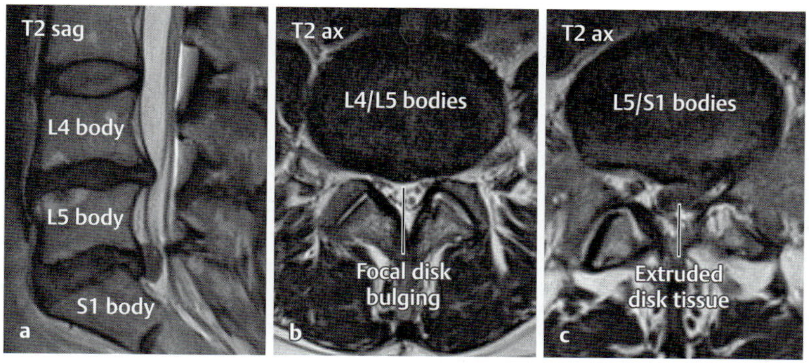

Fig. 10.71 Disk protrusion and extrusion. ▶ For additional images see ▸ Fig. W10.11. **(a)** Protrusion at L4–L5 and extrusion at L5–S1. **(b)** Protrusion in the axial plane. **(c)** Extrusion in the axial plane.

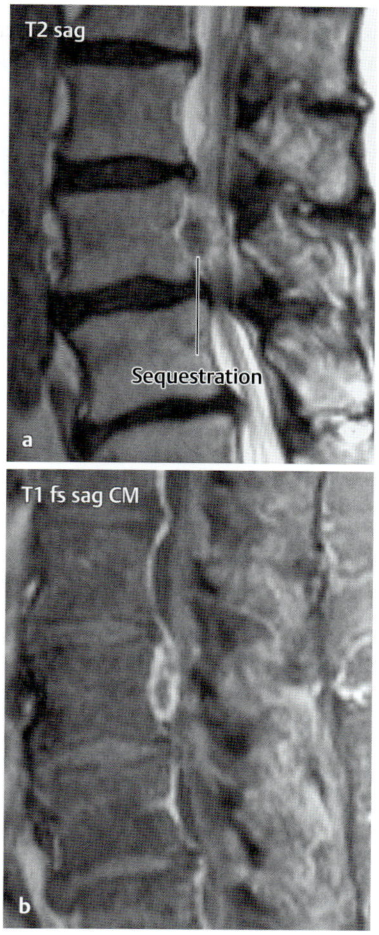

Fig. 10.73 Lumbar disk sequestration. **(a)** Intraspinal space-occupying mass without connection to a disk space. **(b)** No contrast enhancement of the sequestered disk material; only the surrounding tissues take up contrast.

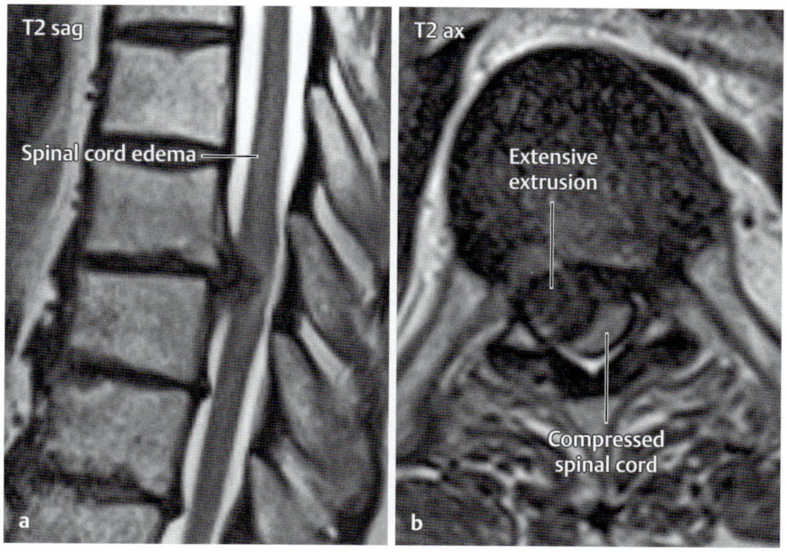

Fig. 10.72 Large disk extrusion T8–T9. **(a)** Myelopathy (increased signal intensity). **(b)** Myelopathy has developed as result of the considerable compression of the spinal cord.

10

Description of the **location of disk herniations** in relation to the vertebral body and pedicles distinguishes between median, paramedian, mediolateral, lateral, (intra-)foraminal, and extraforaminal (▶ Figs. 10.74–10.76).

In the United States the location is often differently described: central (instead of median), paracentral foraminal (instead of intraforaminal). Typically in the United States, a "lateral" disk herniation refers to one in an extraforaminal location.

If imaging morphology allows, a further distinction is made between subligamentous and transligamentous disk hernias in relation to the posterior longitudinal ligament (▶ Fig. 10.77). Very large, space-occupying disk hernias are also known as "massive prolapse" (▶ Fig. 10.78).

Disk tissue that has protruded superiorly or inferiorly into the adjacent vertebra is referred to as a **"Schmorl's node"** (Chapter 10.1.3). Histological evidence has shown that Schmorl's nodes develop when localized osteonecrosis has developed beneath the superior or inferior end plate. According to this idea, therefore, disk material fills up "soft" areas of bone.

As a rule, shrinkage of the protruding disk material occurs **over time** and this is associated with reduction of the space-occupying effect (▶ Fig. W10.12). Observation of increased size supports the case for progression or recurrence of the herniation.

▶ Radiography/CT. Radiographic changes of disk degeneration:

- Narrowing of the intervertebral disk space.
- Vacuum phenomenon within the disk space (see ▶ Fig. 10.78b).
- Calcification in the disk space.
- Development of anterior, lateral as well as dorsal osteophytes (Chapter 10.1.3)
- Bony alterations near the disk (Modic 1 changes).

With appropriate reconstruction and window setting, CT is capable of distinguishing between disk material and the spinal canal with its surrounding soft tissue, allowing the detection of disk herniation (see ▶ Fig. 10.75). Sometimes, however, due to the poor soft tissue contrast of CT (e.g., with extraforaminal herniation) only indirect signs of a disk herniation are evident, such as displacement or loss of epidural and periradicular hypodense fatty tissue (see ▶ Fig. 10.76).

▶ MRI. A normal nucleus pulposus is hyperintense on T2W sequences. The first sign of degenerative alterations is a central, hypointense stripe. The anulus fibrosus is hypointense on T1W and T2W sequences (▶ Fig. 10.79). A normal disk does not enhance with contrast; later, however, contrast enhancement becomes evident due to diffusion. During the process of degeneration the entire disk becomes increasingly hypointense and reduced in height on T2W sequences (disk "dessication"; "black disk"; see ▶ Fig. 10.79). With progression of the degenerative process and involvement of the juxtadiscal parts of the bone, the disk can also display zones of increased signal intensity on T2W images. It may also enhance with contrast as a result of neovascularization (▶ Fig. W10.13). **Annular tears** may appear as linear or comma-shaped zones of high signal intensity (on T2W sequences) in the periphery of the intervertebral disk (see ▶ Fig. 10.68).

In the course of degeneration, **disk calcifications** appear. These are hypointense on T1W and T2W sequences due to a loss of signal. Calcium, however, displays variable signal intensity, depending on its type and concentration: In the early stages of calcification, during the saponification phase, the signal may be hyperintense on T1 (▶ Fig. 10.80), with a hypointense appearance occurring later. In rare cases, liquefaction of the disks is found (strongly hyperintense on T2W images; ▶ Fig. W10.14).

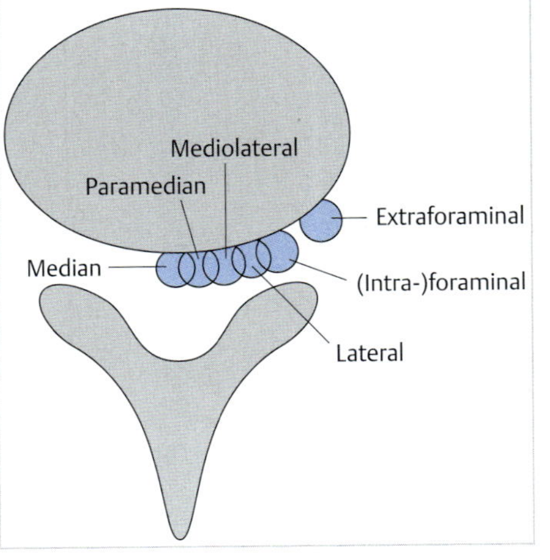

Fig. 10.74 Terms used to describe location of disk hernias. For different uses of terms see text.

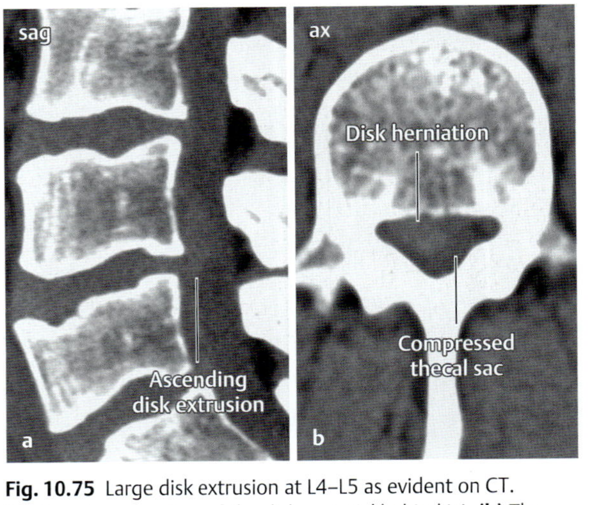

Fig. 10.75 Large disk extrusion at L4–L5 as evident on CT. **(a)** Superior migration of the disk material behind L4. **(b)** The disk tissue is more radiodense than the thecal sac or the nerve roots; it is situated in the right, paracentral region.

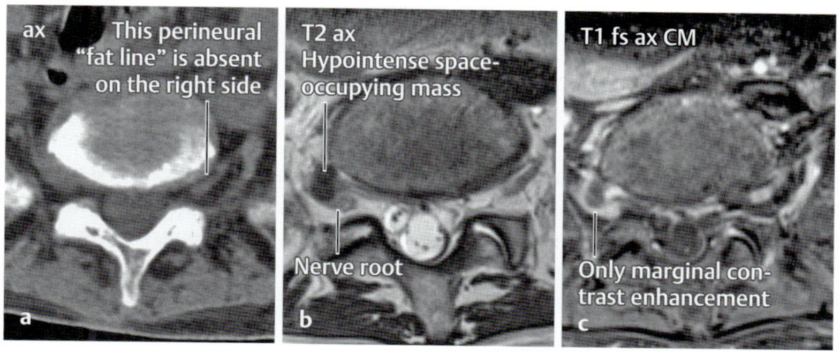

Fig. 10.76 Extraforaminal disk extrusion. **(a)** CT provides only indirect evidence in the form of displacement of the pararadicular fat pad. **(b)** MRI can distinguish between disk hernia and nerve root. **(c)** The extrusion itself does not enhance with contrast.

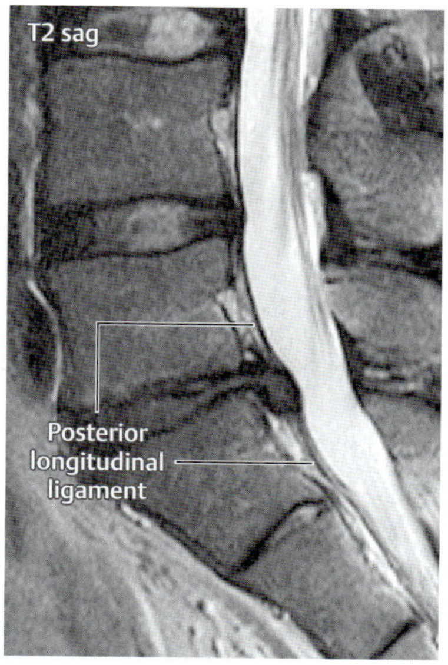

Fig. 10.77 Descending, subligamentous disk extrusion.

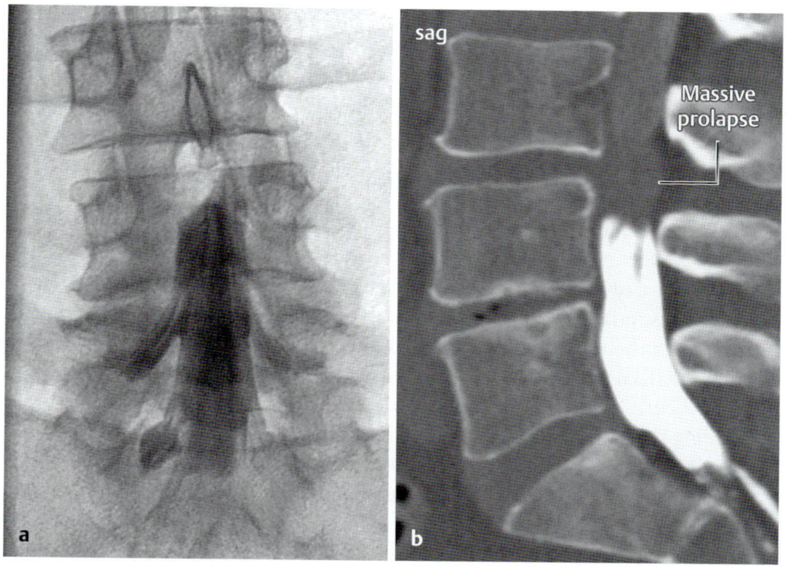

Fig. 10.78 Massive disk prolapse at L3–L4. **(a)** Lumbar myelography: superior block of the contrast column. **(b)** CT myelography: only minimal escape of contrast agent in a cranial direction. Additional finding of osteochondrosis at L4–L5.

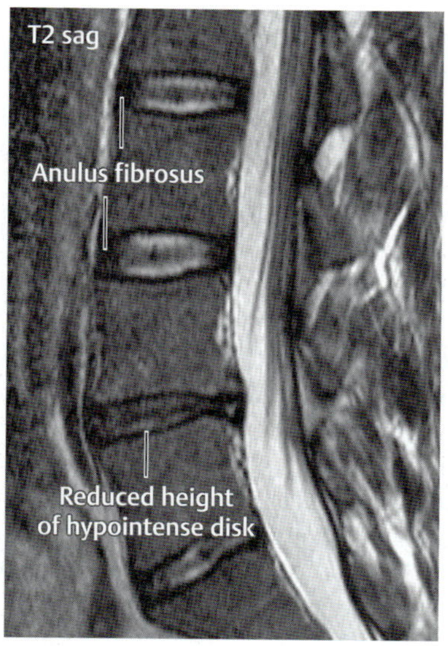

Fig. 10.79 Various signal patterns of intervertebral disks. Early degeneration of the upper two disks, more significant degeneration of the lower dessicated disk.

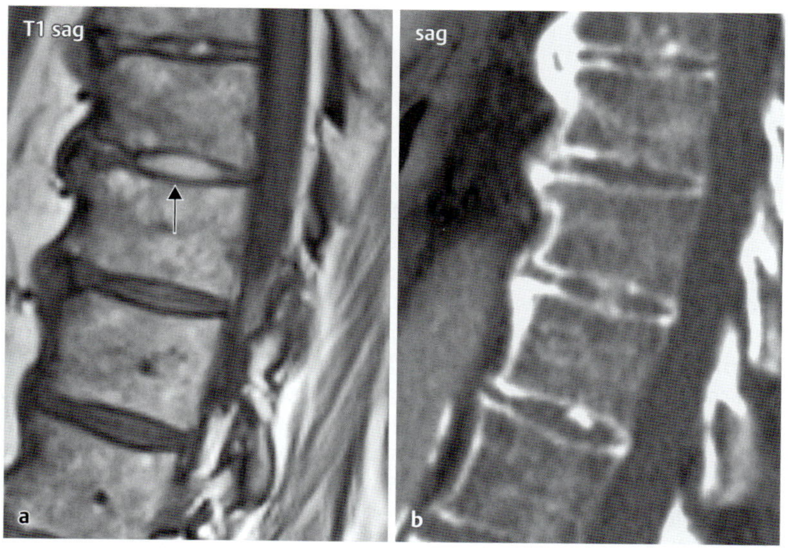

Fig. 10.80 Atypical signal pattern of a disk in the saponification phase (transition stage of calcification). **(a)** Abnormal hyperintense signal on this T1W image (arrow). **(b)** On CT, the corresponding spinal segment displays disk calcification in multiple neighboring segments.

▸ DD. If mechanical compromise is suspected as the cause of nerve irritation but not confirmed as discogenic or osseous, then numerous differential diagnoses should be considered, such as **radiculitis, pseudoradicular pain syndrome,** or **peripheral nerve damage.** Before even considering such rare causes, however, careful examination of the exiting nerve should be performed on axial images so that nerve root compression by an extraforaminal disk herniation is not overlooked (cf. ▸ Fig. 10.76).

The important differential diagnosis of a **spinal tumor** should always be considered (neurinomas and meningiomas in particular may be a source of confusion; ▸ Fig. 10.81). An atypical or unusual level of radiculopathy should be regarded as a warning sign. There is an absolute indication for IV contrast administration in these cases.

MRI Findings after Disk Surgery

▸ MRI. Seromas and hemorrhage, sometimes with significant mass effect, make assessment difficult, especially in the first few days after surgery. Correlation with clinical findings is essential to avoid misinterpretation, especially in such cases. In the majority of cases, the **intervertebral disk** enhances with contrast at its margins after surgery.

Scars along the access route and epidural scarring are difficult to discern from **residual or recurrent herniated disk material**, especially in the first postoperative weeks. Furthermore, distortion of the thecal sac may develop as well as transient radiculitis.

> **Caution**
> Contrast enhancement or increased signal intensity in water-sensitive sequences of the nerves at the level of surgery without clinical signs or symptoms is a common finding after disk surgery.

Initially on T2W sequences, **granulation tissue** usually demonstrates increased signal intensity compared with the anulus or intervertebral disk and becomes hypointense over time (years). Peripheral enhancement of a seroma on T1W images after contrast administration is evident in the first postoperative days; after weeks scar tissue enhances more avidly and more homogeneously. This makes easier differentiation from a nonenhancing recurrent disk herniation. Maximum contrast enhancement is reached 15 minutes after IV contrast administration in a **fibrous scar** (▸ Fig. 10.82); a recurrent hernia, on the other hand, does not take up contrast until after 30 to 45 minutes. Contrast enhancement becomes less as the scar ages, so that contrast enhancement may no longer be detectable after several years.

10.3.4 Juxtadiscal Bony Alterations

Degenerative disk disease and changes in the adjacent vertebrae practically always appear as one entity.

The term **"spondylosis deformans"** describes structural changes in a vertebral body that involve the anulus fibrosus and the adjacent apophyses. These changes are attributed to the physiologic process of aging.

Osteochondrosis, on the other hand, is defined as the additional involvement of the nucleus pulposus and the vertebral end plates. The underlying cause of these alterations, which are not necessarily symptomatic, is assumed to be related to pathologic processes in addition to the physiologic process of aging. The term "erosive osteochondrosis" is used for marked reactive, inflammatory types of osteochondrosis when there is radiographic and/or pathologic evidence of erosions (Latin: *erodere* = to gnaw away).

▸ Pathology. Decreased pressure within the nucleus pulposus leads to ligamentous laxity and associated hypermobility, which in turn causes reactive osteophytic bone proliferation (**osteophytes;** ▸ Fig. 10.83) along the edge of the vertebral body. Osteophytes serve to absorb the stresses related to the increased mobility.

During physiological aging and/or degeneration of the nucleus pulposus, height is lost and internal pressure is reduced, with weight bearing being shifted from the periphery to the center, resulting in laxity of the spinal ligaments. The vertebral bone adjacent to the disk is therefore subjected to increased compressive loads, which can result in recurrent microedema, microhemorrhage, microfractures, and micronecroses similar to the processes occurring in the synovial joints. Subsequently, reactive changes progress in stages, developing areas of pseudo-inflammatory reaction in the juxtadiscal bone, which are classified in **MRI** according to **Modic**:

- **Modic Type 1:** Hyperemia, ingrowth of fibrovascular tissue.
- **Modic Type 2:** Subcortical, juxtadiscal fatty marrow replacement (usually after several months).
- **Modic Type 3:** Subdiscal fibrosis and sclerosis (end stage).

▸ Clinical presentation. Over the years, dorsal osteophytes can lead to narrowing of the neuroforamina and/or spinal canal, especially when associated with hypertrophic osteoarthritis-related alterations of the posterior spinal structures (facet joints, spinous processes). Acute pain is usually caused by local overloading that triggers associated soft tissue hyperemia and/or edema. This produces additional acute entrapment of neural structures within the foramina or spinal canal and may produce pain (acute decompensation of chronic damage) or neurologic deficits.

▸ **Radiography/CT.** Typical findings:

- Bandlike or crescent-shaped sclerosis of the superior or inferior end plates (sometimes of the entire vertebra) (▸ Fig. 10.84). This end plate sclerosis commonly appears irregular and serrated adjacent to the disk space. It is sometimes interspersed with small erosions, in which case it is referred to as "erosive osteochondrosis" (▸ Fig. 10.85).
- Schmorl's nodes are often associated with (osteo-)chondrosis.
- Osteochondrosis can appear as hemispherical bone density located in the anterior or middle third of the vertebra. It is usually situated above the disk space, which can appear radiographically normal or reduced. This is a variant of the normally more bandlike subchondral bony sclerosis.

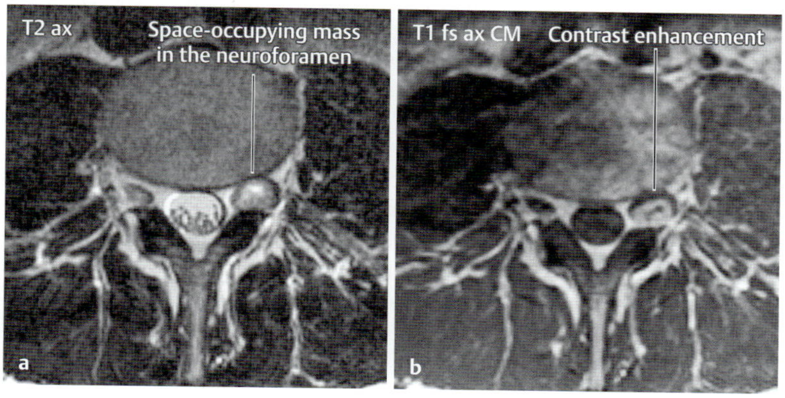

Fig. 10.81 Incidental finding of a foraminal space-occupying lesion at the level of L3–L4. **(a)** Small central cystic component. **(b)** The significant contrast enhancement argues against a sequestered disk fragment. Diagnosis: neurinoma.

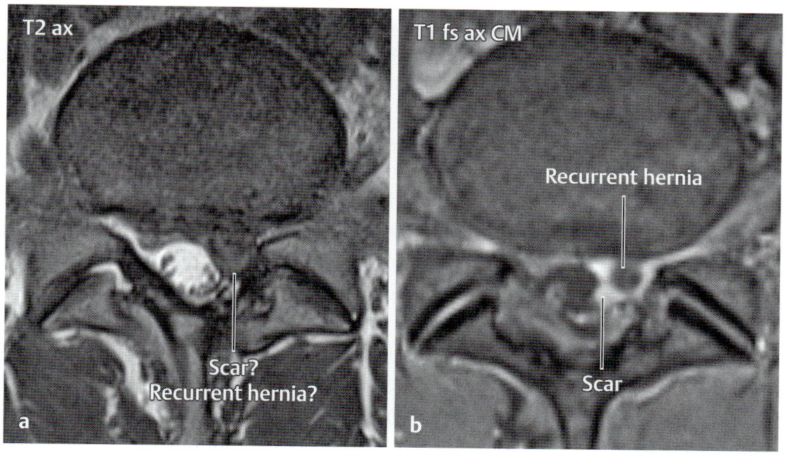

Fig. 10.82 Diagnostic findings after disk surgery for recurrent symptoms. **(a)** Nonspecific tissue in the left paracentral region. **(b)** Postcontrast imaging helps to differentiate between enhancing scar tissue and nonenhancing herniated disk material.

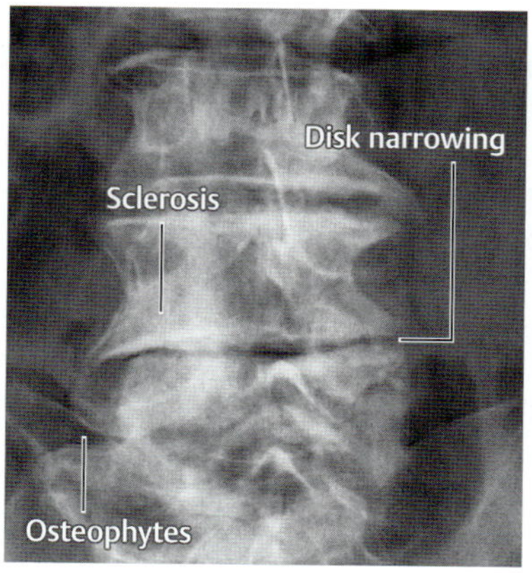

Fig. 10.83

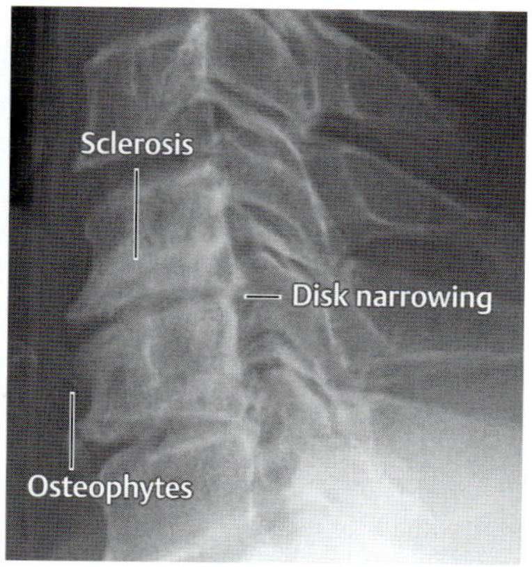

Fig. 10.84

Fig. 10.83 Osteochondrosis and spondylosis deformans of the lumbar spine. The disk space is considerably narrowed.

Fig. 10.84 Osteochondrosis of the cervical spine with marked sclerosis of the adjacent vertebral bodies.

10

▸ **MRI.** According to **Modic** these reactive alterations run a course involving three stages (▸ Fig. 10.86):

- **Stage 1:** The inflammatory (sterile) changes exhibit edemalike signal intensity (hypointense on T1W images and hyperintense on T2W images; ▸ Fig. 10.87), and contrast enhancement.
- **Stage 2:** After resolution of the acute reactive state (usually after a period of several months), subchondral fat is found within the end plate marrow (hyperintense on T1W and T2W sequences without fat suppression; see ▸ Fig. 10.87).
- **Stage 3:** Finally subchondral sclerosis develops, as is commonly seen on conventional radiographs and CT (hypointense on T1W and T2W sequences; ▸ Fig. W10.15).

These stages not only overlap (▸ see ▸ Fig. W10.15), but may also revert to Stage I.

▸ **DD. Differentiation between erosive and activated osteochondrosis and infectious spondylodiskitis** is extremely difficult radiographically, unless marked infectious destruction and vertebral collapse have already occurred. CT often improves diagnostic accuracy by allowing a direct search for irregular end plate destruction without sclerotic margins. If osteochondrosis is combined with "superimposed" infection, as is often the case, the juxtaposition of subchondral sclerosis and more acute-appearing bone destruction is apparent, provided the process is fairly advanced. Bandlike or irregular focal sclerosis is predominant in the late and healing phase of infectious spondylodiskitis, in which case the term "secondary" degenerative changes (osteochondrosis) would be more appropriate. MRI is best suited for differentiation (▸ Fig. 10.88).

The following findings indicate **degenerative changes**:

- Well defined vertebral end plates on the T1W image.
- Hypointense disk on T2W sequences.
- Absent or more bandlike enhancement in the intervertebral disk space after contrast administration.
- Edematous, bandlike signal parallel to the inferior and superior end plates that does not extend to the adjacent disk (the signal may also appear crescent-shaped).
- Nonenhancing or only minimally enhancing soft tissue components.

Nevertheless, in the early stage of spondylodiskitis with preexisting degenerative changes, the diagnosis is often unclear and must be further clarified with a follow-up MRI in 1 to 2 weeks.

Other possible differential diagnoses of erosive osteochondrosis include sterile anterior or posterior spondylitis (**Romanus lesion**) and sterile spondylodiskitis (**Andersson I lesion**) associated with **spondylarthritis** (▸ Fig. 10.89). As a rule, in spondylarthritis additional inflammatory manifestations may be evident in other vertebral components such as the costotransverse, costovertebral, and/or sacroiliac joints, so these areas should be carefully evaluated.

10.3.5 Facet Joint and Uncovertebral Osteoarthritis and Degeneration-based Spondylolisthesis

▸ **Pathology.** Degeneration of the disk with loss of height increases stress on the **facet joints** with consequent craniocaudal subluxation and development of reactive osteoarthritis. As with other synovial joints, the pathologic findings correspond to those of osteoarthritis (cartilage damage, effusion, synovitis, subchondral sclerosis, cyst formation, and deformity). Characteristic features include deformity of the joint surfaces, osteophyte formation, and concomitant hypertrophy of the ligamenta flava. The resultant narrowing of the spinal canal, the lateral recess, and/or the neural foramina can become clinically relevant due to compression of the nerve roots.

The cause of osteoarthritic changes of the **uncovertebral joints** of the cervical spine (uncovertebral osteoarthritis) is based on a compensatory mechanism related to degenerative hypermobility. The cranially extending uncinate processes represent an anatomical peculiarity of the cervical spine. Their sagittal orientation prevents lateral movement of the vertebral body. Uncovertebral joints are not genuine synovial joints.

Degeneration-based spondylolisthesis. Degenerative deformities of the facet joints and disk-space narrowing in association with laxity of ligaments and capsule can result in spondylolisthesis, mainly in the lumbar spine and especially at the L4–L5 level. Initially, this usually results in retrolisthesis and later, via remodeling phenomena (▸ Fig. 10.90), in an anterior slippage of one vertebra over another. Since the term "spondylolisthesis" is already reserved for alterations associated with spondylolysis, i.e., a bony interruption of the interarticular part of the vertebra, the term "**pseudospondylolisthesis**" is used for degenerative anterolisthesis.

Because the neural arch is intact, the degree of slippage is anatomically limited once the inferior articular processes of the anteriorly sliding vertebra reaches the tip of the superior articular processes of the vertebra beneath or its posterior margin. In short, slippage of more than ~30% of the vertebral length is not possible. The result of degenerative spondylolisthesis is **stenosis of the spinal canal**, which is worsened by concomitant hypertrophy of the ligamentum flavum. Additionally, **nerve root compression** occurs in the neuroforamen. Furthermore, the lateral recess is additionally narrowed by hypertrophied and buckled ligaments.

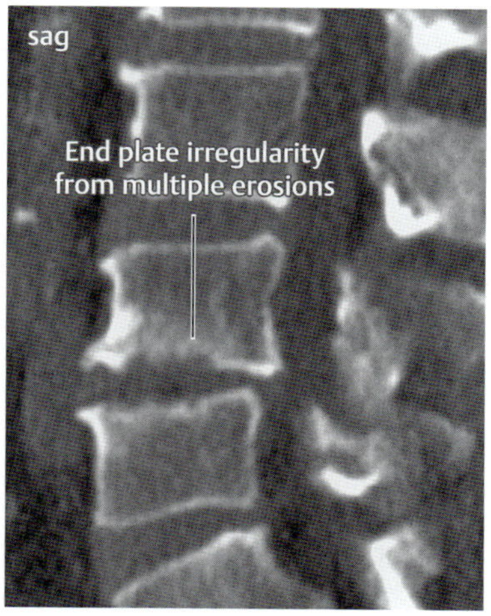

Fig. 10.85 Erosive osteochondrosis.

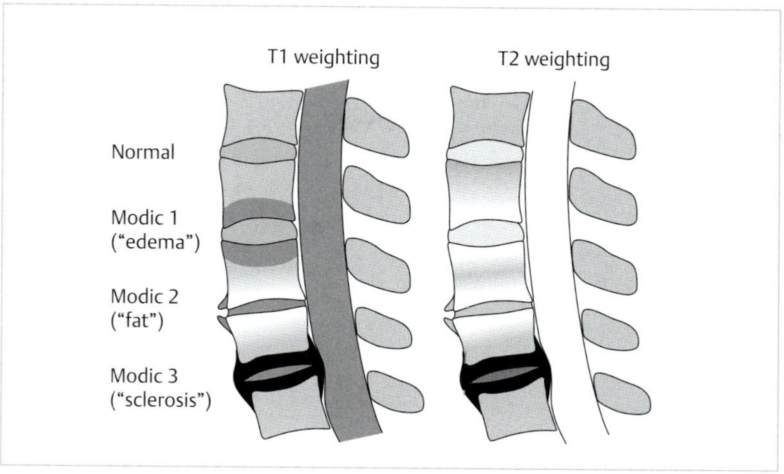

Fig. 10.86 Stages of osteochondrosis (Modic): characteristic signal patterns on MRI.

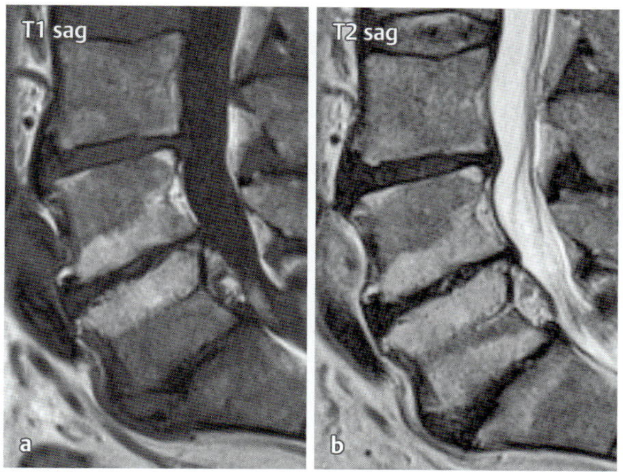

Fig. 10.87 Osteochondrosis of the lumbar spine. Modic Stage 1 at L5–S1 and Modic Stage 2 at L4–L5. **(a)** Hypointense edema at L5–S1. "Fat signal" at L4–L5. **(b)** The T2W image does not allow a definite differentiation between fat signal (L4–L5) and water signal (L5–S1).

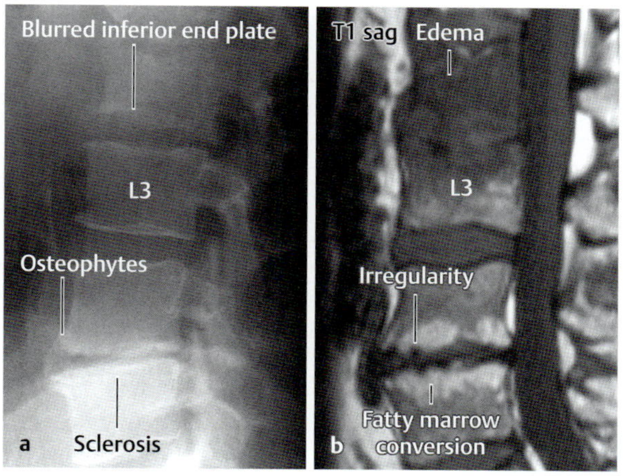

Fig. 10.88 Juxtaposition of spondylodiskitis L2–L3 and erosive osteochondrosis L4–L5. **(a)** Poor definition of the end plates at L2–L3 on the radiograph. **(b)** Typical morphology of osteochondrosis with end plate irregularity and small erosions. Unlike spondylodiskitis, the adjacent vertebral areas are hyperintense in the form of fatty marrow conversion (Modic Type 2).

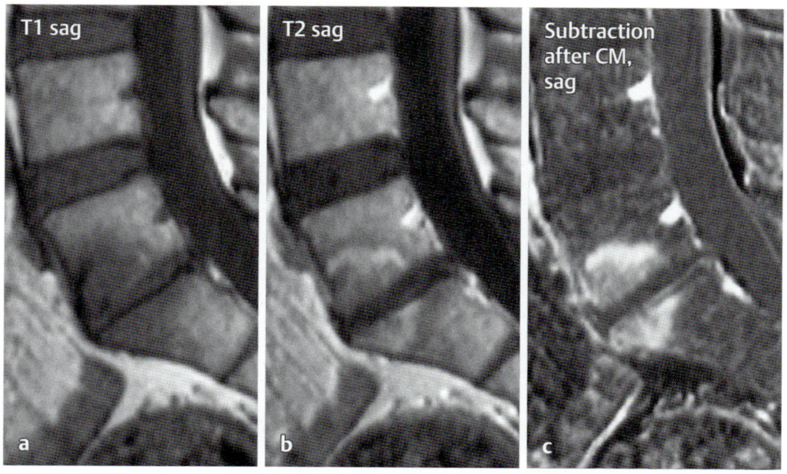

Fig. 10.89 Erosive osteochondrosis (Modic Type 1) in the region of the anterior end plates. Given such a finding, differential diagnosis must include anterior spondylitis (Romanus lesion) with spondylarthritis. **(a)** Sagittal T1W image. **(b)** Sagittal T2W image. **(c)** Sagittal subtraction image after contrast administration.

10

Classification of spondylolisthesis according to Meyerding is purely descriptive and distinguishes four grades, based on the percentage of anterior slippage of the upper over the lower vertebra (▸ Fig. 10.91). Grade 1 corresponds to slippage of less than 25%, Grade 2 slippage of 25 to 50%, Grade 3 slippage of 50 to 75%, and Grade 4 a slippage of more than 75%. Spondyloptosis (▸ Fig. W10.16) is the most extreme form, with complete slippage of one vertebral body over another, and is almost exclusively found at the lumbosacral junction with associated spondylolysis.

Intraspinal synovial cysts. These juxta-articular, extradural **capsular bulges** of osteoarthritic facet joints are of considerable clinical significance. They occur particularly in the lower lumbar spine (most commonly at L4–L5) and are often associated with degenerative spondylolisthesis. They contain joint fluid and may calcify (▸ Figs. 10.92 and ▸ 10.93). Less commonly they may also contain gas or hemorrhage.

▸ **Clinical presentation.** Apart from more nonspecific, dull, and activity-related back pain secondary to facet joint osteoarthritis, **synovial cysts** may also result in radicular symptoms secondary to compression of the adjacent nerve root due to their location in the bony recess or in the neuroforamen of the vertebral body.

▸ **Radiography.** Typically, only increased density and coarsening of the facet joints is seen. The joint space is also scarcely visible on oblique views. The joint appears misshapen and sclerotic with irregular margins (▸ Fig. 10.94).

▸ **CT.** CT better demonstrates the findings in facet joint degeneration (see ▸ Figs. 10.90b and ▸ 10.94b). Apart from the "usual" signs of osteoarthritis (joint space narrowing, subchondral sclerosis, marginal osteophytes, subchondral cysts), the following signs are also typical features:

- Vacuum phenomena.
- Elongation of the articular surface (see ▸ Fig. 10.94b).
- Deformity, widening, and expansion of the joint.
- Thickening (and possible foci of ossification) of the ligamenta flava.

Synovial cysts are evident as rounded, soft tissue density masses within the spinal canal in direct continuity with a facet joint. They can also develop marginal and/or central calcifications (see ▸ Fig. 10.92). It is difficult to differentiate a noncalcified synovial cyst from a space-occupying soft tissue mass, such as herniated disk tissue. MRI is the diagnostic modality of choice in this scenario.

▸ **MRI.** Whereas CT is more suited for assessing bony alterations, MRI is superior for detecting a joint effusion, thickening of the ligamenta flava (▸ Fig. 10.95), and synovial cysts (see ▸ Fig. 10.93). Pathologically increased amounts of fluid in the facet joint are an indication of possible concomitant segmental hypermobility (see ▸ Fig. 10.95).

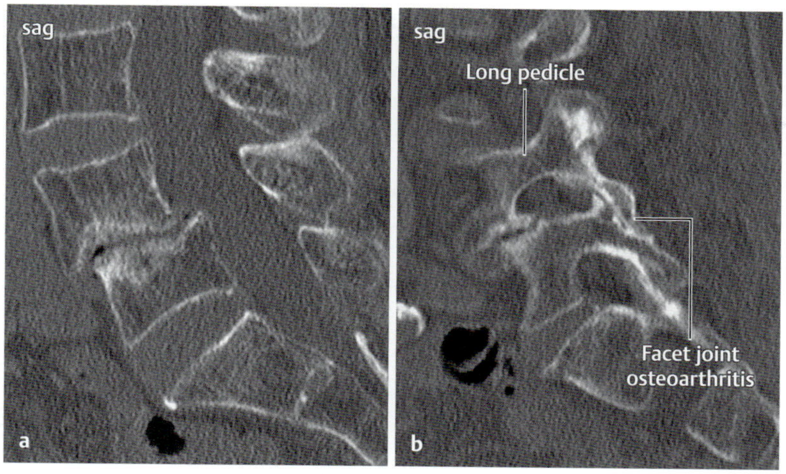

Fig. 10.90 Degenerative spondylolisthesis L4–L5, Meyerding Grade I. **(a)** Loss of disk height, advanced osteochondrosis. **(b)** Remodeling is also evident here from the elongated pedicles.

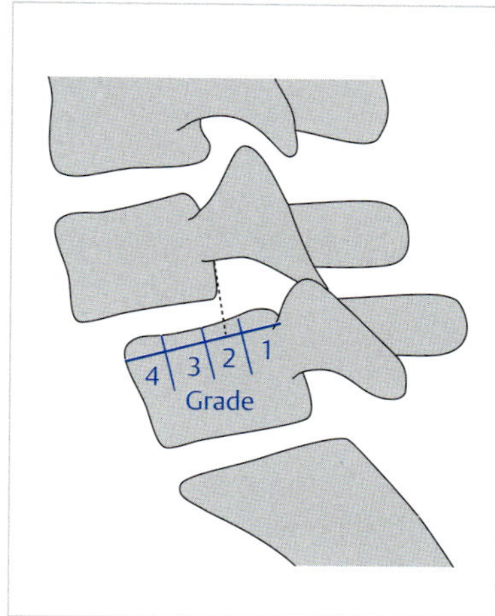

Fig. 10.91 Grading of spondylolisthesis according to Meyerding.

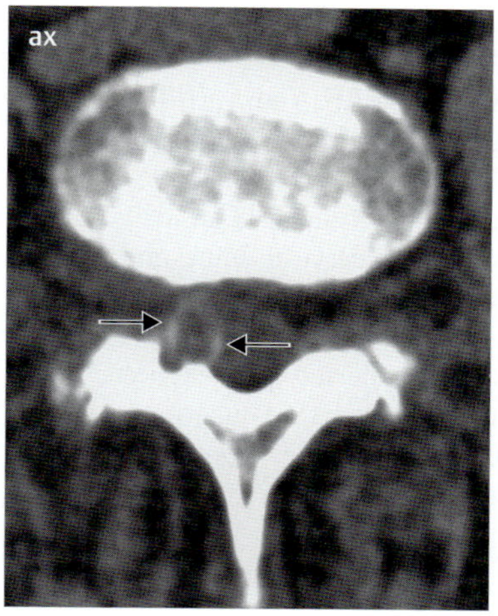

Fig. 10.92 Marginal calcification of a synovial cyst (arrows).

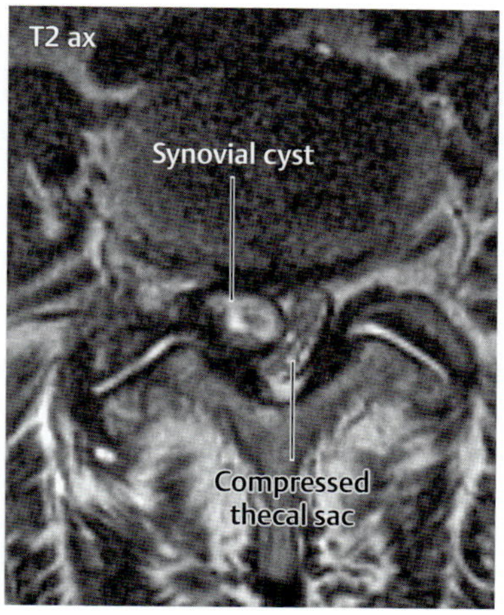

Fig. 10.93 Space-occupying, intraspinal synovial cyst. Characteristic "juxta-articular" location anterior to the facet joint.

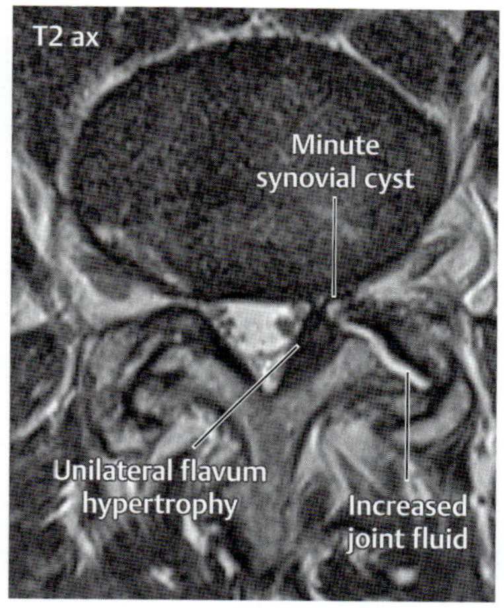

Fig. 10.95 Typical constellation of segmental hypermobility.

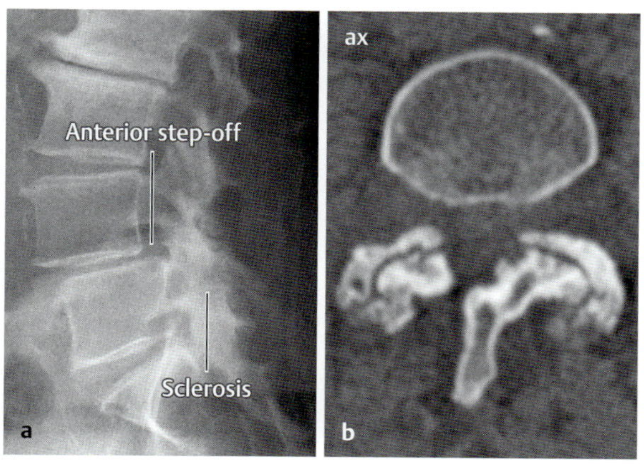

Fig. 10.94 Degenerative spondylolisthesis. **(a)** Meyerding Grade I anterolisthesis. **(b)** The facet joints are sclerotic and considerably hypertrophic.

10.3.6 Ligamentous and Soft Tissue Changes

These include ligamentous hypertrophy, ligamentous calcification, ligamentous ossification and epidural lipomatosis. **Thickening of the ligamentum flavum** is commonly the result of compression or bulging of these ligaments as a result of degenerative narrowing of the disk space. Hypertrophy of the ligament may also develop (see ▶Figs. 10.95 and ▶10.101).

Calcification and ossification of the longitudinal ligaments of the spine (anterior and posterior ligaments) is common. These tend to increase after the age of 50 years, and there also seems to be an ethnic factor (increased incidence of ossification of the posterior longitudinal ligament in Asians, known as the **Japanese disease;** ▶Fig. 10.96) and considerable variability between individuals (possibly genetically determined).

Diffuse idiopathic skeletal hyperostosis (**DISH**) is pathologically and morphologically identical with other forms of ligamentous calcification and ossification, but is defined as a separate entity due to a number of characteristic features (cf. Chapter 10.4).

Epidural lipomatosis refers to a pathologically excessive accumulation of fat within the epidural space of the spinal canal. Its causes include long-term exogenous steroid administration, endocrine diseases (e.g., Cushing's syndrome, underactive thyroid, pituitary adenoma), and obese habitus; some cases remain of idiopathic origin. It extends over several segments, often with a considerable space-occupying effect on the spinal cord or cauda equina (▶Figs. 10.97 and ▶10.98, ▶Fig. W10.17). The mid-thoracic spine and the lower lumbar spine are most often affected; cervical epidural lipomatoses have so far not been reported. MRI is the diagnostic modality of choice. Epidural accumulations of fat of more than 6 to 7 mm in width are regarded as pathologic; the space-occupying effect on the neural structures as displayed by imaging is important. In the lumbar region a Y-shaped compression of the dural sac is a classic feature, known as the Y or stellate sign (see ▶Fig. 10.98).

Degenerative alterations of the cervical or lumbar spine, combined with degeneration of the interspinous ligament and an extreme lordotic position, can result in the abutment of one spinous processes with another ("kissing spine"). Sclerosis and deformity may develop, even to the extent of forming pseudarthroses that are often painful (**Baastrup's syndrome**; Chapter 10.1.3).

10.3.7 Spinal Canal Stenosis

▶Pathology. Factors leading to stenosis of the spinal canal (central stenosis) and to narrowing of the lateral recess (lateral stenosis) are divided into two groups:

Congenital predisposing factors

- Shape, position, and dimension of the facet joints (especially frontal versus sagittal orientation).
- Shape and dimension of the spinal canal (unfavorable clover leaf shape).

Acquired initiating factors

- Spondylarthritis.
- Disk herniation.
- Thickening of the ligamenta flava.
- Subluxation of the facet joints.
- Malalignment secondary to spondylolisthesis.
- Epidural lipomatosis (Chapter 10.3.6).

Reference values for a **normal width** of the bony spinal canal:

- The **sagittal diameter** is at least 13 mm at the level of the cervical spine and at least 15 mm at the level of the lumbar spine.
- The normal **interpedicular distance** in adults is at least 25 mm at the level of the cervical spine and at least 18 mm at the level of the lumbar spine.

Reduction of these values is referred to as "stenosis." However, there are no generally recognized quantitative criteria for grading stenoses as "relative" or "absolute," "mild" or "high-grade," as is often done.

> **Note**
>
> Stenosis of the lumbar spine may be present when there is a sagittal diameter of less than 11 mm or with an interpedicular distance of less than 16 mm. *But* even high-grade stenoses can be asymptomatic. In the cervicothoracic spine, the spinal cord is at risk from stenosis of the spinal canal. This results initially in reversible **cord edema**, and later in irreversible damage with pressure-related **myelomalacic damage** or **secondary ischemic lesions**. Postischemic myelopathic lesions in the territory of the anterior spinal artery are referred to as "snake bites" or "owl-eye phenomenon" because of their pathognomonic appearance (see ▶Fig. 10.100).

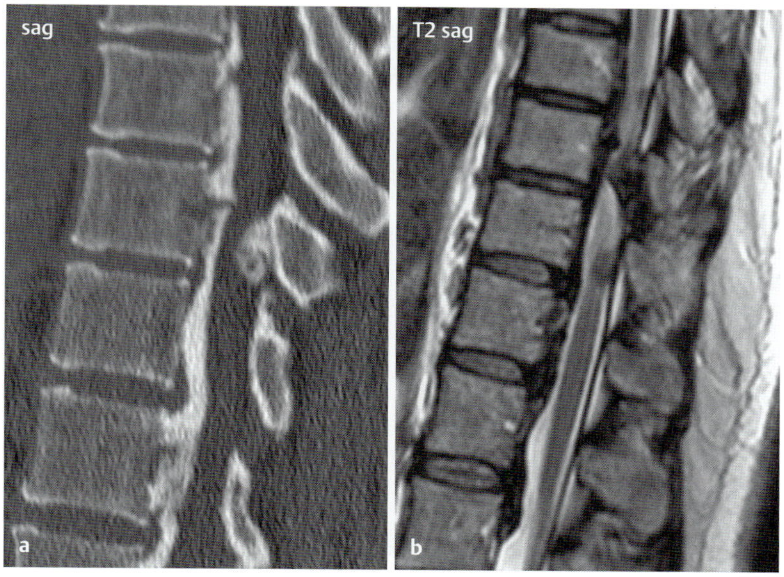

Fig. 10.96 The "Japanese disease." **(a)** Long-segment ossification of the posterior longitudinal ligament. **(b)** Correlative sagittal MR image.

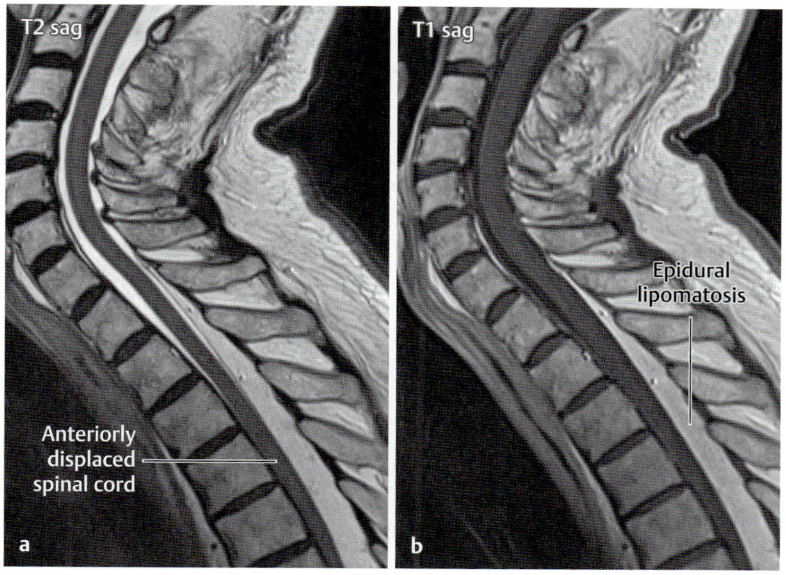

Fig. 10.97 Epidural lipomatosis. Clinically progressive truncal ataxia. **(a)** On the T2W image, the finding is usually only recognizable from displacement of the spinal cord. **(b)** Epidural fat proliferation is clearly evident on the T1W image.

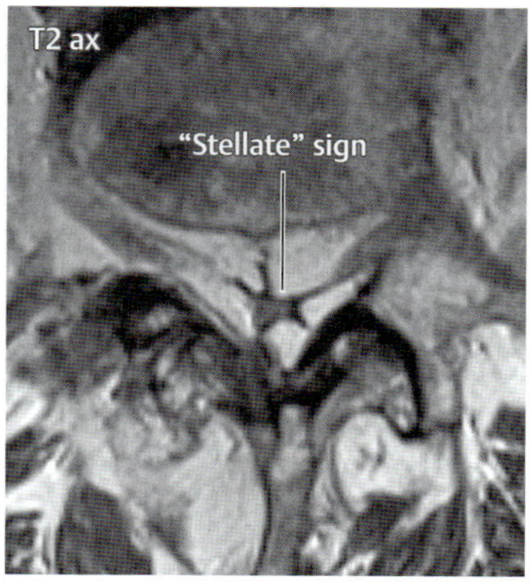

Fig. 10.98 Stellate sign resulting from compression of the thecal sac in a patient with epidural lipomatosis.
For additional images see ▶ Fig. W10.17.

▸ **Clinical presentation.** The classic clinical presentation of **lumbar spinal stenosis** manifests as back pain with pain often radiating down both legs, especially when walking (intermittent spinal claudication), and results in reduced walking tolerance. Radiculopathy presents initially as sensory disturbances. Apart from cervicobrachialgia, with or without concomitant neurologic deficits, **cervical spinal stenosis commonly** presents with disturbances of the "long tracts" associated with gait abnormalities (sense of insecurity when walking associated with ataxia and stumbling), spasticity, hyperreflexia, and pyramidal signs.

▸ **Radiography.** Spinal canal stenosis may be suspected on a lateral radiograph, but confirmation of the diagnosis usually requires axial images using MRI, CT, or CT myelography.

▸ **CT.** CT can most accurately quantify the extent of stenosis and distinguishing between osseous (▸ Fig. 10.99) and soft tissue–related narrowing. Compression of the spinal cord and the nerve roots can also be demonstrated directly by CT myelography.

▸ **MRI.** MRI offers the advantage of displaying the degree of neural element compression without the need for intrathecal administration of contrast while at the same time detecting the presence of any myelopathy (▸ Fig. 10.100; see also ▸ Fig. 10.99). Furthermore, it allows for differentiating the causes of a soft tissue–related narrowing (intervertebral disk, ligamenta flava, space-occupying lesion; ▸ Fig. 10.101).

An MRI protocol should therefore include strongly T2-weighted sequences ("myelosequences") with MIP reconstructions in addition to standard sagittal and transverse sequences (e.g., sagittal and axial T1W and T2W sequences) and an edema-sensitive sequence (e.g., fat-suppressed coronal or sagittal T2W sequences) (see ▸ Fig. 10.97).

▸ **Important findings.** More important than measuring the degree of osseous spinal canal stenosis is a description of the cumulative narrowing (including bone and soft tissue components) and the resulting space-occupying effects on the contents of the spinal canal.

10.3.8 Instability, Segmental Hypermobility, and Functional Studies

The term **"instability"** can be misleading since it may be used to describe traumatic or degenerative alterations of the spine. It should only be used to describe actual mechanical instability of a motion segment that occurs when even a small amount of force results in excessively large displacement of spinal elements (translation or rotation). It usually refers to a sudden, unforeseeable event. Classic examples include traumatic and pathologic fractures.

"Segmental hypermobility" is when a motion segment demonstrates unusually high flexibility or low stability during loading with excessive translation.

> **Note**
> **"Segmental hypermobility"** is the term of choice, rather than "instability" in the context of disk degeneration or spondylolisthesis.

Functional studies can detect segmental hypermobility. But care must be taken since these may be falsely negative due to:

- Insufficient motivation on the part of the radiographer and the patient to produce the maximal motion possible.
- True pain-related restricted range of motion.

There are neither clinically nor radiographically uniform definitions of segmental hypermobility. For example, translation in the sagittal plane by more than 3.5 mm or segmental gaping (more than 11° in the cervical spine, or more than 20° at the level of L4–L5) are pathologic. More important is the difference between intersegmental mobility in comparison with a "healthy" adjacent segment. It should be kept in mind during assessment, however, that there are segmental differences in range of motion. Thus in the lumbar region, physiological angulation is most pronounced at the level L4–L5.

With appropriate technique and patient compliance it is possible to detect segmental hypo- and hypermobility that may indicate pathologic change but the relevance of which is unfortunately not yet defined.

> **Note**
> The value of functional radiographs in cases of segmental hypermobility is controversial for the above reasons. Even if all currently available diagnostic procedures are employed, the objective assessment of segmental hypermobility by imaging is not possible with any degree of confidence.

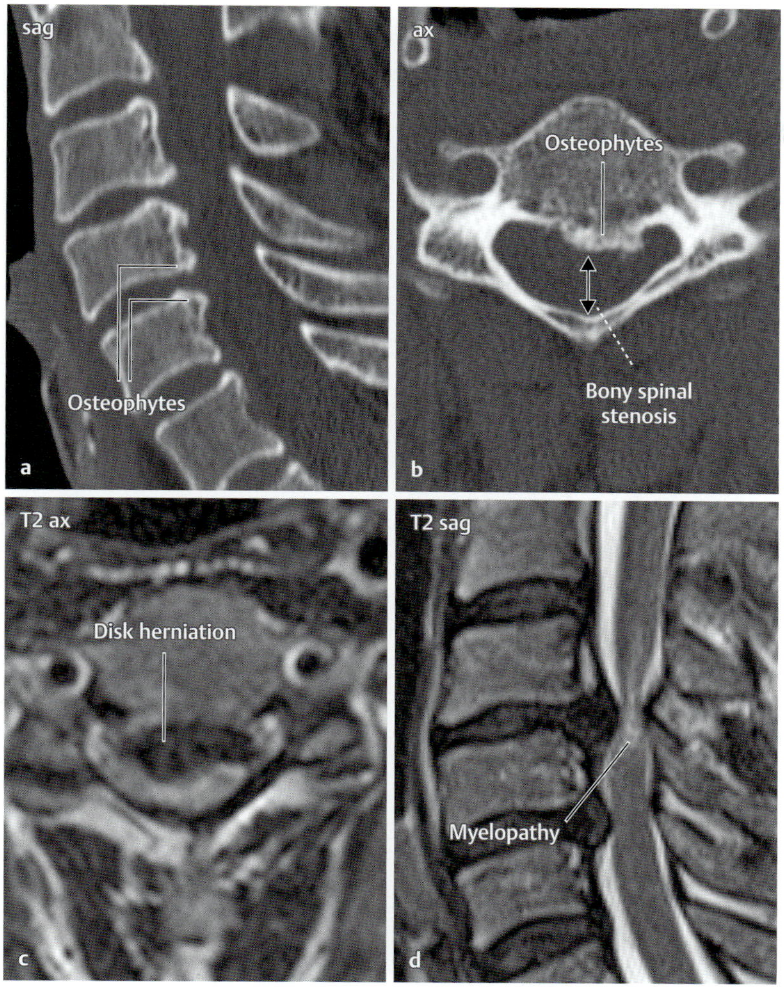

Fig. 10.99 Cervical spinal stenosis. **(a)** CT displays small, dorsal osteophytes. **(b)** Sagittal diameter of the bony spinal canal is reduced to 9 mm. **(c)** In addition, MRI shows superimposed, soft tissue–related discogenic stenosis. **(d)** Spinal cord compression and myelopathy.

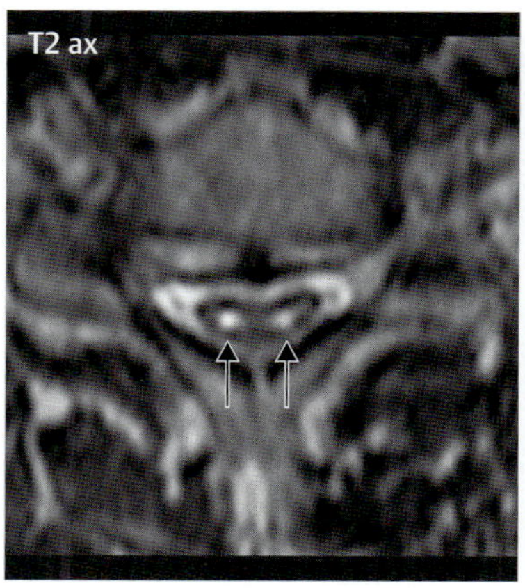

Fig. 10.100 Postischemic myelopathy ("snake bites"; arrows) in a patient with spinal canal stenosis.

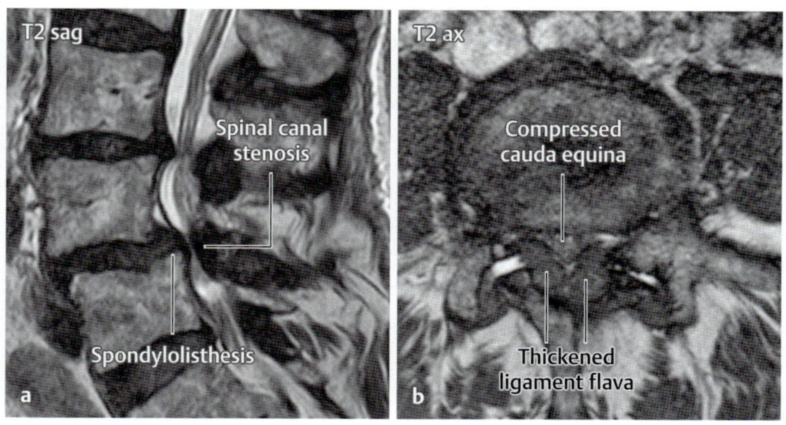

Fig. 10.101 High-grade lumbar spinal stenosis. **(a)** Grade 1 anterolisthesis at the level of the most severe stenosis. **(b)** Thickening of the ligamenta flava is the primary cause of the stenosis.

10.4 Diffuse Idiopathic Skeletal Hyperostosis

DISH (synonym: **Forestier's disease**) is diagnosed when the following criteria are fulfilled:

- Flowing ossification along the anterior longitudinal ligament, extending over at least four segments (lateral involvement possible; ▸ Fig. 10.102).
- Normal height of the intervertebral disk spaces (calcification of the anulus fibrosus is common, however; ▸ Fig. 10.103).
- No ankylosis of the facet joints or erosions of the sacroiliac joints.

▸ **Pathology.** DISH is a noninflammatory condition of unknown etiology. Hyperinsulinemia combined with diabetes mellitus, fluorosis, hypervitaminosis A, among other things, has been associated with DISH.

▸ **Clinical presentation.** The majority of patients are over 50 years of age and complain of progressive limitation of motion in the cervical and lower thoracic regions. As with osteoarthritis, there is often a discrepancy between the severity of the clinical findings and the radiographic features.

▸ **Radiography.** Extensive **"flowing" hyperostoses** along the anterior surfaces of the vertebral bodies is characteristic. Occasionally, a radiolucent line between the ossification and the vertebral bodies is recognizable on the radiograph, differentiating DISH from degenerative osteophytes. Usually the lower cervical spine and the thoracolumbar junction are affected. Intervertebral disks, sacroiliac joints, and facet joints remain normal.

Complications of DISH. Dysphagia secondary to the anterior hyperostosis in the cervical spine is not uncommon (▸ Fig. 10.104). Deformation and **narrowing of the spinal canal,** caused by ligamentous ossification (posterior longitudinal ligament, ligamenta flava), can cause myelopathy. While compression of the spinal cord can be directly recognized on CT, the direct visualization of cord damage requires MRI (bright areas on T2W and contrast-enhanced T1W images). A **stiff spine** due to this type of ossification is vulnerable to injury (cf. Chapter 2.2.4).

▸ **DD. Spondylarthritis.** Ankylosis of the sacroiliac, costovertebral, and facet joints, characteristic of different types of spondylarthritis, is absent in DISH.

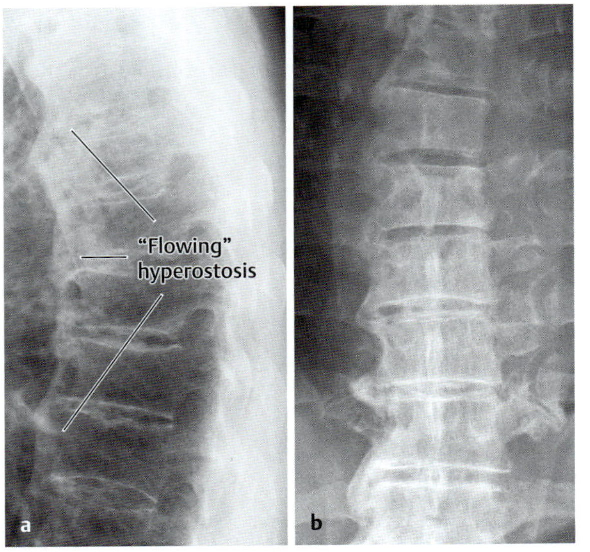

Fig. 10.102 DISH in a 60-year-old woman. **(a)** Typical multisegmental ossification of the anterior longitudinal ligament with preserved intervertebral disk spaces. **(b)** Additional multisegmental, lateral ossification, predominantly on the right, characteristic of DISH.

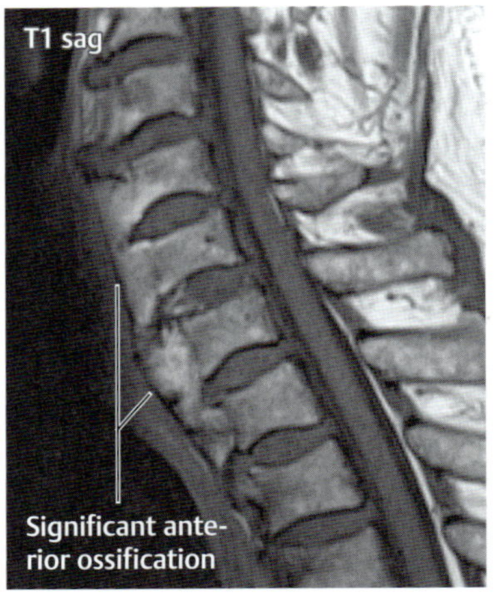

Fig. 10.103 Marked bridging anterior ossification from C4–C7 in a case of DISH. Note also the calcification of the anterior anulus fibrosus.

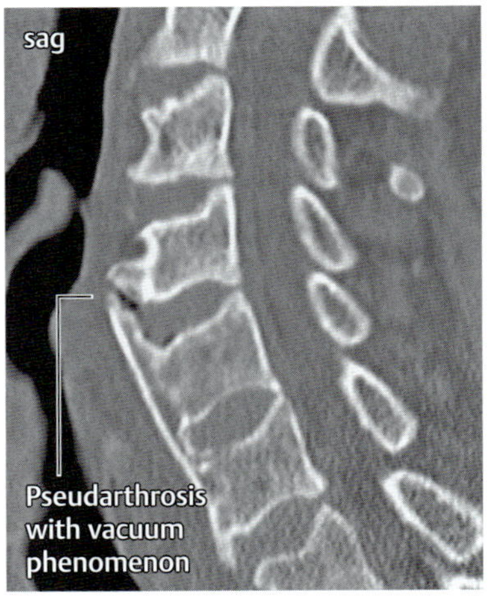

Fig. 10.104 Ankylosis of C4–C6 in a case of DISH. Development of an anterior pseudarthrosis between C4 and C5. The patient suffered from dysphagia.

10.5 Rheumatoid Arthritis and Juvenile Idiopathic Arthritis

10.5.1 Rheumatoid Arthritis

Rheumatoid arthritis (synonym: chronic polyarthritis) is a systemic autoimmune disease that originates primarily in the synovial membrane of affected joints and that progresses if left untreated.

▸ **Pathology.** Patients develop a **progressive joint-destructive autoimmune reaction**, possibly related to a prior infection, and many are found to be carriers of certain HLA-DBRI genes. A subset of T lymphocytes are activated; these stimulate B lymphocytes to produce immunoglobulins (rheumatoid factor and anti-CCP [anti-cyclic citrullinated peptides]) and macrophages to form cytokines (interleukin-1, interleukin-6, and tumor necrosis factor α). This results in the proliferation of mesenchymal tissue elements (fibroblasts) and the influx of inflammatory cells from the blood into the synovial membrane, so that an aggressive granulation tissue (**synovitis** or **pannus**) develops. This pannus passes through three stages, which are particularly evident on contrast-enhanced MRI:

1. **Active-inflammatory synovitis,** associated with a prominent joint effusion.
2. **Partially fibrotic pannus.**
3. **Scar pannus.**

Pannus develops at certain sites of predilection in joints and tendon sheaths that probably depend on the number of synovial B cells present (they react with T lymphocytes), tissue perfusion, and absent or thinned hyaline cartilage covering that portion of bone (bare area). The result is destruction of the cartilage with **joint space narrowing.**

In addition, inflammation stimulates osteoclasts via another cytokine, the RANK ligand (receptor activator of nuclear factor κB). Circumscribed defects, known as **marginal erosions,** develop (▸ Figs. 10.105 and ▸ 10.106). Furthermore, osteoclastic activity results in juxta-articular osteoporosis, known as "**rheumatic osteitis**" (▸ Figs. 10.107 and ▸ W10.18), in addition to a more generalized arthritis-related **osteoporosis** of the entire skeleton.

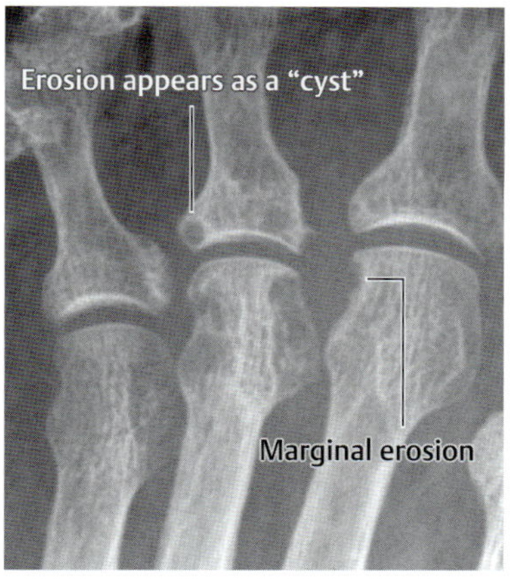

Fig. 10.105 Marginal erosions in a patient with rheumatoid arthritis. Those seen en face appear more like cysts.

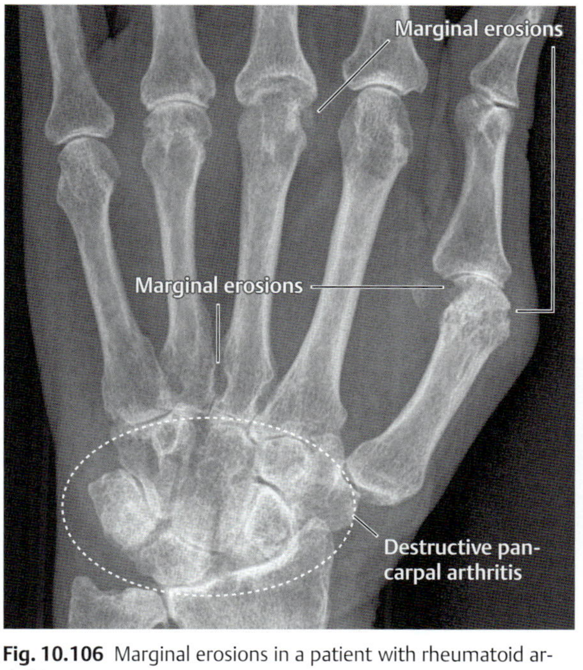

Fig. 10.106 Marginal erosions in a patient with rheumatoid arthritis.

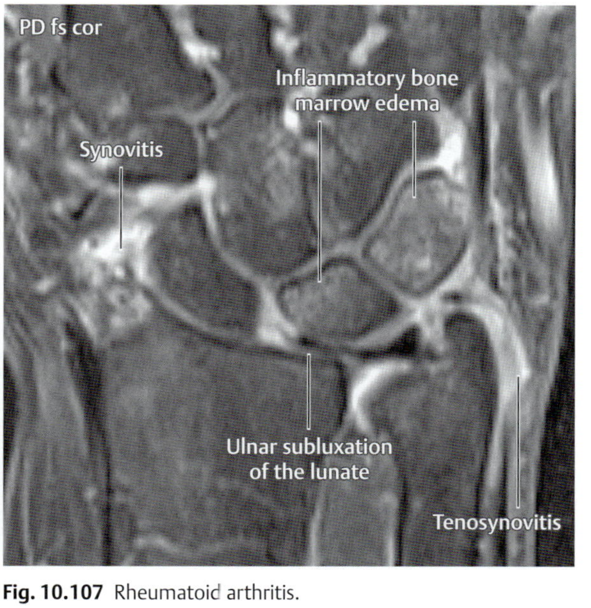

Fig. 10.107 Rheumatoid arthritis.

Collagen-splitting enzymes damage the ligaments, resulting in **subluxation or dislocation**, especially in the hands (▶ Fig. 10.108), the feet, and the atlantodental joint.

Early **secondary osteoarthritis** develops as a result of joint destruction (see ▶ Fig. 10.107). Mutilation and, less commonly, ankylosis occur with complete erosion of the articular surface.

Rheumatoid arthritis is a systemic disease. Numerous **extra-articular manifestations** involving lungs, heart, pericardium, nerves, and salivary glands (secondary Sjögren's syndrome) can also be detected using imaging techniques. Rheumatic nodules may develop in the soft tissues and lungs.

The first 3 months of rheumatoid arthritis are referred to as **early arthritis**. Timely initiation of treatment can favorably affect prognosis in this usually predestructive stage. During this phase, standard radiographs will usually appear normal since the disease is still predominantly confined to the synovial membrane, as can be confirmed by ultrasound and MRI (▶ Fig. 10.109).

▶ Clinical presentation. Clinical presentation and laboratory parameters are documented using the ACR/EULAR scoring system (▶ see References for Chapter 10.5), enabling recognition of early disease with enough confidence to justify effective therapy, despite its enormous clinical variability.

Joint manifestations are characteristically **symmetric** in the wrists, the metacarpophalangeal, the proximal interphalangeal, the metatarsophalangeal, and the interphalangeal joints, with morning stiffness of varying degrees, fusiform swelling, and pain.

10

Variants. In **rheumatoid arthritis of the older adult** (late-onset rheumatoid arthritis) after 60 years of age, classic radiographic features are often combined with signs of osteoarthritis (also known as "superimposed arthritis"; ▶ Fig. 10.110).

Patients with rheumatic disorders of the joints are prone to developing other autoimmune reactions. **Overlap syndrome** refers to the combination of rheumatoid arthritis and scleroderma.

▶ Radiography. To reach an initial diagnosis, radiographs of the hands and feet should include posteroanterior and posteroplantar views, as well as oblique views (with the hand in the modified teacup position). Any other symptomatic joints should be examined, usually including the cervical spine together with functional (flexion/extension) views. Oblique views may be dispensed with on follow-up examinations of the hands and feet.

Typical radiographic signs of rheumatoid arthritis (see also Chapter 10.1 for overview and possible differential diagnoses):

- **In the hand:** Earliest alterations include soft tissue swelling (better recognized using other modalities), juxta-articular decrease in bone density, loss of detail of the subchondral bone plate in joints, and loss of cortical detail (e.g., at the ulnar and radial styloid processes). Another sign is malalignment with ulnar subluxation of the lunate and simultaneous dorsal dislocation of the ulna (▶ Fig. 10.111; see also ▶ Fig. 10.107). More severe forms of malalignment (swan-neck or boutonniere deformity, shoemaker's or hitchhiker's thumb) and rheumatic hand scoliosis (▶ Fig. W10.19) have become rare. Other signs include joint space narrowing and marginal erosions (sometimes appearing as subchondral cysts; see ▶ Figs. 10.105 and ▶ 10.106) and, in late stages, mutilation or, less commonly, ankylosis (as os carpale of the carpus; ▶ see ▶ Fig. W10.19).

Note

Erosions do not develop or are considerably delayed when rheumatoid arthritis is properly treated. When erosions are present, the development of a sclerotic margin around the erosion is an indication of successful treatment (▶ Fig. 10.112). When looking for erosions of the hand, particular attention should be directed toward the index and middle fingers. With the wrist and ankle joint, extra-articular erosions (due to the adjacent inflamed tendon sheath) should also be noted, e.g., at the ulnar styloid process (▶ Fig. W10.20; see also ▶ Fig. 10.108).

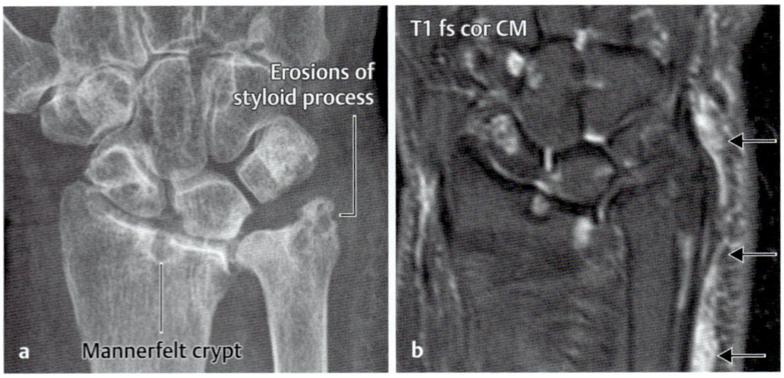

Fig. 10.108 Rheumatoid arthritis. **(a)** Localized widening of the radioscapholunate joint space due to inflammatory destruction of the radioscapholunate ligament with characteristic cyst at the radial ligament insertion (Mannerfelt crypt). **(b)** Tenosynovitis involving the extensor carpi ulnaris tendon (arrows), resulting in erosion of the ulnar styloid process. USP, ulnar styloid process.

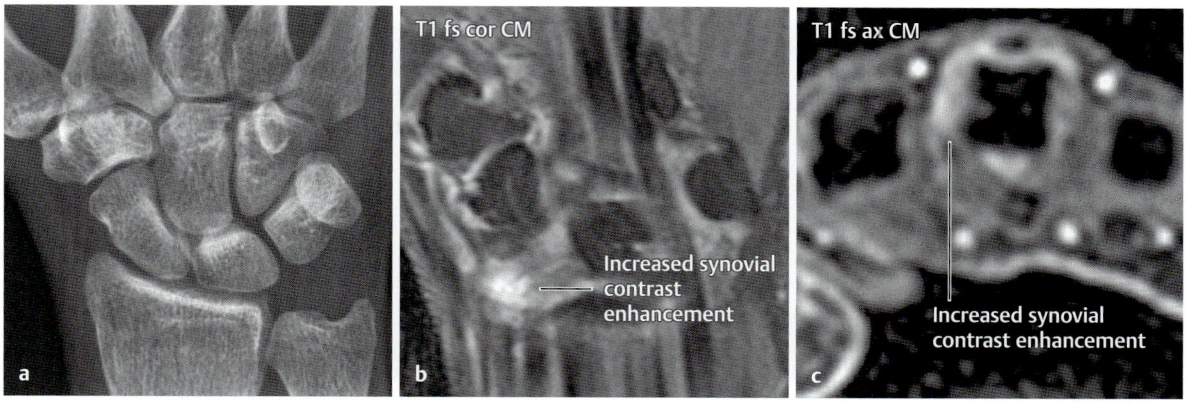

Fig. 10.109 Early arthritis. **(a)** Radiograph shows no abnormality. **(b)** MRI reveals carpal synovitis. **(c)** Evidence of synovitis in the third metacarpophalangeal joint after IV administration of contrast.

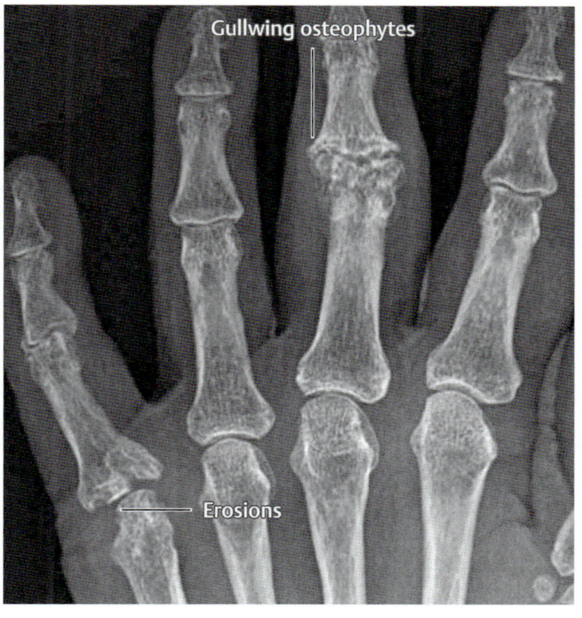

Fig. 10.110 Mixed picture of both rheumatoid arthritis and osteoarthritis ("superimposed arthritis").

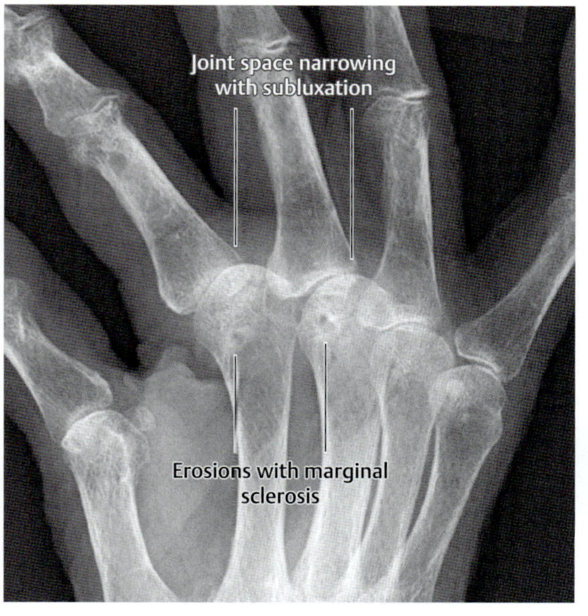

Fig. 10.112 Rheumatoid arthritis. Typical involvement of the second and third metacarpophalangeal joints. Oblique view.

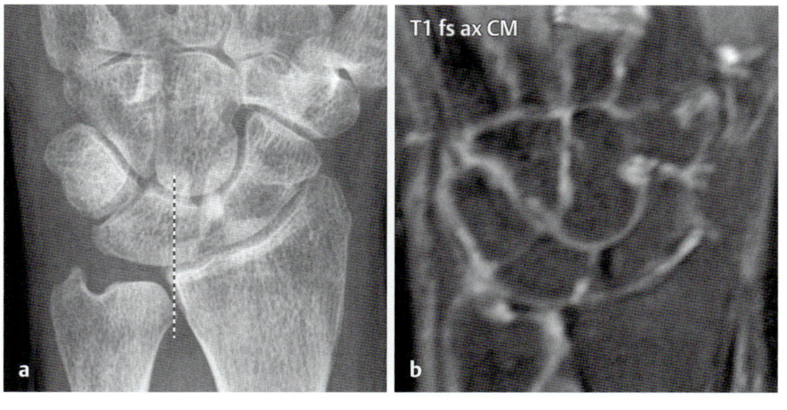

Fig. 10.111 Early signs of rheumatoid arthritis. **(a)** Ulnar subluxation of the lunate (by more than one half of its diameter over the edge of the radius: dashed line). **(b)** The joint spaces are filled with contrast-enhancing inflamed synovium.

10

- **In the foot:** The metatarsophalangeal joints are primarily involved, from lateral to medial.
- **In the cervical spine:** Of prognostic value is **subluxation of the atlantodental joint** with dorsal (▶ Fig. 10.113) or cranial (basilar impression; ▶ Fig. 10.114) subluxation of the odontoid process, as well as the other segments of the cervical spine ("rheumatic stepladder deformity"; ▶ Fig. 10.115). Rupture of the transverse atlantal ligament may be suspected in the presence of widening of the anterior atlantodental joint space by more than 5 mm; values over 3 mm or a significant increase during flexion are to be regarded as suspicious.
- **Soft tissue swelling** of the inflammatory type, i.e., with edema in the para-articular and subcutaneous fat stripes, is characteristically located over the ulnar styloid process (tenosynovitis of extensor carpi ulnaris; see ▶ Figs. 10.107 and ▶ 10.108) and at the second, third, and fifth metacarpophalangeal joints, in the feet at the fifth and second metatarsophalangeal joints, in the interphalangeal joint of the large toe, and as rheumatic pre-Achilles bursitis (▶ Fig. 10.116).
- **Rheumatic osteitis** manifests as circumscribed demineralization of the articular ends of the bone (juxta-articular osteoporosis). Because the accurate detection of this sign depends heavily on technical imaging parameters as well as the amount of overlying soft tissue swelling, this radiographic finding is difficult to conclusively diagnose.

> **Note**
> The Van der Heijde-modified Sharp score is currently used for quantifying radiographic signs of rheumatoid arthritis for treatment studies (see specialized literature).

10

▶ **US.** During the preerosive disease phase, radiographs are supplemented by ultrasound examination using probe frequencies of at least 12 MHz. Hypoechoic synovial swelling and hypoechoic to anechoic effusions of the joints and especially the tendon sheaths are the primary findings. Color Doppler ultrasound allows for grading the severity of the inflammatory process (▶ Fig. W10.21; see References for Chapter 10.5).

▶ **MRI.** T1W and T2W sequences, a fluid-sensitive fat suppression sequence, and as a rule IV contrast administration are employed. MRI serves to detect synovial swelling and enhancement, erosions and in particular juxta-articular bone marrow edema associated with rheumatic osteitis.

> **Note**
> In MRI osteitis does not only appear diffuse (see ▶ Fig. 10.107) but may also appear focal and small (▶ see Fig. W10.18). Given adequate treatment, MRI osteitis may not develop into radiographically visible erosions.

Juxta-articular bursae and synovial sheaths are often also inflamed. On rare occasions they may also contain hypointense low signal foci (rice bodies).

MRI of the upper cervical spine is of particular importance. It will provide information of the extent of pannus within the atlantodental joint and the relationship of the inflammatory tissue to the spinal cord. Destruction of the joint, including the transverse atlantal ligament, results in basilar invagination, which is well demonstrated on MRI (see ▶ Fig. 10.114).

▶ **DD.** The following differential diagnoses should be considered in the presence of synovitis.

Infection. This usually presents as a septic monoarthritis with a tendency toward early bone destruction. This is a typical complication of intensive immunosuppressive therapy. In children the cause may be osteomyelitis of the juxtaarticular bones.

Osteoarthritis with concomitant synovitis. It should be noted that in the hand, involvement of the carpometacarpal joint of the thumb and the distal interphalangeal joints is highly suggestive of osteoarthritis. These joints are rarely involved in rheumatoid arthritis.

Posttraumatic synovitis. This refers to a synovial reaction to a hemarthrosis or the result of synovial entrapment due to subluxation/dislocation, but in a wider sense, any synovial reaction developing after an injury is included under this term.

Crystal arthropathies and periarthropathies. See Chapter 10.9.

Psoriasis. See Chapter 10.6.3.

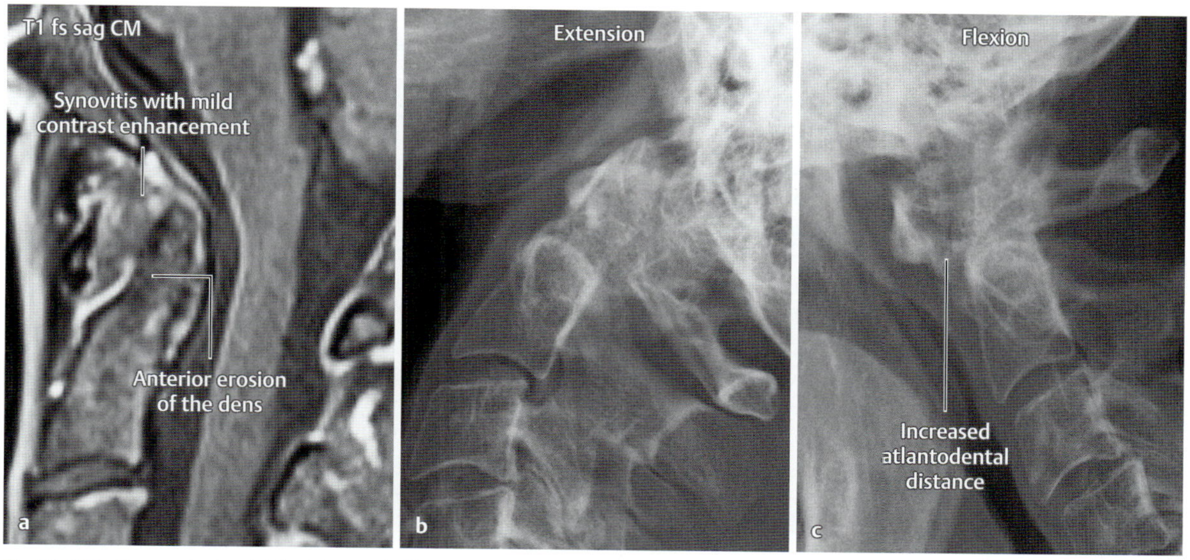

Fig. 10.113 Rheumatoid arthritis. **(a)** Largely fibrous synovitis with increased distance between the anterior arch of the atlas and the odontoid process. **(b)** Extension and **(c)** flexion views demonstrate significant atlantoaxial instability.

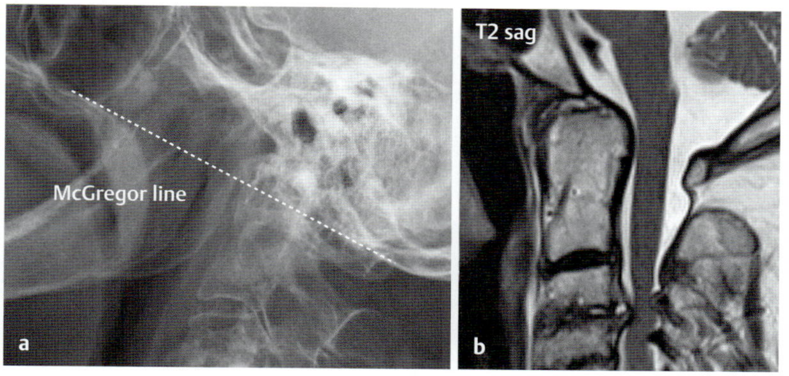

Fig. 10.114 Basilar impression in a patient with rheumatoid arthritis. **(a)** The tip of the odontoid process projects above McGregor's line (the line from the hard palate to the lowest point of the occiput) by more than 5 mm. **(b)** Postinflammatory atlantodental ankylosis with narrowing of the foramen magnum.

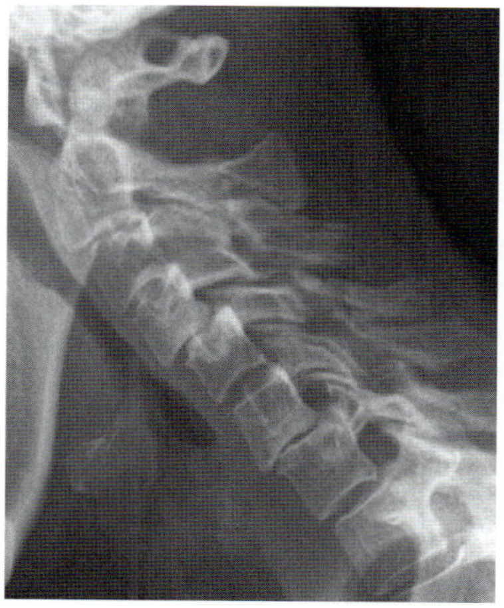

Fig. 10.115

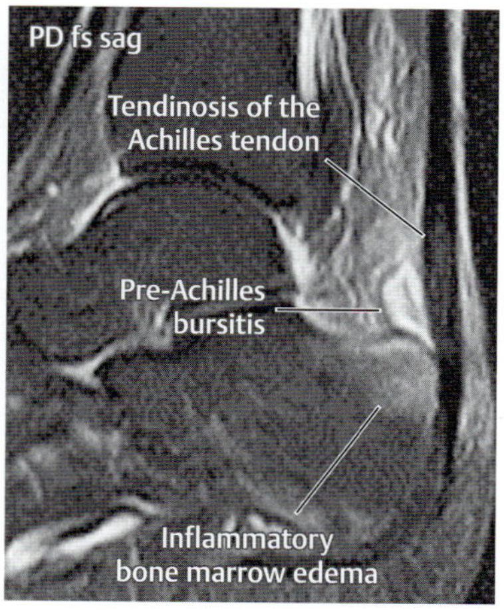

Fig. 10.116

Fig. 10.115 "Rheumatoid stepladder deformity." Multilevel vertebral subluxation secondary to inflammatory destruction of the discoligamentous stabilizers.

Fig. 10.116 Rheumatoid pre-Achilles bursitis.

10.5.2 Juvenile Idiopathic Arthritis

A distinction is made between three types of this heterogeneous group of diseases, which must have begun before the 16th year of life and have persisted for at least 6 weeks:

- **Systemic form (Still's disease):** associated with fever, exanthema, and hepatosplenomegaly (more than two-thirds of cases; the pattern of joint involvement of the hands and major joints is variable).
- **Juvenile idiopathic oligoarthritis:** with up to four inflamed joints, usually the knee and ankle.
- **Juvenile idiopathic polyarthritis:** seropositive or seronegative; with more than five inflamed joints in the early phase.

The disorder usually affects girls in early childhood.

► **Pathology.** The type of disease associated with erosions causes cessation of growth in the acute stage. With a less aggressive clinical course, **hyperemia in and around the growth plates** results in stimulation of growth with "ballooning" of the epiphyses and dysmorphic bone growth (► Fig. 10.117).

► **Radiography.** The appearance significantly differs from that of adult arthritides in the associated growth disturbances and the different significance of various radiographic signs (► Fig. 10.118, ► Figs. W10.22 and W10.23):

- Considerable soft tissue swelling.
- Erosions and joint space narrowings (less common than in the adult form).
- Juxta-articular osteoporosis.
- Periostitis that develops in the growing skeleton more markedly than in adults and can lead to thickening of the phalanges of the hands and feet.

► **US.** Effusions are easily detectable and are helpful for reaching a diagnosis, especially in the early phase, and also assessing progression on follow-up studies.

► **MRI.** Joint effusion and markedly hyperintense synovial membrane enhancement after IV contrast administration are the cardinal findings. Additional findings include cartilage abnormalities such as surface irregularity and thinning, as well as erosions and juxta-articular bone marrow edema.

► **DD.** Joint problems are common in children. Possible differential considerations include **septic arthritis** and **acute hematogenous osteomyelitis.** These infectious diseases are characterized by a monoarthritic involvement and usually pronounced clinical findings.

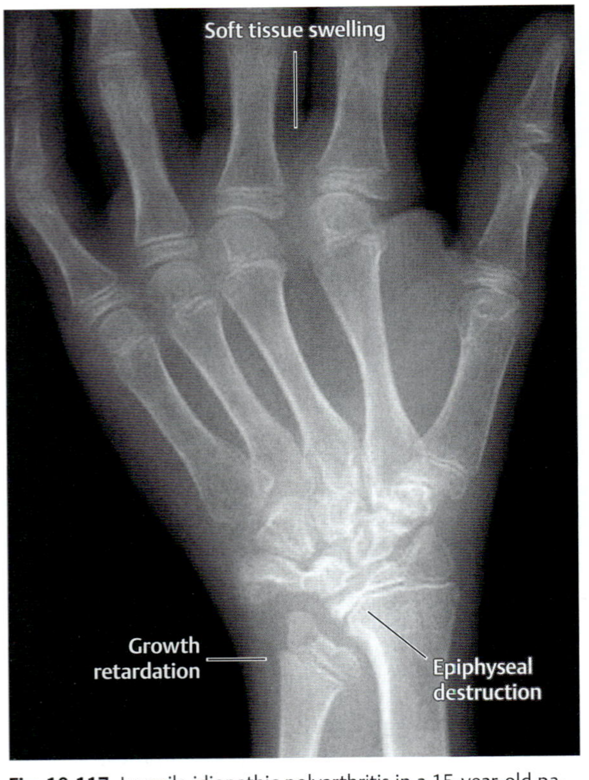

Fig. 10.117 Juvenile idiopathic polyarthritis in a 15-year-old patient who has had arthritis from 2 years of age. Note the associated deformities and interference with growth.

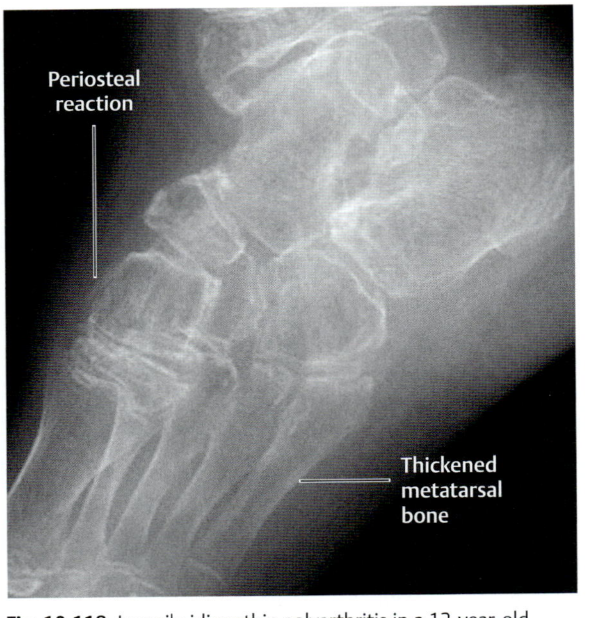

Fig. 10.118 Juvenile idiopathic polyarthritis in a 12-year-old female patient. Inflammatory periostitis and demineralization.

10.6 Spondylarthritis

The terms "seronegative spondylarthritis" and "seronegative spondylarthropathy" are used synonymously (seronegative because the serum rheumatoid factor is not elevated).

The spondylarthritides are a group of rheumatic diseases, each with characteristic clinical findings and a common genetic predisposition, especially for the antigen HLA-B27. Forms of spondylarthritis include **ankylosing spondylitis (Bechterew's disease), (infectious) reactive arthritis, psoriatic arthritis,** the **enteropathic arthropathies, SAPHO syndrome** (Chapter 10.7.2), **Type 2 juvenile oligoarthritis,** and **undifferentiated spondylarthritis.** Chronic, nonbacterial osteomyelitis should also be mentioned, even though it is not included in the official classifications (CRMO; Chapter 10.7.1).

▸**Pathology.** The cause remains hypothetical, possibly taking origin from a bacterial infection. Overloading of the endoplasmic reticulum with misfolded HLA-B27 proteins is believed to result in a proinflammatory response.

Whereas with rheumatoid arthritis the center of the inflammation is located in the synovial membrane and the clinical course, if left untreated, is progressive and destructive, with spondylarthritides the disease is predominantly located in and around the insertions of ligaments and tendons and has an intermittent course with juxtaposed bone destruction and proliferation.

The transitions between the individual forms of spondylarthritis are overlapping and fluid in about one-third of cases. For this reason the various staging systems are under continual development (▸Table W10.2; see References for Chapter 10.6). The current concept of the Spondylarthritis International Society (2009) distinguishes between the following forms:

- **Early (preradiographic) axial spondylarthritis:** This represents about one-half of all initial diagnoses.
- **Axial spondylarthritis:** This is diagnosed by inflammatory back pain plus: either diagnostic imaging findings and one other clinical feature of spondylarthritis are present, or HLA-B27 is positive and two other features of spondylarthritis (such as uveitis, dactylitis, psoriasis, among others) are present. Diagnostic imaging involves either a "positive" or "highly probable" MRI finding (with bone marrow edema or osteitis) or a definitive radiographic diagnosis according to the modified New York criteria (▸Fig. 10.119; ▸ see also ▸Table W10.2).
- **Peripheral spondylarthritis:** ▸Fig. 10.120.

▸**Clinical presentation.** Because the clinical symptoms are intermittent and highly variable, the time until the diagnosis is made averages 7 years. Radiographs are usually negative in the early phases, while correctly formulated case history questions are very sensitive (at just below 80%). The cardinal symptom of axial spondylarthritis is usually inflammatory low back pain. This is a specific form of back pain and presents when four of the following five criteria are fulfilled after 3 months of symptom duration: onset of symptoms before the age of 40 to 45 years; insidious onset; improvement with movement; no improvement with rest; nocturnal pain (improvement on getting up).

- Characteristic extremity symptoms are **oligoarthritis** and **enthesitis** (inflammation of tendon insertions, e.g., in the form of heel pain).
- Specific **organ manifestations** including inflammation of the eyes (such as iridocyclitis), mucosal inflammation (aphthous stomatitis, urethritis), and skin changes (psoriasis-like, among others). Less common findings, detectable by imaging studies include aortitis and interstitial pneumonia.

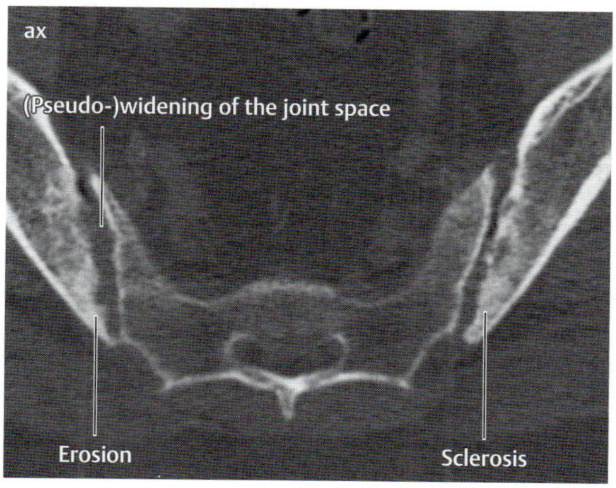

Fig. 10.119 Axial spondylarthritis. CT during the initial diagnostic work-up demonstrates bilateral sacroiliitis, Grade 3 according to the New York criteria (▸ see ▸Table W10.2).

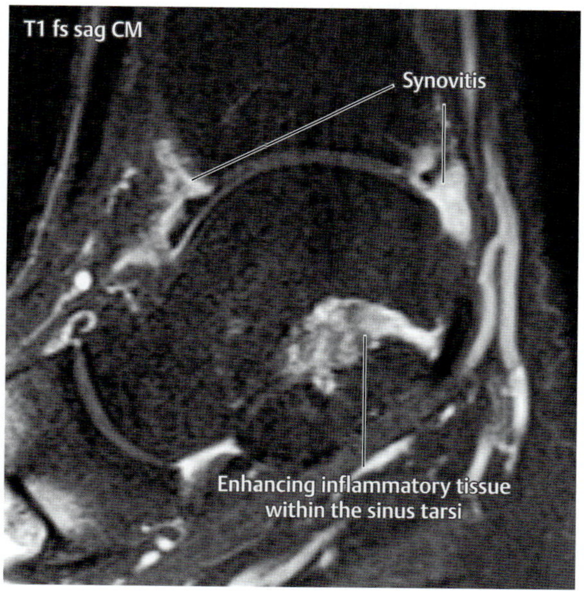

Fig. 10.120 Peripheral spondylarthritis. The same patient as in ▸Fig. 10.119. Inflammatory alterations of the ankle and subtalar joints.

10.6.1 Ankylosing Spondylitis

Ankylosing spondylitis (synonym: Bechterew's disease) is the prototype of spondylarthritis with target areas primarily involving the axial skeleton (especially the sacroiliac joints), the entheses (tendon–bone junction), and the peripheral joints.

▶ **Radiography/CT.** Compare also Chapter 10.1.2 and Chapter 10.1.3.

- **Sacroiliac joints:** The combination of extensive subchondral sclerosis, erosions, osseous bridging and ankyloses is usually present bilaterally (▶ Fig. 10.121). Sometimes these signs are confusing if the ankylosis is complete but with preserved contours (phantom joint) or the erosions become confluent resulting in "pseudo-widening" of the joint space; ▶ Fig. 10.122. CT is superior to conventional radiography for identifying osteoresorptive and osteoproliferative findings (▶ Fig. 10.123).
- **Spine:** Usually originating near the thoracolumbar junction, thin marginal syndesmophytes and shiny corners (Romanus lesion: sclerosis of the vertebral edges, possibly with concomitant erosions; ▶ Fig. 10.124) may be seen. In addition, arthritis of the facet joints and the costovertebral and costotransversal joints are features of spondylarthritis. More severe inflammatory exacerbations result in segmental destruction with noninfectious spondylodiskitis (inflammatory Andersson I lesion). Calcification of the anulus fibrosus and the interspinal ligaments ("double tramlines"), and squared and barrel-shaped vertebrae may develop late. Spondylarthritis-associated osteoporosis promotes the development of fractures of the rigid spine; if suspected, this is a classic indication for CT (▶ Fig. 10.125; Chapter 2.2.4). Insufficiency fractures of the bamboo spine (noninflammatory Andersson lesion II; Chapter 10.1.3) are usually found in the cervicothoracic spine.
- **Peripheral involvement of ankylosing spondylitis:** This typically occurs in the form of enthesitis (fibro-osteitis) with erosion, blurred ossification of tendon insertions or subtendinous sclerosis (see ▶ Fig. 10.122). Arthritis of the ankles or other, usually major, joints (▶ Fig. W10.24; see also ▶ Fig. 10.120) or synchondritis of the symphysis or sternum may also be present.

▶ **MRI.** The examination technique includes T1W, T2W, and fat-suppressed T2W sequences, and usually a fat-suppressed T1W sequence after contrast administration. Signs of active inflammation include subchondral or subtendinous bone marrow edema as an expression of rheumatic osteitis (▶ Fig. 10.126) and strong contrast enhancement in the joint space and in the subchondral bone. Sclerosis or postinflammatory fatty marrow conversion and ankyloses predominate in chronic inflammatory stages (▶ Fig. 10.127).

MRI enables detection of anterior spondylitis (▶ Figs. 10.128 and ▶ W10.25), inflammation of the small vertebral joints, inflammation of the interspinous ligaments (see ▶ Fig. 10.128), and involvement of the costotransverse and costovertebral joints.

▶ **DD.**

Differential diagnosis of sacroiliitis

- **Other forms of spondylarthritis:** Imaging alone does not provide any real differentiating criteria.
- **Septic sacroiliitis:** This usually manifests unilaterally and with abscess formation in the surrounding soft tissues, particularly anteriorly ("lava cleft phenomenon" on CT or MRI).
- **Sacroiliac joint osteoarthritis:** This involves narrow, bandlike subchondral sclerosis associated with osteophytes.
- **Osteitis condensans ilii (hyperostosis triangularis ilii):** This disorder is associated with typical triangular, bilateral, extensive sclerosis without joint destruction, usually after pregnancy.
- **Rheumatoid arthritis:** This rarely involves this location and is diagnosed using clinical and laboratory findings.

Differential diagnosis in cases of inflammatory alterations of the disks

- **Bacterial spondylodiskitis:** This destroys the adjacent vertebral end plates of one segment and is associated with extensive soft tissue inflammation and possibly abscess formation. The inflammatory Andersson I lesion, on the other hand, involves only parts of the superior and inferior end plates. These differences, however, eventually become blurred.
- **Acute intratrabecular herniated disk ("acute Schmorl's node"):** This is not an inflammatory reaction of the intervertebral disk but one within the surrounding bone. In most cases, several older fractures are found together with only one acute lesion.

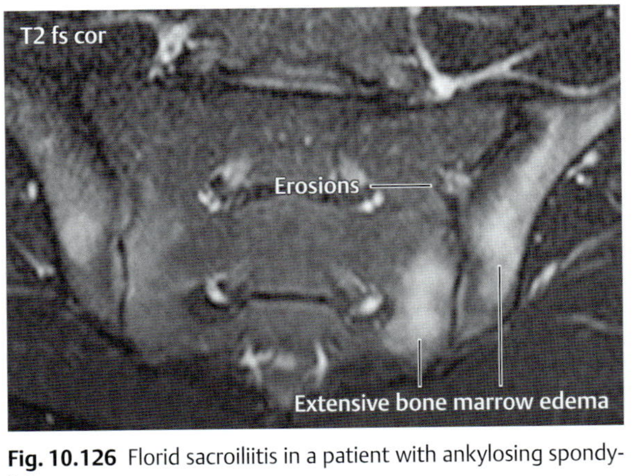

Fig. 10.126 Florid sacroiliitis in a patient with ankylosing spondylitis.

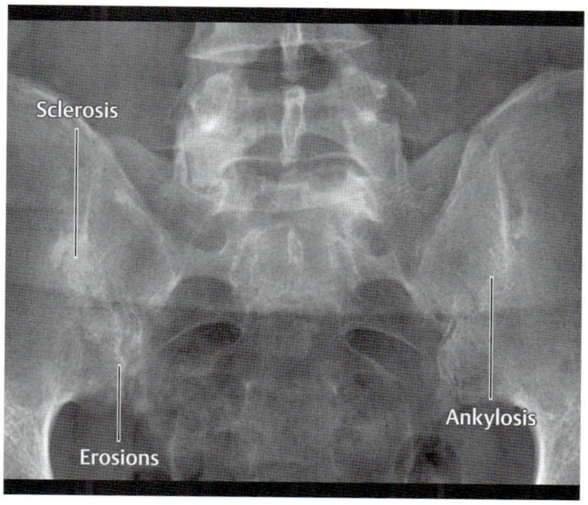

Fig. 10.121 Sacroiliitis in a patient with ankylosing spondylitis.

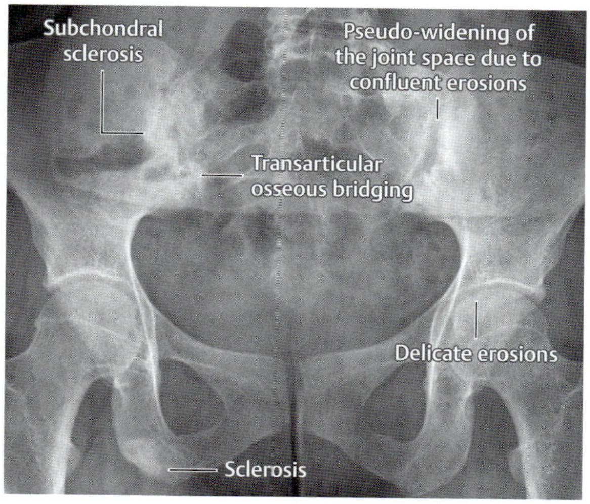

Fig. 10.122 Bilateral sacroiliitis, enthesopathy of the right ischium, and inflammatory arthritis of the left hip in a patient with ankylosing spondylitis.

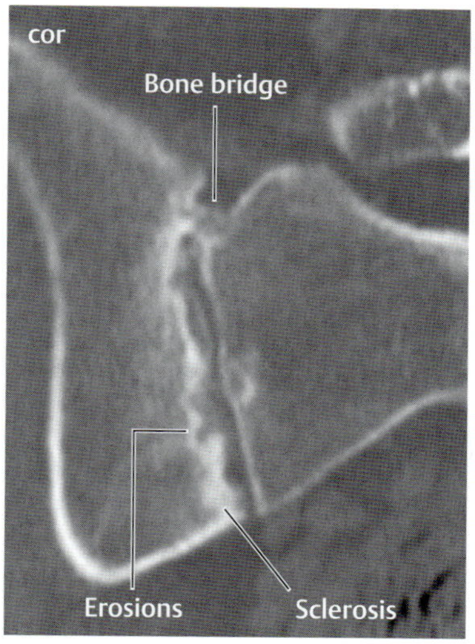

Fig. 10.123 Sacroiliitis in a patient with ankylosing spondylitis.

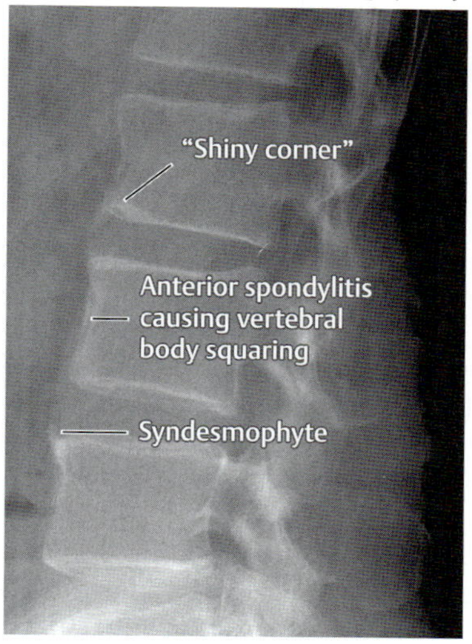

Fig. 10.124 Early anterior manifestations of ankylosing spondylitis.

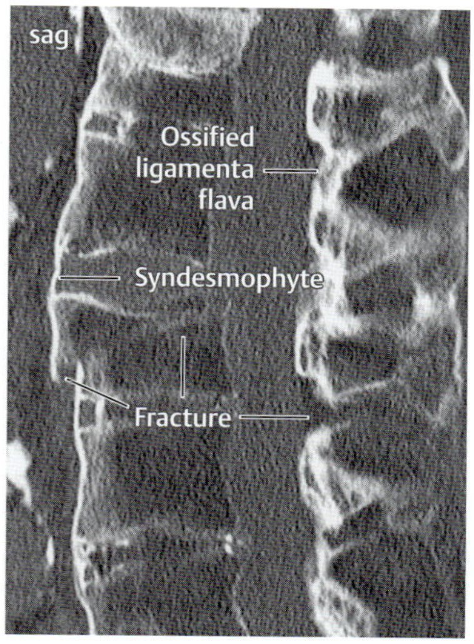

Fig. 10.125 Fracture of the bamboo spine in a patient with ankylosing spondylitis. Compare Chapter 2.2.4.

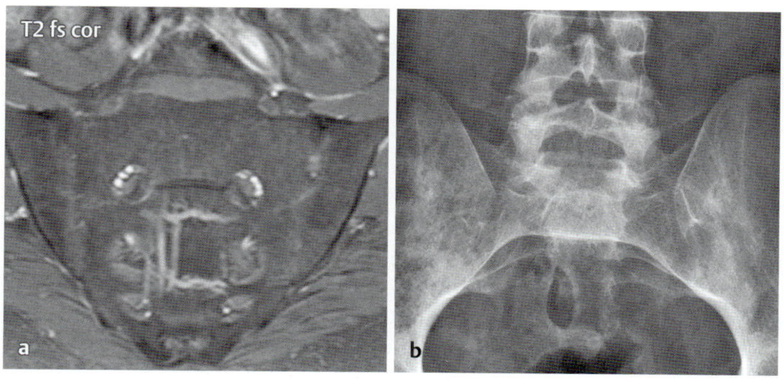

Fig. 10.127 "Burnt-out" bilateral sacroiliitis. **(a)** Postinflammatory diffuse fatty marrow conversion with no bone marrow edema. **(b)** Solid bilateral ankylosis.

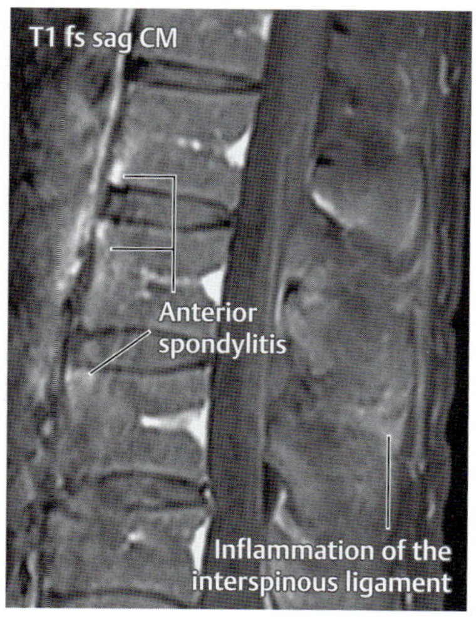

Fig. 10.128 Inflammatory manifestations of the spine in a patient with ankylosing spondylitis.

10.6.2 Reactive Arthritis

Reactive arthritis (synonym: Reiter's syndrome; this term was used formerly for the triad "urethritis, arthritis, and conjunctivitis") is a form of spondylarthritis secondary to a bacterial infection with a self-limiting course covering 3 to 12 months. If no connection can be established with a bacterial infection, then it is referred to as an undifferentiated arthritis or simply spondylarthritis (Chapter 10.6.5).

▶ **Pathology.** In 60% of cases an infection of the urogenital, gastrointestinal, or respiratory tract is diagnosed (most commonly from *Chlamydia* or *Salmonella*) during the month before onset of the disease. Peak incidence is in the 4th decade of life.

▶ **Clinical presentation.** Oligoarthritic involvement of the lower limbs is typical. Monoarthritis is rarely encountered. General symptoms include fever and weight loss. The affected joints are warm to the touch. A "sausage toe" is no rarity. Extra-articular manifestations (skin, urethritis, uveitis) make it clear that distinction from psoriasis and other forms of spondylarthritis is not always easy.

▶ **Radiography.** Significant effusions are found in the peripheral joints, usually without erosions. Associate sacroiliitis is usually bilateral but asymmetric; less commonly nonmarginal syndesmophytes are found in the spine.

▶ **MRI.** MRI reveals signs of synovitis that may be associated with subchondral bone marrow edema of the juxta-articular bones. Enthesitis (involving particularly the Achilles tendon and plantar fascia) is a common finding in reactive arthritis.

10

▶ **DD.**

Septic arthritis. This almost always presents as a monoarthritis and should be differentiated clinically from reactive arthritis.

Lyme arthritis. This is regarded as a variant of reactive arthritis and occurs during the late or chronic stage of borreliosis. Usually the knee is affected and presents with an effusion and soft tissue swelling, rarely with erosions and juxta-articular osteoporosis.

10.6.3 Psoriatic Arthritis

Psoriatic arthritis (synonyms: psoriatic arthropathy, arthritis psoriatica) is associated with underlying psoriasis (in 10% of cases the arthritis is present prior to the onset of the skin abnormalities) involving the joints, the entheses, and even (though less commonly) the spine.

▶ **Pathology.** Genetic, immunologic and environmental factors have been considered as initiating causes as well as numerous medications and mental factors. The arthritis arises particularly at the transition zones between capsule and periosteum with significant vascular involvement. A direct diffusion of proinflammatory cytokines from these structures into the adjacent synovial membrane, periarticular soft tissues (resulting in a sausage digit [dactylitis]), and bone is assumed. Location at the distal interphalangeal joints, which contain less synovial tissue and more prominent fibrous capsular structures, also reinforces the concept of enthesitis as the primary disease manifestation.

▶ **Clinical presentation.** The diverse presentation is subsumed into three flowing pictures: by far the most common is **limb involvement**, then **trunk involvement** (in up to 1 in 4 cases), and **enthesitis** at the insertion sites of tendons and extra-articular ligaments (e.g., on the calcaneus).

Unlike rheumatoid arthritis, limb involvement tends to be asymmetric and occurs in about two-thirds of cases as oligoarthritis, otherwise as polyarthritis, and rarely as monoarthritis. A distinction is made between subtypes of oligoarthritis:

- Axial type involving the hands or feet with uniform soft tissue swelling (dactylitis with sausage digits).
- Transverse type involving the wrists and interphalangeal joints.
- Manifestation involving the knee or other major joints.

The polyarthritic form is in many ways similar to rheumatoid arthritis. This tends to occur later in the course of the disease and has a poor prognosis, i.e., it can result in mutilating arthritis.

Asymmetric sacroiliitis, spondylitis, and occasionally inflammatory alterations of the sternum (arthritis of the sternoclavicular joint or synchondritis manubriosternalis) are often found where involvement of the trunk predominates (psoriatic spondylitis).

▶ **Radiography.** Compare also Chapter 10.1.2 and Chapter 10.1.3.

The joints

- **Soft tissue swelling:** sausage digits (dactylitis).
- Inflammation of the joints at capsular insertions, subperiosteal, short, broad-based proliferations (**protuberances**), and small **erosions,** which are typical for spondylarthritis and together produce the appearance of "mouse ears" (▶ Figs. 10.129–10.131). Massive destruction finally results in "pencil-in-cup" or "pencil-to-pencil" deformities (▶ Fig. W10.26), while complete ankylosis can be seen in the final stage.
- **Periosteal sclerosis** in the form of a protuberance (see ▶ Fig. 10.131); more extensive bony sclerosis produces an "ivory phalanx."

- **Acro-osteolysis** is rare and associated with characteristic findings in the nails (oil-drop, pitting, onycholysis).

Spine

- **Sacroiliitis.**
- In the spine, bull horn–like or comma-shaped nonmarginal syndesmophytes are seen (▶ Fig. 10.132). Less commonly, marginal syndesmophytes are encountered. Compared with those of ankylosing spondylitis, they are more frequently asymmetric and involve the middle and lower lumbar spine rather than the thoracolumbar junction.

▶ US. Signs of strongly vascularized synovitis or enthesitis may be found, even at sites with few clinical symptoms. Tenosynovitis is often detected as well. These findings may be of assistance in specifying clinical oligoarthritis with a characteristic distribution pattern of an axial or transverse involvement (▶ Fig. 10.133).

▶ MRI. An important finding in addition to the radiographic features already mentioned is evidence of rheumatic bone marrow edema (see ▶ Fig. 10.130).

▶ DD.

Osteoarthritis. The associated osteophytes are shorter and usually larger than the osseous protuberances of psoriasis; in the fingers they are gullwinglike and the surrounding soft tissue swelling is nodular. Sometimes the radiographic images look deceptively similar, so the clinical context must also be taken into account.

Rheumatoid arthritis. The imaging findings in the polyarthritic form of psoriatic arthritis can be similar, as can the less common form of psoriasiform rheumatoid arthritis with significant periarticular soft tissue swelling. The clinical presentation is decisive for differentiation.

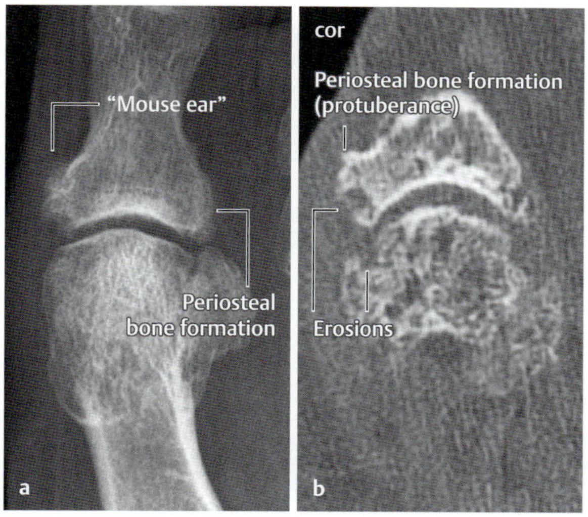

Fig. 10.129 Psoriatic arthritis. **(a)** Involvement of the metatarsophalangeal joint. **(b)** Detailed presentation on CT.

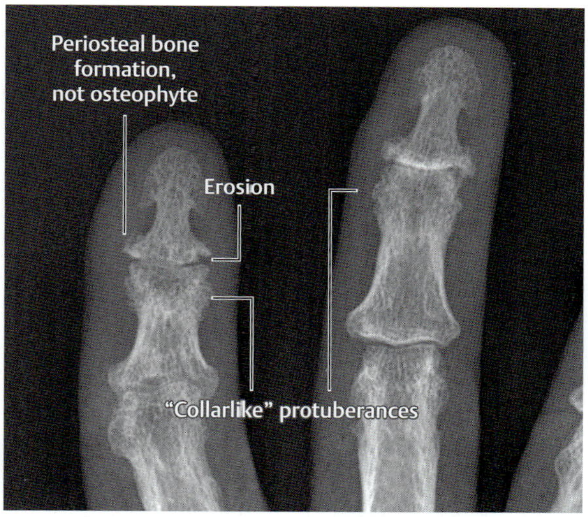

Fig. 10.131 Psoriatic arthritis with oligoarthritic involvement of the fingers.

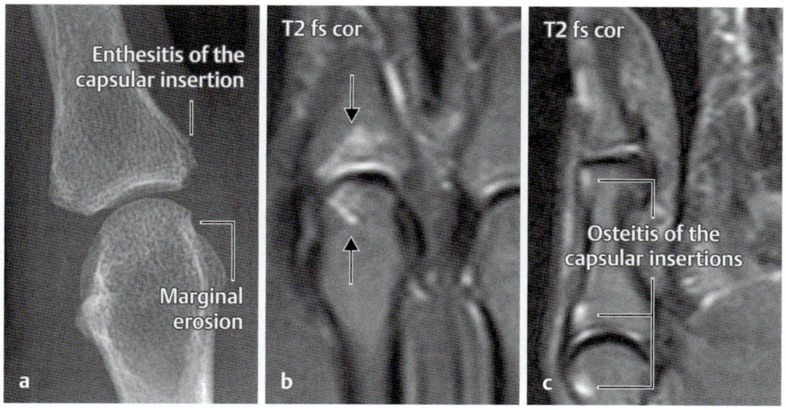

Fig. 10.130 Psoriatic arthritis in a 22-year-old woman. **(a)** Only mild radiographic abnormalities are evident in the second metacarpophalangeal joint. **(b)** MRI reveals bone marrow edema at the second metacarpophalangeal joint (arrows). **(c)** There is also evidence of very early involvement of the first ray.

10.6.4 Enteropathic Arthritis

This disorder is associated with chronic inflammatory bowel diseases, usually Crohn's disease (▶ Fig. 10.134), less commonly ulcerative colitis, and less frequently with other intestinal disorders, such as celiac disease, collagenous colitis, or primary biliary cirrhosis. Involvement of the musculoskeletal system by Whipple's disease (the rod bacterium *Tropheryma whipplei*) is classified under infectious arthritis.

▶ **Clinical presentation.** Since arthralgias often occur with or without mild gastrointestinal symptoms, these clinical pictures should be taken into consideration if such equivocal signs and symptoms develop. Joint and spinal problems tend to be of secondary importance for the disease course and treatment.

▶ **Radiology/CT/MRI.** Sacroiliitis is usually bilateral. Peripheral arthritis is nonspecific and usually confined to juxta-articular osteoporosis and soft tissue findings. Joint-space narrowing is very rare; erosive alterations are occasionally encountered in cases of primary biliary cirrhosis. Areas of lamellated periosteal reaction are common.

▶ **DD. Septic sacroiliitis.** A careful search should be made for any persistent connections (fistulas) leading from a segment of inflamed bowel to the sacroiliac joint, resulting in septic sacroiliitis. A finding of a primarily destructive component of sacroiliitis supports infection.

10.6.5 Undifferentiated Spondylarthritis

▶ **Pathology.** Together with ankylosing spondylitis, undifferentiated spondylarthritis is the most common form of spondylarthritis. The clinical, laboratory, and imaging findings of undifferentiated spondylarthritis, reactive arthritis, and, above all, ankylosing spondylitis overlap.

The diagnosis "undifferentiated spondylarthritis" is made when the clinical criteria suggest spondylarthritis but more specific criteria for ankylosing spondylarthritis, psoriasis, enteropathic spondylarthritis, or a bacterial trigger are absent. There are no pathognomonic clinical or laboratory findings. Some patients with the diagnosis "undifferentiated spondylarthritis" eventually develop more specific signs of ankylosing spondylarthritis and are then reclassified.

▶ **Clinical presentation.** Low back pain, peripheral arthritis, and evidence of enthesopathy of varying degrees are the primary clinical findings.

▶ **Radiology/CT/MRI.** Radiographs of the spine, pelvis, and peripheral joints are often normal. CT is more sensitive than radiography for demonstrating early forms of sacroiliitis (usually unilateral) and—rarely—a syndesmophyte. MRI can diagnose early sacroiliitis, which is evident in ~80% of cases with the initial diagnosis of undifferentiated spondylarthritis. Imaging of peripheral arthritis and enthesitis follows the same rules as for other spondylarthritides.

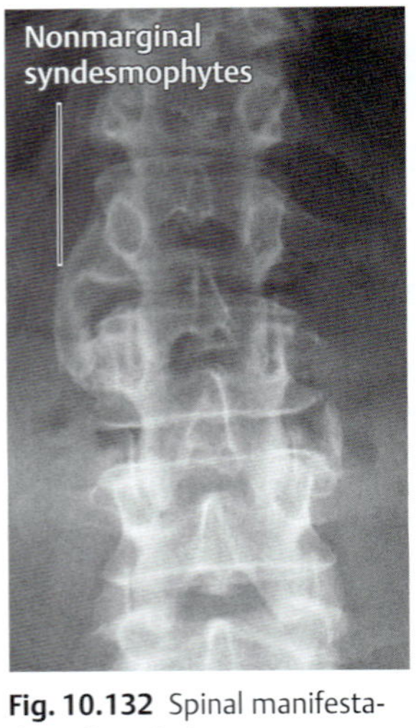

Fig. 10.132 Spinal manifestation of psoriasis.

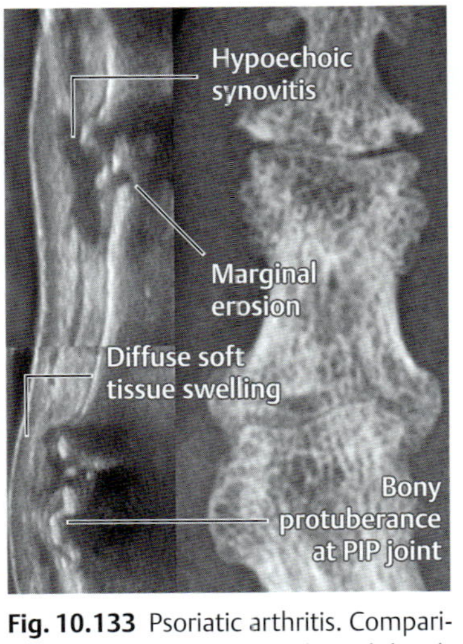

Fig. 10.133 Psoriatic arthritis. Comparison between radiology (enlarged detail from ▶ Fig. 10.131) and ultrasound. The composite image demonstrates the importance of ultrasound in providing a detailed presentation of inflammatory alterations and bone proliferation. PIP joint, proximal interphalangeal joint.

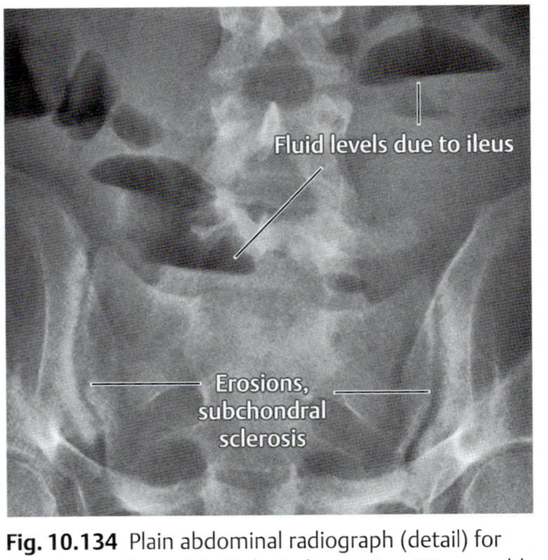

Fig. 10.134 Plain abdominal radiograph (detail) for ileus in a patient with Crohn's disease in a 29-year-old patient. Bilateral enteropathic sacroiliitis as an additional finding.

10.7 Chronic Recurrent Multifocal Osteomyelitis and SAPHO Syndrome

10.7.1 Chronic Recurrent Multifocal Osteomyelitis

CRMO is a nonbacterial form of chronic inflammation of the skeletal system in childhood and adolescence and is classified as a spondylarthritis (Chapter 10.6). There are overlaps with SAPHO (Chapter 10.7.2).

► **Pathology.** A distinction is made between three histological phases:

- Acute granulocytic **initial phase,** which is occasionally difficult to separate histologically from an acute hematogenous osteomyelitis.
- Lymphoplasmacytic **intermediate phase,** which is synonymous with the term "plasma cell osteomyelitis."
- **Healed phase** with marked sclerosis.

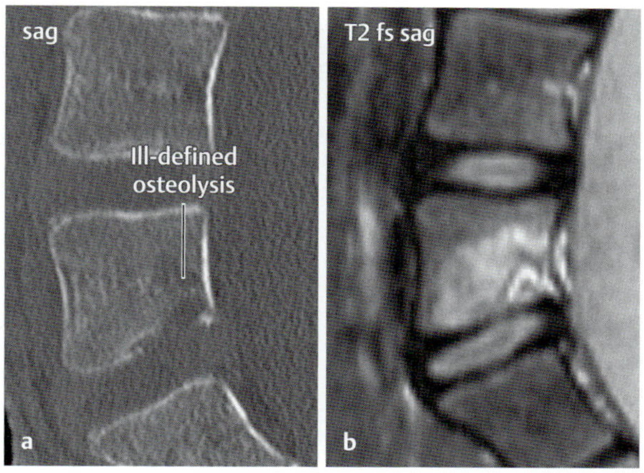

Fig. 10.135 CRMO. **(a)** Osteolytic lesion in L5. **(b)** Classic focus with surrounding edema. The morphological appearance is indistinguishable from bacterial osteomyelitis.

The cause of the inflammation is controversial. Identification of a pathogen is usually unsuccessful; neither pus formation nor fistula formation is seen. The simultaneous presentation of CRMO and a skin disease such as palmoplantar pustulosis or psoriasis vulgaris, is occasionally observed.

► **Clinical presentation.** Intermittent pain and swelling predominate. Fever and elevation of ESR and CRP levels are absent or present to only a mild degree. Children and adolescents are affected. Symptoms can develop at various sites and recur over months or even years. The metaphyses of long bones, the medial portion of the clavicle, the spine, and the sacrum are particularly affected, although any part of the skeleton may be involved. CRMO may start as a monofocal or multifocal disease. At certain intervals, new lesions occur while others have already healed. Simultaneous involvement of bones and joints is not uncommon, and involvement especially of the sacroiliac and sternoclavicular joints may be encountered. Treatment is supportive, on the basis of symptoms; the administration of antibiotics is not necessary.

► **Radiography/CT.** The radiographic appearance depends on the duration of clinical symptoms. If the clinical symptoms have been present for only a short time (less than 3 weeks), osteolytic lesions with blurred margins may be seen and may mimic acute osteomyelitis (► Fig. 10.135a). With more chronic symptoms, the radiographic findings are variable: osteolytic lesions with a sclerotic margin are most common, while mixed lytic and sclerotic lesions (► Figs. 10.136–10.138 and ► Fig. W10.27) and purely osteosclerotic alterations are also seen. Even without treatment, the radiographic course of these lesions is characterized by progressive sclerosis or even complete remission.

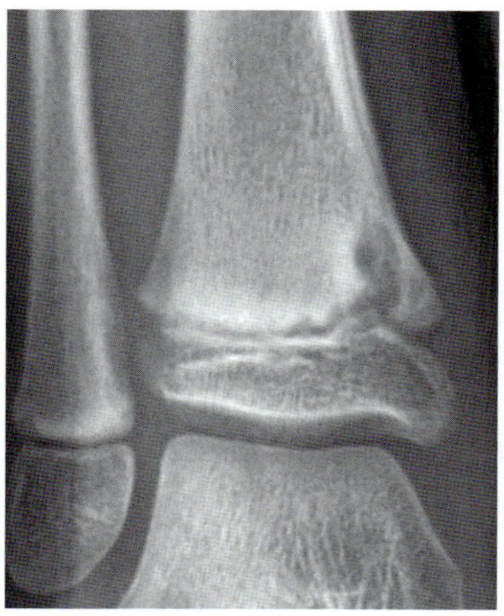

Fig. 10.136 CRMO. Mixed lytic and sclerotic lesion of the distal tibia.

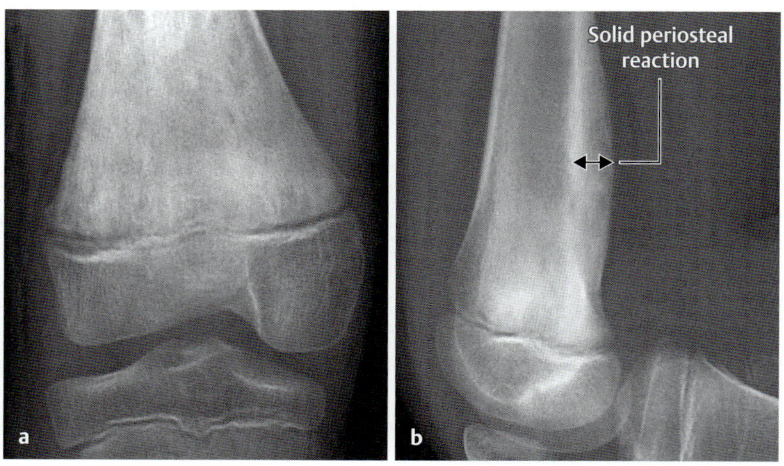

Fig. 10.137 CRMO of the distal femur. **(a)** Mixed lytic and sclerotic alterations of the metaphysis. **(b)** Marked dorsal periosteal reaction.

▸ NUC MED. Triphasic bone scan with technetium 99 m compounds may be utilized to make a diagnosis, and detect clinically silent foci.

▸ MRI. Early on, asymptomatic foci may demonstrate marrow edema (▸ Fig. 10.139). As a rule, the findings at the time of diagnosis are essentially identical with those of acute osteomyelitis (▸ Figs. 10.135b and ▶ W10.28). Osteosclerosis does not become apparent on MRI until much later (see ▸ Fig. 10.138). Moreover, serial MRI examinations can be used to follow activity of the disease (▶ Fig. W10.29); IV administration of gadolinium is useful. Whole-body MRI has clearly diminished the role of nuclear medicine in looking for silent foci.

▸ DD.

Bacterial osteomyelitis. With a solitary focus in a child or adolescent it is difficult, if not impossible, using imaging techniques to distinguish between bacterial osteomyelitis and an early stage of CRMO. The presence of an abscess supports bacterial osteomyelitis. The larger the sclerotic component, the more likely is the diagnosis of CMRO. It is crucial to correlate the imaging findings with the clinical presentation. Mild pain, a slow and undulating clinical course, absent or only slightly elevated inflammatory markers, and signs of sclerosis on the radiograph or CT indicate expectant observation and conservative, supportive treatment.

Malignant lymphoma. Malignant lymphoma should be considered if there are multifocal abnormalities. However, this disease is extremely rare in childhood and adolescence.

Osteoid osteoma. With a solitary finding, differentiation from osteoid osteoma is not always easy using standard radiographic imaging techniques (cf. Chapter 4.2.1); in these cases CT is the best modality. A central radiolucency with a small intralesional calcification supports the diagnosis of osteoid osteoma. A history of pronounced night pain and good response to medication are also supportive findings for osteoid osteoma. A CT-guided biopsy is rarely indicated.

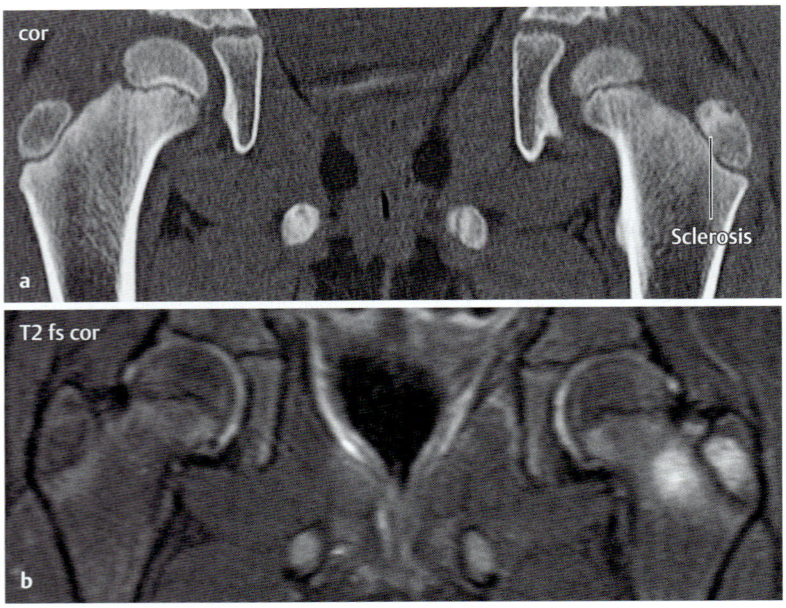

Fig. 10.138 CRMO. **(a)** Focal sclerosis of the left trochanteric apophysis. **(b)** Periphyseal edema on MRI; the sclerosis is not yet visible.

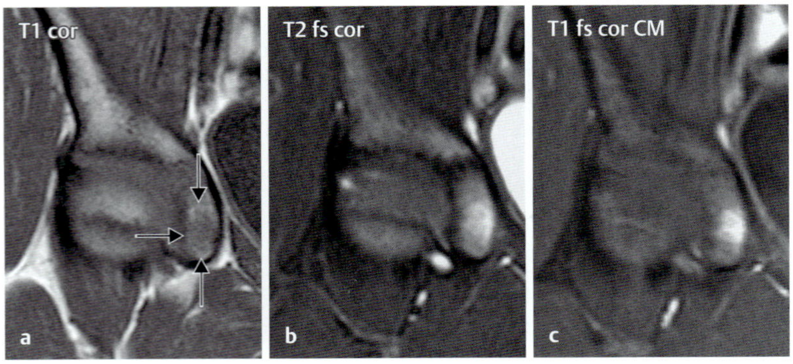

Fig. 10.139 CRMO. Very early, nonspecific periacetabular involvement. **(a)** Hypointense focus on T1W image (arrows). **(b)** Hyperintense edema on the T2W image. **(c)** Strong contrast enhancement.

10

Langerhans cell histiocytosis (eosinophilic granuloma). The radiological morphology of eosinophilic granuloma depends largely on the stage at which the eosinophilic granuloma is diagnosed. Osteolytic lesions are commonly seen in the **spine** and **pelvis** (▸Fig 4.102). The vertebrae can collapse to form a vertebra plana (▸ Fig. W4.17). However, in the majority of cases of CRMO, osteosclerosis is part of the radiological appearance, distinguishing CRMO from eosinophilic granuloma.

Relatively sharply delineated osteolytic rarefactions are found in eosinophilic granuloma in **tubular bones**, as well as moth-eaten osteolytic lesions (▸Fig. 4.103). A sclerotic margin appears if the lesion heals spontaneously.

10.7.2 SAPHO

SAPHO represents a spectrum of abnormalities of the skin, bones, and joints, which can appear simultaneously or consecutively and with different manifestations. SAPHO manifests in the skeleton and joints as **synovitis, hyperostosis,** and **osteitis**. The fundamental component of the SAPHO spectrum is osteitis. A clinical course with remissions and recurrences, its pathohistology, laboratory results, and imaging findings point to the close connection between CRMO (in children and adolescents) and SAPHO (primarily in younger adults).

The term "SAPHO" was coined by Chamot and colleagues in 1987. As early as 1961 an association was reported between acne conglobata and arthritis, and in 1972 between CRMO and palmoplantar pustulosis. The "S" in SAPHO initially stood for "syndrome," but was soon changed to indicate "synovitis." Meanwhile the view has increasingly gained ground that SAPHO in fact is not a syndrome but a spectrum of pathological findings. SAPHO is a chronic disease of the (mostly young) adult with remissions and recurrences. Its clinical course varies greatly from individual to individual. Clinical courses lasting decades have been reported. Clinical signs and symptoms include pain, swelling, and limitation of motion (▸ Fig. W10.30). ESR and CRP values are normal, or only moderately elevated.

SAPHO spectrum

- **Skin disorders:** Acne and palmoplantar pustulosis are typical comorbidities, with incidence in connection with SAPHO reported to be 20 to 60%. Absence of skin changes, therefore, does not exclude SAPHO. Psoriasis vulgaris or pustular psoriasis can also be associated with the osteoarticular SAPHO spectrum, with or without classic signs of psoriatic spondylarthropathy. Skin lesions can precede the osteoarticular manifestations by years, appear simultaneously with them, or occur after them.
- **Hyperostosis and osteomyelitis:** These manifestations are the expression of a chronic inflammation involving cortical and cancellous bone, without a bacterial origin being established. In the early stage, the alterations are not histologically distinguishable from those of a bacteria-induced osteomyelitis. Synovitis is a common finding, while inflammation at osteotendinous junctions ("enthesitis") is rarer. In ~80% of adult cases, joints of the anterior chest wall, the sacroiliac joints, and, less commonly, the peripheral joints are affected. Hyperostosis is found in adults primarily in the articular ends of the clavicles, ribs, and sternum as well as in the vertebral bodies. This is rarely found in the pelvis tubular bones.

▸ **Radiography.**

Anterior chest wall. Every component is involved, especially the sternoclavicular joints and the sternocostal, costochondral, and manubriosternal articulations. The following radiographic features are common:

- Erosive destruction of the articular margins of the joint (▸Fig. 10.140).
- Irregularity and apparent widening of the joint space.
- Enlargement and sclerosis of the articular ends of the bones (see ▸Fig. 10.140).
- Ossification of the ligaments, especially the costoclavicular ligament.
- Ankylosis of the sternocostal articulations.

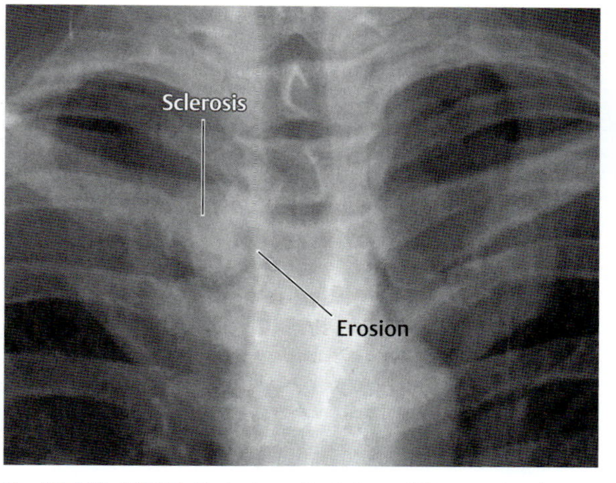

Fig. 10.140 SAPHO. Typical manifestation of the anterior chest wall.

Spine. The thoracic spine is primarily affected. Four main findings are common, occurring individually or in parallel:

- *Abacterial spondylodiskitis:* Erosions with surrounding sclerosis are evident in the superior and inferior end plates. The intervertebral disk space is often narrow.
- *Osteosclerosis* of one or several vertebrae.
- *Paravertebral ossification:* resembles findings in psoriatic spondylarthropathy (▶ Fig. 10.141). Furthermore, bony bridges can develop over a long segment along the anterior vertebral bodies.
- *Involvement of the sacroiliac joints:* Unilateral sacroiliitis is a common component of SAPHO. Osteosclerosis and hyperostosis are found primarily along the iliac side of the sacroiliac joint with concomitant involvement of larger parts of the ilium.

Tubular bones, flat bones. Osteolysis and "moth-eaten" destruction are sometimes found in the early stages, but osteosclerosis and hyperostosis predominate.

Peripheral joints. Juxta-articular osteopenia appears in the acute phase of synovitis. This is eventually followed by erosions (▶ Fig. 10.142). The articular margins of the adjacent bones can become sclerotic in the late phase (▶ Fig. 10.143).

▶ **CT.** The radiographic findings are better displayed by CT; this is especially advantageous in the chest wall, spine, and pelvis as well as in areas of complex anatomy such as the hand and foot (▶ Fig. W10.31; see ▶ Fig. 10.142).

▶ **NUC MED.** Radionuclide scanning is commonly used in cases of suspected SAPHO. There is massive tracer accumulation during the blood pool phase of a triphasic bone scan. The "bull's head sign" at the sternoclavicular and sternocostal joints is pathognomonic (▶ Fig. 10.144). If other areas of abnormal uptake are found in the skeleton apart from the bull's head sign, then a presumptive diagnosis of "SAPHO" may be made.

▶ **MRI.** In many cases MRI can replace a bone scan, since the alterations of the anterior chest wall together with the clinical context allow for a presumptive diagnosis of "SAPHO." Hypointense zones on T1W images and significantly increased signal intensity on fluid-sensitive sequences and in T1W after IV contrast administration are seen. Although these findings are nonspecific, the distribution of involvement (sternoclavicular joint, costosternal, and manubriosternal synchondroses) is an important indication of SAPHO (▶ Fig. 10.145). The precise differentiation from other spondylarthritides will require further clinical and laboratory investigation. SAPHO-related findings of synovitis and osteomyelitis in other regions are nonspecific (▶ Fig. 10.146). In particular, differentiation from other types of arthritic conditions is not possible.

▶ **DD.**

Septic arthritis. Scintigraphy or whole-body MRI provides important clues for differentiation of SAPHO from septic arthritis based on the involvement of the anterior chest wall and other sites (if present). Furthermore, periarticular osteosclerosis predominates in the late stage of SAPHO.

Bacterial spondylodiskitis. With SAPHO there is no evidence of paravertebral abscesses. Significant osteosclerosis is also an indication of SAPHO. In the early stage of SAPHO the intervertebral disk is sometimes not yet affected.

Bacterial osteomyelitis. In the early stage, differentiation of SAPHO from bacterial osteomyelitis is not possible based on imaging findings.

Degenerative alterations of the anterior chest wall. Bone scan and MRI are capable of differentiating between SAPHO and degenerative alterations with their characteristic abnormalities. CT or MRI confirms erosions, which support a diagnosis of SAPHO. Extensive osteosclerotic changes are also supportive of SAPHO and not osteoarthritis.

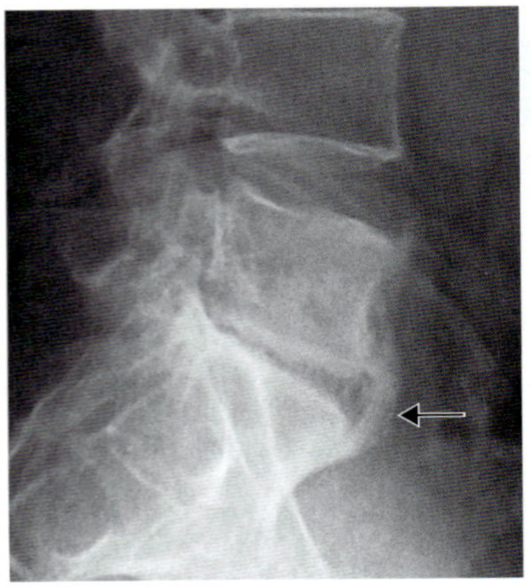

Fig. 10.141 SAPHO. Lumbosacral paravertebral ossification (arrow) and diffuse sclerosis of L5.

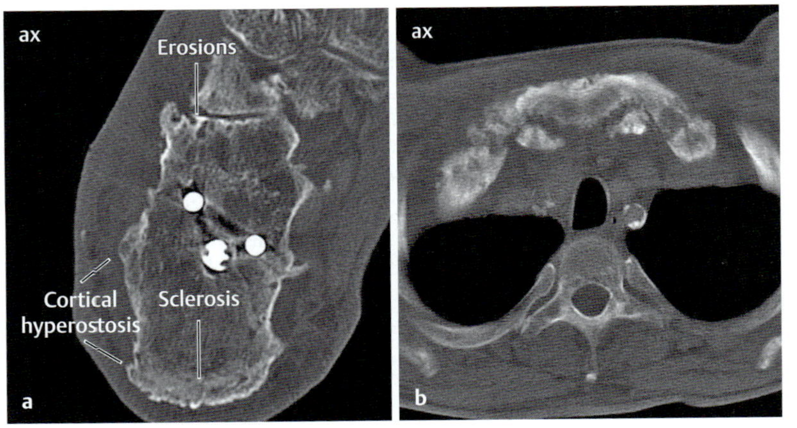

Fig. 10.142 SAPHO. **(a)** Destructive arthropathy that has already resulted in fusion of the subtalar joint. **(b)** In addition there is the typical involvement of the costosternal region (▶ see also ▶ Fig. W10.31).

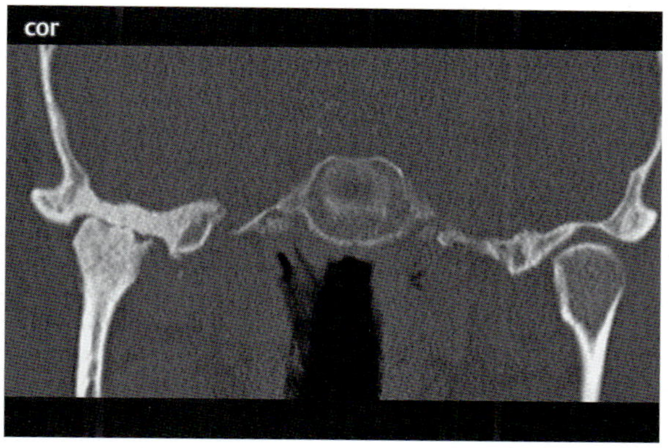

Fig. 10.143 Late stage secondary to arthropathy of the right temporomandibular joint in a patient with SAPHO. Note the significant sclerosis.

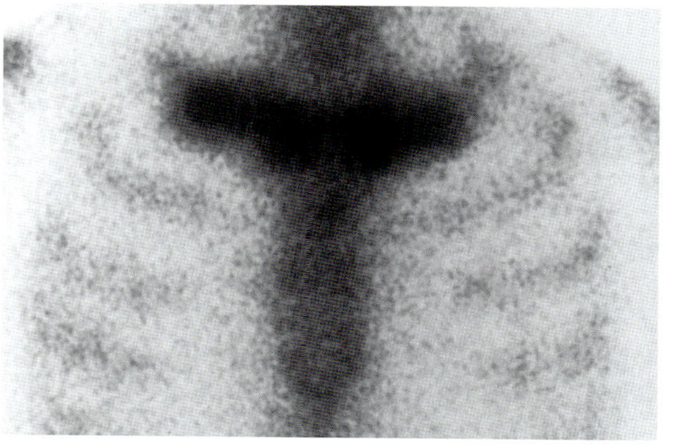

Fig. 10.144 Bull's head sign in the bone scan of a patient with SAPHO.

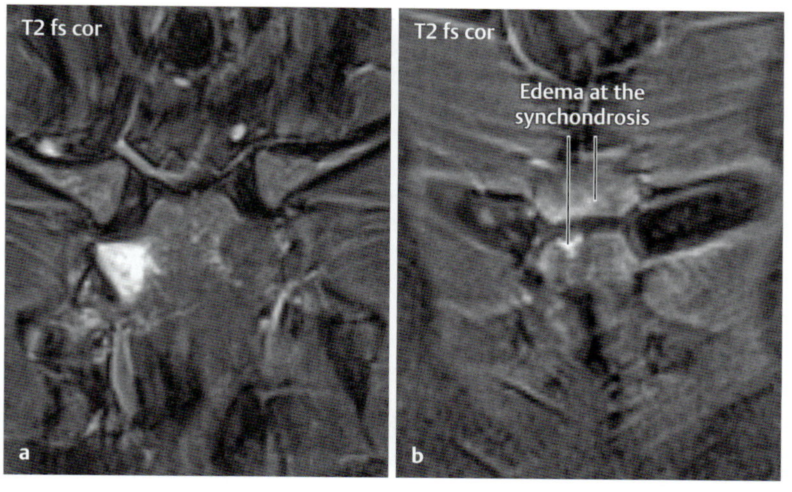

Fig. 10.145 SAPHO. (a) Nonspecific edema in the manubrium sterni without involvement of the clavicle or the sternoclavicular joint. (b) The detection of concomitant involvement of the manubriosternal synchondrosis allows a presumptive diagnosis of SAPHO.

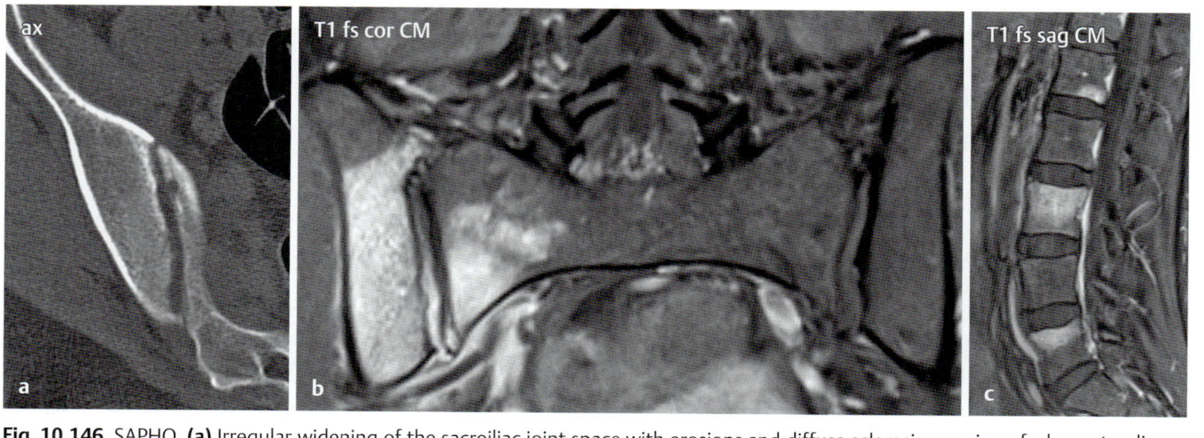

Fig. 10.146 SAPHO. (a) Irregular widening of the sacroiliac joint space with erosions and diffuse sclerosis as a sign of a long-standing process. (b) MRI reveals pronounced enhancement indicating concomitant acute disease. (c) Multiple other lesions in the spine.

10.8 Articular Changes in Inflammatory Systemic Connective Tissue Diseases (Collagenoses)

The primary types of collagenoses (synonym: connectivitis) include systemic lupus erythematosus, progressive systemic sclerosis, dermatomyositis and polymyositis, systemic granulomatous and necrotizing vasculitis, and polyarteritis nodosa and mixed collagenoses (e.g., Sharp's syndrome). Currently, eosinophilic fasciitis and primary and secondary Sjögren's syndrome are also included.

▸ **Pathology.** Classic collagenoses are generalized connective tissue diseases of unknown etiology with systemic damage to vascular and fibrous tissues. Autoimmune phenomena in the form of autoantigen–antibody reactions, which lead to inflammatory changes in the fibrous intercellular substance, are regarded as the common pathogenetic link between these diseases. The individual collagenoses are then defined by their autoantibody profile. The most important autoantibody groups are ANA (antinuclear antibodies) and ANCA (antineutrophilic cytoplasmic antibodies). If these antibody groups overlap, then findings also overlap between the classic collagen diseases, and these are known as undifferentiated or mixed collagenoses.

Although the collagenoses of the joints themselves are usually not destructive, periarticular and muscular soft tissue changes (fibrosis, calcification) can sometimes result in considerable disability. The severe involvement of internal organs often leads to an unfavorable prognosis (▶ see References for Chapter 10.8).

10

10.8.1 Systemic Lupus Erythematosus

▸ **Pathology/clinical presentation.** Systemic lupus erythematosus is a common classic collagenosis and primarily affects younger women (women are 10 times more often affected than men). Severe disease flares are interspersed with longer periods of less pronounced disease activity. About 90% of patients suffer from arthralgias over the course of their illness; typical skin rashes are present in 70% of cases. Involvement of other organs is variable.

Joint involvement typically manifests as symmetrical polyarthritis of the hand and forefoot, usually without any objective radiographic or clinical findings. The knees and shoulders are less commonly involved. Malalignment of joints (without erosions) is common. Tenosynovitis is also an associated finding.

> **Note**
>
> Numerous medications (including antibiotics and cytostatic agents) can cause the development of a lupus erythematosus syndrome with different autoimmune origins and fewer clinical symptoms.

▸ **Radiography.** The discrepancy between the paucity of **radiographic findings** and profound arthralgia is highly characteristic. Over the course of the disease the following signs are found:

- Joint malalignment is common, e.g., swan-neck deformity (▸ Fig. 10.147) and Jaccoud hand (ulnar deviation of the metacarpophalangeal joints; ▸ Fig. 10.148).
- Sometimes Jaccoud hand displays hook-shaped erosions of the metacarpal heads as the *only* sign of destruction (see ▸ Fig. 10.148).
- Epiphyseal necroses (flattening, irregularity, and fragmentation of the joint surfaces) at the metacarpophalangeal and metatarsophalangeal joints and delicate, cystic-appearing radiolucencies in the epiphysis are characteristic, but not very common.
- The juxta-articular osteoporosis of the hands and feet progresses later to generalized osteoporosis.
- Late stage "destruction" and "mutilation" are caused by pressure erosions secondary to muscular and capsular contractures.

▸ **MRI.** Mild capsular swelling and mild synovitis in the joints and tendon sheaths of the hand predominate. Very small erosions may be detected on MRI, usually before they are evident on conventional radiographs.

10.8.2 Progressive Systemic Sclerosis

Progressive systemic sclerosis (synonym: scleroderma) is a chronic, systemic disease of connective tissues. Hence it is also a heterogeneous multisystem disorder in which autoimmune processes (laboratory findings: positive ANAs) play a decisive pathogenetic and diagnostic role.

Variants. CREST syndrome (calcinosis cutis, Raynaud's phenomenon, esophageal dysmotility, sclerodactyly, telangiectasias) is the variation of progressive systemic sclerosis with the most favorable prognosis and usually follows a slower and more protracted course. Subcutaneous calcifications, which occur primarily in those parts of the body subjected to loading, are initially detected on radiographs and appear later on the skin.

More recent Anglo-American classifications

- **lSSc** (limited systemic sclerosis) with acral and fascial involvement but less internal organ involvement, overlaps with CREST syndrome.
- **dSSc** (diffuse systemic sclerosis) with significant involvement of internal organs and a poorer prognosis.

▸ Radiography. Characteristic radiographic findings are most commonly found **in the hand**:

- Soft tissue atrophy with tapering of the terminal phalanges. A reactive osteolysis (acro-osteolysis, ▸ Fig. 10.149), particularly of the nail tuft, but also of the radial and ulnar styloid processes, less commonly of the ribs and the mandible (widening of the periodontal space).
- Interstitial soft tissue calcifications with coarse or "crumbly" radiographic appearance involving the head and limbs or mechanically loaded parts of the body (e.g., elbow). More advanced stages also have periarticular and intra-articular calcifications (▸ Fig. 10.150).
- Another sign is the presence of severe flexion deformities and contractures ("claw hand") as a result of skin shrinkage (▸ Fig. 10.151).
- Predominantly nonerosive arthritis is reported in up to 20% of cases.
- Diffuse demineralization that progresses over the course of the disease.

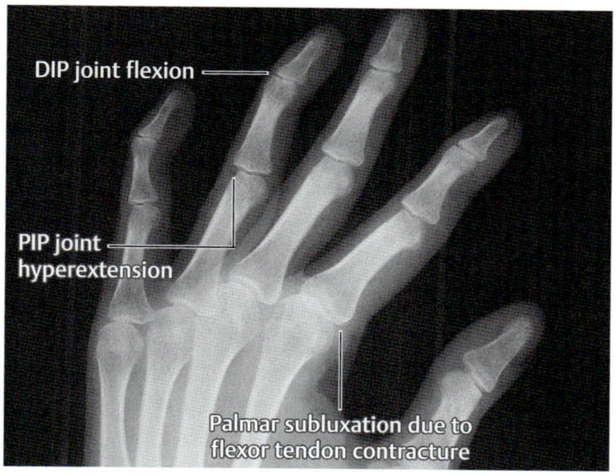

Fig. 10.147 Swan-neck deformity. DIP joint, distal interphalangeal joint. PIP joint, proximal interphalangeal joint.

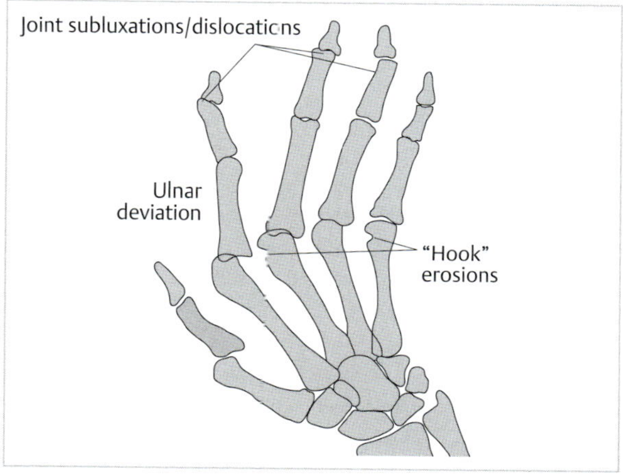

Fig. 10.148 Jaccoud hand.

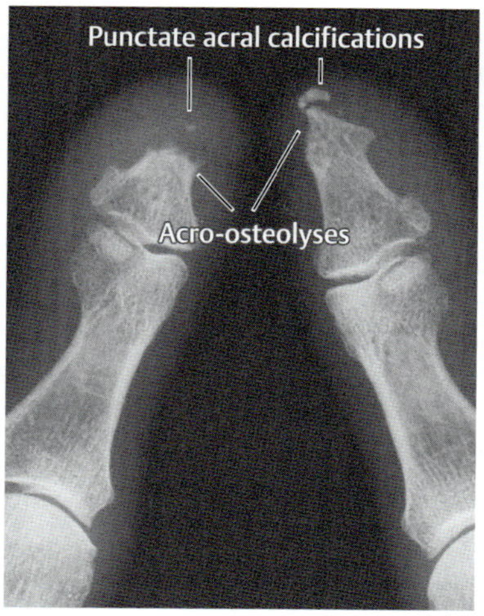

Fig. 10.149 Acro-osteolysis in a patient with progressive systemic sclerosis.

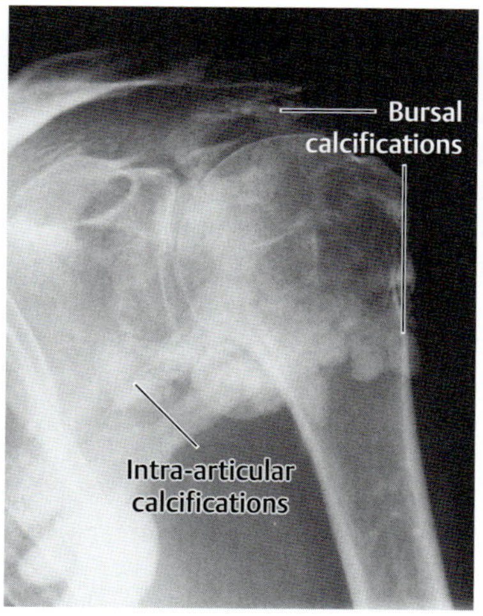

Fig. 10.150 Calcifications of the shoulder in a patient with progressive systemic sclerosis.

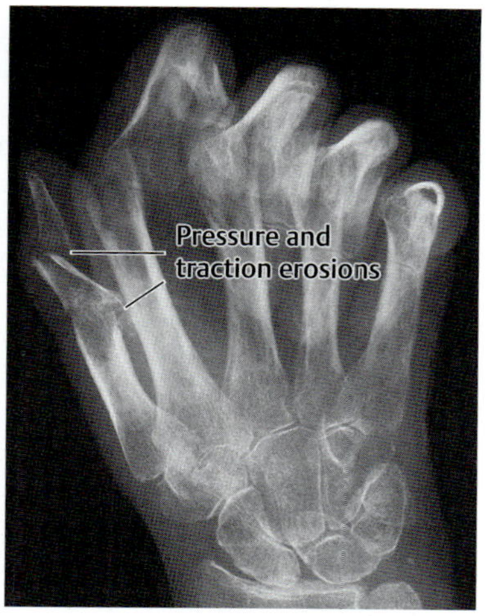

Fig. 10.151 Claw hand in a patient with progressive systemic sclerosis. Note the severe flexion contractures and mechanical erosions.

10

10.8.3 Polymyositis and Dermatomyositis

Polymyositis and dermatomyositis are inflammatory diseases of the skeletal muscles resulting from pathologic (cellular, T cell-mediated) immune mechanisms. The muscles, damaged by inflammation, are infiltrated by fat and become necrotic. In addition, characteristic cutaneous manifestations develop with dermatomyositis. These disorders predominantly affect adults, usually after the second decade of life. Children are affected much less often and in those cases with dermatomyositis. The probability of an underlying paraneoplastic cause increases in patients older than 45 years.

▸ **Radiography.** In more advanced stages, extensive linear calcifications are seen within muscles and fasciae along with lacy reticular subcutaneous calcifications (▸ Fig. 10.152). If there is a concomitant polyarthritis, it is nonerosive.

▸ **MRI.** MRI is extremely useful for identifying **acute myositis** given the prominent muscle edema that demonstrates high signal intensity on water-sensitive sequences (▸ Fig. 10.153). With **chronic myositis**, fat-suppressed sequences help to distinguish between edema and fatty atrophy. MRI is also of particular assistance for selecting a suitable biopsy site (the area of highest signal intensity) and for monitoring therapy.

10.8.4 Mixed Collagenoses

10

Overlap between the different types of collagenosis are common. Mixed collagenosis in its narrower sense (Sharp's syndrome, mixed connective tissue disease) usually demonstrates symptoms of systemic lupus erythematosus, progressive systemic sclerosis, polymyositis/dermatomyositis, and chronic arthralgias or polyarthritis.

▸ **Radiography.** The radiographic findings of **scleroderma** predominate in hands (▸ Fig. 10.154). Polyarthralgias and polyarthritis are typically nonerosive. Erosions are less common and are indistinguishable from those seen in rheumatoid arthritis.

10.8.5 Vasculitis

In the more recent literature, primary systemic vasculitis is no longer included among the collagenoses. With primary systemic vasculitis, inflammatory (and later also granulomatous and necrotizing) vascular alterations associated with microaneurysms trigger the characteristic symptoms and cardinal clinical findings.

Secondary systemic vasculitis can develop in the presence of classic collagenosis and rheumatoid arthritis.

Primary Systemic Vasculitis

Classification is made according to the predominant type of vessel involved as well as the size of vessel (▸ see References for Chapter 10.8). The majority of these types of vasculitis are associated with arthropathies (polyarthralgia; nonerosive as well as erosive arthritic conditions). Areas of radiographically evident, clinically painful periosteal reaction (▸ Fig. 10.155) are the result of an inflammation of the periosteal vessels. The following types of vasculitis are particularly important for the radiologist.

Polyarteritis nodosa. This necrotizing vasculitis affects small and medium-sized arteries. Radiology reveals peripheral arthritides with an episodic and predominantly nonerosive course. Sites of commonly painful periosteal reaction may be detected by conventional radiographs or MRI.

Wegener's granulomatosis. This belongs to the category of granulomatous vasculitis and in this respect displays both clinical as well as immunological similarities (cANCA: classic antineutrophil cytoplasmic antibody) with allergic granulomatosis (**Churg–Strauss syndrome**). Concomitant polyarthralgias and polyarthritis are usually nonerosive in nature. CT of the lungs and paranasal sinuses serves to detect granulomatous lesions.

Polymyalgia rheumatica. This is a disease manifestation of giant cell arteritis. Temporal arteritis also belongs to this group. There is a frequent association with malignancies. At the onset of the disease, swelling commonly develops in the region of the sternoclavicular and acromioclavicular joints, which later demonstrate erosions. Polyarthritis of the hands is rarely of an erosive nature. Even less common is erosive arthritis of the sacroiliac joints or pubic symphysis.

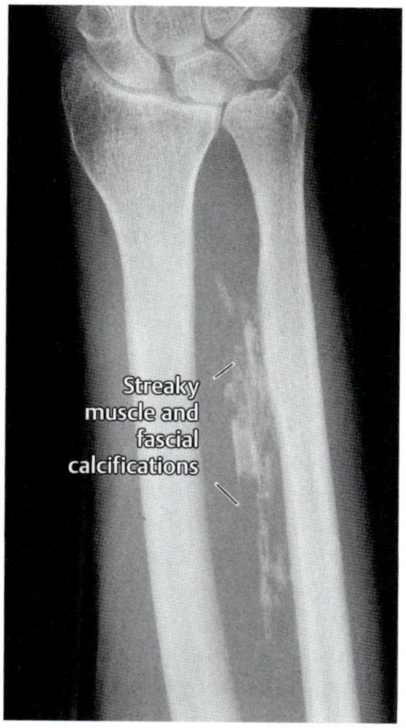

Fig. 10.152 Soft tissue calcifications in a patient with dermatomyositis.

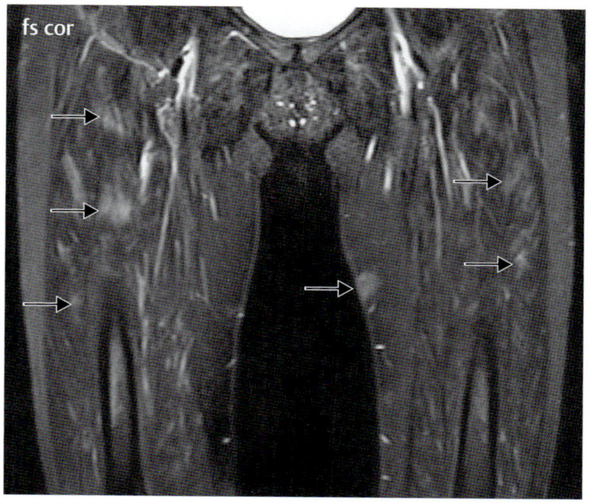

Fig. 10.153 Myositis on MRI Fluid-sensitive fat-suppressed TIRM sequence (turbo inversion recovery magnitude). Multiple hyperintense inflammatory foci (arrows).

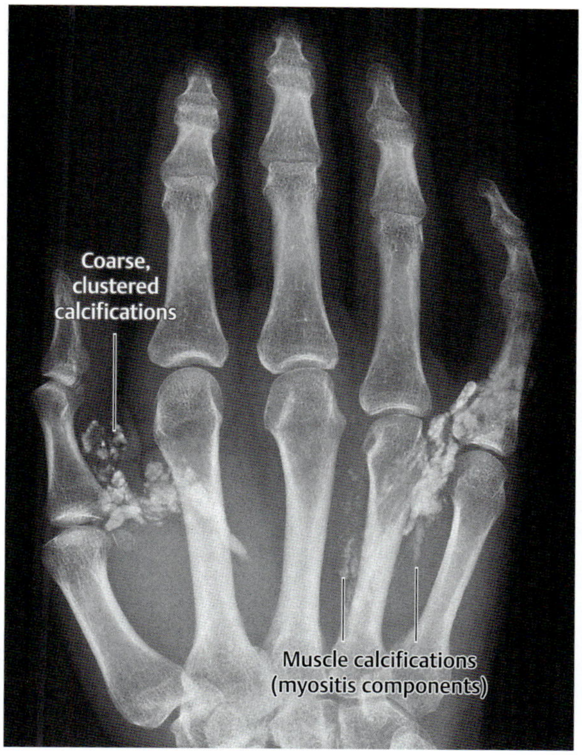

Fig. 10.154 Sharp's syndrome.

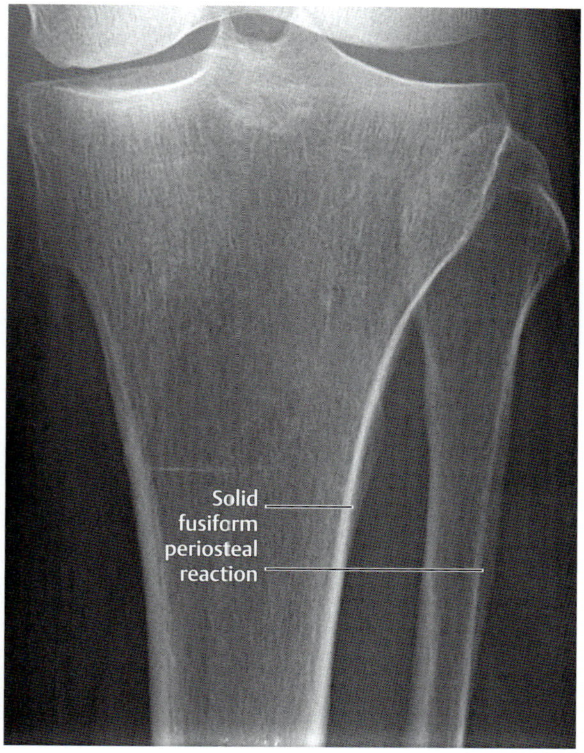

Fig. 10.155 Periosteal reaction of the proximal lower leg in a patient with giant cell arteritis. **Caution:** This nonspecific reaction is much more commonly due to chronic venous insufficiency.

10.9 Crystal-induced Arthropathies, Osteopathies, and Periarthropathies

These are a heterogeneous group of arthropathies characterized by intra-articular and periarticular as well as intraosseous **crystal deposition**. This group includes the following (► Table 10.2):

- **Gout.**
- **CPPD** (calcium pyrophosphate deposition disease).
- **Hydroxyapatite crystal deposition disease.**
- **Secondary forms:**
  - Steroid-induced crystal arthropathy.
  - Secondary gout.
  - Secondary CPPD

Diagnosis is usually based on a combination of radiographic and clinical/laboratory findings. Joint aspiration allows for identification of specific crystals within the aspirate. The standard radiographic examination should assess the following findings:

- **Soft tissue swelling** (e.g., due to soft tissue tophi, joint effusions with increased density).
- **Calcification** (involving cartilage, synovium, tendons, joint capsule, periarticular soft tissues, tophi).
- **Joint morphology** (joint space width, articular destruction, secondary signs of osteoarthritis, subchondral cystic lesions, pattern of joint involvement).
- **Bone** (bone density, lytic lesions, including those distant to the joints, reactive new bone formation).

10

10.9.1 Gout

The symptoms of gout are triggered by localized deposits of monosodium urate crystals.

► **Pathology.** Uric acid is the end product of purine metabolism. Reduced renal excretion of uric acid or, more rarely, its increased production results in hyperuricemia. Genetic alterations of urate transport proteins are regarded as triggers for the impaired renal excretion. The effect of nutrition (protein- and purine-rich nutrition, alcohol consumption) has been confirmed. Over-saturation with uric acid results in precipitation of sodium urate crystals, which induces a local, acute, inflammation-like reaction. Characteristic sites of precipitation include the synovial membrane, joint fluid, tendons sheaths, bursae, subcutaneous tissues, and kidneys. Asymptomatic crystal deposits can precede an acute crystal-induced synovitis. The metatarsophalangeal joint of the large toe is involved in more than 50% of all cases.

Tophi, found in chronic gout, are nodular deposits of urate crystals with a surrounding granulomatous reaction. Tophi may involve the synovial membrane, subchondral bone, and periarticular connective tissues as well as the auricle, tendons, and subcutaneous tissues. These may calcify and enlarge, resulting in compression or erosion of surrounding structures

► **Clinical presentation.** Gout typically manifests clinically for the first time in men aged 40 to 50 years. Only 5 to 10% of cases involve women (usually postmenopausal). Gout passes through three stages or clinical forms:

- **Asymptomatic hyperuricemia:** This stage may last for many years. Only 5% of these patients will eventually develop clinical gout.
- **Acute intermittent gout:** This involves acute episodic attacks of gout with painless ("intercritical") intervals. Over time, the number of attacks increases while the painless intervals become shorter and shorter. In up to 90% of cases, monoarticular involvement of the first metatarsophalangeal joint occurs, followed in descending order of frequency by ankle, knee, and finger joint involvement. During the attack, the affected joint and its surroundings are swollen, erythematous, and painful.
- **Chronic tophaceous gout:** This usually develops 10 or more years after the first attack of gout and is characterized radiographically and clinically by progressive joint destruction, osteolysis, joint deformity, and limitation of motion. Tophi also appear at the fingertips and in tendons and bursae. Complications include kidney stones, early irreversible renal failure, and renal hypertension. Eventually joint involvement tends to be polyarticular, peripheral, and asymmetric. In the foot it affects the first to fifth metatarsophalangeal joints in descending order of frequency. In the hand, the carpus and carpometacarpal joints are primarily involved.

Secondary forms of gout are found most prominently in cases of chronic renal failure, after chemotherapy and radiation therapy, in myelo- and lymphoproliferative disorders, and in hemolytic anemia.

> **Note**
>
> As a rule: no hyperuricemia means no gout. However, if there is clinical, and possibly also radiographic, suspicion of gout, although uric acid levels are normal, then there are two possible explanations:
>
> 1. The diagnosis of "gout" is wrong. Other crystalline arthropathies (Chapter 10.9.2 and Chapter 10.9.3) should be considered.
>
> 2. Acute gout can occur even with normal uric acid levels. This is probably caused by the effect of ACTH (adrenocorticotropic hormone) and adrenaline on the excretory function of the kidney. Episodes of pain, such as in an attack of gout cause the increased release of ACTH and adrenaline.

▶ **Radiography.** In an acute attack of gout:

- Soft tissue swelling may be seen, in some cases with areas of increased density, as a result of crystal deposition (▶ Figs. 10.156 and ▶ 10.157).
- Juxta-articular osteoporosis (though this is rare and nonspecific).

Note

The initial attacks of gout do not have a specific radiographic appearance and, in fact, radiographs are often normal at this stage.

With intermittent and chronic gout:

- Bone density is usually normal, even until the late stages of the disease.
- The joint space width is normal or reduced by secondary (possibly preexisting) osteoarthritis.
- Focal soft tissue masses are the result of soft tissue tophi or gouty bursitis. Tophi may be of dull, mildly increased density (sodium urate deposits) or may display fine calcifications.
- Bony erosions or joint destruction are the result of intraosseous tophi or tophi originating from the synovial membrane (▶ Figs. 10.158–10.160).

Table 10.2 Overview of crystal-induced arthropathies and periarthropathies

Disorder	Composition of the crystals	Site	Common location/main structures
Gout (arthritis urica)	Monosodium urate	Articular, para-articular, intraosseous, parosteal	First metatarsophalangeal joint and surrounding tissues
CPPD	Calcium pyrophosphate dihydrate	Fibrocartilage and hyaline cartilage, fiber-rich connective tissue (joint capsule, tendon insertions), synovial membrane	Wrist: triangular fibrocartilage and hyaline cartilage Knee, hip, shoulder: typically only hyaline cartilage at these sites
Hydroxyapatite crystal deposition disease	Hydroxyapatite	Periarticular soft tissues	Shoulder, hip

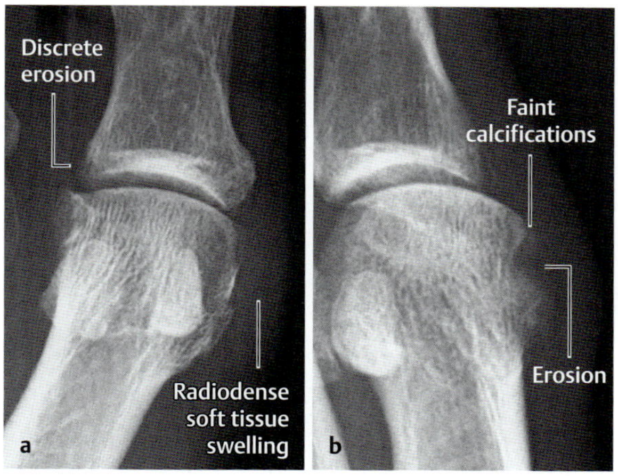

Fig. 10.156 Acute episode of gout. Initial radiographic signs. **(a)** Fine erosion of the proximal phalanx. **(b)** Very subtle alterations on the oblique view.

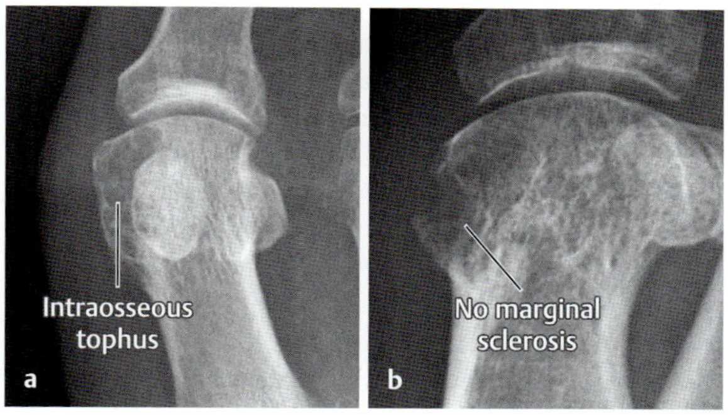

Fig. 10.159 Chronic gout. Typical radiographic morphology. **(a)** Soft tissue swelling with increased density. **(b)** Oblique view. Absent marginal sclerosis is compatible with an acute exacerbation of the patient's long-standing gout.

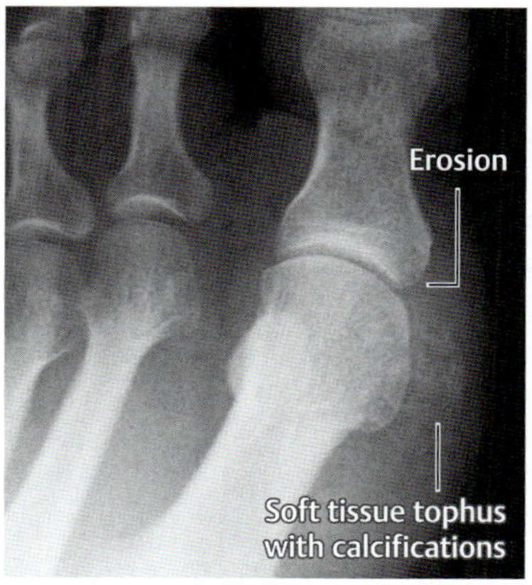

Fig. 10.157 Acute attack in a patient with intermittent gout. Significant soft tissue swelling.

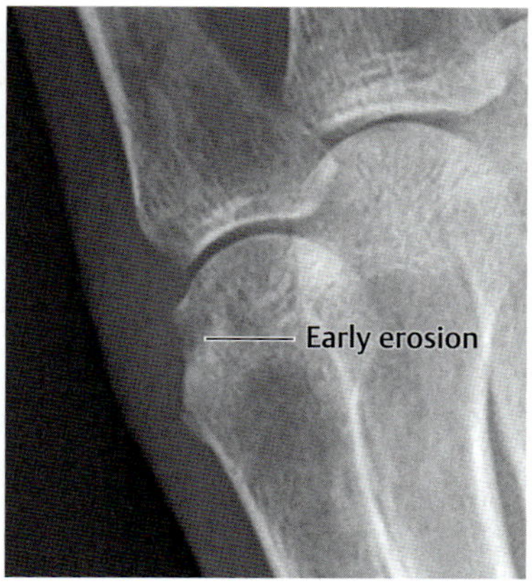

Fig. 10.158 Early erosion in a patient with gout.

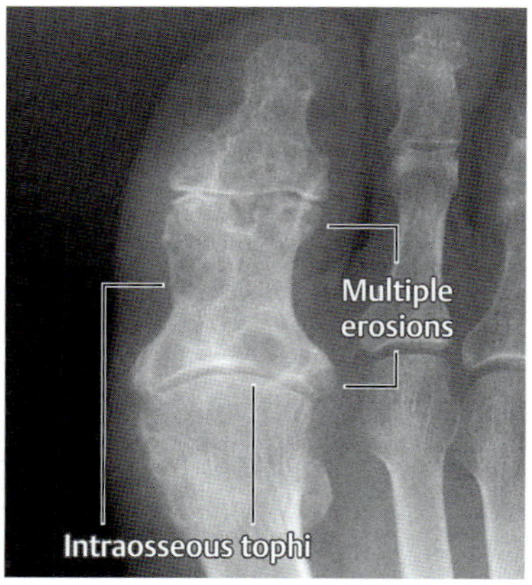

Fig. 10.160 Chronic tophaceous gout with numerous intraosseous tophi.

- Pressure erosions of bone from adjacent parosteal tophi are also seen. They often exceed 5 mm in size and have sclerotic borders if they have not developed acutely.
- Extensive erosions such as tophaceous cupping (► Fig. 10.161) are only rarely encountered these days.

> **Note**
> The "overhanging" bony margin, the "tophaceous spur," and laminated periosteal reaction, usually resulting from a tophus situated immediately adjacent to the bone, represent urate-induced "osteoblastic" bone reactions (► Fig. 10.162 and ► Fig. 10.163). In the case of severe osteoarthritis of the first metatarsophalangeal joint, and in particular hallux rigidus, it is not uncommon to encounter a superimposed case of chronic, slowly developing gout (see ► Fig. 10.163).

► **US.** On ultrasound, tophi appear as sharply delineated space-occupying masses with strong internal echoes (due to the crystals; ► Fig. 10.164). Furthermore, ultrasound displays the double contour sign, a hyperechoic rim along the cartilage surface related to crystal deposition.

► **CT.** Tophi appear as soft tissue masses of increased radiodensity with fine stippled calcifications on CT. Simple punched-out osteolytic lesions and erosions without significant radiodensities may be seen within the bone (► Fig. 10.165). The typical fine sclerotic margin is an indication of the benign nature of the process.

► **MRI.** Tophi appear on T1W images as space-occupying masses that are hypo- to isointense to muscle. On T2W sequences, tophi appear very heterogeneous with areas of decreased and increased signal intensity. Relatively homogeneous areas of hypointense to absent signal are possible. Contrast enhancement is usually very pronounced, particularly in the acute stage, especially in the tissues adjacent to the tophus. Prominent enhancing intra-articular synovitis can develop (► Fig. 10.166). MRI also shows erosions and bone marrow edema.

10

► **DD.**

Differential diagnosis of an initial acute attack of gout

- **Acute bacterial arthritis:** the heterogeneity of the signal on T2W sequences due to the crystals is not seen with septic arthritis.
- **"Articular chondrocalcinosis":** pseudogout attack (**CPPD**) (Chapter 10.9.2).
- **Acute hydroxyapatite disease:** pseudogout attack (Chapter 10.9.3).
- **Iatrogenic crystal-induced synovitis:** after an intra-articular injection of microcrystalline corticosteroid.
- **Psoriatic arthritis or reactive arthritis:** acute sausage digit (dactylitis).

> **Note**
> In 40% of cases, patients with gout also have concomitant CPPD. It is then very difficult to distinguish between the two disorders.

Differential diagnosis of chronic gout osteoarthropathy

- **Rheumatoid arthritis:** especially the cystic form. The crystal deposition results in areas of low signal intensity on MRI that are not seen with rheumatoid arthritis.
- **Activated osteoarthritis psoriatic arthritis.**
- Pyrophosphate tophus and **"tendinosis calcarea"** (periarticular hydroxyapatite deposit): see Chapter 10.9.3.
- **Amyloid deposits.**
- **Sarcoid osteopathy:** rare.

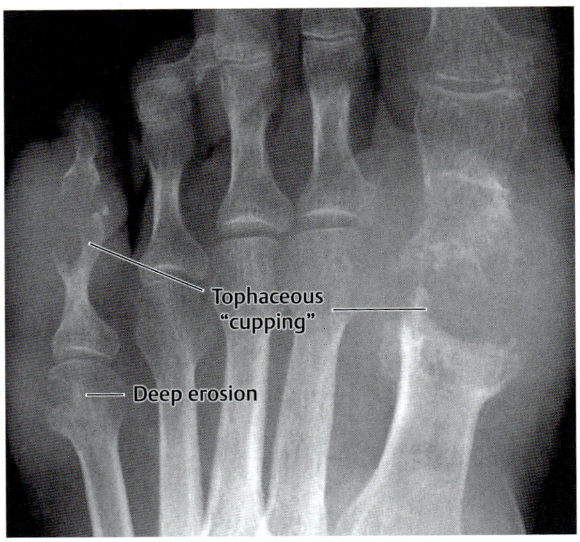

Fig. 10.161 Chronic tophaceous gout at typical location.

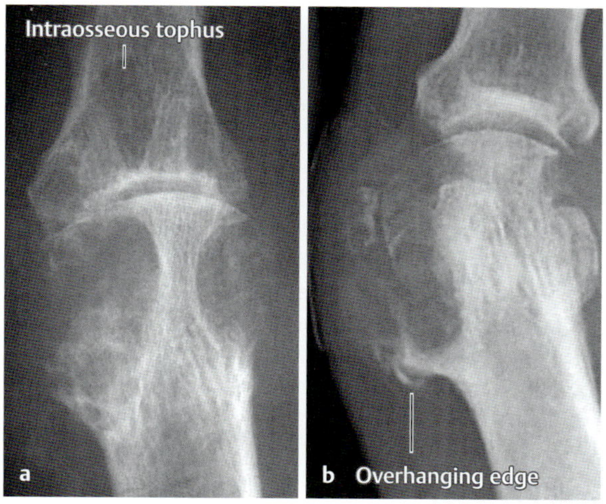

Fig. 10.162 Chronic tophaceous gout. **(a)** Halberdlike appearance from large, characteristically ovoid osteolyses. **(b)** Characteristic overhanging bony margin.

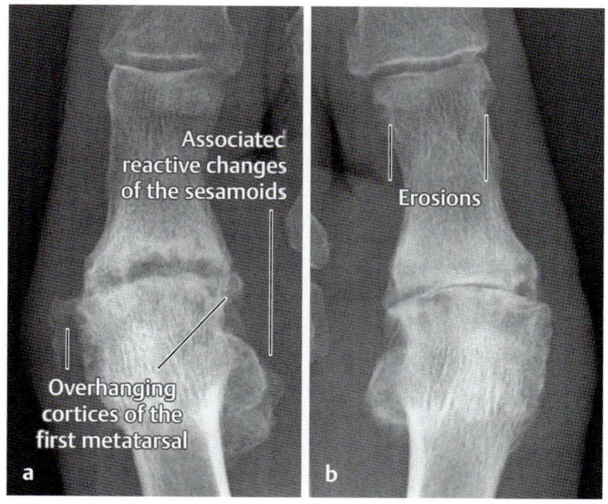

Fig. 10.163 Chronic tophaceous gout. **(a)** Gouty arthritis with severe secondary erosions and reactive sclerosis typical of gout. **(b)** On the contralateral side, the appearance is strongly suggestive of osteoarthritis, but the para-articular erosions are an indication of gout.

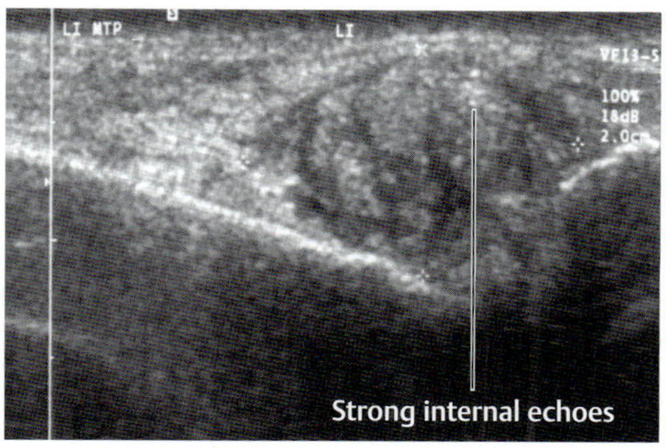

Fig. 10.164 Ultrasound image of a soft tissue tophus.

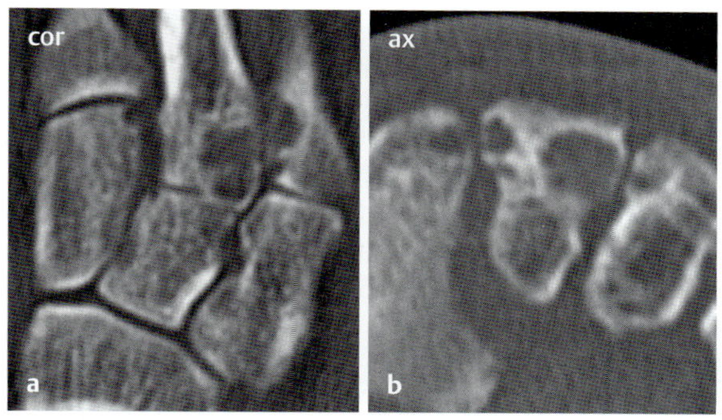

Fig. 10.165 Chronic tophaceous gout. **(a)** Delicate marginal sclerosis of intraosseous tophi in the tarsometatarsal region. **(b)** Additional lesions in the foot exclude the differential diagnosis of PVNS (cf. Chapter 4.6.5).

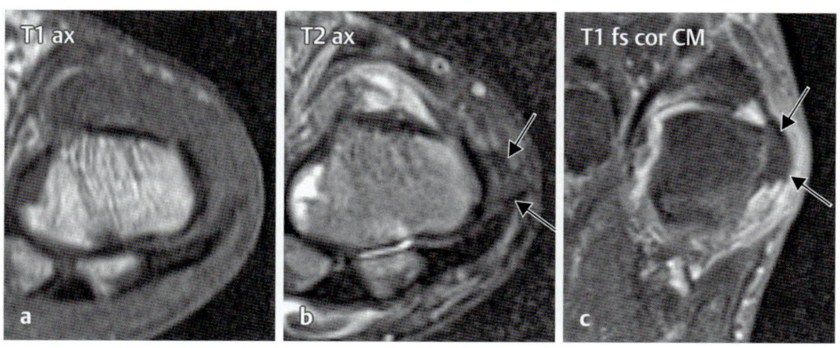

Fig. 10.166 Signal pattern of a synovial tophus (arrows) at the first metatarsophalangeal joint on MRI. **(a)** Isointense to muscle on the T1W image with ill-defined margins. **(b)** Hypointense on the T2W image. **(c)** No contrast enhancement of the tophus, but strong enhancement of the surrounding tissue (synovitis).

10

10.9.2 Calcium Pyrophosphate Deposition Disease (CPPD)

In cases of CPPD, deposition of calcium pyrophosphate dihydrate crystals results in **pyrophosphate arthropathy.**

▸ **Pathology.** The disease probably begins within the hyaline cartilage. The cartilaginous matrix is replaced by chondromucoid material, followed by crystal deposition. The crystals are released into the joint. It is still not clear what actually triggers this process, but there does appear to be a correlation with aging. Additional, unknown factors are also likely involved.

The classification system is based on etiology and distinguishes between three patient groups:

1. **Hereditary** (familial).
2. **Sporadic/idiopathic:** The disorder commonly demonstrates an asymptomatic course and may be discovered in the 5th decade of life, or possibly later as an isolated finding, e.g., in connection with radiographic findings of osteoarthritis, in particular in cases of "activated osteoarthritis."
3. **"Symptomatic"/secondary:** In various underlying endocrine and metabolic conditions, such as hyperparathyroidism, terminal renal failure, long-term hemodialysis, hemochromatosis, and gouty arthritis, there is histological proof of calcium pyrophosphate depositions that is also evident on standard radiological imaging. The post-traumatic/postoperative type is also considered to be a secondary type.

10

▸ **Clinical presentation.** The majority of patients are over 40 years of age; women are more commonly affected than men by a significant margin. Many patients with radiographic signs of CPPD have only a few (or no) symptoms (sporadic type). Clinical manifestations:

- **Pseudogout** (10–20% of cases): This involves recurrent episodes of arthritis associated with swelling and increased skin temperature. The bouts are less painful than with gout and usually involve the knee joint or the hand. Radiographically evident "chondrocalcinosis" in the form of hyaline cartilage calcification can disappear during an attack of pseudogout.
- **Chronic joint disease** (35–60% of cases): This progressive form demonstrates varying degrees of intensity, is predominantly bilateral, and results in secondary osteoarthritis. Characteristic locations include knee (especially the patellofemoral compartment), hip, wrist/hand (radioulnar, radiocarpal, intercarpal, metacarpophalangeal), elbow, ankle, and shoulder.

Disks, ligamentous insertions of the spine, and the symphysis pubis are typically involved with CPPD.

▸ **Radiography.** The detection of calcification is the most important contribution made by radiography.

- **Hyaline cartilage:** The fine linear calcifications run parallel to the articular surface (▸ Fig. 10.167a).
- **Fibrocartilage:** The menisci of the knee and the triangular fibrocartilage are commonly involved (▸ Figs. 10.167b and c). Additional locations include the labra of the hip and shoulder as well as the pubic symphysis.
- **Synovial membrane:** Amorphous calcifications are found, most commonly in the knee, wrist, metacarpophalangeal, and metatarsophalangeal joints.
- **Ligaments, tendons, and joint capsule:** These are affected by thin, linear calcifications that can extend far into the tendons at their insertions (▸ Fig. 10.168; see also ▸ Fig. 10.167a).
- **Extra-articular soft tissues:** Tumorlike calcifications (= tophaceous pseudogout; ▸ Fig. 10.169) are rare.
- **Intervertebral disks:** Here fine, curved marginal calcifications are found (allowing them to be differentiated from syndesmophytes).

Arthropathy associated with CPPD resembles osteoarthritis clinically and radiographically and is often at least a partial cause of osteoarthritis: joint space narrowing, sclerosis, and subchondral cysts are typical findings. Joint involvement is predominantly symmetric. Radiographically visible calcifications may also be (temporarily) absent.

▸ **CT.** CT is the most sensitive modality for detecting cartilaginous and soft tissue calcifications (see ▸ Fig. 10.169). It displays clearly the arthropathy of complex joints (▸ Fig. 10.170a).

▸ **US.** Ultrasound will display the double contour sign (hyperechoic cartilage surface).

▸ **MRI.** Small, hypointense (rarely also hyperintense on T1W) accumulations of calcium pyrophosphate crystals in the menisci, triangular fibrocartilage, hyaline cartilage, and in the anulus fibrosus of the disks are often overlooked on an MRI examination, yet they are—if it at all detectable—characteristic for CPPD. After their release, crystals may also be detected in the joint (▸ Fig. 10.170b).

Caution

MRI is not a suitable modality for diagnosing CPPD. CPPD results in reactive synovitis, which may lead to an erroneous diagnosis of rheumatoid arthritis. In rare cases nonspecific, "inflammatory" soft tissue reactions are also found (▸ Fig. 10.171).

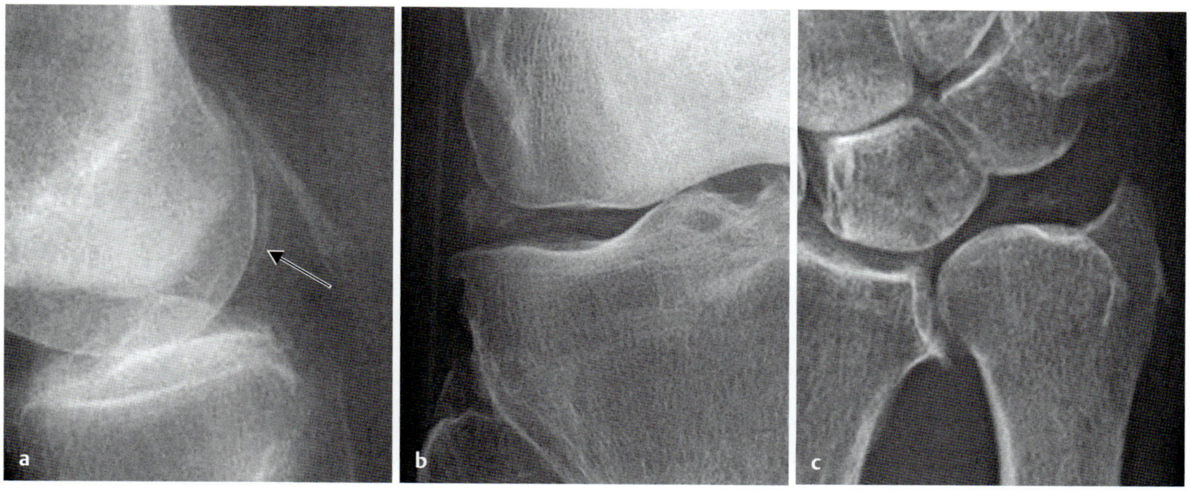

Fig. 10.167 Typical calcifications in CPPD. **(a)** Hyaline cartilage calcification (chondrocalcinosis) posteriorly at the femoral condyle (arrow) and calcification of the gastrocnemius tendon insertion. **(b)** Meniscal calcifications. **(c)** Calcifications of the triangular fibrocartilage.

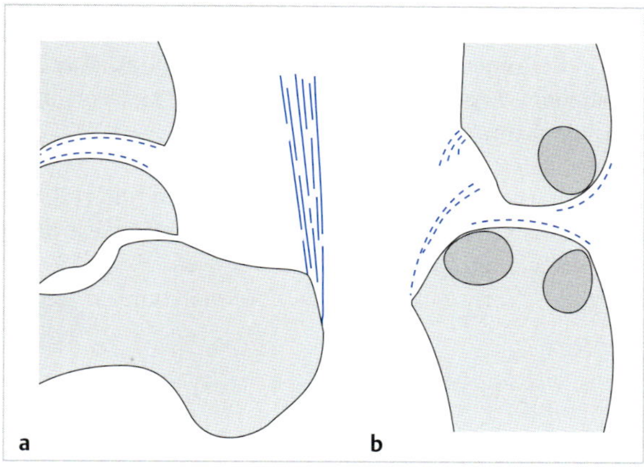

Fig. 10.168 Schematic diagram of the calcifications in CPPD. **(a)** Linear calcifications in the tendons and hyaline cartilage. **(b)** "Cysts" in CPPD with ligamentous and cartilage calcifications.

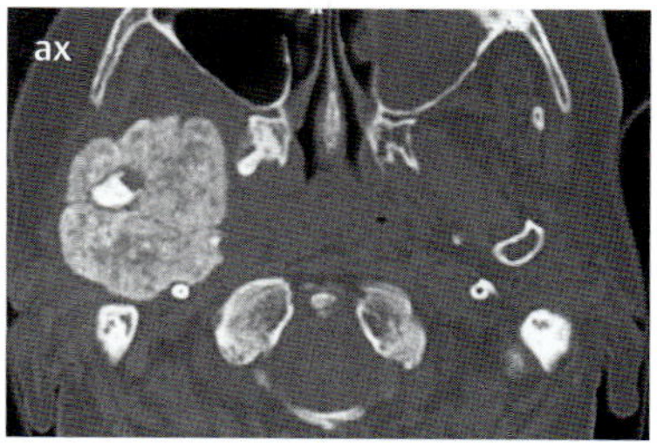

Fig. 10.169 CPPD in the region of the temporomandibular joint.

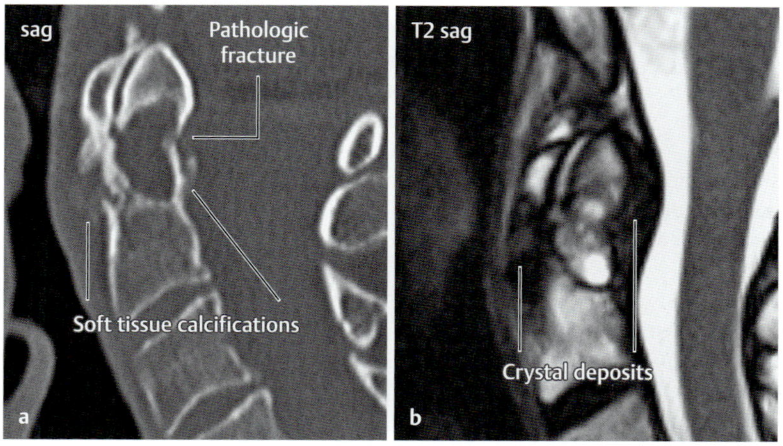

Fig. 10.170 Atlantodental CPPD arthropathy. Pathologic fracture after a minor injury. **(a)** Large "cyst" in the odontoid process, peridental soft tissue calcifications. **(b)** Identification of hypointense crystal deposits and a subchondral cyst. The fracture is not well visualized on this T2W MR image.

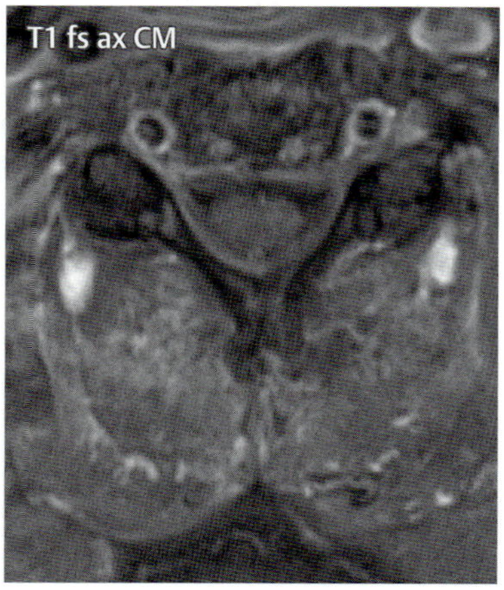

Fig. 10.171 CPPD. Diffusely increased, "inflammatory" contrast enhancement of the posterior paravertebral soft tissues.

> **Note**
> - Advanced osteoarthritis or destructive arthropathy of the radiocarpal, ulnocarpal, and intercarpal joints (late stage of a SLAC wrist; Chapter 2.9.3) and the patellofemoral joints must be reminiscent of pyrophosphate arthropathy, especially when they are disproportionate to adjacent (as yet largely normal) parts of the joint and of course if hyaline or fibrocartilage calcifications are also evident.
> - Calcium deposits within the menisci of the knee are per se nonspecific and represent a not uncommon degenerative finding in the older patient. They are also common after surgery.
> - Clinically, CPPD may mimic severe osteoarthritis, rheumatoid arthritis, neuropathic arthropathy and, of course, pseudogout.

▸ DD.

Osteoarthritis. Particularly severely destructive forms of osteoarthritis can create a similar picture. For decision aids, see the "Note" box above.

Gout. Gout tends to involve more joints than pyrophosphate arthropathy and is characterized by classic erosions and punched-out osteolytic areas. Uric acid and pyrophosphate crystals may also present in the same joint.

Hydroxyapatite crystal deposits. These are usually periarticular and only rarely within a joint.

Rheumatoid arthritis. Rheumatoid arthritis presents a pattern of involvement very similar to that of CPPD, especially in the hand. Cartilage calcification is absent, however.

10

Neuropathic arthropathy. Severe, destructive types of CPPD can create the impression of neuropathic arthropathy.

10.9.3 Hydroxyapatite Crystal Deposition Disease

Deposits of calcium hydroxyapatite crystals in the periarticular connective tissue and in other soft tissues can produce painful inflammatory reactions, but symptomatic deposits within the joints are rare.

▸ **Pathology.** The majority of calcium and phosphate in the body is stored in the skeleton as calcium hydroxyapatite. Deposition of calcium hydroxyapatite in the soft tissues results in necrosis and disintegration of the tissue with associated surrounding inflammatory reaction. More recent research has discovered a familial occurrence with an increased association of certain histocompatibility antigens.

Many areas of symptomatic deposition are **secondary:**
- In the soft tissues, secondary to generalized hypercalcemia or hyperphosphatemia.
- Periarticular, secondary to chronic overuse or an injury (the most common form).
- Intra-articular, secondary to generalized hypercalcemia or hyperphosphatemia or as part of a congenital metabolic disorder.

What is known as **Milwaukee shoulder** is regarded as an intra-articular variant. This results not only in joint space narrowing but also in extensive joint destruction over the course of a few months. Intra-articular hydroxyapatite evidently induces the release of enzymes, which then invade and damage the periarticular soft tissues.

▸ **Clinical presentation.** The clinical literature makes reference to painful, recurrent, juxta-articular calcium deposits under various names, e.g., as peritendinitis calcarea, periarthritis calcarea, bursitis calcarea, and hydroxyapatite rheumatism. The majority of patients are between the ages of 40 and 70 years. These patients may suffer from recurrent, severe episodes of pain or from milder chronic symptoms. The most common clinical picture is that of an attack of pseudogout. Articular hydroxyapatite disease can manifest as acute "arthritis."

Location. The shoulder is the most common location (70% of cases), followed by the hip and the minor joints of the hand and forefoot. The spine may also be involved.

> **Note**
> In hydroxyapatite disease there is no correlation between the size of the deposits and the symptoms. Asymptomatic deposits are not an uncommon incidental radiographic finding.

▸ **Radiography.** **Periarticular calcified deposits** are typically dense, coarse, and well demarcated (in bursae; ▸ Fig. 10.172), but may also be thin, narrow, and delicate (in tendons; ▸ Fig. 10.173). These may remain unchanged for years, enlarge, shrink, or dissolve spontaneously.

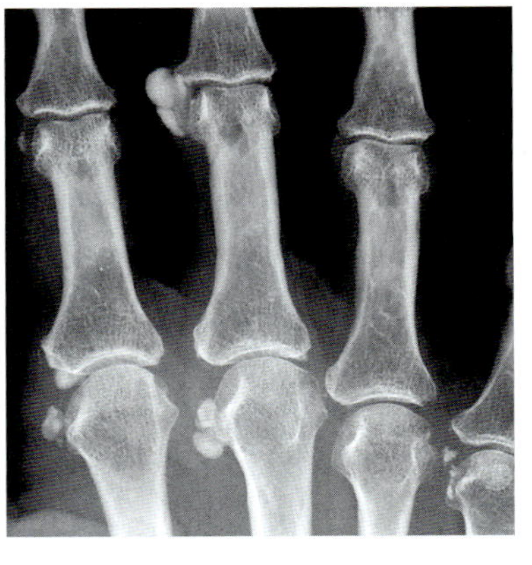

Fig. 10.172 Lobular periarticular calcium hydroxyapatite crystal deposits in the hand.

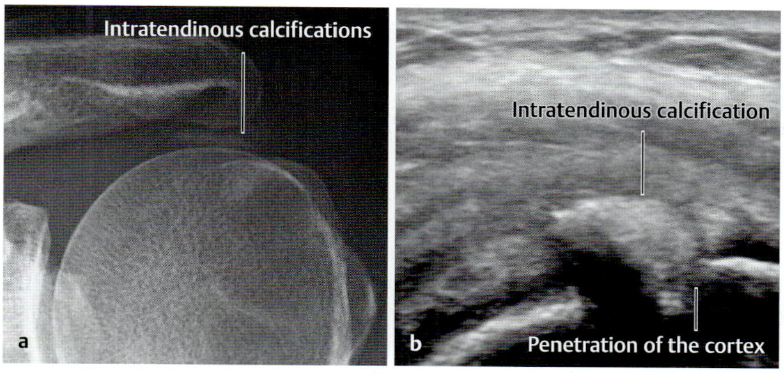

Fig. 10.173 Calcific tendinitis of the rotator cuff. **(a)** Dull calcification near the tendon insertion on the greater tubercle. **(b)** Ultrasound demonstrates penetration of the calcification into the humerus; this presumably triggered the acute episode of pain.

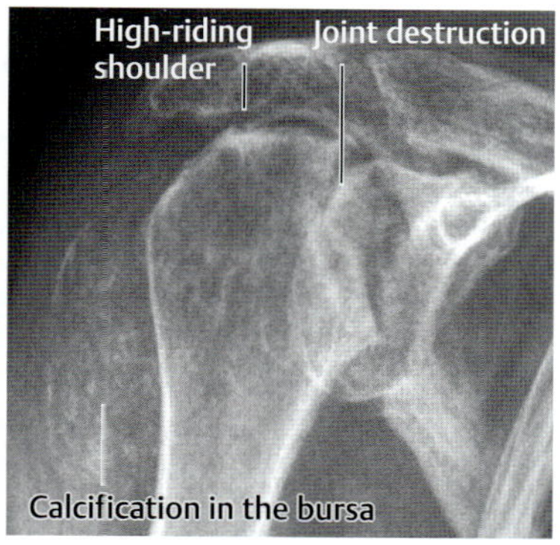

Fig. 10.174 Milwaukee shoulder with extensive destruction.

Intra-articular deposits can remain radiographically occult yet also produce amorphous zones of calcification in the joint capsule. Milwaukee shoulder (▶ Fig. 10.174) results initially in joint space loss, then bony erosions, and finally extensive destruction of the adjacent bones and soft tissues. This is accompanied by a high-riding shoulder, indicating a rotator cuff tear, and a massive joint effusion, which contains calcifications.

▶ **US.** Focal calcifications within a tendon (tendinosis calcarea) and at its insertion are well demonstrated by ultrasound. Calcium deposits are hyperechoic and produce acoustic shadows (see ▶ Fig. 10.173). However, multiple very small calcifications may not demonstrate an acoustic shadow.

▶ **CT.** CT is the most sensitive modality for detecting soft tissue calcifications and can also demonstrate any pressure erosions in adjacent bones.

▶ **MRI.** Calcium is hypointense on all sequences. As a result, it can be very difficult to detect within low signal intensity structures such as tendons when there is no surrounding inflammatory reaction, which will exhibit increased signal intensity on T2W images.

▶ **DD.**

Tendinosis. Intratendinous degeneration may result in ectopic calcification and ossification of tendons. These features are well known for the Achilles tendon and the tendons of abductor pollicis longus and extensor pollicis brevis. Other tendons may also be involved, as well as other flexors and extensors of the hand.

Bursitis. Intrabursal calcification as a sign of degeneration may also be seen, for example, in Haglund syndrome.

Collagenoses. Periarticular, cutaneous, subcutaneous, and muscular calcium deposits are found in collagenoses such as scleroderma, Sharp's syndrome, polymyositis, and dermatomyositis.

Disorders of calcium and phosphorus metabolism. Calcium deposits may be encountered almost anywhere in numerous clinical conditions (primary and secondary hyperparathyroidism, hypervitaminosis D, etc.).

CPPD. Cartilage calcifications are a distinctive feature, but are extremely uncommon in hydroxyapatite disease.

Cortisone-induced crystal deposits. Intra- and periarticular calcifications are sometimes found at the site of prior cortisone injections and are commonly painful. Calcium hydroxyapatite deposits or localized crystallization of steroids may also appear after systemic steroid administration (▶ Fig. 10.175).

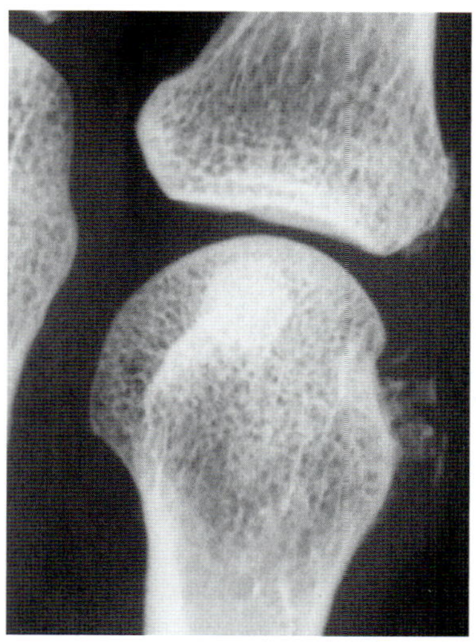

Fig. 10.175 Steroid-induced arthropathy (precipitates of the injected substance) after injection. The finding disappeared after 2 years.

10

11 Miscellaneous Bone, Joint, and Soft Tissue Disorders

11.1 Paget's Disease

▸ **Pathology.** The etiology of Paget's disease (synonym: osteitis deformans) is still unknown. Although a viral infection is commonly cited as its cause, this theory has remained unproven.

Paget's disease is characterized by excessive and pathological bone remodeling, with active and inactive phases. A distinction is made between three characteristic overlapping stages of the disease that form a continuous spectrum: It starts with the **lytic phase**, followed by the **"mixed" lytic and blastic phase**, which ends in the **sclerotic phase**.

▸ **Clinical presentation.** The prevalence of Paget's disease varies worldwide but is generally recognized to be decreasing. The United Kingdom has the highest prevalence (4.6% of the general population). The disorder is also common in Australia, New Zealand, Western Europe, and the United States. The prevalence of the disorder increases with age.

Twenty percent of all patients with Paget's disease are initially asymptomatic. In these patients the disease is often discovered as an incidental finding from a radiograph requested for diagnostic clarification of other signs and symptoms. However, the disease can also become clinically apparent when musculoskeletal, neuromuscular, and cardiovascular complications develop. Laboratory results reveal increased activity of serum alkaline phosphatase (sign of new bone formation) and elevated urine hydroxyproline levels (sign of bone resorption).

Location. Paget's disease is a disease of the axial skeleton, although any bone may be involved. The skull is the most common site. The asymmetric polyostotic type (65–90% of all cases) is more common than the monostotic type.

▸ **Radiography.** A conventional radiograph usually suffices to establish the diagnosis of Paget's disease. The radiographic changes of the disease depend on the duration and stage of the disorder.

- **Lytic phase.** The disorder manifests in the long tubular bones as a well-defined, V-shaped area of osteolysis with a blade-of-grass or candle-flame appearance, starting at an articular surface and extending into the diaphysis (▸ Fig. 11.1). In the tibia, however, the osteolysis can start in the diaphysis without involving the epiphysis or metaphysis. A typical finding in the skull consists of large, well defined, oval-shaped areas of radiolucency without marginal sclerosis that cross the suture lines ("osteoporosis circumscripta"; ▸ Fig. 11.2).
- **Mixed phase.** This phase is characterized by a coarsening and thickening of the trabeculae and cortex (▸ Fig. 11.3). The trabecular thickening is found particularly along the lines of stress (e.g., thickening of the iliopectineal line; ▸ Fig. 11.4). The bones are sometimes enlarged (e.g., the ischium, pubic bone or vertebrae; see ▸ Fig. 11.4). Thickening of the cortical bone of the vertebrae may also be evident in the spine, resulting in a picture-frame vertebral body (▸ Fig. 11.5).
- **Osteosclerotic phase.** Sclerotic areas develop as a result of new bone formation (▸ Fig. 11.6). In the skull, this abnormal bone deposition can appear as a cotton-wool pattern. Marked thickening and sclerosis of the diploic space combined with basilar invagination is known as a "Tam o' Shanter skull" (named for a traditional Scottish cap) (▸ Fig. 11.7). "Ivory vertebrae" can develop in the spine (▸ Fig. 11.8).

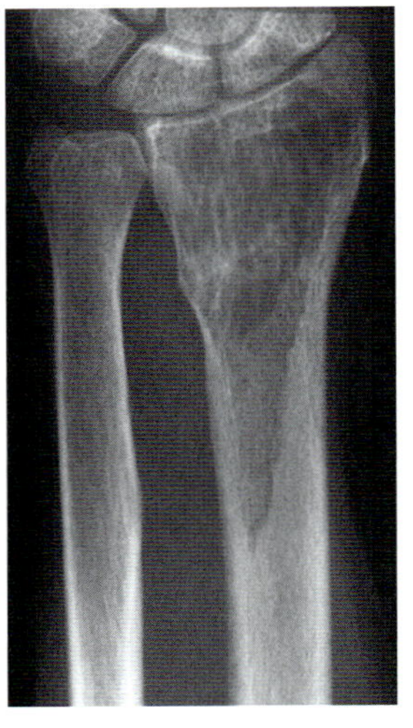

Fig. 11.1 Typical appearance of Paget's disease in the osteolytic phase. Blade-of-grass or candle-flame appearance of osteolysis showing contact with the joint.

Fig. 11.2 Osteoporosis circumscripta of the skull in Paget's disease. ▼

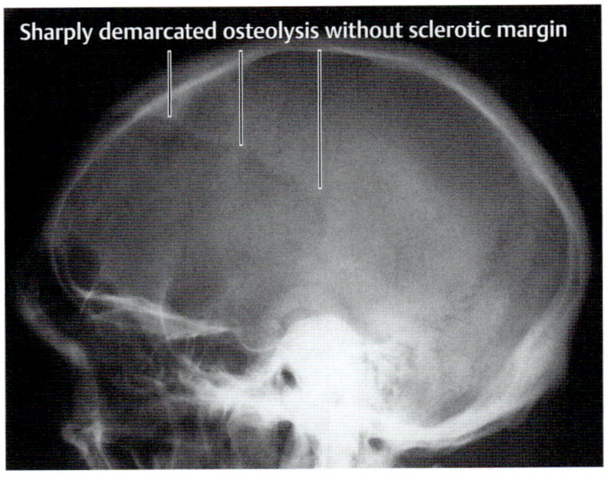

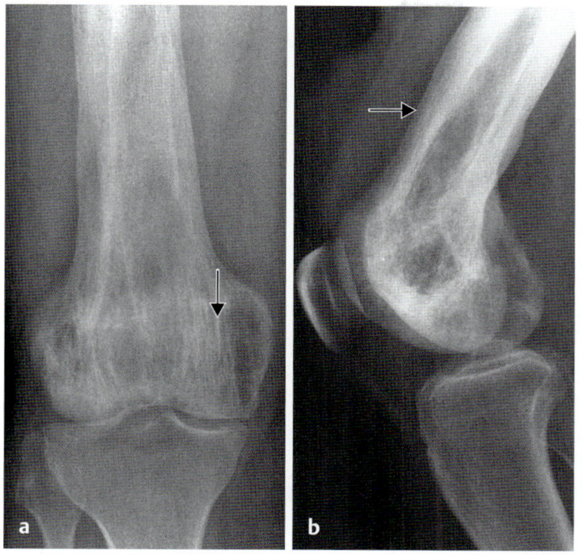

Fig. 11.3 Typical appearance of Paget's disease in the mixed phase. **(a)** Trabecular thickening (arrow). **(b)** Thickening of the cortical bone (arrow).

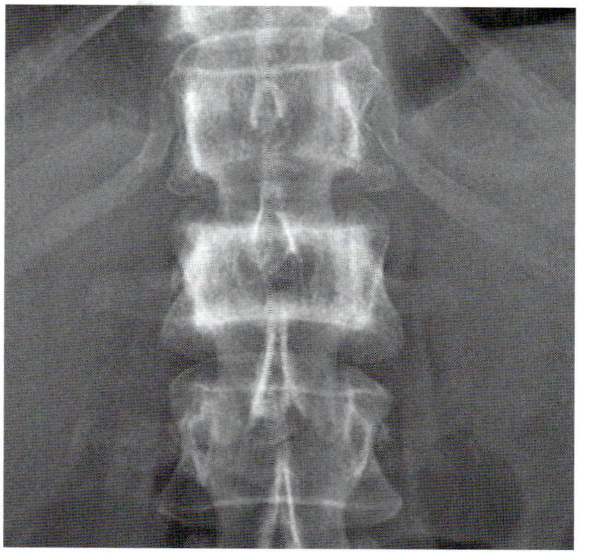

Fig. 11.5 Typical demonstration of Paget's disease with a "picture-frame" vertebral body at L1.

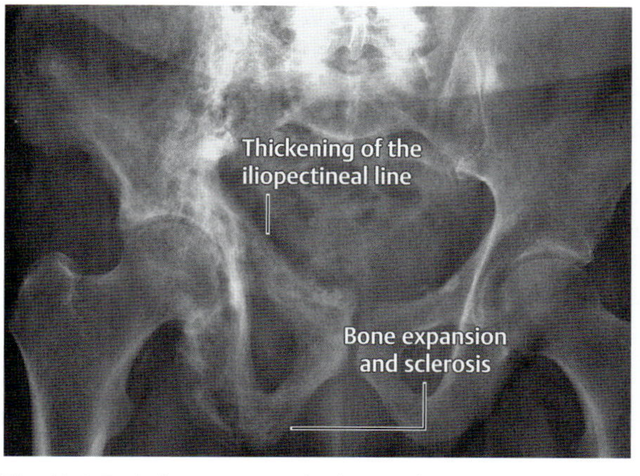

Fig. 11.4 Typical appearance of pelvic involvement in Paget's disease during the mixed phase.

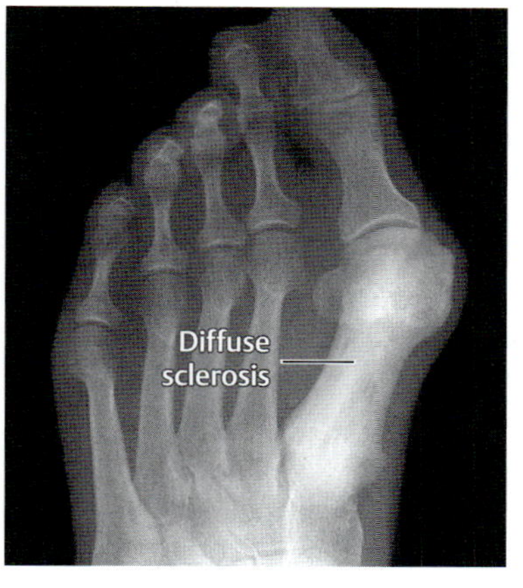

Fig. 11.6 Paget's disease of the first metatarsal in the sclerotic phase.

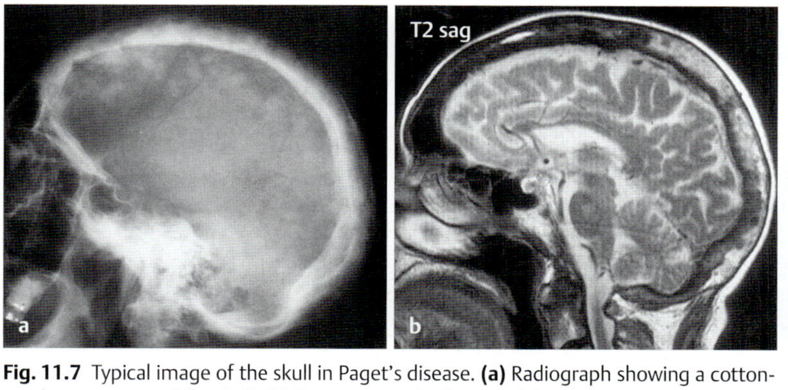

Fig. 11.7 Typical image of the skull in Paget's disease. **(a)** Radiograph showing a cotton-wool appearance of the skull. **(b)** Expansion and sclerosis of the diploic space.

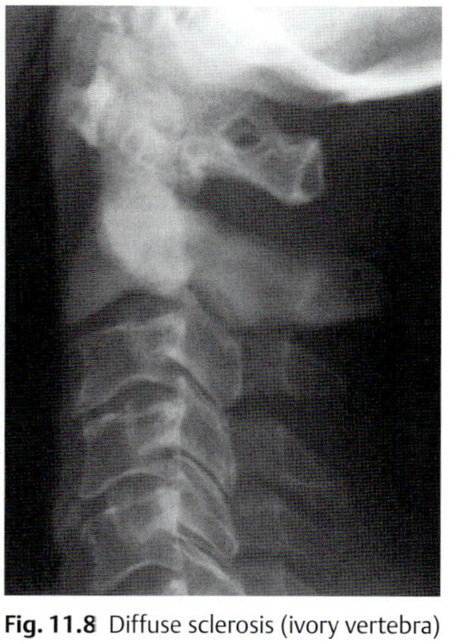

Fig. 11.8 Diffuse sclerosis (ivory vertebra) of C2 in a patient with Paget's disease.

11

▸ CT. The same diagnostic criteria as for conventional radiographs apply and are displayed unobscured by overlying structures (▸ Fig. 11.9).

▸ MRI. Although enlargement of the bone and cortical or trabecular thickening are recognizable on MRI, these findings are better seen on conventional radiographs. The involved bone maintains the signal intensity of fat within its bone marrow (▸ Fig. 11.10). Mild heterogeneity of the bone marrow is still normal. Marked heterogeneity or extensive loss of signal should be an alert for a complication (e.g., pathologic fracture or tumor). Increased bone perfusion results in characteristic contrast enhancement.

▸ NUC MED. An unusually marked increased uptake in all three phases with some expansion of the bone is characteristic on the bone scan (▸ Fig. 11.11). However, the bone scan can also be normal in some cases of metabolically inactive Paget's disease.

Complications of Paget's disease. The complications of Paget's disease can be divided into nonneoplastic and neoplastic complications.

- *Nonneoplastic complications:*
  - **Osseous weakening:** This can result in bowing of the long tubular bones (▸ Fig. 11.12) and basilar impression.
  - **Insufficiency fractures** (see ▸ Fig. 11.12).
  - **Pagetic arthropathy:** The hip and the knee joints are particularly affected (▸ Fig. 11.13).
  - **Neurologic complications:** These can develop as a result of spinal stenosis, stenosis of the neural-exit foramina or cranial nerve compression.
- *Neoplastic complications:* **Pagetic sarcoma** develops in 1% of all patients. Histologically this may be an osteosarcoma, a pleomorphic sarcoma, or uncommonly a chondrosarcoma (▸ Fig. 11.14).

11

Caution

Not every tumor in Paget's disease is a pagetic sarcoma; metastatic spread from other tumors is statistically more common.

▸ DD. In the majority of cases a characteristic radiograph allows the unequivocal diagnosis of Paget's disease.

Metastases. Bony alterations in Paget's disease are better demarcated; cortical bone destruction and soft tissue swelling are not typical. Unlike sclerotic metastases, Paget's disease involving the spine results in thickening of the cortex as well as osseous expansion and often involves the neural arches and spinous processes.

Fibrous dysplasia. Fibrous dysplasia usually affects the outer calvarial table, whereas Paget's disease demonstrates involvement of both the outer and inner tables.

11.2 Sarcoidosis

Sarcoidosis is a systemic, granulomatous, inflammatory condition of unknown origin. Musculoskeletal involvement in sarcoidosis is rare and usually clinically asymptomatic.

Skeletal sarcoidosis classically affects the phalanges of the hands and feet, rarely the long tubular bones and the axial skeleton. Acute **arthropathy** tends to be self-limiting and commonly associated with erythema nodosum and bilateral hilar lymphadenopathy (Löfgren syndrome). As a rule, sarcoid arthropathy affects the ankle joint, the knee, the wrist, and the proximal interphalangeal joints.

▸ Radiography/CT. Skeletal sarcoidosis classically presents as coarse reticular or lacelike honeycomb alterations of the trabeculae in the phalanges of the hands and feet. Cystic lesions are also commonly evident in the phalanges with punched-out cortical erosions. Bone destruction can result in acro-osteolysis, pathologic fractures, and deformity of the phalanges (▸ Figs. 11.15 and ▸ 11.16). Periostitis is characteristically absent and the adjacent joints are usually not affected. Involvement of the soft tissue results in destruction of the cortex from without.

In sarcoidosis, involvement of the joints often exhibits no alterations on the radiograph or merely osteopenia and soft tissue swelling.

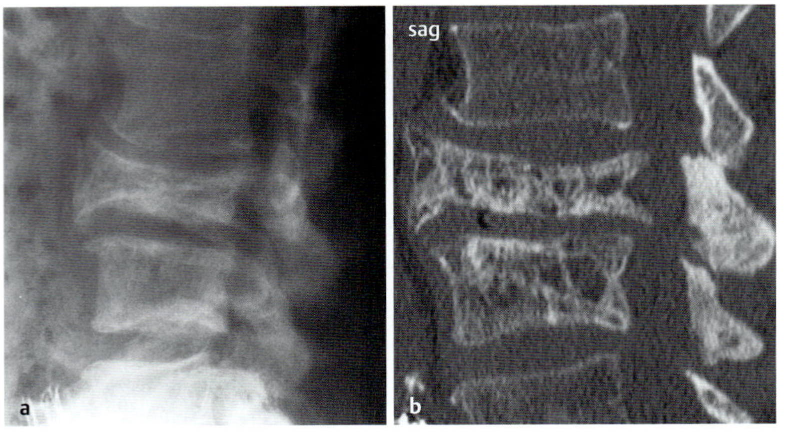

Fig. 11.9 Paget's disease of the lumbar spine. **(a)** Increase in AP diameter of L3 with concomitant loss of height. **(b)** Thickening of the cortex and particularly the cancellous trabeculae.

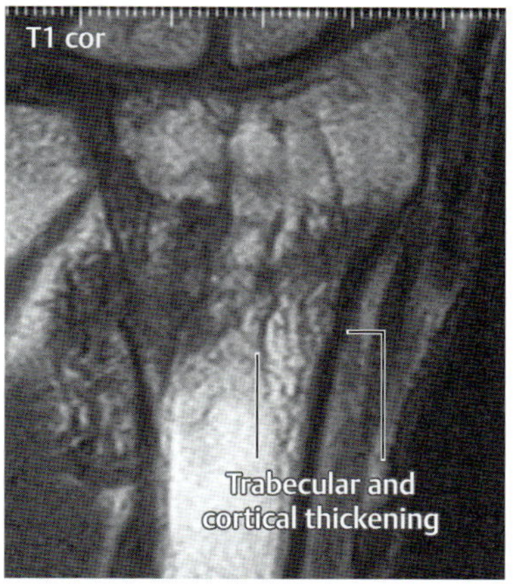

Fig. 11.10 MRI of the radius in a patient with Paget's disease. Note the largely preserved fatty marrow! Same patient as in ▶ Fig. 11.1.

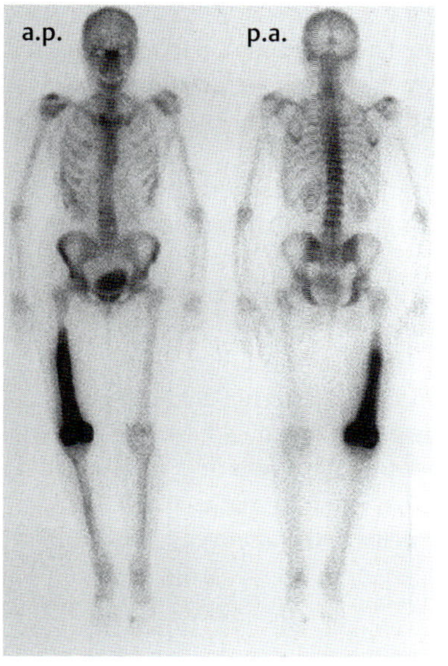

Fig. 11.11 Markedly increased bone metabolism in the right femur of a case of monostotic Paget's disease. Bone scan (late phase).

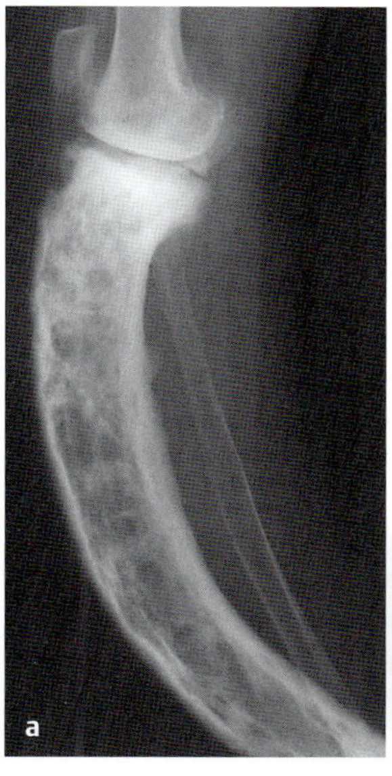

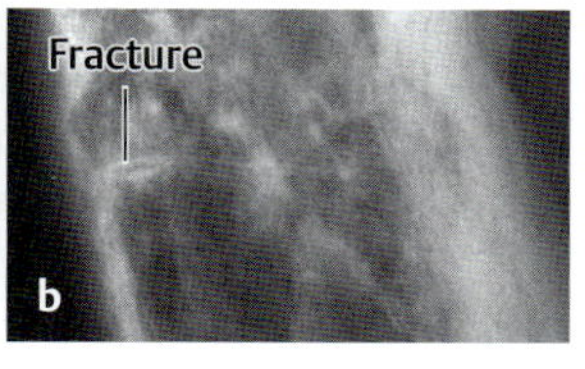

Fig. 11.12 Tibial involvement in Paget's disease. **(a)** Typical anterior bowing (sabre shin). **(b)** The magnified image shows a concomitant insufficiency fracture.

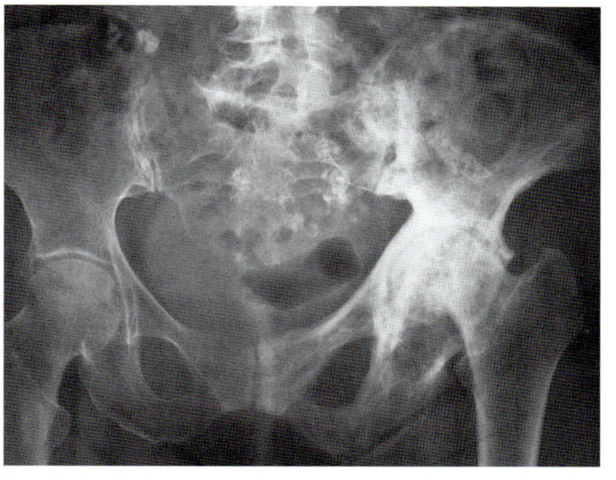

Fig. 11.13 Marked osteoarthritis with acetabular protrusion of the left hip in a patient with Paget's disease.

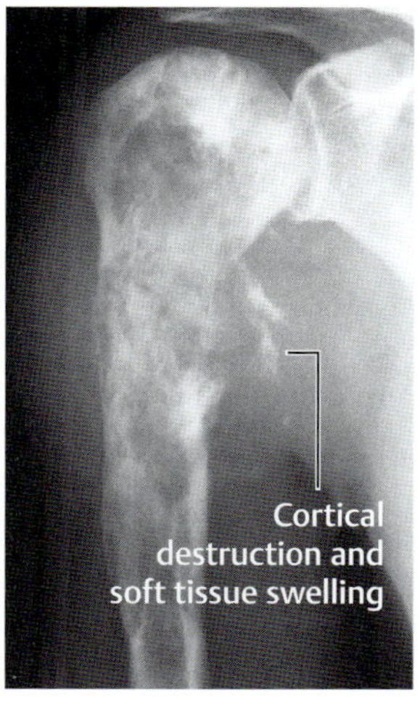

Fig. 11.14 Sarcoma of the right humerus in a patient with Paget's disease.

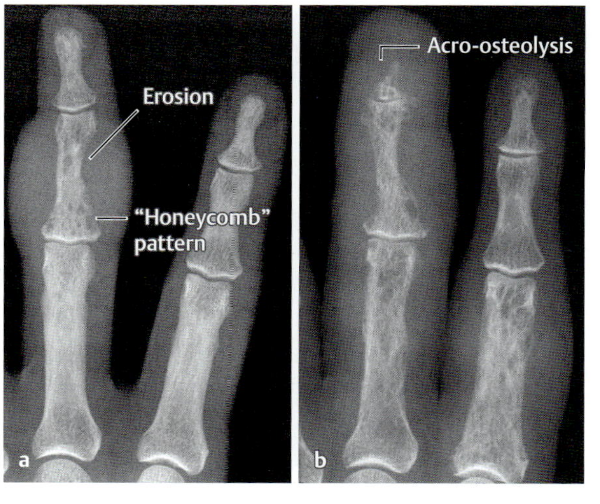

Fig. 11.15 Sarcoidosis of the phalanges. **(a)** Honeycomb-like alterations and soft tissue swelling of the middle phalanx of the middle finger. Involvement of the soft tissue results in destruction of the cortex from without. **(b)** Over time there is progression with acro-osteolysis and involvement of the index finger.

▸ **MRI.** MRI of skeletal sarcoidosis is nonspecific (see ▸ Fig. 11.16) and, without available clinical information, can be mistaken for bone metastases, especially in the long tubular bones and in the axial skeleton. Possible findings of muscular sarcoidosis:

- Diffuse muscle edema may be present in the acute stage.
- Nonspecific muscular atrophy may be identified in the chronic stage.
- A nodular appearance may be evident, albeit rare. The nodular type commonly develops at the musculotendinous junction. It demonstrates a fibrous, central, stellate nodule on all sequences and does not enhance with contrast. On T2W sequences this nodule has a central star-shaped area of decreased signal intensity surrounded by a hyperintense area that enhances diffusely with contrast and is composed of edema and granulomas (the "dark star sign").

11.3 Hypertrophic Osteoarthropathy

▸ **Pathology.** Hypertrophic osteoarthropathy, formerly known as hypertrophic pulmonary osteoarthropathy (synonym: Pierre–Marie–Bamberger disease), was first discovered as a paraneoplastic syndrome associated with bronchial carcinoma. It is divided into a **primary** (rare) and a **secondary form** (~95% of cases). The primary form is also known as **"pachydermoperiostosis"** and represents a congenital disorder. Unlike the primary form, secondary hypertrophic osteoarthropathy is associated with a large number of neoplastic, infectious and inflammatory diseases, with bronchial carcinoma being the most common (▸ Table 11.1). The exact pathogenesis of hypertrophic osteoarthropathy is still unclear, although it is assumed that vascular endothelial growth factor plays a decisive role. Hypertrophic osteoarthropathy occurs almost exclusively bilaterally and always in the tubular bones, with the tibia and fibula being most commonly affected (▸ Fig. 11.17).

> **Note**
> An established diagnosis of (secondary) hypertrophic osteoarthropathy of unknown origin should prompt further diagnostic examinations, especially in search of a tumorous disease (most commonly: bronchial carcinoma).

▸ **Clinical presentation.** Painful swellings in the diaphyseal region of the long tubular bones and clubbing of the fingers are the cardinal symptoms.

▸ **Radiography/CT.** Bilateral and symmetrical, periosteal new bone formations of the tubular bones are characteristic. They appear primarily in the diaphysis and progress toward the metaphysis (▸ Fig. 11.18; see also ▸ Fig. 11.17). Periosteal new bone formation progressing into the epiphysis would suggest a diagnosis of primary hypertrophic osteoarthropathy. The morphology of periosteal new bone formation (lamellated, onion-skin type, solid) can be most varied and depends on the duration of the illness.

▸ **MRI.** MRI demonstrates the nonspecific signs of periostitis.

▸ **NUC MED.** A bone scan is very sensitive; increased tracer uptake precedes radiographic findings (▸ Fig. 11.19).

▸ **DD. Chronic venous insufficiency.** It is possible to differentiate periosteal new bone formation secondary to chronic venous insufficiency from hypertrophic osteoarthropathy by their different clinical presentations.

Thyroid acropachy. This characteristically affects the hands and feet, sparing the long tubular bones.

11.4 Melorheostosis

▸ **Pathology.** Melorheostosis is a rare, nonhereditary, benign mesodermal dysplasia. It primarily involves the long tubular bones and their adjacent soft tissues. All age groups can be affected. The etiology of the disease is unclear. Melorheostosis spreads along so-called sclerotomes (zones of the skeleton that are supplied by an individual, spinal sensory nerve).

▸ **Radiography.** The finding of dense, linear, cortical hyperostosis along the longitudinal axis of the tubular bone is pathognomonic. Its configuration is more undulating, comparable with wax dripping down the side of a burning candle (▸ Fig. 11.20). The hyperostosis may also cross the joint and involve contiguous bone (▸ Fig. 11.21).

> **Note**
> The dripping candle wax sign is indeed pathognomonic of melorheostosis but not always recognizable. Sometimes an osteoma-like appearance predominates (▸ Fig. 11.22). Endosteal hyperostosis can also develop, resulting in partial or complete obliteration of the medullary cavity (see ▸ Fig. 11.21). Juxta-articular ossifications within the soft tissue (▸ Fig. 11.23)—sometimes even at a distance from the bony alterations—have also been reported.

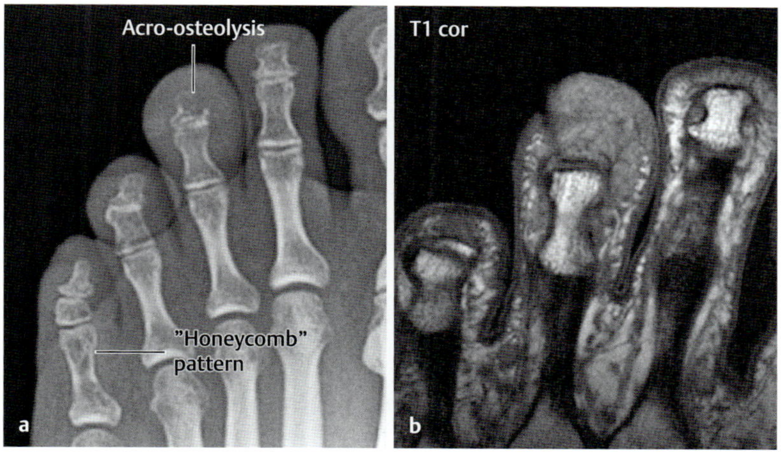

Fig. 11.16 Sarcoidosis of the foot. **(a)** Honeycomblike alterations of the fifth ray with acro-osteolysis of the third toe. **(b)** MRI reveals complete destruction of the distal phalanx of the third toe due to a marked soft tissue component.

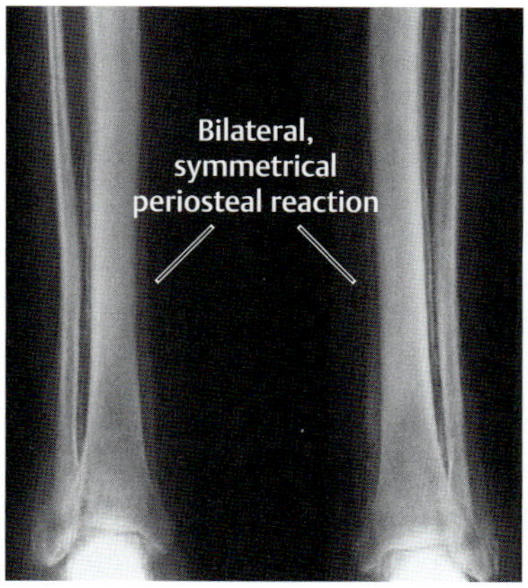

Fig. 11.17 Characteristic appearance of hypertrophic osteoarthropathy involving both lower legs.

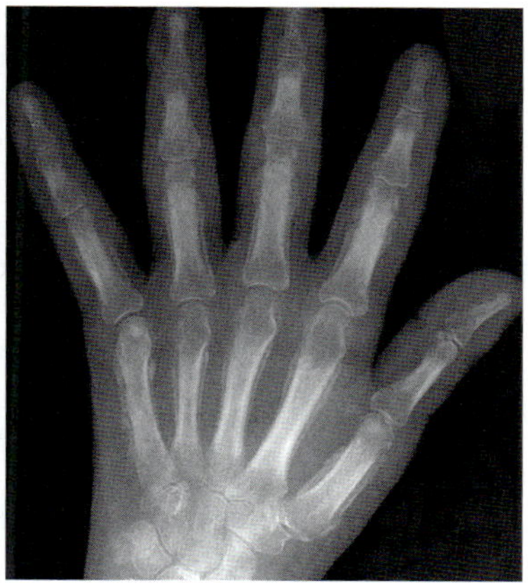

Fig. 11.18 Hypertrophic osteoarthropathy involving the metacarpals and the proximal phalanges.

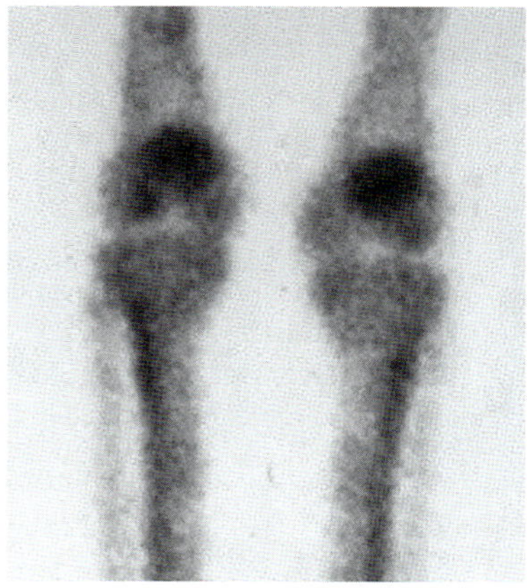

Fig. 11.19 Bone scan of a patient with hypertrophic osteoarthropathy. Typical uptake along both tibiae.

Table 11.1 Causes of secondary hypertrophic osteoarthropathy

Region	Disorders
Lungs and pleura	• Bronchogenic carcinoma • Lymphoma • Abscess • Bronchiectasis • Metastases • Mesothelioma • Pleural fibroma
Gastro-intestinal tract	• Ulcerative colitis • Crohn's disease • Liver cirrhosis • Esophageal cancer • Coeliac disease • Lymphoma • Whipple's disease • Polyposis
Cardiovascular system	• Congenital cyanotic heart disease
Various organ systems	• Nasopharyngeal cancer • AIDS (acquired immune deficiency syndrome)

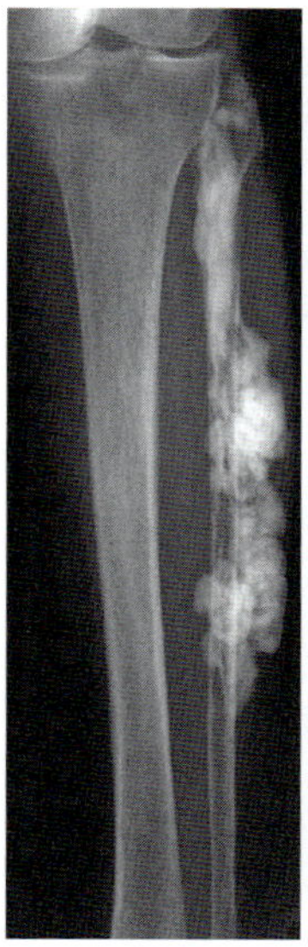

Fig. 11.20 Classic "dripping candle wax sign" in melorheostosis of the fibula.

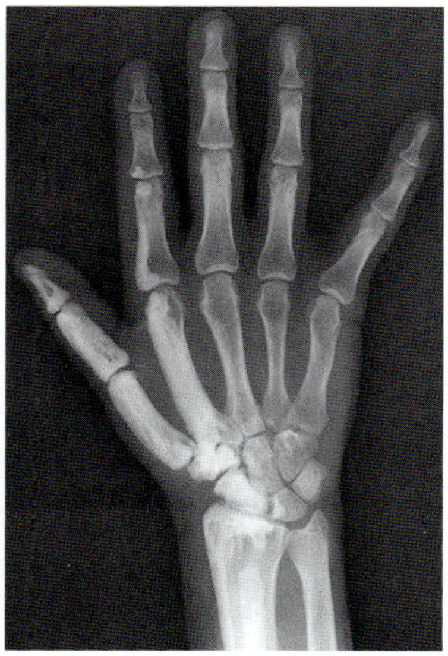

Fig. 11.21 Polyostotic melorheostosis of the radius and the hand. In part, complete obliteration of the medullary cavity.

► CT/MRI. Melorheostosis tends to be an incidental finding on imaging. The findings of projection radiography also apply for CT, where they are unobscured by overlying structures (► Fig. 11.24). On MRI, loss of signal predominates on all sequences. Soft tissue involvement appears on CT as soft tissue density and ossifications within the soft tissue that are characteristically not connected with the adjacent bone (► Fig. 11.25). Unlike CT, the appearance of soft tissue involvement on MRI is most varied and depends on the degree of mineralization.

► DD. **Parosteal osteosarcoma.** This has an irregular pattern, is not as homogeneously dense, and results in bone destruction.

Osteopathia striata. This benign dysplasia of bone involves the medullary cavity of the tubular bones and is usually bilateral. The findings are of epiphyseal and metaphyseal location and appear as more streaked and pillarlike striations. They are vertically orientated ("celery stalk metaphysis").

Note

Osteoma, osteopoikilosis (cf. Chapter 4.3.1), osteopathia striata, and melorheostosis are all mesodermal, benign dysplasias. Demarcation between these pathological conditions is sometimes difficult but clinically not particularly relevant.

11.5 Calcifications and Ossifications of the Soft Tissues

11.5.1 Soft Tissue Calcifications

Soft tissue calcifications may be classified according to location (generalized or localized) or on the basis of their causes:

- Soft tissue calcifications due to disturbances of calcium phosphate metabolism.
- Soft tissue calcifications with normal calcium phosphate metabolism.
- Soft tissue calcifications in dystrophic or necrotic tissue.

A special group comprises the joint-related soft tissue calcifications (hydroxyapatite deposition disease, calcium pyrophosphate deposition disease [CPPD], gout), which are dealt with in detail in Chapter 10.9.

Soft tissue calcifications due to disturbances of calcium phosphate metabolism. The most common causes of soft tissue calcifications secondary to disturbed calcium phosphate metabolism (synonym: metastatic calcification) are renal osteodystrophy and hyperparathyroidism; less common causes are listed in ► Table 11.2. All forms are found, ranging from fine, stippled to coarse calcifications. Hyperparathyroidism demonstrates a predominantly periarticular distribution.

Soft tissue calcifications with normal calcium phosphate metabolism. The most common cause of this form of soft tissue calcification, which is also synonymously known as "idiopathic calcinosis," is collagenosis. A variant is "pseudotumorous" (also: tumoral) calcinosis. It usually occurs in the 20th to 40th years of life (males are more commonly affected than females) and is associated with extensive calcifications, especially in the region of major joints. The radiographic appearance of calcifications is that of a conglomeration of many calcified nodules, ranging in size from 1 to 20 cm, which are demarcated from each other by fine radiolucent lines (see ► Fig. 11.27).

Dystrophic calcification. Dystrophic calcification is caused by any form of tissue necrosis, the most important being burns and frostbite. Additional causes are listed in ► Table 11.2. See also ► Fig. 11.28.

► Radiography/CT. The radiographic appearance of soft tissue calcifications is characterized by stippled, circumferential, extensive densities. The patterns appearing on radiographs and CT do not always allow differentiation of the cause of the calcification. In the first instance, however, distribution pattern and laboratory results are indicative.

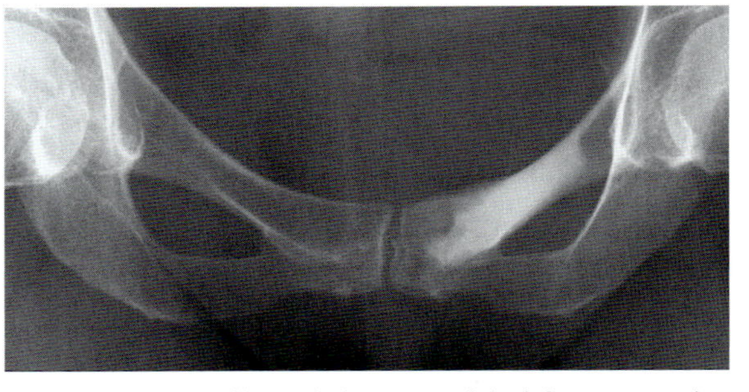

Fig. 11.22 Osteomalike melorheostosis of the left superior pubic ramus.

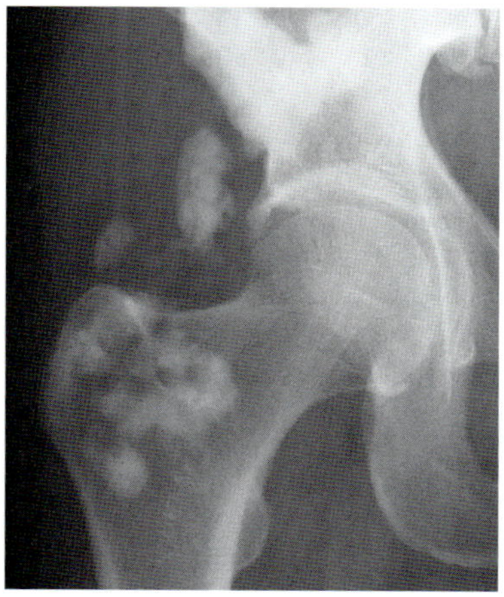

Fig. 11.23 Melorheostosis of the right ilium with juxta-articular soft tissue ossification.

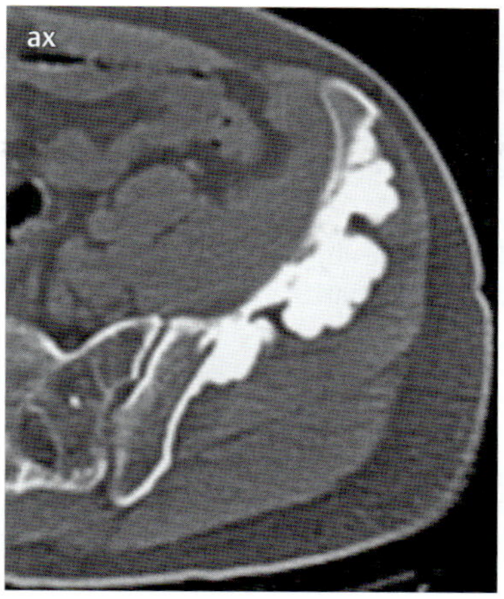

Fig. 11.24 CT image of classic melorheostosis of the ilium.

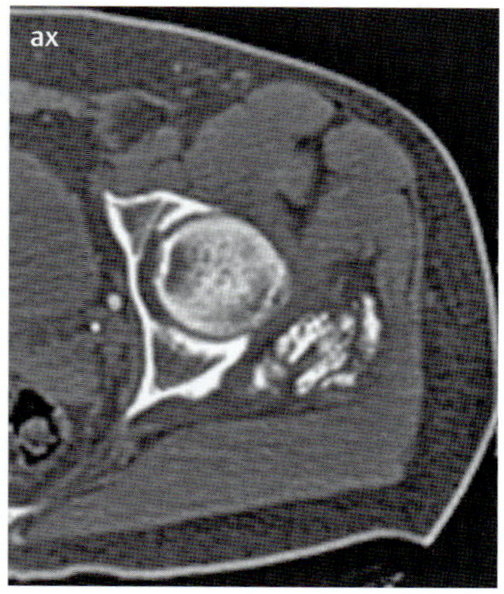

Fig. 11.25 Juxta-articular soft tissue ossification in a case of melorheostosis.

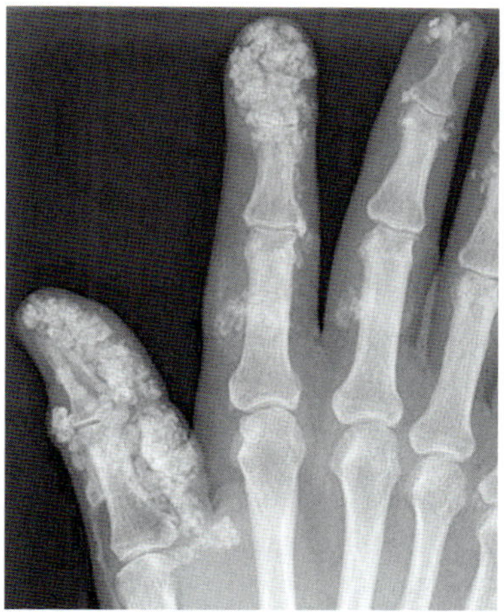

Fig. 11.26 Idiopathic soft tissue calcification in CREST syndrome. (Image courtesy of Herbert Rosenthal, Hannover, Germany.)

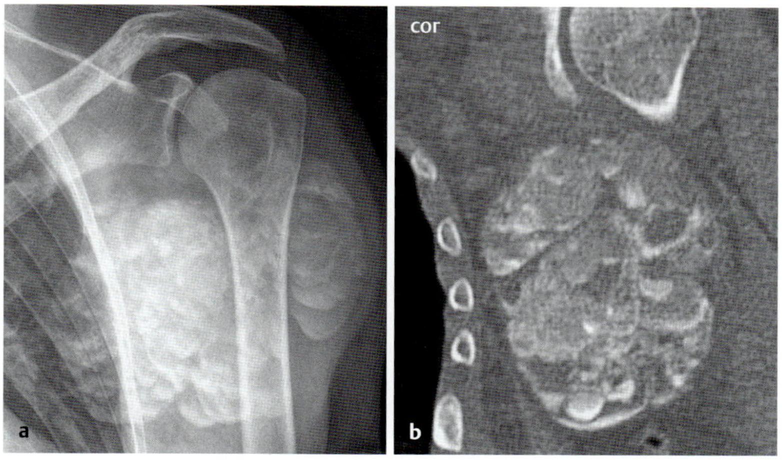

Fig. 11.27 Pseudotumorous calcinosis of the shoulder joint. (Images courtesy of Herbert Rosenthal, Hannover, Germany.) **(a)** Multiple calcified nodules, clearly separated from one another. **(b)** CT image unobscured by overlying structures.

Table 11.2 Overview of the causes of soft tissue calcifications (excluding joint-related soft tissue calcifications, such as hydroxyapatite deposition disease, CPPD and gout; refer to Chapter 10.9)

"Metastatic" calcifications (disturbed calcium and phosphate metabolism)	"Idiopathic" calcifications (normal calcium and phosphate metabolism)	"Dystrophic" calcifications (normal calcium and phosphate metabolism)
• Hyperparathyroidism • Renal osteodystrophy • Hypervitaminosis D • Sarcoidosis • Massive bone destruction in cases of plasmacytoma, leukemia, or extensive metastatic spread	• Collagenoses (e.g., lupus erythematosus, dermatomyositis, CREST syndrome, scleroderma; ▶ Fig. 11.26) • "Pseudotumorous" calcinosis (▶ Fig. 11.27) • Calcinosis universalis (in children)	• Burns • Frostbite • Severe soft tissue injuries • Compartment syndrome • Tumors (without own cartilage or osteoid production; ▶ Fig. 11.28) • Osteonecroses, infarctions • Tuberculosis

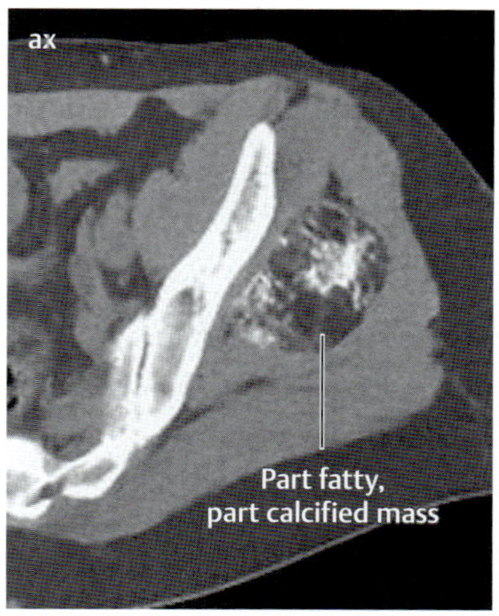

Fig. 11.28 Dystrophic calcification in a gluteal lipoma. (Image courtesy of Herbert Rosenthal, Hannover, Germany.)

11.5.2 Soft Tissue Ossifications

Soft tissue ossifications are new bone formations that, provided they have advanced sufficiently, demonstrate a trabecular structure with bone cortex. Causes include:

- Heterotopic ossification (myositis ossificans).
- Chronic venous insufficiency (▶ Fig. 11.29).
- Tumor matrix (cartilaginous and bony matrix; ▶ Fig. 11.30; cf. ▶ Table 4.1).

> **Note**
> In principle, bone tissue may form from any calcification by the process of secondary ossification. With discrete findings the distinction between ossification and calcification is not always possible from the radiograph, nor is it always reliable using other imaging modalities.

Heterotopic Ossification (Myositis Ossificans)

Heterotopic ossification (synonym: myositis ossificans) is a benign, self-limiting ossifying soft tissue alteration affecting skeletal muscles.

▶ **Pathology.** Trauma is usually the main cause, even if it is not always confirmed by the case history. Heterotopic ossification also complicates the process of rehabilitation in 20 to 30% of patients with spinal cord injuries. Undifferentiated, mesenchymal cells develop whose matrix (a ground substance of osteoid) calcifies and ossifies. This is neither a case of inflammation nor the simple calcification of a hematoma.

▶ **Clinical presentation.** A painful, hyperemic soft tissue swelling appears in the first weeks, followed later by an enlarging induration but with less pain. Laboratory results occasionally reveal elevated inflammatory parameters.

Location. Potentially, heterotopic ossification can develop anywhere, but it has a predilection for the thigh and elbow.

Therapy. Treatment is rarely indicated. In fact, early surgical intervention should be avoided because the lesion tends to recur.

▶ **Radiography.** Heterotopic ossification and its radiographic features follow an evolutionary process of change that can be variable over time:

- **Early signs:** These appear as cloudy, partly extensive and partly linear densities within the musculature (▶ Fig. 11.31a). The densities can extend as far as the bone, although a fine radiolucent line is almost always distinguishable between the bone and the density.
- **Between the 4th and 6th weeks:** The increase in density of the lesion begins at its margin (eggshell appearance). Thus the lesion matures from the periphery to the center (zonal phenomenon; ▶ Fig. 11.32); i.e., while the rim develops a radiodense ring of mature lamellar bone, the less radiodense center displays an irregular osteogenic matrix. The radiograph can also display a relatively homogeneous density (▶ Fig. 11.33).
- **From the 4th month:** The maturation of the ossification progresses (▶ Fig. 11.34) and the lesion becomes denser and smaller.

> **Note**
> In myositis ossificans the cortex of the bone near the lesion remains intact but may also react, with a lamellated or solid periosteal reaction. This form is sometimes referred to as periostitis ossificans.

▶ **US.** A hypoechoic to echo-inhomogeneous space-occupying mass is found in the early stage, while calcifications recognizable on ultrasound may be absent. Color-coded Doppler ultrasound displays increased marginal perfusion. Fine acoustic shadowing artifacts are already evident quite early on and are regarded as signs of incipient calcification or ossification. Their density and homogeneity increases in later (more mature) stages. A wide, hoodlike or caplike echo front with acoustic shadowing is formed that consequently makes assessment of the lesion difficult.

▶ **CT.** Very small disseminated densities are initially found that can be irregularly arranged or even already confluent (▶ Fig. 11.31b). Later the classic zonal phenomenon (dense rim and a less dense center) and the sometimes layered structure are more easily recognizable earlier than on projection radiography. CT—not MRI—is the modality of choice for detailed assessment.

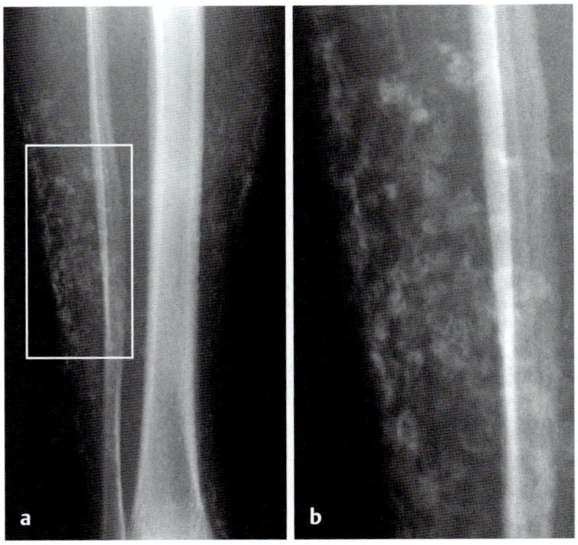

Fig. 11.29 Soft tissue ossifications in chronic venous insufficiency. **(a)** The soft tissue ossifications display a latticelike structure. **(b)** Enlargement of the area marked in (**a**).

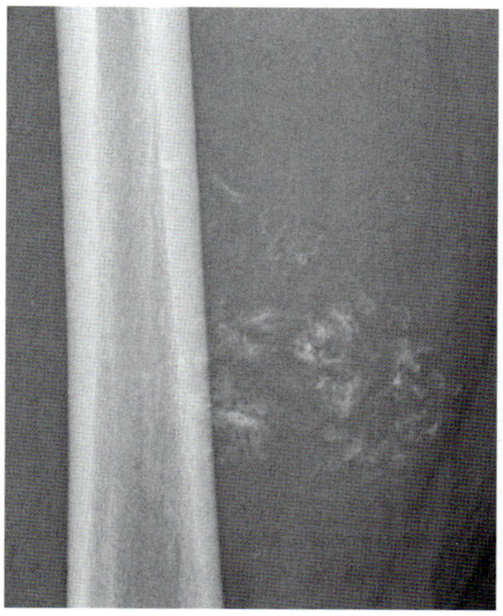

Fig. 11.30 Matrix calcifications of an extraosseous osteosarcoma of the thigh. (Image courtesy of Herbert Rosenthal, Hannover, Germany.)

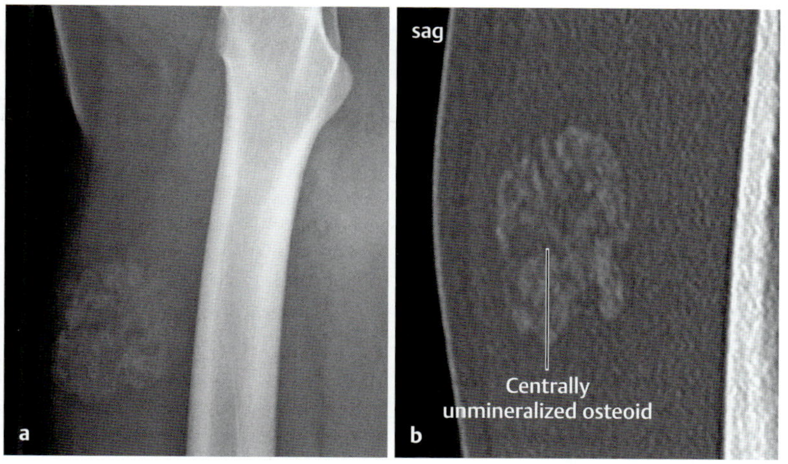

Fig. 11.31 Myositis ossificans. Slowly progressive, mildly painful swelling of the thigh. **(a)** Ossification with irregular contours and quite variable density. **(b)** CT does not yet show the classic zonal architecture.

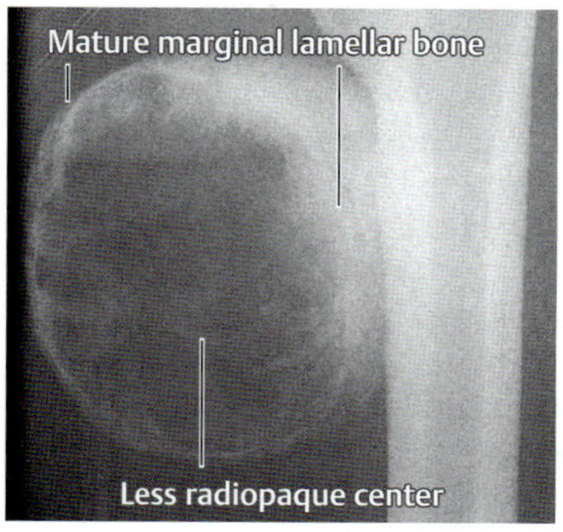

Fig. 11.32 "Mature" myositis ossificans with characteristic zonal phenomenon.

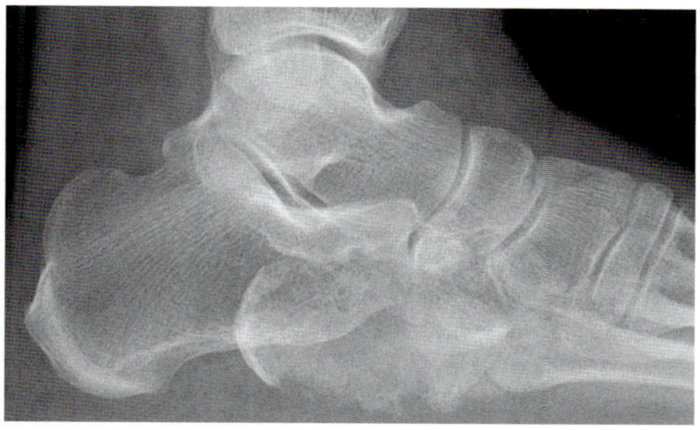

Fig. 11.33 Myositis ossificans. Homogeneous, almost ground-glass density with eggshell-like margin overlying the calcaneus. (Image courtesy of Herbert Rosenthal, Hannover, Germany.)

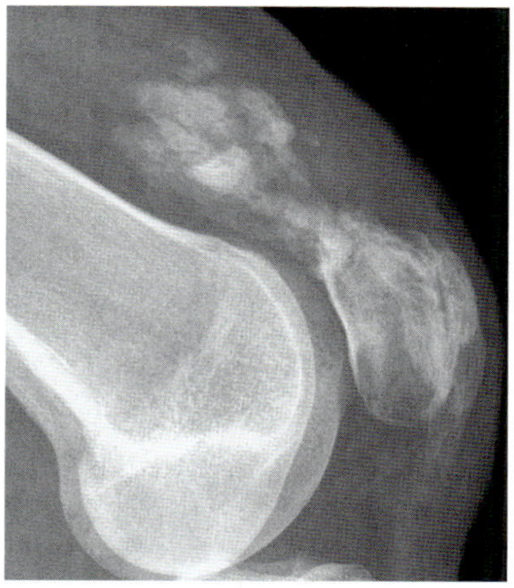

Fig. 11.34 "Mature" myositis ossificans. (Image courtesy of Herbert Rosenthal, Hannover, Germany.)

▸ **MRI.** The alterations found on MRI as well as radiographic and CT signs are dependent on the stage of development. The lesion is usually isointense to normal muscle on T1W images (▸ Figs. 11.35a and ▸ 11.36a). On T2W sequences it appears inhomogeneous, partly with a strong central hyperintensity (▸ Figs. 11.35b and ▸ 11.36b), partly with fluid–fluid levels, as with an aneurysmal bone cyst. In later (more mature) stages a hypointense rim is identifiable on T1W and T2W sequences corresponding to the marginal ossification. GRE sequences can detect small calcifications quite early. The lesion takes up contrast strongly, especially at the margins (▸ Fig. 11.35c). In the early stage, findings have also been reported with a nonenhancing center, accompanied by a strongly enhancing marginal zone. The extensive edema surrounding the lesion is characteristic and sometimes far exceeds the size of the lesion. After ~ 6 to 8 weeks the lesion becomes increasingly demarcated within the decreasing edema. Contrast enhancement also slowly decreases.

▸ **DD. Osteoma and periosteal chondroma.** Heterotopic ossification without an extensive edema is rare (only in the late stage). MRI helps to differentiate from osteochondroma and periosteal chondroma (no edema).

Soft tissue sarcoma. Certain soft tissue sarcomas such as synovial sarcoma and osteosarcoma can calcify. The calcifications are usually distributed throughout the tumor and do not demonstrate a zonal phenomenon (▸ Fig. 11.37).

Chronic venous insufficiency. A distinction is made between the following forms of ossification:

- Nodular or undulating periosteal ossification due to periostitis.
- Genuine soft tissue ossification secondary to metaplastic new bone formation (see ▸ Fig. 11.29).

The diagnosis is usually easily made from the underlying condition, which is generally known, and from the appropriate location of the ossifications.

Muscle hematomas. Secondary ossifications can appear in these hematomas; they are irregular, however, and not only arranged peripherally but also centrally.

Myonecrosis. Amorphous chalklike dystrophic calcifications occur in myonecrosis.

11.6 Compartment Syndrome

Compartment syndromes develop in osteofibrous confined spaces whose anatomy permits only little increase in volume under physiological conditions. Such compartments are typically found in the limbs, although any confined space invested by bone and/or fasciae can develop compartment syndrome under pathological circumstances. Compartment syndromes most commonly occur in the lower leg and the forearm, less frequently in the femoral and gluteal regions.

> **Note**
> Acute compartment syndrome is a surgical emergency requiring immediate diagnosis and treatment.

▸ **Pathology.** The exact pathogenesis is not yet fully understood. It is, however, known that permeability changes, even to the extent of cell membrane destruction, can occur from the effects of a damaging event (e.g., severe tissue contusion, long-standing ischemia, limb fractures), which results in a drastic increase of extracellular fluid volume. This leads to a rapid rise in intracompartmental pressure (over 15–20 mmHg). This in turn exceeds capillary pressure and thus causes capillary stasis, which results in ischemia and nerve damage, triggering off a vicious cycle. If decisive surgical decompressive fasciotomy is delayed or incomplete then muscle necrosis will develop, associated with fibrous remodeling and postischemic contracture.

Exertional compartment syndrome is a separate etiological entity affecting mainly athletes (long-distance runners). A high level of exertion produces a progressively increasing rise in intramuscular pressure that does not return to normal, even under resting conditions, thus resulting in an acute compartment syndrome.

▸ **Clinical presentation.** The clinical presentation is characterized by painful swelling of the affected part of the limb with subsequent neurologic deficit that varies over time (dysesthesia and hypesthesia, later increasing paralysis). The pulse slows down and in rare cases is completely absent. The affected limb feels **cool.**

▸ **Radiography/CT.** Radiographic modalities are noncontributory; on CT there is at best reduced soft tissue differentiation within the compartment and a bulging protrusion of the tense fasciae is recognizable.

▸ **MRI.** Loss of intra- and intermuscular septations is evident on T1W images, with more diffuse increased signal intensity in the affected compartment on T2W sequences (▸ Fig. 11.38). The findings are confined to one compartment, which also applies to (unrecognized) chronic cases that manifest as muscular atrophy and fibrosis. Contrast enhancement patterns are varied: Whereas there is usually a strong muscle contrast enhancement in the acute phase, subacute and chronic compartment syndromes lack any contrast enhancement.

▸ **DD. Neuropathic myopathy (denervation syndrome secondary to nerve entrapment).** Differentiation is occasionally difficult here when based entirely on imaging, but when assessed together with the case history and clinical presentation (trophic alterations?) then the disorders are distinguishable.

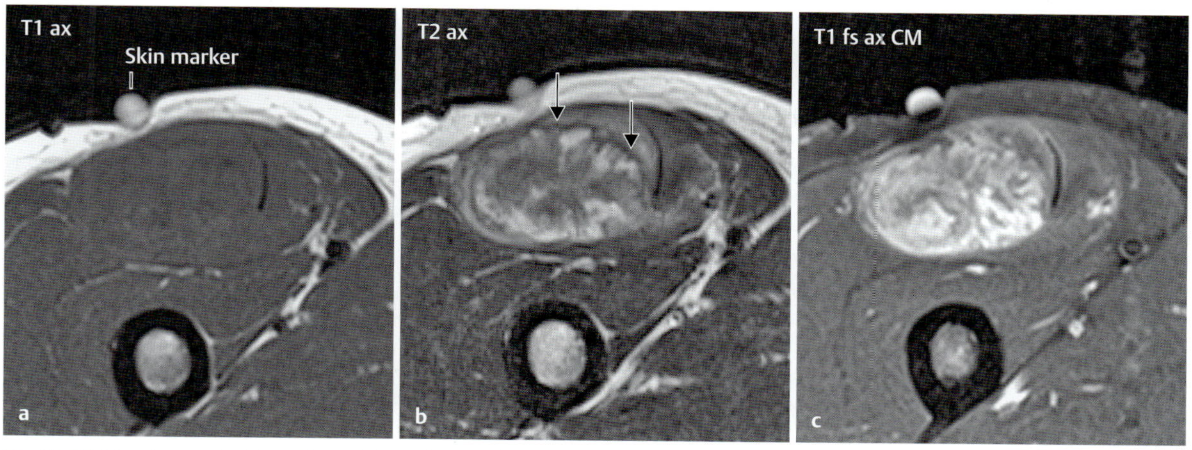

Fig. 11.35 Signal characteristics of myositis ossificans. The same patient as in ▶ Fig. 11.31. **(a)** Almost isointense to normal muscle on the T1W image (later associated with hypointense ossifications). **(b)** Moderately hyperintense and inhomogeneous on the T2W image. A hypointense line is already evident at the margin (arrows). **(c)** Extensive heterogeneous enhancement on T1W fat-saturated image post contrast.

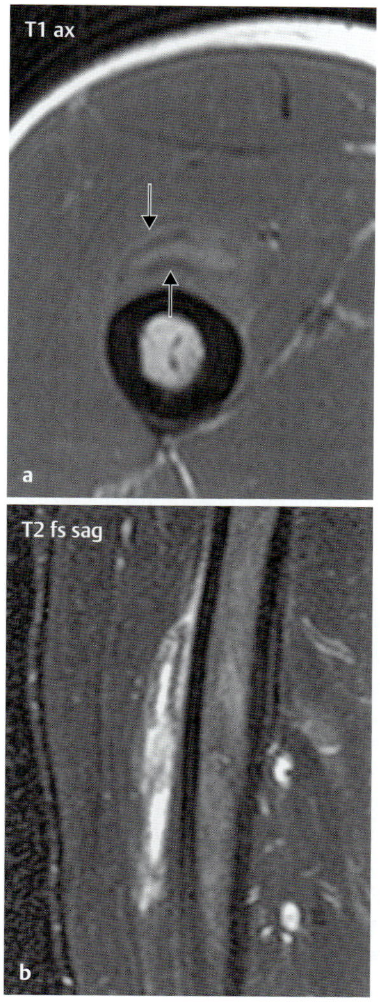

Fig. 11.36 Myositis ossificans. **(a)** Fine, incipient, marginal calcification (arrows). **(b)** Strongly hyperintense fluid components are identified on the T2W image.

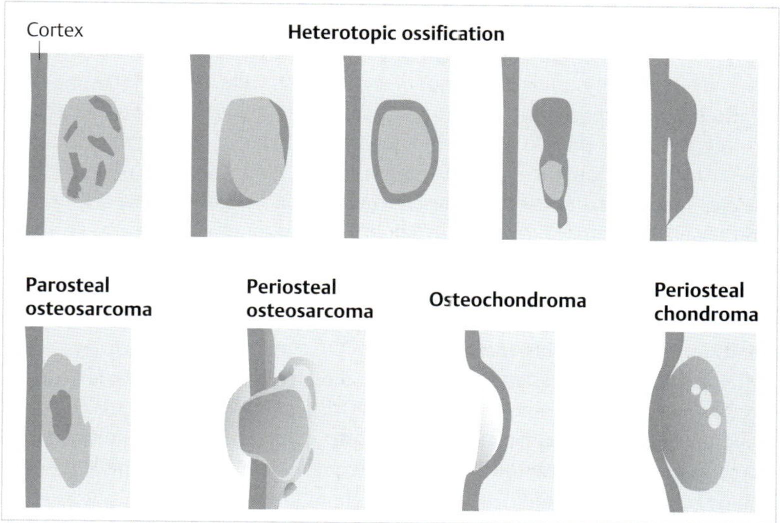

Fig. 11.37 Radiographic signs of heterotopic ossification and differential diagnoses.

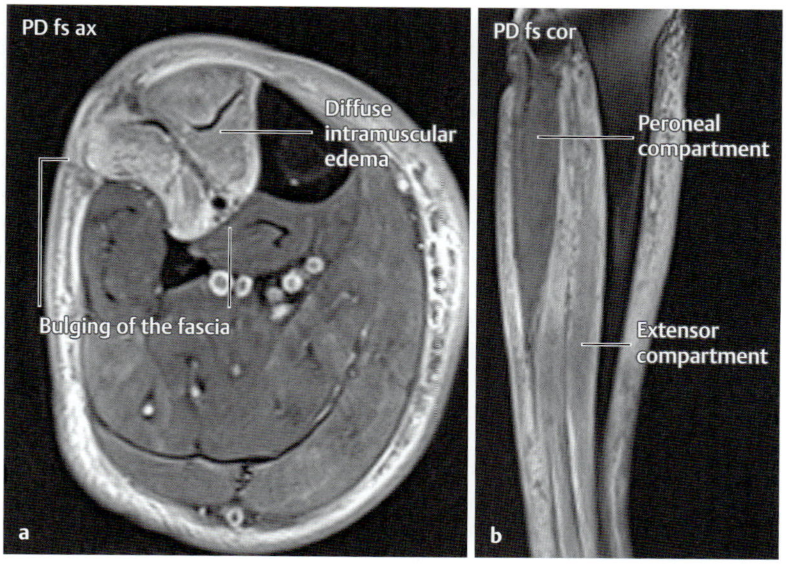

Fig. 11.38 Compartment syndrome of the lower leg secondary to a phlegmonous inflammation. **(a)** Bulging fasciae. Invasive measurement confirmed significantly increased intracompartmental pressure. **(b)** The diffuse intramuscular edema involves the entire extensor compartment.

11

Myositis. Polymyositis is an autoimmune-related disorder and characteristically displays a bilateral and symmetrical distribution pattern (Chapter 10.8.3). Pyomyositis (Chapter 3.2) is recognizable from intramuscular abscess formations. However, compartment-related (ischemic) muscle necrosis does look similar. Ultrasound-guided biopsy is of assistance in unclear cases.

Necrotizing fasciitis. The fasciae and fascial spaces are primarily involved in this potentially life-threatening disorder, which demonstrates extensive edema and enhancement. Adjacent epifascial and subfascial spaces are also involved. Involvement of the deep muscle fasciae and the absence of fascial enhancement are specific for necrotizing fasciitis (Chapter 3.2.1).

Rhabdomyolysis. See Chapter 11.7.

11.7 Rhabdomyolysis

▸ Pathology. Rhabdomyolysis is characterized by the loss of integrity of the muscle cell membranes, which can increase to become an excessive **disintegration of striated muscle**. Mechanical causes of muscle destruction range from localized overuse (exercise myoglobinuria) to extensive soft tissue contusions such as can occur after entrapments and burying (**crush syndrome**). There is also a toxic form of skeletal muscle disintegration caused by alcohol, medications (e.g., hypnosedatives, anesthetic agents, as well as appetite suppressants and statins), addictive drugs (heroin, cocaine), and some snake poisons. Other causes of rhabdomyolysis are hypothermia (e.g., frostbite), hyperthermia (burns), and autoimmune diseases. Less common causes include bacterial infections (e.g., tetanus, typhoid fever) and viral organisms (e.g., flu viruses). And finally there are also hereditary diseases (e.g., McArdle's disease) that induce muscle disintegration.

11

The final common path of all known forms of rhabdomyolysis is nephrotoxic myoglobinuria, which causes obstruction of renal tubules.

▸ MRI. Soft tissue changes of MRI are nonspecific. Early on in the clinical course muscle edema is already identifiable with partly homogeneous, partly heterogeneous increased intramuscular signal intensity on fat-suppressed water-sensitive sequences. These findings appear alone or disseminated in different muscle regions and compartments. Spontaneous hemorrhage occurs and is evident in the form of hyperintense signal alterations on T1W SE sequences (methemoglobin) or strong loss of signal on GRE images (susceptibility artifacts due to hemosiderin deposits). The image can vary after IV administration of contrast, depending on the degree of devitalization. Apart from homogeneous contrast uptake (ubiquitous barrier breakdown), areas with marginal enhancement may also be recognizable.

▸ DD. **Polymyositis, pyomyositis.** See differential diagnosis in Chapter 11.6.

Compartment syndrome. See Chapter 11.6.

Neuropathy-induced soft tissue lesions (nerve entrapment syndromes). See Chapter 11.8.

11.8 Peripheral Nerve Entrapment and Nerve Compression Syndromes

▸ Pathology. Peripheral nerves may be subjected to pathologic intermittent or permanent compression at any site. The terms "nerve compression syndrome" and "nerve entrapment neuropathy" refer to the commonly seen entrapment situations along the course of peripheral nerves.

Peripheral nerve compression syndromes are generally encountered at **atomically recognized bottlenecks,** which are usually located at osteofibrous tunnels or canals. The canals are often slitlike in form, rigid, and nonexpansile and do not allow the nerve any room to avoid imposing forces. Canals can also develop secondary to scar formation (posttraumatic, postoperative), constitutional stenotic tissue tunnels, and additional space-occupying entities (tumors, ganglia, accessory muscles, tendons, and aberrant vessels). Another possible anatomical cause is a **superficial location of the nerve,** which is subsequently directly exposed to external mechanical pressure loads (e.g., repetitive injury of the ulnar nerve at the medial humeral epicondyle; positional injury of the peroneal nerve at the fibular head). Considerably less common causes of peripheral entrapment neuropathies include hypertrophic callus formations (e.g., secondary to radius shaft fractures or scapula neck fractures), exostoses (e.g., supracondylar process of humerus), or bony malunion after fractures and inflammatory processes in the vicinity of peripheral nerves (synovitis, bursitis, tendinopathy).

▸ Tables 11.3 and ▸ 11.4 provide an overview of compression syndromes and entrapment neuropathies.

▸ Radiography/CT. Conventional radiography and CT can always be employed to advantage when dealing with cases where the causes of nerve compression are bone- or calcification-related. Apart from acute diagnostic trauma investigations (fracture, fragment dislocation) and posttraumatic reviews (callus formation, soft tissue calcifications), conventional radiographic examinations play an important role in the assessment of osteophytes, exostoses, bone tumors, and tumorlike lesions.

Table 11.3 Compression syndromes and entrapment neuropathies of the shoulder girdle and upper limbs

Affected nerve	Anatomical region	Syndrome/symptoms
Brachial plexus	Interscalene triangle, costoclavicular space, thoraco-coracopectoral space	*Thoracic outlet syndrome:* most varied etiology and symptoms; often mixed presentation due to association with vascular (arterial/venous) changes; thus no characteristic MRI pathomorphology
	Brachial plexus	*Parsonage–Turner syndrome:* not entrapment, but self-limiting, idiopathic brachial neuritis (neuralgic amyotrophy); sudden onset of painful shoulder girdle, weakness, dysesthesia, and numbness; intramuscular signal changes in the rotators as well as the deltoid and pectoral muscles
Suprascapular nerve	Suprascapular notch, covered by the superior transverse scapular nerve	*Suprascapular notch syndrome:* compression of the suprascapular nerve results in edema or atrophy of the supra- and infraspinatus muscles (► Fig. 11.39)
	Infraspinous fossa, covered by the inferior transverse scapular ligament	"*Spinoglenoid notch syndrome*" (suprascapular nerve entrapment): if only the distal part of the suprascapular nerve is compressed, then only the infraspinatus muscle is involved
Axillary nerve	Lateral axillary hiatus (posttraumatic after shoulder dislocation; fibrous ligaments, hematoma, tumors)	*Lateral axillary hiatus syndrome:* shoulder pain, dysesthesia of the lateral aspect of the upper arm; edema or atrophy of the deltoid muscle (proximal) and/or teres minor (distal)
Ulnar nerve	Medial humeral epicondyle and medial elbow region (arcuate ligament, arcade of Struthers; anconeus epitrochlearis muscle)	*Cubital tunnel syndrome:* compression, dislocation and friction of the nerve may result in edema or atrophy of the flexor carpi ulnaris and flexor digitorum profundus muscles
	Ulnar palm: Guyon's canal (pisohamate canal)	*Ulnar tunnel syndrome (Guyon's canal syndrome):* the interossei and lumbrical muscles are involved, sometimes also the hypothenar muscles and adductor pollicis
Radial nerve	Mid-dorsal aspect of the upper arm (beware in humeral shaft fractures)	Lesion within the radial nerve sulcus (spiral groove) *Entrapment syndrome at the radial hiatus*: all the muscles of the lower arm are affected
Deep branch (posterior interosseous nerve)	Distal and radial cubital fossa: radial tunnel (at the level of the humeroradial joint before division of the radial nerve) and supinator compartment (within the muscle)	*Radial tunnel syndrome:* involves both the motor and sensory part of the radial nerve
		Supinator syndrome (posterior interosseous syndrome): edema or atrophy of all forearm extensors, including supinator (► Fig. 11.40)
Median nerve	Cubital fossa/proximal forearm: between superficial and deep heads of pronator teres	*Pronator teres syndrome:* edema or atrophy of the pronator–flexor muscle group (pronator teres, flexor carpi radialis, flexor digitorum superior, palmaris longus)
	Palmar carpal region (directly beneath the transverse carpal ligament, over or between the radial flexor tendons)	*Carpal tunnel syndrome:* apart from typical sensory deficit there is edema or atrophy of the thenar muscles (except adductor pollicis). Beware: form, thickness, and signal of the median nerve is not particularly specific
Anterior interosseous nerve	Palmar forearm (branches off from the median nerve at the proximal third of the forearm)	*Anterior interosseous syndrome (Kiloh–Nevin syndrome):* edema in pronator quadratus (!); also affected are flexor pollicis longus and radial half of flexor digitorum profundus

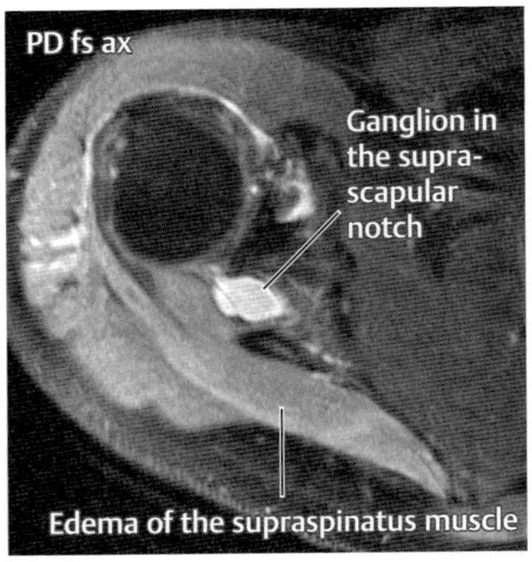

Fig. 11.39 Suprascapular syndrome due to entrapment of the suprascapularis nerve.

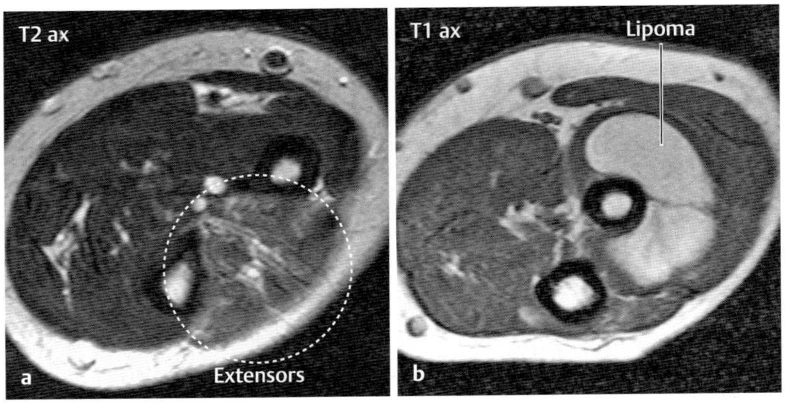

Fig. 11.40 Supinator syndrome. **(a)** Edema of all forearm extensors, including supinator (motion artifacts). **(b)** The cause was a lipoma of the proximal forearm compressing the deep branch of the radial nerve.

Table 11.4 Compression syndromes and entrapment neuropathies of the pelvic girdle and lower limbs

Affected nerve	Anatomical region	Syndrome/symptoms
Sciatic nerve	Lower gluteal region: infrapiriform foramen	*Piriformis syndrome:* nonradicular sciatica; only rarely leads to muscular changes in the distribution area of the sciatic nerve
Obturator nerve	Anterior pubic region (fracture callus; secondary to prostate surgery)	Adductor weakness: edema or atrophy of the thigh adductors (▸ Fig. 11.41) *Howship–Romberg syndrome:* purely sensory
Femoral nerve	Inguinal region (muscular lacuna)	Pain and weakness of anterior thigh: very rarely alterations in muscle signal intensity within quadriceps femoris
Common peroneal nerve	Winds around the fibular head and neck, very superficial position (pressure damage!), joint ganglia, exostoses, proximal fibular fracture	Peroneal nerve compression: the entire extensor and peroneal muscle group may be affected, depending on the level of injury *Fibular tunnel syndrome:* located somewhat farther distally (involves only the deep peroneal nerve); edema or atrophy of the lower leg muscles (most prominently tibialis anterior)
Tibial nerve	Popliteal fossa (tumors of the popliteal surface of the femur, ganglia, popliteal aneurysms)	Plantar flexion weakness: all the calf muscles are involved (edema or atrophy of the superficial and/or deep flexors to varying degrees)
• **Distal tibial nerve and plantar nerves**	Medial perimalleolar region, tarsal tunnel beneath the flexor retinaculum	*(Posterior) Tarsal tunnel syndrome:* the short flexors of the sole of the foot are involved (in particular abducens hallucis, flexor digitorum brevis, abducens digiti minimi, and quadratus plantae)
• **Terminal branches of the medial plantar nerve**	Compression at the level of the knot of Henry (crossing of the flexor digitorum tendon obliquely over the flexor hallucis longus tendon in the midfoot) or at the degenerated first metatarsophalangeal joint	*Jogger's foot:* chronic atrophy of abductor hallucis and flexor hallucis brevis (▸ Fig. 11.42)
• **Inferior calcaneal branch**	Compression of the nerve at the medial border of the heel	*Baxter's neuralgia:* painful myopathy of the abductor digiti minimi muscle (see ▸ Fig. 11.42)
• **Digitorum plantares nerves**	Distal midfoot, bases of the third and fourth toes	*Interdigital Morton's neuroma (Morton's metatarsalgia):* not a true entrapment but rather perineural fibrosis

▶ **US.** Modern high-resolution ultrasound allows assessment of the affected nerve at specific entrapment sites (e.g., hand, wrist, elbow, foot). High-frequency linear probes (13–18 MHz) are even capable of distinguishing individual nerve fascicles. One particular advantage of ultrasound is the option of dynamic examinations and assessment of the nerve along its course and in certain provocation positions. Tendons and tendon sheaths in the vicinity of the nerve, synovial ganglia originating from the adjacent joints, and soft tissue tumors are readily assessed.

▶ **MRI.** It is possible to visualize directly both the affected nerve and its adjacent soft tissue. Important aspects include its high spatial resolution (surface coils, small field of view) and comfortable positioning of the patient (avoidance of motion-generated artifacts). T1W and T2W sequences should be obtained in axial slice angulation, i.e., orthogonal to the course of the nerve. A second view should be obtained as a parallel projection to demonstrate the nerve continuously over a long segment. Fat-suppressed sequences are recommended for identification of neural or perineural edema. The IV administration of gadolinium-containing contrast medium is of importance, particularly for the characterization of tumorous alterations and for a better identification of inflammatory processes (synovitis, arthritis, tendinopathy).

11.9 Neuropathic Osteoarthropathy and Diabetic Foot

11.9.1 Neuropathic Osteoarthropathy

Neuropathic osteoarthropathy (synonym: Charcot joint) is a disorder often associated with excessive destruction of the joints, bone, and/or soft tissues due to a disturbance of neurogenic supply. There are numerous causes (▶ Table 11.5).

This disorder was first described by Charcot and referred to the effects of tabes dorsalis (syphilis). Nowadays neuropathic osteoarthropathy is usually a complication of long-standing diabetes mellitus and involves primarily the foot. The alterations have nothing in common with the sequelae of paralysis or spasticity, which can result in atrophy of the affected muscles or lead to (inactivity) osteoporosis or joint deformities.

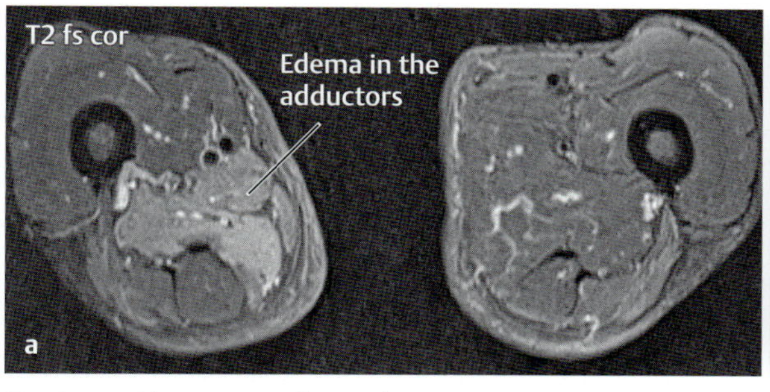

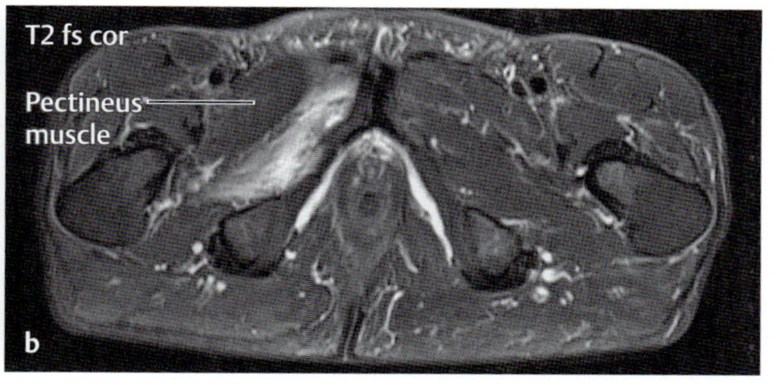

Fig. 11.41 Obturator syndrome due to nerve entrapment after prostate surgery. **(a)** Acute denervation edema in the adductors of the thigh. **(b)** The pectineus muscle is spared (dual innervation by the femoral nerve).

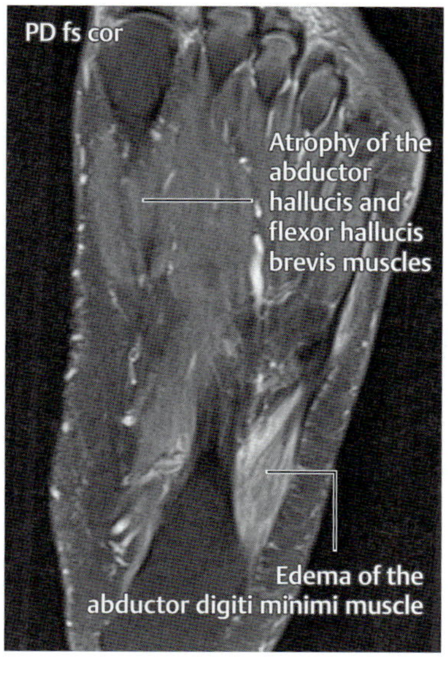

Fig. 11.42 Baxter's neuropathy and jogger's foot.

Table 11.5 Causes and locations of neuro-osteopathies and neuroarthropathies

Causes		Typical location
Metabolic	Diabetes mellitus	Foot, rarely the spine
	Hypercortisolism	Hip, knee, shoulder
	Amyloid neuropathy	Ankle and joints of the foot
Inflammatory	Leprosy	Varied
	Tabes dorsalis	Knee, hip, foot, hands
Congenital	Spinal syringomyelia Dysraphias	Symmetrical involvement of shoulder, elbow, ankle, and joints of the foot
Traumatic		Depending on injury
Unknown (20%)		

▸ **Pathology.** In order to maintain integrity of the joint, regulatory neural circuits must ensure that correct loading of the joint occurs (appropriate control over the muscle system) while the blood supply is adjusted according to the needs of the different tissues. If neuropathy results in disruption of these neural circuits, then the joint is unable to withstand everyday loading, resulting in destruction of the joint that far exceeds the extent of conventional osteoarthritis.

Based on observations of neuropathic joint destruction in bed-ridden patients, it may be assumed that disrupted neural and vascular supply (neurovascular theory) is of greater significance for pathogenesis than faulty loading (neurotraumatic theory).

▸ **Clinical presentation.** Superficial soft tissue changes, such as edema, fistulas, and painless ulcers (mala perforantia), are clinically indicative. The hyposensibility almost always results in a marked discrepancy between the mild subjective symptoms and the gross radiographic findings. One striking feature is the “warm” joint.

The full-blown clinical presentation of neuropathic osteoarthropathy depends on the duration of the disorder and is characterized by a chaotic juxtaposition of bone destruction, by bone formation and fractures of varying degrees, and by the disintegration and subluxation of the joints. Atrophy and osteolysis, as well as hypertrophy and sclerosis predominate (▸ Figs. 11.43–11.45).

The **atrophic changes** include:

- Juxta-articular demineralization, even to the extent of osteolysis, (marginal) erosions; the final appearance is the “worn out” bone.
- Insufficiency fractures (▸ Fig. 11.46), fragmentations.
- Dislocation malalignments.
- Soft tissue swelling, possibly with air inclusions.

11

The **hypertrophic changes** include:

- Cancellous osteosclerosis, apposition of periosteal new bone formation.
- Exuberant callus formation, nonunions, synostoses, osteophytes.
- Hypertrophic soft tissue ossifications (see ▸ Figs. 11.43 and ▸ 11.45).
- Loose joint bodies.

▸ **DD. Insufficiency fractures.** The majority of these fractures are not the result of a neuropathic disease yet are also part of the pattern of findings of Charcot disease. The diagnosis of neuropathic osteoarthropathy is based on the involvement of several joints located closely together. Furthermore, Charcot disease is almost always associated with destruction of the entire joint, which is not typical for an insufficiency fracture even if it is located near to the joint.

Osteoarthritis. Cystic findings do indeed appear in osteoarthritis and may be interpreted as osteolysis and erosions, but osteoarthritis rarely demonstrates a destructive character, unless additional insufficiency fractures are present. Also the pattern of involvement is different. Charcot disease appears more clusterlike at several joints in close vicinity to each other (e.g., in the midfoot).

11.9.2 Diabetic Foot

“Diabetic foot” is defined as the foot of a person with diabetes associated with characteristic soft tissue, joint, and bone alterations caused by neuropathy, faulty mechanical weight-bearing, and angiopathy. A dreaded complication of the diabetic foot is superadded bacterial infection (Chapter 3.1.3). Diabetic osteoarthropathies located in areas other than the foot are rare.

▸ **Pathology.** Metabolic damage to the peripheral nerves and microangiopathy of the vasa nervorum are regarded as the most important causes among the pathogenetic factors.

▸ **Radiography/CT.** On the whole, the radiographic signs of a Charcot joint are present (see ▸ Figs. 11.43–11.45). The Chopart and Lisfranc joints and the tarsometatarsal joints are most commonly involved. The radiographic signs often develop in stages, initially with periosteal new-bone appositions at the diaphyses and metaphyses of the metatarsal bones (▸ Fig. 11.47b) and then as an acute exacerbation associated with osseous fragmentation and erosions (▸ Fig. 11.47a). Insufficiency fractures of varying ages are also seen (see ▸ Fig. 11.49). The further clinical course is marked by the disintegration of the joint (see ▸ Fig. 11.48). Reparative bone processes can be observed during a consolidation phase lasting over a period of months, which can then turn into a healing phase with smoothed bony contours.

> **Note** !
>
> A “Charcot foot” without diabetes is possible. A “diabetic foot” without “Charcot” on the other hand is not.

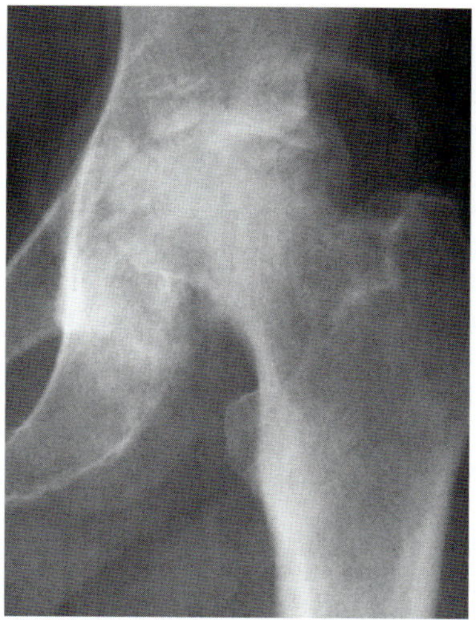

Fig. 11.43

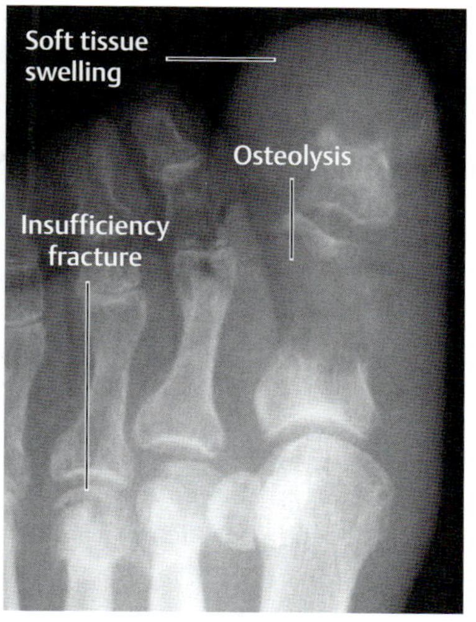

Fig. 11.44

Fig. 11.43 Classic Charcot joint with "melting away" of the femoral head. Soft tissue calcifications. The cause was tabes dorsalis (syphilis). The differential diagnosis from destructive osteoarthropathy (based on insufficiency fractures) was made because of the additional involvement of the knees and feet.

Fig. 11.44 Neuropathic osteoarthropathy secondary to traumatic nerve damage (war injury). Diabetes mellitus was excluded.

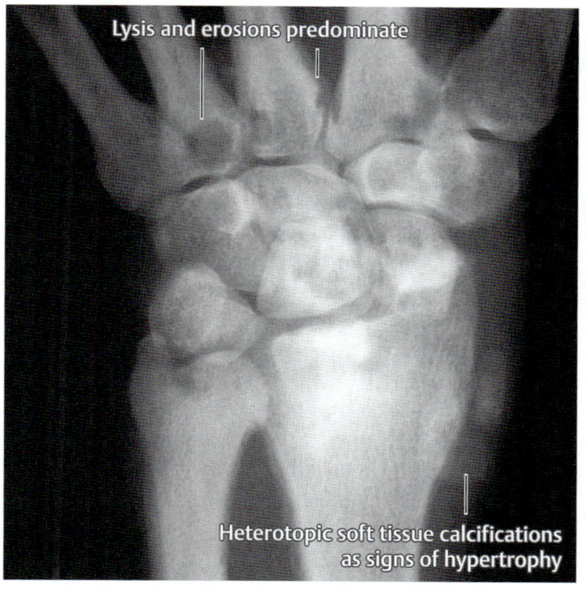

Fig. 11.45 Patient with syringomyelia. Mixed form of neuropathic osteoarthropathy.

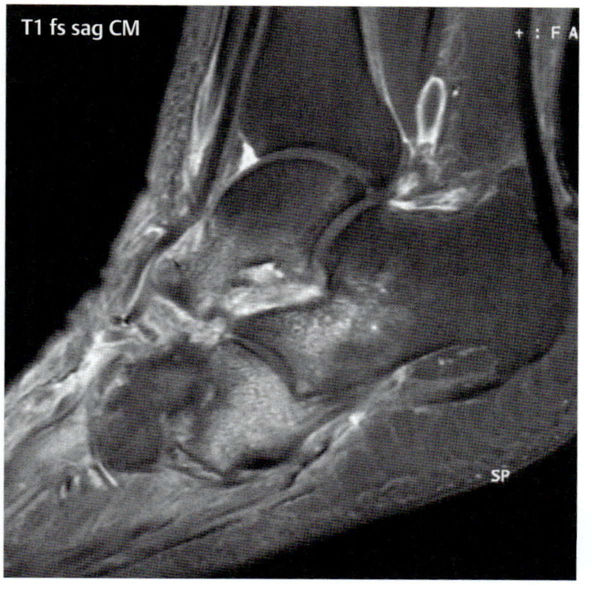

Fig. 11.46 Neuropathic osteoarthropathy. The trabecular enhancement is due to insufficiency fractures.

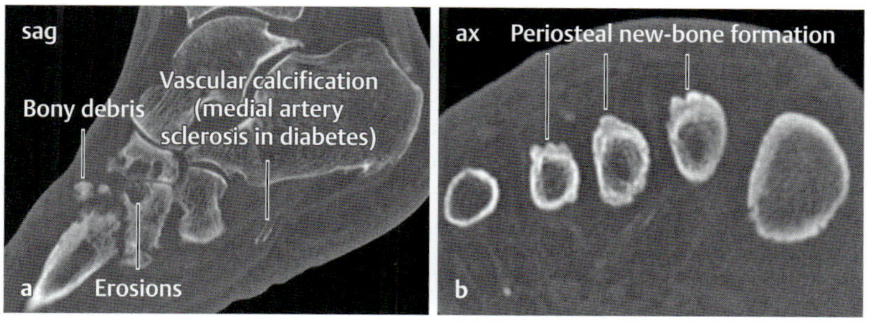

Fig. 11.47 Charcot foot in a diabetic patient. **(a)** Typical finding with joint destruction and debris. **(b)** Reactive periosteal new-bone appositions are seen along the metatarsals.

11

Radiographs are capable of distinguishing whether an atrophic (early or active phase: a "decompensated" foot; ▶ Fig. 11.48) or a **hypertrophic form** (late or reparative phase: a "stabilized" foot; ▶ Fig. 11.49) is present. Mixed forms are usually found (▶ Fig. 11.50).

Media calcifications of the pedal arteries are a common finding and help distinguish from other forms of neuroarthropathy.

Signs of superinfection

- Erosions and osteolyses even to the stage of "melting away" of the bone, which are superimposed onto the osteosclerosis of the Charcot foot.
- Lamellated periosteal reactions.
- Gas inclusions in the soft tissues.

▶ **NUC MED.** The bone scan is characterized by a strong, nonspecific nuclide uptake.

Only a leukocyte scintigram will increase specificity for a superadded infection. However, it is not used routinely for confirming or excluding superinfection because this method is also not sufficiently specific. Nor is ^{18}F-FDG-PET an established method for diagnosing infection because it is not capable of making a safe distinction between infection and a nonspecific inflammatory reaction as part of the constant repair and remodeling processes of the diabetic foot.

▶ **MRI.** Areas of soft tissue edema (bright on T2W fat-suppressed TSE or STIR sequences) are the predominant and nonspecific result of neuropathy and angiopathy (insufficiency) fractures and nonunions, joint destruction, and infections. The detection of fluid accumulation with strong, perifocal edema formation, possibly in continuity with a fistula, is the only relatively sure sign of a superinfection (T1W image with fat suppression after IV contrast administration).

11

11.10 Adhesive Capsulitis

Adhesive capsulitis (synonym: frozen shoulder) is a common disorder of the shoulder whose etiology remains unknown. It presents in stages and is characterized by pain and stiffness of the shoulder.

▶ **Pathology.** Primary, or genuine, shoulder stiffness without recognizable cause is distinguished from a secondary form. An association with diabetes mellitus is recognized but immobilization (e.g., postoperatively) can also result in a frozen shoulder. The disorder commonly takes on a staged course and can be subdivided pathogenically into the following phases:

- **Stage 1:** Capsulitis and synovitis.
- **Stage 2:** Capsular fibrosis.
- **Stage 3:** Resolution of the fibrosis.

Such a classification of this usually self-limiting disorder is only a rough guide. The individual stages (4–6 months per stage) follow in succession, but their time course can be variable. Some cases may persist without resolution.

▶ **Clinical presentation.** Adhesive capsulitis is a disorder of adulthood. The range of motion of the shoulder is restricted in all directions. At the onset of the disorder, the cardinal symptom, however, is the relatively sudden pain without a recognizable cause. The self-healing tendency is less common in the secondary forms, especially in patients with diabetes. Steroids, administered orally or intra-articularly, relieve the clinical symptoms in the short term.

▶ **Radiography.** Pathologic findings are not to be expected. Imaging, however, is important for differential diagnostic considerations (osteoarthritis? calcifications?).

▶ **US.** US is capable of estimating the thickness of the coracohumeral ligament (structure reinforcing the capsule and forming the "roof" of the rotator interval), thus contributing toward reaching a diagnosis.

▶ **MRI.** MRI will detect a thickened (more than 3 mm) coracohumeral ligament that displays increased signal intensity on fluid-sensitive sequences and increased contrast enhancement in the parasagittal plane, extending over the biceps tendon, which has an intra-articular course (▶ Fig. 11.51). Thickening of the inferior glenohumeral ligament, which forms the axillary recess, is also a characteristic feature. This is best demonstrated on coronal oblique images. MRI is particularly capable of showing inflammation of the pericapsular structures (▶ Fig. 11.52). Clinical practice has shown that IV administration of contrast raises the chances of detection of the often very subtle findings. Direct MR arthrography does not contribute at all to reaching a diagnosis.

> **Caution**
> Referrals for MRI of the shoulder rarely specify the indication "frozen shoulder"; rotator cuff pathology is more likely to be suspected. This diagnosis should also be considered where there is any restriction of shoulder movement.

▶ **DD.** Often the clinical diagnosis of adhesive capsulitis is not as simple as presented in text books. Pathological conditions of the acromioclavicular joint, the biceps tendon, and the rotator cuff are not only mistaken for a frozen shoulder but may also be associated with it.

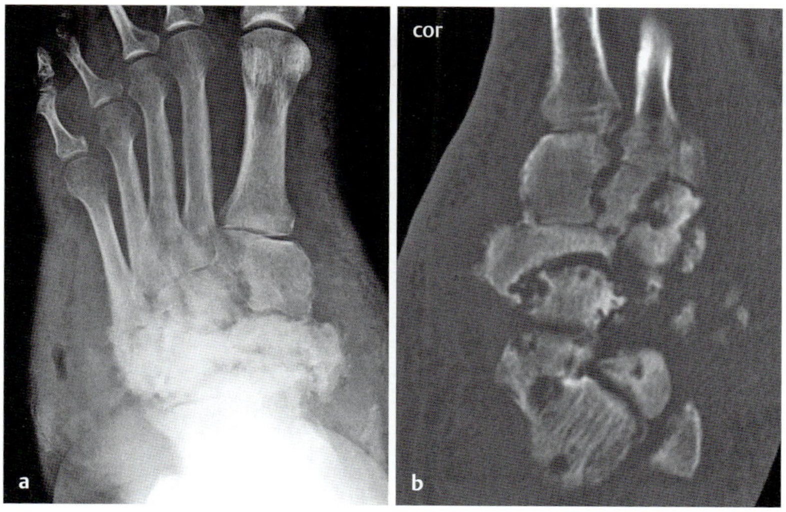

Fig. 11.48 Charcot foot in a diabetic patient. **(a)** Destruction of the tarsal bones; significant soft tissue swelling. **(b)** Predominantly atrophic changes; no consolidation.

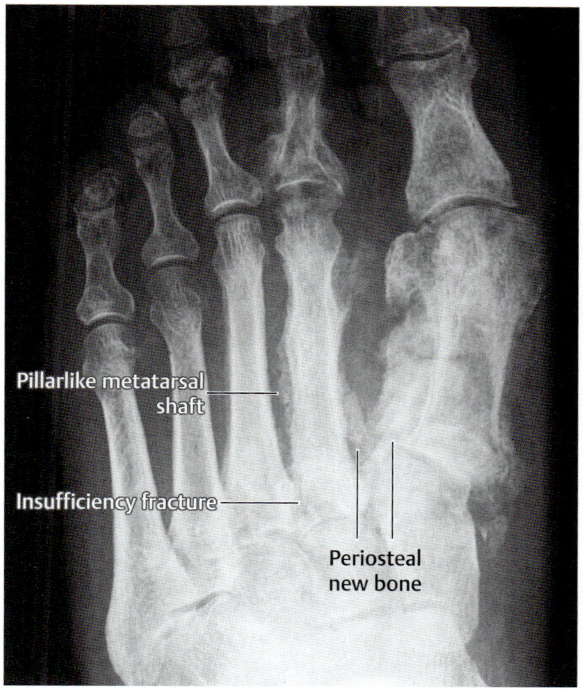

Fig. 11.49 Charcot foot; hypertrophic form.

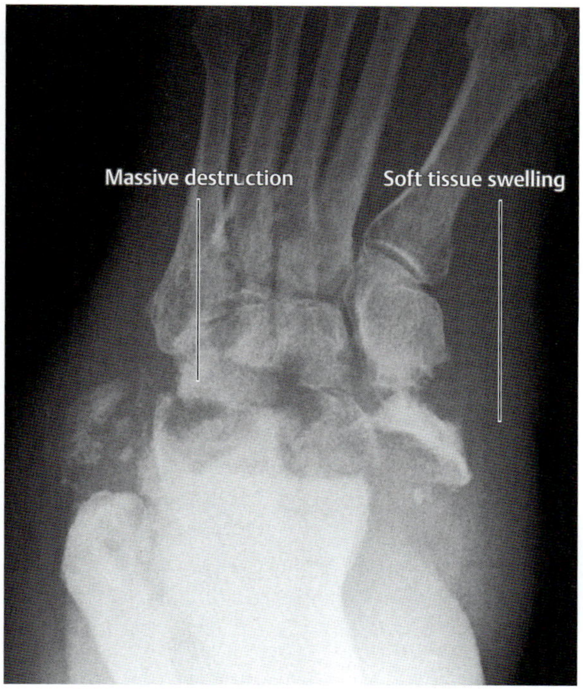

Fig. 11.50 Charcot foot; predominantly mixed atrophic form.

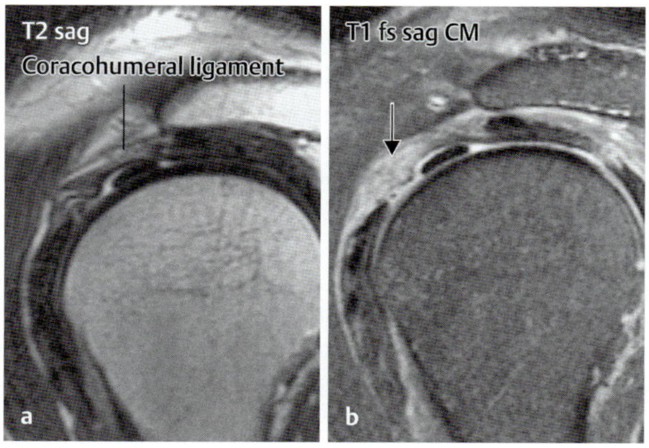

Fig. 11.51 Adhesive capsulitis. **(a)** Thickening of the coracohumeral ligament. **(b)** The diagnosis of adhesive capsulitis is confirmed by the strong contrast enhancement of the ligament (arrow) and the pericapsular tissue.

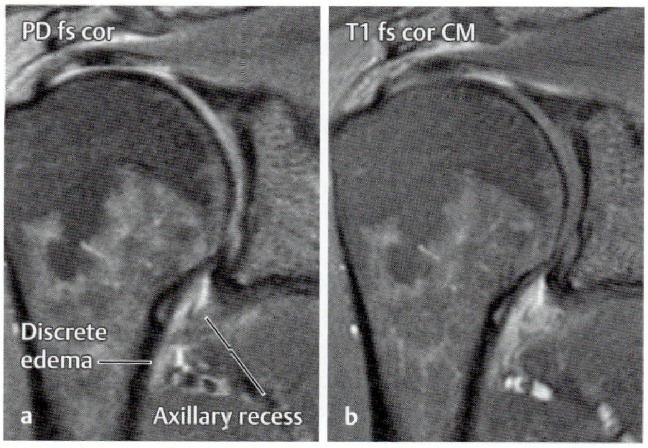

Fig. 11.52 Adhesive capsulitis. **(a)** It is difficult to recognize the inflammation. **(b)** The administration of contrast clearly improves the detection of the pericapsular inflammation.

12 Interventions Involving the Bone, Soft Tissues, and Joints

12.1 Arthrography

12.1.1 Indications

Despite the introduction and technical improvement of sectional imaging (CT and MRI), direct arthrography is still an important tool in the diagnosis of musculoskeletal disorders. It should always be combined with CT or MRI to maximize diagnostic information.

Advantages of direct arthrography (in combination with sectional imaging)

- The injected fluid distends the joint and so allows better assessment of articular structures.
- Visualization of contrast imbibition or leakage provides increased sensitivity for tears involving ligaments, menisci, or disks.
- High image contrast between cartilage and joint interior improves the assessment of cartilaginous lesions.

In addition, direct arthrography may be augmented by the diagnostic and/or therapeutic injection of a local anesthetic and/or an anti-inflammatory steroid. Analysis of aspirated joint fluid, prior to the contrast injection, can also contribute to obtaining a diagnosis (septic arthritis, crystal arthropathy, etc.).

> **Note**
> Following appropriate informed consent, direct arthrography must be performed under strictly aseptic conditions.

12.1.2 Contraindications

- Infected soft tissue along the access path.
- Pathologic clotting profile (INR > 1.5, PTT [partial thromboplastin time] > 50 seconds, platelet count < 50 000/μL), anticoagulation therapy.

12.1.3 Technique

The injection for direct arthrography is usually performed under imaging guidance using ultrasound or fluoroscopy (▶ Figs. 12.1 and ▶ 12.2). This ensures that the contrast agent is accurately injected into the joint. In addition, functional images and/or dynamic studies can be obtained under an image intensifier before or after the injection. Arthrography is also possible under CT or MRI control or by using anatomical landmarks for guidance ("blind technique").

The following contrast medium dilutions are recommended to achieve optimum image contrast:

- **Image intensifier/CT:** Iodine-containing contrast medium, diluted 1 : 1 with normal saline or local anesthetic.
- **MRI:** Gadolinium-based contrast agent, dilution 1 : 200.

The reader should refer to the specialized literature for the exact technique of intra-articular injections of individual joints.

12.1.4 Complications

- **Septic arthritis:** This risk is minimal when a consistent sterile method of working is adopted (~ 1/20 000 arthrographies).
- **Allergic reactions:** These are extremely rare after intra-articular drug administration.
- **Localized pain and limitation of motion:** These depend on the amount of injected fluid and are reversible; local cooling and rest may be indicated.
- **Extra- or intra-articular hemorrhage:** Knowledge of vascular anatomy and attention to contraindications regarding coagulation (Chapter 12.1.2) help to minimize this risk.

12.2 Biopsy

12.2.1 Indications

Any biopsy of the musculoskeletal system requires a **precise indication** in consultation with the responsible clinician and an experienced pathologist. The main indications are:

- Histological examination of a (solitary) suspicious finding for metastasis.
- Confirmation, exclusion, and subtyping of (solitary or oligo-ostotic) plasmacytoma and malignant lymphoma.
- Differentiation between tumor-related and osteoporotic fracture.
- Confirmation of infection and its classification.
- Classification of primary bone and soft tissue tumors.

Lesions that have been unequivocally classified with imaging, especially those that can be identified as "leave-me-alone" lesions, need no histological clarification.

If the finding relates to a primary bone or a soft tissue tumor, then the following conditions should be fulfilled prior to biopsy:

- Establishing the indication (especially the question whether an open biopsy is an alternative) is best accomplished after consultation in a multidisciplinary tumor conference.
- The pathologist should be experienced in bone and soft tissue tumors.

12.2.2 Contraindications

- Bleeding risk (INR > 1.5, PTT > 50 seconds, platelet count < 50 000/µL).
- Hypervascularized lesion in the immediate vicinity of the spinal cord.
- Infected access path to a noninfected lesion.
- Unfavorable location (e.g., atlas, odontoid process).

12.2.3 Technique

The **biopsy access route** should be agreed upon in consultation with the operating surgeon in order to protect uninvolved compartments and neurovascular bundles for subsequent curative surgery.

In most cases **analgesia and sedation** is adequate for percutaneous biopsy. Usually CT is employed as the **imaging modality for guiding** a percutaneous biopsy where the anatomy is complex (possibly using CT fluoroscopy; ▶ Figs. 12.3 and ▶ 12.4). Depending on location and tissue contrast, the procedure may be possible with, or may necessitate, the use of ultrasound (▶ Fig. 12.5) or MRI guidance. The type of **biopsy needle** depends strongly on the nature of the lesion; a distinction is made between aspiration, cutting, and trephine biopsy needles. A combination of several types of needles is often chosen via a **coaxial needle technique**; for example, an aspiration needle for fluid components, a cutting biopsy needle for soft tissue components, and a trephine biopsy needle for hard bone.

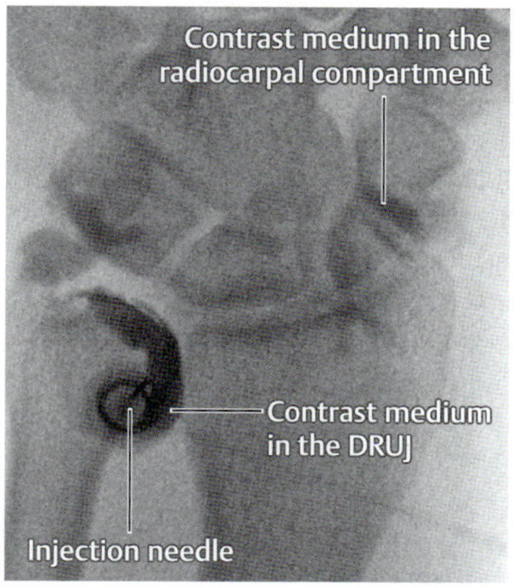

Fig. 12.1 Bicompartmental arthrogram of the wrist performed under fluoroscopic guidance. DRUJ, distal radioulnar joint.

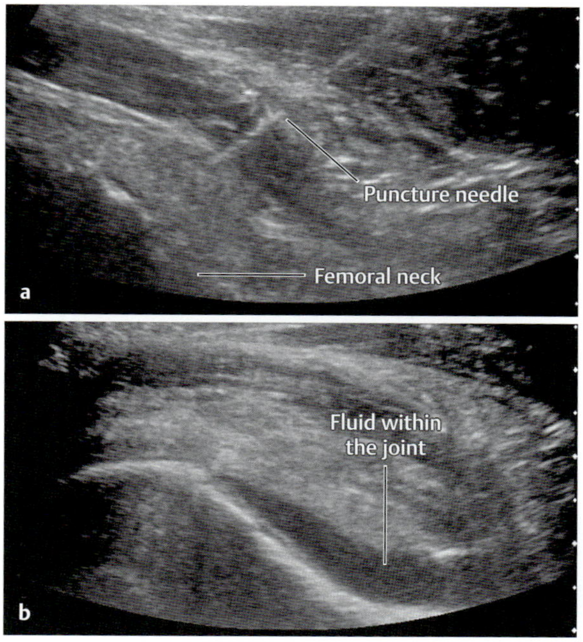

Fig. 12.2 Ultrasound-guided arthrography of the hip. **(a)** The illustration shows the position of the puncture needle. **(b)** The fluid within the joint is clearly visible.

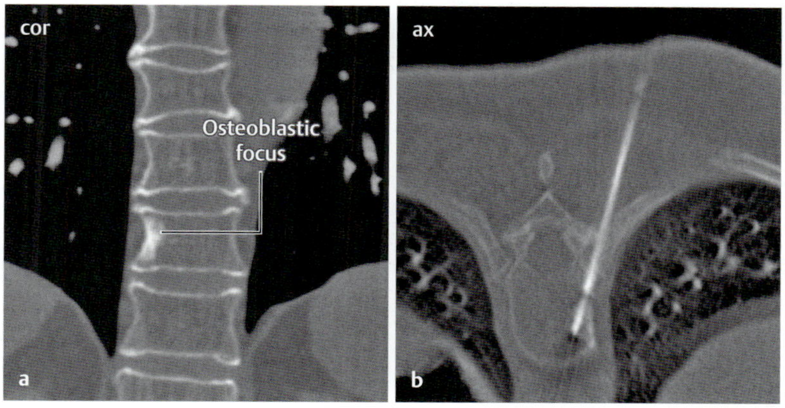

Fig. 12.3 CT-guided bone biopsy. **(a)** Single osteoblastic focal lesion in T10. **(b)** Biopsy under CT fluoroscopy. Histology confirmed metastatic breast cancer.

Direct assessment of the tissue sample by an on-site pathologist is ideal. If this is not practical, then three cores should be sampled if at all possible. It should be borne in mind when **selecting the biopsy site** that sclerotic components have less prospect of success than osteolytic areas, while necrotic parts should be avoided. A specimen should always be sent for microbiological examination as infection may mimic tumor and vice versa.

12.2.4 Complications

The complication rate for percutaneous biopsy depends mainly on the site and type of needle used. The literature reports complication rates as ranging between 0 and 10% of cases. Serious complications occur in less than 1% of biopsies. These include hemorrhage requiring blood transfusion, infection, neurologic deficits, pneumothorax during thoracic spine procedures, and (rarely) fractures.

12.2.5 Results

Image-guided percutaneous biopsy has several advantages over open biopsy: lower complication rate, earlier initiation of therapy after biopsy, and reduced costs. It has also been shown that the accuracy of percutaneous biopsy at 81 to 97% is comparable with that of open biopsy. The distinction between benign and malignant, taken on its own, has a success rate of approximately 98%.

12.3 Drains

12.3.1 Indications

Percutaneous drainage should be considered as a primary step for all soft tissue abscesses. However, insertion of a drain is only advocated for an abscess with a larger diameter (> 3 cm); smaller abscesses can be punctured or aspirated (▸ Fig. 12.6). The indication for the procedure should be established by interdisciplinary consultation.

12.3.2 Contraindications

Hemorrhage (INR > 1.5, PTT > 50 seconds, platelet count < 50000/μL).

12.3.3 Technique

Choice of the suitable image-guided modality: CT lends itself for anatomically complex regions, while ultrasound is also suitable for easily accessible sites, possibly combined with fluoroscopy.

A distinction is made between two techniques for placing a drain:

- **Trocar technique:** After applying local anesthetic down to the abscess and making a trial aspiration, the drain is inserted directly into the abscess with the aid of the provided guide needle and the pointed central stylet. The approach requires a safe access route.
- **Seldinger technique:** The abscess is punctured under local anesthesia using an 18G needle. After a trial aspiration, a steel wire is inserted into the abscess via the 18G needle, which is then removed. The access route may be dilated over the wire before insertion of the drain (▸ Fig. 12.7).

Large-bore drains (for soft tissue abscesses usually 14F) should be used for viscous, purulent material; smaller-bore drains (8 to 10F) are adequate for more liquid material. More important than drain size is the ability to **empty the abscess completely at the first attempt** and to **carefully irrigate the abscess cavity several times** with sterile saline solution (irrigation volume = half of the aspiration volume). After several irrigations the aspirated irrigation fluid should be as clear as possible and of low viscosity.

The intervention is completed with the careful contrast filling of the abscess cavity using diluted contrast agent and confirmation by CT. In case of ultrasound-guided drain insertion, a fluoroscan may be used in adjunct. If there are still noncontrasted abscess areas present, then a decision should be considered regarding a further drain placement or aspiration. Securing the drain to the skin with a cutaneous

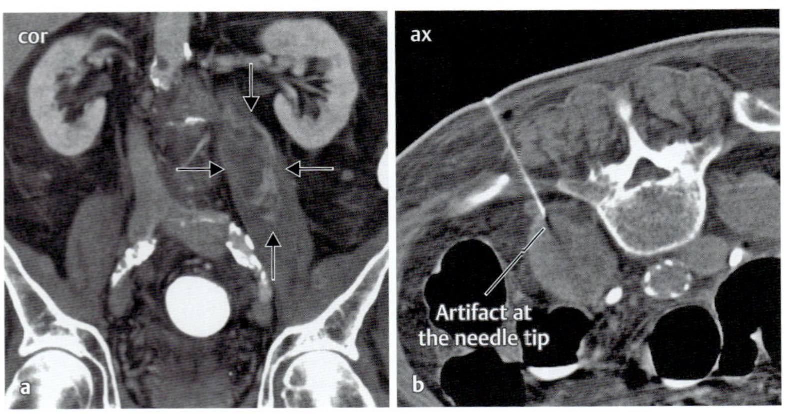

Fig. 12.4 CT-guided soft tissue biopsy. **(a)** Marginal contrast-enhancing, space-occupying lesion (arrows) in the left psoas muscle (abscess). **(b)** The tip of the needle is advanced to the lesion before performing the punch biopsy.

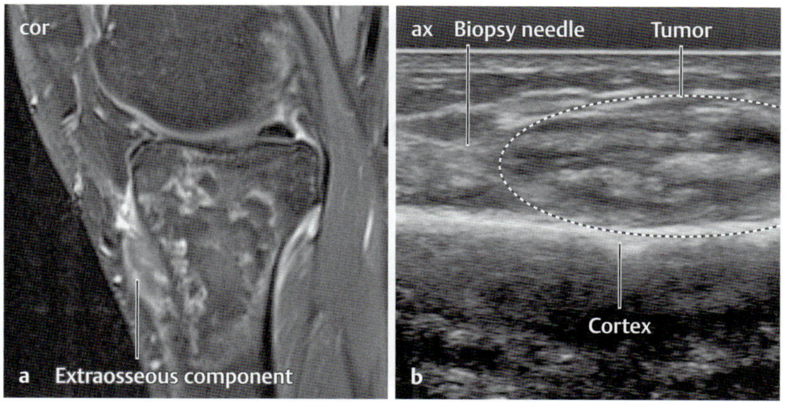

Fig. 12.5 Ultrasound-guided soft tissue biopsy. **(a)** MRI demonstrated an intra- and extraosseous space-occupying lesion in the proximal tibia. **(b)** The biopsy revealed an aggressive non-Hodgkin's lymphoma.

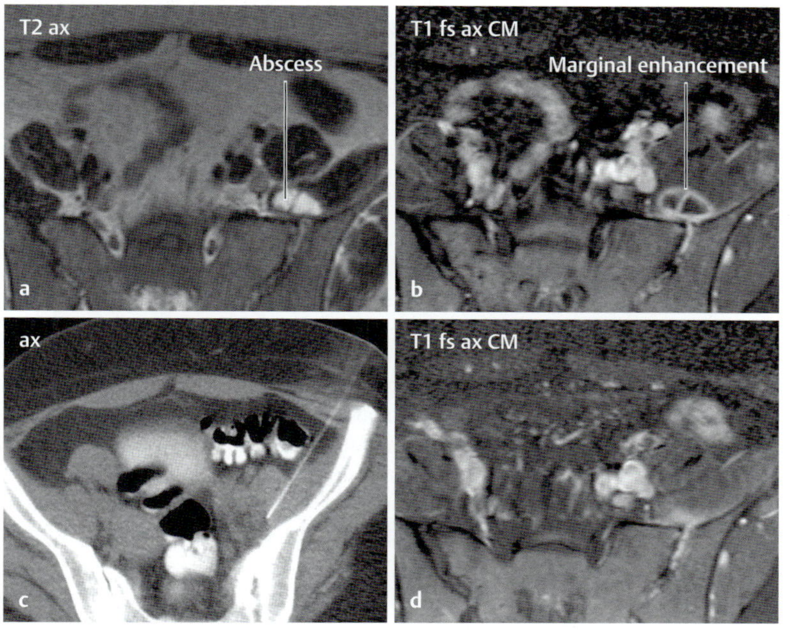

Fig. 12.6 Abscess aspiration anterior to the left sacroiliac joint. **(a)** The collection is too small to require a drain. **(b)** Typical marginal contrast enhancement. **(c)** CT-guided abscess aspiration. **(d)** MRI follow-up confirmed complete drainage; the residual mild contrast enhancement is a sign of the inflammation.

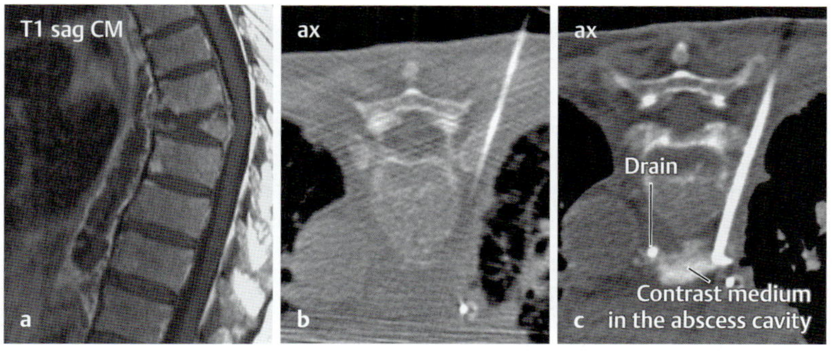

Fig. 12.7 CT-guided drain placement. **(a)** Prevertebral abscess extending over several segments. **(b)** Puncture directed toward the abscess under CT fluoroscopy. **(c)** After placement of the drain and drainage of the abscess, contrast is applied via the drain to assess the abscess cavity.

suture is recommended, as is a customized plaster to avoid kinking. Do not forget to send a specimen to microbiology for culture and determination of the sensitivity of the pathogen.

Providing the ward with an **irrigation plan** is essential, as is follow-up imaging of the abscess cavity in the subsequent days.

Drain removal may be considered once the patient is completely afebrile with normal inflammatory parameters, discharge from the drain has almost completely ceased (less than 10 mL/day), and imaging has confirmed reduced volume of the abscess cavity. On average this is usually accomplished after about 2 to 3 weeks; the patient should already be afebrile within the first 24 to 48 hours. Prolonged drainage time should be anticipated, however, in the presence of additional fistula communication with intestinal structures.

12.3.4 Complications

Possible complications depend on location: organ injury, hemorrhage, spread of infection, sepsis secondary to overinjection of the abscess cavity.

12.3.5 Results

This is a good and safe procedure that often renders surgical drainage superfluous. Healing rates following percutaneous abscess drainage in larger cumulative patient populations with various abscess sites total around 80%; morbidity ranges between 5 and 10%.

12.4 Nerve Root Block

Nerve root block is an interventional, imaging-guided form of treatment for the symptomatic management of radicular pain syndromes. It involves injecting local anesthetic together with a steroid in crystal suspension (triamcinolone) into the direct vicinity of the affected nerve root (periradicular). Treatment may be repeated at intervals of at least 2 weeks, with approximately three treatment sessions being required.

12.4.1 Indications

The classic indication is **radicular pain** arising from mechanical nerve root compression that, in turn, may be caused by disk herniation, foraminal stenosis, spinal stenosis, or scar tissue. Compression by scar tissue in postdiskectomy syndrome in particular is a common indication, given that revision surgery often produces disappointing results.

12.4.2 Contraindications

Nerve alterations expected to result in permanent neurologic deficits usually represent an indication for surgery. Borderline cases (e.g., sensory deficit and discrete motor weakness) require interdisciplinary discussion, together with the patient, as to whether nerve root block is justified. Further contraindications include tumor-related alterations to the roots and inflammation. Finally, the general contraindications for needle drainage apply (no patient consent, coagulopathy, etc.).

Since cortisone is administered, diabetes mellitus and gastrointestinal ulcers are mentioned as relative contraindications, as are allergy to contrast medium and hyperthyroidism due to the local application of contrast.

12.4.3 Procedure

A suitable puncture site is determined with the aid of transverse slices without tilting the gantry (▶ Fig. 12.8a). After application of local anesthetic, a 22G needle is advanced until close to the affected nerve root. For this purpose, a co-axial technique using an 18G cannula can be employed, as this allows more precise guidance of the very flexible 22G needle (▶ Figs. 12.8b and ▶ 12.9).

This is followed by administration of the local anesthetic (e.g., 1.5–2 mL of a 0.25% bupivacaine solution). This is mixed with a little contrast agent to allow subsequent control of the fluid distribution (▶ Fig. 12.8c). On confirmation of distribution around the nerve roots and, if required, in the intraspinal epidural space, 20 mg triamcinolone is then administered.

12.4.4 Complications

The local anesthetic can produce transient leg paralysis. The patient must be informed of this prior to the procedure (accompanying person; inability to drive). Drug-related anaphylactic reactions and hyperthyroidism are possible. Serious specific complications are extremely rare. Nerve injury with permanent damage is theoretically possible as is damage to the spinal cord from an intra-arterial injection into a spinal artery.

12.4.5 Trial Nerve Root Block

A trial nerve root block dispenses with the administration of steroid, with only a local anesthetic injected. It serves to test whether radicular pain syndrome is indeed present and, in clinically equivocal cases, to locate the level of the affected root. A trial nerve root block is commonly undertaken before embarking on a series of therapy sessions. It may, however, be dispensed with if there is a clear correlation between symptoms and the morphological imaging results.

12.5 Facet Block

Facet block is a form of pain management for symptomatic facet joint osteoarthritis. Here, the afferent pain fibers of the medial branch of the dorsal ramus are numbed (blocked) or denervated.

For this purpose a 22G needle is inserted posteriorly, somewhat medial to the affected facet joint. Approximately 4 mL bupivacaine 0.5% is applied as a diagnostic block, supplemented with a little contrast agent. The fluid should be distributed around the joint (▶ Fig. 12.10).

If success is confirmed by repeated diagnostic blocks, then denervation may be undertaken with 96% ethanol (1.5–2 mL) after renewed local anesthesia. Denervation by thermocoagulation is less painful. It does, however, require appropriate equipment.

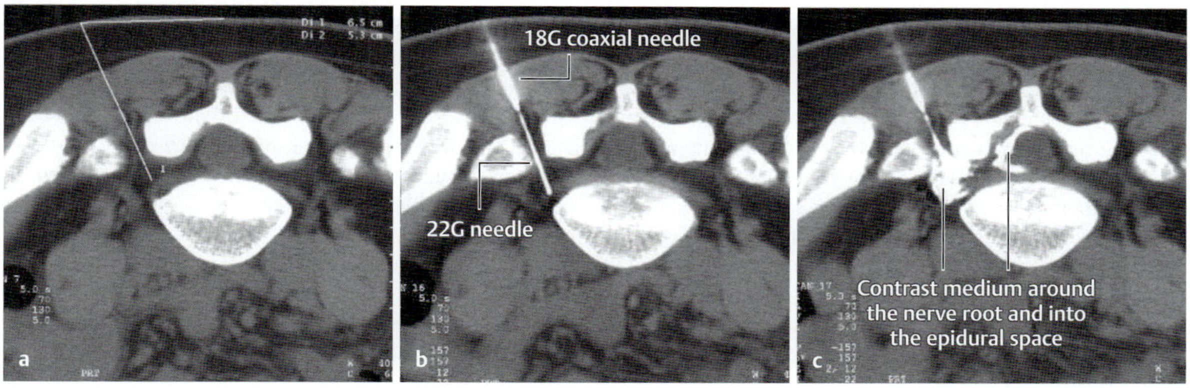

Fig. 12.8 Procedure for CT-guided therapy at the level of L4–L5. **(a)** Selection of the access route, obliquely lateral to the neural foramen. **(b)** Approach using coaxial technique under CT guidance. **(c)** Favorable distribution of the fluid around the nerve root, extending intraspinally into the epidural space.

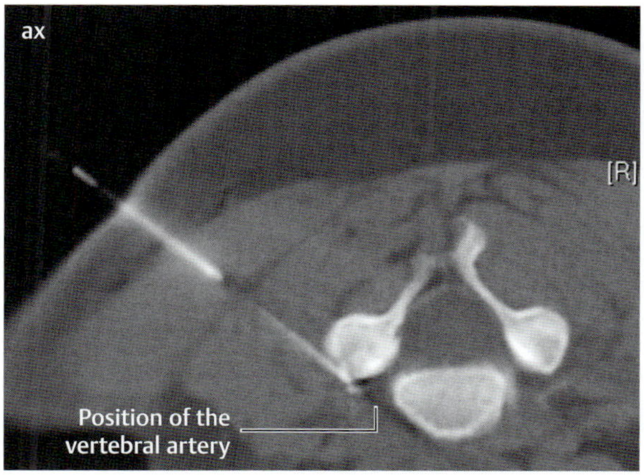

Fig. 12.9 CT-guided cervical nerve root block performed at C5/C6. The tip of the needle is positioned in front of the facet joint. In the cervical spine, attention should be paid to the immediate vicinity of the vertebral artery.

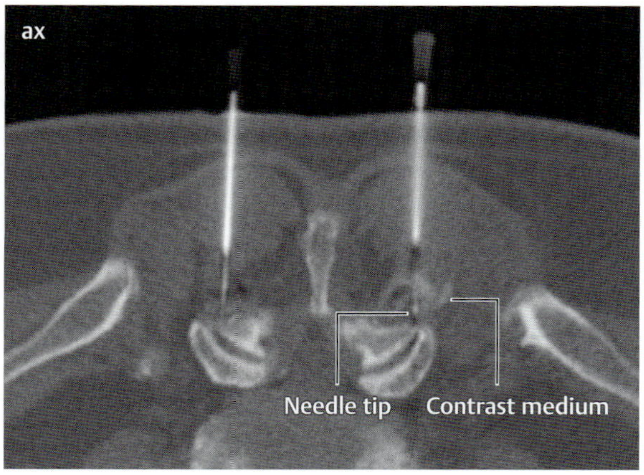

Fig. 12.10 CT-guided lower lumbar facet block.

12

12.6 Vertebroplasty, Kyphoplasty, and Sacroplasty

Vertebroplasty and kyphoplasty are forms of pain therapy using polymethylmethacrylate (bone cement) for fractured vertebrae. The mechanism of action has not yet been clarified. With kyphoplasty, and to a lesser extent also with vertebroplasty, an attempt is also made to restore the physiological position of the spine by reducing spinal deformity.

Sacroplasty utilizes the vertebroplasty principle in the sacrum.

12.6.1 Indications

- Painful vertebral osteoporotic fracture/compression fracture with only minor or absent trauma in patients with failed, or impractical for any reason, conservative management (▶Fig. 12.11; the interval between onset of pain and interventional therapy must take into account the individual patient's circumstances).
- Painful, traumatic, stable fracture associated with osteoporosis in patients with failed, or impractical, conservative treatment that does not present an indication for standard surgery as based on defined criteria.
- Painful osteolytic lesions of disseminated malignant tumors (secondary tumors and malignant hematologic disorders) as a palliative measure and a supplement to oncological therapy (▶Fig. 12.12).
- Perioperative or intraoperative vertebroplasty or kyphoplasty during surgical measures of stabilization.

The health impact of both procedures in nonosteoporotic and fresh traumatic fractures as compared with conservative management with analgesia is currently unclear.

> **Caution**
> The indication for vertebroplasty or kyphoplasty should be made with due consideration—not every vertebral fracture is an indication for intervention or surgery. The majority of vertebral fractures will heal spontaneously and without residual symptoms within 2–4 weeks.

12.6.2 Imaging Procedures before Diagnosis

Radiographs of the affected, painful spinal segment in two projections are obtained. An MRI of the affected segment allows old fractures to be distinguished from fresh ones and to confirm the level of the vertebra causing the pain. Alternatively, in the presence of contraindications to MRI, a bone scan may be obtained.

12.6.3 Contraindications

Absolute contraindications

- Recalcitrant coagulopathy or bleeding diathesis.
- Bacterial infection of the affected vertebral segment.
- Osteoblastic metastases.
- Asymptomatic vertebral fracture.
- "Prophylactic" vertebroplasty or kyphoplasty.

Relative contraindications

- Neurologic symptoms originating from the spinal segment to be treated.
- Unstable posterior margin, fragment displacement into the spinal canal.
- More than three vertebrae in one session.
- Allergy to the components used.
- Younger patients (depending on the individual situation).

12.6.4 Complications

Severe complications are rare and usually the result of faulty technique and lack of experience. This applies particularly for (pulmonary) cement embolism and marked cement leakage into the spinal canal and intervertebral disk space. The patient should also be informed about local and systemic infections and hemorrhage. Spinal cord injury, injury to spinal nerves or nerve roots, pneumothorax, and fractured ribs are extremely rare.

12.6.5 Technique

The vertebra is punctured under fluoroscan or CT guidance using a thick (11–8G), beveled cannula via a transpedicular, costotransversal (▶Fig. 12.13), or direct access. Then ~2–6 mL polymethylmethacrylate is injected under fluoroscopic guidance. High-viscosity cements with the possibility of longer processing times (over 15 minutes) are becoming increasingly established ("radiofrequency kyphoplasty"). The aim of kyphoplasty is to restore vertebral height using various techniques. CT fluoroscopic guidance is obligatory for sacroplasty in order to observe exactly the distribution of the cement in relation to the neural-exit foramina (▶Fig. 12.14).

12

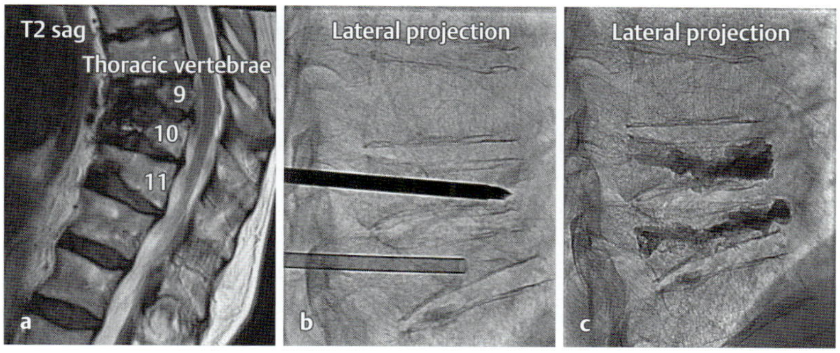

Fig. 12.11 Radiofrequency kyphoplasty with multiple osteoporotic vertebral body collapses. **(a)** Initial finding: vertebra plana T9 and T10, older inferior end plate compression T11. **(b)** Fluoroscan-guided transpedicular approach to T9 and T10. **(c)** Final check: correct cement distribution. Small, insignificant anterior leak at T10.

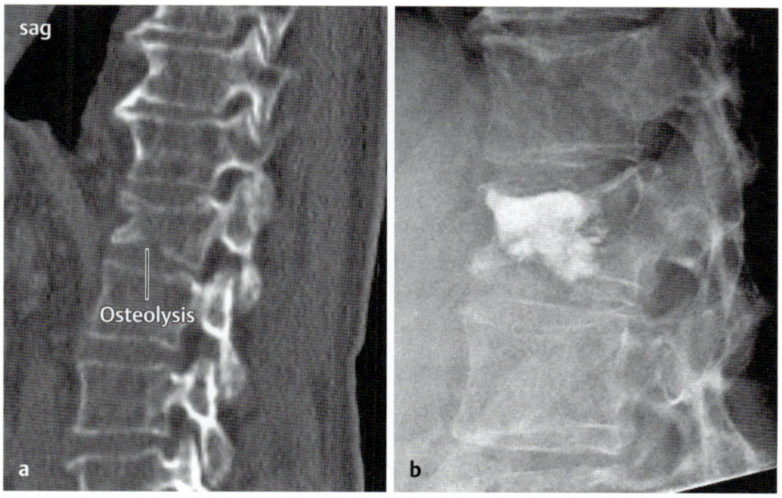

Fig. 12.12 Radiofrequency kyphoplasty. **(a)** Painful osteolysis of L1; known plasmacytoma. **(b)** Result after kyphoplasty.

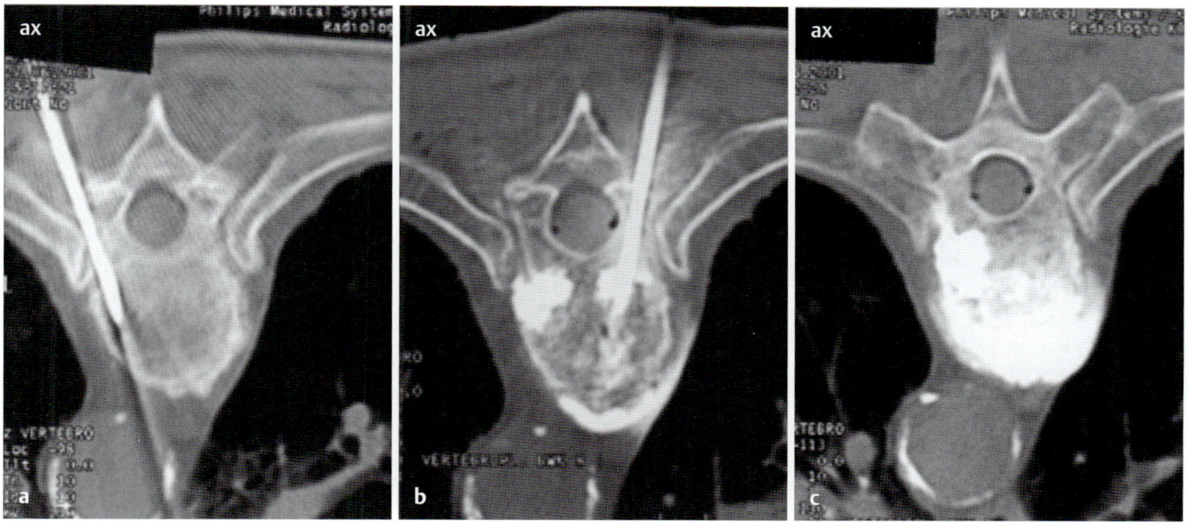

Fig. 12.13 Access routes for vertebroplasty. **(a)** Costotransverse approach. **(b)** Transpedicular approach. **(c)** Final result with correct distribution of the bone cement.

12.6.6 Results

Significant improvement of symptoms or absence of pain is achieved in 80 to 90% of treated osteoporotic fractures. The results of pain treatment are the same for vertebroplasty and kyphoplasty. Pain reduction for malignant destructions is successful in ~ 50 to 70% of cases.

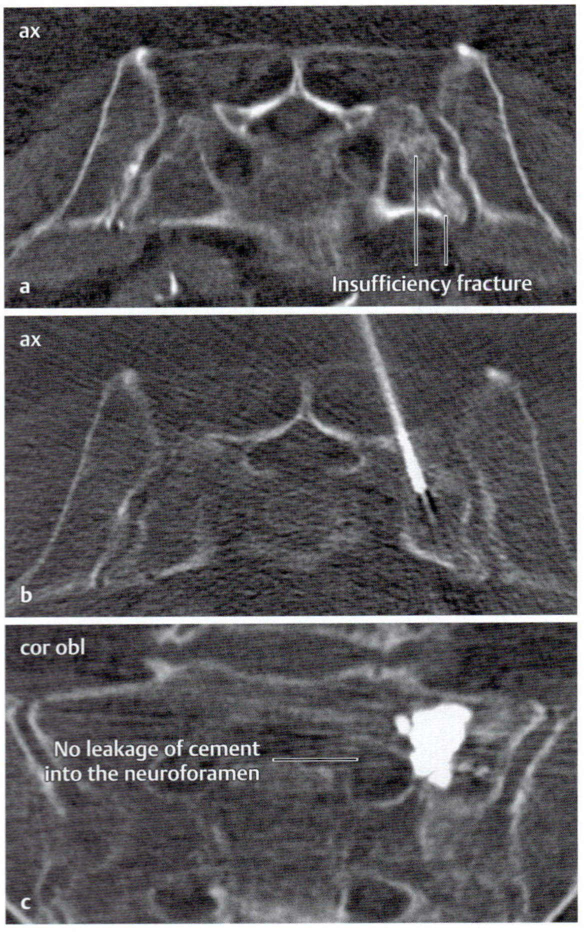

Fig. 12.14 CT-guided sacroplasty. **(a)** Initial finding: chronic insufficiency fracture of the lateral ala. **(b)** CT-guided sacroplasty. **(c)** Final review: correct cement distribution.

12.7 Laser Therapy and Radiofrequency Ablation

Both laser therapy and radiofrequency ablation are thermal ablation procedures in which the local generation of heat induces tissue necrosis.

In the skeleton the procedure is primarily used for the treatment of osteoid osteomas (▶ Figs. 12.15 and ▶ 12.16), with success rates of 75 to 100% being reported. It is increasingly being used for the treatment of small chondroblastomas in the epiphyses rather than curettage. Other indications (e.g., palliative ablation of metastases) have not yet been routinely established.

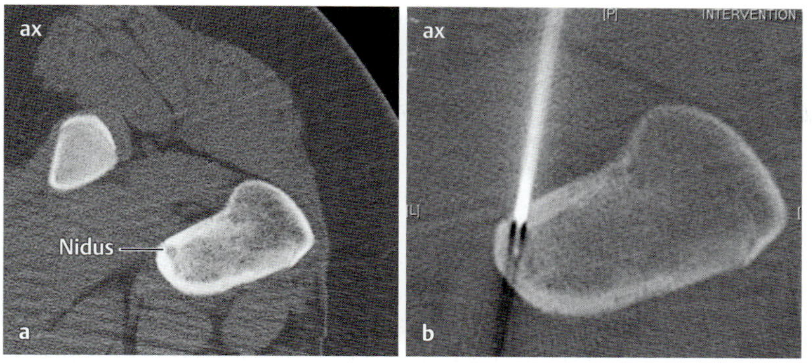

Fig. 12.15 Laser therapy of an osteoid osteoma of the femoral neck. **(a)** Characteristic CT morphology with nidus and surrounding sclerosis. **(b)** Laser thermoablation.

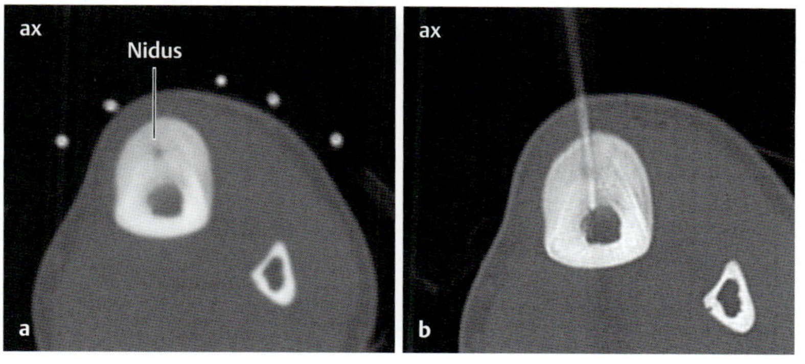

Fig. 12.16 Laser therapy of an osteoid osteoma of the tibia. **(a)** Thick sclerotic margin around the nidus. **(b)** Laser thermoablation.

Index

Page numbers in *italics* refer to illustrations

A

C

D

E

F

I

J

K

L

O

T

U